Mosby's
DENTAL
DICTIONARY

Mosby's
DENTAL
DICTIONARY

*With **395** illustrations*

 Mosby

An Affiliate of Elsevier

Mosby
An Affiliate of Elsevier

11830 Westline Industrial Drive
St. Louis, Missouri 63146

MOSBY'S DENTAL DICTIONARY   ISBN 0-323-02510-2
Copyright © 2004, Mosby, Inc. All rights reserved.

Library of Congress Cataloging in Publication Data

Mosby's dental dictionary.
     p. ; cm.
    Includes bibliographical references.
    ISBN 0-323-02510-2
    1. Dentistry—Dictionaries. 1. Title: Dental dictionary.
    [DNLM: 1. Dentistry—Dictionary—English. WU 13 M8941 2003]
RK27.M672 2003
617.6'003—dc22

                             2003059395

Publishing Director: Linda Duncan
Executive Editor: Penny Rudolph
Senior Developmental Editor: Jaime Pendill
Publishing Services Manager: Linda McKinley
Senior Project Manager: Jennifer Furey
Design Manager: Gail Morey Hudson

Printed in China

Last digit is the print number: 9 8 7 6 5 4 3

Editorial Consultants

Thomas Zwemer, DDS, MSD, FACD, FICD
Vice President for Academic Affairs, Emeritus
Professor of Orthodontics, Emeritus
School of Dentistry, Medical College of Georgia
Augusta, Georgia

Margaret J. Fehrenbach, RDH, MS
Dental Hygienist and Oral Biologist
Adjunct Faculty, Marquette University, Milwaukee, Wisconsin;
Educational Consultant and Private Practice
Seattle, Washington

Mary Emmons, CDH, Med
Co-Director of Dental Hygiene Program
School of Dental Hygiene, Parkland College
Champaign, IL

Mary Ann Tiedemann, BS Home Economics, AAS Dental Hygiene
Adjunct Faculty
School of Dental Hygiene, Parkland College
Champaign, IL

Key staff members of Publication Services, Inc. worked cooperatively to expand the concentration subject areas in the realm of dental hygiene and dental assisting:
Project Coordinators: Elisa Laird and Theodore Young
Editor: Scott Stocking
Associate Editor: Jyothimai Gubili
Pronunciation Editor: Jerome Colburn
Database Design: Richard Bronson
Audio CD Producers: Brian Martinez and Louise B. Toft
Elocutionist: Greg Whitlock

Preface

The expanding realm of dentistry has placed ever-increasing demands on the entire dental team; therefore, whether you have been in the field for a decade or have just graduated from a dental program, *Mosby's Dental Dictionary* is an essential tool to help you meet these additional responsibilities and expectations.

In response to increasing demands on dentists, dental hygienists, and assistants, *Mosby's Dental Dictionary* contains approximately 2100 definitions that have become relevant to these fields. Definitions for words commonly used in immunology, microbiology, radiography, special needs dentistry, pediatric dentistry, anesthesiology, and common medicine, as well as terminology from the legal and insurance fields with which a hygienist or assistant should be familiar are included. Pronunciations for key entries ensure accuracy of speech. Synonyms are included where applicable to help users understand terms.

Another exciting feature of *Mosby's Dental Dictionary* is the accompanying mini CD-ROM. Every copy of the dictionary includes a mini CD-ROM that contains the entire dictionary text, and an audio feature that allows users to hear the correct pronunciation of the most complex terms (approximately 30% of all terms). Words that include a bold pronunciation indicate which terms can be heard on the mini CD-ROM. This mini CD-ROM will work only when placed into tray-loaded CD-ROM drives. If your computer is set to autorun, just load the CD-ROM into the drive. The CD-ROM will do the rest!

More than 350 diagrams, photographs, and line drawings help bring these terms to life before your eyes. As you flip through *Mosby's Dental Dictionary*, you will find full-color examples of conditions, some extremely rare, that you may encounter throughout your dental career.

Extensive appendices provide quick, easy-to-use resources for vital information. From the most updated American Dental Association (ADA) dental codes to an overview of the Health Insurance Portability and Accountability Act (HIPAA) of 1996, the appendices serve as an invaluable guide for dental professionals and those working in dental-oriented businesses and insurance.

Health care workers in dentistry are being subjected to higher standards and need continued education in order to remain marketable in the dental world. If you are affiliated with the dental profession, you know that the role of the dental team is moving beyond initial care and cleaning, requiring expertise in immunology, microbiology, radiology, nutrition, and basic medical principles. *Mosby's Dental Dictionary* provides those in the dental profession with a comprehensive, hands-on resource that will be used on a daily basis.

345111

Contents

Pronunciation Guide

VOWEL SOUNDS

Print	Key words
a	hat
ä	father
ā	play, fate, feign
e	flesh
ē	she, sweet
er	air, ferry
i	sit
ī	eye, kind, mine
ir	ear, weird
o	proper
ō	nose, coal
ô	saw, fawn
oi	coin, (German) feuer
o͞o	moon, move
o͝o	put, book
ou	out
u	cup, love
Y	(German) grün, Führer; (French) tu
ur	fur, first
ə	ago, career
œ	(German) schön, Goethe
N	This symbol does not represent a sound but indicates that the preceding vowel is nasal, as in (French) bon.

CONSONANTS

Print	Key words
b	book
ch	chew, watch
d	day, dead
f	fast, phone, enough
g	good
h	happy
j	jump, gem
k	cook, quick
l	late
m	mammal
n	noon
ng	sing, drink
ng-g	finger
p	pulp
r	ready, rely

s	sassy
sh	shine, sure, lotion
t	to
th	thin (voiceless)
th	than, with (voiced)
v	valve
w	work
y	yes
z	zeal, has
zh	azure, vision
(h)w	when, while
kh	(Scottish) loch, (German) Bach
kh	(German) ich
nyə	onion, (Spanish) señor, (French) Boulogne

a nativitate (ä′ nətiv′itāt, -tä′tā), *adj* existing at birth or from infancy; denotes a congenital disability.

A point, *n* See point, A.

A-P discrepancy, *n* See anterior-posterior discrepancy.

A:G ratio, *n* See ratio, A:G.

aa, *adv* an abbreviation for the Greek term ana, used in prescription writing, meaning "of each."

A-alpha fibers, *n.pl* See fibers, nerve.

ab (antecedent), *prep* beforehand; a notice given previously or a condition existing earlier.

abacterial (ā′baktir′ē-əl), *adj* nonbacterial; free from bacteria.

abandonment (of a patient), *n* withdrawing a patient from treatment without giving reasonable notice or providing a competent replacement.

abatement (əbāt′ment), *n* a decrease in severity of pain or symptoms.

Abbé-Estlander operation (ab′ē-est′landur), *n* See operation, Abbé-Estlander.

abdomen, *n* the portion of the body between the thorax and the pelvis.

abdominal thrust, *n* See Heimlich maneuver.

abduct (abdukt′), *v* to draw away from the median line or from a neighboring part or limb.

abduction (abduk′shən), *n* the process of abducting; opposite of adduction.

aberrant (aber′ənt), *adj* deviating from the usual or normal course, location, or action.

A-beta fibers, See fibers, nerve.

abfraction (ab′frakshən), *n* a mechanism that explains the loss of dentin tissue and tooth enamel caused by flexure and ultimate material fatigue of susceptible teeth at locations away from the point of loading. The breakdown is dependent on the magnitude, duration, frequency, and location of the forces.

ablation, *n* an amputation or excision of any part of the body, or a removal of a growth or harmful substance.

abnormal, *adj* departing from the norm, however defined; departing from the mean of a distribution (statistics); departing from the usual, from a state of integration or adjustment.

abnormal tooth mobility, *n* excessive movement of a tooth within its socket as a result of changes in the supporting tissues caused by injury or disease.

abrade (əbrād), *v* to wear away by friction.

abrasion (əbrā′zhən), *n* **1.** the abnormal wearing away of a substance or tissue by a mechanical process. *n* **2.** the grinding or wearing away of tooth substance by mastication, incorrect brushing methods, bruxism, or similar causes.

Abrasion. (Sapp/Eversole/Wysocki, 2004)

abrasion, dentifrice, *n* the wearing away of the cementum and dentin of an exposed root by an abrasive-containing dentifrice.

abrasive (əbrā′siv), *n* a substance used for grinding or polishing that will wear away a material or tissue.

abrasive disk, *n* See disk, abrasive.

abrasive point, rotary, *n* See point, abrasive, rotary.

abrasive polishing agent, *n* a paste containing sharp-edged particles that are moved over the surface of a material with varying pressure and speed. The movement abrades the surface with microscopic scratches, which creates a polished finish.

abrasive strip, *n* See strip, abrasive.

abrasive system, *n* materials used for

A

polishing and cleansing. Common materials include calcium carbonate (calcite, chalk, whiting), diamond particles (for porcelain), some aluminum derivatives (not for enamel), rouge (jeweler's rouge; applied to gold and precious metal alloys), and tin oxide (putty powder, stannic oxide).

abscess (ab′ses), *n* a localized accumulation of pus in a cavity formed by tissue disintegration.

Abscess. (Regezi/Sciubba/Jordan, 2003)

abscess, alveolar, n See periapical abscess.

abscess, apical, n See periapical abscess.

abscess, dentoalveolar, n See periapical abscess.

abscess, gingival, n a superficial periodontal abscess occurring within the free gingival sulcus surrounding the tooth, frequently caused by the impaction of food. A hull of popcorn is a frequent culprit.

abscess, lateral, n See periodontal abscess.

abscess, periapical, n an abscess involving the apical region of the root, alveolus, and surrounding bone as a sequela of pulpal disease.

abscess, pericoronal, n See pericoronitis.

abscess, periodontal, n an abscess involving the attachment tissues and alveolar bone as a sequela of periodontal disease.

abscess, pulpal, n an abscess occurring within pulpal tissue.

abscess, staphylococcal, n an abscess caused by the bacteria *Staphylococcus aureus,* an infectious agent that can be transmitted via saliva and other discharges of the body. The incubation period is 4 to 10 days; the duration of the abscess varies and is indefinite. The bacteria are communicable throughout the drainage period of the lesions and while the carrier state continues.

absorb (əbzôrb′), *v* **1.** etymological: to suck up. *v* **2.** to incorporate or assimilate a liquid or gas into tissue or cells.

absorbable gelatin sponge, *n trade name:* Gelfoam; *drug class:* hemostatic; *action:* absorbs blood and provides area for clot formation; *uses:* hemostasis during and following surgery.

absorbefacient (abzôr′bifā′shənt), *adj/n* causing absorption, or an agent that promotes absorption.

absorbent (abzôrb′ənt), *adj* a substance that causes absorption of diseased tissue; taking up by suction.

absorptiometry, dual energy x-ray, *n* standard technique that uses two x-ray beams to diagnose osteoporosis and to assess the efficacy of treatment.

absorption (abzôrp′shən), *n* **1.** the passage of a substance into the interior of another by solution or penetration. *n* **2.** the taking up of fluids or other substances by the skin, mucous surfaces, absorbent vessels, or dental materials. *n* **3.** the process by which radiation imparts some or all of its energy to any material through which it passes.

absorption coefficient, n the ratio of the linear rate of change of intensity of roentgen rays in a given homogeneous material to the intensity at a given point within the same mass.

absorption, drug, n in dental terms, one of the factors that determines the speed and duration of response to a local anesthetic. The faster the absorption, the higher the chance of systemic toxicity and the lower the duration of effectiveness. The rate is altered by route of administration.

abstinence, *n* **1.** self-restraint, especially from harmful substances or morally questionable behaviors. *n* **2.** the intentional decision to refrain from sexual activity, especially by unmarried persons. See also withdrawal.

abstraction (abstrak′shən), *n* indicates teeth or other maxillary and mandibular structures that are inferior to (below) their normal position; away from the occlusal plane.

abuse, *n* the improper use of program benefits, resources, and/or services by either dentists, institutions, or patients.

abuse, child, *n* See child abuse.

abuse, nitrous oxide, *n* deliberate inhalation of nitrous oxide to produce mood-altering effects.

abuse, polysubstance, *n* physical dependence on at least three substances that have been classified as habit forming, but without any one of the substances having greater importance or influence than the others. The concept does not include caffeine or nicotine.

abuse, sexual, *n* sexual acts performed with children or with nonconsenting adults in a criminal manner.

abutment (əbut′mənt), *n* a tooth, root, or implant used for support and retention of a fixed or removable prosthesis.

Abutment. (Daniel/Harfst, 2002)

abutment, intermediate, *n* an abutment located between the abutments that form the ends of the prosthesis.

abutment, multiple, *n* abutments splinted together as a unit to support and retain a fixed prosthesis.

a.c., *adv* the abbreviation for ante cibum, a Latin phrase used in prescription writing meaning "before eating."

Academy of General Dentistry, *n.pr* a nonprofit, international organization dedicated to serving the needs and representing the general interests of dentists.

acanthesthesia (əkan′thesthē′zē-ə, zhə), *n* a form of paresthesia experienced as numbness, tingling, or "pins and needles."

acanthion (əkan′thē-on), *n* the tip of the anterior nasal spine.

acantholysis, *n* the loosening, separation, or disassociation of individual prickle cells within the epithelium from their neighbor, often seen in conditions such as pemphigus vulgaris and keratosis follicularis.

acanthosis (ak′ənthō′sis), *n* an increase in the number of cells in the prickle cell layer of stratified squamous epithelium, with thickening of the entire epithelial cell layer and a broadening and fusing of rete pegs.

acapnia (akap′nē-ə), *n* a condition characterized by diminished carbon dioxide in the blood.

acarbia (akär′bē-ə), *n* a condition in which the blood bicarbonate level is decreased.

acarbose, *n* *trade name:* Precose; *drug class:* oligosaccharide, glucosidase enzyme inhibitor; *action:* inhibits α-glucosidase enzyme in the GI tract to slow the breakdown of carbohydrates to glucose; *uses:* a single drug or in combination with others when diet control is ineffective in controlling blood glucose levels.

acatalasemia (ə′katələsē′mē-ə), *n* a congenital lack of the enzyme catalase in blood and other tissues that leads to a progressive necrosis of the oral tissues (Takahara's disease).

accelerator (aksel′ərātur), *n* **1.** that which increases rapidity of action or function. *n* **2.** a catalyst or other substance that hastens a chemical reaction (for example, NaCl added to water and plaster to hasten the set). *n* **3.** a film-developing solution of potassium hydroxide or sodium carbonate used to enlarge the emulsion and to establish an alkaline medium.

accelerator, platelet thrombin, *n* See factor, platelet 2.

accelerator, prothrombin conversion, I, *n* (factor V, labile factor, plasma accelerator globulin, proaccelerin, serum accelerator globulin), considered by some to be a factor in serum and plasma that catalyzes the conversion of inactive prothrombin to an active form.

accelerator, prothrombin conversion, II, *n* (extrinsic thromboplastin, factor VII, serum prothrombin conversion accelerator [SPCA], stable factor), considered by some to be one of the factors in the blood that accelerates the conversion of active prothrombin to thrombin by thromboplastin. Vitamin K deficiency reduces the activity of this factor.

accelerator, serum, *n* See factor V.

accelerin, *n* See factor V.

acceptability, *n* overall assessment of the dental care available to a person or group; includes accessibility, cost, quality, results, convenience, and attitudes of dentists and patients.

acceptance, *n* the act of a person to whom something is offered or tendered by another, whereby he receives that which is offered with the intention of retaining it. A contract is not valid without the acceptance of an offer by the party to whom the offer is made, either expressly or by conduct.

acceptance, absolute, *n* an express and positive agreement to pay a bill according to its text.

acceptance, conditional, *n* an agreement to pay a bill on the fulfillment of a condition.

acceptance, implied, *n* an acceptance interpreted by law from the acts or conduct of the patient.

access (ak′ses), *n* **1.** means of approach. *n* **2.** surgical preparation of hard or soft tissue to allow entrance to a treatment site and adequate space for visualization and instrumentation of the field.

access, cavity, *n* a coronal opening required for effective cleaning, shaping, and filling of the pulp space.

access, computer, *n* **1.** the process of transferring information into or out of a storage location. *n* **2.** the time required to begin and complete the read and write functions of a specified piece of data.

access flap, *n* a periodontal surgical technique that provides visualization of the root in conjunction with curettage and root planing. Types of access flaps include supracrestal, subcrestal-full thickness, and partial thickness flaps.

access, form, *n* the surgical removal of tooth structure sufficient for visualization and instrumentation of a restorative preparation.

accessibility standards, *n.pl* requirements designed by the Americans with Disabilities Act (ADA), by which public places must provide disabled individuals with barrier-free access to buildings, forms of communication, and modes of transportation.

accessory, *adj* providing complementary or supplementary assistance.

accessory canal (akses′ərē), *n* See canal, accessory root.

accident, *n* **1.** an unusual, unforeseen event. *n* **2.** an unusual or unexpected result attending the performance of a usual or necessary act or event. *n* **3.** occurring without intent or happening by chance. The term does not have a precise legal definition but is generally used to indicate that an occurrence was not the result of negligence.

accident, cerebrovascular (CVA), *n* apoplexy resulting from hemorrhage into the brain or occlusion of the cerebral vessels resulting from embolism or thrombosis.

accident, unavoidable, *n* an accident not occasioned, either remotely or directly, by the want of such care or skill as the law holds every person bound to exercise; occurring without fault or negligence.

accident prevention, *n* a set of precautionary measures taken to avoid possible bodily harm. Devices that can be especially important in preventing damage to the dentofacial area are seat belts and bicycle helmets; the use of these should be encouraged in all patients.

accidental exposure management, *n* a set of regulations followed in case of inadvertent exposure to hazardous materials.

account, *n* a basic storage unit in an accounting system. Individual accounts accept debit and credit entries that reflect the different types of transactions made by the practice.

account book, *n* a book in which the financial transactions of a business or profession are entered. Such books may be admitted as evidence.

account, open, *n* a straightforward arrangement between the dentist and the patient for the handling of financial payments due the dentist and owed by the patient.

account, payable, *n* a dollar amount owed to creditors for items or services purchased from them.

accountability, *n* an obligation to

periodically disclose appropriate information in adequate detail and consistent form to all contractually involved parties.

accreditation, *n* a process of formal recognition of a school or institution attesting to the required ability and performance in an area of education, training, or practice.

accretions (əkrē′shənz), *n.pl* accumulations of foreign material such as mucinous plaque, materia alba, and calculus on teeth.

accrual, *n* continually recurring short-term liabilities. Examples are accrued wages, taxes, and interest.

accrued interest, *n* the interest accumulated on a bond since the last payment was made. The buyer of the bond pays the market price plus accumulated interest. Exceptions include bonds that are in default and income bonds.

accrued needs, *n.pl* the amount of treatment needed by an individual or a group at any given time. In dental plans, usually refers to conditions present at the time of enrollment. Synonym: accumulated needs.

acebutolol HCl, *n trade names:* Monitan, Sectral; *drug class:* antihypertensive, selective β_1 blocker; *action:* produces fall in blood pressure without reflex tachycardia or significant reduction in heart rate; *uses:* mild-to-moderate hypertension and ventricular dysrhythmias.

acellular, *adj* not composed of or having cells.

acenesthesia (əsen′esthē′zē-ə, zhə), *n* the loss, or lack, of the normal perception of one's own body; absence of the feelings of a physical existence, a symptom that is common with many psychiatric disorders.

acentric relation (āsen′trik), *n* See relation, jaw, eccentric.

acesulfame-K, *n* a synthetic nonnutritive sweetener.

acetabulum, *n* cup-shaped attachment site located laterally on the hip bone for the head of the femur.

acetaminophen, *n trade names:* Tylenol, Anacin-3; *drug class:* nonnarcotic analgesic; *action:* thought to block initiation of pain impulses by inhibition of prostaglandin synthesis; *uses:* mild-to-moderate pain, fever;

also used in combination with narcotic analgesics.

acetate (as′ətāt), *n* **1.** a salt of acetic acid. *n* **2.** short for cellulose acetate, the film base for x-rays.

acetazolamide/acetazolamide sodium, *n trade names:* Dazamide, Acetazolam, Apo-Acetazolamide; *drug class:* diuretic; carbonic anhydrase inhibitor; *action:* inhibits carbonic anhydrase activity in proximal renal tubular cells to decrease reabsorption of water, sodium, potassium, bicarbonate; *uses:* open-angle glaucoma, epilepsy, drug-induced edema.

acetic acid, *n* a clear, colorless, pungent liquid that is miscible with water, alcohol, glycerin, and ether and that constitutes 3% to 5% of vinegar.

acetohexamide, *n trade names:* Dimelor, Dymelor; *drug class:* sulfonylurea; antidiabetic; *action:* causes functioning β cells in the pancreas to release insulin, leading to a drop in blood glucose level; *uses:* stable adult-onset diabetes mellitus (type II).

acetone (as′ətōn), *n* Dimethylketone; an organic solvent normally present in urine in small amounts but in increased amounts in individuals who have diabetes.

acetone abuse, *n* deliberate inhalation of acetone to produce mood-altering effects.

acetyl groups, *n.pl* carbon- and hydrogen-containing groups required for synthesis of lipids.

acetylcholine (as′ətilkō′lēn, əsē′til), *n* **1.** an acetate ester of choline that serves as a neurohumoral agent in the transmission of an impulse in autonomic ganglia, parasympathetic postganglionic fibers, and somatic motor fibers. *n* **2.** an ester of choline actively involved as a chemical mediator at the neuromuscular junction, at autonomic ganglia, and between parasympathetic nerve endings and visceral effectors.

acetylcysteine, *n trade name:* Mucosil; *drug class:* mucolytic; *action:* decreases viscosity of pulmonary secretions by breaking disulfide links of mucoproteins; *uses:* acetaminophen toxicity, bronchitis, pneumonia, cystic fibrosis, emphysema, atelecta-

A

sis tuberculosis, and complications of thoracic surgery.

achlorhydria (ā'klôrhī'drē-ə), *n* the absence of free hydrochloric acid in the stomach, even with histamine stimulation.

achondroplasia (ākon'drōplā'zē-ə, -zhə), *n* a hereditary disturbance of endochondral bone formation transmitted as a mendelian dominant factor and resulting in dwarfism. Malocclusion and prognathism may occur.

achromatopsia (əkrōm-ətōp'sē-ə), *n* total color blindness.

Achromycin V, *n.pr* a proprietary name for the antibiotic tetracycline hydrochloride.

achylia, *n* the absence or lack of hydrochloric acid and the enzyme pepsinogen in the stomach.

acid (as'id), *n* a chemical substance that, in an aqueous solution, undergoes dissociation with the formation of hydrogen ions; pH levels range from 0 to 6.9.

acid, acetic, n the acid of vinegar, sometimes used as a solvent for the removal of calculus from a removable dental prosthesis. See also solvent.

acid, ascorbic, n See vitamin C.

acid, carbolic, n See phenol.

acid, cevitamic, n See vitamin C.

acid etchant, n an application of phosphoric acid used to prepare enamel surfaces to aid sealant placement.

acid etching, n treating the tooth enamel, generally with phosphoric acid, by removal of approximately 40 mm of rod cross-section to provide retention for resin sealant, restorative material, or orthodontic bracket.

acid, folic, n See vitamin B complex.

acid, hydroxypropionic, n See acid, lactic.

acid, lactic (hydroxypropionic acid), n a monobasic acid, $C_3H_6O_3$, formed as an end product in the intermediary metabolism of carbohydrates. The accumulation of lactic acid in the tissues is in part responsible for the lowering of pH levels during inflammatory states; that is, the drop in pH level is believed to hasten bone resorption in periodontitis because the minerals in the bone are stable

within the matrix only at the normal tissue pH level of 7.4.

acid, nicotinic, n **1.** one of the vitamins of the B complex group and its vitamer, niacinamide, specific for the treatment of pellagra. Niacinamide functions as a constituent of coenzyme I (DPN) and coenzyme II (TPN). Nicotinic acid is found in lean meats, liver, yeast, milk, and leafy green vegetables. *n* **2.** an acid (C_5H_4N [COOH]) that forms part of the B complex group of vitamins. The body requires this acid as a cofactor in intermediary carbohydrate metabolism. This acid is a constituent of certain coenzymes that function in oxidative-reductive metabolic systems. With niacinamide, nicotinic acid is a pellagra-preventive factor. Also called *niacin, P.-P. factor, pyridine 3-carboxylic acid, vitamin P.-P.*

acid, orthophosphoric, n See acid, phosphoric.

acid, pantothenic, n **1.** one of the B complex vitamins, the importance of which has not been established in human nutrition. Pantothenic acid is a constituent of coenzyme A and as such is presumed to be involved in adrenocortical function. *n* **2.** a vitamin of the B complex that is widely distributed in food and tissues and important for normal development in certain animals such as chickens and rats. Pantothenic acid deficiency in rats produces retrograde changes in alveolar and supporting bone.

acid phosphatase, n an enzyme found in the kidneys, serum, semen, and prostate gland. Acid phosphatase is elevated in serum blood levels in individuals with prostate cancer and in individuals who have recently experienced trauma.

acid, phosphoric (H_3PO_4, orthophosphoric acid), n the principal ingredient of silicate and zinc phosphate cement liquids.

acid, pteroylglutamic, n See vitamin B complex.

acid salt, n a salt containing one or more replaceable hydrogen ions.

acid, strong, n an acid that is completely ionized in aqueous solution.

acid-base balance, *n* in metabolism, the balance of acid to base necessary to keep the blood pH level normal (between 7.35 and 7.43).

acidemia (as′idē′mē-ə), *n* a decreased pH level of the blood, irrespective of changes in the blood bicarbonate.

acidemia, isovaleric, *n* a genetic disorder of amino acid metabolism in which isovaleric acid accumulates in the blood and urine at abnormally high levels; may respond to a low-protein diet and the administration of synthetic amino acids. See also homocystinuria.

acidifier (əsid′iff′ur), *n* a chemical ingredient (acetic acid) that maintains the required acidity of the fixer and stop-bath solutions in the photographic development process.

acidogenic, *adj* generating acid or acidity.

acidophilic (as′idōfil′ik), *adj* **1.** readily stained with acid dyes. *adj* **2.** growing well in an acid medium.

acidosis (as′idō′sis), *n* a pathologic disturbance of the acid-base balance of the body characterized by an excess of acid or inadequate base. Causes include acid ingestion, increased acid production such as that seen in diabetes or starvation, or loss of base through the kidneys or intestine.

acidosis, compensated, *n* a condition of acidosis in which the body pH level is maintained within the normal range through compensatory mechanisms involving the kidneys or lungs.

acidosis, respiratory, *n* acidemia resulting from retention of an excess of CO_3 caused by hypoventilation

acidosis, uncompensated, *n* acidosis in which compensatory mechanisms are unable to maintain the body pH level within the normal range.

acidulated phosphate fluoride, *n* topical agent used in prevention of dental caries.

Acinetobacter, *n* a genus of nonmotile, aerobic bacteria of the family *Neisseriaceae* that often occurs in clinical specimens.

acinus, *n* saclike cavity present in a gland or the lungs.

Ackerman-Proffit orthogonal analysis, *n.pr* a taxonomy of malocclusion based on set theory or Boolean algebra, which is organized using combinations and permutations of malocclusions within the three planes of space. See also Appendix F.

acne, *n* an inflammatory, papulopustular skin eruption occurring most often in or near the sebaceous glands on the face, neck, shoulders, and upper back.

acne rosacea, *n* a condition of the facial skin typically indicated by blushing, swelling, and the appearance of broken blood vessels in a "spider web" pattern.

acne vulgaris, *n* a common form of acne seen predominantly in adolescents and young adults. Acne vulgaris is probably an effect of the rise of androgenic hormones.

Acne rosacea. (Regezi/Sciubba/Jordan, 2003)

acoustic coupler, *n* a connection between a phone line and a data set, or modem. The coupler makes use of an ordinary telephone and headset and requires no modification to the normal phone.

acoustic turbulence, *n* agitation observed in fluids by mechanical vibrations of an ultrasonic tip; used to disrupt bacterial cell walls.

acquired centric relation (sen-′trik), *n* See relation, centric, and relation, jaw, eccentric.

acquired immunodeficiency syndrome (AIDS), *n* a disease caused by a retrovirus known as human immunodeficiency virus type 1 (HIV-1). A related but distinct retrovirus (HIV-2) has recently appeared in a limited number of patients in the United States. Patients are considered to have AIDS when one or more indicator diseases, as defined by the Centers for Disease Control (CDC), are present. The CDC has classified stages of the disease as follows:

Group I: acute HIV infection, *n* within one month of exposure, the first clinical evidence of HIV infection may appear as an acute retroviral syndrome. This is a mononucleosis-like syndrome with symptoms including fever, rash, diarrhea, lymphadenopathy, myalgia, arthralgia, and fatigue. Development of antibodies usually follows.

Group II: asymptomatic HIV infection, *n* most persons develop antibodies to the HIV within 6 to 12 weeks after exposure. Although individuals may remain asymptomatic for months or years, they can transmit the virus.

Group III: persistent generalized lymphadenopathy (PGL), *n* HIV-infected patients in this group develop persistent generalized lymphadenopathy that lasts longer than 3 months.

Group IV: HIV-associated diseases, *n* patients in this group are clinically variable and have signs and symptoms of HIV infection other than or in addition to lymphadenopathy. Based on clinical findings, patients in Group IV may be assigned to one or more of the following subgroups: (A) constitutional disease, also known as wasting syndrome. This subgroup is characterized by fever that lasts more than one month, involuntary weight loss of greater than 10% for baseline, or diarrhea persisting for more than one month, (B) neurological disease, (C) secondary infectious disease, (D) secondary cancers, and (E) other conditions resulting from HIV infections.

acridine, *n* a dibenzopyridine compound used in the synthesis of dyes and drugs.

acroanesthesia
(ak′rō-an′esthē′zē-ə, -zhə), *n* anesthesia of the extremities.

acrocephalia (ak′rōsefal′ē-ə), *n* a deformity of the head characterized by an upward and forward bulge of the frontal bones and a flat occiput. Synonym: oxycephalia.

acrodermatitis, *n* any eruption of the skin of the hands and feet caused by a parasitic mite, which is a member of the order Acarina.

acrodynia (ak′rōdī′nē-ə), *n* (erythredema polyneuropathy, Feer's syndrome, pink disease, Swift's syndrome, Selter's disease), a disease that occurs in infants and young children in which manifestations occur with the eruption of the primary teeth. Symptoms include raw-beef

hands and feet, superficial sensory loss, photophobia, tachycardia, muscular hypotonia, changes in temperament, stomatitis, periodontitis, and premature loss of teeth. The etiology has been related to mercury and deficiency of vitamin B6 and essential fatty acids. See also erythredema polyneuropathy.

acroesthesia (ak′rō-esthē′zē-ə, -zhə), *n* **1.** increased sensitivity. *n* **2.** pain in the extremities.

acromegaly (akrəmeg′əlē), *n* (Marie's disease), a condition caused by hyperfunction of the pituitary gland in adults. Characterized by enlargement of the skeletal extremities, including the feet, hands, mandible, and nose.

Acromegaly. (Proffit/White/Sarver, 2003)

acrosclerosis (ak′rōsklerō′sis), *n* a special form of scleroderma that affects the extremities, head, and face and is associated with Raynaud's phenomenon. There may be significant thickening of the periodontal membrane.

acrylic (/əkril′ik), *adj* formed from acrylic acid; for example, acrylic resin, acrylic resin denture, and acrylic resin tooth. See also denture, acrylic resin; and tooth, acrylic resin.

acrylic resin, *n* See resin, acrylic.

ACTH (adrenocorticotropic hormone), *n* hormone produced by basophilic cells of the anterior lobe of the pituitary gland that exerts a reciprocal regulating influence on the production of corticosteroids by the adrenal cortex.

actinic cheilitis (aktin′ik), *n* See cheilitis, actinic.

Actinobacillus, *n* a genus of nonmobile, gram-negative aerobic and facultatively anaerobic bacteria of the family Brucellaceae that is pathogenic to cattle, sheep, horses, and pigs.

Actinomyces israelii, *n.pl* a normally occurring oral bacteria that aggressively causes infection (actinomycosis) when oral health is compromised.

Actinomyces naeslundii, *n* a specific strain of bacteria resident in open sores in the mouth.

Actinomyces viscosus, *n* a species of *Actinomyces* occurring in high numbers in the dental plaque, cemental caries, and tonsillar crypts.

actinomycetemocomitans (aktinōmīsē′temokom′itanz), *n* a microorganism found in and considered responsible for some periodontal infections.

actinomycetes (ak′tinōmīse′tēz), *n.pl* filamentous microorganisms that have been implicated in the formation of dental calculus and serve as a mode of attachment of dental calculus to the tooth surface. These microorganisms have also been found in pathologic lesions of the alveolar processes (actinomycosis).

actinomycosis (ak′tinōmīkō′sis), *n* (lumpy jaw), an infection of humans and some animal species caused by species of *Actinomyces,* which are gram-positive, filamentous, microaerophilic microorganisms.

Actinomycosis. (Regezi/Sciubba/Jordan, 2003)

action potential, *n* **1.** an electric impulse consisting of a self-propagating series of polarizations and depolarizations, transmitted across the cell membranes of a nerve fiber during the transmission of a nerve impulse and across the cell membranes of a muscle cell during contraction. *n* **2.** the electrical potential developed in a muscle or nerve during activity.

activate (ak′tivāt), *v* to adjust an appliance so that it will exert effective force on the teeth and jaws.

activated resin, *n* See resin, auto polymer.

activator (ak′tivātur), *n* **1.** an alkali, sodium carbonate, which is a component of photographic developing solution that softens and swells the gelatin of the film emulsion and provides the necessary alkaline medium for the developing agents to react with the sensitized silver halide crystals. *n* **2.** a removable orthodontic appliance intended to function as a passive transmitter and sometimes stimulator of the forces of the perioral muscles. One in the myofunctional category of appliances also known by such names as *Andresen, Bimler, Monobloc,* and *Frankel.*

active, *adj* pertaining to the condition of an orthodontic appliance that has been adjusted to apply effective force to the teeth or jaws.

active reciprocation, *n* See reciprocation, active.

acts, practice, *n.pl* the statutory requirements of a sovereign state for the education, training, examination, credentialing, supervision, and accountability of a wide range of health care providers, including dental hygienists.

acuity (əkyōōitē), *n* sharpness; clearness; keenness.

acuity, auditory, *n* the sensitivity of the auditory apparatus; sharpness of hearing. The ability to hear a given tone with respect to the degree of intensity required to produce a sensation that is just perceptible.

acuity, visual, *n* sharpness, acuteness, clearness of vision. Visual acuity may be defective because of optical or neurologic dysfunction.

acupuncture, *n* a method of producing analgesia or altering the function of a system of the body by inserting fine, wire-thin needles into the skin at specific sites on the body along a series of lines or channels called meridians. The needles may be twirled, energized electrically, or warmed. Acupuncture originated in the Far East and has gained increasing attention in the West since the early 1970s.

acute, *adj* pertaining to a traumatic, pathologic, or physiologic phenomenon or process having a short and relatively severe course. Antonym: chronic.

acute phase reactions, n.pl abnormalities in the blood associated with acute and chronic inflammatory and necrotic processes and detected by a variety of tests, including erythrocyte sedimentation rate, C-reactive protein, serum hexosamine, serum mucoprotein, and serum nonglucosamine polysaccharides.

acyclovir (āsī′klōvir), *n* an antiviral drug active against herpes viruses. Used as a 5% ointment; may be used systemically. Drug of choice in immunocompromised patients with candidiasis. *Trade name:* Zovirax.

acyclovir sodium, n trade name: Zovirax; *drug class:* antiviral; *action:* see **acyclovir, topical;** *uses:* as above, plus *herpes. zoster* and *varicella* (chickenpox).

acyclovir, topical, n trade name: Zovirax; *drug class:* antiviral; *action:* interferes with viral DNA replication; *uses:* simple mucocutaneous herpes simplex, in immunocompromised patients with initial herpes genitalis.

ADA, *n* **I.** the abbreviation for *American Dental Association,* the national professional organization for dentists in the United States. *n* **2.** the abbreviation for the *American Dairy Association. n* **3.** the abbreviation for **adenosine deaminase,** an enzyme that breaks down toxic biological products. The absence of this enzyme causes a rare disease called *severe combined immunodeficiency.*

ADA Seal of Acceptance, *n.pr* the insignia of the American Dental Association's Council on Scientific Affairs given to safe and effective consumer and professional products used in all aspects of oral health and maintenance, from toothpaste and

dental floss to orthodontic surgical instruments and prosthodontic devices.

ADA Seal of Acceptance.

adamantinoma (adəman′tinō′mə), *n* See ameloblastoma.

adamantoblastoma (adəman′tōblastō′mə), *n* See ameloblastoma.

Adams' clasp, *n* a retention clasp designed by C. Philip Adams to stabilize removable appliances by engaging the mesiobuccal and distobuccal surfaces of buccal teeth.

adaptation, *n* **I.** an alteration that an organ or organism undergoes to adjust to its environment. **2.** a close approximation of a tissue flap, an appliance, or a restorative material to natural tissue. **3.** an accurate adjustment of a band or a shell to a tooth. **4.** a condition in reflex activity marked by a decline in the frequency of impulses when sensory stimuli are repeated several times.

adaptation, instrument, n the process of manually adjusting and positioning the functional end, edge, or surface of a dental instrument for safe and effective use according to its purpose and relative to the shape of the tooth.

adapter, band, *n* an instrument used as an aid in fitting an orthodontic band to a tooth.

adaptive functioning, *n* the relative ability of a person to effectively interact with society on all levels and care for one's self; affected by one's willingness to practice skills and pursue opportunities for improvement on all levels. Often used to describe levels of mental retardation.

addict (ad′ikt), *n* an individual who has developed physiologic or psychologic dependence on a chemical such as alcohol or other drugs.

addiction (ədik′shən), *n* the state of being addicted. Although there is no universally accepted definition, addiction is generally considered a condition involving two factors: (1) a compulsive behavior pattern, and (2) an altered physiologic state that requires continued use of the drug to prevent withdrawal symptoms.

addictive (ədik′tiv), *adj* pertaining to a drug whose repeated use may produce addiction. Present federal regulations place greater emphasis on the broader designation of potential for abuse.

Addison's disease, *n.pr* See disease, Addison's.

Addison-Biermer anemia (ad′isən bir′mur), *n.pr* See anemia, pernicious.

additive, *n* an ingredient added to a food, drug, or other preparation to produce a desired result, such as color or consistency, unrelated to the primary purpose of the preparation.

adduct (ədukt′), *v* to draw toward the center or midline.

adduction (əduk′shən), *n* the process of bringing two objects toward each other; the opposite of abduction.

A-delta fibers, *n.pl* See fiber, nerve.

adenine, *n* a component of the nucleic acids, DNA and RNA, and a constituent of cyclic AMP and the adenosine portion of AMP, ADP, and ATP.

adenitis (ad′əni′tis), *n* an inflammation of glandular tissue, often accompanied by pain.

adenoameloblastoma (ad′ənō′-amel′ōblastō′mə), *n* an epithelial neoplasm with a basic structure resembling enamel organs and glandular (adenomatous) tissue. It is generally benign.

adenocarcinoma (ad′ənōkarsinō′mə), *n* any one of a large group of malignant epithelial cell tumors of the glands. Specific tumors are diagnosed and named by the cell type of the tissue affected.

adenocarcinoma, acinar cell, *n* a malignant tumor whose cells appear as glandular tissue.

adenoid, *adj* **1.** having a glandular appearance, particularly lymphoid. *n.pl* **2.** adenoids refer to the pharyngeal tonsils located on the posterior wall of the nasopharynx.

adenoid facies, *n* an archaic term used to describe patients who exhibit a long, narrow face, short upper lip, open-mouth breathing, and a hyperactive swallowing pattern.

adenoidectomy, *n* the removal of the lymphoid tissue in the nasopharynx, usually in conjunction with the surgical removal of the tonsils.

adenoma (ad′ənō′mə), *n* a benign epithelial neoplasm or tumor with a basic glandular (acinar) structure, suggesting derivation from glandular tissue.

Adenoma. (Regezi/Sciubba/Jordan, 2003)

adenoma, acidophilic, *n* See oncocytoma.

adenoma, oxyphilic, *n* See oncocytoma.

adenomatosis oris (ad′ənōmətō′sis), *n* an enlargement of the mucous glands of the lip without secretion or inflammation.

adenopathy (ad′ənop′əthē), *n* an enlargement or increase in size of glandular organs or tissues usually resulting from disease processes.

adenosine, *n* a compound derived from nucleic acid, composed of adenine and a sugar, D-ribose. Adenosine is the major molecular component of nucleotides and the nucleic acids.

adenosine monophosphate (AMP), *n* an ester, composed of adenine, D-ribose, and phosphoric acid, that affects energy release in work done by a muscle.

adenosine triphosphate (ATP), *n* a compound consisting of the nucleotide adenosine attached through its ribose group to three phosphoric acid molecules. It stores energy in muscles, which is released when it is hydrolized to adenosine diphosphate.

Adenoviridae, *n* family of unenveloped, 20-sided DNA viruses found in mammals (Mastadenovirus) and birds (Aviadenovirus). The human variety can cause a number of diseases, from conjunctivitis to urinary tract infection.

adequacy, velopharyngeal, *n* a functional closure of the velum to the postpharyngeal wall that restricts air and sound from entering the nasopharyngeal and nasal cavities.

adequate intake (AI), *n* the consumption and absorption of sufficient food, vitamins, and essential minerals necessary to maintain health. See also dietary reference intakes; estimated average requirement; recommended dietary allowances; and upper intake levels, tolerable.

ADH, *n* See hormone, antidiuretic.

adhesion (adh'zhən), *n* **1.** the attraction of unlike molecules for one another. **2.** the molecular attraction existing between surfaces in close contact. **3.** the condition in which a material sticks to itself or another material. **4.** the abnormal joining of tissues, generally by fibrous connective tissue, to each other after repair of an injury.

adhesion, bacterial, *n* microbial surface antigens that frequently exist in the form of filamentous projections and bind to specific receptors on epithelial cell membranes.

adhesive foil, *n* See foil, adhesive.

adhesion, sublabial, *n* the abnormal union of the sublabial mucosa of the upper lip to the alveolar process; usually present in a unilateral or bilateral cleft of the lip.

adhesive, *n* an intermediate material that causes two materials to stick together; a luting agent.

adhesives, bonding, for desensitization, *n* sealant materials applied to the open ends of dentinal tubules which block the stimuli linked to tooth sensitivity.

adipose tissue, *n* a connective tissue composed of a collection of fat cells.

adjudicate, *v* the final step in dental peer review at which the dental peer review committee renders a formal, nonlegal decision on a case.

adjunct (aj'ungkt), *n* a drug or other substance that serves a supplemental purpose in therapy.

adjust (əjust'), *v* to make correspondent, comfortable, or to fit.

adjustment (əjust'ment), *n* a modification of a restoration or of a denture after insertion in the mouth.

adjustment, occlusal, *n* a grinding of the occluding surfaces of teeth to develop harmonious relationships between each other, their supporting structures, muscles of mastication, and temporomandibular joints.

adjuvant (aj'əvənt), *n* in a prescription, an auxiliary active ingredient that supports the action of the basic drug. See also basis.

administration, *n* the giving of, dispensing of, or application of medicines, drugs, or remedies to relieve or cure an illness.

administration, buccal, *n* the delivery of a medication by application to the buccal mucosa.

administration, inhalation, *n* the delivery of a medication by breathing it.

administration, intranasal, *n* See administration, inhalation.

administration, oral, *n* the delivery of a medication by mouth.

administration, rectal, *n* the delivery of a medication through the rectum.

administration, sublingual, *n* the delivery of a medication by placing it under the tongue for dissolution and absorption through the mucous membrane.

administration, topical, *n* the delivery of a medication by application to the skin.

administrative costs, *n.pl* the overhead expenses incurred in the operation of a dental benefits program, excluding costs of dental services provided.

administrative services only (ASO), *n* an arrangement in which a third party, for a fee, processes claims and handles paperwork for a self-funded group. This frequently includes almost all insurance company services, including actuarial services, underwriting, and benefit description, and excluding assumption of risk.

administrator, *n* a person who manages or directs a dental benefits program on behalf of the program's sponsor. See also third-party administrator and dental benefits organization.

admission, *n* the voluntary concession or admission that a fact or allegation is true.

admission, hospital, n **1.** full stay. The formal acceptance by a hospital or other inpatient health care facility of a patient who is to be provided with room, board, and continuous nursing service in an area of the hospital or facility where patients generally reside at least overnight. *n* **2.** surgicenter with short stays. Day bed only with nursing; patient does not stay overnight. *n* **3.** outpatient admission. Pertains to a patient who enters the hospital but requires no bed; the patient enters for treatment and leaves after treatment.

adnexa (adnek´sə), *n* conjoined anatomic parts, or tissues adjacent to or contained within a nearby space.

adolescence, *n* the period of human development between the onset of puberty and adulthood. This period is generally marked by the appearance of secondary sex characteristics, usually from 11 to 13 years of age, and spans the teen years.

adolescent growth spurt, *n* a period of rapid increase in height, weight, and muscle mass which, for boys, takes place at age 12 to 16 and, for girls, at age 11 to 14. See also adolescence.

adrenal cortex, *n* the greater portion of the adrenal gland fused with the gland's medulla and producing mineralocorticoids, androgens, and glucocorticoids, hormones essential to homeostasis. The outer cortex is normally a deep yellow; the inner part is dark red or brown.

adrenal corticoid, *n* See corticoid, adrenal.

adrenal crisis, *n* See crisis, adrenal.

adrenal steroids, *n.pl* See corticoid, adrenal.

adrenalectomy, *n* the surgical removal of one or both of the adrenal glands or the resection of a portion of one or both of the adrenal glands.

Adrenalin (ədren´əlin), *n* the trade name for epinephrine. See also epinephrine.

adrenaline (ədren´əlin), *n* the British term for epinephrine.

adrenergic (ad´rinur´jik), *adj* **1.** transmitted by norepinephrine or activated by norepinephrine or the other sympathomimetic agents. *n* **2.** a term applied to nerve fibers that liberate epinephrine or norepinephrine at a synapse when a nerve impulse passes. *n* **3.** a drug that mimics the action of adrenergic nerves.

adrenergic agonists, n.pl drugs which mimic the actions of norepinephrine, a neurotransmitter resulting in stimulation of the sympathetic nervous system.

adrenergic blocking agent, n See agent, adrenergic blocking.

adrenergic fibers, n.pl See fibers, adrenergic.

adrenergic receptors, n.pl See receptors, adrenergic.

adrenic (ədrē´nik), *adj* pertaining to the adrenal gland.

adrenocortical insufficiency (ədrē´ nōkôr´tikəl), *n* acute or chronic adrenocortical hypofunction, as in Waterhouse-Friderichsen syndrome or Addison's disease. See hypoadrenocorticalism.

adrenocorticotropin (ədrē´nōkôr´ tikōtrō´pin), *n* See ACTH.

adrenolytic (ədrē´nōlit´ik), *adj* capable of impeding the action of epinephrine, levarterenol (norepinephrine), or both (sympatholytic).

adrenolytic agent, n See agent, adrenergic blocking.

adrenotropic (ədrē´nōtrōp´ik), *adj* having a special affinity for the adrenal gland.

adsorb, *v* to attract molecules of a substance to the surface of another solid substance.

adsorbent, *adj* a substance that adsorbs, such as activated charcoal and clay.

adsorption, *n* a natural process whereby molecules of a gas or liquid adhere to the surface of a solid.

adult, *n* **1.** a person who is fully developed and who has attained the intellectual capacity and the emotional and psychologic stability characteristic of a mature person. *n* **2.** a person who has reached full legal age.

adumbration (ad´əmbrā´shən), *n* a geometric lack of sharpness of the x-ray shadow. See also penumbra, geometric.

advances, *n.pl* monies paid before the scheduled time of payment.

adverse drug effect, *n* a harmful, unintended reaction to a drug administered at normal dosage.

adverse reaction, *n* any harmful, unintended effect of a medication, diagnostic test, or therapeutic intervention.

adverse reactions, *n.pl* unfavorable reactions resulting from administration of a local anesthetic; responsible factors include the drug used, concentration, and route of administration.

adverse selection, *n* a statistical condition within a group when there is a greater demand for dental services and/or more services necessary than the average expected for that group.

advertising, *n* any paid form of nonpersonal presentation and promotion of ideas, goods, or services by an identified sponsor.

aeration (erā′shən), *n* the passage of air or gases into liquid (for example, the passage of oxygen from pulmonary alveoli into the blood).

aerobiosis, *n* life occurring in the presence of oxygen.

aerodontalgia (er′ōdontal′jə), *n* pulpal pain with decreased barometric pressure.

Aeromonas, *n* a genus of bacteria usually found in water.

aerosol (er′əsôl), *n* **1.** the suspension of materials in a gas or vapor (for example, saliva vaporized in airwater spray from a high-speed handpiece). **2.** a substance dispensed as a constituent of a gas or vapor suspension.

aesthetic factors, *n.pl* See esthetic dentistry.

affect (af′ekt), *n* **1.** the feeling of pleasantness or unpleasantness produced by a stimulus. *n* **2.** the emotional complex influencing a mental state. *n* **3.** the feeling experienced in connection with an emotion.

affective domain, *n* the area of learning involved in appreciation, interests, and attitudes.

afferent (af′ərənt), *adj* conveying from a periphery to a center.

afferent impulse, *n* an impulse that arises in the periphery and is carried into the central nervous system. An afferent nerve conducts the impulse from the site of origin to the central nervous system.

afferent nerves, *n.pl* See nerves, afferent, in pulp.

afferent neurons, *n.pl* See neuron, afferent. See also afferent impulse.

affiliation (əfil′ē-ā′shən), *n* the incorporation or formation of a partnership by two or more dentists for the purpose of practicing the profession of dentistry.

afflux (af′luks), *n* the rush of blood to a body part.

affricative (əfrik′ətiv), *n* a fricative speech sound initiated by a plosive.

aflatoxins, *n.pl* a group of carcinogenic and toxic factors produced by *Aspergillus flavus* food molds.

afterperception, the perception of a sensation after the stimulus producing it has ceased. (not current)

agar, hydrocolloid (ä′gär), *n* a reversible hydrocolloid made from agar-agar.

age, *n* the period of time a person has existed since birth or an object has existed since its beginning.

age, chronologic, *n* age determined by the passage of time since birth.

age determination, *n* (by teeth) an estimate of age from the stage of tooth development and/or pattern of wear.

age distribution, *n* a grouping of the persons within a population on the basis of birth date.

age factors, *n.pl* variables affected by time since birth.

age hardening, *n* See hardening, age.

age of onset, *n* the chronologic age of the patient at which the disease, affliction, or disability appeared.

aged, *n* a state of having grown older or more mature than others of the population. See also geriatrics.

agenesis (ājen′əsis), *n* the defective development or congenital absence of parts.

agent(s), *n* **1.** a person or product that causes action. *n* **2.** a person authorized to act for, or in place of, another.

agent, adrenergic blocking, *n* a drug that blocks the action of the neurohormones norepinephrine and/or epinephrine or of adrenergic drugs at sympathetic neuroeffectors.

agent, adrenolytic blocking, n an uncertain term sometimes used in reference to adrenergic blocking agents.

agent, anesthetic, n a drug that produces local or general loss of sensation.

agent, antianxiety, n any medication prescribed to relieve anxiety disorder symptoms, primarily stress and insomnia. The most common forms are benzodiazepine derivatives.

agent, antiarrhythmic, n.pl substance used to prevent or relieve an irregular rhythm of heartbeat. Also mistakenly called *antidysrhythmic.*

agent, antigingivitis, n any compound that inhibits, controls, or kills organisms associated with the formation of gingivitis.

agent, antihypertensive, n medication used to lower elevated blood pressure (e.g., diuretics, beta-blockers, and vasodilators).

agent, antiinflammatory, n a drug that reduces inflammation.

agent, antimanic, n a substance used to treat various nervous system and psychiatric disorders; possible effects on fetal development include sluggishness, oxygen deficiency, and physical malformations.

agent, antiparasitic, n an antimicrobe that specifically targets pathogenic microorganisms.

agent, bleaching, n an agent used in the modification or removal of discoloration.

agent, blocking, n an agent that occupies or usurps the receptor site normally occupied by a drug or a biochemical intermediary (for example, acetylcholine or epinephrine).

agent, chemotherapeutic, n a chemical of natural or synthetic origin used for its specific action against disease, usually against infection.

agent, cholinergic blocking, n **1.** a drug that inhibits the action of acetylcholine or cholinergic drugs at the postganglionic cholinergic neuroeffectors. *n* **2.** an anticholinergic agent.

agent, cleaning, n.pl an abrasive substance contained in toothpastes, gels, and powders which polishes teeth and aids in the removal of stains and plaque. See also abrasion, dentifrice.

agent, coloring, n.pl any substance contained in toothpastes, gels, and powders purely to make the product more appealing.

agent, ganglionic blocking, n a drug that prevents passage of nerve impulses at the synapses between preganglionic and postganglionic neurons.

agent, myoneural blocking, n a drug that prevents transmission of nerve impulses at the junction of the nerve and the muscle.

agent, oxidizing, n an agent that provides oxygen in reaction with another substance or, in the broader and more definitive chemical sense, a chemical capable of accepting electrons and thereby decreasing the negative charge on an atom of the substance being oxidized.

agent, polishing, n an abrasive that produces a smooth, lustrous finish.

agent, postganglionic sympathetic blocking, n.pl pharmacologic agents used to treat hypertension by blocking the release of the naturally occurring hormone norepinephrine.

agent, reducing, n a category of chemicals used in film processing which brings out the gray tones of an image by creating black metallic silver from silver halide crystals.

agent, wetting, n any agent that will reduce the surface tension of water. Generally used in investing wax patterns.

agents, antiadrenergic, centrally acting, n.pl antihypertensive drugs used to lower blood pressure, specifically those that operate by stimulating α-receptors in the central nervous system and arterioles.

agents, antianginal, n one of several types of medication used to treat heart disease; alleviates pain associated with angina by lowering blood pressure during systole. See also vasodilator.

agents, oxygenating, n.pl substances, such as hydrogen peroxide, which, when used as mouthrinses, release oxygen into gingival tissues and reduce inflammation. It has not proved to reduce the bacteria causing the inflammation. Long-term use may cause tissue damage.

agents, sympathetic, n.pl pharmacologic agents which stimulate the sympathetic nervous system by imitating the actions of naturally occurring norepinephrine and epinephrine. They may be used to treat cardiac arrest, nasal congestion, asthma, glaucoma, and attention deficit hyperactivity disorder. They may cause anxiety, loss of appetite, and arrythmias. Also called *adrenergic agents*.

ageusia (əgōō′sē-ə), *n* a loss or impairment of the sense of taste.

agglutination (əglōō′tinā′shən), *n* the aggregation or clumping together of cells as a result of their interaction with specific antibodies called agglutinins, commonly used in blood typing and in identifying or estimating the strength of immunoglobulins or immune sera.

agglutinin (əglōō′tinin), *n* **1.** a specific kind of antibody whose interaction with antigens is manifested as agglutination. **2.** an antibody that agglutinates red blood cells or renders them agglutinable.

aging, *n* in human development, the process of growing old. Physically, aging is marked by the reduction in the ability of cells to function normally or to produce new body cells at an optimal rate.

aging schedule, *n* a report showing how long accounts receivable have been outstanding. It gives the percentage of receivables not past due and the percentage past due by 1 month, 2 months, or other periods.

agitation, *n* **1.** the shaking of a substance, either for mixing ingredients or to remove debris or buildup from an object within the substance, such as a removable oral prosthetic. **2.** the intentional, usually mild, disturbance of the skin, mucosa, or other surface (e.g., with a wooden interdental cleaner or probe instrument) to determine if infection or disease is present. If agitated surfaces bruise or bleed easily, or are otherwise disrupted (e.g., develop a lesion), the presence of a pathology should be suspected. **3.** a psychosomatic condition represented by uncontrollable or excessive body movements. The psychological aspect may often indicate the presence of unresolved stress.

aglossia (aglôs′ē-ə), *n* a developmental anomaly in which a portion or all of the tongue is absent.

agnathia (agnath′ē-ə), *n* an absence of the lower jaw.

agnosia (agnō′zē-ə, -zhə), *n* a loss of ability to recognize common objects (that is, a loss of ability to understand the significance of sensory stimuli [for example, tactile, auditory, or visual] resulting from brain damage).

agonist (ag′ənist), *n* **1.** an organ, gland, muscle, or nerve center that is so connected physiologically with another that the two function simultaneously in forwarding a given process, such as when two muscles pull on the same skeletal member and receive a nervous excitation at the same time. Antonym: antagonist. **2.** a drug or other substance having a specific cellular affinity that produces a predictable response.

agony, *n* **1.** severe pain or extreme suffering. **2.** the death struggle.

agoraphobia, *n* an anxiety disorder characterized by a fear of being in an open, crowded, or public place where escape may be difficult or help may not be available if needed.

agranulocytosis (āgran′yŏŏlōsītō-′sis), *n* a decrease in the number of granulocytes in peripheral blood resulting from bone marrow depression by drugs and chemicals or replacement by a neoplasm. Oral lesions are ulceronecrotic, involving the gingivae, tongue, buccal mucosa, or lips. Regional lymphadenopathy and lymphadenitis are prevalent.

Agranulocytosis. (Regezi/Sciubba/Jordan, 2003)

agreement, *n* the coming together in accord of two minds on a given proposition; a concord of understanding and intention with respect to the effect on relative rights and duties.

AH-26, *n* an epoxy resin root canal sealer.

AHF, *n* the abbreviation for antihemophilic factor. See also factor VIII.

aid, *n* assistance; support.

aid in physiotherapy, *n* an agent used by the patient to cleanse the teeth and oral tissues and provide pseudofunctional stimulation of the gingival tissues to maintain periodontal health.

aid, speech therapy, *n* a restoration, appliance, or electronic device used to improve speech.

aid, visual, *n* any model, drawing, or photograph used to help the patient understand proposed treatment.

AIDS, *n* the abbreviation for acquired immunodeficiency syndrome.

AIDS-related complex (ARC), *n* See acquired immunodeficiency syndrome.

air, *n* the invisible, odorless, gaseous mixture that makes up the earth's atmosphere.

air, ambient, *n* the encircling or enveloping environment; surrounding air.

air chamber, *n* See chamber, relief.

air, complemental, *n* See volume, inspiratory reserve.

air, functional residual, *n* See capacity, functional residual.

air, minimal, *n* the volume of air in the air sacs themselves (that is, part of the residual air).

air reserve, *n* See volume, expiratory reserve.

air, residual, *n* See volume, residual.

air, supplemental, *n* See volume, expiratory reserve.

air syringe, *n* See syringe, air.

air, tidal, *n* See volume, tidal.

air turbine handpiece, *n* See handpiece, air turbine.

air application in calculus identification, *n* See calculus, identification of, by air application.

air bubbles on radiographic film, *n* See film fault, white spots.

air embolism, *n* an obstruction of a blood vessel caused by the entrance of air into the bloodstream. See also embolism.

air tip, *n* part of a compressed air syringe, with an angled end that facilitates dental examination procedures.

air-powder polisher, *n* an instru-ment for plaque and stain removal which propels sodium bicarbonate particles and water against the teeth in a regulated flow using air and water pressure. Also called *airabrasive* or *airbrasive.*

airborne contaminants, *n.pl* materials in the atmosphere that can affect the health of persons in the same or nearby environment. Also referred to as *air pollution.*

airway, *n* **1.** a clear passageway for air into and out of the lungs. **2.** a device for securing unobstructed respiration during general anesthesia or in states of unconsciousness.

airway, chin lift, *n* a method of opening the trachea of an individual by manually changing the position of his or her head in order to perform rescue breathing.

airway obstruction, *n* an abnormal condition of the respiratory pathway characterized by a mechanical impediment to the delivery or to the absorption of oxygen in the lungs, as in choking, bronchospasm, obstructive lung disease, or laryngospasm.

airway obstruction, chest thrust, *n* an alternate method of removing an obstacle lodged in the airway by compressing the sternum; used when pregnancy or a patient's body size render the Heimlich maneuver impossible or inappropriate. See Heimlich maneuver.

airway obstruction, infant chest thrust, *n* a method of removing an obstacle lodged in the airway of an infant by placing the child face down along the forearm and striking the child's back with the opposite hand. See Heimlich maneuver.

airway resistance, *n* the ratio of pressure difference between the mouth, nose, or other airway opening and the alveoli to the simultaneously measured resulting volumetric gas flow rate.

akinesia, *n* a loss of controllable motion and feelings of exhaustion.

akinesthesia, *n* a loss of the power to perceive the sensation of movement resulting from dearangement of deep sensibility. (not current)

Al-Anon, *n.pr* group connected to Alcoholics Anonymous specifically organized for spouses, adult children, siblings, parents, and other individuals connected to the recovering alcoholic.

ala (ā′lə), *n* any winglike process (for example, the ala of the nose is the cutaneous-covered cartilaginous structure on the lateral aspect of the external naris).

alanine, *n* a nonessential amino acid found in many proteins in the body. Alanine is metabolized in the liver to produce pyruvate and glutamate.

ALARA concept, *n* acronym for As Low As Reasonably Achievable; pertains to radiation exposure encountered when taking x-rays. This idea requires that every possible precaution is taken to limit radiation levels when exposing the patient or technician to radiation.

alarm reaction, *n* See reaction, alarm and syndrome, general adaptation.

Alateen, *n.pr* group connected to Alcoholics Anonymous specifically organized for teenage children of recovering alcoholics.

albendazole, *n* an antiparasitic anthelmintic (especially effective against *Taenia solium* and *Echinococcus granulosus* larvae) that denies the parasites energy through the disruption of ATP production. Effective against neurocysticercosis and hydatid cyst diseases in about 75% of cases.

Albers-Schönberg disease (al′berz shœn′berg), *n.pr* See osteopetrosis.

Albright's syndrome, *n.pr* See syndrome, Albright's.

albumin (albyōō′min), *n* the primary protein of plasma (4.5% g) that aids in maintaining capillary osmotic pressure.

albuminuria (albyōō′minyōō′rē-ə), *n* (hyperproteinuria, proteinuria, proteuria), the presence of clinically detectable amounts of protein in the urine. Usually less than 100 mg/24 hr may be found normally by special methods. The usual protein is albumin, although globulins, Bence Jones protein, and fibrinogen may be present and may exceed the amount of albumin. The condition may be caused by prerenal or renal disease or by inflammation of the urinary tract.

albuterol, *n trade names:* Proventil, Proventil Repetabs, Nova-Salmol, Ventodisk, Ventolin, Ventolin Rotacaps; *drug class:* adrenergic β_2-agonist; *action:* causes bronchodilation; *uses:* prevents exercise-induced asthma, bronchospasm.

Alcaligenes (al′kə-lij′ə-nēz), *n.pl* (literally, "alkali-generating") aerobic, gram-negative eubacteria, commonly found in invertebrate intestinal tracts and normally occurring on the skin.

alcohol (al′kəhôl), *n* a transparent, colorless liquid that is mobile and volatile. Alcohols are organic compounds formed from hydrocarbons by the substitution of hydroxyl radicals for the same number of hydrogen atoms.

alcohol, absolute, *n* alcohol containing no more than 1% H_2O.

alcohol abuse, *n* frequent intake of large amounts of alcohol, typically distinguished by decreased health and physical and social functioning impairment.

alcohol blood level, *n* See blood alcohol concentration.

alcohol dependence, *n* a mental and physical need to consume alcohol in order to prevent the pains of withdrawal and obtain certain results; causes a limited capacity to control actions during consumption of alcohol. See also alcohol abuse.

alcohol hallucinosis, *n* a complication of the last stage of withdrawal from alcohol occurring within 48 hours of sudden decrease or halt of increased consumption after a lengthy period of dependence. It is indicated by severely impairing visual and auditory hallucinations similar to schizophrenia symptoms that may persist for weeks or months.

alcohol withdrawal delirium, *n* a complication of the last stage of withdrawal from alcohol occurring within one week of sudden decrease or halt of increased consumption after a lengthy period of dependence; indicated by dramatic auditory, visual, and tactile hallucinations, confusion, delusions, disorientation, tremors, nervous actions, sweating, and rapid heart beat. Also called *DTs* or *delirium tremens.*

Alcoholics Anonymous, *n.pr* a group program in which the members help themselves and each other defeat alcoholism. Members address each other only on a first-name basis, and group confidentiality is highly guarded. Also called *AA*.

alcoholic group therapy, *n* an association of men and women devoted to helping each other treat alcohol dependence. Participants and facilitators may use psychotherapy, behavior therapy, and the recruitment of family members and friends to achieve objectives.

alcoholic, recovering, *n* a person who is attempting to refrain from the compulsive consumption of alcohol and thereby escape the physiological, psychological, and social impairments associated with it.

alcoholism, *n* the continued extreme dependence on excessive amounts of alcohol, accompanied by a cumulative pattern of deviant behaviors. The most frequent medical consequences of alcoholism are chronic gastritis, central nervous system depression, and cirrhosis of the liver, each of which can compromise the delivery of dental care.

aldehyde, *n* any of a large category of organic compounds derived from a corresponding alcohol by the removal of two hydrogen atoms, as in the conversion of ethyl alcohol to acetaldehyde.

aldesleukin, *n* (interleukin-2, IL-2), *trade name:* Proleukin; *drug class:* antineoplastic; *action:* enhancement of lymphocyte mitogenesis and stimulation of IL-2-dependent cell lines; *uses:* metastatic renal cell carcinoma in adults.

aldosterone (aldos'tərōn), *n* an adrenal corticosteroid hormone that acts primarily to accelerate the exchange of potassium for sodium in the renal tubules and other cells. Aldosterone is a potent mineralocorticoid but also has some regulatory effect on carbohydrate metabolism.

aldosteronism, primary (aldos'tərō'nizəm), *n* a hyperadrenal syndrome caused by abnormal elaboration of aldosterone and characterized by excessive loss of potassium and resultant muscle weakness. The symptoms suggest tetany. The condition is often associated with an adenoma or cortical hyperplasia of the adrenal glands.

alendronate sodium, *n trade name:* Fosamax; *drug class:* amino biphos-phonate; *action:* acts as a specific inhibitor of osteoclast-mediated bone resorption; *uses:* osteoporosis in postmenopausal women, Paget's disease of bone.

alganesthesia (algan'esthē'zhə), *n* the absence of a normal sense of pain.

algesia (aljē'zē-ə), *n* sensitivity to pain; hyperesthesia; a sense of pain.

algesic (aljē'sik), *adj* painful.

algesimetry (aljəsim'etrē), *n* the measurement of response to painful stimuli.

algetic (aljet'ik), *adj* painful.

alginate (al'jināt), *n* a salt of alginic acid (for example, sodium alginate), which, when mixed with water in accurate proportions, forms an irreversible hydrocolloid gel used for making impressions. See also hydrocolloid, irreversible.

algorithm, *n* an explicit protocol with well-defined rules to be followed in solving a complex problem.

align (əlīn), *v* to move the teeth into their proper positions to conform to the line of occlusion.

alignment, tooth (əlīn'ment), *n* the arrangement of the teeth in relation ship to their supporting bone (alveolar process), adjacent teeth, and opposing dentition.

alkali (al'kəlī), *n* a strong water-soluble base. A chemical substance that, in aqueous solution, undergoes dissociation, resulting in the formation of hydroxyl (OH) ions.

alkaline (al'kəlin), *adj* having the reductions of an alkali. A pH level of 7.1 to 14 designates an alkaline solution.

alkaline diet, *n* See diet, alkaline.

alkaline phosphatase, *n* an enzyme present in bone, the kidneys, the intestine, plasma, and teeth. It may be elevated in the serum in some diseases associated with disturbances in bone, liver, or other tissues.

alkaline reserve, *n* See reserve, alkaline.

alkaloid (al'kəloid), *n* any one of the many nitrogen-containing organic bases derived from plants. The alkaloids are bitter and physiologically active. A number are useful therapeutic agents.

alkaloid, synthetic, *n* a synthetically prepared compound having the chemical characteristics of the alkaloids.

alkalosis (alkəlō′sis), *n* a disturbance of acid-base balance and water balance, characterized by an excess of alkali or a deficiency of acids.

alkalosis, compensated, n a condition in which the blood bicarbonate is usually higher than normal but compensatory mechanisms have kept the pH level within normal range. See also alkalosis, uncompensated.

alkalosis, hypochloremic, n a metabolic abnormality caused by an increase in blood bicarbonate after significant chloride loss.

alkalosis, respiratory, n alkalemia produced by hypoventilation. Plasma bicarbonate is therefore decreased in respiratory alkalosis but raised in metabolic alkalosis.

alkalosis, uncompensated, n alkalemia usually accompanied by an increased blood bicarbonate.

allele (əlēl′), *n* (allelomorph), one or more genes occupying the same location in a chromosome but differing because of a mutational change of one.

allergen (al′urjen), *n* a substance capable of producing an allergic response. Common allergens are pollens, dust, drugs, and foods.

allergy (al′urjē), *n* a hypersensitive reaction of the body to an allergen; an antigen-antibody reaction is manifested in several forms—anaphylaxis, asthma, hay fever, urticaria, angioedema, dermatitis, and stomatitis.

Manifestations of allergies. (Regezi/Sciubba/Pogrel, 2000)

allergy, cross-reactive, n condition in which a patient allergic to one ester will experience an allergic reaction to all other esters and their derivatives. See also resistance, cross.

allergy, "spontaneous" clinical, n See atopy.

allied health personnel, *n.pl* health professionals, other than physicians, dentists, clinical psychologists, pharmacists, and nurses, with education, training, and experience to serve as members of the health care delivery team.

allochiria (al′ōkī′rē-ə, al′ōkir′ē-ə), *n* the tactile sensation experienced at the side opposite its origin.

allografts, *n.pl* the transplantation of tissue between genetically nonidentical individuals of the same species. Also known as *homoplastic grafts,* or *homografts.*

alloplast (al′lōplast), *n* a transplant (implant) consisting of material originating from a nonliving source that is surgically inserted to replace missing tissue.

alloplastic (al′ōplas′tik), *adj* nonbiologic material such as metal, ceramic, and plastic.

alloplasty (al′ōplas′tē), *n* a plastic surgical procedure in which material not from the human body is used.

allopurinol, *n trade names:* Lopurin, Zyloprim; *drug class:* antigout drug; *action:* inhibits the enzyme xanthine oxidase, reducing uric acid synthesis; *uses:* chronic gout, hyperuricemia associated with malignancies.

allowable benefits, *n.pl* any necessary, reasonable, and customary items of service or treatments covered in whole or in part under an insurance plan.

allowable charge, *n* the maximum dollar amount on which benefit payment is based for each dental procedure.

allowable expenses, *n.pl* the dollar amounts allowable for each dental procedure covered by a dental insurance policy.

alloxan(əlok′san), *n* a substance, mesoxalyl urea, capable of producing experimental diabetes by destroying the islet cells of the pancreas.

alloy (al′oi), *n* **I.** a solution composed of two metals dissolved in each other when in the liquid state. *n* **2.** the product of the fusion of two or more metals.

alloy, amalgam, *n* the alloy or product of the fusion of several metals, usually supplied as filings, that is mixed with mercury to produce dental amalgam.

alloy, cobalt-chromium, *n* (chromecobalt amalgam), base metal alloys. Used in dentistry for metallic denture bases and partial dentures.

alloy, dental amalgam, *n* See amalgam.

alloy, dental gold, *n* an alloy in which the principal ingredient is gold.

alloy, eutectic, *n* any combination of metals the melting point of which is lower than that of any of the individual metals of which it consists. An alloy in which the components are mutually soluble in the solid state. A eutectic alloy has a nonhomogeneous grain structure and is therefore likely to be brittle and subject to tarnishing and corrosion.

alloy, nickel-chromium, *n* a stainless steel.

alopecia (al'əpē'shə), *n* normal or abnormal deficiency of hair. Baldness.

alpha-adrenergic blockers, *n.pl* drugs prescribed for hypertension which impede α-receptors, which in turn halts sympathetic autonomic nervous system action. See also agent, adrenergic blocking.

alpha-amylase, *n* a starch-splitting enzyme used in the treatment of inflammatory conditions and edema of soft tissues associated with traumatic injury.

alpha-estradiol (al'fə-estrədī'-ôl), *n* an estrogenic steroid, prepared by dehydrogenation of estrone, which is one of the factors responsible for the maintenance of the epithelial integrity of the oral tissues. A deficiency results in epithelial desquamation.

alpha-glucosidase inhibitors, *n.pl* an orally administered agent used in the treatment of type 2 diabetes. Examples include acarbose, which slows the digestion and absorption of glucose into the bloodstream.

alpha-hemihydrate (al'fəhem'ēhī'drāt), *n* a physical form of the hemihydrate of calcium

sulfate $(CaSO_4)$-H_2O; dental artificial stone.

alpha-interferon, *n* See interferon, alpha.

alpha-selective blockers, *n.pl* antihypertensive drugs which lower blood pressure by blocking α-receptors in the arterioles and venules.

alpha-tocopherol, *n* See vitamin E.

alphabet, international phonetic, *n* a set of internationally agreed upon alphabetical symbols, one for each sound; supplements the existing alphabet to fill out needed representation of sounds.

alphanumeric, *adj* pertaining to a character set that contains letters and numerals and usually other special characters.

alprazolam, *n trade names:* Xanax, Apo-Alpraz, Novo-Alprazol, Nu-Alpraz; *drug class:* benzodiazepine (Controlled Substance Schedule IV); *action:* produces CNS depression; *uses:* anxiety, panic disorders, anxiety with depressive symptoms.

alprostadil, *n trade name:* Caverject; *drug class:* naturally occurring prostaglandin; *action:* induces erection by relaxation of trabecular smooth muscle and by dilation of cavernosal arteries; *uses:* treatment of erectile dysfunction caused by neurogenic, vasculogenic, psychogenetic, or mixed etiology.

alternate benefit, *n* a provision in a dental plan contract that allows the third-party payer to determine the benefit based on an alternative procedure that is generally less expensive than the one provided or proposed.

alternate treatment, *n* contract provisions that authorize the insurance carrier to determine the amount of benefits payable, giving consideration to alternate procedures, services, or courses of treatment that may be performed to accomplish the desired result. The attending dentist and the patient have the option of which procedure to use, although payment for the procedure may be based on the alternate treatment principle.

alternative benefit plan, *n* a plan other than a traditional (fee-forservice, freedom of choice) indemnity or service corporation plan for reimbursing a participating dentist for providing treatment to an enrolled patient population.

A

alternative delivery system, *n* an arrangement for the provision of dental services in other than the traditional way (for example, licensed dentist providing treatment in a fee-for-service dental office).

alternative plan, *n* a compromise plan of treatment deviating from the ideal plan in scope and financial investment.

altitude, *n* pertaining to any location on earth with reference to a fixed surface point, which is usually sea level. The higher the altitude, the lower the oxygen concentration and the greater the ultraviolet radiation, both of which can cause health problems.

altretamine, *n trade name:* Hexalen; *drug class:* antineoplastic; *action:* products of metabolism interact with tissue macromolecules, including DNA, which may be responsible for cytotoxicity; *uses:* palliative treatment of recurrent, persistent ovarian cancer.

alumina (əlōōminə), *n* aluminum oxide, an abrasive sometimes used as a polishing agent.

aluminum, *n* a widely used metallic element and the third most abundant of all the elements. Aluminum is a principal component of many compounds used in antacids, antiseptics, astringents, and styptics. Aluminum hydroxychloride is the most commonly used agent in antiperspirants.

aluminum carbonate gel, *n trade name:* Basajel; *drug class:* antacid; *action:* neutralizes gastric acidity, binds phosphates in GI tract; *uses:* antacid, prevention of phosphate stones, phosphate binder in chronic renal failure.

aluminum filters/disks, *n.pl* extremely thin (0.05 cm) pieces of aluminum which are placed over the aperture of the x-ray tube to eliminate x rays over a certain wavelength.

aluminum hydroxide, *n trade names:* AlternaGEL, Alu-Cap, Alu-Tab, Amphojel, Dialume; *drug class:* antacid; *action:* neutralizes gastric acidity, binds phosphates in GI tract; *uses:* antacid, hyperphosphatemia in chronic renal failure.

aluminum oxide, *n* an aluminum compound found in many polishing agents.

Aluwax (al'yəwaks), *n* a commer-cially prepared wax wafer containing aluminum that is used to register jaw relationship.

alveolalgia (al'vē-ōlal'jē-ə), *n* See socket, dry.

alveolar (alvē'-ōlär), *adj* pertaining to an alveolus.

Alveolar mucosa
Alveolar mucosa. (Liebgott, 2001)

alveolar bone loss, *n* See bone loss, periodontal.

alveolar crest, *n* See crest, alveolar.

alveolar process, *n* See process, alveolar.

alveolar ridge, *n* See ridge, alveolar.

alveolar ridge augmentation, *n* a surgical procedure to improve the shape and size of the alveolar ridge(s) in preparation to receive and retain a dental prosthesis.

alveolectomy (al'vē-əlek'təmē), *n* the excision of a portion of the alveolar process to aid in the removal of teeth, modification of the contour after the removal of teeth, and preparation of the mouth for dentures.

alveolitis, *n* in dentistry, the inflammation of a tooth socket.

alveoloplasty, *n* the surgical shaping and smoothing of the margins of the tooth socket after extraction of the tooth, generally in preparation for the placement of a prosthesis.

alveolus (alvē'əlus), *n* **1.** an air sac of the lungs formed by terminal dilations of the bronchioles. *n* **2.** the socket in the bone in which a tooth is attached by means of the periodontal ligament.

Alzheimer's disease, *n.pr* (Alois Alzheimer, German neurologist, b. 1854), a presenile dementia characterized by confusion, memory failure, disorientation, restlessness, agnosia, hallucinosis, speech disturbances, and the inability to carry out purposeful movement. The disease usually begins in later middle life with slight defects in memory and behavior that become progressively more severe. Also known as primary progressive aphasia.

amalgam (əmal′gəm), *n* (dental amalgam alloy), an alloy, one of the constituents of which is mercury.

amalgam carrier, n See carrier, amalgam.

amalgam carver, n See carver, amalgam.

amalgam condenser, n See condenser, amalgam.

amalgam, copper, n an alloy composed principally of copper and mercury. See also amalgam.

amalgam, dental, n an amalgam used for dental restorations and dyes.

amalgam matrix, n See matrix, amalgam.

amalgam pigmentation, n See amalgam tattoo.

amalgam plugger, n See condenser, amalgam.

amalgam, silver, n a dental amalgam, the chief constituent of which is silver. The ADA composition specifications are as follows: silver, 65% minimum; tin, 25% minimum; copper, 6% maximum; zinc, 2% maximum.

amalgam squeeze cloth, n a piece of linen used to hold plastic amalgam from which excess mercury is to be squeezed.

amalgam tattoo, n a solitary discrete gray, blue, or black discoloration of tissue usually located in the gingiva, alveolar ridge, or buccal mucosa caused by minute amounts of dental amalgam that became embedded under the surface. The asymptomatic lesion is static and requires no treatment. If doubt exists about the lesion or if the lesion is unsightly, excisional biopsy is recommended.

Amalgam tattoo. (Sapp/Eversole/Wysocki, 2004)

amalgamation (əmal′gəmā′shən), *n* the formation of an alloy by mixing mercury with another metal or other metals. See also trituration.

amalgamation amalgamator (əmal′gəmātur), *n* a mechanical device used to triturate the ingredients of dental amalgam into a plastic mass.

Amantadine (əman′tidān), *n.pr* an antiviral that prevents uncoating and replication of the influenza A virus; most effectively used in the early stages of exposure.

ambulatory care, *n* health services provided on an outpatient basis to those who can visit a health care facility and return home the same day.

ambulatory surgery, *n* surgical care provided to persons who do not require overnight nursing care.

amcinonide, *n trade name:* Cyclocort; *drug class:* topical fluorinated corticosteroid, group II high potency; *action:* antipruritic, antiinflammatory; *uses:* psoriasis, eczema, contact dermatitis, pruritus.

amelia (əmel′ē-ə, əmē′lē-ə), *n* a congenital abnormality characterized by the absence of one or more limbs.

ameloblast, *n* an epithelial cell associated with the tooth bud which, during tooth formation, secretes the tooth enamel.

ameloblast atrophy, n a wasting of or decrease in the epithelial cells, which form tooth enamel; may occur as the result of a deficiency in vitamin A. See also atrophy, periodontal.

ameloblastic fibroma, *n* See fibroma, ameloblastic.

ameloblastic sarcoma, *n* See sarcoma, ameloblastic.

ameloblastoma (am′əlōblastō′mə), *n* an epithelial neoplasm with a basic structure resembling the enamel organ and suggesting derivation from ameloblastic cells. It is usually benign but aggressive. Also called *adamantinoblastoma* or *adamantinoma*.

ameloblastoma, acanthomatous, n an epithelial odontogenic tumor that differs from the simple ameloblastoma in that the central cells within the cell nests are squamous and may be keratinized rather than stellate.

The peripheries of the cell nests are composed of ameloblastic cells. See also ameloblastoma.

amelogenesis, *n* the process during which tooth enamel is formed. See also ameloblast.

amelogenesis imperfecta **(am'əlōjen'əsis),** *n* a severe hypoplasia or agenesis of enamel that is inherited as a dominant characteristic.

Amelogenesis imperfecta. (Regezi/Sciubba/Pogrel, 2000)

amenorrhea (əmen'ōrē'-ə), *n* the absence or abnormal cessation of the menstrual cycle.

American Cancer Society (ACS), *n.pr* a national advocacy and fundraising organization, headquartered in Atlanta, Georgia, that is dedicated to raising public awareness about cancer and to providing support for cancer patients and their families.

American Dental Association (ADA), *n.pr* a nonprofit professional association whose membership is made up of dentists in the United States. Its purpose is to assist its members in providing the highest professional and ethical care to the citizens of the United States and to serve as an advocate for the advancement of the profession.

American Dental Hygienists Association (ADHA), *n.pr* a nonprofit professional association of dental hygienists in the United States created to assist its members in providing the highest professional and ethical care to the citizens of the United States and to serve as an advocate for the advancement of the profession.

American Foundation for the Blind, *n.pr* an advocacy group for individuals with visual disabilities.

American Hospital Association (AHA), *n.pr* a nonprofit national organization of individuals, institutions, and organizations engaged in direct patient care. The association works to promote the improvement of health care services.

American manual alphabet, *n.pr* a representation of alphabet letters using a variety of finger positions.

American Medical Association (AMA), *n.pr* a nonprofit professional association of physicians in the United States, including all medical specialties. Its purpose is to assist its members in providing the highest professional and ethical medical care to the citizens of the United States and to serve as an advocate for the advancement of the profession.

American Sign Language (ASL), *n.pr* a mode of communication using gestures and visuals with a unique grammatical structure. ASL is used by individuals with limited or no hearing ability and by those who communicate regularly with such individuals.

Americans with Disabilities Act, *n.pr* a federal law enacted on July 26, 1990, that defines a private dental office as a place of public accommodation, thereby requiring, as of January 26, 1992, that dentists serve persons with disabilities.

amiloride HCl, *n trade name:* Midamor; *drug class:* potassium-sparing diuretic; *action:* acts primarily on the distal renal tubule, increasing the retention of potassium; *uses:* edema in chronic heart failure in combination with other diuretics, for hypertension, with INH solution for cystic fibrosis.

amines, *n.pl* organic compounds that contain nitrogen.

amino acid, *n* an organic acid in which one of the CH hydrogen atoms has been replaced by NH_2. Amino acids are the building blocks of proteins.

amino acid, essential, *n* the group of amino acids that cannot be synthesized by the organism but are required by the organism. They must be supplied by the diet. Isoleucine,

leucine, lysine, methionine, phenylalanine, threonine, tryptophan, and valine are essential for adults; these eight plus arginine and histidine are considered essential for infants and children.

amino acid, glucogenic (glōōkōjen'ik), *n* the group of amino acids that produce enzymes that may be converted to glucose if necessary.

amino acid, ketogenic (kē'tōjen'ik), *n* an amino acid that produces ketone bodies following chemical alteration of its carbon skeleton.

amino acid, nonessential, *n* the group of amino acids that can be synthesized by the organism and are not required in the diet.

amino acid pool, *n* an accumulation of amino acids in the liver and blood that adjusts to meet the body's need for protein and amino acids.

aminocaproic acid, *n trade name:* Amicar; *drug class:* hemostatic; *action:* inhibits fibrinolysis by inhibiting plasminogen activator substances; *uses:* hemorrhage from hyperfibrinolysis; adjunctive therapy in hemophilia; unapproved, hemorrhage following dental surgery in hemophilia.

aminoglutethimide, *n trade name:* Cytadren; *drug class:* antineoplastic, adrenal steroid inhibitor; *action:* acts by inhibiting the enzymatic conversion of cholesterol to pregnenolone, thereby blocking synthesis of all adrenal steroids; *uses:* suppression of adrenal function in Cushing's syndrome, metastatic breast cancer, and adrenal cancer.

aminoglycosides, *n.pl* bacteriocidal antibiotics obtained from *Streptomyces* that inhibit protein synthesis in bacterial ribosomes and are effective against aerobic gram-negative bacilli.

aminophylline (theophylline ethylenediamine), *n trade names:* Phyllocontin; *drug class:* xanthine; *action:* relaxes smooth muscle of the respiratory system; *uses:* bronchial asthma, bronchospasm, Cheyne-Stokes respirations.

amiodarone HCl, *n trade name:* Cordarone; *drug class:* antidysrhythmic (drug class III); *action:* prolongs action potential duration and effective refractory period; *uses:* documented life-threatening ventricular tachycardia.

amitriptyline HCl, *n trade names:* Apo-Amitriptyline, Elavil, Emitrip, Endep, Enovil, Levate, Novotriptyn; *drug class:* tricyclic antidepressant; *action:* inhibits both norepinephrine and serotonin (5-HT); *uses:* major depression.

amlodipine besylate, *n trade name:* Norvasc; *drug class:* calcium channel blocker; *action:* inhibits calcium ion influx across cell membrane during cardiac depolarization; produces relaxation of coronary vascular smooth muscle and dilates coronary arteries, decreases SA/AV node conduction; *uses:* hypertension as a single agent or in combination with other antihypertensives, chronic stable angina pectoris, vasospastic angina.

ammeter (am'ētur), *n* a contraction of amperemeter. An apparatus that measures the amperage of an electric current.

ammonia, *n* a colorless aromatic gas consisting of nitrogen and hydrogen, produced by the decomposition of nitrogenous organic matter. Some of its many uses are as an aromatic stimulant, a detergent, and an emulsifier.

ammonia thiosulfate (əmō'nyə thī-ōsul'fāt), *n* an ingredient of the photographic fixing solution that acts as a solvent for silver halides.

ammoniacal silver nitrate, *n* See silver nitrate, ammoniacal.

ammonium chloride, *n* the chlorine salt of the ammonium ion. Ammonium chloride is a popular deliquescent agent (that is, it attracts and absorbs water from the atmosphere).

amnesia (amnē'zē-ə, -zhə), *n* the lack or loss of memory.

amnesiac (amnē'zē-ak), *n* a person affected by amnesia.

amnesic (amnē'zik), *n/adj* See sedative.

amnestic (amnes'tik), *adj* amnesic; causing amnesia.

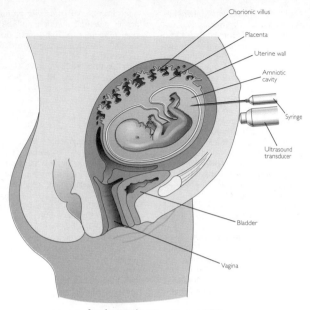

Amniocentesis. (Moore/Persaud, 2003)

Labels on figure:
- Chorionic villus
- Placenta
- Uterine wall
- Amniotic cavity
- Syringe
- Ultrasound transducer
- Bladder
- Vagina

amniocentesis (am´nē-ōsentē´sis), *n* a procedure in which fluid is drawn from the amniotic sac by a hollow needle and tested, especially to determine the sex of the fetus and the presence of any genetic or chromosomal abnormalities.

amniotic fluid (am´nē-ot´ik), *n* a serum within the amniotic sac in which the embryo is immersed and cushioned.

amniotic sac, *n* a thin membrane that completely surrounds the embryo and contains a protective fluid in which the embryo is immersed. Also called the *amnion.*

amobarbital/amobarbital sodium, *n trade name:* Amytal; *drug class:* barbiturate sedative-hypnotic (Controlled Substance Schedule II); *action:* nonselective depression of CNS ranging from sedation to hypnosis to anesthesia to coma, depending on dose administered; *uses:* sedation, preanesthetic sedation, insommia, anticonvulsant, adjunct in psychiatry, hypnotic.

amoeba (əmē´bə), *n* a Rhizopod protozoa that uses extensions of its cytoplasm, called pseudopodia, to move. Some varieties of amoebae are implicated in human infection. Also spelled *ameba(s).*

amorphous (āmôr´fus, əmôr´fus), *adj* a substance having no specific space lattice, the molecules being distributed at random.

amortization, *n* a generic term that includes various specific practices, such as depreciation, depletion, write-off of intangibles, prepaid expenses, and deferred charges.

amoxapine, *n trade name:* Asendin; *drug class:* tricyclic antidepressant; *action:* inhibits both norepinephrine and serotonin (5-HT) uptake in brain; *uses:* depression.

amoxicillin trihydrate, *n trade names:* Amoxil, Apo-Amoxi, Novamoxin, Nu-Amoxi and others; *drug class:* aminopenicillin; *action:* interferes with cell wall replication of susceptible organisms; *uses:* sinus infections, pneumonia, otitis media, skin, urinary tract infections. This is a drug of choice for antibiotic premedication for patients at risk for bacterial endocarditis unless there is an allergy to penicillin-related antibiotics.

amoxicillin/clavulanate potassium, *n trade names:* Augmentin, Clavulin; *drug class:* aminopenicillin with a β-lactamase inhibitor; *action:* interferes with cell wall replication of susceptible organisms; *uses:* sinus infections, pneumonia, otitis media, skin, urinary tract infections; effective for strains of *E. coli, H. influenzae, S. pneumoniae,* and β-lactamase-producing organisms.

ampere (am′pir), *n* (Amp), a unit of measurement of the quantity of electric current, equal to a flow of 1 coulomb per second or 6.25 time 10^{18} electrons per second. The current produced by 1 volt acting through a resistance of 1 ohm.

amphetamines, *n.pl* a group of nervous system stimulants that are subject to abuse because of their ability to reduce appetite and produce wakefulness and euphoria. Abuse of amphetamines may lead to compulsive behavior, paranoia, hallucinations, and suicidal tendencies.

amphotericin, *n* an antibiotic and antifungal agent used extensively in the treatment of systemic mycoses. **amphotericin B, topical,** *n trade name:* Fungizone; *drug class:* polyene antifungal; *action:* increases cell membrane permeability in susceptible organisms by binding to sterols; *uses:* cutaneous, mucocutaneous infections caused by *Candida.*

ampicillin, *n* an acid-stable semisynthetic penicillin antibiotic with a broader spectrum of effectiveness than penicillin G.

amputation neuroma, *n* See neuroma, traumatic.

amputation, pulp, *n* See pulpotomy.

amputation, root, *n* the removal of a root of a multirooted tooth.

amylase (am′ilās), *n* an enzymatic protein essential for changing starches into sugars.

amyloid, *n* a starchlike protein-carbohydrate complex that is deposited abnormally in some tissues during certain chronic disease states, such as amyloidosis, rheumatoid arthritis, and tuberculosis.

amyloidosis (am′iloidō′sis), *n* a condition in which amyloid, a glycoprotein, is deposited intercellularly in

tissues and organs. Four types of amyloidosis are recognized, two of which, primary amyloidosis and amyloid tumor, frequently produce nodules in the tongue and gingiva.

Amyloidosis. (Regezi/Sciubba/Jordan, 2003)

amyloidosis, primary, n amyloidosis occurring without a known predisposing cause. Amyloid deposits are found in the tongue, lips, skeletal muscles, and other mesodermal structures. The disease may be manifested by polyneuropathy, purpura, hepatosplenomegaly, heart failure, and the nephrotic syndrome.

amyloidosis, secondary, n amyloidosis occurring secondary to chronic diseases such as tuberculosis, leprosy, rheumatoid arthritis, multiple myeloma, and prolonged bacterial infections. Amyloid deposits are found in parenchymal organs. The disease is usually manifested by proteinuria and hepatosplenomegaly.

amyotonia (ā′mī-ōtō′nē-ə), *n* an abnormal flaccidity or flabbiness of a muscle or group of muscles.

amyotrophic lateral sclerosis, *n* a degenerative disease of the motor neurons, characterized by atrophy of the muscles of the hands, forearms, and legs, and spreading to involve most of the body. It is commonly known as Lou Gehrig's disease.

anabolic steroids, *n.pl* a group of compounds derived from testosterone or prepared synthetically to promote general body growth. Anabolic steroids are used in the treatment of aplastic anemia, anemias associated with renal failure, myeloid metaplasia, and leukemia. Anabolic steroids are subject to abuse to promote muscle mass in athletes.

anabolism (ənab′əlizəm), *n* the constructive process by which substances are converted from simple to complex forms by living cells; constructive metabolism.

A

anaerobe (an'ərōb), n a microorganism that can exist and grow only in the partial or complete absence of molecular oxygen.

analeptic (an'əlep'tik), n **1.** an agent that acts to overcome depression of the central nervous system. n **2.** a strong central nervous system stimulant that is used to restore consciousness, especially from a drug-induced coma.

analgesia (an'əljē'zē-ə), n insensibility to pain without loss of consciousness; a state in which painful stimuli are not perceived or interpreted as pain; usually induced by a drug, although trauma or a disease process may produce a general or regional analgesia.

analgesia, diagnostic, n the administration of a local anesthetic to determine the location, source, or cause of pain.

analgesia, endotracheal, n an inhalation technique in which the anesthetic agent and respiratory gases are passed through a tube inserted in the trachea via either the nose or mouth.

analgesia, infiltration, n the arrest of the sensory responses of nerve endings at the surgical site by injections of an anesthetic at that site.

analgesia, insufflation, n the delivery of anesthetic gases or vapors directly to the airway of a patient while he or she is breathing room air. Insufflation is usually an open drop method.

analgesia, intranasal, n the delivery of an analgesic agent to the membrane of the nose by either topical application or insufflation.

analgesia, nonnarcotic, n drugs that relieve pain by action at the site of the pain. Generally, nonnarcotic analgesics do not produce tolerance or dependence.

analgesia, patient-controlled, n mechanisms by which the patient can administer and/or control the application of an analgesic agent to an area of the body. One such mechanism is the use of transcutaneous electric nerve stimulation (TENS) to control facial pain. The TENS unit is a variable controlled device designed to deliver a controlled electrical stimulus to the skin surface overlying a painful muscle.

analgesia, regional, n the reversible loss of pain sensation over an area of the body by blocking the afferent conduction of its innervation with a local anesthetic agent.

analgesic (anəljē'zik), adj (analgetic), **1.** the property of a drug that enables it to raise the pain threshold. n **2.** an analgesic may be classified in one of two groups: an analgesic that blocks the sensory neural pathways of pain (for example, procaine and its derivatives) or an analgesic that acts directly on the thalamus to raise the pain threshold.

analgetic (anəljet'ik), adj See analgesic.

analgia (anal'jē-ə), n an absence of pain.

analysis (ənal'isis), n a separation into component parts.

analysis, anthropometric (an'thrōpōmet'rik), n a study of the human body which uses such tools as body mass index, basal metabolic rate, bioelectrical impedance, and dual energy x-ray absorptiometry, along with measurements of skinfold thickness and arm muscle circumference, to assess the structure, form, and composition of the body for purposes of comparison.

analysis, bite, n See analysis, occlusal.

analysis, cephalometric (sef'əlōmet'rik), n the evaluation of the growth pattern or morphologic conoval of teeth, modification of the contour after the removal of teeth, and preparation of the mouth for dentures.

analysis, dietary, n a comparison of an individual's typical food choices with those recommended in the Food Guide Pyramid; deviations are noted, and recommendations are given.

analysis, occlusal, n a study of the relations of the occlusal surfaces of the opposing teeth and their functional harmony.

analyzing rod, n See rod, analyzing.

anamnesis (an'amnē'sis), n a past history of disease or injury based on the patient's memory or recall at the time of dental and/or medical interview and examination.

anaphylactic (an'əfilak'tik), adj pertaining to decreasing, rather than increasing, immunity.

anaphylactic hypersensitivity, n (Arthus' reaction), a local tissue response that is the result of an Ag-AB reaction caused by repeated intradermal injections with one antigen, resulting in inflammation and necrosis.

anaphylactoid (an'əfilak'toid), adj resembling anaphylaxis; pertaining to a reaction, the symptoms of which resemble those of the anaphylactic response produced by the injection of serum and other nonspecific proteins.

anaphylactoid reaction, n See reaction, anaphylactoid.

anaphylaxis (an'əfilak'sis), n a violent allergic reaction characterized by sudden collapse, shock, or respiratory and circulatory failure after injection of an allergen.

anaplasia (an'əplā'zhə), n a regressive change in cells toward a more primitive or embryonic cell type. Anaplasia is a prominent criterion of malignancy in tumors.

anasarca (an'əsär'kə), n (dropsy), generalized edema.

anastomosis, n the joining together of two blood vessels or other tubular structures to furnish a direct or indirect communication between the two structures.

anastomosis graft, n the connection of two autogenous tubular structures as a part of reconstructive surgery.

anatomic (anətom'ik), adj pertaining to the anatomy of a structure.

anatomic crown, n See crown, anatomic.

anatomic dead space, n the actual capacity of the respiratory passages that extend from the nostrils to and including the terminal bronchioles.

anatomic form, n See form, anatomic.

anatomic height of contour, n See contour, height of.

anatomic impression, n See impression, anatomic.

anatomic landmark, n See landmark, anatomic.

anatomic teeth, n.pl See tooth, anatomic.

anatomical root, n See root.

anatomy (ənat'ōmē), n the science of the form, structure, and parts of animal organisms.

anatomy, dental, n the science of the structure of the teeth and the relationship of their parts. The study involves macroscopic and microscopic components.

anatomy, radiographic, n the images on a radiographic film of the combined anatomic structures through which the roentgen rays (x-rays) have passed.

anatomy, subgingival, n structures located beneath the gums and between the base of the crown and the gums.

ANB angle, n a cephalometric measurement of the anterior-posterior relationship of the maxilla with the mandible.

anchorage, n **1.** the supporting base for orthodontic forces applied to stimulate tooth movement. n **2.** the area of application of the reciprocal forces generated when corrective forces are applied to teeth. Anchorage units may be one tooth or more or may include a portion of the neck or cranium.

anchorage bends, n.pl bends placed in an orthodontic wire to enhance the resistance to the anterior displacement of teeth during orthodontic treatment; primarily used in the Tweed and Begg techniques.

anchorage, cervical, n an extraoral anchorage based at the back of the neck.

anchorage, cranial, n an extraoral anchorage based at the back of the skull.

anchorage, extraoral, n an orthodontic anchorage based outside the mouth. Dental attachments are typically linked to a wire bow or hooks extending between the lips and attached elastically to a cap, a strap around the neck, or another extraoral device.

anchorage, facial, n an extraoral anchorage based on the face, usually the chin or forehead.

anchorage, intermaxillary, n an anchorage based in the opposite jaw.

anchorage, intramaxillary, n an anchorage based on teeth within the same jaw.

anchorage, intraoral, n an anchorage based within the mouth (intermaxillary, intramaxillary, or myofunctional).

anchorage, occipital, n a cranial anchorage based in the occipital area.

anchorage, reciprocal, n all anchorage is reciprocal; sometimes used to describe a force system in which the resistance units are similar.

anchorage, simple, *n* the use of a tooth as a resistance unit without tipping control.

anchorage, stationary, *n* a genus of Nematoda commonly known as *hookworm.*

Andresen appliance, *n.pr* See appliance, Andresen.

androgen (an'drōjen), *n* any substance that possesses masculinizing qualities, such as testosterone.

anemia (ənē'mē-ə), *n* a term indicating that the concentration of hemoglobin or the number of red blood cells is below the accepted normal value with respect to age and sex. In true anemia the total concentration of hemoglobin, or the total number of erythrocytes, is below normal regardless of concentration values. Symptoms, which may not be evident, include weakness, pallor, anorexia, and those related to the cause of the anemia.

anemia, Addison-Biermer, *n.pr* See anemia, pernicious.

anemia, aplastic, *n* an anemia characterized by a decrease in all marrow elements, including platelets, red blood cells, and granulocytes.

anemia, Biermer's, *n.pr* See anemia, pernicious.

anemia, Cooley's, *n.pr* See thalassemia major.

anemia, displacement, *n* See anemia, myelophthisic.

anemia, erythroblastic, *n* See thalassemia major.

anemia, hemolytic, *n* an anemia characterized by an increased rate of destruction of red blood cells, reticulocytosis, hyperbilirubinemia, and/or increased urinary and fecal urobilinogen, and, generally, splenic enlargement. Hereditary hemolytic anemias include congenital hemolytic jaundice, sickle cell anemia, oval cell anemia, and thalassemia. Acquired hemolytic anemias include paroxysmal nocturnal hemoglobinuria and those caused by immune mechanisms (erythroblastosis fetalis), transfusions of incompatible blood, infections, drugs, and poisons. Autoimmune hemolytic anemias are acquired hemolytic anemias associated with antibody-like substances that may not

be true autoantibodies or even antibodies; they may be primary (idiopathic), or they may be secondary to lymphoma, lymphatic leukemia, disseminated lupus erythematosus, or sensitization to drugs and pollens.

anemia, hemorrhagic, *n* a deficiency in red blood cells and/or hemoglobin resulting from excessive bleeding.

anemia, hyperchromic, *n* an anemia in which the erythrocytes are larger than normal in size so that the content but not the concentration of hemoglobin is increased.

anemia, hypochromic, *n* an anemia caused by impaired hemoglobin synthesis resulting from a deficiency of iron or pyridoxine and from chronic lead poisoning.

anemia, iron deficiency, *n* an anemia resulting from a deficiency of iron, characterized by hypochromic microcytic erythrocytes and a normoblastic reaction of the bone marrow. Iron deficiency may result from an increased demand during growth or repeated pregnancies, chronic or recurrent hemorrhage such as from menstrual abnormalities, hemorrhoids, or peptic ulcer, a low intake of iron, or impaired absorption, as often occurs with chronic diarrhea.

anemia, macrocytic normochromic, *n* an anemia related to a failure of nucleoprotein synthesis caused by a deficiency of vitamin B_{12}, folic acid, or related substances.

anemia, Mediterranean, *n* See thalassemia major.

anemia, megaloblastic, *n* an anemia characterized by hyperplastic bone marrow changes and maturation arrest resulting from a dietary deficiency, impaired absorption, impaired storage and modification, or impaired use of one or more hematopoietic factors. Included are pernicious anemia, nutritional macrocytic anemias associated with gastrointestinal disturbances, anemias associated with impaired liver function (for example, macrocytic anemia of pregnancy), hypothyroidism, leukemia, and achrestic anemia.

anemia, microcytic hypochromic, *n* an anemia in which the mean corpuscular volume (MCV), mean corpuscular hemoglobin (MCH) content, and mean corpuscular hemoglobin concentration (MCHC) are all low (for example, iron deficiency anemia, hereditary leptocytosis, hemoglobin C anemia, and anemias resulting from pyridoxine deficiency and chronic lead poisoning).

anemia, myelophthisic, n (displacement anemia), an anemia resulting from displacement or crowding out of erythropoietic cells of the bone marrow by foreign tissue, as in leukemia, metastatic carcinoma, lymphoblastoma, multiple myeloma, osteoradionecrosis, and xanthomatosis.

anemia, normocytic normochromic, n an anemia associated with disturbances of red cell formation and related to endocrine deficiencies, chronic inflammation, and carcinomatosis.

anemia, nutritional macrocytic, n macrocytic normochromic anemia occurring as a result of a deficiency of substances necessary for deoxyribonucleic acid synthesis; for example, vitamin B_{12} and folic acid deficiency may result from a lack of intrinsic factors, sprue, or regional enteritis. Folic acid deficiency may occur in chronic alcoholism, as a result of a diet deficient in meats and vegetables, and in diseases causing intestinal malabsorption.

anemia, oval cell, n See elliptocytosis.

anemia, pernicious, n (Addison-Biermer anemia), a macrocytic normochromic (megaloblastic) anemia associated with achlorhydria and lack of a gastric intrinsic factor necessary for the binding and absorption of vitamin B_{12}, which is an erythrocyte maturing factor. In addition to hematologic findings, atrophic glossitis and gastrointestinal and nervous disorders occur.

Pernicious anemia. (Sapp/Eversole/Wysocki, 2004)

anemia, physiologic, n an anemia characterized by lowered blood values resulting from an increase in plasma volume that occurs most markedly during the sixth and seventh months of pregnancy.

anemia, sickle cell, n (drepanocythemia, sicklemia), a hereditary hemolytic anemia in which the presence of an abnormal hemoglobin (hemoglobin S) results in distorted, sickle-shaped erythrocytes. Manifestations include episodic crises of muscle, joint, and abdominal pain; neurologic symptoms; and leg ulcers. Sickle cell anemia occurs almost exclusively in African Americans. See also trait, sickle cell.

anemia, spherocytic, n See jaundice, congenital hemolytic.

anergy (an′urjē), *n* in terms of hypersensitivity, an inability to react to specific antigens (that is, lack of reaction to intradermally injected antigens in measles, Hodgkin's sarcoma, and overwhelming tuberculosis).

anesthesia (an′esthē′zē-ə, an′esthē′zhə), *n* the loss of feeling or sensation, especially loss of tactile sensibility, with or without loss of consciousness.

anesthesia, basal, n a state of narcosis, induced before the administration of a general anesthetic, that permits the production of states of surgical anesthesia with greatly reduced amounts of general anesthetic agents.

anesthesia, block, n an anesthesia induced by injecting the drug close to the nerve trunk, at some distance from the operative field. See also anesthesia, infiltration.

anesthesia, conduction, n an anesthesia induced by injecting the drug close to the nerve trunk, at some distance from the operative field.

anesthesia, general, n an irregular, reversible depression of the cells of the higher centers of the central nervous system that makes the patient unconscious and insensible to pain.

anesthesia, glove, n an anesthesia with a distribution corresponding to the part of the skin covered by a glove.

anesthesia, infiltration, n an anesthesia induced by injecting the anesthetic solution directly into or around the tissues to be anesthetized; used for operative procedures on the maxillary premolar, anterior teeth, and mandibular incisors. See also anesthesia, block.

The process of infiltration anesthesia.
(Bird/Robinson, 2002)

anesthesia, intraosseous, *n* an anesthesia produced by the injection of an anesthetic agent into the cancellous portion of a bone.

anesthesia, intrapulpal, *n* the injection of a local anesthetic directly into pulpal tissue under pressure.

anesthesia, local, *n* (regional anesthesia), the loss of pain sensation over a specific area of the anatomy without loss of consciousness.

anesthesia, regional, *n* a term used for local anesthesia. See also anesthesia, local.

anesthesia, topical, *n* a form of local anesthesia whereby free nerve endings in accessible structures are rendered incapable of stimulation by applying a suitable solution directly to the surface of the area.

anesthesiologist (an′əsthē′zē-ol′əjist), *n* a physician specializing in the administration of anesthetics.

anesthesiology, *n* the branch of medicine concerned with the relief of pain and the administration of medication to relieve pain during surgery or other invasive procedures.

anesthetic (an′esthet′ik), *n* a drug that produces loss of feeling or sensation generally or locally.

anesthetic, aerosol spray topical, *n* application of an aerosol spray directly on the surface of a mucous membrane, resulting in loss of nerve conduction.

anesthetic agent, *n* See agent, anesthetic.

anesthetic, allergy to, *n* hypersensitivity to a locally administered anesthetic agent, which is fairly common with esters but rarely occurs with amides. Persons allergic to bisulfites should avoid anesthetics containing vasoconstrictors.

anesthetic, amide (am′id), *n* a local anesthetic made from a specific class of chemical compounds that are broken down in the body by the liver and are generally considered more effective and longer-lasting than esters. This type of anesthetic rarely causes allergic reactions.

anesthetic, antioxidants in, *n* a preservative substance added by the manufacturer to a local anesthetic cartridge containing a vasoconstrictor. Metabisulfite and sodium bisulfite are the most common antioxidants used.

anesthetic, carpule (kär′pyōōl), *n* a capsule-like vessel containing the local anesthetic solution that is inserted into the syringe in preparation for an injection.

anesthetic, ester, *n* a short-acting local anesthetic made from a specific class of chemical compounds that are broken down in the body by blood enzymes. They are less effective than amide anesthetics and more likely to cause allergic reactions.

anesthetic, local, *n* a drug that, when injected into the tissues and absorbed into a nerve, will temporarily interrupt its property of conduction.

anesthetic, topical, *n* a drug applied to the surface of tissues that produces local insensibility to pain.

anesthetist (ənes′thətist), *n* a person who administers anesthetics.

anesthetize (ənes′thətīz), *v* to place under anesthesia.

aneurysm (an′yōōrizəm), *n* a localized dilation of an artery in which one or more layers of the vessel walls are distended.

aneurysm, arteriovenous, *n* See shunt, arteriovenous.

angiitis, visceral (an′jē-ī′tis), *n* See disease, collagen.

angina (anjīnə), *n* a spasmodic, choking pain. The term is sometimes applied to the disease producing the pain (for example, Ludwig's angina).

angina, agranulocytic, n See agranulocytosis.

angina, Ludwig's, n.pr a cellulitis involving the submandibular space and characterized clinically by a firm swelling of the floor of the mouth, with elevation of the tongue.

angina, monocytic, n a "sore throat" associated with infectious mononucleosis.

angina pectoris, n frequently a symptom of cardiovascular diseases; characterized by a severe, viselike pain behind the sternum that sometimes radiates to the arms, neck, or mandible. Symptoms may also include a sense of constriction or pressure of the chest. Angina pectoris is caused by exertion or excitement and is relieved by rest.

angina, Vincent's, n an incorrect term for involvement of the pharynx by the spread of acute necrotizing ulceromembranous gingivitis.

angioedema (an'jē-ō-əde'mə), n See edema, angioneurotic.

angiography, n the radiographic visualization of the internal anatomy of the heart and blood vessels after the intravascular introduction of radiopaque contrast medium.

angioma (an'jē-ō'mə), n a benign tumor of vascular nature. See also hemangioma and lymphangioma.

angioneurotic edema (an'jē-ōnyōōrot'ik), n See edema, angioneurotic.

angle, n the degree of divergence of two or more lines or planes that meet each other; the space between such lines. Measured in degrees of an arc.

angle, bayonet former, n a hoe-shaped, paired cutting instrument; biangled with the blade parallel with the axis of the shaft. The cutting edge is not perpendicular to the axis of the blade. Used to accentuate angles in an "invisible" class 3 cavity.

angle, Bennett, n the angle formed by the sagittal plane and the path of the advancing condyle during lateral mandibular movement, as viewed in the horizontal plane.

angle board, n a device used to facilitate the establishment of reproducible angular relationships between a patient's head, the x-ray beam, and the x-ray film.

angle, cavosurface, n the angle in a prepared cavity, formed by the junction of the wall of the cavity with the surface of the tooth.

angle, cranial base, n the angle formed by a line representing the floor of the anterior cranial fossa intersecting a line representing the axis of the clivus of the base of the skull.

angle, cusp, n **1.** the angle made by the slopes of a cusp with the plane that passes through the tip of the cusp and is perpendicular to a line bisecting the cusp; measured mesiodistally or buccolingually. Half of the included angle between the buccolingual or mesiodistal cusp inclines. n **2.** the angle made by the slopes of a cusp with a perpendicular line bisecting the cusp; measured mesiodistally or buccolingually.

angle, facial, n an anthropometric expression of the degree of protrusion of the lower face, assessed by measuring the inclination of the facial plane relative to a horizontal reference plane.

angle, former, n one of a series of paired, hoe-shaped cutting instruments having the cutting edge at an angle other than a right angle in relation to the axis of the blade.

angle, Frankfort-mandibular incisor (FMIA), n a measure of the mandibular incisor to the Frankfort horizontal plane.

angle, incisal (insī'zal), n the degree of slope between the axis-orbital plane and the palatal discluding skidway of the maxillary incisor.

angle, incisal guidance, n the angle formed with the occlusal plane by drawing a line in the sagittal plane between the incisal edges of the maxillary and mandibular central incisors when the teeth are in centric occlusion.

angle, incisal guide, n the inclination of the incisal guide on the articulator.

angle, lateral incisal guide, n the inclination of the incisal guide in the frontal plane.

angle, line, n an angle formed by the junction of the two walls along a line; designated by combining the names of the walls forming the angle.

angle, occlusal rest, *n* the angle formed by the occlusal rest with the upright minor connector.

angle of mandible, *n* the gonial angle. The relation existing between the body of the mandible and the ramus of the mandible.

angle, point, *n* an angle formed by the junction of three walls at a common point; designated by combining the names of the walls forming the angle.

angle, prophylaxis, *n* clinical jargon for an angled instrument which holds a rubber cup or bristle brush used to polish teeth. It may be either contra- or right-angled. May also be called a *prophy angle.*

angle, protrusive incisional guide, *n* the inclination of the incisal guide in the sagittal plane.

angle, rest, *n* See angle, occlusal rest.

angle, symphyseal, *n* the angle of the chin, which may be protruding straight or receding, according to type.

Angle's classification modified, *n.pr* a classification of the different forms of malocclusion set up by Edward Hartley Angle, American orthodontist (1855-1930).

Class I, *n* the normal anteroposterior relationship of the mandible to the maxillae. The mesiobuccal cusp of the permanent maxillary first molar occludes in the buccal groove of the permanent mandibular first molar; special class I-mutilated.

Type I, *n.pr* all teeth in linguoversion.

Type II, *n.pr* narrow arches; labioversion of the maxillary anterior teeth and linguoversion of the mandibular anterior teeth.

Type III, *n.pr* linguoversion of the maxillary anterior teeth; bunched; lack of development in the proximal region.

Class II, *n.pr* the posterior relationship of the mandible to the maxillae. The mesiobuccal cusp of the permanent maxillary first molar occludes mesial to the buccal groove of the permanent mandibular first molar.

Division 1, *n.pr* labioversion of the maxillary teeth.

Subdivision, *n.pr* signifies a unilateral condition.

Division 2, *n.pr* linguoversion of the maxillary central incisor teeth.

Subdivision, *n.pr* signifies a unilateral condition.

Class III, *n.pr* the anterior relationship of the mandible to the maxillae, may have a subdivision. The mesiobuccal cusp of the permanent maxillary first molar occludes distal to the buccal groove of the permanent mandibular first molar.

Type I, *n.pr* good alignment generally but arch relationship abnormal.

Type II, *n.pr* good alignment of the maxillary anterior teeth but linguoversion of the mandibular anterior teeth.

Type III, *n.pr* an underdeveloped upper arch; linguoversion of maxillary anterior teeth; good mandibular alignment.

angled shank, *n* an adaptation to the design of a hand-held instrument in order to allow easier access to posterior teeth or to individual tooth surfaces which might otherwise be difficult to reach. See also instrument, hand.

angstrom (Å) unit, *n* See unit, angstrom.

angular cheilitis, *n* a disease that most often occurs among the elderly but is caused by parasitic fungi or a deficiency in vitamin B rather than age; angular cheilitis appears as skin lesions on the lips, particularly as breaks in the tissue at the corners of the mouth. Often occurs in conjunction with reduced mobility and strength in the mouth. See perlèche.

angular cheilosis, *n* See cheilosis, angular.

angular thickening, *n* a widening of the space between the periodontal ligament and the root of a tooth which indicates the presence of periodontal infection. This shows up on x-rays as a thick black line next to the root.

angulation (instrumental) (ang′gyōōlā′shən), *n* the angle formed between the blade of an instrument and a tooth or tissue to provide increased access and more effective treatment.

Instrumental angulation. A, Ideal initial placement. **B,** Too close to effectively remove calculus. **C,** Ideal for debridement. **D,** Too open. (Daniel/Harfst, 2002)

angulation, bisecting error, n See bisecting-the-angle error.

angulation, bisecting-angle technique, n the proper angle to take a periapical survey x-ray using the bisecting angle technique. Horizontally angled so that the ray passes through the interproximal space as close to the center of the area being radiographed as possible, and vertically angled so that the ray travels perpendicular to the bisection of the angle formed by the x-ray film and the long axes of the targeted teeth.

angulation for air-powder polishing, n the correct angle at which the polisher's handpiece must be positioned in order to reduce the backflow of aerosol spray during treatment. The position varies according to tooth position and surface.

angulation, horizontal, n the angle measured within the occlusal plane at which the central ray of the x-ray beam is projected relative to a reference point in the vertical or sagittal plane.

angulation, mandibular midline projection, n the proper angle to take a mandibular midline x-ray. The position-indicating device should be pointed at the end of the chin at a −55° angle to the film for a view of the incisal region. To view the mouth floor, the position-indicating device should be perpendicular to the film, directly below the chin.

angulation, maxillary midline projection, n the proper angle to take a maxillary midline x-ray. The position-indicating device should be aimed at a +65° angle at the bridge of the nose.

angulation of central ray/beam, n the horizontal and vertical angles at which the central ray is aimed. Too much horizontal angulation causes superimposed images, while too much vertical angulation causes foreshortening. Also, too little vertical angulation causes elongation of the image.

angulation, paralleling technique, n the proper angle for taking a periapical x-ray using the paralleling technique. The central ray should be directed through the interproximal area roughly at the center of the film while the vertical angle should be at a precise right angle to the film. This technique is sometimes preferable because, unlike the bisecting angle technique, no x-rays are directed at the thyroid.

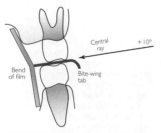

Vertical angulation. (Haring/Jansen, 2000)

angulation, vertical, n the angle measured within the vertical plane at which the central ray of the x-ray beam is projected relative to a reference in the horizontal or occlusal plane.

angulation (radiographic) (ang′-gyōōlā′shən), n the direction of the primary beam of radiation in relation to object and film.

anhidrosis (an′hīdrō′sis), n an abnormal deficiency in the production of sweat; may be associated with an odontia in ectodermal dysplasia.

anhidrotic ectodermal dysplasia, n See hypohidrotic ectodermal dysplasia.

anhydrous (anhī′drus), adj without water.

anion (an′ī-ən), n a negatively charged ion.

anionic detergent (an′ī-on′ik), n See detergent, anionic.

anirodia, n the absence of the iris. Usually a congenital condition.

anisocytosis (anī′sōsītō′sis), n an inequality in cell size, especially of red blood cells.

anisognathous (an′īsog′nathəs), adj a condition in which the maxillary and mandibular dental arches or jaws are of different sizes.

anisotropy, n not having properties or characteristics that are the same in all directions.

ankyloglossia (ang′kilōglôs′ē-ə), n tongue-tie; an abnormally short lingual frenum that limits movement of the tongue.

ankylosis (ang′kilō′sis), n an abnormal fixation and immobility of a joint.

ankylosis, bony, n a joining of bone with tooth or bone with bone that causes total loss of movement. See also tooth, ankylosed.

ankylosis, false, n an inability to open the mouth because of trismus rather than disease of the joint.

ankylosis, fibrous, n the fixation of a joint by fibrous tissue.

ankylosis of tooth, n See tooth, ankylosed.

anlage (on′lägə), n the first cells in the embryo that form any distinct part or organ of the body.

anneal (anēl′), n (homogenizing heat treatment, softening heat treatment), the softening of a metal by controlled heating and cooling.

anneal foil, n a process of subjecting noncohesive foil to heat to volatilize a protective gaseous coating on its surface, thus leaving the surface clean, making it cohesive.

anneal glass, n a process of regulated heating and subsequent cooling to remove strain hardening or work hardening of glass.

anneal metal, n a process of regulated heating and subsequent cooling to remove strain hardening or work hardening of metal.

announcement, n a communication, usually printed, that states office policies or practice limitations to the public and profession.

annual reports, *n.pl* statistical, fiscal, and descriptive yearly reports used to inform a constituency of the status of the institution or organization.

annual statement, n the report of an insurer or carrier showing assets and liabilities, receipts and disbursements, and other information for a specified 12-month period (fiscal or calendar year).

annuity, n a series of payments of a fixed amount for a number of years.

anochromasia (an′ōkrōmā′zē-ə, -zhə), n a variation in the staining quality of cells, particularly of degenerating red blood cells.

anoclassociation (ənō′sē-əsōsē-ā′shən), n the blocking of neuroses, fear, pain, and harmful influences or associations to prevent shock.

anode (an′ōd), n the electrically positive terminal of a roentgen ray (x-ray) tube; a tungsten block embedded in a copper stem and set at an angle of 20 or 45 degrees to the cathode. The anode emits roentgen rays (x-rays) from the point of impact of the electronic stream from the cathode.

anode, rotating, n an anode that rotates during x-ray production to present a constantly different focal spot to the electron stream and to permit use of small focal spots or higher tube voltages without overheating the tube.

anodontia (an′ōdon′tē-ə), n (aplasia of dentition), the failure of teeth to form; may be partial or complete.

anodontia, partial, n the absence of parts of the dentition resulting from arrested tooth development.

Anodontia (partial). (Sapp/Eversole/Wysocki, 2004)

anodontia, total, n a complete absence of teeth resulting from arrested tooth development.

anodyne (an′ōdīn), n an agent or drug that relieves pain; milder than analgesia.

anomaly (ənom′əlē), n an aberration or deviation from normal anatomic growth, development, or function.

anomaly, dental, n an abnormality in which a tooth or teeth have deviated from normal in form, function, or position.

anomaly, dentofacial, n a term indicating an oral or dysgnathic abnormality.

anomaly, dysgnathic, n an abnormality that extends beyond the teeth and includes the maxillae, the mandible, or both.

anomaly, eugnathic, n an abnormality limited to the teeth and their immediate alveolar supports.

anomaly, gestant, n See odontoma.

anomaly, maxillofacial, n a distortion of normal development of the face and jaws; a dysgnathic anomaly.

anomaly, oral, n an abnormal structure of the mouth and jaws other than of the teeth.

anophaxia (anōfax′ē-ə), n a tendency for one eye to turn upward.

anophthalmos, n a congenital absence of all tissues of the eyes.

anorexia (anōrek′sē-ə), n the partial or complete loss of appetite for food.

anorexia nervosa, n a psychoneurotic disorder characterized by a prolonged refusal to eat, resulting in emaciation, amenorrhea in women, emotional disturbance concerning body image, and an abnormal fear of becoming fat.

A

anoxemia (an'oksē'mē-ə), n a deficient aeration of the blood; a total lack of oxygen content in the blood.

anoxia (anok'sē-ə), n a condition of total lack of oxygen; a term frequently misused as a synonym of hypoxia.

anoxic hypoxia, n See hypoxia, anoxic.

antagonist, n **1.** a drug that counteracts, blocks, or abolishes the action of another drug. n **2.** a muscle that acts in opposition to the action of another muscle (for example, flexor vs. extensor). n **3.** a tooth in one jaw that occludes with a tooth in the other jaw.

antagonist, narcotic, n a narcotic drug that acts specifically to reverse depression of the central nervous system.

antagonists, insulin, n.pl circulating hormonal and nonhormonal substances that stimulate glyconeogenesis (for example, 11-oxysteroids and S hormones).

ante cibum (an'tē sī'bum), adv See a.c.

antegonial notch, n the notch or concavity usually present at the junction between the ramus and body of the mandible, near the anterior margin of the masseter muscle attachment.

anterior, adj **1.** situated in front of. adj **2.** a term used to denote the incisor and canine teeth or the forward region of the mouth. adj **3.** the forward position.

anterior cranial base, n the anterior cranial fossa, sometimes identified by related landmarks such as the sella turcica and nasion.

anterior determinants of occlusion, n.pl See occlusion, anterior determinants of cusp.

anterior guide, n See guide, anterior.

anterior nasal spine, n See spine, anterior nasal.

anterior palatal bar, n See connector, anterior palatal major.

anterior tooth arrangement, n See arrangement, tooth, anterior.

anterior-posterior discrepancy, n an anterior-posterior morphologic imbalance between the maxilla and mandible and consequently between structures attached to either.

anterocclusion, n a malocclusion of the teeth, in which the mandibular teeth are in a position anterior to their normal position relative to the teeth in the maxillary arch.

anteversion, n the tipping or tilting of teeth or other maxillary and mandibular structures too far forward (anterior) from the normal or generally accepted standard.

anthelmintic (an'thelmin'tik), n a drug that acts against parasitic worms, especially intestinal worms.

anthrax (an'thraks), n an infectious disease in herbivorous animals caused by a spore-forming *Bacillus* organism. Primary lesions in human beings may be on the lips or cheeks.

anthrocyclanins, n.pl a group of floral pigments existing as glycosides that may be used as hematoxylin substitutes.

anthropology, n the science of human beings ranging from physical characteristics to cultural, social, and environmental aspects.

anthropology, cultural, n the study of the interpersonal and community mores of a society or isolate.

anthropology, physical, n the study of the physical attributes of a society or isolate.

anthropometry, n the measurement of the human body and its parts.

anti-HAV, n a passively acquired antibody to the hepatitis A virus which provides protective immunity against recurrences of the infection. It may be detected in the blood of infected individuals within 14 days after they show the first symptoms of hepatitis A.

anti-HBc, IgM, n an antibody to the core antigen of the hepatitis B virus. Its presence in the blood indicates a previous infection with the hepatitis B virus.

anti-HBe, n an antibody to the e antigen of the hepatitis B virus. Its detection in the blood indicates the presence of a low titer hepatitis B infection and decreased ability of the infected person to pass the virus on to another person.

anti-HBs, n an antibody to the surface antigen of the hepatitis B virus; indicative of either active immunity to the hepatitis B virus as a result of prior infection or passive immunity from the presence of hepatitis B immunoglobulin in the blood. It may also be an immune response triggered as the result of having received vaccination against the hepatitis B virus.

anti-HCV, *n* an antibody to the hepatitis C virus. Its presence in the blood is indicative of an active or chronic hepatitis C infection.

anti-HDV, *n* an antibody to the hepatitis D virus. Its presence in the blood is indicative of a hepatitis D infection that may be either active, chronic, or under control.

anti-HSV antibodies, *n.pl* immunoglobulin contained in the fluid of the gingival sulcus which may or may not provide immunity to recurrent attacks of the herpes simplex virus.

antibiotic (an'tibī-ot'ik), *n* an organic substance produced by one of several microorganisms, especially certain molds, that is capable, in low concentration, of destroying or inhibiting the growth of certain other microorganisms.

antibiotic, oral reactions to, *n* manifestations on the oral mucous membrane of reactions to antibiotics; characterized by glossitis, angular cheilosis, and/or a hairy tongue. Reactions may result from an imbalance of oral flora produced by the antibiotics or from hypersensitivity to the antibiotics.

antibiotic prophylaxis, *n* the use of an antibiotic to protect a patient from an anticipated bacterial invasion associated with a medical or dental invasive procedure, particularly patients with a compromised cardiovascular system.

antibiotic, subgingival placement, *n* the efficient administration of antimicrobials in the subgingival region to control bacterial infections.

antibiotic therapy, *n* See therapy, antibiotic.

antibody (an'tibodē), *n* **1.** a specific substance that is produced by an animal as a reaction to the presence of an antigen and that reacts specifically with an antigen in some observable way. *n* **2.** an immunoglobulin, essential to the immune system, produced by lymphoid tissue in response to bacteria, viruses, or other antigenic substances. Each antibody is identified by its action, agglutinins, bacteriolysins, opsonins, and precipitins.

antibody, antinuclear, *n* having an affinity for the cell nuclei.

antibody formation, *n* the response of the lymphatic system to the presence of foreign substances in the body such as bacteria, viruses, food substances, pollens, and other antigens.

antibody, monoclonal, *n* produced by a clone or genetically homogeneous population of hybrid cells.

antibody, specificity, *n* the lymphatic system produces antibodies specific to each antigen. Viruses have the capacity to alter an antigen's genetic makeup, thereby creating a mutant antigen that requires new antibodies to combat it.

antibody-mediated hypersensitivity, *n* **1.** anaphylactic (Type I), also known as "immediate," allergen-induced IgE antibodies that remem-

Antibiotic: mode of action

Mode of action	Representative antibiotics
Inhibition of bacterial cell wall synthesis	Penicillins
Alteration of membrane permeability	Cephalosporins
Inhibition of microbial DNA translation and transcription	Bacitracins
	Polymyxin B
Inhibition of essential metabolite synthesis	Amphotericin B
	Nystatin
	Erythromycin
	Tetracyclines
	Streptomycin
	Lincomycin
	Kanamycin
	Chloramphenicol
	Paraminosalicylic acid
	Sulfonamides

ber the target antigen and proliferate against it, producing mediators such as histamines. *n* **2.** cytotoxic (Type II), antigens and antibodies that come together on the surface of a cell, causing lysis of the cell or other cell membrane damage. *n* **3.** immune complex (Type III), a complex of antigens and antibodies that is attracted to tissue.

anticariogenic (an′tīker′ē-ōjen′ik), *adj* term used to describe foods that tend to contribute favorably to dental health by remineralizing teeth and discouraging the acid that causes dental caries.

anticariogenic agents, *n.pl* inhibiting or arresting dental caries formation. See also flourides, sealants.

anticholinergic (an′tīkō′linur′jik), *n* (parasympatholytic, cholinolytic), a drug that acts to inhibit the effects of the neurohormone acetylcholine or to inhibit its cholinergic neuroeffects. A cholinergic blocking agent.

anticholinesterase (an′tīkō′lines′ tərās), *n* a drug or chemical that inhibits or inactivates the enzyme cholinesterase, resulting in the actions produced by the accumulation of acetylcholine at cholinergic sites.

anticoagulant (an′tīkō-ag′yələnt), *n* a drug that delays or prevents coagulation of blood.

anticonvulsive (an′tīkonvul′siv), *adj* relieving or preventing convulsion.

antidepressants, *n.pl* agents used to counteract or treat depression.

antidepressants, tricyclic, n.pl a classification of antidepressant drugs used to treat a variety of psychiatric conditions, including severe depression, social phobia, and mood, panic, or obsessive-compulsive disorders. The substance may be toxic in large amounts.

antidiabetes mellitus agents, *n.pl* drugs used to combat diabetes mellitus, particularly insulin; also drugs which combat the common side effects of diabetes mellitus, hypoglycemia, and hyperglycemia.

antidiarrheals, *n.pl* drugs which combat diarrhea by decreasing gastrointestinal motility; may cause sedation of the central nervous system and xerostomia.

antidote (an′tidōt), *n* a substance that acts to antagonize the toxic

effects of a drug, especially in overdose, or of a poison.

antidysrhythmics (an′tīdisrith′miks), *n.pl* a misnomer for antiarrhythmia. See antiarrhythmia.

antiemetic (an′tē-əmet′ik, an′tī- əmet′ik), *n* drug used to prevent, stop, or relieve nausea and emesis (vomiting).

antiepileptic drugs, *n.pl* agents that inhibit or control seizures associated with epilepsy.

antiflux, *n* a material that prevents and confines the flow of solder (for example, graphite).

antifungal agents, *n.pl* agents that inhibit, control, or kill fungi. The most common yeastlike fungus occurring in or near the oral cavity is *Candida albicans.*

antigen (an′tijen), *n* a substance, usually a protein, that elicits the formation of antibodies that react with it when introduced parenterally into an individual or species to which it is foreign.

antigenic drift, *n* the ability of viruses to alter their genetic makeup, thereby creating mutant antigens and bypassing the antibody barrier of the host.

antihemophilic factor (an′tīhē′mōfil′ik), *n* See factor VII.

antihistamine (an′tīhis′təmin), *n* a drug that counteracts the release of histamine such as occurs in allergic reactions; also has topical anesthetic and sedative effects, as well as a drying effect on the nasal mucosa.

antihistaminic (an′tīhistəmin′ik), *adj* referring to a drug that acts to prevent or antagonize the pharmacologic effects of histamine released in the tissues.

antihypertensive drugs, *n.pl* agents that lower or reduce high blood pressure.

antihypnotic (an′tīhipnot′ik), *adj* preventing or hindering sleep. (not current)

antiinflammatory agents, *n.pl* compounds that counteract or reduce inflammation.

antileptic (an′tilep′tik), *adj* assisting, supporting, revulsive.

antimicrobial, systemic, *n* an antimicrobial agent, usually in the form of an antibiotic, that is generally administered orally and absorbed into the blood stream through the intestine. Systemic antimicrobials move from the circulatory system to the body tissues where they reach the periodontal pocket through the gingival sulcus fluid.

antimony, *n* a bluish crystalline metallic element occurring in nature both free and as salts. Antimony compounds are used in the treatment of filariasis, leishmaniasis, and other parasitic diseases. Antimony is also used as an emetic.

antineoplastic agent, *n* a drug that prevents the development, maturation, or spread of neoplastic cells.

antiodontalgic, *adj* pertaining to a toothache remedy.

antioxidants, *n.pl* agents that reduce or prevent oxidation, such as occurs in the deterioration of fats, oils, and nonprecious metals.

antiphlogistic (an'tĭflōjis'tik), *adj* an obsolete term for antiinflammatory or antipyretic.

antiplaque agents, *n.pl* compounds that inhibit, control, or kill organisms associated with dental plaque formation.

antipruritic (an'tĭprōōrit'ik), *adj* relieving or preventing itching.

antipsychotics, *n.pl* medications used to decrease hallucinations, delusions, and other symptoms associated with schizophrenia and other psychotic disorders; enables functioning in daily life for individuals.

antipyretic (an'tĭpĭret'ik), *n* a drug that reduces fever primarily through action on the hypothalamus, thereby resulting in increased heat dissipation through augmented peripheral blood flow and sweating.

antipyrine, *n* an analgesic and antipyretic used in conjunction with salicylates.

antisepsis (an'tĭsep'sis), *n* the prevention of infection of a body surface, usually skin or oral mucosa, through the application of an antimicrobial agent.

antiseptic (an'tisep'tik), *n* an antimicrobial agent for application to a body surface, usually skin or oral mucosa, in an attempt to prevent or minimize infection at the area of application.

antisialic (an'tĭsĭ-al'ik), *adj* checking or that which checks salivary secretions.

antisialogogue (an'tĭsĭ-al'əgog), *n* a drug that reduces, slows, or prevents the flow of saliva.

antispasmodic (an'tĭspazmod'ik), *n* (antispastic), a drug that relieves muscle spasms.

antispastic, *adj* See antispasmodic.

antistreptolysin O (an'tĭstreptol'əsin), *n* an antibody against streptolysin O, a hemolysin produced by group A streptococci. A high titer is supporting evidence of rheumatic fever.

antithermic, *adj* reducing temperature. See also antipyretic.

antitoxin, *n* a subgroup of antisera usually prepared from the serum of horses immunized against a particular toxin-producing organism, such as botulism antitoxin and diphtheria antitoxin given prophylactically to prevent those infections.

antitragus (an'tĭtrā'gus), *n* the structure located opposite the tragus, a cartilaginous prominence in front of the external opening of the ear.

antitussive (an'tĭtus'iv), *n* a drug that relieves or prevents cough.

antrodynia (an'trōdĭ'nē-ə), *n* pain in the maxillary antrum. (not current)

antrostomy (antros'təmē), *n* a surgical opening into an antrum, either through the medial wall into the nose or through the lateral wall into the oral cavity.

antrum (an'trum), *n* a maxillary sinus. A cavity in the maxilla, lined by ciliated columnar epithelium, the inferior border of which approximates the apices of the roots of the maxillary posterior teeth.

antrum, maxillary, *n* See sinus, maxillary.

antrum of Highmore, *n.pl* See sinus, maxillary.

ANUG, *n* the abbreviation for acute necrotizing ulcerative gingivitis. A distinct, recurrent periodontal disease primarily involving the interdental papillae, which undergo necrosis and ulceration.

anxiety, *n* a condition of heightened and often disruptive tension accompanied by an ill-defined and distressing aura of impending harm or injury. Anxiety can disrupt physiologic functions through its effect on the autonomic nervous system. The patient may assume a tense posture, show excessive vigilance, move the hands and feet restlessly, and speak with a strained, uneven voice. The pupils may be widely dilated, giving the appearance of unrestrained fright, and the hands and face may perspire excessively. In extremely acute forms the patient may have generalized visceral reactions of respiratory, cardiac, vascular, and gastrointestinal dysfunction. The dentist must recognize the existence of anxiety, seek its etiology and relation to dental treatment, and determine ways that the patient's defenses against anxiety can be used to facilitate rather than inhibit treatment.

anxiety control, n the combination of measures which are used to eliminate patient apprehension and control pain during the performance of a dental procedure. The determination of the appropriate measures to be taken depends on the patient's overall periodontal health and tolerance for pain, as well as the specific treatment to be delivered.

anxiety neurosis, n an extreme manifestation of anxiety characterized by acute anxiety attacks (sympathetic overreactivity) and phobias, causing avoidance of the anxiety-provoking situations.

anxiolytic medication (angk′sē-ōlit′ik), n drug used to decrease emotional stress or anxiety. Also called *antianxiety agent.*

aorta, n the main arterial trunk of the systemic circulation. Consists of four parts: the ascending aorta, the arch of the aorta, the thoracic portion of the descending aorta, and the abdominal portion of the descending aorta.

aortic aneurysm, n a localized dilatation or ballooning of the wall of the aorta caused by atherosclerosis, hypertension, or a combination.

aortic valve, n a valve in the heart between the left ventricle and the aorta; also known as the tricuspid valve.

apathic (əpath′ik), adj without sensation or feeling.

apathism (ap′əthizm), n the state of being slow in responding to stimuli.

apatite (ap′ətīt), n the inorganic mineral substance of teeth and bone. See also carbonate hydroxyapatite.

APC, n See aspirin, phenacetin, caffeine.

Apert's syndrome, n.pr See syndrome, Apert's.

apertognathia (əpur′tōnath′ē-ə), n "open-bite" deformity. An occlusion characterized by a vertical separation between the maxillary and mandibular anterior teeth. Incorrectly called an *open bite.*

aperture, n an opening.

apex, n the end of the root.

apex blunderbuss, n an open or everted apex of a tooth, resembling the divergent form of the barrel of a blunderbuss rifle.

apexification (āpek′sifikā′shə), n the process of induced root development or apical closure of the root by hard tissue deposition.

apexigraph (āpek′sigraf), n a device for determining the position of the apex of a tooth root.

APF, n the abbreviation for **acidulated phosphate fluoride,** an agent used as a dental caries preventive and suggested by some for the control of plaque.

aphagia (əfā′jē-ə), n the inability to swallow.

aphasia (ə-fa′zhə), n a loss of power of expression through speech, writing, or signs of comprehension of spoken or written language resulting from disease or injury of the brain centers.

aphtha (af′thə), n (aphthous stomatitis), **1.** a small ulcer on the mucous membrane. -hae n.pl **2.** vesicles that undergo subsequent ulceration and are surrounded by a raised erythematous area.

aphtha, Bednar's (bed′närz), n.pr (pterygoid ulcer), an ulcer on the soft palate near the greater palatine foramen; seen in newborns.

aphtha, Mikulicz' (mik′ulich), n.pr a recurrent ulceration of the oral mucosa, resembling herpes. See also periadenitis mucosa necrotica recurrens.

aphtha, recurrent, n See stomatitis, herpetic and ulcer, aphthous, recurrent

aphtha, recurrent scarring, n See periadenitis mucosa necrotica recurrens.

aphthosis, n a clinical manifestation of apthae.

aphthous fever, n a fever associated with aphthosis.

aphthous pharyngitis, n aphthosis of the pharynx.

aphthous stomatitis (af'thus), n See aphtha and stomatitis, aphthous

aphthous, adj characterized by aphthae or aphthosis.

apical (ap'ikəl), adj pertaining to the end portion of the root.

apical curettage, n surgical removal of diseased tissue surrounding a root apex.

apical fiber, n See fiber, apical.

apicectomy, See apicoectomy.

apicoectomy (ap'ikō-ek'təmē), n (apicectomy, apiectomy, root amputation, root resection), the surgical removal of the apex or apical portion of a root.

Apicomplexa **protozoa (ap'ikomplek'sə),** n a parasitic group that sometimes needs multiple hosts to survive. Some varieties are implicated in diarrhea and malaria.

aplasia (əplā'zhə), n a lack of origin or development (for example, aplasia of dentition associated with ectodermal dysplasia).

aplasia of dentition, n See anodontia.

apnea (apnē'ə, ap'nē-ə), n a temporary cessation of respiratory movements.

apneumatic (apnōōmat'ik), adj free from air; used to describe something accomplished with the exclusion of air, such as an apneumatic operation. (not current)

apoplexy (ap'ōplek'sē), n a stroke caused by acute vascular lesions of the brain.

apoptosis, n cell reduction by fragmentation into membrane bound particles that are phagocytosed by other cells.

apostematosa, cheilitis glandularis, n See cheilitis glandularis apostematosa.

apothecaries' system, n See system, apothecaries'.

apoxesis (ap'əksē'sis), n See curettage, apical.

apparatus (ap'ərat'us), n an arrangement of a number of parts that act together to perform some special function.

apparatus, attachment, n the tissues that invest and support the teeth for function: the cementum, periodontal ligament, and alveolar bone.

apparatus, masticating, n the structures involved in chewing (that is, the teeth, mandibular musculature, mandible and its temporomandibular joints, accessory mandibular and facial musculature, and tongue), which are controlled by an exquisitely functioning neuromuscular mechanism. See also system, stomatognathic.

appellant (əpel'ənt), n the party who, dissatisfied with the disposition of a case on the trial level, appeals to a higher court.

appendicitis, n an inflammation of the vermiform appendix, usually acute, which, if undiagnosed and not surgically removed, leads rapidly to perforation and peritonitis.

appendix, n an accessory part of a main structure; in human anatomy, generally refers to the *vermiform appendix,* which is located at the junction of the small and large intestines.

appetite, n a natural or instinctive desire for food.

appetite suppressant, n an agent that diminishes the desire for eating.

appliance (əplī'-əns), n a device used to provide function or therapeutic effect. See also restoration.

appliance, Andresen removable orthodontic, n.pr an appliance intended to function as a passive transmitter and sometimes stimulator of the forces of the perioral muscles. One of the activator types of orthodontic appliances that induces or directs oral forces to contribute to improved tooth position and jaw relationship.

appliance, Begg fixed orthodontic, n.pr an appliance developed by P.R. Begg, based on a modified ribbon-arch attachment.

appliance, Bimler removable orthodontic, n.pr an activator-type appliance.

appliance, chin cup extraoral orthodontic, n an extraoral traction appliance used to restrain the forward positioning of the mandible and/or the forward growth of the mandible.

appliance, Crozat removable orthodontic, n.pr a wrought wire appliance originally introduced by George Crozat.

appliance, edgewise fixed orthodontic, n an orthodontic appliance, the last of those developed by E.H.

Angle, characterized by attachment brackets with a rectangular slot for engagement of a round or rectangular arch wire.

appliance, extraoral orthodontic, n a device that uses a portion of the face, neck, or back of the head as a base from which to deliver traction force to the teeth or jaws.

appliance, fixed orthodontic, n an appliance that is cemented to the teeth or attached by an adhesive material.

appliance, fracture, n (biphase pin fixation, external pin fixation, Stader splint), any one of the various devices for extraoral reduction and fixation of fractures in which pins, clamps, or screws are placed in the fractured segments, the fractured parts are aligned, and then the pins, clamps, or screws are joined with metal bars or rigid plastic connectors (for example, the Stader splint or Roger-Anderson pin-fixation appliance).

appliance, Frankel removable orthodontic, n.pr an activator-type appliance developed by Rolf Frankel.

appliance, Hawley retaining orthodontic, n.pr See retainer.

appliance, hay rake fixed orthodontic, n a device used to limit abnormal swallowing excursions of the tongue. In this manner, harmful effects of tongue thrusting are mitigated until the patient learns a new swallowing pattern.

appliance, intraoral orthodontic, n a device placed inside the mouth to correct or alleviate a malocclusion.

appliance, Kloehn cervical extraoral orthodontic, n.pr the classical cervical extraoral traction appliance introduced by S.J. Kloehn. Uses a relatively light and flexible (0.045 inch; 1.15 mm) inner arch rigidly attached to a long outer bow.

appliance, labiolingual fixed orthodontic, n an appliance using the maxillary and mandibular first permanent molars as anchorage, with labial arches 0.036 to 0.040 inch (0.090 to 0.10 cm) in diameter introduced into horizontal buccal tubes attached to the anchor bands and lingual arches of the same diameter fitted into vertical or horizontal tubes

fastened to the lingual side of the anchor bands.

appliance, orthodontic, n a device used for influencing tooth position. Orthodontic appliances may be classified as fixed or removable, active or retaining, and intraoral or extraoral.

appliance, pin and tube fixed orthodontic, n a labial arch with vertical posts that insert into tubes attached to bands on the teeth.

appliance, prosthetic, n (archaic term; generally not used to refer to a prosthesis), a complete or partial denture for children when groups of teeth are lost or are congenitally missing. Used to maintain space or masticatory function or for esthetic reasons.

appliance, removable orthodontic, n an appliance designed so that it can be removed and replaced by the patient.

appliance, retaining orthodontic, n an orthodontic device used to hold the teeth in place, following orthodontic tooth movement, until the occlusion is stabilized.

appliance, straight-wire fixed orthodontic, n a variation of the edgewise appliance in which an effort is made to obviate the need for many arch-wire adjustments by reorientation of the arch-wire slots. The first such modifications were introduced by E.H. Angle; L.M. Andrews first proposed such variations in all planes of space.

appliance, therapeutic, n a vehicle used to transport and retain some agent for therapeutic purposes (for example, a radium carrier).

appliance, twin-wire fixed orthodontic, n an orthodontic appliance developed by J.E. Johnson, typically using a pair of 0.010-inch (0.25-mm) wires to form the midsection of the arch wire.

appliance, universal fixed orthodontic, n an orthodontic appliance developed by S.R. Atkinson, combining some of the principles of edgewise and ribbon-arch appliances with very light arch wires.

application program, *n* a standard and frequently used computer program tailored to medical and dental needs. It may be supplied to the user by the manufacturer, purchased from a software house, or written by the user.

applicator, *n* a device for applying medication; usually a slender rod of glass or wood, used with a pledget of cotton on the end.

appointment, *n* a mutually agreed-on time reserved for the patient to receive treatment.

appointment book, *n* a ledger or table of workdays divided into segments of time to enable the dentist to reserve specified lengths of time for patient treatment.

appointment card, *n* a small card given to the patient as a reminder of the time reserved for the appointment.

apposition (ap′əzish′ən), *n* **1.** the condition of being placed or fitted together; juxtaposition; coaptation. *n* **2.** layered formation of a firm or hard tissue such as cartilage, bone, enamel, dentin, and cementum.

appropriate, *adj* **1.** the determination that the service provided is suited for the condition. *adj* **2.** suitable for a particular person, group, community, condition, occasion, and/or place. *adj* **3.** proper.

approved services, *n.pl* **1.** all services provided in a dental plan. In some plans, authorization must be obtained before approved service is provided; other plans make exception for treatment of emergency needs; still others require no prior authorization for any treatment approved under the program. *n.pl* **2.** dental services that meet quality standards maintained in a dental plan.

approximal, *adj* (approximating), contiguous; adjacent; next to each other.

approximating, *adj* See approximal.

apraclonidine, *n trade name:* Iopidine; *drug class:* selective α_2-adrenergic agonist; *action:* reduces intraocular pressure; *uses:* control or prevention of increases in intraocular pressure related to laser surgery of eye.

apraxia (əprak′sē-ə), *n* a loss of ability to execute a purposeful, goal-oriented, or skilled act resulting from selective damage to certain high-level brain centers, either sensory, motor, or both.

apron, *n* a piece of clothing worn in front of the body for protection.

apron band, *n* a labioincisal or gingival extension of an orthodontic band that aids in retention of the band and in proper positioning of the bracket.

apron, lead, *n* an apron made of materials containing metallic lead or lead compounds used to reduce radiation hazards.

apron, lingual, *n* See connector, linguoplate major.

apron, rubber dam, *n* a small strip of rubber dam, perforated to fit over an implant abutment that is used to inhibit introduction of cement into the periimplant space.

aprotinin, *n* a protease and kallikrein inhibitor useful in the treatment of pancreatitis.

aptitude, *n* a natural ability. Usually refers to the quickness to learn, understand, or acquire a skill.

aqueous (ā′kwē-us), *adj* containing or relating to water.

arachidonic acid, *n* an essential fatty acid that is a component of lecithin and a basic material for the biosynthesis of some prostaglandins.

Arachnia propionica, *n* an opportunistic, naturally occurring organism in the human body, especially in body cavities and on the skin. It is sometimes implicated in actinomycosis, especially in open wounds.

arboviruses, *n.pl* an acronym for hemophagic **ar**thropod-**bo**rne viruses, passed on to the host by a bite; implicated in viral encephalitis. The term is not accepted as an official taxonomic nomenclature.

ARC, *n* the abbreviation for **AIDS-related complex.** See also acquired immunodeficiency syndrome.

arc, reflex, *n* a system of nerves used in a reflex or involuntary act, consisting primarily of an afferent nerve with sensory receptor, a nerve center, and an efferent nerve that stimulates the effector muscle or gland.

arch (pl. es), *n* a structure with a curved outline.

arch bar, *n* See bar, arch.

arch, basal, *n* See base, apical.

arch, dental, *n* the composite structure of the dentition and alveolar ridge or the remains thereof after the loss of some or all of the natural teeth.

arch, dental, contraction, *n* See contraction.

arch, dentulous dental, *n* a dental arch containing natural teeth.

arch, edentulous dental, *n* a dental arch from which all natural teeth are missing. The residual alveolar ridge.

arch expansion, *n* See expansion.

arch form, See form, arch.

arch, high labial, *n* a labial arch wire adapted so that it lies gingival to the anterior tooth crowns; it has auxiliary springs extending downward in contact with the teeth to be moved.

arch length, *n* the length of a dental arch, usually measured through the points of contact between adjoining teeth.

arch length, available, *n* the space available for all teeth.

arch length, deficiency, *n* the difference between required and available arch length.

arch length, required, *n* the sum of the mesiodistal widths of all teeth.

arch, ovoid, *n* an arch that curves continuously from the molars on one side to the molars on the opposite side so that two such arches placed back to back describe an oval.

arch, palatine, *n* (glossopalatine arch), the pillars of the fauces; the two arches of mucous membrane enclosing the muscles at the sides of the passage from the mouth to the pharynx.

arch, partially edentulous dental, *n* a dental arch from which one or more but not all teeth are missing.

arch, passive lingual, *n* an orthodontic appliance effective in maintaining space and preserving arch length when bilateral primary molars are prematurely lost.

arch, pharyngeal, *n* the branchial arches of the fetus.

arch, removable lingual, *n* an arch wire designed to fit the lingual surface of the teeth. It has two posts soldered on each end that fit snugly into the vertical tubes of the molar anchor bands.

arch, stationary lingual, *n* an arch wire designed to fit the lingual sur-

face of the teeth and soldered to the anchor bands.

arch, tapering, *n* a dental arch that converges from molars to central incisors to such an extent that lines passing through the central grooves of the molars and premolars intersect within 1 inch (2.5 cm) anterior to the central incisors.

arch, trapezoidal, *n* an arch that has the same convergence as a tapering arch but to a lesser degree. The anterior teeth are somewhat square to abruptly rounded from canine tip to canine tip. The canines act as corners of the arch.

arch, U-shaped, *n* a dental arch in which there is little difference in diameter (width) between the first premolars and the last molars; the curve from canine to canine is abrupt, so a dental arch in the shape of a capital U is formed.

arch width, *n* the width of a dental arch. The width, which varies in all diameters between the right and left opposites, is determined by direct measurement between the canines, between the first molars, and between the second premolars. These intercanine, interpremolar, and intermolar distances can be cited as arch width.

arch wire, *n* a wire applied to two or more teeth through fixed attachments to cause or guide orthodontic tooth movement.

arch wire, full, *n* a wire extending from the molar region of one side of an arch to the other.

arch wire, sectional, *n* a wire extending to only a few teeth, usually on one side or in the anterior segment.

architecture, *n* in medicine and dentistry, usually refers to the framework of a structure or system.

architecture, gingival, *n* See gingival architecture.

archiving, *n* the storage of older, rarely required data or patient information in a cheaper and/or more compact form.

arcus senilis (är′kəs senil′is), *n* an opaque, grayish-white ring at the periphery of the cornea occurring in older adults.

area, *n* region.

area, apical, *n* See base, apical.

area, basal seat, *n* (denture-bearing

area, denture-supporting area, stress-bearing area, stress-supporting area), the portion of the oral structures available to support a denture.

area, contact, n See point, contact.

area, denture-bearing, n See area, basal seat.

area, denture-supporting, n See area, basal seat.

area, impression, n the surface of the oral structures recorded in an impression.

area, pear-shaped, n See pad, retromolar.

area, post dam, n See area, posterior palatal seal.

area, posterior palatal seal, n the soft tissues along the junction of the hard and soft palates on which compression, within the physiologic limits of the tissues, can be applied by a denture to aid in its retention.

area, postpalatal seal, n See area, posterior palatal seal.

area, pressure, n an area of excessive displacement of soft tissue by a prosthesis.

area, recipient, n the portion of the body on which a skin, bone, tooth, or other graft is placed.

area, relief, n the portion of the surface of the mouth under prosthesis on which pressures are reduced or eliminated.

area, rest (rest seat), n the prepared surface of a tooth or fixed restoration into which the rest fits, giving support to a removable partial denture.

area, rugae (rōō'jē), n (rugae zone), that portion of the hard palate in which rugae are found.

area, saddle, n See area, basal seat.

area, stress-bearing, n See area, basal seat.

area, stress-supporting, n See area, basal seat.

area, supporting, n the areas of the maxillary and mandibular edentulous ridges best suited to carry the forces of mastication when the dentures are in use. See also area, basal seat.

area, work, n the entire space in which the dental hygienist moves and works while treating a patient. This includes the instrument tray and dental chair, unit, and light.

Arenaviridae, *n* a grouping of enveloped, helix-shaped RNA viruses implicated in a relatively benign form of meningitis (lymphoctyic choriomeningitis; severe encephalitic forms do occur rarely) that affects young adults.

arginine, *n* one of the essential amino acids for infants and children. See also amino acid.

Argyll Robertson pupil (ärgil'), *n.pr* See pupil, Argyll Robertson.

argyria (ärjir'ē-ə), *n* a bluish color of the skin or mucous membranes produced by the deposition of silver salts in collagen fibers after prolonged use of silver salts.

argyria, local, n a localized blue pigmentation of the oral mucosa from the deposition of silver amalgam in the submucosal connective tissue.

argyrosis (ärjirō'sis), *n* a pathologic bluish-black pigmentation in a tissue resulting from the deposition of an insoluble albuminate of silver.

ariboflavinosis (ərī'bōflāvinō'sis), *n* a nutritional disease resulting from a deficiency of riboflavin (vitamin B_2); characterized by angular cheilosis, seborrheic dermatitis, a magenta tongue, and ocular disturbance.

Arkansas stone (är'kənsô), *n* See stone, Arkansas.

arm, *n* an extension or projection of a removable partial denture framework.

arm, neutral position of, n a body position to be assumed while treating a patient which prevents cumulative trauma to the arm; incorporates proper placement of the wrist, elbow, and shoulder.

arm, reciprocal, n a clasp arm used on a removable partial denture to oppose any force arising from an opposing clasp arm on the same tooth. See also arm, retention.

arm, retention, n an extension or projection that is part of a removable partial denture and is used to aid in the retention and stabilization of the restoration. See also retainer divet.

arm, truss, n See connector, minor.

arm, upright, n See connector, minor.

armamentarium (är'məmenter'ē-əm), *n* the equipment and materials of a practitioner.

arrangement, *n* the pattern into which a group of things is organized.

arrangement, financial, n an agreement between the dentist and patient on the method of handling the patient's account.

arrangement, tooth, *n* the placement of teeth on a denture or temporary base with definite objectives in mind.

arrhythmia (ərith′mē-ə), *n* a variation from the normal rhythm of the heart.

art, *n* in medicine and dentistry, usually refers to the skill, craftsmanship, or facility in one's work.

arteriole (ärtir′ē-ōl), *n* a minute arterial branch proximal to a capillary.

arteriosclerosis (ärtir′ē-ōsklerō′sis), *n* a term applied to a group of diseases that affect the elasticity of the blood vessels. It may refer to atherosclerosis, hyperplastic arteriosclerosis, or Mönckeberg's sclerosis. These degenerative processes generally affect only the tunica media and tunica intima. The effect is narrowing of the lumen of a blood vessel, causing rupture of the blood vessel or ischemia of an area of tissue that the vessel supplies.

arteriosclerotic heart disease (ärtir′ē-ōsklerot′ik), *n* See disease, heart, arteriosclerotic.

arteriovenous shunt (ärtir′ē-ōvē′nus), *n* See shunt, arteriovenous.

arteritis (ärtərī′tis), *n* an inflammatory condition of the inner layers or the outer coat of one or more arteries. It may occur as a separate clinical entity or accompanying another disorder, such as rheumatoid arthritis, rheumatic fever, or systemic lupus erythematosus.

arteritis, temporal, *n* an inflammation of the temporal artery that produces a nodular, tortuous swelling of the temporal artery accompanied by a burning, throbbing pain, initially in the teeth, temporomandibular joint, and eye, but ultimately localized over the artery. This disorder occurs primarily in persons over 55 years of age.

artery, *n* a blood vessel through which the blood passes from the heart to the various structures of the body. There are three layers of tissue in every artery: the inner coat (tunica intima), composed of an inner endothelial lining, connective tissue, and an outer layer of elastic tissue (inner elastic membrane); the middle coat (tunica media), composed chiefly of muscle tissue; and the outer coat (tunica adventitia), composed chiefly of connective tissue. The structure of the three layers varies with the location, size, and purpose of the blood vessel.

artery arthograms, n.pl x-rays of a joint usually with the introduction of a contrast compound into the joint capsule. In dentistry, an arthogram usually involves the temporomandibular joint.

artery, large, *n* an elastic artery with an abundant supply of elastic tissue and a great reduction of smooth muscle. The tunica intima is thick, and the endothelial cells are round or polygonal. The tunica media is the thickest of the three layers. It contains few smooth muscle fibers, and its outer border has a special concentration of elastic fibers—the external elastic membrane. The tunica adventitia is relatively thin and ill defined and is continuous with the loose connective tissue surrounding the vessel.

artery, medium-sized, *n* most of the arteries in the body (for example, facial, maxillary, radial, ulnar, and popliteal). Thick muscular bands are found in the tunica media. Thin elastic fibers course circularly in the tunica media and run longitudinally in the tunica adventitia. The tunica adventitia is as thick as the tunica media, and its outer layer gradually blends with the connective tissue that supports the artery and surrounding structures.

arthralgia (ärthral′jē-ə), *n* pain in a joint or joints.

arthritis (ärthrī′tis), *n* any of a number of types of inflammation of a joint or joints.

arthritis, allergic, *n* arthralgia, swelling, and stiffness of joints associated with food and drug allergies and serum sickness.

arthritis, atrophic, *n* See arthritis, rheumatoid.

arthritis, bacterial, *n* See arthritis, infective.

arthritis, hypertrophic, *n* See osteoarthritis.

arthritis, infective, *n* (bacterial arthritis), a primary and secondary bacterial infection of the joints (for example, by staphylococcal, gonococcal, streptococcal, or pneumococcal organisms).

arthritis, rheumatic **(rōōmat′ik),** *n* an acute polyarticular and migratory arthritis of unknown cause but assumed to be related to group A streptococcal infection of the upper respiratory tract.

arthritis, rheumatoid **(rōō′mətoid),** *n* a chronic destructive inflammation of the joints of unknown origin, with associated constitutional manifestations. Chronic synovitis and regressive changes in the articular cartilage occur with pain, swelling, deformity, limitation of motion, and occasionally ankylosis of the joints. Variable systemic manifestations include weakness, loss of weight, anemia, leukopenia, splenomegaly, lymphadenopathy, and the formation of subcutaneous nodules. Small joints are principally affected. In most instances, onset is in the third or fourth decade of life.

arthritis, senile, *n* arthritis occurring in persons of advanced age.

arthritis, specific infectious, *n* arthritis caused by direct invasion and subsequent infection of joint structures by microorganisms from the bloodstream. Nearly all pathogenic bacteria have been isolated as etiologic agents.

arthritis, traumatic, *n* an acute or chronic inflammation of a joint as a result of acute or chronic injury.

Arthrobacter, *n* a genus of a strictly aerobic gram-positive bacteria found in soil and present in dental caries.

arthroplasty (är′thrəplas′tē), *n* the surgical correction of a joint abnormality.

arthroplasty, gap, *n* See gap arthroplasty.

arthroplasty, interposition, *n* See interposition arthroplasty.

arthroscope, *n* an instrument used to view the inside of a joint.

arthrostomy (ärthros′təmē), *n* the surgical formation of an opening into a joint.

articaine, *n* a local anesthetic drug of the amide group that is used to anesthetize the treatment site during a dental procedure. The drug is now available in the United States.

articular cartilage, *n* See cartilage, articular.

articulare, *n* the point of intersection of the dorsal contour of the mandibular condyle and the temporal bone.

articulate (ärtik′yōōlāt), *v* **I.** to arrange or place in connected sequence. See also arrangement, tooth. *v* **2.** to connect by articulating strips, paper, or cloth coated with ink-containing or dye-containing wax, used for marking or locating occlusal contacts.

articulation (ärtik′yōōlā′shən), *n* **I.** a joint. See also joint. *n* **2.** the relationship of cusps of teeth during jaw movement.

articulation, anatomic, *n* a rigid or movable junction of a bony part.

articulation, articulator, *n* the use of a device that incorporates artificial temporomandibular joints that permit the orientation of casts in a manner duplicating or simulating various positions or movements of the mandible.

articulation, balanced, *n* the simultaneous contacting of the maxillary and mandibular teeth as they glide over each other when the mandible is moved from centric relation to the various eccentric relations. See also occlusion, balanced.

articulation, mandibular, *n* See articulation, temporomandibular.

articulation, temporomandibular, *n* (temporomandibular joint, mandibular joint), **I.** the joint formed by the two condyles of the mandible. *n* **2.** the bilateral articulation between the glenoid or mandibular fossae of the temporal bones and condyles (condyloid processes) of the mandible. The structures that make up the temporomandibular joint include the mandibular fossae of the temporal bones, articular disks, mandibular condyles, and articular tubercles of the zygomatic process of the temporal bone.

articulation, temporomandibular, capsule, *n* the ligamentous covering of the temporomandibular joint.

articulation, temporomandibular, collagen disease, *n* rheumatoid arthritis in which the joint may be so involved because of bone changes that the mandibular condyle is fused to the articular fossa in the base of the cranium.

articulation, temporomandibular, hormonal disturbances, n.pl hormonal disorders that frequently affect growth patterns of the skeleton, involving the temporomandibular joint (for example, acromegaly).

articulation, temporomandibular, neuromuscular disorders, n.pl neuromuscular disorders involving the temporomandibular joint in which the patient is unable to maintain appropriate patterns of mandibular closure consistent with good dental occlusion. The natural teeth degenerate rapidly and are frequently lost prematurely; when dentures are substituted, they cause the residual tissues to deteriorate rapidly. In addition to the chronic masticatory disability, the deglutitive mechanism functions poorly because of incoordinated lip and tongue action.

articulation, temporomandibular, pain-dysfunction syndrome, n See temporomandibular joint pain-dysfunction syndrome.

articulator, adjustable (ärti-k'yōōlātur), *n* an articulator that may be adjusted to permit movement of the casts into various recorded eccentric relationships.

artifact (är'təfakt), *n* a blemish or image in the radiograph that is not present in the roentgen image of the object.

artificial intelligence (A-I), *n* a system that makes it possible for a machine to perform functions similar to human intelligence. Computer technology produces many systems and functions that mimic and surpass some human capabilities, such as the ability to play chess.

artificial organs, *n.pl* devices used to support life because of the failure or limited capacity of the human organ. The most effective is the artificial kidney, which consists of a set of tubes that pass the blood through a dialysate solution where wastes are removed by osmosis and diffusion.

artificial respiration, *n* See respiration, artificial.

artificial stone, *n* See stone, artificial.

arytenoepiglottic (er'ətē'nō-ep'iglot'ik), *adj* pertaining to the arytenoid cartilage and the epiglottis.

ASA classification, *n* a system de-

veloped by the American Society of Anesthesiologists for categorizing a patient's physical status. See also health ASA classification.

asbestos, *n* a group of fibrous impure magnesium silicate minerals. Inhalation of the fibers can lead to pulmonary fibrosis.

Ascaris, *n* a genus of large parasitic intestinal roundworms such as *Ascaris lumbricoides.*

Aschheim-Zondek (AZ) test (ash'hīm tson'dek), *n* See test, pregnancy.

ascites (əsī'tēz), *n* an abnormal accumulation of serous fluid, containing large amounts of protein and electrolytes, in the peritoneal cavity. Ascites is a complication of cirrhosis, congestive heart failure, nephrosis, malignant neoplastic disease, and various fungal and parasitic diseases.

ascorbic acid (vitamin C), *n trade name:* generic; many brand names; *drug class:* vitamin C, water-soluble vitamin; *action:* needed for wound healing, collagen synthesis, antioxidant, carbohydrate metabolism; *uses:* vitamin C deficiency, scurvy, delayed wound and bone healing, chronic disease, urine acidification, before gastrectomy.

asepsis (əsep'sis), *n* the condition of being without infection; of being free of viable pathogenic microorganisms.

asepsis, chain of, *n* a series of tasks, each step of which is performed in a bacteria-free environment, which serves to maintain the sterility of the entire process.

aseptic, *adj* not producing microorganisms or free from microorganisms.

asialia (əsē-ā'lē-ə), *n* See asialorrhea.

asialorrhea (əsī'-əlōrē'-ə), *n* (asialia), a decrease in or lack of salivary flow. See also hyposalivation.

asparagine, *n* a nonessential amino acid found in many proteins in the body.

aspartame, *n* a low-calorie sweetening agent about 200 times as sweet as sucrose.

aspect, buccal, *n* the facial surface or cheek side of posterior teeth.

aspergillosis, *n* an infection caused by a fungus of the genus *Aspergillus.* Most commonly affects the ear but is capable of causing inflammatory, granulomatous lesions on or in any organ.

Aspergillosis. (Neville/Damm/Allen/Bouquot, 2002)

Aspergillus, *n* a genus of fungi that is a common contaminant in the laboratory and a cause of nosocomial infection. See also aspergillosis.

asphyxia (asfik′sē-ə), *n* a condition of suffocation resulting from restriction of oxygen intake and interference with the elimination of carbon dioxide.

aspirate (as′pirāt), *v* **1.** to draw or breathe in. *v* **2.** to remove materials by vacuum. *n* **3.** a phonetic unit whose identifying characteristic is the sound generated by the passage of air through a relatively open channel; the sound of *h;* a sound followed by or combined with the sound of *h.*

aspirated materials, managing, *n* steps taken to keep a patient from ingesting tools or materials during treatment, for example, a rubber dam. See also risk management.

aspiration (as′pirā′shən), *n* **1.** the act of breathing or drawing in. *n* **2.** the removal of fluids, gases, or solids from a cavity by means of a vacuum pump.

aspiration biopsy, *n* See biopsy, aspiration.

aspiration pneumonia, *n* pneumonia produced by aspiration of foreign material into the lungs.

aspirator (as′pərātur), *n* an apparatus used for removal of fluids, gases, or solids from a cavity by vacuum.

aspirin, *n* *trade name:* ASA, Aspirin, Ecotrin; *drug class:* nonnarcotic analgesic salicylate; *action:* inhibits prostaglandin synthesis, possesses analgesic, antiinflammatory, antipyretic properties; *uses:* mild-to-moderate pain or fever.

aspirin burn, *n* See burn, aspirin.

aspirin, phenacetin, caffeine (APC,

PAC), *n* a pharmaceutical preparation used as an analgesic.

assault, *n* an intentional, unlawful offer of bodily injury to another by force or unlawfully directing force toward another person to create a reasonable fear of imminent danger, coupled with the apparent ability to do the harm threatened if not prevented. A completed assault is a battery. In a medical setting, the unconsented touching of the body would be an assault and battery.

assertiveness, *n* a form of behavior that is directed toward claiming one's rights without denying the rights of others.

assessment, *n* the qualified opinion of a healthcare provider, informed by patient feedback and examination results, with regard to a specific health issue, whether critical, pending, or routine.

assessment, extraoral, *n* a preliminary examination of the head, neck, and face, usually made in conjunction with an intraoral examination, to recognize anomalies that might impact the patient's health; may require observation, listening, touch, and smell.

assessment, risk, *n* process of evaluating a potential hazard, likelihood of suffering, or any adverse effects.

assessment stroke, *n* the light movement of an instrument against a tooth to detect calculus, caries, overhangs, or other surface irregularities; the movement of a probe to determine pocket depth. Also called *exploratory stroke.*

assets, *n.pl* everything a business owns or that is owned. Cash, investments, money due, materials, and inventories are current assets. Buildings and equipment are fixed assets. Goodwill is an intangible asset.

assignment of benefits, *n* a procedure whereby a beneficiary or patient authorizes the administrator of the program to forward payment for a covered procedure directly to the treating dentist.

assistant, *n* an agent or employee.

assistant, dental, *n* an auxiliary to the dentist. See also certified dental assistant.

assistant's stool, *n* an adjustable chair with additional base support and footrest used to maintain the comfort of the individual assisting the clinician during an examination.

association, *n* a connection, union, joining, or combination of things.

astemizole, *n trade name:* Hismanal; *drug class:* antihistamine, H_1-histamine antagonist; *action:* decreases allergic response by blocking pharmacologic effects of histamine; *uses:* rhinitis, allergy symptoms.

asthenia (asthē´nē-ə), *n* the loss of vitality or strength; a condition of debility; weakness.

asthenic (asthēn´ik), *adj* describing an individual with a long, slender appearance who is thin and flat-chested and has long limbs and a short trunk; comparable to the ecto-morph in Sheldon's classification.

asthma (az´mə), *n* paroxysmal wheezing and difficulty in breathing resulting from bronchospasms. Frequently has an allergic basis and occasionally an emotional origin. See also status asthmaticus.

asthma, cardiac, *n* shortness of breath (paroxysmal dyspnea), sonorous rales, and expiratory wheezes that resemble bronchial asthma; related to cardiac failure.

astigmatism (əstig´mətizəm), *n* a defective curvature of the refractive surfaces of the eye, resulting in a condition in which a ray of light is not focused sharply on the retina but is spread over a more or less diffuse area.

astringent (əstrin´jənt), *n* styptic; an agent that checks the secretions of mucous membranes and contracts and hardens tissues, limiting the secretions of glands.

astrocytes, *n* a large, star-shaped cell found in certain tissues of the nervous system. A mass of astrocytes is called astroglia. See also astrocytoma.

astrocytoma, *n* a primary tumor of the brain composed of astrocytes and characterized by slow growth, cyst formation, invasion of surrounding structures, and often, the development of a highly malignant glioblastoma within the primary tumor mass.

asymmetric (āsimet´rik), *adj* unevenly arranged; out of balance; not the same on both sides; not a mirror image on both sides.

asymmetry, *n* an inharmonious relationship between the maxillary and mandibular teeth during closure or functional jaw movements.

asymptomatic carrier, *n* an individual who serves as host for an infectious agent but who does not show any apparent signs of the illness; may serve as a source of infection for others.

asynergy (āsin´urjē), *n* a lack of muscular coordination in special functions (for example, hand-to-mouth movements for feeding).

asystole (āsis´təlē), *n* the faulty contraction of the ventricles of the heart, resulting in incomplete or imperfect systole.

ataractic (at´ərak´tik), *n* (ataraxic, tranquilizer), one of a poorly defined group of drugs designed to produce ataraxia. The former concept, that the use of ataractics involved no mental or motor impairment, is subject to question.

ataraxia (at´ərak´sē-ə), *n* a state of complete serenity without impairment of mental or physical functions.

ataxia (ātak´sē-ə), *n* a muscular incoordination characterized by irregular muscle activity.

ataxia, locomotor, *n* See tabes dorsalis.

atelectasis (at´ilek´təsis), *n* the complete or partial collapse of a lung.

atenolol, *n trade name:* Nova-Atenol, Tenormin; *drug class:* antihypertensive, selective β_1 blocker; *action:* produces fall in blood pressure without reflex tachycardia or significant reduction in heart rate; *uses:* acute myocardial infarction, mild-to-moderate hypertension, prophylaxis of angina pectoris.

atheroma, *n* a fatty, fibrous deposit developing on the artery lining. Also called *atheromatous plaque.*

atherosclerosis (ath´ərōsklərō´sis), *n* a degenerative disease principally affecting the aorta and its major branches, the coronary artery, and the larger cerebral arteries. The arterial changes include narrowing of the lumen of the vessels; weakening of the arterioles, leading to rupture; an increased tendency toward development of atheromatous plaques; and thrombi. Atherosclerosis is a common cause of coronary thrombosis, congestive heart failure, aneurysms, hemorrhage, cerebral infarcts, and apoplexy.

athetosis (ath′əto′sis), *n* a neuromuscular impairment in which extensive twisting and swaying spasms of the skeletal musculature interfere with voluntary control of movement; the spasms are especially conspicuous and disconcerting during emotional stress and on initiation of conscious voluntary acts.

athiaminosis (əthī′-əminō′sis), *n* a deficiency of thiamine. See also beriberi.

athletic (athlet′ik), *adj* pertaining to a bodily constitution characterized by a strong, muscular, robust appearance.

athletic injuries, n.pl injuries sustained by persons while engaged in sports, more frequently while engaged in contact sports such as football.

atlantooccipital joint, *n* one of a pair of condyloid joints formed by the articulation of the atlas of the vertebral column with the occipital bone of the skull.

atlas, *n* the first cervical vertebra articulating above with the occipital bone and below with the axis (second cervical vertebra).

atmosphere (atm), *n* the natural body of air, composed of approximately 20% oxygen, 78% nitrogen, and 2% carbon dioxide and other gases, that covers the surface of the earth.

atom (at′əm), *n* the smallest part of an element capable of entering into a chemical reaction.

atomic (ətom′ik), *adj* pertaining to the atom.

atomic energy, n See energy, atomic.

atomic mass number, n (symbol: A), the total number of nucleons (protons and neutrons) of which an atom is composed.

atomic number (Z), n **1.** the number of electrons outside the nucleus of a neutral atom. *n* **2.** the number of protons in the nucleus.

atomic structure theory, n the theory that matter is composed of a vast number of particles, or atoms, bound together by a force of attraction of electrical charges.

atomic weight, n the weight of one atom of an element as compared with the weight of an atom of hydrogen.

atomizer (at′əmīzur), *n* an apparatus for changing a jet of liquid into a spray.

atonia, in cerebral palsy, *n* an inability to stand or lift the head and diminished capacity to speak or swallow due to weak muscular tone.

atonic, *adj* lacking rigidity or regular tone.

atopy (ā′tōpē), *n* (atopic hypersensitivity, "spontaneous" clinical allergy), a group of "allergic" disorders showing a marked familial distribution; although the susceptibility appears to be inherited, contact with the antigen must occur before hypersensitivity can develop. Disorders include asthma or hay fever resulting from pollens and gastrointestinal tract and skin reactions resulting from food.

atovaquone, *n trade name:* Mepron; *drug class:* antipneumocystic; *action:* unknown, may inhibit synthesis of ATP and nucleic acids; *uses:* treatment of *Pneumocystis carinii* pneumonia in patients who are intolerant of trimethoprim-sulfamethoxazole.

atresia (ətrē′zē-ə), *n* the congenital absence or occlusion of a normal opening of one or more ducts in an organ.

atresia, aural, n the absence of closure of the auditory canal.

atrial fibrillation, *n* a heart condition characterized by rapid random contractions of the atria at the rate of 130 to 150 ventricular beats per minute.

atrophy (at′rōfē), *n/v* a progressive, acquired decrease in the size of a normally developed cell, tissue, or organ. Atrophy may result from a decrease in cell size, number of cells, or both.

atrophy, adipose, n atrophy resulting from a reduction in fatty tissue.

atrophy, alveolar, n a depletion of the size of the alveolar process of the jaws from disuse, overuse, or pathologic disturbance of the bone.

atrophy, bone, n **1.** bone resorption internally (in density) and externally (in form) (for example, of residual ridges). *n* **2.** a loss of bone substance or volume. Atrophy of bone ordinarily occurs without a corresponding change in the volume or external dimensions of bone, but the mass of bone tissue may be reduced by as much as 75%. The internal architecture of the bone gradually becomes attenuated and finally disappears. Atrophied bone is brittle and has a more spongy consistency than normal bone. In cross-section the cortex is thin, and the periosteal surface is smooth and unchanged, but the intramedullary substance is composed of a yellow, fatty, cancellous bone tissue. Bone atrophy may be systemic, regional, or local.

atrophy, central papillary, n lesion on the central dorsum of the tongue, possibly due to a fungal infection, not a developmental disorder; it may be raised or flat. Formerly called *median rhomboid glossitis.*

atrophy, diffuse alveolar, n See periodontosis.

atrophy, facial, n the failure of facial development. If it is bilateral, it may produce brachygnathia; unilateral types, although rare, are more common than the bilateral type. Causes include physical injury, neurovascular disease, and paralysis.

atrophy, gerodontic mucosal, n oral degenerations in which the tissue of the epithelium in the mouth thins and loses some of its vascular structure and elasticity.

atrophy, muscular, n a wasting of muscle tissue, especially resulting from lack of use. There are numerous causes for simple atrophy of muscle, such as chronic malnutrition, immobilization, and denervation.

atrophy, of disuse, n atrophy resulting from a lack of function of a tissue, organ, or body part.

atrophy, periodontal, n the quantitative degenerative changes that occur in the attachment apparatus and supporting bone of a tooth as a result of disease or disuse. When a tooth loses its antagonist, osteoporotic changes in the supporting bone, an afunctional change in the direction of periodontal fibers, and a narrowing of the periodontal membrane space occur.

atrophy, postmenopausal, n a thinning of the oral mucosa after menopause.

atrophy, pressure, n the tissue destruction and reduction in size as a consequence of prolonged or continued pressure on a local area or group of cells.

  atrophy, pressure, by epithelial attachment, n a theoretical type of atrophy. The theory, advanced to explain destruction of gingival fibers during gingival inflammation, states that gingival fiber degeneration is produced by pressure exerted by the proliferating pocket epithelium. It is now generally conceded that proteolytic substances produced in the tissues during inflammation are responsible for gingival fiber destruction; subsequently, the epithelium can proliferate apically.

atrophy, senile, n the atrophy or diminution of all tissues characteristic of advanced age.

atropine (at′rō̄pēn), n an alkaloid that annuls parasympathetic effects and antagonizes the effects of pilocarpine. It acts directly on the effector cells, preventing the action but not the liberation of acetylcholine. It suppresses sweat and other glandular sections.

atropine sulfate, n trade name: Sal-Tropine; *drug class:* anticholinergic; *action:* inhibits muscarinic actions of acetylcholine at postganglionic parasympathetic neuroeffector sites; *uses:* reduction of salivary and bronchial secretions.

attached gingiva, n See gingiva, attached.

attachment, n 1. fastener, connector, associated part. *n* **2.** a mechanical device for retention and stabilization of a dental prosthesis.

attachment, abnormal frenum (frē′nəm), n aberrant insertions of labial, buccal, or lingual frena capable of initiating or perpetuating periodontal disease, such as creating diastemata between teeth, limiting lip or tongue movement.

attachment, epithelial, n the epithelial device that connects the junctional epithelium to the tooth surface.

attachment, gingival, n the fibrous attachment of the gingival tissues to the teeth.

attachment, intracoronal, n (precision attachment, slotted attachment). See retainer, intracoronal.

attachment level, clinical (CAL), n the amount of space between attached periodontal tissues and a fixed point, usually the cementoenamel junction. A measurement used to assess the stability of attachment as part of a periodontal maintenance program.

attachment, migration of epithelial, *n* the apical progression of the epithelial attachment along the tooth root.

attachment, orthodontic, n a device, secured to the crown of a tooth, that serves as a means of attaching the arch wire to the tooth.

attachment, parallel, n a prefabricated device for attaching a denture base to an abutment tooth. Retention is provided by friction between the parallel walls of the two parts of the attachment.

attachment, precision, n See retainer, intracoronal

attachment, slotted, n See retainer, intracoronal.

attack, heart, *n* See thrombosis, coronary.

attending dentist's statement, *n* a form used to report dental procedures to a third-party payer. The claim form was developed by the American Dental Association. Also called *dental claim form.*

attention, *n* the element of cognitive functioning in which the mental focus is maintained on a specific issue, object, or activity. The length of time of such focus is called *attention span.*

attention deficit hyperactivity disorder (ADHD), *n* a childhood neurologic disorder that manifests itself as excessive movement, irritability, immaturity, and an inability to concentrate or control impulses. It affects learning and skill acquisition.

attenuation (**ǝten′yōō-ā′shǝn**), *n* the process by which a beam of radiation is reduced in energy when passing through some material.

attitude, *n* a person's mental set, opinion, or disposition.

attrition (**ǝtrish′ǝn**), *n* the normal loss of tooth substance resulting from friction caused by physiologic forces.

Attrition. (Sapp/Eversole/Wysocki, 2004)

attritional occlusion, *n* See occlusion, attritional.

atypical (**ātip′ikǝl**), *adj* pertaining to deviation from the basic or typical.

Au, *n* See unit, angstrom.

audiogram (**ô′dē-ǝgram**), *n* a graphic summary of the measurement of hearing loss showing the number of decibels lost at each frequency tested.

audiologist, *n* individual trained to identify, diagnose, measure, and rehabilitate hearing impairments.

audiology (**ô′dē-ol′ǝjē**), *n* the study of the entire field of hearing, including the anatomy and function of the ear; impairment of hearing; and evaluation, education or reeducation, and treatment of persons with hearing loss.

audiometer (**ôdē-om′ǝtǝr**), *n* a device for testing hearing; calibrated to register hearing loss in terms of decibels.

audit, *n* **1.** an examination of records or accounts to check accuracy. *n* **2.** a posttreatment record review or clinical examination to verify information reported on claims.

audit of treatment, n **1.** an administrative or professional review of a participating dentist's treatment recommendations (peer audit). *n* **2.** the review of reimbursement claims for service performed (postaudit).

auditory stimuli, *n.pl* irregularities or deposits on the surface of a tooth which may be detected by ear during examination and probing. The movement of an instrument across clean enamel makes no sound, while calculus and metallic restorations are noisy when scraped.

augmentation (**ôg′mentā′shǝn**), *n* **1.** assistance to respiration by the application of intermittent pressure on inspiration. *n* **2.** an increase in size beyond the existing size, such as an implant placed over the mandibular or maxillary ridges.

aura, *n* the brief period of heightened sensory activity that immediately precedes the onset of a seizure. It may be characterized by numbness, nausea, or unusual sensitivity to light, odor, or sound.

aural, *adj* relating to the ear.

auranofin, *n* *trade name:* Ridaura; *drug class:* gold salt; *action:* specific antiinflammatory action unknown; *uses:* rheumatoid arthritis.

Aureomycin (ô'rē-ōmī'sin), *n* the trade name for chlortetracycline.

auricle (ô'rikəl), *n* **1.** pinna, the external part of the ear. *n* **2.** atrium, the chamber of the heart that receives the blood: on the right, from the general circulation, and on the left, from the pulmonary circulation.

auricular fibrillation, *n* See fibrillation, auricular.

auricular tags, *n* rudimentary appendages of auricular tissue on the face along the line of union of the first branchial arch.

Auricular tags. (Zitelli/Davis, 2002)

auriculotemporal syndrome, *n* See syndrome, auriculotemporal.

aurothioglucose/gold sodium thiomalate, *n trade name:* Solganal/ Myochrisine; *drug class:* antiinflammatory gold compound; *action:* unknown; may decrease phagocytosis, lysosomal activity, prostaglandin synthesis; *uses:* rheumatoid arthritis; juvenile arthritis.

auscultation (ôskultā'shən), *n* the examination procedure of listening for sounds produced by the body to detect or judge an abnormal condition.

authorization, *n* a written consent to release protected health information.

autism, *n* a developmental disorder that appears in children before the age of 3 that is characterized by communication, behavioral, and sensory impairments, including the inability to interact with others in a socially acceptable manner. The con-

dition is not directly linked to oral health, but may require a special approach when teaching dental care.

autoantibody, *n* an immunoglobulin that reacts against a normal constituent in a person's body.

autoclave (ô'tōklāv), *n* an apparatus for effecting sterilization by steam under pressure.

autogenous, *adj* self-originated; springing from within.

autogenous bone graft, *n* See graft, autogenous bone.

autograft, *n* See graft, autogenous.

autoimmune (ô'tō-imyōōn'), *adj* the development of an immune response to one's own tissues.

autoimmune disease, n See disease, autoimmune.

automatic condenser, *n* See condenser, mechanical.

automatic mallet, *n* See condenser, mechanical.

automation, *n* the use of a machine designed to follow repeatedly and automatically a predetermined sequence of individual operations. Automation is used extensively in preparing tissue for microscopic examination.

automatism (ôtom'ətiz'əm), *n* a tendency to take extra or superfluous doses of a drug when under its influence.

autonomic, *n* See autonomic nervous system.

autonomic drugs, n agents that act on the autonomic nervous system.

autonomic dysreflexia/hyperreflexia, n an emergent, typically life-threatening, medical condition resulting from a dramatic increase in blood pressure occurring in individuals with traumatic lesions at or above T6. Symptoms may include a throbbing headache, blushing, chills, sweating, stuffy nose, and fidgetiness.

autonomic nervous system, n the part of the nervous system that regulates involuntary vital function, including the activity of the cardiac muscle, the smooth muscle, and the glands. The autonomic nervous system has two parts: the sympathetic nervous system, which accelerates heart rate, constricts blood vessels, and raises blood pressure; and the parasympathetic nervous system, which slows heart rate, increases intestinal peristalsis and gland activity, and relaxes sphincters.

autonomic nervous system, fibers of, in pulp, n.pl nerve fibers of the sympathetic autonomic system which enter the pulp tissue and function in regulating blood flow.

autonomic symptoms, n indications of pathology or trauma including paleness, sweating, blushing, dilation of pupils, irregular cardiac rhythm, and lack of bladder control.

autopolymer (ô'tōpol'imur), *n* a resin to which certain chemicals have been added to initiate and propagate polymerization without addition of heat.

autopolymer resin, n See resin, autopolymer.

autopolymerization (ô'tōpol' imərizā'shən), *n* (cold-curing), the accomplishment of polymerization by chemical means without external application of heat or light.

autoprothrombin I (ô'tōprōthrom'bin), *n* See factor VII.

autoprothrombin II, *n* See factor IX.

autopsy, *n* a postmortem examination performed to confirm or determine the cause of death.

autoradiography (ô'tōrādē-og'rəfē), *n* 1. a photographic recording of radiation from radioactive material, obtained by placing the surface of the radioactive material in close proximity to a photographic emulsion. *n* 2. the use of radioactive substances introduced into tissue followed by the placement of a photographic plate on the surface of the tissue preparation, usually employed in cytology and histology.

autosomal dominant disorders, *n.pl* genetic disorders that are transmitted by a dominant gene within an autosomal chromosome as opposed to a sex chromosome.

autosomal recessive disorders, *n.pl* genetic disorders carried by a recessive gene within an autosomal chromosome as opposed to a sex chromosome.

autotransformer, *n* a transformer with a single winding, having a large number of connections, or taps. Used to deliver a precise voltage to the high-tension primary circuit.

autotransplant, *n* See graft, autogenous.

auxiliary, *adj* supporting or assisting; supplementary; secondary.

auxiliary personnel, n.pl nonprofessional aides who assist the responsible professional in the provision of professional services. Dental hygienists are formally trained and may be licensed or certified by state authorities. Dental assistants, laboratory technicians, and other auxiliaries may be formally trained.

auxiliary wires, n.pl orthodontic wires that support or augment the action of the main or primary arch wire in an orthodontic appliance. The Begg technique and the segmental technique make frequent and regular use of auxiliary wires.

AV, *n* 1. the abbreviation for atrioventricular. *n* 2. the abbreviation for auriculoventricular.

availability, *n* the supply in terms of type, volume, and location of health resources and services relative to the demands of a given individual or community.

average life (mean life), *n* the average of the individual lives of all of the atoms of a particular radioactive substance; 1.443 times radioactive half-life. See also half-life.

avidin, *n* a glycoprotein in nondenatured egg whites (raw) that binds biotin and prevents its absorption, causing biotin depletion.

avitaminosis (āvī'təminō'sis), *n* a disease or condition resulting from a deficiency of one or more vitamins in the diet (for example, scurvy, which results from ascorbic acid deficiency, and beriberi, which results from a thiamine deficiency).

avitaminosis, fat-soluble, n a disease resulting from deficiency of the fat-soluble vitamins (that is, A, D, E, and K).

avoidance behavior, *n* a conscious or unconscious defense mechanism by which a person tries to escape from unpleasant situations or feelings, such as anxiety and pain.

avoirdupois system, *n* See system, avoirdupois.

avulse, *v* to tear off forcibly, as when a tooth is lost in an accident.

avulsed tooth, *n* See tooth, evulsed.

avulsion (əvul'shən), *n* See evulsion.

avulsion, nerve, n See evulsion, nerve.

axial filaments (ak'sē-əl), *n.pl* the means of mobility for the spirochete-type bacteria.

axial inclination, *n* See inclination, axial.

axial plane, *n* See plane, axial.

axial wall plane, *n* See plane, axial wall.

axilla, *n* a pyramid-shaped space forming the underside of the shoulder between the upper part of the arm and the side of the chest.

axiopulpal (ak'sē-ōpul'pəl), *adj* relating to the angle formed by the axial and pulpal walls of a prepared cavity.

axis (ak'sis), *n* **1.** a straight line around which a body may rotate. *n* **2.** the second cervical vertebra.

axis, cephalometric, n See axis, Y.

axis, condylar, n an imaginary line through the two mandibular condyles around which the mandible may rotate during a part of the opening movement.

> *axis, condylar, determination, n* the location of the condylar axis by fixing a face-bow rigidly to the lower teeth, having the patient open and close the jaws, and recording the most posteriosuperior points of pure rotation with tattoo ink on the outer skin. See also face-bow and hinge-bow.

axis, condyle, n one of three axes of the jaw condyles: (1) the hinge axis, an intercondyle imaginary line across the face through both condyles; whenever either condyle is chosen to be a rotator, it will display (2) a vertical axis, and (3) a sagittal axis. The hinge axis is a moving center for the opening and closing movements. The vertical axis is the center for the horizontal components of orbital movements. The sagittal axis is the center for the vertical components of orbital movements.

axis, hinge, -orbital plane, n a craniofacial plane determined by three tattooed points. Two are located with one on each side of the face at the point of exit through the skin in front of the tragus of the imagined extended rearmost mandibular hinge axis. The third point is located on the right side of the nose at the level of the orbital rim just beneath the pupil when the patient is gazing directly forward. This plane corresponds to the anthropologic Frankfort plane.

axis, horizontal, n See axis, hinge.

axis, long, n an imaginary line passing longitudinally through the center of a body.

axis, mandibular, n See axis, condylar.

axis of preparation, n the path taken by a restoration as it slides on or off the preparation.

axis, opening, n See axis, condylar.

axis, orbital movements of, n.pl movements projected on the axis-orbital plane in gathering the input data for an articulator.

axis, sagittal, n the imaginary line around which the working condyle rotates in the frontal plane during lateral mandibular movement. The sagittal and vertical axes function concurrently.

axis shift, n the imprecise term used before the nine different directionalized laterotrusions were discovered and named.

axis, vertical, n the imaginary line around which the working condyle rotates in the horizontal plane during lateral mandibular movement. The sagittal and vertical axes function concurrently.

axis, Y, n (cephalometric axis), the angle of a line connecting the sella turcica and the gnathion and related to a horizontal plane. An indicator of downward and forward growth of the mandible.

axon (ak'son), *n* an extension of a nerve cell body that conducts impulses away from the cell. Generally there is only one axon to a cell, and it may extend up to 3 feet (0.9 m) in length.

azatadine maleate, *n trade name:* Optimine; *drug class:* antihistamine; *action:* decreases allergic response by blocking histamine; *uses:* allergy symptoms, rhinitis, chronic urticaria, pruritus.

azathioprine, *n trade name:* Imuran; *drug class:* immunosuppressant; *action:* inhibits purine synthesis in cells, thereby preventing RNA and DNA synthesis; *uses:* renal transplants to prevent graft rejection, refractory rheumatoid arthritis, bone marrow transplants, glomerulonephritis.

azdiothymidine (AZT), *n* a drug used to lengthen or extend the median incubation period of the human immunodeficiency virus. *Brand name:* Retrovir.

azelaic acid, *n trade name:* Azelex; *drug class:* a naturally occurring straight-chain dicarboxylic acid; *action:* has antimicrobial activity against *Propionibacterium acnes* and *Staphylococcus epidermidis;* *use:* topical therapy of mild-to-moderate inflammatory acne vulgaris.

azithromycin, *n trade name:* Zithromax; *drug class:* macrolide antibiotic; *action:* binds to 50S ribosomal subunits of susceptible bacteria and suppresses protein synthesis; similar spectrum of activity to erythromycin; *uses:* mild-to-moderate infections of the upper respiratory tract, lower respiratory tract, uncomplicated skin and skin structure infections.

AZT, *n* the abbreviation for azidothymidine. See also azidothymidine.

B point, *n* See *point, B.*
Babesia microti, *n.pl* parasitic protozoan microbes from the Apicomplexa phylum, spread primarily by ticks. They are implicated in babesiosis, a disease with malaria-like manifestations.
babesiosis (bə-bē'zē-o'sis), *n* a disease caused by *Babesia microti* which is evidenced by malaria-like symptoms. Also called *babesiasis* or *piroplasmosis.*

Baby bottle tooth decay. (Zitelli/Davis, 2002)

baby bottle tooth decay, *n* a dental condition that occurs in children from 1 to 3 years of age as a result of being given a bottle at bedtime, resulting in prolonged exposure of the teeth to milk, formula, or juice with a high sugar content. Dental caries results from the breakdown of sugars to lactic acid and other decay-causing substances.

bacampicillin HCl, *n trade names:* Penglobe, Spectrobid; *drug class:* aminopenicillin; *action:* interferes with cell-wall replication of susceptible organisms; *uses:* respiratory tract, skin, and urinary tract infections; effective for gram-positive cocci.

bacillary dysentery (bas'i-ler'ē), *n* a gastrointestinal tract infection contracted from food or water contaminated by infected individuals. Also called *shigellosis.* See also *Shigella.*

Bacillus, *n* a genus of gram-positive, spore-producing bacteria in the family Bacillaceae, order Eubacteriales, including three that are pathogenic (the rest are saprophytic soil forms). Many microorganisms formerly classified as *Bacillus* are now classified in other genera.

Bacillus anthracis, *n* a species of gram-positive facultative anaerobes that causes anthrax. The spores of this organism, if inhaled, can cause a pulmonary form of anthrax; the spores can live for many years in animal products such as hides and wool, as well as in the soil.

Bacillus stearothermophilus (stē-er'ōthurmof'əlus), *n* a type of biologic spore, the absence of which is tested for to verify proper sterilization of equipment in the dental environment; used with steam autoclave sterilizing or chemical vapor sterilizer methods.

Bacillus subtilis, *n* a *Bacillus* species found in grass and hay. Some strains produce the antibiotic bacillomyxin.

bacitracin (bas'i-trā'sin), *n* an antibiotic produced by a gram-positive, spore-forming organism of the *Bacillus licheniformis* group; usually administered topically.

bacitracin, topical, *n trade names:* Baciguent, Bacitin; *drug class:* local antiinfective; *action:* interferes with bacterial cell-wall function by inhibiting protein synthesis; *uses:* topical

B

for nonserious infections caused by staphylococci and streptococci.

back, *n* the posterior or dorsal portion of the trunk of the body between the neck and the pelvis. The skeletal portion of the back includes the thoracic and lumbar vertebrae and both scapulae. The nerves that innervate the muscles of the back include some branches of the dorsal primary divisions of the spinal nerves, the lateral branches of the dorsal primary division of the middle and lower cervical nerves, and some branches of the ventral primary division of the spinal nerves.

back pain, *n* a pain in the lumbar, lumbosacral, or cervical regions of the back, varying in sharpness and intensity. Causes may include muscle strain or pressure on the root of a nerve.

back-action clasp, *n* See *clasp, back-action.*

backing, *n* a metal support used to attach a facing to a prosthesis.

baclofen, *n trade name:* Lioresal; *drug class:* central-acting skeletal muscle relaxant; *action:* inhibits both monosynaptic and polysynaptic reflexes in the spinal cord; *uses:* treatment for skeletal muscle spasticity in multiple sclerosis and spinal cord injury.

bacteremia (bak´tirē´mē-ə), *n* **1.** presence of bacteria in the bloodstream. It may be transient, intermittent, or continuous. Transient bacteremia may result from dental procedures such as root planing or tonsillectomy, or it may accompany the early phases of many infections. Continuous bacteremia is a feature of endocarditis. *n* **2.** presence of bacteria in the blood (for example, as occurs during root planing of the tooth of a patient with rheumatism who has not been prophylactically premedicated with antibiotics).

bacteria, *n.pl* **1.** small, unicellular microorganisms of the kingdom Monera. The genera vary morphologically, being spheric (cocci), rod-shaped (bacilli), spiral (spirochetes), or comma-shaped (vibrios). *n* **2.** The phylum in which these microorganisms are classified.

bacteria, aerobic, *n.pl* bacteria that require the presence of oxygen to live and grow.

bacteria, anaerobic, *n.pl* bacteria that can survive and grow without the presence of free oxygen in their immediate environment.

bacteria, resident (oral), *n.pl* the microorganisms constant in the oral flora of an individual.

bacterial culture, *n* See *culture, bacterial.*

bacterial spore, *n* a bacteria that, because of its thick outer wall, is easily able to survive in hostile environments otherwise not conducive to bacterial growth and reproduction.

bacterial toxin, *n* any poisonous substance produced by a bacterium. Two general types of toxins are common: those formed within the cell (endotoxins) and those formed within the cell and excreted (exotoxins).

bactericide (bak-tir´i-sīd), *n* a substance that kills bacteria. See also bacteriophage.

bacteriology, *n* the scientific study of bacteria.

bacteriolytic action (bak-tir´ē-ō-lit´ik), *n* the breaking down of bacteria by an enzyme or other agent (for example, by antibacterial factors in saliva).

bacteriophage, *n* any virus that causes lysis of host bacteria.

bacteriostatic (bak-tir´e-ō-stat´ik), *adj* preventing bacteria from growing and multiplying.

Bacteroides **(bak´tər-oi´dēz),** *n* a genus of *Schizomycetes* made up of rod-shaped, highly pleomorphic, gram-negative, nonspore–forming obligate anaerobic bacteria sometimes associated with periodontitis.

B. endodontalis, *n* a strain of *B. melaninogenicus* associated with papal infections.

B. forsythus, *n* a recently identified anaerobic gram-negative species of *Bacteroides* found in periodontal pockets.

B. fragilis, *n* the most common and virulent strain of a genus of obligate anaerobic bacilli normally found in the mouth, upper respiratory system, colon, and genital tract.

B. gingivalis, *n* a strain of *B. melaninogenicus* associated with acute periodontitis.

B. intermedius, *n* a strain of *B. melaninogenicus* associated with acute necrotizing ulcerative gingivitis.

B. melaninogenicus, *n* a small, gram-negative diplobacillus, also known as *Bacterium melaninogeni-*

cum, found in the mouth and pharynx; an anerobic organism sometimes associated with periodontitis.

bad-faith insurance practices, *n.pl* **1.** the failure to deal with a beneficiary of a dental benefits plan fairly and in good faith. *n.pl* **2.** an activity that impairs the right of the beneficiary to receive the appropriate benefits of a dental benefits plan or receive them in a timely manner. Some examples of bad-faith insurance practices include evaluating claims based on standards significantly at variance with the standards of the community, failure to investigate a claim for benefits properly, and unreasonably and purposely delaying or withholding payment of a claim.

badge, film, *n* See *film badge.*

bailment, *n* the delivery of personal property by one person to another in trust for a specific purpose with an expressed or implied contract that after the purpose has been fulfilled the property shall be returned, duly accounted for, or kept until reclaimed.

balance, *n* **1.** equilibrium or harmony. *n* **2.** occlusal equilibrium or facial esthetic harmony.

balance, acid-base, n in metabolism, the balance of acid to base necessary to keep the blood pH level normal (between 7.35 and 7.43).

balance billing, n billing a patient for the difference between the dentist's actual charge and the amount reimbursed under the patient's dental benefits plan.

balance sheet, n a condensed statement showing the nature and amount of a company's assets, liabilities, and capital on a given date. In dollar amounts the balance sheet shows the assets the company owns, the money it owes, and the ownership interest in the company of its stockholders.

balanced articulation, *n* See *occlusion, balanced.*

balanced bite, See *occlusion, balanced.*

balanced occlusion, *n* See *occlusion, balanced.*

balancing contacts, *n.pl* the contacts of teeth on the side opposite the bolus side. See also *contact, balancing.*

balancing occlusal surfaces, See *surfaces, occlusal, balancing.*

balancing side, *n* the side opposite

the working side of the dentition or denture.

balloon payment, *n* a final payment larger than the preceding payments when a debt is not fully amortized.

balloon, sinus, *n* a hollow rubber structure expandable with liquid or air that is used to support depressed fractures of the walls of the maxillary sinus.

balsam (bôl′səm), *n* any of many viscous, sticky, aromatic fluids derived from plants; consists of resins plus oils.

BANA, *n.pr* an acronym for benzolarginine naphthylamide. See also *benzol-arginine naphthylamide.*

band, *n* **1.** a cord, tie, chain, or metal collar by which something is bound. *n* **2.** a contrasting strip or strip of material running through or along the edge of a material.

band adapter, n See *adapter, band.*

band, adjustable orthodontic, n a band provided with an adjusting screw to permit alteration in size.

band, apron, n See *apron band.*

band, orthodontic, n a thin metal ring, usually stainless steel, that secures orthodontic attachments to a tooth. The band, with orthodontic attachments welded or soldered to it, is closely adapted to fit the contours of the tooth and then is cemented into place.

band, pusher, n an instrument used to adapt the metal band to the tooth.

band remover, n an instrument used to remove bands from the teeth.

band, rubber, n See *elastic.*

band, slip, n a band formed when a metal is placed under a load and one grain tends to slip or slide on another.

band, striated, n See *striations, muscle.*

bandage, *n* a strip of material wrapped about or applied to any body part.

bandage, Barton's, n.pr a figure-eight bandage passing below the mandible and around the cranial bone to give upward support to the mandible.

bandage, thyroid, n a large bandage consisting principally of a towel applied around the neck that exerts moderate pressure to the anterolateral part of the neck.

bank plan, *n* a financial arrangement made between the dentist, patient, and bank for financing dental accounts; the bank provides the capital for a rate of interest that enables the patient to pay the dental account over a longer period than would otherwise be possible—usually 12 to 18 months.

bankruptcy, *n* the legal process by which a person, business, or corporation is declared to be insolvent and unable to pay creditors.

bar, *n* a metal segment of greater length than width. See also *bar, connector.*

bar, anterior palatal, *n* See *connector, major, anterior palatal.*

bar, arch, *n* any one of several types of wires, bars, and splints conforming to the arch of the teeth and used for the treatment of fractures of the jaws and the stabilization of injured teeth (for example, *Erich, Jelenko, Niro,* or *Winter*).

bar, buccal, *n* an orthodontic appliance auxiliary consisting of a rigid metal wire extending from the buccal side of the molar band anteriorly.

bar clasp, *n* See *clasp, bar.*

bar, connector, *n* a connector of greater thickness and reduced width as compared with a platelike connector, which has greater width and is thinner.

bar, fixable-removable cross arch, *n* See *connector, cross arch bar splint.*

bar, Gilson fixable-removable, *n.pr* See *connector, cross arch bar splint.*

bar, Kennedy, *n* See *connector, minor, secondary lingual bar.*

bar, labial, *n* a major connector located labial (or buccal) to the dental arch that joins bilateral parts of a mandibular removable partial denture.

bar, lingual, *n* a major connector located lingual to the dental arch that joins bilateral parts of a mandibular removable partial denture. See also *connector, major, lingual bar.*

bar, palatal, *n* a major connector that crosses the palate and unites bilateral parts of a maxillary removable partial denture. See also *connector, major.*

bar, posterior palatal, *n* See *connector, major, posterior palatal.*

bar, secondary lingual, *n* See *connector, minor, secondary lingual bar.*

barb-, *comb* combining form used to indicate derivatives of barbituric acid.

barbiturate (bär-bich′ŏŏr-āt), *n* a derivative of barbituric acid that acts as a sedative or hypnotic. Barbiturates are controlled substances that have addictive potentials.

barbiturates, ultrashort-acting, *n.pl* drugs administered to bring on rapid anesthesia; examples include thiopental sodium (Pentathol) and methehexital sodium (Brevital); rapid onset is countered by a abbreviated period of duration.

barium (Ba) (ber′ē-əm), *n* a pale yellow, metallic element classified with the alkaline earths.

barium sulfate, *n* a white, finely ground, tasteless powder that is insoluble in water, solvents, and solutions of acids and alkalis; used in radiography as a contrast medium because of its opacity to roentgen rays and as a protective barrier in plaster walls.

barodontalgia (barē-ō-don-tal′jē-ə), *n* sudden, sharp tooth pain that may occur in response to a decrease in atmospheric pressure such as that experienced during flight at high altitudes. Also called *aerodontalgia.*

barosinusitis, *n* the painful symptoms related to the maxillary sinus resulting from a change in barometric pressure.

barrier, protective, *n* material of a composition that greatly absorbs radiation (for example, lead or concrete).

barrier techniques, *n.pl* protocols used in infection control to prevent cross-contamination between healthcare worker and patient, between patient and healthcare worker, and between patients. Strict barrier techniques are recommended by the Centers for Disease Control and Prevention (CDC) and the American Dental Association (ADA) to prevent the transmission of hepatitis B virus and human immunodeficiency virus types 1 and 2. However, any number of bacterial, viral, and fungal microorganisms can be transferred through improper or inadequate infection control procedures.

basal, *adj* **1.** describing the minimal functions necessary for life. *adj* **2.** located at or forming the base of a structure. *n* **3.** the fundamental structures from which an organism is derived.

basal bone, *n* See *bone, basal.*

Basal layer of the epidermis. (Moore/Persaud, 2003)

basal layer, *n* innermost layer of the epidermis made up of cuboidal-shaped cells that proliferate by mitosis to produce new cells.

basal metabolic rate (BMR) (bā′səl met′ə-bol′ik), *n* the basal rate, or energy exchange, determined by means of a clinical test of oxygen consumption in a subject who has had a good night's rest, has fasted for 12 to 14 hours, and has been physically, mentally, and emotionally at rest for 30 minutes; usually indicated as a percentage of the normal calorie production per surface area, the normal values ranging between plus and minus 20%.

basal metabolism, *n* See *basal metabolic rate.*

basal seat, *n* the oral tissues and structures that support a denture.

basal seat area, *n* See *area, basal seat.*

basal seat outline, *n* an outline on the mucous membrane or on a cast of the entire area that is to be covered by a denture.

basal surface, *n* See *surface, basal.*

base, *n* **1.** the foundation or support on which something rests; the point of attachment of a part; the principal ingredient of a material. *n* **2.** a compound that yields hydroxyl ions in water solution and causes neutralization of acid to form a salt and water.

base, acrylic resin, *n* a denture base made of an acrylic resin.

base, apical (basal arch), *n* the portion of the jawbone that gives support to the teeth.

base, cement, *n* a layer of insulated, sometimes medicated dental cement placed in the deep portions of a cavity preparation to protect the pulp, reduce the bulk of the metallic restoration, or eliminate undercuts in a tapered preparation.

base, denture, *n* **1.** the part of a denture that fits the oral mucosa of the basal seat, restores the normal contours of the soft tissues of the dentulous mouth, and supports the artificial teeth. *n* **2.** the portion of a denture that overlies the soft tissue, usually fabricated of resin or combinations of resins and metal.

base, extension (free-end), *n* a unit of a removable prosthesis that extends anteriorly or posteriorly, terminating without end support by a natural tooth.

base, film, *n* a thin, flexible, transparent sheet of cellulose acetate or similar material.

base, mandibular, *n* the body of the mandible, on which the teeth and alveolar tissues are situated.

base, material, *n* any substance from which a denture base may be made (for example, acrylic resin, vulcanite, polystyrene resin, and metal).

base, metal, *n* the basal surface of a denture constructed of metal (for example, aluminum, gold, and cobalt-chromium) to which the teeth are attached.

base, plastic, *n* a denture base, baseplate, or record base made of a plastic material.

base, record, *n* See *baseplate.*

base, shellac, *n* resinous material adapted to maxillary or mandibular casts to form baseplates.

base, sprue, *n* See *crucible former.*

base, temporary, *n* See *baseplate.*

base, tinted denture, *n* a denture base that simulates the coloring and shading of natural oral tissues.

base, trial, *n* See *baseplate.*

Basedow's disease (baz′ə-dōz), *n.pr* See goiter, exophthalmic.

baseplate, *n* a temporary form representing the base of a denture and used for making maxillomandibular (jaw) relation records, arranging artificial teeth, or facilitating trial placement in the mouth.

baseplate, stabilized, *n* a baseplate lined with plastic or other material to improve its adaptation and stability.

baseplate wax, *n* See *wax, baseplate.*

basic life support (BLS), *n* fundamental emergency treatment consisting of cardiopulmonary resuscitation (CPR) or emergency cardiac care (ECC) that is provided until more precise medical treatment can begin.

basic metabolic rate, *n* See *basal metabolic rate.*

basic services, *n.pl* frequently insurance companies split dental procedures into basic and major categories. Basic services usually consist of diagnostic, preventive, and routine restorative dental services. The plan may provide different deductibles, coinsurance, and maximums for basic versus major services as incentives to good dental care.

basion (bā′sē-on), *n* the midline point at the anterior margin of the occipital foramen.

basis, *n* the principal active ingredient in a prescription.

basophil (bā′sə-fil), *n* See *leukocyte.*

basophilia (bā′sō-fil′ē-ə), *n* an aggregate of blue-staining granules found in erythrocytes; seen in lead poisoning, leukemia, malaria, severe anemias, and certain toxemias.

basophilic line (bā′sō-fil′ik), *n* See *line, basophilic.*

batch processing, *n* data processing in which a number of similar input data items are grouped together and processed during a single machine run with the same program.

Battle's sign, *n* See *sign, Battle's.*

bayonet, *n* a binangled instrument, the nib or blade of which is generally parallel to the shaft; resembles a bayonet. See also *angle former, bayonet* and *condenser, bayonet.*

beading, *n* the scribing of a shallow groove (less than 0.5 mm in width or depth) on a cast that outlines the major connector. It is used to transfer the design to the investment cast and ensure tissue contact of the major connector.

beam, *n* a stream or approximately unidirectional emission of electromagnetic radiation or particles.

beam, central, *n* the center of the beam of roentgen rays emitted from the tube.

beam, useful, *n* the part of the primary radiation that passes through the aperture, cone, or other collimator.

beauty, *n* the quality of an attribute that is pleasing to the senses or the mind.

beclomethasone dipropionate, *n* *trade names:* oral—Beclovent, Vanceril; nasal—Vancenase AQ Nasal, Beconase AQ Nasal, *drug class:* corticosteroid, synthetic; *action:* prevents inflammation by depression of migration of polymorphonuclear leukocytes and fibroblasts and reversal of increased capillary permeability; *uses:* chronic asthma and rhinitis.

bedsheet, for body enclosure, *n* a blanket used to stabilize, support, and provide comfort for patients; typically used with children.

beeswax, *n* a wax that melts at low heat, which is an ingredient of many dental waxes.

Begg's appliance, *n.pr* See *appliance, Begg's.*

behavior, *n* the manner in which a person acts or performs; any or all of the activities of a person, including physical action learned and unlearned, deliberate or habitual.

behavior management, *n* techniques used to control or modify an action or performance of a subject. In dentistry, usually associated with the management of oral hygiene behavior, dietary behavior, or patient behavior under stress.

behavior modification, *n* alterations, changes, or transfers from a socially unacceptable and destructive act to a socially acceptable, nondestructive one. In dentistry, usually associated with oral habits such as finger or thumb sucking, mouth breathing, nail biting, and smoking.

behavior therapy, *n* a kind of psychotherapy that attempts to modify observable, maladjusted patterns of behavior by the substitution of a new response or set of responses to a given stimulus.

behavioral medicine, *n* a branch of clinical psychology that deals with behavior modification and may involve assertiveness training, aversion therapy, contingency management, operant conditioning, and systemic desensitization.

behavioral sciences, *n.pl* those sciences devoted to the study of human and animal behavior.

Behçet's syndrome, *n* See *syndrome, Behçet's.*

bell stage, *n* developmental stage of odontogenesis during which the cup-shaped enamel organ is transformed into a bell-shaped structure.

Bell's palsy, sign, palsy test, *n.pr* See *palsy, Bell's; sign, Bell's; and palsy test, Bell's.*

belladonna alkaloids, *n trade name:* Bellafoline; *drug class:* gastrointestinal anticholinergic; *action:* inhibits muscarinic actions of acetylcholine at postganglionic parasympathetic neuron effector sites; *uses:* treatment of peptic ulcer disease and irritable bowel syndrome in combination with other drugs.

Benadryl, *n.pr* trade name for diphenhydramine hydrochloride, an antihistamine with anticholinergic (drying) and sedative side effects.

benazepril, *n trade name:* Lotensin; *drug class:* angiotensin-converting enzyme (ACE) inhibitor; *action:* selectively suppresses renin-angiotensin-aldosterone system; *uses:* treatment of hypertension, alone or in combination with thiazide diuretics.

Bence Jones protein, *n.pr* See *protein, Bence Jones.*

Benedict's test, *n.pr* See *test, Benedict's.*

beneficiary, *n* **1.** a person eligible for benefits under a dental plan. *n* **2.** a person who receives benefits under a dental benefit contract. See also *covered person; insured; member;* and *subscriber.*

benefit booklet, *n* a booklet or pamphlet provided to the subscriber that contains a general explanation of the benefits and related provisions of the dental benefits program. Also known as a *summary plan description.*

benefit plan summary, *n* the description or synopsis of employee benefits required by the Employee Retirement Income Security Act (ERISA) to be distributed to employees.

benefits, *n.pl* **1.** the monies paid and discounts applied for various procedures performed. *n.pl* **2.** the dental services or procedures covered by the insurance policy, also known as the *schedule of benefits.*

benign (bē-nīn′), *adj* describing a neoplasm unable to metastasize.

Bennett angle, movement, *n* See *angle, Bennett* and *movement, Bennett.*

benzathine penicillin G, *n* a benzathine salt of natural penicillin that forms a slowly absorbable injectable antibiotic effective against penicillin-susceptible organisms.

benzene, abuse of, *n* improper, recreational inhaling of the chemical hydrocarbon C_6H_6. Benzene is found in gasoline and adhesives.

benzocaine, *n* a local anesthetic agent derived from aminobenzoic acid, used in many over the counter compounds for pruritus and pain. A minimum of 5% benzocaine is required for a compound to be effective.

benzocaine (topical), *n trade names:* 20% liquid—Anbesol Maximum Strength, Orajel Mouth Aid; 20% gel—Anbesol Maximum Strength, Hurricaine, Orajel Brace-Aid; 10% gel—Denture Orajel, Baby Orajel Nighttime; *drug class:* topical ester local anesthetic; *action:* inhibits conduction of nerve impulses from sensory nerves; *uses:* treatment of oral irritation, toothache, cold sores, canker sores, teething pain, and pain caused by dental prostheses or orthodontic appliances.

benzodiazepine (ben′zō-dī-az′ə-pēn), *n* a drug used to decrease emotional stress, lessen anxiety, and bring about sleep.

benzol-arginine naphthylamide, *n* a bacterial enzyme that mimics the activity of trypsin. It is used as a marker of bacterial growth in dental plaque or as a marker for the diagnosis of periodontal disease involving *Bacteroides gingivalis, B. forsythus,* and *Treponema denticola.*

benzonatate, *n trade name:* Tessalon; *drug class:* antitussive, nonnarcotic; *action:* inhibits cough reflex by anesthetizing stretch receptors in respiratory system; *uses:* nonproductive cough relief.

benzoyl peroxide, *n* **1.** a chemical incorporated into the polymer of res-

B

ins to aid in the initiation of polymerization. *n* **2.** an antibacterial, keratolytic drying agent prescribed in the treatment of acne.

benztropine mesylate, *n* *trade names:* Apo-benzotropin, benztropine mesylate; *drug class:* anticholinergic, antidyskinetic; *action:* blocks central acetylcholine receptors; *use:* treatment of Parkinson's disease symptoms.

bepridil HCl, *n* *trade names:* Vascor, Bepadin; *drug class:* calcium channel blocker; *action:* inhibits calcium ion influx across cell membrane during cardiac depolarization; *uses:* treatment of stable angina, alone or in combination with propranolol or nitrates.

beriberi (asjike, athiaminosis, endemic multiple neuritis, endemic polyneuritis, hinchazon, inchacao, kakke, loempe, panneuritis endemica, perneiras), *n* a nutritional disease resulting from a deficiency of thiamine. Classically it is characterized by multiple neuritis, muscular atrophy, weakness, cardiovascular changes, and progressive edema.

beryllium (Be), *n* a steel-gray, lightweight metallic element with an atomic number of 4 and an atomic weight of 9.01218. Alloys of beryllium are used in fluorescent powders. Inhalation of beryllium fumes or particles may cause the formation of granulomas in the lungs, skin, and subcutaneous tissues.

beta-blocker, non-specific, *n* any drug that targets either of the two β-receptors, $β_1$ or $β_2$, of the effector organs, which in turn blocks the sympathetic autonomic nervous system action.

beta-blocker, specific, *n* a drug that specifically blocks either $β_1$ or $β_2$ receptors of the effector organs, which in turn block the sympathetic autonomic nervous system action.

betamethasone (valerate, betamethasone benzoate, betamethasone dipropionate), *n* *trade names:* Uticort, Beben, and others; *drug class:* topical corticosteroid; *action:* interacts with steroid cytoplasmic receptors to induce antiinflammatory effects; possesses antipruritic, antiinflammatory actions; *uses:* treat-

ment of psoriasis, eczema, contact dermatitis, pruritus, and oral ulcerative inflammatory lesions.

betatron (bā′tə-tron), *n* a machine that produces high-speed electrons through magnetic induction.

betaxolol HCl, *n* *trade name:* Kerlone; *drug class:* antihypertensive, selective $β_1$-blocker; *action:* produces fall in blood pressure without reflex tachycardia or significant reduction in heart rate; *uses:* treatment of hypertension.

bethanechol chloride, *n* *trade names:* Duvoid, Urecholine, Urebeth; *drug class:* cholinergic stimulant; *action:* stimulates muscarinic acetylcholine receptors directly; stimulates gastric motility; *uses:* treatment of postoperative or postpartum urinary retention and neurogenic atony of bladder with retention.

bevel, *n* the inclination that one surface makes with another when not at right angles; in cavity preparation, a cut that produces an angle of more than 90 degrees with a cavity wall.

bevel, cavosurface, *n* the incline or slant of the cavosurface angle of a prepared cavity wall in relation to the plane of the enamel wall.

bevel, contra, *n* blade placement toward the base of the periodontal pocket to separate the sulcular from the external epithelium. Also known as a *reverse,* or *internal, bevel.*

bevel, instrument, *n* the sloping keen edge of a cutting instrument.

bevel, reverse, *n* See *bevel, contra.*

BHN, *n.pr* See *number, Brinell hardness* and *test, Brinell hardness.*

bias, *n* **I.** a prejudiced or subjective attitude. *n* **2.** in statistics, the systematic distortion of a statistic caused by a particular sampling process.

bibulous (bib′yōō-lus), *adj* pertaining to absorption; a material's ability to absorb fluids.

bibulous pad (saliva absorber), *n* a permeable cotton pad placed inside the cheek during the application of a sealant to staunch the flow of saliva and keep the treatment field dry.

bicarbonate, *n* a salt resulting from the incomplete neutralization of carbonic acid such as from passing excess carbon dioxide into a base solution.

Bicillin, *n.pr* trade name for penicillin G benzathine.

bicuspid (bī-kus'pid), *n* See *premolar.*

b.i.d., *adv* the abbreviation for *bis in die,* a Latin phrase meaning "twice a day."

bidigital palpation (bī-dij'i-təl), *n* a tactile method of oral examination in which the examiner uses the thumb and forefinger of one hand to rule out abnormalities.

Biermer's anemia (bir'murz), *n.pr* See *anemia, pernicious.*

bifid (bī'fid), *adj* divided in two.
bifid tongue, *n* See *tongue, bifid.*
bifid uvula, *n* See *uvula, bifid.*

Bifidobacterium, *n* a genus of anaerobic bacteria containing gram-positive rods of highly variable appearance. Pathogenicity for human beings or for animals has not been reported although these bacteria have been isolated from the feces of infants and older people.

bifurcation (bī'fur-kā'shən), *n* the division into two parts or branches such as any two roots of a tooth.

biguanides (bīg-wan'īdz), *n.pl* orally administered agents used in the treatment of type 2 diabetes, which prevents the liver from breaking down glycogen into glucose and increases the sensitivity body tissues have to insulin. See *metformin HCl.*

bilateral (bī-lat'ər-əl), *adj* pertaining to both sides.

bilharziasis (bil'här-zī'-ə-sis), *n* See *schistosomiasis.*

biliary atresia, *n* a congenital absence or underdevelopment of one or more of the biliary structures, causing jaundice and early liver damage.

bilirubinemia (bil'i-rōōbi-nē'mē-ə), *n* the presence of bilirubin in the blood. It may result from obstruction inside or outside the liver or from increased hemolysis. The total serum bilirubin in an adult is 0.2 to 0.7 mg/100 mL.

bilirubinuria (bil'i-rōō-bi-nyōō'rē-ə), *n* the presence of bilirubin in the urine. More often, an excess of bilirubin in the urine resulting from excessive hemolysis.

billing, *n* the procedure of preparing a financial statement.

bimanual palpation, *n* a tactile method of oral examination in which the examiner uses both hands to examine the patient's mouth from both the inside and outside at the same time.

bimaxillary (bī-mak'si-ler-ē), *adj* pertaining to the right and left maxillae; sometimes incorrectly used to refer to the maxillae and mandible.
bimaxillary protrusion, *n* See *protrusion, bimaxillary.*

bimeter (bī-mē'tur), *n* a gnathodynamometer with a central bearing point adjustable to varying heights. See also *gnathodynamometer.*

Bimler's appliance, *n.pr* See *appliance, Bimler's.*

binangle (bin'ang-gəl), *n* an instrument having two offsetting angles in its shank. The angles keep the cutting edge or the face of the nib within 3 mm of the axis of the shaft.

binder, *n* a substance, usually sticky, that holds the solid particles in a mixture together, thus aiding in the preservation of the physical form of the mixture.

binding, *n* a reversible combination of various drugs with body constituents such as plasma proteins.

binding site, *n* the location on the surface of a cell or molecule where other cell fragments or molecules attach to initiate a chemical or physiologic action.

binge-eating and purging, *n* one type of anorexia nervosa in which an individual consumes a large amount of food and then forces vomiting or uses enemas, laxatives, or diuretics to avoid additional weight gain.

binocular loupe, *n* See *loupe, binocular.*

bioburden, *n* the number of bacteria living on a surface before it is sterilized.

biochemistry, *n* the chemistry of living organisms and life processes.

biocidal (bī'-ō-sī'dəl), *adj* capable of destroying microorganisms.

biocompatible material, *n* a substance that does not threaten, impede, or adversely affect living tissue.

biodegradability, *n* the natural ability of a chemical substance to be broken down into less complex compounds with fewer carbon atoms by bacteria or other microorganisms.

bioelectrical impedance (bī-ō-e-lek'trik-əl im-pē'dəns), *n* a method of measuring total body fat that uses electrical current and is based on the premise that lean body mass is a better conductor of electricity than fat. See also *body mass index calculation.*

bioethics, *n* the study of social and moral issues raised in the field of biology, including medicine and dentistry.

biofeedback, *n* the instrumented process or technique of learning voluntary control over automatically regulated body functions; useful in the treatment of bruxism, temporomandibular joint dysfunction, and pain, and in facilitating anxiety control in the dental setting.

biofeedback,   electromyographic (EMG), *n* an instrumented process that helps patients learn control over muscle tension levels previously under automatic control; especially useful in treatment of dental disorders such as bruxism, temporomandibular joint dysfunction, tension headaches, and other disorders involving the muscles of mastication. In addition to neuromuscular education, electromyographic biofeedback is useful in treating dental phobias and anxiety and facilitating pain control by helping patients learn deep-muscle relaxation techniques.

biofeedback, temperature, *n* an instrumented learning process whereby a patient learns to control temperature of body parts. Training in self-controlled vasodilation (handwarming) technique has been found useful in treating migraine headaches and anxiety in dental patients.

biofilm, *n* a very thin layer of microscopic organisms that covers the surface of an object.

biofilm, plaque, *n* See *film on teeth.*

biofilm,   waterline, *n* microbial growth that adheres to the waterlines used in dental procedures. Poses a serious risk for immunocompromised individuals.

bioflavonoids, *n.pl* naturally occurring flavone or coumarin derivatives having the activity of so-called vitamin P. Their use in controlling gingival bleeding remains controversial.

bioglass, *n* a fused silica-containing aluminum oxide that presents a surface-reactive glass film compatible with connective and epithelial tissues. Bioglass is used as a surface coating in blade and endosteal implants.

biologic, *adj* pertaining to biology.

biologic factors, *n* the variables that influence life and living tissues.

biologic (permucosal) seal, *n* refers to the health-protecting zone between the living soft tissue and the post or implant in patients with full replacement dental work. Works to prevent bacteria and any other health-threatening organisms from breaching healthy tissue.

biologic science, *n* the science that deals with life processes.

biologic value (BV), *n* a number reached by comparing the amount of nitrogen retained with the amount absorbed to aid in determining protein quality.

biologic vector, *n* the live carrier, usually an arthropod, in which an infectious organism matures prior to infecting a receiver.

biological age, *n* age determined by physiology rather than chronology; factors of biological aging include changes in the physical structure of the body as well as changes in the performance of motor skills and sensory awareness.

biology, *n* the science of life or living matter in all its forms and phenomena.

biomarker, *n* a short-lived radioactive molecule that can be used as a marker to follow a condition or a process.

biomass, *n* the total quantity of living organisms in a particular volume of matter.

biomechanics (bī′-ō-mə-kan′iks), *n* See *biophysics.*

biomedical engineering, *n* a system of techniques in which knowledge of biologic processes is applied to solve practical medical problems and answer questions in biomedical research.

biometrics (bī′-ō-met′riks), *n* the science of the application of statistical methods to biologic facts.

bionator, *n* a removable orthodontic appliance designed to correct functional and skeletal anteroposterior discrepancies between the maxilla and mandible.

biophysics (bī-ō-fiz′iks), *n* the science dealing with the forces that act on living cells of the body, the relationship between the biologic behavior of living structures and the physical influences to which they are subjected, and the physics of vital processes. Also known as *biomechanics.*

biophysics, dental, n the branch of biophysics that deals with the biologic behavior of oral structures as influenced by dental restorations.

biopsy (bī´-op-sē), n the removal of a tissue specimen or other material from the living body for microscopic examination to aid in establishing a diagnosis.

biopsy, aspiration, n the procedure of obtaining a biopsy specimen by aspiration through a needle; used for diagnosing bone or deep soft tissue lesions. Also known as a *needle biopsy.*

biopsy, brush, n a noninvasive procedure used to detect early oral cancer during which a sterile brush is rotated against the suspected lesion to obtain a tissue sample.

biopsy, excisional, n the removal of an entire lesion, usually including a significant margin of contiguous normal tissue, for microscopic examination and diagnosis.

biopsy, exploratory, n exploration combined with biopsy to determine method and degree of local extension, usually of bone or deep soft-tissue lesions.

biopsy, incisional, n the surgical removal of a selected mass of a lesion and adjacent normal tissue for microscopic examination and diagnosis.

biopsy, needle, n See biopsy, aspiration.

biopsy, punch, n biopsy material obtained by use of a punch.

biosynthesis, n the formation of a chemical compound by enzymes.

biotechnology, n **1.** the study of the relationships between humans or other living organisms and machinery. n **2.** the industrial application of the results of biologic research such as recombinant deoxyribonucleic acid (DNA) and gene splicing that permit the production of synthetic hormones or enzymes.

biotin (bī´-ə-tin), n See vitamin, biotin.

biotransformation, n the chemical and physical changes produced in drugs after they enter the body (for example, hydrolysis, conjugation).

biperiden lactate, n trade name: Akineton; *drug class:* anticholinergic; *action:* centrally acting competitive anticholinergic; *use:* treatment of Parkinson's disease symptoms.

bird face, n See brachygnathia; retrognathism.

birth control, n oral contraceptives, usually a mixture of a steroid having progestational activity and an estrogen.

birth, premature, n a birth in which the child is delivered before it has reached the full period of gestation (37 weeks).

birth weight, n the measured heaviness of a baby when born, the average of which is about 3500 g, or 7.5 lb. A baby weighing less than 5 lb is considered premature or underdeveloped.

bis-, pref a prefix meaning that two like or mirror-image moieties are joined together to form a chemical compound.

bisacodyl, n trade names: Dulcolax, Fleet Bisacodyl, Bisacodyl Uniserts, Fleet Laxative; *drug class:* laxative, stimulant; *action:* acts directly on intestine by increasing motor activity; *uses:* short-term treatment of constipation, and bowel or rectal preparation for surgery or examination.

biscuit, n firing bakes, or stages (referred to as *low, medium,* and *high*), during the fusing of dental porcelain preceding the final, or glaze, bake.

bisecting-angle technique, n See angulation, bisecting angle technique.

bisecting-angle technique, central ray direction for, n when taking a periapical survey using this technique, the ray should be directed through the apical third of the targeted teeth. The maxillary apices can be determined by imagining a line from the tragus of the ear to the ala of the nose, which is roughly the level where the apices are located. The manibular apices are located about a half an inch above the bottom of the mandible.

bisecting-angle technique, film placement and position for, n when taking a periapical survey using the bisecting angle technique, the film center should be centered on the teeth being radiographed, except for a maxillary canine film, which is arranged slightly farther from the front and center of the jaw; the film should be kept flat as much as possible.

bisecting-angle technique, patient position for, *n* for taking a periapical survey using the bisecting-angle technique, the patient should be positioned so that their sagittal plane is at a right angle to the floor, and the occlusal plane is parallel to the floor.

bisecting-the-angle error, *n* error in which the vertical angulation is not well controlled, resulting in either very long or short images. See also *distortion, film-fault.*

bisexual, *n* a person who engages in or desires sexual contact with persons of both sexes.

Bismarck brown (Easlick's disclosing agent), *n.pr* one of a variety of dental applications, reveals deposits on the teeth by temporarily coloring them. Characterized by its brown color and licorice flavor.

bismuth (biz´məth), *n* a reddish, crystalline, trivalent metallic element that in combination with other elements forms salts that are used in the production of many pharmaceutical compounds.

bismuth poisoning, *n* See *bismuthosis.*

bismuth subsalicylate, *n* *trade names:* Bisamatrol, Pepto-Bismol; *drug class:* antidiarrheal; *action:* mechanism of action unknown; *uses:* treatment of diarrhea, prevention of diarrhea when traveling.

bismuthia (biz-myōō´thē-ə), *n* the discoloration of mucous membranes and skin from bismuth poisoning.

bismuthism, *n* See *bismuthosis.*

bismuthosis (biz´məth-ō´sis), *n* acute or chronic bismuth intoxication resulting from the ingestion or injection of bismuth salts. Possible manifestations include albuminuria, exfoliative dermatitis, gastrointestinal disturbances, and stomatitis. Also known as *bismuth poisoning,* or *bismuthism.* See also *stomatitis, bismuth.*

bisoprolol fumarate, *n trade name:* Zebeta; *drug class:* antihypertensive,

selective β_1 blocker; *action:* produces fall in blood pressure without reflex tachycardia or significant reduction in heart rate; *uses:* treatment of hypertension as a single agent or in combination.

bisphosphonate (bis-fos´fə-nōt), *n* **1.** an anion, ester, or salt component of diphosphonic acid. *n* **2.** any group of these compounds, currently undergoing experimental investigation for hindrance of bone resorption in animals and the control of periodontal infections in humans. Also called *diphosphonate.*

bisulfite, allergy to, *n* a hypersensitive reaction to certain antioxidant substances, such as the preservatives sodium metabisulfite, acetone sodium bisulfite, and sodium or potassium bisulfite, which are used in local anesthetics containing vasoconstrictors. Persons allergic to bisulfites should avoid all local anesthetics that contain vasoconstrictors.

bite, *n* **1.** the part of an artificial tooth on the lingual side between the shoulder and the incisal edge of the tooth. *n* **2.** an interocclusal record or relationship. See also *denture space; distance, interarch; record, interocclusal;* and *record, maxilloman.*

bite analysis, *n* See *analysis, occlusal.*

bite, balanced, *n* See *occlusion, balanced.*

bite block, *n* **1.** in intraoral radiography, a film holder that the patient bites to provide stable retention of the film packet. *n* **2.** occlusion rim. *n* **3.** a commercially available device, usually made of rubber, which can be used to prop open a patient's mouth during a prolonged treatment session.

Styrofoam-type disposable bite block.
(Bird/Robinson, 2002)

bite, close, n See distance, small interarch.

bite, closed, n **1.** an abnormal overbite. *n* **2.** a decrease in the occlusal vertical dimension produced by factors such as tooth abrasion and loss or failure of eruption of supportive posterior teeth. See also *distance, reduced interarch.*

bite closing, n See *dimension, vertical decrease.*

bite, convenience, n See *occlusion, acquired, eccentric.*

bite, edge-to-edge, n an occlusion in which the incisal edge of the maxillary incisors meets the incisal edge of the mandibular incisors. See also *occlusion, edge-to-edge.*

bite force, n the interocclusal force produced in jaw closure, usually measured in grams or pounds.

bite fork, n See *fork, face-bow.*

bite guard, n See *guard, bite.*

   bite guard splint, n See *splint, acrylic resin bite-guard.*

bite, human, n a puncture or laceration of tissue caused by human teeth. The markings may be distinctive and useful in forensic pathology to determine the person responsible. Human bite wounds may become infected, requiring antibiotic treatment and tetanus toxoid injection.

bite, locked, n See *occlusion, locked.*

bite marks, n.pl distinctive tooth patterns in a wound that may have forensic or legal implications.

bite, normal, n See *occlusion, normal.*

bite, open, n a malformation in which the anterior teeth do not occlude in any mandibular position.

bite opening bends, n.pl bends made in maxillary and mandibular light round wires mesial to the molar tubes in orthodontics.

bite plate, n See *plate, bite.*

bite pressure, n the pressure produced by jaw closure per unit of area, usually measured in grams per square millimeter. See also *pressure, occlusal.*

bite raising, n See *dimension, vertical, increasing occlusal.*

bite record, n See *path, generated occlusal.*

bite rest, n See *position, rest, physiologic.*

bite rim, n See *rim, occlusion.*

bite, working, n See *occlusion, working.*

biteplane (bīt′plān), *n* a removable appliance that covers the occlusal surfaces of the teeth to prevent their articulation.

bite-wing film, *n* See *film, bite-wing.*

bite-wing radiograph, *n* See *radiograph, bite-wing.*

biting, cheek, *n* See *habit.*

biting, lip, *n* See *habit.*

biting, nail, *n* See *habit.*

biting pressure, *n* See *pressure, occlusal.*

biting strength, *n* See *strength, biting.*

bitolterol mesylate, *n trade name:* Tornalate; *drug class:* adrenergic beta-2-agonist; *action:* causes bronchodilation; *uses:* treatment or prophylaxis of asthma, bronchitis, bronchospasm.

blackout, *n* brief impairment of short- and long-term memory occurring during episodes of excessive alcohol consumption or of other substance abuse; consciousness is retained.

blade, *n* See *specific instrument parts.*

blanching, gingival, *n* See *gingival blanching.*

Blandin and Nuhn's gland, *n.pr* See *gland, Blandin and Nuhn's.*

blanket stitch, *n* See *suture, blanket.*

blastomatoid lesion (blas-tō′mə-toid), *n* an overzealous reactive process that because of tumescence has some features of neoplasia. Specific tissue elements, such as fibroblasts, endothelial cells, osteoblasts, osteoclastic giant cells, or nerves, predominate in a specific lesion to form granuloma pyogenicum, giant cell reparative granuloma, traumatic fibroma, tori, or traumatic neuroma.

Blastomyces dermatitidis **(blas-tō-mī′sēz dur′mə-tit′ə-dis),** *n* a species of fungus causing North American blastomycosis.

blastomycosis (blas-tō-mī-kō′sis), *n* an infection resulting from the fungus *Blastomyces dermatitidis* (North American blastomycosis) or *Blastomyces brasiliensis* (South American blastomycosis); characterized by chronic suppurative lesions. The disseminated form is usually fatal.

B

Blastomycosis. (Neville/Damm/Allen/ Bouquot, 2002, Courtesy of Dr. William Welton)

blastomycosis, South American, n a fungous infection that often begins when organisms enter the body through the oral mucosa, producing local ulcers, or through an extraction site, producing papillary lesions. Dissemination leads to granulomatous lesions of the lymph nodes, gastrointestinal tract, liver, and lungs and to microabscesses of the skin. The causative agent is *Blastomyces brasiliensis.*

bleaching, *n* the use of a chemical oxidizing agent (sometimes in combination with heat) to lighten tooth discolorations. See also *agent, bleaching.*

bleeding, *n* the flowing of blood.
bleeding disorders, n.pl hemorrhagic disorders including capillary abnormalities, platelet deficiencies, and blood clotting defects characterized by spontaneous and sometimes uncontrollable bleeding.
bleeding, gingival, n See *gingival bleeding.*
bleeding, occult, n hemorrhage of such small proportions that the blood can be detected only by chemical test, microscope, or spectroscope.
bleeding points, n.pl a series of puncture points made through the gingival tissue; used as a guide for making the gingivectomy incision.
bleeding time, n the time required

for blood to stop flowing from a tiny wound. Normal bleeding time is from 2 to 6 minutes. Bleeding time is increased in disorders of platelet count, uremia, and ingestion of aspirin and other antiinflammatory medications.

blepharophimosis, *n* a decrease in the size of the palpebral opening without a fusion of the eyelid margins.

blepharoptosis, *n* a drooping of the upper eyelid.

blindness, color, *n* defective color vision characterized by decreased ability to detect differences in color. See also achromatopsia.
blindness, color, blue-yellow, n a color disability in which the spectrum is seen in reds and greens; a form of protanopia.
blindness, color, red-green, n the more common form of color disability, in which the entire spectrum is constituted by yellows and blues; a form of protanopia.

blindness, legal, *n* a condition distinguished by having less than 20/200 vision with the use of eyeglasses to correct vision.

blister, *n* a vesicle or bulla, usually a consequence of a burn or friction.

blisterform oral lesions, *n* well-defined, fluid-filled abnormalities in the mouth; may appear as pustules, vesicles, or bullae; characterized by elevation above the level of the surface where they are found, blisterform oral lesions are typically see-through and soft. Color varies according to content of blister, which may include blood, serum, mucin, or pus; ranges in size from less than 1 cm in diameter to larger than 1 cm in diameter.

Bloch-Sulzberger syndrome, *n.pr* See *syndrome, Bloch-Sulzberger.*

block, *n* a mental obstacle that prohibits a patient from having favorable responses to the dentist and suggested treatment plans.
block, data, n a physical unit of data that can be conveniently stored by a computer on an input or output device. The block is normally composed of one or more logical records or a portion of a logical record. Synonymous with *physical record.*
block, field, n the reversible inter-

ruption of nerve conduction over terminal branches by infiltration of a suitable agent into the area.

block, nerve, n See *nerve block.*

blocking, n the process of obstructing or deadening, as a nerve.

blocking agent, n See *agent, blocking.*

blockout, n elimination of undesirable undercut areas on a cast to be used in the fabrication of a removable denture. Also known as *waxout.*

blood, n the fluid circulating through the heart, arteries, capillaries, and veins; carries nutrients and oxygen to body tissues.

blood alcohol concentration (BAC), n the amount of ingested alcohol absorbed into the body's cells and intercellular fluid, measured by a percentage based on milligrams of alcohol per deciliter of blood. The higher the BAC, the greater the physical and mental impairment. Most states have a legal limit of 0.10% (100 mg/dL) or lower for intoxication.

blood, arterial, n oxygen-rich blood taken away from the heart through the arteries and used as nourishment for the tissues of the body.

blood, bad, n the lay term for syphilis.

blood-borne pathogens, n.pl pathogenic microorganisms that are present in human blood and cause disease in humans.

blood-borne pathogens exposure control plan, n a plan that is compliant with Occupational Safety and Health Administration (OSHA) regulations and that explains ways to minimize or eliminate exposure of humans to blood-borne pathogens.

blood-brain barrier, n an anatomic-physiologic feature of the brain thought to consist of walls of capillaries in the central nervous system and surrounding glial membranes. The blood-brain barrier prevents or slows the passage of some drugs, other chemical compounds, radioactive ions, and disease-causing organisms such as viruses from the blood into the nerve tissues of the central nervous system.

blood calcium, n the level of calcium in the blood plasma, generally regulated by parathyroid gland activity in conjunction with the degree of calcium ingestion, absorption, use, and excretion. Normal value is 8.5 to 11.5 mg/100 mL of blood serum.

blood cell count, n an estimation of the number and types of circulating blood cells (for example, red blood cells [erythrocytic series], white blood cells, differential).

blood cells, n.pl any of the formed elements of the blood, including red cells (erythrocytes), white cells (leukocytes), and platelets (thrombocytes).

blood chemistry, n the determination of the chemical constituents of blood by assay in a clinical laboratory as part of a diagnostic protocol.

blood circulation, n the circuit of blood through the body from the heart through the arteries, arterioles, capillaries, venules, and veins and back to the heart.

blood clot, n See *clot, blood.*

blood clotting, n the conversion of blood from a free-flowing liquid to a semisolid gel. Within seconds of injury to a blood vessel wall, platelets clump at the site. If normal amounts of calcium, platelets, and tissue factors are present, prothrombin will be converted to thrombin. Thrombin acts as a catalyst for the conversion of fibrinogen to a mesh of insoluble fibrin in which all the formed elements of blood are immobilized. Also called *blood coagulation.*

blood coagulation disorder, n any disturbance in the normal clotting mechanism of the blood.

blood, color index of, n a figure gained by dividing the hemoglobin percentage by the red blood cell percentage. In most anemias the result is lower than 1, but in pernicious anemia it is characteristically higher than 1.

blood, components of, n.pl a cellular fraction consisting of erythrocytes, leukocytes, and platelets, and a noncellular fraction made up of plasma.

blood component transfusion, n the administration of one or more elements of blood rather than the whole blood. May include red blood cells, platelets, and other elements.

blood disorders, n.pl hematologic dyscrasias that affect the component cells and plasma elements of the blood. Blood disorders are generally divided into two broad groups: those in which an increase in bulk occurs (for example, plethora, hydremia, polycythemia) and those in which a decrease in bulk occurs (for example, anhydremia, dehydration, anemia).

blood dyscrasias, *n* pathologic conditions or disorders such as leukemia or hemophilia in which any of the constituents of the blood are abnormal or are present in abnormal quantity.

blood gas analysis, *n* the study of gas dissolved in the liquid part of the blood. Blood gases include oxygen, carbon dioxide, and nitrogen, all components of inspired air.

blood glucose level, *n* the concentration of sugar (chiefly glucose-"true blood sugar") in the blood. It is usually kept within a narrow range by an interplay of many factors: glycogenolysis, glyconeogenesis, intestinal absorption, insulin, insulin antagonists, and other hormones. In the testing of total reducing substances, the normal range of concentration of fasting blood sugar is 80 to 120 mg/mL; in the testing of true blood sugar, the normal range of concentration is 70 to 100 mg/mL.

blood glucose levels, *n.pl* the amount of the simple sugar glucose in the blood at any given time. An unusually low level results in hypoglycemia, whereas an abnormally high level causes hyperglycemia; an important level to monitor in diabetic patients, because changes in insulin levels can adversely affect glucose levels.

blood groups, *n.pl* the division of blood into types on the basis of the compatibility of the erythrocytes and serum of one individual with the erythrocytes and serum of another individual. The groups are immunologically and genetically distinct.

blood pressure, *n* See *pressure, blood.*

blood pressure classification, *n* the rating system for blood pressure levels in millimeters of mercury (mm Hg), given as the systolic over the diastolic pressure. The diastolic pressure is the indicator of concern for cardiovascular problems. Normal is

less than 130 over 85; high normal is 130 to 139 over 85 to 89 diastolic; and hypertension is diagnosed at levels greater than 140 over 90.

blood pressure cuff, *n* part of a sphygmomanometer that fits over the patient's arm. The cuff comes in four sizes, for children up to obese adults. It should be made of a nonelastic material, and the cuff used should be about 20% bigger than the arm it fits over—an undersized cuff will cause the blood pressure reading to appear higher than it is in reality, whereas an oversized cuff will cause the reading to appear too low.

blood products, *n* constituents of whole blood such as plasma or platelets that are used in replacement therapy.

blood transfusion, *n* the administration of whole blood or a component such as packed red cells to replace blood lost through trauma, surgery, or disease.

blood urea nitrogen (BUN), *n* nitrogen in the form of urea in whole blood or serum. Its concentration is a gross measure of renal function. The upper limit of the normal range is 25 mg/100 mL.

blood, venous, *n* the deoxygenated blood that is returned from tissues throughout the body to the heart, then pumped into the lungs for reoxygenation.

blood vessel(s), *n* any one of the network of muscular tubes that carry blood. The kinds of blood vessels are arteries, arterioles, capillaries, venules, and veins.

blood vessels, periodontal ligament, *n.pl* part of a well-developed vascular system that enters the periodontal ligament and supplies blood to all the regions surrounding the tooth.

blood vessels, pulp, *n.pl* part of a well-developed vascular system that enters the apical foramen of the tooth and supplies blood to the pulp tissue.

blood, volume index of, *n* the volume of red blood cells divided by the total volume of blood times 100 times the volume percent of packed red blood cells (hematocrit index). A value greater than 1 indicates an abnormally large number or size of erythrocytes.

blower, chip, *n* See *syringe, air, hand.*

blowpipe, *n* a torch that employs gas-oxygen, or oxygen and acetylene, to melt metal in dental casting and soldering procedures.

blue, methylene (meth′ə-lēn), *n* **1.** a dye used to color bacteria for microscopic examination. *n* **2.** an aniline dye often used as an antiseptic and topical analgesic in the treatment of lesions of the oral mucous membranes and skin.

blue nevus, *n* See *nevus, blue.*

BMR, *n* See *basal metabolic rate.*

board certification, *n* the examination program that establishes the clinical proficiency of a dental specialist according to the procedures established by the individual specialty certification board under the rules and authority of the Council on Dental Education of the American Dental Association.

board certified, *adj* the status of a dental specialist such as an orthodontist who has become a board diplomate by successfully completing the certification program of the recognized certification board in that area of practice.

board diplomate, *n* a dental specialist who has achieved certification by the recognized certifying board in that specialty, as attested by a diploma from the board.

board eligible, *adj* the status of a dental specialist whose educational qualifications have been verified by acceptance of an application for certification by the recognized certifying board. Board eligibility depends on advanced education in the specialty and timely progress toward completion of the certification procedure. Regular renewal is required to maintain eligibility until the examination is completed.

board qualified, *adj* an unrecognized term used variously and inaccurately to identify any of the stages from educational qualification to certification.

bodily movement, *n* See *movement, body.*

body, *n* any mass or collection of material.

body burden, *n* the activity of a radiopharmaceutical retained by the body at a specified time after administration.

body fluid, *n* any liquid portion of the body such as plasma, lymph, tears, saliva, and urine.

body, foreign, *n* any object or material that is not normal for the area in which it is located.

body height, *n* the overall length of the body from the crown to the bottom of the feet, usually taken in the standing position. Body length refers to the overall length taken in the supine position.

body image, *n* a person's subjective concept of personal physical appearance. The loss of a limb, breast, or tooth may cause psychologic trauma because of unresolved conflict in the change of body image. A distorted body image may be a causal factor in anorexia nervosa and bulimia.

body, ketone, *n* any of the compounds acetoacetic acid, betahydroxybutyric acid, and acetone that are formed in the liver and released in the blood. Elevated levels occur during excessive fat use such as in diabetes or starvation.

body mass index (BMI) calculation, *n* a method for assessing obesity and determining optimal weight, which involves dividing body weight in kilograms by height in square meters.

body mechanics, *n* the field of physiology that investigates actions and functions of the muscular system relating to body posture maintenance.

body, Schaumann's (shou′mänz), *n.pr* a round to oval cytoplasmic inclusion composed of concentric deposits of an amorphous material. Seen in the giant cells of sarcoidosis, in beryllium lesions, and sometimes in other giant cells.

body shields, *n.pl* patients are sometimes legally required to wear protective coverings during x-ray examinations; usually a leaded apron containing lead 0.25 mm thick. The protective surface covers the torso and gonads; the covering should never be folded, or cracks might occur.

B

body temperature, n the level of heat produced and sustained by body processes. Variations and changes in body temperature are major indicators of disease and other abnormalities.

Boeck's disease (bœks), *n.pr* See *sarcoidosis.*

Boeck's sarcoid, *n.pr* See *sarcoidosis.*

Bogarad's syndrome, *n.pr* See *syndrome, auriculotemporal.*

Bohn's nodules, n See *nodules, Bohn's.*

boil (furuncle), n localized swelling; oral boils are usually located on the alveolar process at the apex of a root.

Boil. (Thibodeau/Patton, 2002)

Boley gauge, *n.pr* See *gauge, Boley.*

Bolton analysis, *n.pr* a computation developed by Wayne Bolton for the evaluation of tooth size discrepancies between upper and lower arches.

Bolton-nasion plane, *n.pr* See *plane, Bolton-nasion.*

Bolton plane, *n.pr* See *plane, Bolton-nasion.*

Bolton point, triangle, *n.pr* See *point, Bolton* and *triangle, Bolton.*

bolus (bō′ləs), n a mass of food ready to be swallowed or a mass passing through the intestines.

bond, n the force that holds two or more units of matter together.

bond, peptide, n.pl the linking mechanisms that bind together the amino acid building blocks of proteins.

bond, primary, n a chemical bond that requires some change in structure of matter. Primary bonds are ionic, covalent, or metallic.

bond, secondary, n a physical bond (sometimes called *van der Waals forces*) that involves weak inter-

atomic attractions such as variations in physical mass or location of electrical charge.

bond strength, n the force with which a sealant holds fast to the surface of a tooth.

bonding, n adhesion of orthodontic attachments to the teeth without use of an interposed band.

bonding, direct, n individual placement of attachments on the teeth at the time of adhesion.

bonding, indirect, n the positioning of attachments on a dental cast and transfer of them to the teeth en masse for adhesion by means of a molded matrix bone.

bone, n **1.** the material of the skeletons of most vertebrate animals; the tissue composing bones. n **2.** dense, hard, and slightly elastic connective tissue in which the fibers are impregnated with a form of calcium phosphate similar to hydroxyapatite. Bone tissue makes up the 206 bones of the human skeleton. n **3.** any single element of the skeleton such as a rib or femur.

bone, alveolar, n the specialized bone structure that contains the alveoli or sockets of the teeth and supports the teeth.

bone, alveolar, architecture, n the structural pattern of the alveolar bone and its subjacent latticework of supporting bone. The alveolar bone is thin and compact adjacent to the periodontal membrane. The trabecular bone connects and reinforces the individual alveoli. The architecture of a bone is the result of functional stimuli to that bone; the stimuli vary according to type, intensity, and duration.

bone, alveolar, metabolism, n the metabolic activity occurring within alveolar bone, which is generally slower than that occurring within metaphyseal bone but more rapid than that of diaphyseal bone.

bone apposition, n See *bone deposition.*

bone, basal, n that part of the mandible and maxilla from which the alveolar process develops.

bone, bundle, n the bone forming the immediate bone attachment of the numerous bundles of collagen fibers of the periodontal ligament that have been incorporated into the bone.

bone bur, *n* a drill designed to cut into bone.

bone calcium content, *n* the amount of calcium stored in bone tissue. Plasma calcium is in constant exchange with the calcium of the extracellular fluid and bones. The parathyroid gland maintains the constancy of the calcium concentration in the plasma. The bones serve as a reservoir of calcium and phosphate to provide for the other needs of the body and supply minerals for deposition in the skeleton.

bone, cancellous (spongiosa, spongy bone, supporting bone, trabecular bone), *n* the bone that forms a trabecular network, surrounds marrow spaces that may contain either fatty or hematopoietic tissue, lies subjacent to the cortical bone, and makes up the main portion of a bone.

> **bone, cancellous, atrophy of disuse,** *n* wasting of bone tissue occurring with loss of function of a part (for example, a tooth). The supporting bone assumes an osteoporotic nature, and the marrow remains fatty or hematopoietic.

bone cells, *n.pl* osteoblasts, osteocytes, osteoclasts, and osteoprogenitor cells.

bone changes, mechanical factors, *n.pl* pressure and tension forces that play an important role in determining bone structure. Improperly controlled appliances can resorb bone faster than deposition can occur, causing mobile teeth and traumatic occlusion. Poor vascularity is a concomitant cause of undue pressure and tension and may inhibit repair and cause necrosis.

bone chips, *n.pl* small pieces of cancellous bone generally used to fill in bony defects and precipitate recalcification.

bone, compact, *n* hard, dense bone composing the outer cortical layer and consisting of a variety of periosteal bone, endosteal bone, and haversian systems.

bone conduction, *n* See *conduction, bone.*

bone crest, *n* the most coronal portion of alveolar bone.

bone cyst, *n* **1.** a vascular cyst ec-

centrically placed within a bone. *n* **2.** ostitis fibrosa cystica, a parathyroid disorder characterized by cyst formation and the replacement of bone tissue with fibrous connective tissue.

bone defects, angular, *n.pl* usually localized anomalies that occur in the crestal bone as the result of both periodontal inflammation and occlusive trauma.

bone density, *n* the compactness of bone tissue. The demonstration of bone density by means of radiographs directly depends on the quantity of inorganic salts contained in the bone tissue.

bone deposition, *n* the apposition or formation of new bone as a normal physiologic process.

bone development, *n* B See *bone, endochondral, formation; bone formation;* and *bone, membrane, formation.*

bone, effect of external radiation to, *n* damage to the bones of adults is most often seen after heavy and localized x-ray treatment.

bone, endochondral (en′dō-kon′drəl), *n* a bone that is developed in relation to antecedent cartilages (for example, long bones, mandible). See also *bone, membrane.*

> **bone, endochondral, formation,** *n* primarily a replacement of previously formed embryonic cartilage with an adult bony structure; a more complex bone formation than membrane bone. The actual replacement of cartilage by bone is only part of the process, however; much of the bone is laid down directly external to the embryonic cartilage. See also *bone, membrane, formation.*

bone formation, *n* the deposition of an organic mucopolysaccharide matrix (osteoid) that is subsequently mineralized with calcium salts. See also *bone apposition* and *bone deposition.*

bone graft, autogenous, *n* See *graft, autogenous bone.*

bone graft, donor site, *n* See *donor site.*

bone graft, onlay, *n* See *graft, onlay bone.*

bone graft, recipient site, *n* See recipient site.

bone groove, *n* osteotomy into or

near the crest of the alveolar ridge for placement of an endosteal blade type of implant.

bone groove, canted, *n* an osteotomy sloped to avoid the mandibular canal or keep the implant infrastructure within the medullary confines.

bone, horizontal loss of, *n* a shrinkage of bone caused by periodontal inflammation in which the bone crest remains even with the cementoenamel junctions of two adjoining teeth. The condition may be localized or generalized.

Horizontal bone loss. (Regezi/Sciubba/Pogrel, 2000)

bone, internal reconstruction of, *n* the formation of bone on the tensional side of the periodontal ligament with concurrent resorption from the marrow space; contralaterally, resorption of alveolar bone with apposition from the endosteum in the marrow space.

bone, interproximal, *n* the bone that forms the septa between the teeth; consists primarily of a spongiosa of supporting bone covered by a layer of cortical bone. See also *septum, interdental.*

bone involvement, *n* changes in the alveolar and supporting bone occurring as a sequel to or accompanying inflammatory or dystrophic disease; usually of a resorptive nature.

bone lamella, *n* bone having the appearance of layers of thin leaves or plates. This appearance is produced by lines representing periods of inactivity of bone formation.

bone, malar (zygomatic bone), *n* a quadrangular bone on each side of the face that unites the frontal and superior maxillary bones with the zygomatic process of the temporal bone. It forms the cheek prominence, a portion of the lateral wall and floor

of the orbit, and parts of the temporal fossa and infratemporal fossa.

bone, marble, *n* See *osteopetrosis.*

bone marrow, *n* the soft vascular tissue that fills bone cavities and cancellous bone spaces and consists primarily of fat cells, hematopoietic cells, and osteogenetic reticular cells.

bone marrow transplant, *n* the transplantation of bone marrow from healthy donors to stimulate production of formed blood cells. It is used in treatment of hematopoietic or lymphoreticular diseases such as aplastic anemia, leukemia, immune deficiency syndromes, and acute radiation syndrome.

bone, membrane, *n* a bone developed within a membrane but having no antecedent cartilage (for example, parietal, frontal, bones of upper face). See also *bone, endochondral.*

bone, membrane, formation, *n* membrane bone forms directly from the mesenchyme, first as a thin, flattened, irregular bony plate or membrane in the dermis and gradually expanding at its margins and becoming thickened by the deposition of successive layers of additional bone on the inner and outer surfaces. See also *bone, endochondral, formation.*

bone membranes, *n.pl* membrane structures associated with the growth, development, and repair of bone. They include the periosteum, a connective tissue layer adjacent to bone surfaces; periodontal membrane, a modified periosteum associated with tooth structure; and endosteum, a thin layer of connective tissue lining the walls of the bone marrow spaces.

bone, microscopic appearance of, *n* the composition of bone tissue as viewed under a microscope. Microscopically, bone is composed of osteocytes embedded within lacunae in a calcified intercellular matrix. Extending from the lacunae are minute canals called canaliculi, which communicate with canaliculi of adjacent lacunae. Through this system of canals, nutrient material reaches the osteocytes and provides avenues for the removal of waste products of metabolism. Bone is deposited in incremental layers (lamellae) around haversian canals, the lamellae toward the surface of the bone being more or less parallel to it.

bone mineral content, chemistry of, *n* the hardness of bone results from its mineral content in the organic matrix. The minerals (commonly designated as bone salts) and the organic matrix make up the interstitial substance of bone. The bone salts consist essentially of hydroxyapatite $(Ca_{10}[PO_4]_6[OH_2])$, carbon dioxide, and water, with small amounts of other ions.

bone, normal level of, *n* the distance from the interdental bone crest to the cementoenamel junction in healthy teeth, usually 1 to 1.5 mm.

bone onlay, *n* See *graft, onlay bone.*

bone, perichondrial, *n* bone that is deposited in concentric layers around the long shaft of the bone in a manner similar to that of the growth of endochondral bone.

bone, physical properties of, *n* compact bone has the following physical characteristics: specific gravity, 1.92 to 1.99; tensile strength, 13,000 to 17,000 psi; compressive strength, 18,000 to 24,000 psi; compressive strength parallel to the long axis, 7150 psi; compressive strength at right angles to the long axis, 10,800 psi. These physical characteristics make bone particularly suitable for carrying out its functions of weight bearing, leverage, and protection of vulnerable viscera.

bone rarefaction, *n* a decreased density of bone such as a decrease in weight per unit of volume.

bone recession, *n* See *recession, bone.*

bone, resorption and repair of, *n* an adaptive physiologic mechanism occurring as long as the individual retains the natural dentition. See also *resorption of bone.*

bone, resting lines in, *n.pl* lines created by alternating periods of bone formation and rest, giving a tierlike appearance to lamellar bone.

bone, reversal lines in, *n.pl* irregular lines containing concavities directed away from the bundle bone and serving as histologic indications that resorption has taken place up to that line from the marrow side.

bone sequestrum, *n* See *sequestrum.*

bone, sphenoid, *n* an irregular, wedge-shaped bone located at the base of the skull in front of the temporal bone and the basilar portion of the occipital bone. It is composed of a cuboidal body hollowed out interiorly to form the sphenoidal air sinuses. Extending from the body laterally are two large wings and two small wings. Projecting below the body are two pterygoid processes. The lateral surfaces of the pterygoid processes give origin to the external pterygoid muscles, whereas the medial surfaces give origin to the internal pterygoid muscles.

bone, spongy, *n* See *bone, cancellous.*

bone support, *n* the amount of alveolar and trabecular bone adjacent to a tooth that can provide attachment, investment, and support for the tooth.

bone, supporting, *n* See *bone, cancellous.*

   bone, supporting, atrophy of disuse, *n* See *bone, cancellous, atrophy of disuse.*

bone surgery, *n* See *surgery, osseous.*

bone, thickened margin of, *n* widening of the crest of the alveolus, primarily on the buccal and lingual aspects, varying from a thick ledge to a "beading" of the bone margin; results in a more or less bulbous contour of the gingival tissue overlying it.

bone, trabecular, *n* See *bone, cancellous.*

bone, vertical loss of, *n* a usually localized shrinkage of bone caused by periodontal inflammation and occlusal trauma in which the bone crest is below the cementoenamel junctions of two adjoining teeth.

bone volume (mass), age-affecting, *n* decreases that occur in human body bone mass after age 40. Diet and exercise may be contributing factors.

bone wax, *n* See *wax, bone.*

bone, woven, *n* a character and pattern of bone resulting from the interweaving of broad bands of bone.

bone, zygomatic, *n* See *bone, malar.*

Bonwill-Hawley chart, *n.pr* See *chart, Hawley.*

Bonwill's triangle, *n* See *triangle, Bonwill's.*

B

bony crater, *n* a concave resorptive defect in the alveolar crest, usually occurring interdentally.

bony crepitus, *n* See *crepitus, bony.*

borax, *n* often a principal ingredient in casting fluxes. Used in gypsum products as a retardant for the setting reaction and a strengthener for hydrocolloids.

border, *n* a circumferential margin or edge.

border, denture (denture edge, denture periphery), *n* the limit, boundary, or circumferential margin of a denture base.

border, mandibular (mandibular plane), *n* tangent to the lower border of the mandible. A line joining point gonion to point gnathion.

border molding, *n* the shaping of an impression material by the manipulation or action of the tissues to determine the denture border position.

border movement, *n* See *movement, border.*

border seal, *n* the contact of the denture border with the underlying or adjacent tissues to prevent the passage of air or other substances.

border structures, *n.pl* the oral structures that bound the borders of a denture.

border tissues, movement, *n* the action of the muscles and other structures adjacent to the borders of a denture.

Bordetella pertussis,* *n.pl the infectious bacteria responsible for whooping cough (pertussis), which is spread from person to person by direct contact with mucosal discharges.

boutons terminaux, *n.pl* See *endfeet.*

Bowen's disease, *n.pr* See *carcinoma in situ.*

box, light, *n* See *illuminator.*

boxing, *n* the building up of vertical walls, usually in wax, around an impression to produce the desired size and form of the base of the cast.

boxing strip, *n* See *strip, boxing.*

brace, *n* an orthotic device to support and hold any part of the body in the correct position to allow function, such as a leg brace that permits walking and standing. Sometimes used to describe orthodontic appliances.

brachycephalic (brak′i-səf-al′ik), *adj* descriptive term applied to a broad, round head having a cephalic index of more than 80.

brachydactyly, *n* abnormal shortness of the fingers, usually associated with some congenital syndrome.

brachygnathia (bird-face, micrognathia) (brak′ig-nā′thē-ə), *n* marked underdevelopment of the mandible. *adj* brachygnathous. See also *retrognathism.*

bracing, *n* a resistance to the horizontal components of masticatory force.

bracket, *n* a small metal attachment fixed to a band that serves as a means of fastening the arch wire to the band.

bradycardia (brad′i-kär′dē-ə), *n* abnormal slowness of the heart as evidenced by a slowing of the pulse rate (less than 50 beats per minute).

bradydiastole (brad′i-dī-as′tōle), *n* abnormal prolongation of diastole.

bradykinesia (brad′i-kinē′zh-ə), *n* an irregular slowness in motions and reflexes.

bradykinin, *n* one of a number of plasma kinins, a potent vasodilator; one of the physiologic mediators of an anaphylactic reaction.

bradypnea (brad′ip-nē′-ə), *n* abnormal slowness of breathing.

Respiration patterns. (Kinn/Woods, 1999)

Braille (brāl), *n.pr* a printing and writing system, developed by Louis Braille, using elevated dots to represent letters. The system allows those individuals with limited or no visual ability to read via touch.

brain death, *n* an irreversible form of unconsciousness characterized by a complete loss of brain function while the heart continues to beat.

brain, electrical activity of, *n* electrical energy that can be observed as waves with electroencephalographic equipment. These rhythms and patterns have been organized into a system that imputes values for the state of health and disease. Electrical evidence of brain activity in the cerebral cortex reveals that different potential patterns are produced by different states of mental activity (for example, tension, mental work, sleep).

brainstem, *n* the portion of the brain comprising the medulla oblongata, pons, and mesencephalon. It performs motor, sensory, and reflex functions.

branchial nerve, *n* See *nerve, branchial.*

Branemark technique, *n.pr* See *osseointegration.*

breach of contract, *n* See *contract, breach of.*

break-even point, *n* the level of patient visits or net revenues at which the revenues for a period are equal to the expenses incurred in that period.

breath, *n* air inhaled and exhaled in respiration.

breath, bad (offensive), *n* See *halitosis.*

breathing check, *n* a series of steps, based on the pneumonic ABCD (Airway, Breathing, Circulation, Disability), used to determine the respiratory status of a patient in respiratory distress.

breathing, Kussmaul, *n.pr* a deep, slow breathing that requires great effort, which often occurs during a diabetic coma.

breathing, mouth, *n* the process of inspiration and expiration of air primarily through the oral cavity. It is commonly seen in nasal conditions such as deviated septum, hypertrophied adenoids, and allergies and may produce excessive drying of the oral mucosa with a tendency to gingival hyperplasia.

breathing, rescue, *n* an emergency treatment aimed at restoring natural respiration in a person who has stopped breathing in which the rescuer inflates the victim's lungs by breathing air into his or her mouth or nose directly or through a ventilation device. The technique may be combined with cardiac compressions if the victim has no pulse.

bregma (breg'mə), *n* the point at which the sagittal and coronary sutures meet.

Breuer's reflex, *n.pr* See *reflex, Hering-Breuer.*

bridge, *n* a colloquial expression for a fixed partial denture. See also *denture, partial, fixed.*

bridge, cantilever, *n* See *denture, partial, fixed, cantilever.*

bridge, fixed, *n* See *denture, partial, fixed.*

bridge, removable, *n* a colloquial expression for a removable partial denture. See also *denture, partial, removable.*

bridge splint, *n* See *splint, fixed.*

Brill-Symmers disease, *n.pr* See *lymphoma, giant follicular.*

Brinell hardness number, *n.pr* See *number, Brinell hardness.*

Brinell hardness test, *n.pr* See *test, Brinell hardness.*

brittle, friable, *adj* Technically a brittle material is one in which the proportional limit and ultimate strength are close together in value. See also *ductility.*

broach, *n* an instrument with numerous barbs protruding from a metal shaft. It is generally used to engage the dental pulp for extirpation.

broach, barbed, *n* See *broach.*

broach holder, *n* an instrument similar to a pin vise used to hold a broach.

broach, pathfinder, *n* See *broach, smooth.*

broach, smooth (pathfinder, pathfinder broach), *n* an instrument used for locating the orifice of a root canal and exploring the canal to determine the accessibility of the root end.

broad spectrum, *adj* indicates that a chemical can be used for its intended function with a wide variety of microbes.

Broders' classification, *n.pr* See *index, Broders'.*

bromide (brō'mīd), *n* a broad-acting chemical agent used to disinfect surfaces in the dental environment; comes in tablet form and is for use on hard surfaces only.

bromine, *n* a toxic, red-brown, liquid

element of the halogen group. Bromine is widely used in industry, photography, the manufacture of organic chemicals, and pharmaceuticals.

bromism (brō′miz-əm), *n* the toxic state induced by excessive exposure to or ingestion of bromine or bromine-containing compounds.

bromocriptine mesylate, *n trade name:* Parlodel; *drug class:* dopamine receptor agonist, ovulation stimulant; *action:* inhibits prolactin release by activating postsynaptic dopamine receptors; *uses:* treatment of female infertility, Parkinson's disease, amenorrhea.

bromodeoxyuridine, *n* a compound that competes with uridine for incorporation in ribonucleic acid.

bromopnea (brə-mop′nē-ə), *n* See *halitosis.*

brompheniramine maleate, *n trade names:* Bromphen, Dehist, Veltane; *drug class:* antihistamine, H_1-receptor antagonist; *action:* acts on blood vessels and gastrointestinal and respiratory systems by competing with histamine for H_1-receptor sites; *uses:* treatment of allergy symptoms, rhinitis.

bronchia (brong′kē-ə), *n.pl* bronchial tubes smaller than bronchi and larger than bronchioles.

bronchiarctia (brong′kē-ärk′shē-ə), *n* the stenosis of a bronchial tube.

bronchiectasis (brong′kē-ek′tə-sis), *n* a chronic disease characterized by dilation of the bronchi and bronchioles, clinically recognizable by fetid breath and purulent matter; dilation of the bronchi, either local or general.

bronchiocele (brong′kē-ō-sēl), *n* a dilation or swelling of a branch smaller than a bronchus.

bronchiole (brong′kē-ōl), *n* a terminal division of a bronchium.

bronchitis, *n* an acute or chronic inflammation of the mucous membranes of the tracheobronchial tree.

bronchium (brong′kē-əm), *n* one of the subdivisions of a bronchus.

bronchoalveolar, *adj* referring to both the bronchia and alveoli of the lungs.

bronchoconstriction (brong′kō-kən-strik′shən), *n* the reduction of the caliber of the bronchi.

bronchodilation (brong′kō-dī-lā′shən), *n* the dilation of a bronchus; the operation of dilating a stenosed bronchus.

bronchodilator (brong′kō-dī-lā′tur), *n* a drug that dilates, or expands, the size of the lumina of the air passages of the lungs by relaxing the muscular walls.

bronchopneumonia, *n* an acute inflammation of the lungs and bronchioles characterized by chills, fever, high pulse and respiratory rates, bronchial breathing, cough with purulent bloody sputum, severe chest pain, and abdominal distension.

bronchoscope, *n* a curved flexible tube for visual examination of the bronchi.

bronchoscopy, *n* the visual examination of the tracheobronchial tree using a standard rigid, tubular metal bronchoscope or a narrower, flexible, fiberoptic bronchoscope. Bronchoscopy is used to secure a biopsy, aspirate fluids, and diagnose such conditions as lung abscess, bronchial obstruction, and localized atelectasis.

bronchospasm (brong′kō-spaz′əm), *n* a spasmodic contraction of the muscular coat of the bronchial tubes such as occurs in asthma.

bronchostenosis (brong′kō-stən-ō′sis), *n* stenosis of the bronchi; bronchiarctia.

bronchus, *n* one of the subdivisions of the trachea serving to convey air to and from the lungs.

Brooke's tumor, *n.pr* See *epithelioma adenoides cysticum.*

brown dental stains, *n* dark, mottled spots on teeth that may indicate fluorosis; may be caused by a prolonged exposure to a high concentration of fluoride during a crucial time in tooth development.

brown pellicle, *n* See *pellicle, brown.*

bruise, *n* in medical terminology, a contusion; an injury made on the flesh by an instrument, without breaking the skin.

bruit (brōō′-ē), *n* an extracardiac blowing sound heard at times over peripheral vessels; generally denotes cardiovascular disease.

brush, bristle polishing, *n* a polishing brush with natural or synthetic bristles.

brush, clasp, *n* a uniquely conceived

tool, made to clean the clasps that connect a prosthesis to the natural teeth. Because the clasps are in a critical and difficult to reach position, the 2- to 3-inch tool features a twisted, tapered brush that removes plaque and other debris.

brush, Dixon bristle, *n* a soft brush used to polish the nonmetal parts of removable dentures.

brush, polishing, *n* an instrument consisting of natural, synthetic, or wire bristles mounted on a mandrel or in a hub to fit on a lathe chuck; used to carry abrasive or polishing media to polish teeth, restorations, and prosthetic appliances.

brush, wheel polishing, *n* a polishing brush with bristles mounted similar to spokes of a wheel.

brush, wire polishing, *n* a polishing brush with bristles of wire, usually steel or brass.

brushing, *n* See *abrasion, denture.*

bruxism (bruk′siz-əm), *n* the involuntary gnashing, grinding, or clenching of teeth. Bruxism is usually an unconscious activity, whether the individual is awake or asleep; often associated with fatigue, anxiety, emotional stress, or fear, and frequently triggered by occlusal irregularities, usually resulting in abnormal wear patterns on the teeth, periodontal breakdown, and joint or neuromuscular problems.

Bruxism. (Christensen, 2002)

BSP test, *n* See *test, Bromsulphalein.*

bubo (byoo′bo), *n* a lymph node that is enlarged as a result of an infection. The process may lead to suppuration; seen in primary syphilis, chancroid, plague, malaria, and other infectious processes.

buccal (buk′əl), *adj* pertaining to or adjacent to the cheek.

buccal aspect, n See *aspect, buccal.*

buccal contour, n See *contour, buccal.*

buccal flange, n See *flange, buccal.*

buccal mucosa, n See *mucosa, oral.*

buccal notch, n See *notch, buccal.*

buccal shelf, n See *shelf, buccal.*

buccal splint, n See *splint, buccal.*

buccal surface, n See *surface, buccal.*

buccal tube, n See *tube, buccal.*

buccal vestibule, n See *vestibule, buccal.*

buccocclusion (buk′ō-kloo′zhən), *n* an occlusion in which the dental arch or group of teeth is buccal to the normal position.

buccolingual relationship, *n* See *relationship, buccolingual.*

buccolingual stress, *n* See *stress, buccolingual.*

buccoversion (buk′ō-vur′zhən), *n* any deviation from the normal line of occlusion toward the cheeks.

buck knife, *n* See *knife, buck.*

buckling, *n* the crowding of anterior teeth in the dental arch.

buclizine HCl, *n trade name:* Bucladin-S; *drug class:* antihistamine, H_1-receptor antagonist; *action:* acts centrally by blocking chemoreceptor trigger zone; *uses:* treatment for motion sickness.

budesonide, *n trade names:* Rhinocort Nasal Inhaler, Pulmicort; *drug class:* corticosteroid, synthetic; *action:* interacts with steroid cytoplasmic receptors to induce antiinflammatory effects; *uses:* management of symptoms of allergic rhinitis in adults and children; perennial nonallergic rhinitis in adults.

budget plan, *n* a method of financing dental accounts in which arrangements are made for the patient to pay a series of small amounts on an account, usually over a period of 12 to 18 months.

buffer, *n* any substance in a fluid that tends to lessen the change in hydrogen ion concentration that otherwise would be produced by adding acids or alkalis.

buffering capacity, *n* the body's ability to neutralize the acids that play a role in the decalcification of teeth; may be enhanced by eating firmly textured foods which improve chewing and stimulate the flow of saliva.

bug, *n* an error in a computer program.

bulb, speech, *n* See *aid, speech, prosthetic, pharyngeal section.*

bulimarexia (bōō-lim′ə-rek′sē-ə), *n* an eating disorder distinguished by a combination of the symptoms prevalent in both anorexia nervosa and bulimia nervosa; develops primarily in teenage and young adult females.

bulimia, *n* repeated secretive bouts of excessive eating followed by self-induced vomiting, purging, and anorexia, usually accompanied by feelings of guilt, depression, and self-disgust. Oral signs may include dental erosion of the lingual aspect of the maxillary anterior teeth.

Bulimia. (Sapp/Eversole/Wysocki, 2004)

bulla (bŏŏl′ə), *n* a circumscribed, elevated lesion of the skin containing fluid and measuring more than 5 mm in diameter.

bumetanide, *n* trade name: Bumex; *drug class:* loop diuretic; *action:* acts on the loop of Henle to decrease reabsorption of chloride and sodium with resultant diuresis; *uses:* treatment of edema in chronic heart disease, renal disease, pulmonary edema, ascites, and hypertension.

BUN, *n* See *blood urea nitrogen.*

Bunnell test, *n.pr* See *test, Paul-Bunnell.*

Bunyaviridae (bun′yəv-ir′i-dā), *n* a grouping of enveloped, helix-shaped ribonucleic acid (RNA) viruses, implicated in certain forms of encephalitis and sandfly fever.

Buonocore, Dr. Michael, *n.pr* the head of a team of researchers at the Eastman Dental Center in Rochester, New York, responsible for developing dental sealants.

bupivacaine HCl (local), *n* trade *names:* Marcaine, Senorcaine; *drug class:* amide local anesthetic; *action:* inhibits ion fluxes across membranes, particularly sodium transport across cell membranes; decreases rise of depolarization phase of action potential; blocks nerve action potential; *uses:* local dental anesthesia, epidural anesthesia, peripheral nerve block, caudal anesthesia.

bupropion, *n* trade name: Wellbutrin, Zyban; *drug class:* antidepressant; *action:* weak uptake inhibitor of dopamine, serotonin, norepinephrine; mechanism unknown; *uses:* treatment of depression and anxiety disorders; smoking cessation.

bur, *n* a rotary cutting instrument of steel or tungsten carbide, supplied with cutting heads of various shapes.

bur, carbide, *n* a bur made of tungsten carbide; used at high rotational speeds.

bur, crosscut, *n* a bur with blades slotted perpendicularly to the axis of the bur.

bur, end-cutting, *n* a bur that has cutting blades only on the end of its head.

bur, excavating, *n* a bur used to remove dentin and debris from a cavity.

bur, finishing, *n* a bur with numerous fine-cutting blades placed close together; used to contour metallic restorations.

bur, intramucosal insert base-preparing, *n* See *insert, intramucosal.*

bur, inverted cone, *n* a bur with a head shaped like a truncated cone, the larger diameter being at the terminal (distal) end.

bur, plug-finishing, *n* See *bur, finishing.*

bur, round, *n* a bur with a sphere-shaped head.

bur, straight fissure, *n* a bur without crosscuts that has a cylindrical head.

bur, tapered fissure, *n* a bur having a long head with sides that converge from the shank to a blunt end.

burden of proof, *n* in a legal proceeding, the duty to prove a fact or facts in dispute.

Burkitt's tumor (African lymphoma), *n.pr* a type of lymphosarcoma seen in African children. About half the patients have lesions in the jawbones. Recent evidence suggests a possible viral cause.

Burlew wheel, *n.pr* a trade name for an abrasive-impregnated, knife-edged, rubber polishing wheel; used on a mandrel in the dental handpiece to smooth metallic restorations and tooth surfaces.

Burlew wheel, high luster, n Burlew wheel in which jeweler's rouge or iron peroxide is used as the abrasive agent.

Burlew wheel, midget, n a miniature form of Burlew wheel.

Burlew wheel, sulci, n See *Burlew wheel, midget.*

burn, *n* a lesion caused by contact of heat, radiation, friction, or chemicals with tissue. Thermal burns are classified as follows: first degree, manifested by erythema; second degree, manifested by formation of vesicles; third degree, manifested by necrosis of the mucosa or dermis; and fourth degree, manifested by charring into the submucous or subcutaneous layers of the body.

burn, aspirin, n an irregularly shaped, whitish area on the mucosa caused by the topical application of acetylsalicylic acid.

Aspirin burn. (Neville/Damm/Allen/Bouquot, 2002)

burnisher, *n* an instrument shape with rounded edges used to burnish, polish, or work-harden metallic surfaces.

burnisher, ball, n a burnisher with a working point in the form of a ball.

burnisher, beaver-tail, n See *burnisher, straight.*

burnisher, fishtail, n a burnisher that slightly resembles a fish's tail in shape.

burnisher, straight, n a burnisher that resembles a beaver's tail in shape; the broad, flat blade is smoothly continuous with the shank,

meeting it in a slight curve; the edges and the point are smoothly rounded.

burnishing, *n* a process related to polishing and abrading; the metal is moved by mechanically distorting the normal space lattice. Commonly accomplished during the polishing of soft golds.

burnout, *n* the elimination by heat of an invested pattern from a set investment to prepare the mold to receive casting metal.

burnout, high heat, n the use of temperatures higher than 1100° F (593.5° C) to effect wax elimination and prepare the mold to receive casting metal.

burnout, inlay (wax), n the elimination of wax from an invested inlay flask. See also *wax elimination.*

burnout, job, n the condition of having no energy left to care, resulting from chronic, unrelieved job-related stress and characterized by physical and emotional exhaustion and some times by physical illness.

burnout, radiographic, n excessive penetration of the x-ray beam of an object or part of an object, producing a totally black, or overexposed, area on the radiograph.

burnout, wax, n See *burnout, inlay* and *wax elimination.*

business area, *n* the area adjacent to the reception room in which the receptionist conducts the business affairs of the office and directly through which patients must pass to enter and leave the dental office.

business hours (office hours), *n.pl* those hours of the day during which professional, public, and other kinds of business are ordinarily conducted.

business office, *n* the room reserved for the dentist in which the business of the dental practice is conducted.

buspirone HCl, *n trade name:* BuSpar; *drug class:* antianxiety agent; *action:* unknown, may inhibit 5-HT receptors or dopamine receptors; *use:* management and short-term relief of anxiety disorders.

busulfan, *n trade name:* Myleran; *drug class:* antineoplastic; *action:* changes essential cellular ions to covalent bonding with resultant alkylation, which interferes with biologic function of deoxyribonucleic acid; *uses:* treatment of chronic myelocytic leukemia.

butoconazole nitrate, *n trade name:* Femstat; *drug class:* antifungal; *action:* binds sterols in fungal cell membrane, which increases permeability; *use:* treatment of vulvovaginal infections caused by *Candida.*

butt, *v* to place directly against the tissues covering the residual alveolar ridge; to bring any two square-ended surfaces into contact, as a butt joint.

button, *n* the excess metal remaining from the casting and sprue; located at the end of the sprue, opposite the casting.

button, implant, n See *insert, intramucosal.*

buttonhole approach, *n* a method of surgical treatment of a periodontal abscess in which, after an incision is made in the fluctuant abscess, an additional attempt is made to curet the area adjoining the root and the fundus of the abscess through the destroyed portion of the alveolar plate or bone.

cachexia (kəkek′sē-ə), *n* weakness, loss of weight, atrophy, and emaciation caused by severe or chronic disease.

cachexia, hypophysial, n See disease, Simmonds'.

cachexia hypopituitary, n See disease, Simmonds'.

cadaver, *n* a dead body, most often used in reference to a body used for dissection and study.

cadaverine, *n* a foul-smelling diamine formed by bacterial decarboxylation of lysine. It is poisonous and irritating to the skin.

cadmium, *n* a bluish-white metallic element that resembles tin. Cadmium bromide, used in engraving, lithography, and photography, can cause severe gastrointestinal symptoms if ingested.

Caesarean section, *n* a procedure in which a child is delivered through a surgical incision made in the walls of the abdomen and uterus. Also called a *Caesarean* or *C-section.*

café-au-lait spots, *n.pl* See spots, café-au-lait.

cafeteria plan, *n* employee benefits plan in which employees select their medical insurance coverage and other nontaxable fringe benefits from a list of options provided by the employer. Cafeteria plan participants may receive additional, taxable cash compensation if they select less expensive benefits.

caffeine (kafēn′, kaf′ē-in), *n* a white, odorless, bitter compound isolated from tea and coffee that is used as a stimulant of the central nervous system. See also aspirin, phenacetin.

CAGE questionnaire, *n.pr* four-question survey used to identify potential alcohol dependence. CAGE is an acronym for the four areas identified (felt need to Cut back, Annoyance by critics, Guilt about drinking, and Eye-opening morning drinking).

calcific metamorphosis (of dental pulp), *n* a frequently observed reaction to trauma, characterized by partial or complete obliteration of the pulp chamber and canal.

calcification (kal′sifikā′shən), *n* the process whereby calcium salts are deposited in an organic matrix. The condition may be normal, as in bone and tooth formation, or pathologic in nature.

calcification, dystrophic, n the pathologic deposition of calcium salts in necrotic or degenerated tissues.

calcification, ectopic oral, n the displaced accumulation of hardened calcium salts in the mouth; stones found in pulp or saliva.

calcification, metastatic, n the pathologic deposition of calcium salts in previously undamaged tissues. This process is caused by an excessively high level of blood calcium, such as in the hyperparathyroid.

calcifying epithelial odontogenic tumor (Pindborg tumor), *n* an uncommon tumor arising from odontogenic epithelium characterized by focal areas of calcification. It has the same age, gender, and site distribution as the ameloblastoma.

calcination (kal′sinā′shən), *n* a process of removing water by heat; used in the manufacture of plaster and stone from gypsum.

calcinosis (kal'sənō'sis), *n* **1.** the deposition of calcium salts in various tissues because of hypercalcemia and tissue degeneration. **2.** the presence of calcification in or under the skin. The condition may occur in a localized (calcinosis circumscripta) or generalized (calcinosis universalis) form.

calcipotriene, *n* *trade name:* Dovonex; *drug class:* vitamin D3 derivative (synthetic); *action:* regulation of skin cell production and development; *use:* moderate plaque psoriasis.

calcite, *n* an abrasive agent made from crystallized natural calcium carbonate.

calcitonin, *n trade names:* Calcitonin, Calcimar, Miacalcin; *drug class:* synthetic polypeptide calcitonins; *action:* inhibits bone resorption, reduces osteoclast function, reduces serum calcium levels in hypercalcemia; *uses:* Paget's disease, postmenopausal osteoporosis, hypercalcemia.

calcitriol, *n* *trade name:* Calcijex; *drug class:* vitamin D3 hormone; *action:* increases intestinal absorption of calcium and phosphorus; *uses:* hypocalcemia in chronic renal dialysis and rickets, nutritional supplement.

calcium (Ca) (kal'sē-əm), *n* a basic element, with an atomic weight of 40.07, found in nearly all organized tissues. Essential for mineralization of bone and teeth. The normal level of calcium in the blood is 9 to 11.5 mg/100 ml. A deficiency of calcium in the diet or in use may lead to rickets or osteoporosis. Overexcretion in hyperparathyroidism leads to osteoporotic manifestations. See also factor IV.

calcium binding protein, *n* See calmodulin.

calcium, blood, *n* See blood calcium.

calcium carbonate, *n trade names:* Maalox Antacid, Rolaids Calcium Rich, Tums E-X; *drug class:* antacid; *action:* neutralizes gastric acidity, supplies calcium; *uses:* antacid, calcium supplement.

calcium carbonate and magnesium hydroxide, *n* *trade name:* Rolaids; *drug class:* antacid; *action:* neutralizes gastric acidity; *use:* antacid.

calcium channel blocker, *n* a drug that inhibits the flow of calcium ions across the membranes of smooth muscle cells. The reduction of calcium flow relaxes smooth muscle tone and reduces the risk of muscle spasms. Calcium channel blockers are used in the prevention and treatment of coronary artery spasms.

calcium, dietary, *n* the amount of absorbable calcium ingested daily.

calcium fluoride, *n* a compound that is used as a flux in the manufacture of some silicate cements.

calcium hydroxide, *n* a white powder that is mixed with water or another medium and used as a base material in cavity liners and for pulp capping.

calcium oxalate, *n* an insoluble sediment in the urine and urinary calculi.

calcium phosphate, *n* an odorless, tasteless white powder, the various forms of which are sometimes used as abrasives in dentifrices.

calcium salts, *n pl* calcium present in salivary fluid as phosphates and carbonates. They are believed to form dental calculus on their precipitation from saliva.

calcium sulfate, *n* See alpha-hemihydrate, beta-hemihydrate, gypsum.

calcium tungstate, *n* a chemical substance used in crystal form to coat screens; the screens fluoresce when struck by roentgen rays.

calculogenesis (kal'kyōōlōjen'əsis), *n* the process during which calculus is formed.

calculogenic (kal'kyōōlōjen'ik), *adj* pertaining to the formation of calculus on tooth surfaces.

calculus, *n* a concretion composed of calcium phosphate, calcium carbonate, magnesium phosphate, and other elements within an organic matrix composed of desquamated epithelium, mucin, microorganisms, and other debris.

Calculus. (Bird/Robinson, 2002)

calculus, dental, n a salivary deposit of calcium phosphate and carbonate with organic matter on the teeth or on a dental prosthesis.

calculus, identification of, by air application, n the use of compressed air to dry the periodontal region and visualize minimal amounts of calculus, which are otherwise difficult to see.

calculus record, n a written accounting of the number and distribution of calculus deposits on tooth surfaces that becomes part of the patient's permanent chart and is used to monitor progress and plan treatment.

calculus, serumal, n See calculus, subgingival.

calculus, subgingival, n calculus deposited on the tooth structure and found apical to the gingival margin within the confines of the gingival cervix, gingival pocket, or periodontal pocket. Usually darker, more pigmented, and denser than supragingival calculus.

calculus, supragingival, n calculus deposited on the teeth occlusal or incisal to the gingival crest.

calibrated probe, n See probe, periodontal.

calibration, n the process of comparing a measurement instrument against a verified standard instrument. The US Bureau of Standards maintains the national calibration instruments for weights and measures.

calibration of x-ray unit, n See unit, x-ray calibration.

Caliciviridae (kal′isēvir′idā), n a grouping of nonenveloped, 20-sided RNA viruses, whose most notorious member is the Norwalk gastroenteritis virus, named for the Ohio city where an outbreak was isolated.

caliper, axis-orbital, n a caliper used to record facial measurements and transfer them to an adjustable articulator. It consists of the following: (1) a hinge-bow, (2) a bite fork covered with compound, (3) an indicator of the axis-orbital plane, (4) an upright rod to hold the orbital indicator in place, (5) a toggle to freeze the bow's base to the bite fork, and (6) a toggle to attach and allow adjustments for the support of the indicator. Also called *hinge-bow transfer recorder.*

Callahan's method, *n.pr* See method, chloropercha.

callus (kal′əs), n the tissue near and about the broken fragments of a bone that becomes involved in the repair of the fracture through various stages of exudate, fibrosis, and new bone formation.

calmodulin, n a calcium-binding protein that mediates a variety of biochemical and physiologic processes, including the contraction of muscles and the release of norepinephrine.

calorie, n the amount of heat required to raise 1 g of water 1° C at atmospheric pressure, also called gram calorie or small calorie. A great calorie, or kilocalorie, consists of 1000 small calories. The kilocalorie is the unit used to denote the heat expenditure of an organism and the fuel or energy value of food.

calorimetry, n the measurement of the amounts of heat radiated and absorbed.

Camper's line, *n.pr* See line, Camper's.

camphorated opium tincture, n *trade name:* Paregoric; *drug class:* antidiarrheal; *action:* antiperistaltic and analgesic with activity related to morphine content; *use:* diarrhea.

camphorated parachlorophenol (per′əklôr′ōfē′nol), n a mixture of 35% parachlorophenol and 65% camphor; used to treat root canals and periapical infections.

Campylobacter, n.pr a microorganism associated with progressive periodontal destruction and refractory forms of periodontitis.

Campylobacter gastroenteritis, n a gastrointestinal tract infection with typical symptoms, caused by *Campylobacter jejuni* bacteria.

Campylobacter jejuni, n.pl microaerophilic bacteria naturally occurring in humans and other mammals; pathogenic forms of the bacteria may cause a form of gastroenteritis.

canal, n the portion of the root that contains the pulp tissue and is bounded by dentin.

canal, accessory root, n a lateral branching of the main root canal, usually occurring in the apical third of the root.

C

canal, branching, n See canal, collateral pulp.

canal, collateral pulp (branching canal), n a dental pulp canal branch that emerges from the root at a place other than the apex.

canal, interdental (nutrient canal), n the nutrient channels that pass upward through the body of the mandible. Seen as radiolucent lines on radiographs.

canal, mandibular, n a channel extending from the mandibular foramen on the medial surface of the ramus of the mandible to the mental foramen. It contains mandibular blood vessels (arteries and veins) and a portion of the mandibular branch of the trigeminal nerve.

canal, nutrient, n See canal, interdental.

canal, pulp, n the space in the radicular portion of the tooth occupied by the pulp.

canal, root, n See canal, pulp.

canal, root, measurements, n.pl a technique employing the use of radiographs to determine the length of the root canal.

canaliculus (kan′əlik′yəlus), n a minute channel that extends from or to the lacunae of bone and cementum and contains filamentous processes of the cells that occupy the lacunae; interconnects with canaliculi extending from neighboring lacunae.

cancer (kan′sur), n a malignant neoplasm. The term is sometimes incorrectly used to include any neoplasm, whether benign or malignant. Carcinoma and sarcoma are more limiting terms.

cancer, oral, n malignancies indicative of unchecked cell growth that may be found in and around the oropharynx, gingiva, alveolar and buccal mucosae, lower mouth, lips and tongue.

cancrum oris (kang′krəm ôr′is), n See stomatitis, gangrenous.

Candida albicans **(kan′didə al′bəkanz),** n.pr a budding, yeast-like fungus present in the normal flora of the mucous membrane of the female genital tract and human respiratory and gastrointestinal tracts (including the mouth) that is capable of assuming a pathogenic role in the production of oral and systemic moniliasis, such as thrush and monilial infection.

candidiasis (kan′didī-əsis), n an infection by *Candida albicans.* See also moniliasis; thrush.

Chronic hyperplastic candidiasis. (Ibsen/Phelan, 2000)

candidiasis, angular cheilitis, n forms fissures or ulcers radiating from the angles of the mouth often accompanied by white plaques. Usually observed in elderly patients, although when observed in a young person, it may be an indicator of HIV infection. Candidiasis of the esophagus, trachea, bronchi, or lungs is associated with group IV human immunodeficiency virus (HIV) infection. See also acquired immunodeficiency syndrome; AIDS.

candidiasis, erythematous (atrophic), n forms smooth red patches on the hard or soft palate, buccal mucosa, or dorsal surface of the tongue.

candidiasis, hyperplastic, n forms white plaques that cannot be removed by wiping or scraping.

candidiasis, pseudomembranous, n forms loosely adherent (wipeable), yellowish-white plaques on the oral mucosal surface.

canine (kā′nīn), n (cuspid), one of the four pointed teeth in human beings, situated one on each side of each jaw, distal to the lateral incisor; forms the keystone of the arch. The term *canine* is increasingly preferred to *cuspid.*

canine eminence, n bony projection that covers the root of the canine tooth on the labial surface of both the jaws.

canine fossa, n See fossa, canine.

canine guidance, n a concept of

occlusal function in which the canine teeth are assigned a major control role in the excursive movements of the mandible.

canker (kang´kur), *n* See herpes labialis.

canker sore, n See sore, canker.

cannabis, *n* a psychoactive herb derived from the flowering tops of a variety of hemp, *Cannabis sativa.* It is the active ingredient of marijuana. Cannabis has no currently acceptable clinical use in the United States but has been employed in the treatment of glaucoma and as an antiemetic in some cancer patients to counter the nausea and vomiting associated with chemotherapy. Cannabis is controlled under Schedule I of the Comprehensive Drug Abuse Prevention and Control Act of 1970.

cannula (kan´yələ), *n* a tube for insertion into the body; its caliber is usually occupied by a trocar during the act of insertion.

cannula, nasal, n a small, half-moon shaped plastic tube, the ends of which fit into the nostrils of an individual.

canthus, lateral (kan´thus), *n* lateral angle between the upper and lower eyelids.

canthus, medial, *n* medial angle between the upper and lower eyelids.

cantilever bridge, *n* See denture, partial, fixed, cantilever.

cantilever partial denture, *n* See denture, partial, cantilever fixed.

capacity, *n* legal qualification, competency, power, or fitness.

capacity, functional residual, n (normal capacity), the volume of gas in the lungs at resting expiratory level.

capacity, iron-binding, n a measure of the binding capacity of iron in the serum; helps to differentiate the causes of hypoferremia. This capacity tends to increase in iron deficiency and diminishes in chronic diseases and during infection.

capacity, normal, n See capacity, functional residual.

capacity, total lung (TLC), n the volume of air in the lungs at the end of maximal inspiration.

capacity, vital (VC), n the maximum volume of air that can be expired after maximal inspiration.

capillarity (kap´iler´itē), *n* the phenomenon by which a film of fluid is drawn and held between two closely approximating surfaces.

capillary (kap´ilerē), *n* the terminal vessels uniting the arterial with the venous systems of the body. Capillaries are organized into extensive branching reticular beds to provide a maximal surface for exchange of fluids, electrolytes, and metabolites between tissues and the vascular system. The capillary bed has the largest cross-sectional area of the entire vascular system.

capillary attraction, n the quality or state that, because of surface tension, causes elevation or depression of the surface of a liquid that is in contact with a solid. Considered to be one of the factors in retention of complete dentures.

capillary disorder, n hemorrhagic disorder caused by increased fragility of the blood vessels that may cause hemorrhages in the skin and mucous membranes

capital budgeting, *n* the process of planning expenditures on assets, the returns of which are expected to extend beyond 1 year.

capitation, *n* **1.** the practice of dentistry financed by a set fee per person per given period of time. A form of contracted dental care, usually by a corporation, institution, or other group. **2.** a system by which the contracting dentist, assuming the financial risk, is compensated at a fixed per capita rate, usually on specific, predetermined dental services as appropriate and necessary to eligible subscribers. **3.** a dental benefits program in which a dentist or dentists contract with the program's sponsor or administrator to provide all or most of the dental services covered under the program to subscribers in return for payment on a per capita basis.

capitation fee, n a predetermined per-person charge made by the carrier for benefits available under an insurance plan.

capitulum (kəpich´əlum), *n* a small head. The term used by some European writers instead of *head* or *condyle.*

capitulum mandibulae, n See process, condyloid.

Capnocytophaga, *n* species of gram-negative facultatively anaerobic bacteria belonging to the genus *Capnocytophaga.* It is present in both normal and diseased oral cavities of humans.

capnophilic (kap′nōfil′ik), *adj* the ability to thrive in conjunction with carbon dioxide.

capping, direct pulp, *n* application to the exposed pulp of a drug or material for the purpose of stimulating repair of the injured pulpal tissue.

capping, indirect pulp, *n* a chemical (usually calcium hydroxide) placed over a layer of carious dentin remaining over the potentially exposed pulp to protect the pulp from external irritants.

capping, pulp, *n* the covering of an exposed dental pulp with a material that protects it from external influences.

capsaicin, *n trade names:* Zostrix, Capzasin-P, Axsain; *drug class:* topical analgesic for selected pain syndromes; *action:* depletes and prevents reaccumulation of substance P in peripheral sensory neurons; *uses:* neuralgia associated with herpes zoster, rheumatoid arthritis, temporomandibular joint (TMJ) pain.

capsule, joint, *n* a fibrous sac or ligament that encloses a joint and limits its motion. It is lined with synovial membrane.

capsule, temporomandibular joint, *n* See articulation, temporomandibular, capsule.

captopril, *n trade name:* Capoten; *drug class:* angiotensin-converting enzyme; *action:* dilation of arterial and venous vessels; *uses:* hypertension.

carat, *n* a standard of fineness of gold, 24 carats being taken as expressing absolute purity.

carbamazepine, *n trade names:* Apo-Carbamazepine, Epitol, Novo Carbamaz; *drug class:* anticonvulsant; *action:* inhibits nerve impulses by limiting influx of sodium ions across cell membrane in motor cortex; *uses:* tonic-clonic complex-partial, mixed seizures, a specific analgesic for trigeminal neuralgia, sometimes used in the treatment of herpes zoster.

carbaminohemoglobin, *n* hemoglobin compounded with CO_2.

carbenicillin, *n* a semisynthetic penicillin that is acid resistant and rapidly absorbed from the small intestine and thus suitable for oral administration.

carbide bur, *n* See bur, carbide.

carbohemia (kär′bōhē′mē-ə), *n* an imperfect oxygenation of the blood.

carbohydrates, *n.pl* a group of organic compounds with the class name saccharides, which are the aldehydic or ketonic derivatives of polyhydric alcohols. Carbohydrates such as sugar, starch, cellulose, and gum are generally synthesized by green plants. Carbohydrates constitute the main energy source in the diet and are classified as mono-, di-, tri-, and polysaccharides.

carbohydrate tolerance, *n* See tolerance, carbohydrate.

carbon, *n* a nonmetallic tetravalent element that occurs in pure form in diamonds and graphite. It occurs as a component of all living tissue. Most of the study of organic chemistry focuses on the vast number of carbon compounds.

carbon coated, adj a vitreous carbon coating applied to either an endosteal or blade implant to improve tissue compatability.

carbon dioxide, n a colorless, odorless gas produced by the complete oxidation of carbon. Carbon dioxide is a product of cell respiration and is carried by the blood to the lungs and exhaled. The acid-base balance of body fluids and tissues is affected by the level of carbon dioxide and its carbonate compounds.

carbon monoxide, n a colorless, odorless, poisonous gas produced by the combustion of carbon or organic fuels in a limited oxygen supply. Carbon monoxide combines irreversibly with hemoglobin, preventing the formation of oxyhemoglobin and reducing the oxygen supply to the tissues.

carbonate, *n* a mineral salt of carbonic acid.

carbonate hydroxyapatite (kär′bənāt hīdrok′sē-ap′ətīt), n the composition and crystal structure of hard tissues.

carbonic acid, *n* an unstable acid formed by dissolving carbon dioxide in water. It is the basis of carbonated beverages and contributes the negative ion to carbonate salts.

carbonic anhydrase, *n* an enzyme that plays a role in transferring carbon dioxide from tissue cells to the lungs by turning carbon dioxide into carbonic acid in red blood cells. Also called *carbonate dehydratase.*

Carborundum stone, *n.pr* See stone, Carborundum.

carboxylate, *n* a carboxylic acid salt, ester, or ion.

carboxylation, *n* the chemical process by which a carboxyl group (COOH) is added or displaces a hydrogen atom.

carboxypeptidase (kärbok'sēpep-'tidās), *n* an exopeptidase that stimulates the hydrolytic cleavage of the last or second to last peptide bond at the C-terminal end of a peptide or polypeptide.

carcinogen, *n* a substance or agent that causes the development or increases the incidence of cancer.

carcinoma (kär'sinō'mə), *n* a malignant epithelial tumor. Also called *cancer.*

carcinoma, adenoid cystic (**cylindroma, adenocystic carcinoma, adenocystic basal cell carcinoma, basaloid mixed tumor**), *n* a pseudoadenomatous basal cell carcinoma originating from salivary glands, the cells of which resemble basal cells and form ductlike or cystlike structures. It grows slowly but is malignant.

carcinoma, basal cell (**basal cell epithelioma, rodent ulcer, turban tumor**), *n* an epithelial neoplasm with a basic structure resembling the basal cells of the epidermis. It develops from basal cells of the epidermis or from the outer cells of hair follicles or sebaceous glands, particularly the middle third of the face. It rarely, if ever, metastasizes but is locally invasive. It does not arise from oral mucosa.

carcinoma, basosquamous, *n* carcinoma that histologically exhibits both basal and squamous elements. It may occasionally be seen in the oral cavity; considered to have a greater tendency to metastasize than does basal cell carcinoma.

carcinoma, epidermoid, *n* a malignant epithelial neoplasm with cells resembling those of the epidermis. The term *squamous cell carcinoma* is used for intraoral lesions of this nature.

carcinoma, exophytic, *n* a malignant epithelial neoplasm with marked outward growth similar to a wart or papilloma.

carcinoma in situ, *n* a dysplastic epithelial disease involving the skin and mucous membranes and considered to be precancerous. Dyskeratosis is evident, but no invasion has yet occurred.

carcinoma, intraepithelial, *n* See carcinoma in situ.

carcinoma, mucoepidermoid, *n* a malignant epithelial tumor of the salivary gland characterized by acini with mucus-producing cells.

carcinoma, squamous cell, *n* See carcinoma, epidermoid.

Squamous cell carcinoma. (Regezi/Sciubba/Pogrel, 2000)

carcinoma, transitional cell, *n* a malignant tumor arising from a transitional type of stratified epithelium.

carcinoma, verrucous, *n* a squamous cell carcinoma, usually intraoral, that is exophytic and has a papillary appearance.

cardia, *n* the opening between the esophagus and the cardiac portion of the stomach; characterized by the absence of acid cells. Also an archaic term formerly used to describe the heart and the region surrounding it.

cardiac, *adj* relating to the heart.

cardiac arrest, *n* a stopping of heart action; a complete cessation of heart function.

cardiac massage, *n* See massage, cardiac.

cardiac output, *n* the volume of blood put out by the heart per minute; the product of the stroke volume and the heart rate per minute.

cardiac pacemaker, *n* See pacemaker.

cardiac surgery, n operative procedure used to treat a disease of the heart or its blood vessels.

cardioinhibitory (kär´dē-ōinhib´itôrē), *adj* restraining or inhibiting the movements of the heart.

cardiokinetic (kär´dē-ōkinet´ik), *adj* exciting the heart; a remedy that excites the heart.

cardiology, n the scientific study of the anatomy, normal function, and disorders of the heart.

cardiomyopathy, hypertrophic, n a disease of the heart in which the heart is enlarged.

cardiopulmonary, *adj* pertaining to the heart and lungs.

cardiopulmonary resuscitation (CPR), n a basic emergency procedure for life support, consisting of artificial respiration and manual external cardiac massage.

cardiovascular disease, n any one of a number of abnormal conditions that involve dysfunction of the heart and blood vessels, including but not limited to systemic hypertension, atherosclerosis and coronary heart disease, and rheumatic heart disease.

cardiovascular system, n the network of structures, including the heart and blood vessels, that convey the blood throughout the body.

care, n as a legal term, the opposite of negligence.

care, reasonable, n such care as an ordinarily prudent person would exercise under the conditions existing at the time that person is called on to act.

caregiver, n a person providing treatment or support to a sick, disabled, or dependent individual.

caries (ker´ēz), n in general medicine, the decay or death of a bone.

caries, arrested dental, n the state existing when the progress of the decay process has halted.

caries, cemental (root surface), n decay of the cementum that occurs as a result of gingival recession and exposure of the root surface. See also caries, cervical (root surface).

caries, cervical (root surface), n decay that appears on the root at the neck of the tooth as a result of gingival recession and exposure of the root surface. See also caries, cemental (root surface).

caries, dental, n an infectious disease with progressive destruction of tooth substance, beginning on the external surface by demineralization of enamel or exposed cementum.

caries, enamel, n decay that occurs in the enamel of a tooth because of a fissure or the collection of bacterial plaque. It appears first as white spots which later darken to brown.

caries, healed dental, n See caries, dental, arrested.

caries, incipient dental, n a decayed part of a tooth in which the lesion is just coming into existence.

caries, pit-and-fissure dental, n See cavity, pit and fissure and sealant, pit and fissure.

Dental/pit-and-fissure caries. (Sapp/Eversole/Wysocki, 2004)

caries, proximal dental, n decay occurring in the mesial or distal surface of a tooth.

caries, rampant dental, n a suddenly appearing, widespread, rapidly progressing type of caries.

caries, recurrent dental, n the extension of the carious process beyond the margin of a restoration.

caries, residual dental, n (residual carious dentin), the decayed material left in a prepared cavity and over which a restoration is placed.

caries, root dental, n tooth decay occurring on a portion of the root that is exposed.

caries, senile dental (senile decay), n caries noted particularly in old age when supporting tissues have receded; occurs in cementum, usually on proximal surfaces of the teeth.

caries, smooth surface dental, n decay that occurs on the smooth surfaces of the tooth. See also caries, proximal dental.

cariogenesis (ker´ē-ōjen´əsis), n the process during which cavities develop in teeth.

cariogenic challenge, *n* episode in which tooth enamel is exposed to acid, a byproduct of cariogenic foods and plaque bacteria.

cariogenicity, *n* the ability of a substance to induce or potentiate the formation of dental caries.

cariostatic, *adj* pertaining to the oils in fats that provide a protective coating for teeth to keep food particles from sticking and to prevent sugars and acids from entering or leaving plaque. See anticariogenic.

carious (ker′ē-us), *adj* pertaining to caries or decay.

carious dentin, adj pertaining to caries or decay. See wax, carious.

carisoprodol, *n trade names:* Soma, Vanasom; *drug class:* skeletal muscle relaxant, central acting; *action:* nonspecific central nervous system sedation; *uses:* adjunct for relief of muscle spasm in musculoskeletal conditions.

carnauba wax, *n* See wax, carnauba.

Carnoy's solution, *n.pr* See solution, Carnoy's.

carotene (ker′ətēn), *n* an orange pigment found in carrots, leafy vegetables, and other foods that may be converted to vitamin A in the body.

carotenemia (ker′ətēnē′mē-ə), *n* excess carotene in the blood, producing a pigmentation of the skin and mucous membranes that resembles jaundice.

carotid (kərot′id), *n* either one of the two main right and left arteries of the neck.

carotid stenosis, n the narrowing and hardening of the carotid artery.

carpal tunnel syndrome, *n* an irritation and inflammation of the synovials surrounding the tendons controlling the fingers. Carpal tunnel syndrome is a disabling condition for persons who work with their hands, particularly those engaging in keyboard activities in music, typing, and data management.

carrier, *n* **1.** a person harboring a specific infectious agent without clinical evidence of disease and who serves as a potential source or reservoir of infection for others. May be a healthy or convalescent carrier. *n* **2.** the party of the dental plan contract who agrees to pay claims or provide service. Also called *insurer, under-*

writer, and administrative agent. See also third party.

carrier, amalgam, *n* an instrument used to carry plastic amalgam to the prepared cavity or mold into which it is to be inserted.

carrier, foil, *n* See foil passer.

carteolol, *n trade name:* Cartrol; *drug class:* nonselective β-adrenergic blocker; *action:* competitively blocks stimulation of β-adrenergic receptors within vascular smooth muscle, decreases rate of sinoatrial (SA) node discharge, increases SA node recovery time; *use:* mild-to-moderate hypertension.

carteolol HCl, n trade name: Ocupress; *drug class:* β-adrenergic blocker; *action:* nonselective β-adrenergic blocking agent, reduces production of aqueous humor by unknown mechanisms; *uses:* chronic open/angle glaucoma, ocular hypertension.

cartilage, *n* a derivative of connective tissue arising from the mesenchyme. Typical hyaline cartilage is a flexible, rather elastic material with a semitransparent, glasslike appearance. Its ground substance, or matrix, is a complex protein (chondromucoid) through which is distributed a large network of connective tissue fibers. Distributed throughout the matrix are cartilage cells that are rounded and do not have the branching characteristics of bone cells. The cells are isolated in the matrix they have secreted and normally have no blood vessels. Therefore nutrients and metabolites are exchanged with the circulation by passage through the matrix.

cartilage, articular, n a thin layer of hyaline cartilage located on the joint surfaces of some bones. Not usually found on articular surfaces of temporomandibular joints, which are covered with an avascular fibrous tissue.

cartilage, cricoid, n the lowest cartilage of the larynx.

cartilage, Meckel's, n.pr the cartilaginous process in the embryo derived from the mesenchymal tissue of the mandibular process.

cartilage, Reichert's (rī′kherts), n.pr the cartilaginous process located laterally in the embryonic tympanum; gives rise to styloid processes, stylohyoid ligaments, and lesser horns of hyoid bone.

caruncle, submandibular, *n* the orifice of the sublingual (Wharton's) duct that opens into the mouth on small papillae bilateral to the lingual frenum.

carvedilol, *n* *trade name:* Coreg; *drug class:* nonselective β-adrenergic blocking agent with α-blocking activity; *action:* produces fall in blood pressure without reflex tachycardia or significant reduction in heart rate; *use:* essential hypertension alone or with other antihypertensives.

carver (carving instrument), *n* an instrument used to shape a plastic material such as wax or amalgam.

carver, amalgam, *n* an instrument used to shape plastic amalgam.

carving, *n* shaping and forming with instruments.

case, *n* the term often incorrectly used instead of the appropriate noun (for example, *patient, flask, denture, casting*). Case is not synonymous with patient because the latter is the human being affected with the disease.

case charting, *n* the recording of a patient's status of health or disease.

case dismissal, *n* the technique of illustrating to the patient the results of treatment, usually done during the last appointment of a series.

case history, *n* See history, case.

case management, *n* the monitoring and coordination of treatment rendered to patients with specific diagnoses or requiring high cost or extensive services.

case presentation, *n* explanation of dental needs to the patient.

case summary, *n* enumeration of all the services to be performed for an estimated amount of money.

case-control study, *n* an investigation employing an epidemiologic approach in which previously existing incidents of a medical condition are used in lieu of gathering new information from a randomized population. Control is obtained by comparing known cases of the medical condition with a group of persons who have not developed the medical problem.

cash budget, *n* a schedule showing cash flows (receipts, disbursements, net cash) for a firm over a specified period.

cash cycle, *n* the length of time between the purchase of raw materials and the collection of accounts receivable generated in the sale of the final product.

cash flow, *n* the reported net income of a corporation plus amounts charged off for depreciation, depletion, amortization, and extraordinary charges to reserves, which are bookkeeping deductions not paid out in actual dollars and cents. A measurement tool used in recent years to offer a better indication of the ability of a company to pay dividends and finance expansion from self-generated cash than the conventional reported net income figure.

cassette (kəset´), *n* a light, tight container in which x-ray films are placed for exposure to x-rays; usually backed with lead to eliminate the effect of backscattered radiation.

cassette, cardboard (**cardboard film-holder**), *n* a cardboard envelope of simple construction suitable for use in making radiographs on "direct exposure" or "no-screen" types of x-ray films.

cassette, screen-type, *n* a cassette usually made of metal, with the exposure side of low-atomic number material, such as Bakelite, aluminum, or magnesium, and containing intensifying screens between which a "screen type" of film or films may be placed for exposure to x-rays.

cast, *n* **1.** an object formed by pouring plastic or liquid material into a mold in which it hardens. *v* **2.** to throw metal into an impression to form the casting.

cast, bar splint, *n* See splint, cast bar.

cast, corrected master, *n* a dental cast that has been modified by the correction of the edentulous ridge areas as registered in a supplemental, correctable impression.

cast, dental, *n* a positive likeness of a part or parts of the oral cavity reproduced in a durable hard material.

cast, diagnostic, *n* a positive likeness of dental structures for the purpose of study and treatment planning.

cast, diagnostic, anatomic portion, *n* the section of a finished cast that contains the actual impression of the teeth and surrounding tissue. It should account for approximately 65% of the cast's total height.

cast, diagnostic, double-pour method, n a method of forming the base of a cast in which the inverted impression is held against the surface of prereadied stone while the sides and edges of the cast are shaped; eliminates the possibility of inverting the impression before the stone has set. Also called *two-step method.*

cast, diagnostic, implant, n a cast made from a conventional mucosal impression on which the wax trial denture and surgical impression trays are made or selected.

cast, gnathostatic, n a cast of the teeth trimmed so that the occlusal plane is in its normal position in the mouth when the cast is set on a plane surface. Such casts are used in the gnathostatic technique of orthodontic diagnosis.

cast, implant, n a positive reproduction of the exposed bony surfaces made in a surgical bone impression and on which an implant frame is designed and fabricated.

cast, investment, n See cast, refractory.

cast, keying of, n the process of forming the base (or capital) of a cast so that it can be remounted accurately. Also referred to as the split-cast method of returning a cast to an articulator.

cast, master, n an accurate replica of the prepared tooth surfaces, residual ridge areas, or other parts of the dental arch reproduced from an impression from which a prosthesis is to be fabricated.

cast, preextraction, n a cast made before the extraction of teeth. See also cast, diagnostic.

cast, preoperative, n See cast, diagnostic.

cast, record, n a positive replica of the dentition and adjoining structures, used as a reference for conditions existing at a given time.

cast, refractory, n a cast made of materials that can withstand high temperatures without disintegrating and that, when used in partial denture casting techniques, expand to compensate for metal shrinkage.

cast, trimming diagnostic, n a set of finishing steps for a study cast in which the bases, posterior borders,

sides, heels, and anterior surfaces are smoothed and shaped to ensure a finished product that is attractive, well proportioned, and useful as a diagnostic tool. The treatment is best accomplished using a mechanical model trimmer.

cast, working, n an accurate reproduction of a master cast; used in preliminary fitting of a casting to avoid injury to the master cast.

casting, n **1.** a metallic object formed in a mold. **2.** forming a casting in a mold.

casting flask, n See flask, refractory.

casting machine, n a mechanical device used for throwing or forcing a molten metal into a refractory mold.

casting machine, air pressure, n a casting machine that forces metal into the mold via compressed air.

casting machine, centrifugal, n a casting machine that forces the metal into the mold via centrifugal force.

casting machine, vacuum, n a casting machine in which the metal is cast by evacuation of gases from the mold. Atmospheric pressure actually forces metal into the mold.

casting model, n See cast, refractory.

casting ring, n See flask, refractory.

casting temperature, n See temperature, casting.

casting, vacuum, n the casting of a metal in the presence of a vacuum. See also casting machine, vacuum.

casting wax, n See wax, casting.

Castle's intrinsic factor, *n.pr* See factor, Castle's intrinsic.

castration, n the surgical excision of one or both testicles or ovaries, usually to reduce the production and secretion of certain hormones that may stimulate the proliferation of malignant cells in women with breast cancer and men with prostate cancer. Surgically referred to as *orchidectomy* and *oophorectomy.*

castration anxiety, n **1.** the fantasized fear of injury to or loss of the genital organs. **2.** a general threat to the body image of a person or the unrealistic fear of bodily injury or loss of power or control.

casualty insurance, n insurance against loss caused by accidents; usually applied to property but may apply to bodily injury or death from accident.

cat-scratch disease, n See fever, cat-scratch.

catabolism (kətab'ōlizəm), n the destructive processes (opposite of the anabolic-metabolic processes) by which complex substances are converted into more simple compounds. A proper relation between anabolism and catabolism is essential for the maintenance of bodily homeostasis and dynamic equilibrium.

catabolism of energy, n dissipation of energy in living tissues as work or heat (one phase being metabolism, the other being anabolism).

catabolism of substance, n destructive metabolism; the conversion of living tissues into a lower state of organization and ultimately into waste products.

catalase reaction (kat'əlās), n the response of bubbling in the presence of hydrogen peroxide given by blood exudates or transudates.

catalysis (kətal'əsis), n the increase in rate of a chemical reaction, induced by a substance called a *catalyst,* which takes no part in the reaction and remains unchanged.

catalyst (kat'əlist), n a substance that induces an increased rate of a chemical reaction without entering into the reaction or being changed by the reaction.

catamenia (kat'əmē'nē-ə), n menstruation. Frequently used to designate age at onset of menses.

cataract, n an abnormal progressive condition of the lens of the eye, characterized by loss of transparency.

catatonia (kat'ətō'nē-ə), n a form of schizophrenia characterized by alternating stupor and excitement. A patient's arms often retain any position in which they are placed.

catecholamine, n any one of a group of sympathomimetic compounds composed of a catechol molecule and the aliphatic portion of amine. Some catecholamines (epinephrine and norepinephrine) are produced naturally by the body and function as key neurologic chemicals.

catechol-o-methyl transferase (COMT), n an enzyme that deactivates epinephrine and norepinephrine.

catgut, n sheep's intestine prepared as a suture and used for ligating vessels and closing soft tissue wounds.

catheter, n a hollow, flexible tube that can be inserted into a vessel or cavity of the body to withdraw or instill fluids.

catheter, balloon-tip, n a tube with a balloon at its tip that can be inflated or deflated without removal after insertion.

catheter, indwelling, n a catheter left in place in the bladder; usually a type of balloon catheter.

catheterization, n the process of introducing a hollow, flexible tube into a blood vessel or body cavity to withdraw or instill fluids.

cathode, n a negative electrode from which electrons are emitted and to which positive ions are attracted. In x-ray tubes, the cathode usually consists of a helical tungsten filament, behind which a molybdenum reflector cup is located to focus the electron emission toward the target of the anode.

cathode ray tube (CRT), n a vacuum tube in which a beam of electrons is focused to a small point on a luminescent screen and can be varied in position to form a pattern.

cathode-anode circuit, high-voltage, n one of the two electrical circuits required to take x-rays, provides the power to accelerate electrons enough to create x-ray photons.

cation (kat'īon), n a positive ion carrying a charge of positive electricity, therefore attracted to the negatively charged cathode.

cationic detergent, See detergent, cationic.

causalgia (kôzal'jə), n a postextraction localized pain phenomenon usually characterized by a continuous burning sensation.

causality, n a relationship between one event or action that precedes and initiates a second action or influences the direction, nature, or force of a second action. In scientific study, causality must be observable, predictable, and reproducible and thus is difficult to prove.

cause of action, n generally, a ground or reason for a legal action; a wrong that is subject to legal redress.

cause of death, n the immediate or proximate agent or act that resulted in the loss of life.

caustic, *adj* destroying living tissue by chemical burning action.

cauterize (kô′tərīz), *v* to sear or burn living tissue in order to stop bleeding; a corrosive agent, hot metal, or electricity may be used.

cavernous sinus, *n* one of a pair of irregularly shaped, bilateral venous channels located below the base of the brain between the sphenoid bone of the skull and the dura mater.

cavernous sinus thrombosis, n infection of the cavernous venous sinus.

cavitation (kav′itā′shun), *n* the formation and collapse of bubbles in the fluid spray released by a mechanized instrument used for debridement.

cavity, *n* a carious lesion or hole in a tooth.

cavity, access, n See access cavity.

cavity, amniotic, n the space between the developing fetus and the amnion, consisting of amniotic fluid.

cavity, axial surface, n a cavity occurring in a tooth surface in which the general plane is parallel to the long axis of the tooth.

cavity classification, n carious lesions are classified according to the surfaces of a tooth on which they occur (for example, labial, buccal, occlusal), type of surface (that is, pit, fissure, or smooth surface), and nu-

merical grouping (G. V. Black's classification).

cavity classification, artificial (G. V. Black), n classification of cavities.

cavity, complex, n a cavity that involves more than one surface of a tooth.

cavity, compound, n See cavity, complex.

cavity floor, n the base-enclosing side of a prepared cavity. See also cavity, prepared.

cavity, gingival (gingival third cavity), n a cavity occurring in the gingival third of the clinical crown of the tooth (G. V. Black's Class 5).

cavity lining, n material applied to the prepared cavity before the restoration is inserted to seal the dentinal tubules for protection of the pulp.

cavity medication, n a drug used to clean or treat a cavity before inserting a dressing, base, or restoration.

cavity, nasal, n two irregular spaces that are situated on either side of the midline of the face, extend from the cranial base to the roof of the mouth, and are separated from each other by a thin vertical septum. In radiographs the nasal cavity appears over the roots of the maxillary incisors as a large, segmented, radiolucent area. Also called *nasal fossa.*

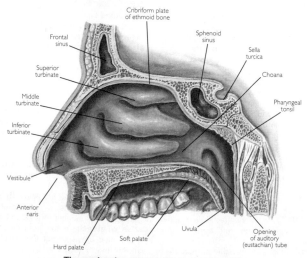

The nasal cavity. (Seidel/Ball/Dains/Benedict, 2003)

cavity, pit and fissure, *n* a cavity that begins in minute faults in the enamel. Caused by imperfect closure of the enamel.

cavity preparation, *n* the orderly operating procedure required to remove diseased tissue and establish in a tooth the biomechanically acceptable form necessary to receive and retain a restoration.

cavity, prepared, *n* the form developed in a tooth to receive and retain a restoration.

cavity, prepared, floor of, *n* the flat bottom or enclosing base wall of a prepared cavity; on an axial plane it is called the *axial wall,* and on the horizontal plane it is called the *pulpal wall.*

cavity, prepared, impression, *n* a negative likeness of a tapered type of prepared cavity.

cavity, proximal, *n* a cavity occurring on the mesial or distal surface of a tooth.

cavity, pulp, *n* the space in a tooth bounded by the dentin; contains the dental pulp. The part of the pulp cavity within the coronal portion of the tooth is the pulp chamber, and the part found within the root is the pulp canal, or root canal.

cavity, simple, *n* a cavity that involves only one surface of a tooth.

cavity, smooth surface, *n* a cavity formed by decay beginning in surfaces of teeth that are without pits, fissures, or enamel faults.

cavity toilet, *n* G. V. Black's final step in cavity preparation. Consists of freeing all surfaces and angles of debris.

cavity varnish, *n* See varnish, cavity.

cavity wall, *n* See wall, cavity.

cavosurface angle, *n* See angle, cavosurface.

cavosurface bevel, *n* See bevel, cavosurface.

CBC, *n* the abbreviation for *complete blood count,* a procedure in which all the blood cells are counted per cubic millimeter, including a differential counting of the white blood cells (leukocytes).

CD-ROM, *n* the acronym for compact disk/read-only memory. These disks are used to store program information (software) for computer programs. Information and instructions can be retrieved from these disks, but information cannot be added or revised without destruction of the existing data.

CD4 (T4) lymphocyte, *n* an immunologically important white cell that is responsible for cell-mediated immunity. It is the cell invaded by the human immunodeficiency virus and in which the virus replicates itself.

CDC, *n.pr* the acronym for the Centers for Disease Control and Prevention.

cecum, *n* a cul-de-sac constituting the first part of the large intestine. It forms the junction between the ileum and the large intestine.

cefaclor, *n* *trade names:* Ceclor, Ceclor CD; *drug class:* antibiotic second generation cephalosporin; *action:* inhibits bacterial cell wall synthesis; *uses:* eradication of gram-negative bacilli from the upper and lower respiratory tract and treatment of urinary tracts and skin infections and otitis media.

cefadroxil, *n* *trade names:* Duricef, Ultracef; *drug class:* first generation cephalosporin; *action:* inhibits bacterial cell wall synthesis, rendering cell wall osmotically unstable; *uses:* eradication of gram-negative bacilli from the upper and lower respiratory tracts, and treatment of urinary tract and skin infections and otitis media.

cefazolin sodium, *n* *trade names:* Ancef, Kefzol, Zolicef; *drug class:* first-generation cephalosporin; *action:* inhibits bacterial cell wall synthesis, rendering cell wall osmotically unstable; *uses:* eradication of gram-negative bacilli from the upper and lower respiratory tract, and treatment of urinary tracts, skin, bone, joint, biliary, genital infections, endocarditis, surgical prophylaxis, and septicemia.

cefepime, *n* trade name: Maxipime; *drug class:* fourth-generation cephalosporin; *action:* inhibits cell wall synthesis in sensitive organisms and is bactericidal; *uses:* respiratory tract, urinary tract, and skin and other soft tissue infections associated with gram-negative organisms.

cefixime, *n* trade name: Suprax; *drug class:* third-generation cephalosporin; *action:* inhibits bacterial cell wall synthesis, rendering cell wall osmotically unstable; *uses:* uncomplicated urinary tract infections, pharyngitis and tonsillitis, otitis media, acute bronchitis, and acute exacerbations of chronic bronchitis.

cefpodoxime proxetil, *n* trade name: Vantin; *drug class:* second-generation cephalosporin; *action:* inhibits bacterial cell wall synthesis, rendering cell wall osmotically unstable; *uses:* upper and lower respiratory tract infections, pharyngitis and tonsillitis, gonorrhea, urinary tract infections, skin structure infections.

cefprozil monohydrate, *n* trade name: Cefzil; *drug class:* second-generation cephalosporin; *action:* inhibits bacterial cell wall synthesis, which renders cell wall osmotically unstable; *uses:* pharyngitis and tonsillitis, otitis media, secondary bacterial infection of acute bronchitis, skin and skin structure infections.

ceftibuten, *n* trade name: Cedax; *drug class:* third-generation cephalosporin; *action:* causes cell death by attaching to the bacterial membrane wall; *uses:* lower respiratory and urinary tract infections, gynecologic and enteric infections, pharyngitis, tonsillitis, and otitis media caused by susceptible organisms.

cefuroxime axetil, *n* trade name: Ceftin; *drug class:* second-generation cephalosporin; *action:* inhibits bacterial cell wall synthesis, rendering cell wall osmotically unstable; *uses:* eradication of gram-negative bacilli and gram-positive organisms; treatment of serious lower respiratory tract, urinary tract, skin, and gonococcal infections, septicemia, and meningitis.

cell(s), *n* the basic unit of vital tissue. One of a large variety of microscopic protoplasmic masses that make up organized tissues. Each cell has a cell membrane, protoplasm, nucleus, and a variety of inclusion bodies. Each type of cell is a living unit with its own metabolic requirements, functions, permeability, ability to differentiate into other cells, reproducibility, and life expectancy.

cell, beta, *n* any cell that produces insulin in the islets of Langerhans region of the pancreas.

cell, bone-forming, *n.pl* See osteoblast.

cell, centrioles of (sen′trē-ōl), *n.pl* cylinder-shaped organelles that contain microtubules. Function is to organize spindle fibres during cell division.

cell, connective tissue, *n* the fibroblast, which for purposes of clarity is characterized by such terms as *perivascular connective tissue cell* or *young connective tissue cell.*

cell count, *n* the number of cells contained in a unit volume, usually refers to red and/or white blood cells in a unit volume of blood.

cell culture, *n* living cells that are maintained in vitro in artificial media of serum and nutrients for the study and growth of certain strains, experiments in controlling diseases, or study of the reaction to certain drugs or agents.

cell cycle, *n* the sequence of events that occur during the growth and division of tissue cells.

cell, cytoplasm of (sī′tōplazəm), *n* aqueous part of the cell in which are suspended all the organelles and inclusions. Site of all metabolic activities in the cell.

cell death, *n* the point in the process of dying at which vital functions have ceased at the cellular level. Cell death precludes the use of tissue or organs as transplant donors.

cell, defense, *n* a cell, mobilized within inflamed, irritated, or otherwise diseased tissue, that acts as a protective element to neutralize or wall off the foreign irritant. Defense cells include plasma cells, polymorphonuclear leukocytes, and the cells of the reticuloendothelial system.

cell differentiation, *n* the development of the cells into the various basic cell units of tissue: the epithelial cell and the nerve cell, which arise from the ectodermal tissue layer of the embryo; and the blood, muscle, bone, cartilage, and other connective tissue cells, which arise from the mesodermal tissue of the embryo. The mature tissue cell has many intermediary, transitional forms that are sequential in their development from the primitive, less differentiated anlage cell forms. These intermediary forms are evident clinically in disease in blood dyscrasias, tumors, and inflammation and in health in the normal processes of growth, development, healing, and repair.

cell, endoplasmic reticulum of, n See endoplasmic reticulum.

cell, endosteal, n a reticular cell that is modified and identified by its location; the endosteum is a condensation of the stroma of the bone marrow.

cell, filaments of, n.pl threadlike structures the function of which is to support the cytoskeleton; also integral parts of intercellular junctions.

cell, germ, n a cell of an organism the function of which is to reproduce an entity similar to the organism from which the germ cell originated. Germ cells are characteristically haploid.

cell, giant, n a large cell frequently having several nuclei.

cell, Golgi complex in, n See Golgi apparatus.

cell homeostasis, n See homeostasis, cell.

cell, homeostasis of (hō′mē-ōstā′sls), n See homeostasis, cell.

cell, inclusions of, n.pl nonliving bodies, by-products of cellular metabolism present in the cytoplasm.

cell, Langerhans', n.pr star-shaped cells of unknown function that appear to be permanent residents of the epithelium.

cell, lysosomes in (lī′sōsōm), n.pl membranous organelles produced from the Golgi complex; contain hydrolytic enzymes, which aid intracellular digestion.

cell membrane, n the outer covering of a cell. The membrane controls the exchange of materials between the cell and its environment.

cell, membrane of, transport through, n movement of biomolecules into and out of cells. See diffusion, osmosis, active transport, phagocytosis.

cell, mesenchymal, n an embryonic connective tissue cell with an outstanding capacity for proliferation and capable of further differentiation into reticular cells or osteoblasts. When persisting in the adult organism, the cells are usually arranged in loose connective tissue along the small blood vessels or in reticular fibers. They are identified by their location and capacity to differentiate into other cell types, such as smooth muscle cells in the formation of new arteries, phagocytes in inflammatory processes, and bone cells in the formation of new bone tissue.

cell, microtubules of, n.pl See microtubule.

cell, mitochondria of, n.pl See mitochondria.

cell, nucleus of, n See nucleus.

cell, plasma, n a cell of disputed origin (lymphatic versus undifferentiated mesenchymal cell) that is seen in chronic inflammation and certain disease states and tumors but not normally in the circulating blood. The cell is larger than a lymphocyte and has an eccentric nucleus with basophilic nuclear chromatin peripherally located, like figures on a clock face. Currently, the cells are believed to produce and carry antibodies.

cell, replication, n See mitosis.

cell, reticular, n a cell of reticular connective tissue, such as in the stroma of the bone marrow, that retains both osteogenic and hematopoietic potencies; it is identified by its location, morphology, potency, and direct origin from mesenchymal cells.

cell, stem, n.pl the cells in the bone marrow from which all blood cells originate.

cell, typical, n See cell.

cell wall, n See cell membrane.

cells, radiosensitivity of, n the amount of sensitivity of a particular cell, determined by three factors: cell metabolism—the higher the metabolic rate, the more sensitive, cell differentiation—less mature cells are more sensitive than specialized cells, and mitotic activity—cells are more sensitive when they are dividing or rapidly reproducing.

cellulitis (sel′yōōlī′tis), n a diffuse inflammatory process that spreads along fascial planes and through tissue spaces without gross suppuration.

Cellulitis. (Zitelli/Davis, 2002)

celluloid strip, *n* See strip, plastic.

cellulose, *n* the primary component of plant cell walls; provides the fiber and bulk necessary for optimal functioning of the human digestive tract.

cellulose, oxidized (sel′yōōlōs), *n* cellulose, in the form of cotton, gauze, or paper, that has been more or less completely oxidized.

cement, *n* a material that produces a mechanical interlocking effect on hardening.

cement, acrylic resin dental, *n* a dental cement, dispensed as a powder and a liquid, that is mixed as is any other cement. The powder contains polymethyl methacrylate, a filler, plasticizer, and polymerization initiator. The liquid monomer is methyl methacrylate with an inhibitor and an activator.

cement, copper dental, *n* a zinc phosphate cement to the powder of which has been added a copper oxide.

cement, dental, *n* any one of the materials used in dentistry as luting agents, bases, and temporary restorations. See also cement, acrylic resin dental; cement, zinc.

cement, dental base, *n* an insulating layer of cement placed in the deeper portion of a prepared cavity to insulate the pulp.

cement dressing, *n* postoperative dressing applied after periodontal surgery.

cement dressing, dental, Kirkland, *n.pr* See dressing, Kirkland cement.

cement, Kryptex dental, *n.pr* See cement, silicophosphate.

cement line, *n* See line, cement.

cement, polycarboxylate, *n* a dental cement used for cementation of cast restorations and orthodontic appliances and as bases. Prepared by mixing a zinc oxide powder with a liquid of polycarboxylic acid.

cement sealer, *n* a compound used in filling a root canal; it is inserted in a plastic condition, solidifies after placement, and fills any irregularities in the surface of the canal.

cement, silicate, *n* a relatively hard, translucent restorative material used primarily in anterior teeth. Prepared by mixing a liquid and a powder. The powder is an acid-soluble glass prepared by the fusion of CaO, SiO, Al_2O_3, and other ingredients with a fluoride flux. The liquid is a buffered phosphoric acid solution.

cement, silicious dental, *n* See cement, silicate.

cement, silicophosphate, *n* (Kryptex cement), a combination zinc phosphate and silicate cement. Less translucent, less irritating, and less soluble than silicate and stronger than zinc phosphate cement.

cement, zinc oxide–eugenol dental, *n* least irritating of the cements. The powder is essentially zinc oxide with strengtheners and accelerators. The liquid is basically eugenol.

cement, zinc phosphate, *n* a material used for cementation of inlays, crowns, bridges, and orthodontic appliances; occasionally used as a temporary restoration. Prepared by mixing a powder and a liquid. The powders are composed primarily of zinc oxide and magnesium oxides. The principal constituents of the liquid are phosphoric acid, water, and buffer agents.

cemental repair, *n* See repair, cemental.

cemental tear, *n* a small portion of cementum forcibly separated, either partially or completely, from the underlying dentin of the root as a result of occlusal force; seen on the tension side in occlusal traumatism.

cementation (sē′mentā′shən), *n* attachment of an appliance or a restoration to natural teeth or attachment of parts by means of a cement.

cementicle (səmen′tikəl), *n* a calcified body sometimes found in the periodontal ligament of older individuals. Degenerated epithelial cells are presumed to form the nidus for this calcification.

cementifying fibroma, *n* See fibroma, cementifying.

cementing line, *n* See line, cemental.

cementoblast (səmen′tōblast), *n* the cell that forms the organic matrix of cementum. Derived from the inner aspect of the dental sac during the initial formation of cementum or from the mesenchymal cell of the periodontal membrane after completion of primary cementogenesis. The cementoblast, trapped within cellular cementum, becomes a cementocyte.

cementoclasia (səmen′tōklā′zhə, -zē-ə), *n* destruction of cementum by cementoclasts.

cementocyte (səmen′tōsīt), *n* the cell found within lacunae of cellular cementum; possesses protoplasmic processes that course through the canaliculi of the cementum; derived from cementoblasts trapped within newly formed cementum.

cementoenamel junction, *n* See junction, cementoenamel.

cementogenesis (sēmen'tōjen'əsis), *n* formation of cementum, the calcified connective tissue that envelops the roots of teeth, from the epithelial root sheath. See also cementoblast.

cementoid, *n* the most recent uncalcified layer covering the surface of cementum.

cementoma (sementō'mə), *n* (traumatic osteoclasia), an endontogenic tumor associated with the apices of teeth. It may be present as a mass of fibrous connective tissue, fibrous connective tissue with spicules of cementum, or a calcified mass resembling cementum and having few cellular elements.

cementoma, first-state, *n* See fibroma, periapical.

cementopathia (səmen'tōpath'ē-ə), *n* the concept wherein necrotic, diseased cementum and lack of productivity of cementum are implicated in the causation of periodontitis and periodontosis.

cementum (səmen'tum), *n* a specialized, calcified connective tissue that covers the anatomic root of a tooth, giving attachment to the periodontal ligament.

cementum, abnormalities of, *n.pl* reversal lines in the cementum, which represent bone tissue resorption or cementum resorption. Cementicles are calcified epithelial cells found in older persons. Hypercementosis is cementum overgrowth on the roots. See also reversal lines, cementicle, and hypercementosis.

cementum, acellular, *n* cementum that contains no cementocytes.

cementum, cellular, *n* the portion of the calcified substance covering the root surfaces of the teeth. It is bonelike and contains cementocytes embedded within lacunae, with protoplasmic processes of the cementocytes coursing through canaliculi that anastomose with canaliculi of adjacent lacunae. The lacunae are dispersed through a calcified matrix arranged in lamellar form. Cellular cementum is localized primarily at the apical portion of the root but may deposit over the acellular cementum or serve to repair areas of cemental resorption.

cementum, collagen fibrils of, *n* fibrils that penetrate the cementum surface and are continuous with the periodontal fibers necessary for tooth support.

cementum, lamellar, *n* cementum in which layers of appositional cementum are arranged in a sheaflike pattern, the layers of cementum being more or less parallel to the cemental surface and demarcated by incremen-

Cementum. (Bird/Robinson, 2002)

Labels: Crown, Neck, Root, Enamel, Dentin, Gingiva, Pulp within pulp cavity, Cementum, Root canal, Bone (alveolar process), Apical foramen

C

tal lines that represent periods of inactivity of cementum formation.

cementum, necrotic, n nonvital cementum that is situated coronal to the bottom of the periodontal pocket.

cementum, properties of, n.pl calcified, avascular connective tissue that is derived from the dental follicle and functions in protecting the roots of teeth.

cementum, secondary, n the term used to describe all subsequent layers of cementum formed after the primary layer. It may be cellular or acellular.

center of rotation, n a point or line around which all other points in a body move.

Centers for Disease Control and Prevention (CDC), n the federal facility for disease eradication, epidemiology, and education, headquartered in Atlanta, Georgia.

central bearing, n the application of forces between the maxilla and mandible at a single point located as near as possible to the center of the supporting areas of the upper and lower jaws. The purpose is to distribute the closing forces of the jaws evenly throughout the areas of the supporting structures during the registration and recording of maxillomandibular (jaw) relations and the correction of occlusal errors.

central bearing device, n a device that provides a central point of bearing or support between upper and lower occlusion rims. It consists of a contracting point attached to one occlusion rim and a plate on the other rim that provides the surface on which the bearing point rests or moves.

central bearing point, n See point, central-bearing.

central nervous system, n that portion of the nervous system consisting of the brain and spinal cord. The portion of the nervous system beyond the brain and cord is known as the *peripheral nervous system.*

central occlusion, n See occlusion, centric.

central processing unit (CPU), n the primary processor of a computer, containing the internal memory unit (memory), arithmetic logic unit (ALU), and input/output control unit (I/O control).

central tendency, n the tendency of a group of scores to cluster around a central representative score. The statistics most frequently used for measures of central tendency are the mean, median, and mode.

centric (sen′trik), *adj* (objectionable as a noun) describing jaw and tooth relationships. See also position, centric; relation, centric; occlusion, centric.

centric checkbite, n See record, occluding, centric relation.

centric occlusion, n See occlusion, centric.

centric position, n See position, centric.

centric relation, n See relation, centric.

centrifugal force (sentrif′əgəl), n See force, centrifugal.

cephalexin, *n trade names:* Ceporex, Keftab, Keflex; *drug class:* first-generation cephalosporin; *action:* inhibits bacterial cell wall synthesis, rendering cell wall osmotically unstable; *uses:* eradication of gram-negative bacilli from the upper and lower respiratory tracts, urinary tract, and skin; treatment of bone infections and otitis media.

cephalic index, n an anthropometric value based on the ratio between the width and length of the head.

cephalogram (sef′əlōgram), n a cephalometric radiograph. On tracings of these films, anatomic points, planes, and angles are drawn that assist in the evaluation of the patient's facial growth and development.

cephalometer (sef′əlom′ətur), n See cephalostat.

cephalometer, radiographic, n See cephalostat.

cephalometric analysis, n See analysis, cephalometric.

cephalometric landmark, n See landmark, cephalometric.

cephalometric radiograph, n a radiograph of the head made with precise reproducible relationships between x-ray source, subject, and film. The generally accepted distances between x-ray source and the center of the subject are 5 feet (152.4 cm) or 150 cm. The distance between subject and film is usually 12 cm but may be standardized at a different value or varied with patient size and recorded for each exposure. The two standard orientations are lateral (profile) and posteroanterior.

cephalometric skeletal analysis, *n* an assessment of the facial type of a skeleton; the relationship of the parts to each other, to the skull, and to an estimated "normal."

cephalometric tracing, *n* a tracing of selected structures from a cephalometric radiograph made on translucent drafting paper or film for purposes of measurement and evaluation.

cephalometrics (sef′əlōmet′riks), *n* the scientific study of the measurements of the head.

cephalometry (sef′əlom′ətrē), *n* the measurement of the bony structure of the head using reproducible lateral and anteroposterior radiograms.

cephalophore (sef′əlō′fōr), *n* a cephalostat designed to take in-sequence-oriented facial photographs and gnathostatic models.

cephalosporins, *n* semisynthetic derivatives of an antibiotic originally derived from the microorganism *Cephalosporium acremonium.* Cephalosporins are similar in structure to penicillins.

cephalostat (sef′əlōstat), *n* a head-positioning device that ensures reproducibility of the relations between an x-ray beam, a patient's head, and an x-ray film in radiography.

cephradine, *n trade name:* Velosef; *drug class:* first-generation cephalosporin; *action:* inhibits bacterial cell wall synthesis, rendering cell wall osmotically unstable; *uses:* eradication of gram-negative bacilli and gram-positive organisms from serious respiratory tract, urinary tract, and skin infections and otitis media.

ceramics, *n* the art of making dental restorations or parts of restorations from fused porcelain.

ceramics, orthoclase, *n* See feldspar.

cerebellum (ser′əbel′um), *n* a major division of the brain, behind the cerebrum and above the pons and fourth ventricle, consisting of a median lobe, two lateral lobes, and major connections through pairs of peduncles to the cerebrum, pons, and medulla oblongata. The cerebellum is intimately connected with the auditory vestibular apparatus and the proprioceptive system of the body and hence is involved in maintenance of body equilibrium, orientation in space, and muscular coordination and tonus.

cerebral arteries, *n.pl* arteries to the brain that supply the cerebrum.

cerebral cortex, *n* a thin layer of gray matter on the surface of the cerebral hemisphere, folded into gyri with about two-thirds of its area buried in fissures. The cerebral cortex integrates higher mental functions, general movement, visceral functions, perception, and behavioral reactions.

cerebral hemorrhage, *n* a medical condition indicated by the rupturing of a blood vessel in the brain and the subsequent bleeding into the tissues of the brain.

cerebral infarction, *n* the blockage of the flow of blood to the cerebrum, causing or resulting in brain tissue death. Blockage may be caused by a thrombosis, an embolism, a vasospasm, or a rupture of a blood vessel.

cerebral ischemia, *n* the reduction or loss of oxygen to the cerebrum; prolonged ischemia may lead to cerebral infarction.

cerebral palsy, *n* See palsy, cerebral.

cerebrospinal fluid, *n* the fluid that flows through and protects the four ventricles of the brain, subarachnoid space, and spinal canal.

cerebrovascular accident (CVA/ stroke), signs and symptoms of, *n* a complete paralysis on one side of the body or various parts (e.g., face, arm, or leg), a diminished capacity to see, speak, swallow, or control saliva, an increase or decrease in sensitivity to touch and pain, and an alteration in mental processes and personality; depends on the degree of involvement and the area of the brain damage.

cerebrum (ser′əbrum, sərē′brum), *n* the largest portion of the brain. Operating at the highest functional level and occupying the upper part of the cranium, the cerebrum consists of two hemispheres united at the bottom by commissures of large bundles of nerve fibers. As with all parts of the nervous system, each part of the cerebrum has highly specific functions (for example, a specific outer cortical area controls voluntary chewing, whereas certain inner subcortical areas are involved in involuntary jaw posture).

cerium, *n* a ductile, gray rare-earth element. Cerium oxalate is used as a sedative, an antiemetic, and an antitussive.

certificate holder, *n* **1.** the person, usually the employee, who represents the family unit covered by the dental benefits program; other family members are referred to as *dependents.* **2.** generally refers to a subscriber of a traditional indemnity program. **3.** in reference to the program for dependents of active-duty military personnel, the certificate holder is called the *sponsor.* See also subscriber. Synonyms: subscriber, enrollee.

certificate of eligibility, *n* an official identification card or similar document issued to program beneficiaries as evidence of entitlement to services.

certificate of insurance, *n* a statement issued to a group member describing in general terms the policy provisions for eligibility, deductibles, coinsurance, allowances, and maximums. Used in lieu of issuing copies of the group or master contract to each individual employee member of an insured group.

certification, *n* a process by which an individual, institution, or educational program is evaluated and recognized as meeting certain predetermined criteria and standards.

certified dental assistant, *n* a person who has completed the Certification Board of the American Dental Assistant Association.

cervical (sur′vikəl), *adj* relating to the neck, or cervical line, of a tooth.
cervical appliance, n See appliance, cervical.
cervical convergence, n See convergence, cervical.
cervical fibers, n See nerve fibers.
cervical line, n See junction, cemento-enamel.
cervical vertebrae, n the first seven segments of the vertebral column that defines the neck.

cervical chain (lymph nodes), *n* one of three serially linked groups of lymph nodes located in the neck, including the superficial, deep, and posterior chains.

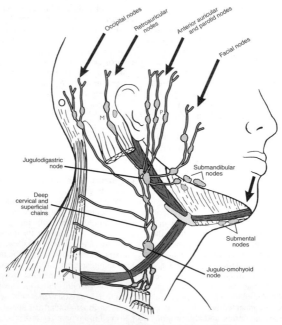

Lymphatic drainage of the face. (Liebgott, 2001)

cervical collar, *n* a leaded device positioned over the throat roughly midway between the chin and collarbones. Used because extended exposure of the thyroid gland to x-rays can cause thyroid cancer.

cervical lymphadenectomy (limfad′ ənek′tōmē), *n* See neck dissection.

cesium, *n* an alkali metal element used in photoelectric cells and television cameras.

cestode (ses′tōd), *n* a tapeworm that resides in the small intestine or other vital organs (including the brain). It can be passed on to humans through contaminated or improperly cooked meats, including fish. Symptoms of infection, when they occur, are similar to mild food poisoning.

cetirizine HCl, *n* trade names: Reactine, Zyrtec; drug class: antihistamine; action: competitive antagonist for peripheral H1 receptors; uses: treatment of symptoms of seasonal allergic rhinitis, perennial allergic rhinitis, chronic urticaria.

Cetylpyridinium chloride (sē′tilpir′ idin′ē-um), *n* an anti-infective agent used as a topical disinfectant and as a preservative in prepared pharmaceutical compounds.

Chagas' disease, *n.pr* a parasitic disease caused by *Trypanosoma cruzi* transmitted to humans by the bite of bloodsucking insects.

chalazion forceps (kəlā′zē-on), *n* See forceps, chalazion.

chalk, *n* an abrasive agent made from compact calcite.

chamber, *n* an enclosed area.

chamber, air-equivalent ionization, *n* a chamber in which the materials of the wall and electrodes produce ionization essentially similar to that produced in a free-air ionization chamber.

chamber, air-wall ionization, *n* an ionization chamber with walls of material of low atomic number, having the same effective atomic number as atmospheric air.

chamber, extrapolation ionization, *n* an ionization chamber with electrodes of which the spacing can be adjusted and accurately determined to permit extrapolation of its reading to zero chamber volume.

chamber, free-air ionization, *n* an ionization chamber in which a delimited beam of radiation passes between the electrodes without striking them or other internal parts of the equipment. The electric field is maintained perpendicular to the electrodes in the collecting region; as a result the ionized volume can be accurately determined from the dimensions of the collecting electrode and limiting diaphragm. This is the basic standard instrument for dosimetry within the range of 5 to 400 kV.

chamber, ionization, *n* an instrument for measuring the quantity of ionizing radiation, in terms of the charge of electricity associated with ions produced within a defined volume of air.

chamber, monitor ionization, *n* an ionization chamber used for checking the constancy of performance of roentgen-ray apparatus.

chamber, pocket ionization, *n* a small, pocket-sized ionization chamber used for monitoring radiation exposure of personnel. Before use it is given a charge, and the amount of discharge is a measure of the quantity of radiation received.

chamber, pulp, *n* (pulp cavity), the space occupied by the pulp.

chamber, relief, *n* a recess in the impression surface of a denture created to reduce or eliminate pressure from the corresponding area of the mouth.

chamber, standard ionization, *n* See chamber, ionization, free-air.

chamber, suction, *n* See chamber, relief.

chamber, thimble ionization, *n* a small cylindrical or spherical chamber, usually with walls of organic material.

chamber, thin-wall ionization, *n* an ionization chamber having walls so thin that nearly all secondary corpuscular rays reaching them from external materials can penetrate them easily.

chamber, tissue-equivalent ionization, *n* a chamber in which the walls, electrodes, and gas are selected to produce ionization essentially equivalent to the characteristics of the tissue under consideration.

chamfer (cham′fu), *n* in extracoronal cavity preparations, a marginal finish that produces a curve from an axial wall to the cavosurface.

chancre (autochthonous ulcer) (shang′kur), *n* the primary lesion of syphilis, located at the site of entrance of the spirochete into the body, occurring about 3 weeks after contact. It begins as a papule and then develops into a clean-based shallow ulcer. Secondary infection may produce suppuration. Has the appearance of a buttonlike mass because of the contiguous induration and rolled border. Weeping characteristics also are present.

chancre of lip, *n* the primary lesion of syphilis that often appears as an ulcerated or crusted, indurated lesion with a brownish or copper-colored weeping base when located on the lip. The lesion is teeming with *Treponema pallidum.*

chancre, soft, *n* See chancroid.

chancroid (shang′kroid), *n* (soft chancre), a venereal disease caused by *Haemophilus ducreyi.* It is characterized by a soft chancre that is a necrotic draining ulcer similar to a chancre but without characteristic induration. A regional bubo may occur.

channel, *n* a definite furrow, groove, or tubelike passage.

channel, vascular, *n* a blood or lymph vessel through which inflammatory infiltrate and periodontitis proceed from a localized superficial area to involve the deeper structures of the periodontium.

character, *n* one of a set of elementary symbols that may be arranged in groups to express information. They may include the decimal digits 0 to 9, the letters A to Z, punctuation marks, operation symbols, and any other single symbol that a computer may read, store, or write.

characteristics, acquired, *n.pl* environmentally influenced attributes that manifest after birth.

characteristics, sex, *n.pl* **1.** primary sex characteristics are those organs concerned with reproduction such as the gonads and genitalia. **2.** secondary sex characteristics include differences in voice range and timbre, muscularity, and distribution of hair and adipose tissue.

charcoal, *n* a carbonized reduction of wood used as fuel and as an adsorptive substance to cleanse the air; it is used in some medical products.

Charcot's joint, *n.pr* See joint, Charcot's.

charges, *n.pl* the financial obligation made to a patient's account for services rendered, usually on a quoted fee for explicit services provided.

charlatan, *n* a quack, a person who pretends to have skills or knowledge that he or she does not possess.

Charles' law, *n* See law, Charles'.

chart, *n* a sheet of paper or pasteboard that presents a graphic representation of a condition or state.

chart, Bonwill-Hawley, n.pr See chart, Hawley.

chart, dental, *n* a diagrammatic chart of the teeth on which the findings from the clinical and radiographic examinations are recorded.

chart, Hawley, n.pr (Bonwill-Hawley chart), graded outlines of dental arch sizes based on the mesiodistal diameters of the six anterior teeth.

chart, health, *n* See chart, history.

chart, history, *n* forms and records for obtaining a thorough medical and oral history combined with a complete record of findings that enable the practitioner to gather and have on hand the necessary records to render total patient care.

chart, tooth, *n* See chart, dental.

Charters' method, *n.pr* See method, Charters'.

charting, *n* the tabulation of the progress of a disease; the compilation of a clinical record.

charting, computerized, *n* an automated method for documenting a patient's dental health, utilizing such computer innovations as voice activation and mouse-activated software to ensure accuracy and save time.

charting symbols, *n.pl* commonly accepted notations that are made to the patient's chart to indicate the condition, position, and restorative history of individual teeth.

Chayes' attachment (shāz), *n.pr* believed to be the first internal precision attachment. See also attachment, intracoronal.

Cheadle's disease (chē′dəl), See scurvy, infantile.

checkbite, *n* See record, interocclusal.

checkbite, centric, n See record, interocclusal, centric and record, maxillary.

checkbite, eccentric, n See record, interocclusal, eccentric.

checkbite, lateral, n See record, interocclusal.

checkbite, protrusive, n See record, interocclusal, protrusive.

cheek, n a fleshy prominence, especially the fleshy protuberances on each side of the face below the eye and between the ear, nose, and mouth.

cheek biting, n the chewing of one's cheek (buccal mucosa) because of malocclusion, oral habit, or lack of coordination in the chewing cycle.

cheilion (kīlē′-ən), n the corner of the mouth.

cheilitis (kīlī′tis), n an inflammation of the lip.

Cheilitis. (Regezi/Sciubba/Pogrel, 2000)

cheilitis, actinic (solar cheilitis), n crusting, desquamation, ulceration, atrophy, and inflammation of the lips, more especially the lower lip, caused by chronic exposure to the elements and actinic rays of sunlight.

cheilitis, cigarette paper, n focal areas of inflammation of the lips caused by cigarette paper sticking to the surface and injury produced by efforts to remove it.

cheilitis, glandularis apostematosa, n chronic diffuse nodular enlargement of the lower lip associated with purulent inflammatory hyperplasia of the mucous glands and ducts. Rare; unknown etiology.

cheilitis, solar, n See cheilitis, actinic.

cheiloplasty (kī′əplastē), n corrective surgery or restoration of the lips.

cheilorraphy (kīlôr′əfē), n surgical repair of a congenital cleft lip.

cheilosis (kīlō′sis), n a noninflammatory condition of the lip usually characterized by chapping and fissuring. It is characteristic of either vitamin B complex deficiency of the mouth orifice or monilial infection.

cheilosis, angular, n See perleche.

cheilotomy (kīlôt′əmē), n incision into or excision of a part of the lip.

chelating agents, n.pl chemical compounds used to bind or inactivate metal poisons in the body.

chelation (kēlā′shən), n chemical reaction of a metallic ion (for example, calcium ion) with a suitable reactive compound (for example, ethylenediamine tetra-acetic acid) to form a compound in which the metal ion is tightly bound.

chelation therapy, n the use of a chelating agent to bind firmly and sequester metallic poisons.

chemamnesia (kem′amne′zhə, -zē-ə), reversible amnesia produced by a chemical or drug.

Chemclave, n.pr the brand name for chemical vapor sterilizer that uses a mixture of alcohols, ketones, formaldehyde, and water heated to approximately 127° C under a pressure of at least 20 pounds per square inch. American Dental Association accepted.

chemical cure, n a type of treatment in which a chemical process begins when the ingredients are completely mixed. The setting time depends on temperature and any added accelerator.

chemical dependence, n psychological or physical reliance on any number of drugs, both legal and illegal, prescription and over the counter. The individual may experience withdrawal symptoms if the chemical is no longer taken into the body.

chemical solutions, darkroom, n.pl developer, fixer and distilled water use to mix the chemicals for processing radiographic films.

chemically induced, adj initiating biologic action or response by the introduction of a chemical.

chemistry, n the science dealing with the elements, their compounds, and the molecular structure and interactions of matter.

chemoreceptor (kē′mōrēsep′tər), n a specialized sensory end organ adapted for excitation by chemical substances (for example, olfactory and gustatory receptors) or specialized sense organs of the carotid body that are sensitive to chemical changes in the bloodstream.

chemotaxis, *n* a response involving movement that is positive (toward) or negative (away from) to a chemical stimulus.

chemotaxis, leukocyte, *n* the phagocytic activity of neutrophils and monocytes in response to chemical factors released by invading microorganisms.

chemotherapeutic agent, *n* See agent, chemotherapeutic.

chemotherapy, *n* a cancer treatment method which uses chemical agents to modify or destroy cancer cells; dental patients who are undergoing chemotherapy may have increased needs for certain nutrients. See also agent, chemotherapeutic.

chemotherapy, local, for gingivitis, *n* the treatment of gingivitis with a topical antibiotic agent. The most effective antigingivitis chemotherapeutic agent is chlorhexidine.

chenodiol, *n* trade name: Chenix; *drug class:* anticholelithic; *action:* increases amount of bile acids in relation to cholesterol; *use:* dissolving gallstones.

cherubism (familial intraosseous swelling) (cher′əbiz′əm), *n* **1.** a fibroosseous disease of the jaws of genetic nature. The swollen jaws and raised eyes give a cherubic appearance; multiple radiolucencies are evident on radiographic examination. **2.** a familial form of fibrous dysplasia characterized by unilateral or, more often, bilateral swelling of the jaws in children. See also dysplasia, fibrous.

Cherubism. (Regezi/Sciubba/Pogrel, 2000)

chest pain, *n* a physical complaint that requires immediate diagnosis and evaluation. Chest pain may be symptomatic of cardiac disease such as angina pectoris, myocardial infarction, or pericarditis or disease of the lungs and its linings. It also may be referred from the gastrointestinal tract or elsewhere. The differential diagnosis of chest pain is a crucial element of medical practice.

chew-in record, functional, *n* the method by which the dentist records a patient's occlusal paths in the wax patterns to be used in making restorations. In making the grooves and ridges in the wax patterns directly, the dentist asks the patient to make right-and-left and fore-and-aft sliding occlusal strokes to generate the paths of the opposite prominences. See also path, generated occlusal.

chewing, *n* the movements of the mandible during mastication; controlled by neuromuscular action and limited by the anatomic structure of the temporomandibular joints.

chewing cycle, *n* See cycle, chewing.

chewing force, *n* See force, chewing.

chewing tobacco, *n* See smokeless tobacco and nicotine stomatitis.

Cheyne-Stokes reflex, *n.pr* See respiration, Cheyne-Stokes.

Cheyne-Stokes respiration, *n.pr* See respiration, Cheyne-Stokes.

chi square, *n* a nonparametric statistic used with discrete data in the form of frequency count (nominal data) or percentages or proportions that can be reduced to frequencies. Used to determine differences between categories (for example, yes-no; visits dentist every 6 months, 1 year, 2 years, 5 years); compares the observed results with the expected results to determine significant differences. May be used with many categories of response.

chickenpox, *n* See varicella.

child, *n* **1.** a person of either gender between the time of birth and adolescence, or puberty. **2.** in the law of negligence and in laws for the protection of children, a term used as the opposite of *adult* (generally under the age of puberty) without reference to parentage and distinction of gender.

child abuse, n the physical, sexual, or emotional maltreatment of a person under 18 years of age. Child abuse occurs predominantly with children under 3 years of age. Symptoms include bruises and contusions, medical record of repeated trauma, radiographic evidence of fractures, emotional distress, and failure to thrive.

child neglect, n a form of child abuse in which proper care is denied or withheld.

chin, n the raised triangular extension of the anterior portion of the mandible below the lower lip. It is formed by the mental protuberance of the mandible.

chin cup, n See cup, chin.

chip, n a logic element containing electronic circuit components, both active and passive, embedded in a cohesive material of any shape.

chip blower, n See syringe, air, hand.

chiropractic, n a branch of the healing arts dealing with the nervous system and its relationship to the spinal column and interrelationship with other body systems in health and disease. The primary spinal and paraspinal structural derangements with which chiropractors are concerned are known as *chiropractic subluxations.* Treatment is referred to as *chiropractic management* or *adjustment.*

chisel, n an instrument modeled after a carpenter's chisel intended for cutting or cleaving hard tissue. The cutting edge is beveled on one side only; the shank may be straight or angled.

chisel, contra-angle (binangle chisel), n a chisel-shaped, binangled, paired cutting instrument whose blade meets the shank at an angle greater than 12°.

chisel, posterior, n See chisel, contra-angle.

chisel, Wedelstaedt, n.pr a chisel with a blade that is continuous with the shank, has no constricting neck, curves rather than angles into the shank, and is available in varying widths.

Chlamydia, n.pr a genus of microorganisms that live as intercellular parasites and have a number of prop-

erties in common with gram-negative bacteria. Two species of Chlamydia organisms have been identified; both are pathogenic to humans.

Chlamydia psittaci, n.pr an organism that infests birds and causes a type of pneumonia in humans (psittacosis).

Chlamydia trachomatis, n.pr an organism that lives in the conjunctivae of the eye and the epithelium of the urethra and cervix and is responsible for conjunctivitis, lymphogranuloma venereum, and trachoma.

chloral hydrate, n *trade names:* Aquachloral Supprettes, Novo-chlorhydrate; *drug class:* sedative hypnotic chloral derivative, controlled substance schedule IV, schedule F; *action:* produces central nervous system depression; *uses:* sedation, treatment of insomnia, anesthesia adjunct.

chlorambucil, n *trade name:* Leukeran; *drug class:* antineoplastic alkylating agent; *action:* inhibits enzymes that allow synthesis of amino acids in proteins; *uses:* chronic lymphocytic leukemia, Hodgkin's disease, breast carcinoma, ovarian carcinoma.

chloramine solution, n See solution.

Chloramphenicol, n a broad-spectrum antibacterial and antirickettsial agent that should be reserved for serious infections in which other agents are ineffective.

chlordiazepoxide HCl, n *trade names:* Librium, Novopoxide; *drug class:* benzodiazepine antianxiety; *action:* produces central nervous system depression; *uses:* short-term management of anxiety, acute alcohol withdrawal, preoperatively for relaxation.

chlorhexidine gluconate, n *trade names:* Peridex, PerioGard; *drug class:* antiinfective oral rinse; *action:* absorbed by tooth surfaces, dental plaque, and oral mucosa; sustained reduction of plaque organisms; *uses:* as a rinse between dental visits as a part of treatment of gingivitis; unlabeled use—denture stomatitis.

chloride shift (klôr′ĭd), n the exchange of a chloride ion for a bicarbonate ion across the erythrocyte membrane as part of the buffering system in the blood. It accounts for the greater chloride content of venous erythrocytes than arterial erythrocytes.

chlorine, *n* a yellowish-green gaseous element of the halogen group. Chlorine has a strong, distinctive odor that is irritating to the respiratory tract and is poisonous if ingested or inhaled. It occurs chiefly as a compound of sodium chloride. Chlorine is used as a bleach and disinfectant. Chlorine compounds are used in solvents, cleaning fluids, and chloroform and formerly in general use as an anesthetic.

chlorine dioxide, *n* an oxidizing agent used in oral care to decrease amounts of volatile sulfur compounds that may cause halitosis.

chloroform, *n* a nonflammable, volatile liquid that was the first inhalation anesthetic to be discovered. It is no longer in general use because of its inherent risk factors and low margin of safety.

chloroformization (klôr´əfôrm´izā´shən), *n* the administration of chloroform.

Chloromycetin, *n.pr* the brand name for chloramphenicol. See also chloramphenicol.

chloropercha (klôr´ōpur´chə), *n* a solution obtained by mixing various amounts of chloroform with gutta-percha.

chloropercha method, *n* See method, chloropercha.

chlorophyll (klôr´ōfil), *n* the pigment required for photosynthesis in plants.

chlorophyllin (klôr´əfilin), *n* any one of a number of products resulting from the reaction of certain decomposition products of chlorophyll with copper and other metallic ions.

chloroquine HCl/chloroquine phosphate, *n trade names:* Aralen HCl, Aralen Phosphate; *drug class:* antimalarial; *action:* inhibits parasite replication; *uses:* malaria, rheumatoid arthritis, amebiasis.

chlorothiazide, *n trade name:* Diuril; *drug class:* thiazide diuretic; *action:* acts on distal tubule by increasing excretion of water, sodium chloride, potassium; *uses:* edema and hypertension, diuresis.

chlorotrianisene, *n trade name:* TACE; *drug class:* nonsteroidal synthetic estrogen; *action:* required for the development, maintenance, and adequate function of the female reproductive system, decreases release of gonadotropin-releasing hormone, inhibits ovulation, and helps maintain bone structure; *uses:* prostatic cancer, menopause, female hypogonadism, atrophic vaginitis.

chlorpheniramine maleate, *n trade names:* Chlor-Trimeton, Novopheniram; *drug class:* antihistamine H1-receptor antagonist; *action:* acts on blood vessels, gastrointestinal system, respiratory system by competing with histamine for H1-receptor site; *uses:* relief of allergy symptoms, rhinitis.

chlorphensin carbamate, *n trade name:* Maolate; *drug class:* skeletal muscle relaxant, central acting; *action:* unknown; may be related to sedative properties; does not directly relax muscle or depress nerve conduction; *use:* adjunct for relieving pain in acute, painful musculoskeletal conditions.

chlorpromazine HCl, *n trade name:* Thorazine; *drug class:* antipsychotic; *action:* blocks neurotransmission at dopaminergic synapses in the cerebral cortex, hypothalamus, and limbic system; *uses:* psychotic disorders, mania, schizophrenia, anxiety, intractable hiccups, nausea, vomiting, preoperatively for relaxation, behavioral problems in children.

chlorpropamide, *n trade names:* Apo-Chlorpromide, Diabinese; *drug class:* antidiabetic, first generation sulfonylurea; *action:* causes functioning beta-cells in pancreas to release insulin, leading to drop in blood glucose levels; *uses:* stable adult-onset diabetes mellitus type II.

chlortetracycline (klôr´tetrəsī´klēn), *n* (Aureomycin) a broad-spectrum antibiotic possessing bacteriostatic properties of some value in the treatment of disease produced by large viruses (the psittacosis and lymphogranuloma inguinale groups).

chlorthalidone, *n trade names:* Novothalidone, Apo-Chlorthalidone, Thalitone; *drug class:* diuretic with thiazide-like effects; *action:* acts on distal tubule by increasing excretion of water, sodium, chloride, potassium; *uses:* edema, hypertension, diuresis, chronic heart disease.

chlorzoxazone, *n trade names:* Paraflex, Parafon Forte DSC; *drug class:* skeletal muscle relaxant, central acting; *action:* depresses multi-synaptic pathways in the spinal cord; *uses:* adjunct for relief of muscle spasm in musculoskeletal conditions.

choice of path of placement, *n* See placement, choice of path of.

cholagogue (kō′ləgog), *n* a substance that stimulates emptying of the gallbladder and flow of bile.

cholera, *n* an acute bacterial infection of the small intestine characterized by severe diarrhea and vomiting, muscular cramps, dehydration, and depletion of electrolytes. The disease is spread by water and food that have been contaminated by feces of infected persons.

cholera toxin, n (choleragen), an exotoxin produced by the cholera vibrio that stimulates the secretion of electrolytes and water into the small intestine, draining body fluids and weakening the patient.

cholera vaccine, n an active immunizing agent against cholera.

choleretic (kō′ləret′ik), *n* a substance that stimulates production of bile by the liver.

cholestasis, *n* the interruption in the flow of bile through any part of the biliary system from the liver to duodenum.

cholesteatoma, *n* a cystic mass composed of epithelial cells and cholesterol that is found in the middle ear and occurs either as a congenital defect or as a serious complication of chronic otitis media.

cholesterol (kəles′tərōl), *n* a lipid common to all animal, but not plant, cells. As a sterol, it contains the cyclopentanophenanthrene nucleus. High levels are found in nerve tissue, atheromas, gallstones, and cysts. Normally 140 to 220 mg are present in 100 ml of blood.

cholestyramine, *n* *trade names:* Questran, Cholybar; *drug class:* antilipemic; *action:* absorbs, combines with bile acids to form insoluble complex that is excreted through the feces; lowers cholesterol levels; *uses:* primary hypercholesterolemia, pruritus associated with biliary obstruction, diarrhea caused by excess bile acid, digitalis toxicity, xanthomas.

choline, *n* a lipotropic or transmethylation factor found in most animal tissue either free or in combination as lecithin, acetylcholine, or as cytidine diphosphate. Its acetate form (acetylcholine) is essential for synaptic transmission. Administration of choline appears to improve memory and has shown some beneficial use in Alzheimer's disease.

choline salicylate, n trade name: Arthropan; *drug class:* salicylate analgesic; *action:* inhibits prostaglandin synthesis by interfering with cyclooxygenase need for biosynthesis; *uses:* relief of mild-to-moderate pain from fever, arthritis, juvenile rheumatoid arthritis.

cholinergic (parasympathomimetic) (kō′linur′jik), *adj* producing or simulating the effects of acetylcholine.

cholinergic blocking agent, n See agent, blocking, cholinergic.

cholinergic crisis, in myasthenia gravis, n a medical condition resulting from an administration of too much anticholinesterase, indicated by an immediate increase in muscle weakness, excessive secretion of pulmonary matter, diarrhea, and cramps.

cholinesterase (kō′lines′tərās), *n* an esterase that hydrolyzes acetylcholine. It is an enzyme that is widely distributed throughout the muscles, glands, and nerves of the body and that converts acetylcholine into choline and acetic acid.

cholinolytic (kō′linōlit′ik), *n/adj* See anticholinergic.

chondrodysplasia punctata, *n* an inherited form of dwarfism characterized by skin lesions, radiographic epiphyseal stippling, and a pug nose. Two types are most often seen: a benign type marked by mild asymmetric limb shortening that is transmitted by an autosomal dominant gene, and a lethal type with marked proximal limb shortening that is transmitted by an autosomal recessive gene.

chondroectodermal dysplasia (Ellis-van Creveld syndrome) (kon′drō-ek′tōdur′məl displā′zhə), *n* a syndrome characterized by the following tetrad: (1) bilateral polydactyly; (2) chondrodysplasia of the long bones resulting in acromelic dwarfism; (3) anomalies of the teeth, nails, hair, and maxillary and mandibular region anteriorly; and (4) heart malformation.

chondroitin, *n* a mucopolysaccharide present in the ground substance or matrix of connective tissue, particularly cartilage.

chondroiton sulfate (kondrō´-itin, kondroi´tin), *n* a mucopolysaccharide contained in skin, bones, teeth, and cartilage.

chondroma (kondrō´mə), *n* a benign tumor of cartilage. However, many chondrosarcomas arise in preexisting chondromas.

chondromyxosarcoma (kon´drōmik´sōsärkō´mə), *n* chondrosarcoma that exhibits an appreciable amount of myxomatous degeneration. See also chondrosarcoma.

chondrosarcoma (kon´drōsärkō´mə), *n* a malignant neoplasm composed of cartilage-like tissue.

Chondrosarcoma. (Sapp/Eversole/Wysocki, 2004)

chorda tympani nerve, *n* a nerve branching from the facial nerve that passes through the tympanic cavity to join the lingual branch of the mandibular nerve; it conveys taste sensation from the anterior two-thirds of the tongue and carries parasympathetic preganglionic fibers to the submandibular and sublingual salivary glands.

chorea (kôrē´ə) (St. Vitus' dance), *n* a disorder of the central nervous system resulting in purposeless, involuntary athetoid (writhing) movements of the muscles of the face and extremities. It may be associated with or follow rheumatic fever (Sydenham's chorea), hysteria, senility, or infections or it may be a hereditary disorder (Huntington's chorea).

choriamnionitis, *n* an inflammatory reaction in the amniotic membranes caused by bacteria or viruses in the amniotic fluid.

Christian's disease, *n.pr* See disease, Hand-Schüller-Christian.

Christmas disease, *n.pr* See hemophilia B.

chromatin (krō´mətin), *n* genetic material present in the nucleus, consisting of DNA and associated proteins, seen as irregular clumps in quiescent cells.

chromatography, *n* any one of several processes for separating and analyzing various gaseous or dissolved chemical materials according to differences in their absorbency with respect to a specific substance.

chromium, (Cr), *n* a hard, brittle, metallic element with an atomic number of 24 and an atomic weight of 51.996. Chromium strongly resists corrosion and is used extensively to plate other metals and as an alloy to harden steel. Stainless steels are more than 10% chromium.

chromium-cobalt-molybdenum, *n* a stainless alloy used in interosseous implants for dental prostheses.

chromogenic (krō´mōjen´ik), *adj* pertaining to color production.

chromosome (krō´məsōm), *n* one of a number of small, dark-staining, and more or less rod-shaped bodies situated in the nucleus of a cell. At the time of cell division, chromosomes divide and distribute equally to the daughter cells. They contain genes arranged along their length. The number of chromosomes in the somatic cells of an individual is constant (the diploid number), whereas just half this number (the haploid number) appears in germ cells.

chromosome aberration, n any rearrangement of chromosome parts as a result of breakage and reunion of broken ends.

chronic, *adj* characterized by a long, slow course, as opposed to *acute*.

chronic pulmonary emphysema, *n* a condition in which breathing is made difficult by an accumulation of mucus in the bronchioles and a loss of elasticity in the lungs.

chronology, *n* the arrangement of events in a time sequence, usually from the beginning to the end of an event.

chylomicrons (kī´lōmī´kronz) *n.pl* tiny lipoproteins of approximately 2% protein that convey dietary fat throughout the body.

cicatricial pemphigoid, *n* See pemphigoid, benign mucous membrane.

cicatrix (sik′ətriks) (scar), *n* the result of healing by secondary intention; characterized microscopically by excessive collagenation of the granulation tissue.

cicatrization (sikətrizā′shən), *n* the conversion of granulation tissue into scar tissue.

ciclopirox olamine (topical), *n trade name:* Loprox; *drug class:* topical antifungal; *action:* interferes with fungal cell membrane; *uses:* tinea cruris, tinea corporis, tinea pedis, tinea versicolor, cutaneous candidiasis.

ciliophora protozoa (sil′ē-of′ōrə), *n* the only human ciliate parasite *(Balantidium coli)* implicated in a type of dysentery and contracted from fecal contamination of water supplies.

cimetidine, *n trade names:* Tagamet, Apo-Cimetidine; *drug class:* H₂-histamine receptor antagonist; *action:* inhibits histamine at H₂-histamine receptor site in parietal cells, which inhibits gastric acid secretion; *uses:* short-term treatment of duodenal and gastric ulcers by the control of hyperacidity.

cineradiography (sin′irā′dē-og′rəfē), *n* the making of motion pictures by means of roentgen rays and image intensification. Studies are used for diagnosis and research purposes. Speech patterns can be studied during the process of phonation; the action of the tongue, jaws, and palate can be studied during mastication and deglutition.

cingulum (sing′gyōōlum), *n* the portion of the incisor teeth and canines, occurring on the lingual or palatal aspects, that forms a convex protuberance at the cervical third of the anatomic crown. Represents the lingual or palatal developmental lobe of these teeth.

cingulum modification, *n* the alteration of the lingual form of an anterior tooth to provide a definite seat for the support of a rest unit of a removable partial denture.

cinoxacin, *n trade name:* Cinobac; *drug class:* urinary tract antibacterial; *action:* interferes with deoxyribonucleic acid replication; *use:* urinary tract infections.

ciprofloxacin, *n trade name:* Cipro;

drug class: fluoroquinolone antiinfective; *action:* a broad-spectrum bactericidal agent that inhibits enzyme deoxyribonucleic acid (DNA) gyrase needed for replication of DNA; *uses:* adult urinary tract infection, uncomplicated gonorrhea, typhoid fever, effective against some periodontal organisms.

circuit voltmeter, *n* the device on the x-ray machine that records the line voltage on the circuit prior to the voltage being augmented by the transformer. Also may be used to measure the kilovoltage produced by the action of the transformer.

circuits, in x-ray machine, *n.pl* an x-ray machine contains two circuits, the low-voltage filament circuit and the high-voltage cathode-anode circuit. The low-voltage circuit uses a step-down transformer to form an electron cloud by heating up the filament. The high-voltage circuit uses a step-up transformer to increase the current enough to accelerate the electrons to the point that they create x-ray photons.

circulation, *n* the movement of blood through blood vessels.

circulation, peripheral, *n* the passage of fluids, electrolytes, and metabolites through the walls of terminal vessels of the vascular tree into and out of the tissue spaces.

circulation, pulmonary, *n* the circulation of venous blood from the right ventricle of the heart to the lungs and back to the left atrium of the heart.

circulation, systemic, *n* the circulation of oxygenated blood from the left ventricle of the heart to the various tissues and of venous blood back to the right atrium of the heart.

circulatory system, *n* the system for the circulation of blood, consisting of the heart, arteries, arterioles, capillaries, venules, and veins.

circulatory system, head and neck, *n* the network of arteries and veins running throughout the head and neck that carries oxygen, blood, and other fluids to and from the heart.

circumferential fibers, *n.pl* See fibers, circular.

circumferential probing, *n* an examination technique in which the probe remains in the sulcus or periodontal pockets while it is "walked" around the mouth; prevents excessive

C

trauma to the gingiva that can occur from repeated probe insertion and withdrawal.

circumferential wiring, *n* See wiring, circumferential.

circumpubertal (sur′kumpyōō′burtəl), *adj* relating to or occurring during the period of puberty.

cirrhosis, *n* a chronic degenerative disease of the liver in which blood flow is restricted and metabolic and detoxification functions are impaired or destroyed. Cirrhosis is most commonly the result of chronic alcohol abuse.

cisapride, *n trade name:* Propulsid; *drug class:* oral prokinetic; *action:* enhancement of acetylcholine release; *uses:* symptomatic treatment and prophylaxis of nocturnal heartburn caused by gastroesophageal reflux disease.

cisplatin, *n* an antineoplastic prescribed in the treatment of a wide variety of neoplasms such as metastatic testicular, prostatic, and ovarian tumors.

citric acid, *n* a white, crystalline, organic acid freely soluble in water and alcohol. It can be extracted from citrus fruits or through a fermentation of sugars. Citric acid is a key intermediary in metabolism. See also citric acid cycle.

citric acid cycle, *n* a sequence of enzymatic reactions involving the metabolism of carbon chains of sugars, fatty acids, and amino acids to yield carbon dioxide, water, and high-energy phosphate bonds. Also called *Krebs' citric acid cycle* or *tricarboxylic acid cycle.*

citrin (sit′rin), *n* See factor, platelet 1.

civil action, *n* a noncriminal legal action.

civil law, *n* a statutory law, as opposed to common law or judge-made law (such as case law). The Dental Practice Act is a civil law.

claim, *n* **1.** in a juridic sense, a demand of some type made by one person or another. **2.** a request for payment under a dental benefits plan. **3.** a statement listing services rendered, the dates of services, and itemization of costs. Includes a statement signed by the beneficiary and treating dentist that services have

been rendered. The completed form serves as the basis for payment of benefit.

claim form, *n* the form used to file for benefits under a dental benefits program; includes sections for the patient and the dentist to complete.

claimant, *n* a person who files a claim for benefits. May be the patient or the certificate holder.

claims payment fraud, *n* the intentional manipulation or alteration of facts submitted by a treating dentist, resulting in a lower payment to the beneficiary or the treating dentist than would have been paid if the manipulation had not occurred.

claims reporting fraud, *n* the intentional misrepresentation of material facts concerning treatment provided and charges made to cause a higher payment.

claims review, *n* **1.** in dental prepayment, the routine examination by a carrier or intermediary of the claim submitted to it for payment or predetermination of benefits; may include determination of eligibility, coverage of service, and plan liability. **2.** in quality assurance, examination by organizations of claims as part of a quality review or use review process.

clamp, *n* a device used to effect compression or retention.

clamp, cervical, *n* See clamp, gingival.

clamp, Ferrier 212 gingival, *n.pr* a purposely unbalanced gingival rubber dam clamp for retracting gingival tissue from the field of operation. It must be stabilized to position with modeling compound. Developed by W. I. Ferrier.

clamp, gingival, *n (cervical clamp),* a rubber dam clamp intended to retract gingival tissues.

clamp, Hatch gingival, *n.pr* an adjustable gingival rubber dam clamp.

clamp, root rubber dam, *n* a clamp with jaws designed to fit on the root surfaces of a tooth; usually used for the retention of a rubber dam.

clamp, rubber dam **(rubber dam retainer),** *n* a device made of spring metal and used to retain a rubber dam in place or improve the operating field by isolating it from the oral environment.

clarithromycin, *n trade name:* Biaxin; *drug class:* macrolide antibiotic; *action:* binds to 50S ribosomal subunits of susceptible bacteria and suppresses protein synthesis; *uses:* treatment of mild-to-moderate infections of the upper and lower respiratory tracts, otitis media, acute maxillary sinusitis.

Clark's rule, *n.pr* See rule, Clark's.

clasp, *n* an extracoronal direct retainer of a removable partial denture, usually consisting of two arms, a retentive arm and a reciprocal arm, joined by a body that may connect with an occlusal rest.

clasp, Adams, *n.pr* a formed wire clasp of modified arrowhead design using the buccomesial and distoproximal undercuts of a tooth for retention.

clasp, arm, *n* clasp extensions, usually from minor connectors, that provide retention, reciprocation, or stabilization.

clasp, arm, fatigue of, *n* a situation in which the retentive arm of a clasp metal has undergone flexure at the same point repeatedly, and fracture has resulted. Tapering the clasp arm tends to distribute the flexure and reduce such tendency to fracture.

clasp, arm, reciprocal, *n* an arm of a clasp, usually at or occlusal to the height of contour, located in such a manner as to reciprocate any force arising from an opposing clasp arm on the same tooth.

clasp, arm, retentive (**retention terminal**)**,** *n* a clasp arm that is flexible and engages the infrabulge area at the terminal end of the arm.

clasp, arrowhead, *n* a wire clasp, for retention of removable appliances, whose active elements are in the shape of an arrowhead and engage the mesioproximal and distoproximal undercuts on the buccal aspects of adjacent teeth.

clasp, back-action, *n* a clasp that originates on one surface of a tooth and traverses the suprabulge area to another surface, where it is supported by an occlusal rest; it then continues to encircle the tooth on the third surface, where it terminates in the infrabulge area beyond the opposite angle of the tooth surface where it originated.

clasp, bar, *n* a clasp with arms that are bar-type extensions from major connectors or from within the denture base; the arms pass adjacent to the soft tissues and approach the point of contact on the tooth in a cervicoocclusal direction.

clasp, bar, arm, *n* a clasp arm that originates from the denture base or from a major or minor connector. It consists of the arm, which traverses but does not contact the gingival structures, and a terminal end, which approaches its contact with the tooth in a cervicoocclusal direction.

clasp, cast, *n* a clasp made of an alloy that has been cast into the desired form and retains its crystalline structure.

clasp, circumferential, *n* a clasp that encircles more than 180 degrees of a tooth, including opposite angles, and usually contacts the tooth throughout the extent of the clasp, at least one terminal being in the infrabulge area (cervical convergence).

clasp, circumferential arm, *n* a clasp arm that has its origin in a minor connector and follows the contour of the tooth approximately in a plane perpendicular to the path of placement of the removable partial denture.

clasp, combination, *n* a clasp that employs a wrought-wire retentive arm and a cast reciprocal or stabilizing arm. A clasp that employs a bar type of retentive arm and a cast reciprocal or stabilizing arm.

clasp, continuous, *n* a secondary lingual bar.

clasp design, *n* the determination of the shape and construction of a clasp with its position outlined on the cast.

clasp, embrasure (**embrā′zhur**)**,** *n* a clasp used where no edentulous space exists. It passes through the embrasure, using two occlusal rests, and clasps the two teeth with circumferential clasps that have a common body.

clasp flexibility, *n* the property of a clasp that enables it to be bent without breaking and to return to its original form. Factors that affect the flexibility of a retentive clasp arm are its length, diameter, cross-section form, structure, and the alloy of which it is made.

clasp flexure, *n* See flexure, clasp.

clasp, formed, *n* See clasp, wrought.

C

clasp, mesiodistal, n a type of clasp that embraces the distolingual and mesial surfaces of a tooth and takes its retention in either or both mesial and distal undercuts.

clasp, reciprocal, circumferential arm, n an arm of a clasp located in such a manner as to reciprocate any force arising from an opposing clasp arm on the same tooth.

clasp, retentive circumferential arm (**retention terminal**), n a circumferential clasp arm that is flexible and engages the infrabulge area at the terminal end of the arm.

clasp, Roach, n See clasp, bar.

clasp, stabilizing circumferential arm, n a circumferential clasp arm that is rigid and contacts the tooth at or occlusal to the surveyed height of contour.

clasp, stress-breaking action of, n relief for the abutment teeth from all or part of torquing occlusal forces; partially achieved by having a retentive arm of maximum flexibility that will provide adequate retention.

clasp, wrought (**formed clasp**), n a clasp made of an alloy that has been drawn into various forms of wire.

classification, n the systematic arrangement according to characteristics of groups or classes.

classification, Angle's, n See Angle's classification, modified.

classification, Broders', n See index, Broders'.

classification, cavity, n See cavity, classification.

classification, Kennedy, n See Kennedy classification.

classification of habits, n a compilation of habits that may cause periodontal disease. Habit neuroses include lip biting, cheek biting, biting of foreign objects, and abnormal tongue pressure against the teeth. Occupational habits include thread biting, musician's habits, holding nails in the mouth, etc. Miscellaneous habits include thumb sucking, pipe smoking, incorrect toothbrushing habits, cracking nuts with the teeth, and mouth breathing.

classification of motion, n a classification system that identifies the extent of involvement of the body in completing a dental motor task.

classification of partial dentures, n grouping of partially edentulous situations based on various conditions (for example, location of the edentulous space, location of remaining teeth, position of direct retainers, and ability of oral structures to support a partial denture).

classification of periodontal diseases, n the division of periodontal diseases into three classes: (1) inflammation-gingival abrasion, gingivitis, marginal periodontitis; (2) dystrophy-disuse atrophy, occlusal traumatism, periodontosis; and (3) combinations of inflammatory and dystrophic diseases-periodontosis and periodontitis, and occlusal traumatism.

classification of pockets, n the division of pockets into two classes: (1) suprabonygingival and periodontal and (2) infrabony, according to the number of osseous walls (that is, three osseous walls, two osseous walls, one osseous wall).

clavicle, n a long, curved, horizontal bone just above the first rib, forming the ventral portion of the shoulder girdle. It articulates medially with the sternum and laterally with the scapula.

cleansing, biomechanical, n the process of cleaning and shaping a root canal with endodontic instrumentation in conjunction with irrigating solutions.

cleansing solution, n See solution, cleansing.

clearance, n **1.** a condition in which moving bodies may pass without hindrance. **2.** removal from the blood by the kidneys (for example, urea or insulin) or by the liver (for example, certain dyes).

clearance, interocclusal, n the difference in the height of the face when the mandible is at rest and when the teeth are in occlusion. This is determined by measuring the amount of space between the maxillary and mandibular teeth when the mandible is in the position of physiologic rest. The difference between the rest vertical dimension and the occlusal vertical dimension of the face, as measured in the incisal area. See also distance, interocclusal.

clearance, occlusal, n a condition in which the mandibular teeth may pass the maxillary teeth horizontally without contact or interference.

clearance time, *n* the time taken for a cariogenic exposure to pass from the mouth; depends largely upon type of food ingested, efficiency of the lips, teeth, and tongue, and the amount of saliva present in an individual's mouth.

cleat, *n* a fixed point of anchorage, usually in the form of a metal spur or loop embedded in the acrylic resin base of a Hawley retainer or soldered onto an arch wire, to which a rubber dam elastic or other device is attached during orthodontic tooth movement.

cleft, *n* a longitudinal fissure of opening.

cleft, facial, *n* fissures along the embryonal lines of the junction of the maxillary and lateral nasal processes; usually extend obliquely from the nasal ala to the outer border of the eye.

cleft, gingival, *n* a cleft of the marginal gingiva; may be caused by many factors, such as incorrect toothbrushing, a breakthrough to the surface of pocket formation, or faulty tooth positions, and may resemble a V-shaped notch.

cleft lip, *n* a congenital anomaly of the face caused by the failure of fusion between embryonic maxillary and medial nasal processes.

Cleft lip and palate. (Zitelli/Davis, 2002)

cleft, occult, *n* See submucous cleft.
cleft, operated, *n* (postoperative cleft), a cleft that has been surgically repaired.
cleft palate, *n* a congenital anomaly of the oral cavity caused by the failure of fusion between the embryonic palatal shelves.

cleft palate, alveolar graft, *n* a bone graft placed at the site of a hard palate cleft before teeth have an opportunity to break through the gingiva tissue. It creates the architecture necessary for normal eruption of the top teeth and provides support for adjacent teeth. It may also eliminate the need for prosthetic intervention in the future.

cleft palate, hard palate graft, *n* a bone graft used to block the oronasal passage in order to facilitate breathing in children with hard palate clefts.

cleft palate prosthesis, *n* See prosthesis, cleft palate.

cleft, postoperative, *n* See cleft, operated.

cleft, Stillman's, *n* small fissures extending apically from the midline of the gingival margin in teeth subjected to trauma. Although these clefts may be found in traumatism, they are not necessarily diagnostic of occlusal trauma.

cleft, submucous, *n* See submucous cleft.

cleft, unoperated, *n* a cleft of the palate that has not been surgically repaired.

cleidocranial dysostosis, *n* See dysostosis, cleidocranial.

clemastine fumarate, *n* *trade names:* Tavist, Tavist-1; *drug class:* antihistamine, H1-receptor antagonist; *action:* acts on blood vessels and gastrointestinal and respiratory systems by competing with histamine for H1-receptor sites; *uses:* allergy symptoms, rhinitis, angioedema, urticaria.

clenching, *n* the nonfunctional, forceful intermittent application of the mandibular teeth against the maxillary teeth.

cleoid (klē'-oid), *n* a carving instrument having a blade shaped like a pointed spade or claw, with cutting edges on both sides and tip.

Cleoid blade. (Roberson/Heymann/Swift, 2002)

clicking, *n* a sound associated with dysfunction of the temporomandibular joint; also the sound made by poorly fitting dentures.

clidinium bromide, *n trade name:* Quarzan; *drug class:* gastrointestinal anticholinergic; *action:* inhibits muscarinic actions of acetylcholine at postganglionic parasympathetic neuroeffector sites; *use:* treatment of peptic ulcer disease in combination with other drugs.

climacteric (klīmak′tərik, klī′makter′ik), *n* the period during which women gradually lose their reproductive capabilities as a result of aging. Also used as an adjective to describe this period.

climate, occlusal, *n* the new occlusal relationship and environment produced by occlusal adjustment, orthodontic tooth movement, or a periodontal prosthesis.

clindamycin HCl/clindamycin palmitate HCl, *n trade names:* Cleocin, Dalacin C.; *drug class:* lincomycin derivative antiinfective; *action:* binds to 50S subunit of bacterial ribosomes, suppresses protein synthesis; *uses:* infections caused by staphylococci, streptococci, pneumococci, topically for acne, bacterial vaginosis.

clinic, table, *n* a display or demonstration of a topic, limited in scope, for transmitting information to a small number of persons at a time.

clinical, *adj* pertaining to a clinic, direct patient care, or materials used in the direct care of patients.

clinical clerkship, n the assignment of medical and other health professionals to a tour of active learning in the direct care of patients.

clinical crown, n See crown, clinical.

clinical crown:clinical root ratio, n See ratio, clinical crown:clinical root.

clinical diagnosis, n See diagnosis, clinical.

clinical medicine, that aspect of medicine that deals with direct patient care.

clinical protocol, n the detailed outline of the steps to be followed in the treatment of a patient.

clinical trials, n organized studies to provide large bodies of clinical data for statistically valid evaluation of treatment.

clinical trial, *n* a trial based upon the scientific method in which a control group and a test group are compared

over a period of time in order to study a single, differing factor.

clinician, *n* a licensed primary-care professional who provides preventative, therapeutic, and educational services that promote oral health.

clinoidale (klinoid′al), *n* the most superior point on the contour of the anterior clinoid.

clioquinol, *n* an antifungal ointment or cream used topically to treat angular cheilitis. Brand name Vioform.

clobetasol propionate, *n trade names:* Dermovate, Temovate, Temovate Emollient Cream; *drug class:* topical corticosteroid group I potency; *action:* possesses antipruritic and antiinflammatory actions; *uses:* psoriasis, exzema, contact dermatitis.

clock system, *n* system in which the dental instrument and the sharpening tool are held in such a way that the optimum angle required for sharpening is achieved.

clocortolone pivalate, *n trade name:* Cloderm; *drug class:* topical corticosteroid, group III medium potency; *action:* possesses antipruritic and antiinflammatory actions; *uses:* psoriasis, eczema, contact dermatitis, pruritus.

clofibrate, *n trade names:* Abitrate, Atromid-S, Claripex, Novofibrate; *drug class:* antipherlipidemic; *action:* inhibits biosyntheis of VLDA and LDL, which are responsible for triglyceride development; increases excretion of neutral steroids; *use:* hyperlipidemia types III, IV, V.

clomiphene citrate, *n trade names:* Clomid, Serophene, Milphene; *drug class:* nonsteroidal ovulatory stimulant; *action:* binds to estrogen receptors, resulting in increase of LH and FSH release from pituitary; *use:* female infertility.

clomipramine, *n trade name:* Anafranil; *drug class:* tricylic antidepressant; *action:* inhibits both norepinephrine and serotinin (5-HT) uptake in brain; *uses:* obsessive-compulsive disorder, panic disorder, neurogenic pain.

clonazepam, *n trade names:* Klonopin, Rivotril; *drug class:* anticonvulsant, benzodiazepine derivative, controlled substance schedule IV; *action:* inhibits spike-wave formation; *uses:* akinetic myoclonic seizures.

clonic (klon′ik), *n* the alternating pattern of releasing and tightening a muscle.

clonidine HCl/clonidine transdermal, *n trade names:* Catpres, Dixarit, Catapres-TTS; *drug class:* antihypertensive, central α-adrenergic agonist; *action:* inhibits sympathetic vasomotor center in central nervous system; *uses:* hypertension, nicotine withdrawal, vascular headache.

clonus (klō′nəs), *n* alternating muscular spasm and relaxation in rapid succession.

clorazepate dipotassium, *n trade names:* Tranxene, Gen-Xene, Apo-Chlorazepate, Tranxene-SD; *drug class:* benzodiazepine, controlled substance schedule IV; *action:* produces central nervous system depression; *uses:* anxiety, acute alcohol withdrawal.

closed bite, *n* See bite, closed.

closed panel, *n* **1.** in a prepayment plan, a group of dentists sharing office facilities who provide stipulated services to an eligible group for a set premium. For beneficiaries of plans using closed panels, choice of dentists is limited to panel members. Dentists must accept any beneficiary as a patient. **2.** a closed-panel dental benefits plan exists when patients eligible to receive benefits can receive them only if services are provided by dentists who have signed an agreement with the benefits plan to provide treatment to eligible patients. As a result of the dentist reimbursement methods characteristic of a closed-panel plan, only a small percentage of practicing dentists in a given geographic area are typically contracted by the plan to provide dental services.

closed procedure, *n* the reduction of a fracture of the jaw or placement of an implant without surgical flap retraction.

closed reduction, for jaw fracture, *n* a process by which the broken portions of the jaw are approximated and stabilized without surgically opening the mucosal covering. The fixation of the reestablished approximation of the parts is accomplished with preformed bars attached to the teeth with ligatures or elastic bands.

Clostridium, *n* a genus of spore-forming anaerobic bacteria of the Bacillaceae family.

Clostridium bifermentans, *n* found in gaseous gangrene.

Clostridium botulinum, *n* causes botulism.

Clostridium perfringens, *n* the main cause of gas gangrene in humans; also causes food poisoning, cellulitis, and wound infections.

Clostridium tetani, *n* causes tetanus.

closure, *n* the act or condition of being brought together or closed up.

closure adjustive arcs of, *n.pl* arcs of jaw closure found in deflective malocclusion caused by an intercusping of the teeth that does not coincide with a centrically related jaw closure.

closure, arcs of mandibular, *n.pl* circular or elliptic arcs created by closure of the mandible.

closure, centric path of, *n* the path traversed by the mandible during closure when its associated neuromuscular mechanism is in a balanced state of tonus.

closure, velopharyngeal, *n* the closure of nasal air escape by the knee-action elevation of the soft palate and contraction of the posterior pharyngeal wall.

closure, voluntary arcs of, *n.pl* jaw closure directions consciously made by a patient.

clot, *n* coagulated blood, plasma, or fibrin.

clot, blood, *n* a coagulum formed of blood of a semisolidified nature.

clotrimazole, *n trade names:* Lotrimin, Canesten, Gyne-Lotrimin, Mycelex-7, Mycelex Troches; *drug class:* imidazole antiinfective; *action:* interferes with fungal DNA replication; *uses:* tinea pedis, tinea cruris, tinea corporis, tinea vesicolor, and *Candida albicans* infection of the mouth, throat, vulva, and vagina.

clotting factors, *n.pl* chemical and cellular constituents of the blood responsible for the conversion of fibrinogen into a mesh of insoluble fibrin causing the blood to coagulate or clot.

cloxacillin sodium, *trade names:* Apo Cloxi, Cloxapen, Novo-cloxin, Tegopen; *drug class:* penicillinase-resistant penicillin; *action:* interferes with cell-wall replication of susceptible organisms; *uses:* effective

C

for gram-positive cocci when penicillinase-producing organisms are the confirmed pathogens.

clozapine, *n* *trade name:* Clozaril; *drug class:* antipsychotic, atypical; *action:* interferes with binding of dopamine at D_1 and D_2 receptors; acts as adrenergic, cholinergic, histaminergic, and serotonergic antagonist; *uses:* management of psychotic symptoms in schizophrenic patients for whom other antipsychotics have failed.

clubbing (pulmonary osteoarthropathy), *n* a deforming enlargement of the terminal phalanges of the fingers. It is usually acquired and may be associated with certain cardiac and pulmonary diseases.

cluster, *n* in epidemiology, a composite of confirmed cases of a disease, defect, or disability that occur in close proximity to one another with regard to time or space.

cluster analysis, *n* A complex statistical technique of data analysis of numeric scale scores, producing clusters of variables related to one another.

cluster headache, *n* See histamine headache.

clutch, *n* a device made for gripping the teeth in a dental arch, to which face-bows or tracing devices may be attached rigidly enough to behave in space relations during the movements as if they were jaw outgrowths.

CMV, *n* the abbreviation for **cytomegalovirus.** See also cytomegalovirus.

coagulating current, *n* See current, coagulating.

coagulation (kō-ag′yōōlā′shən), *n* causing a liquid to solidify; clotting.

coagulation time, *n* See time, coagulation.

coal tar, *n* an extract of coal used in combination with other compounds for the treatment of chronic skin diseases, such as eczema and psoriasis. Also a derivative of tobacco smoke that may act as an irritant and carcinogen.

coalescing (kō-əles′ing), *n* a joining or fusing of parts.

coaptation (kō′-aptā′shən), *n* the bringing together of two parts so as to create a seamless alignment.

coated tongue, *n* See tongue, coated.

coating, enteric (enter′ik), *n* a tablet covering that resists the action of the fluids and enzymes in the stomach but dissolves readily in the upper intestine.

coating material, *n* a biologically acceptable, usually porous nonmetal applied over the surface of a metallic implant with the expectation that tissue ingrowth will occur in the pores. Often a carbon polymer or ceramic substance.

cobalamin, *n* See vitamin, cobalamin.

cobalt-chromium alloy, *n* See alloy, cobalt-chromium.

cocaine (C, Cadillac, Charlie, coke, freebase, gold dust, joy powder, snow), abuse of, *n* illegal recreational use of cocaine hydrochloride or one of its derivatives. Medically prescribed for its anesthetic properties. Psychological addiction may result from continued, compulsive use, typically by sniffing, injecting, applying topically, or smoking. See also crack cocaine.

Coccidioides immitis, n a dustborne fungus endemic to the windblown desert dust of southwest United States. It is the chief culprit in coccidioidomycosis.

coccidioidomycosis, *n* an infectious fungal disease caused by the inhalation of spores of the bacterium *Coccidioides immitis,* which is carried on windborne dust particles. Although endemic in the southeastern United States, coccidioidomycosis is considered among the opportunistic infections that are indicators of AIDS.

Coccobacilli, **morphologic form of,** *n.pl* the uniformly scattered small ovals that are characteristic of *Coccobacilli* bacteria.

code, *n* **1.** a system of recording information by symbols so that only selected people will know the meaning. Used also to conserve space. **2.** a systematic statement.

code of ethics, n a series of principles used as a guide in assisting a dentist to fulfill the moral obligations of professional dental practice.

codeine (kō′dēn), *n* a crystalline alkaloid, morphine methyl ether that is used as an analgesic and antitussive.

codeine sulfate/codeine phosphate, n generic codeine; *drug class:* narcotic analgesic controlled substance schedule II, Canada N; *action:* depresses pain impulse transmission in central nervous system by interacting with opioid receptors; *uses:* mild-to-moderate pain, nonproductive cough.

coding, *n* writing instructions for a computer either in machine language or nonmachine language.

Coecal (kō′kôl), *n* the trade name for dental stone (hydrocal).

coefficient, absorption, *n* See absorption coefficient.

coefficient of thermal expansion, *n* See expansion, thermal coefficient.

coefficient, phenol, *n* the ratio of potency of a given germicide to that of phenol under standard conditions.

coenzyme, *n* a nonprotein substance, such as a B-complex vitamin, that combines with enzymes to assist in the catabolic process.

coenzyme A (CoA), *n* an important metabolite in the citric acid cycle. Although not a true enzyme, it plays a significant role in the transfer of acetyl groups and the metabolism of acids and amino acids.

cofactor V, *n* See factor VII.

cognition (cognish′ən), *n* the higher mental processes, including understanding, reasoning, knowledge, and intellectual capacity.

cognitive (cog′nitiv), *adj/n* pertaining to the mental processes of knowing, perceiving, or being aware; an expression of intellectual capacity.

cognitive domain, *n* area of study that deals with the processes and measurable results of study, as well as the practical ability to apply intelligence.

cognovit note, *n* a written authority of a debtor granting entry of a judgment against the debtor if the amount set forth in the note is not paid by the debtor when due. A cognovit note sets aside every defense that the maker of the note may otherwise have had.

cohere, *v* to stick together, to unite, to form a solid mass.

coherent (Thompson/unmodified) scattering, *n* the dispersing of low-energy x-rays without losing photon energy, caused by elastic collision.

cohesion, the ability of a material to adhere to itself.

cohesive, *n* the capability to cohere or stick together to form a mass.

cohort, *n* in statistics, a collection or sampling of individuals who share a common characteristic, such as the same age or sex.

cohort study, *n* a scientific study that focuses on a specific subpopulation, such as children born on a certain date in a specific environment.

coinsurance, *n* **1.** a means of sharing, dividing, or splitting the cost of dental services between the dental plan and the insured patient. A common division is 80/20. This means the insurance company will pay 80% of the cost of the dental service and that the patient will pay 20%. Percentages vary and may be applied to scheduled or usual, customary, and reasonable fee plans. **2.** a provision of a dental benefits program by which the beneficiary shares in the cost of covered services, generally on a percentage basis. **3.** the percentage of a covered dental expense that a beneficiary must pay (after the deductible is paid). A typical coinsurance arrangement is one in which the third party pays 80% of the allowed benefit of the covered dental service and the beneficiary pays the remainder of the charged fee. Percentages vary and may apply to a table of allowance plans, usual, customary, and reasonable plans; and direct reimbursement programs.

coinsurance clause, *n* a provision in an insurance contract stipulating that the insurer will pay a specified share of dental expenses covered by the plan.

coitus (kō′-itus), *n* the act of sexual intercourse.

col (kôl), *n* refers to a depression in the gingival tissue of the interdental papilla inferior to the contact.

colchicine, *n* generic colchicine; *drug class:* antigout agent; *action:* inhibits deposition of ureate crystals in soft tissues; *uses:* gout, gouty arthritis, arrest progression of neurologic disability in multiple sclerosis.

cold, clinical applications of, *n.pl* clinical uses of cold to treat cold injury such as frostbite, relieve pain in burn injury, relieve pain in severe and acute inflammation (pulpitis), and relieve pain and swelling in contusions, abrasions, and sprains. See also heat, applied, and cold.

cold, physiologic effects of, *n* in reference to application of cold to a local area, marked vasoconstriction followed by vasodilation and edema. In extreme exposure the effects include a significant drop in temperature on the surface and a lesser drop in deeper tissue layers, depending on the degree of cold and duration of application; decreased phagocytosis; a decrease in local metabolism; and analgesia to varying degrees of anesthesia of the part exposed to cold.

cold sore, *n* See sore, canker, and herpes labialis.

cold welding, *n* See welding, cold.

cold work, *n* a deformation of the space lattice of metals by mechanical manipulation at room temperature. The process alters certain properties (for example, ductility).

cold-curing resin, *n* See resin, autopolymer.

colestipol HCl, *n trade name:* Colestid; *drug class:* antihyperlipidemic; *action:* absorbs, combines with bile acids to form insoluble complex that is excreted through feces; loss of bile acids lowers cholesterol levels; *uses:* primary hypercholesterolemia, xanthomas, digitalis toxicity, pruritus caused by biliary obstruction, diarrhea caused by bile acids.

colic, *n* a sharp visceral pain resulting from torsion, obstruction, or smooth muscle spasm of a hollow or tubular organ, such as a ureter or an intestine.

colitis, *n* an inflammatory condition of the large intestine. Most of the diseases of this group are of unknown origin.

collagen, *n* an intercellular constituent of connective tissue and bone consisting of bundles of tiny reticular fibrils, most noticeable in the white, glistening, inelastic fibers of tendons, ligaments, and fascia.

collagenase, *n* an enzyme capable of depolymerizing collagen, found in some microorganisms and believed to contribute to periodontal disease.

collapse, *n* a state of extreme prostration and depression with failure of circulation; abnormal falling in of the walls of any part or organ; with reference to a lung, an airless or fatal state of all or part of the lung.

collar, *n* the small part of the root of a tooth that is a part of an artificial tooth (denture).

collective bargaining, *n* the negotiations between organized labor and employers on matters such as wages, hours, working conditions, and health and welfare programs.

collimating film holder, *n* a stainless steel holder for x-ray film that provides rectangular lining-up (collimation) of the x-ray beam; useful when employing the paralleling technique for periapical survey. May also be called *precision film holder.*

collimation (kol'imā'shən), *n* literally, making parallel. In radiology, collimation refers to the elimination of the peripheral (more divergent) portion of a useful x-ray beam by means of metal tubes, cones, or diaphragms interposed in the path of the beam. See also diaphragm.

collimation, rectangular, *n* a method for minimizing a patient's exposure to unnecessary radiation during treatment by using a rectangular position-indicating device (PID) to reduce the size of the radiation beam.

collimator (kol'imātur), *n* a diaphragm or system of diaphragms made of an absorbent material and designed to define the dimensions and direction of a beam of radiation.

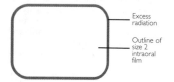

Excess radiation

Outline of size 2 intraoral film

Rectangular collimator. (Haring/Jansen, 2000)

collision tumor, *n* See tumor, collision.

colloid (kol'oid), *n* a suspension of particles in a dispersion medium. The particles generally range in size from 1 to 100 mm. Hydrocolloids and silicate cements are examples of dental colloids.

colon, *n* the body of the large intestine between the cecum and rectum.

color blindness, *n* See blindness, color.

color, temper, *n* the color produced by the thickening of the oxide coating on carbon steel as temperature is increased. Used as an indication of the degree of tempering.

coloring, extrinsic, coloring from without, as in the application of color to the external surface of a prosthesis.

coloring, intrinsic, *n* coloring from within. The incorporation of pigment within the material of a prosthesis.

Coloumb per kilogram (C/kg) (kŏŏ′lŏm pur kil′əgram), *n* the unit of measurement for radiation exposure from the French Système International d'Unités, can be converted to the traditional Roentgen (R) by the formula 1 R = 2.58 × 10⁻⁴ C/kg.

coma (kō′mə), *n* a state of unconsciousness from which the patient cannot be aroused, even by powerful stimulation. It is gradual in onset, prolonged, and not spontaneously reversible.

coma, diabetic, n unconsciousness accompanying severe diabetic acidosis. It may develop from omission of insulin, surgical complications, or disregard of dietary restrictions. Premonitory symptoms include weakness, anorexia, dry skin and mouth, drowsiness, abdominal pain, and fruity breath odor. Late symptoms are coma, air hunger, low blood pressure, tachycardia, dehydration, soft and sunken eyeballs, glycosuria, hyperglycemia, and a high level of ecetoacetic acid. See also shock, insulin.

comatose (kō′mətōs), *adj* relating to the state of being unconscious and unable to wake.

combination clasp, *n* See clasp, combination.

command, *n* the portion of a computer-related instruction that specifies the operation to be performed. A term used with hardware operations.

comminution of food, *n* See food, comminution of.

commissure (kəmish′ur), *n* the lateral angle located at the outer edge of the eye or mouth.

common deductible, *n* a deductible amount that is common to the dental and another health insurance policy (usually a major medical policy). In a major medical policy with a $100 common deductible, once $100 of medical or dental expense has been

incurred under either policy or both, no further deductible is required.

common law, *n* judge-made law, as contrasted with statutory law. This body of law originated in England and was in force at the time of the American Revolution; modified since that time on a case-by-case basis in the courts.

communicable disease, *n* any disease transmitted from one person or animal to another directly or by vectors.

communicable period, *n* the period of time when the infectious agent that causes a communicable disease may be transmitted to a susceptible host, such as in diseases that initially involve the mucous membrane (for example, diphtheria and scarlet fever). The period of communicability is from the time of exposure to the disease until termination of the carrier state, if one develops.

communication, *n* the technique of conveying thoughts or ideas between two people or groups of people.

communication, privileged, n certain classes of communications between persons who stand in a confidential or fiduciary relationship to each other that the law will not permit to be divulged in court. Examples of confidential relationships are those of psychiatrist and patient and attorney and client. Confidentiality of communications depends on the law in each state.

community dentistry, *n* a branch, discipline, or specialty of dentistry that deals with the community and its aggregate dental or oral health rather than that of the individual patient. Formal recognition of dentists engaged in community dentistry is through the American Board of Public Health Dentistry.

community health aides, *n.pl* paraprofessionals who assist in the treatment or support of patients (in their residential setting) within the patient's community environment.

Community Periodontal Index of Treatment Needs (CPITN), *n.pr* an assessment tool used to establish periodontal treatment priorities for individual children and adults or groups.

compact, *v* to form by uniting or

condensing particles with the application of pressure (for example, the progressive insertion and welding of foil and the building up of plastic amalgam in a preparation).

compacter, *n* a rotary instrument used in the McSpadden endodontic technique to condense the guttapercha cone into the root canal.

compaction, *n* the act of compacting or the state of being compact.

compensating curve, *n* See curve, compensating.

compensation, *n* the monetary reward for rendering a service; insurance providing financial return to employees in the event of an injury that occurs during the performance of their duties and that prohibits work. Compulsory in many states.

compensation, unemployment, *n* insurance covering the employee so that compensation may be provided for loss of income as a result of unemployment.

competence, *n* a measure of the degree of a person's ability to cope with all aspects of the environment.

competent, *adj* having legal capacity, ability, or authority.

compiler, *n* a computer program that translates a high-level language program into a corresponding machine instruction. The program that results from compiling is a translated and expanded version of the original program.

complaint, *n* any ailment, problem, or symptom disclosed by the patient.

complaint, chief, *n* the symptom or reason for which the patient seeks treatment. The most troublesome ailment, problem, or symptom.

complement, *n* one of 11 complex, enzymatic serum proteins. In an antigen-antibody reaction, complement causes lysis. Complement is also involved in anaphylaxis and phagocytosis.

complement fixation, *n* an immunologic reaction in which an antigen combines with an antibody and its complement, causing the complement factor to become inactive, or "fixed."

complement-fixation test (C-F test), a serologic test in which complement fixation is detected, indicating the presence of a particular antigen. The

Wassermann test for syphilis is a C-F test, used to detect amebiasis, Rocky Mountain spotted fever, tryanosomiasis, and typhus.

complemental air, *n* See volume, inspiratory reserve.

complete blood count, *n* See count, blood, complete.

complete denture, *n* See denture, complete.

complex, *n* a combination of a number of things; the sum or total of various things.

complex, craniofacial, *n* the bones and surrounding soft structure of the cranium and face.

complex, dentofacial, *n* referring to the dentition and surrounding structures.

compliance, *n* **1.** the fulfillment by the patient of the caregiver's prescribed course of treatment. **2.** the fulfillment of oversight criteria and/or standards of care necessary for licensure, certification, and accreditation.

complication, *n* a disease or injury that develops during the treatment of an earlier disorder. An example is a bacterial infection acquired by a person weakened by a viral infection.

component(s), *n* a part or element.

component, A, *n* See factor II.

component of force, *n* See force, component of.

component of partial denture, *n* See denture, partial, components of.

component, salivary, *n* See lysozyme.

component, thromboplastic cellular (TCC), *n* See factor, platelet, 3.

composite cement, *n* a dental adhesive made of colloidal silica powder combined with the matrix monomer dimethacrylate.

composite odontoma, *n* See odontoma, composite.

composite resin, *n* See resin, composite.

composites, hybrid, *n.pl* resins made from a combination of macrofill and microfill particles that are generally considered easy to polish and highly resistant to fracture and wear. They may be used for either anterior or posterior applications. See also resin, composite and resin-filled.

composites, macrofilled, *n.pl* strong resins made from small particles filled with either glass or quartz. They may be difficult to polish. See also resin, composite and resin-filled.

composites, microfilled, n.pl filled resins made from finely ground silica used for anterior esthetic restorations because they polish well and retain their shine. See also resin, composite and resin-filled.

compound, *n* **1.** a combination of elements held together in a well-defined pattern by chemical bonds. In pharmacy, a mixture of drugs. **2.** a thermoplastic substance used as a nonelastic impression material.

compound A, B, E, F, S, n See corticoid, adrenal.

compound cone, n a compound in the form of a cone or pyramid; used for impressions of individual preparations.

compound, impression (modeling compound), n See compound.

compound, intermetallic, n a compound of two metals in which the metals are only partially soluble in one another; exhibits a homogeneous grain structure, but the atoms do not intermingle randomly in all proportions.

compound, modeling, n See compound, impression.

compound, phenolic, n mouthwashes made from essential oils in combination with alcohol which is available over the counter and approved by the American Dental Association for use in controlling plaque and gingivitis. Also called *essential oils mouthrinses.*

compound tracing stick, n a compound dispensed in stick form.

compound, tray, n a compound similar to impression compound but with less flow and more viscosity when soft and more rigidity when chilled.

comprehensive dental care, *n* the coordinated delivery of the total dental care required or requested by the patient.

comprehensive health care, *n* the coordinated delivery of the total health care required or requested by the patient.

comprehensive orthodontic therapy, *n* a coordinated approach to improvement of the overall anatomic and functional relationships of the dentofacial complex, as opposed to partial correction with more limited objectives such as cosmetic improvement. Usually but not necessarily uses fixed orthodontic attachments as a part of the treatment appliance. Includes treatment and adjunctive procedures, such as extractions, maxillofacial surgery, other dental services, nasopharyngeal surgery, and speech therapy, directed at malrelationships within the entire dentofacial complex. Optimal care requires periodic evaluation of patient needs, especially during the growing years. Treatment is most effective when begun in the deciduous or mixed dentition and accomplished in successive phases as the face matures. Active correction in the adult dentition can usually be accomplished in one phase.

compressed gas cylinders, *n.pl* the color-coded storage cylinders containing either nitrous oxide (light blue) or oxygen (green or white) under pressure; used in controlled combination to induce conscious sedation.

compression, *n* the act of pressing together or forcing into less space.

compression molding, n See molding, compression.

compression of tissue, n See tissue, displaceability.

compressive strength, *n* See strength, compressive.

compromise (käm′prəmīz′), *n* an arrangement arrived at, in or out of court, for settling a disagreement on terms considered by the parties to be fair.

Compton scatter radiation, *n.pr* incidental radiation that is energized enough to break an electron bond, but instead strikes a weak bond. The leftover energy then continues in an altered direction.

compulsion (kəmpul′shən), *n* a repetitive, stereotyped, and often trivial motor action, the performance of which is compelled even though the person does not wish to perform the act. Oral habits such as bruxism and clenching may become compulsions.

computed tomography (CT), *n* a radiographic body scanning technique in which thin or narrow layer sections of the body can be imaged for diagnostic purposes. The technique uses a computer-linked x-ray machine to focus the x-rays on a particular section of the body to be viewed.

computer, *n* a device capable of accepting data in the form of facts and figures, manipulating them in a prescribed way, and supplying the results of these processes as meaningful information. This device usually consists of input and output devices, storage, arithmetic and logic units, and a control unit. Usually an automatic, stored-program machine is implied.

computer, digital, *n* a computer that operates on discrete data by performing arithmetic and logic processes on them.

computer graphics, *n* the use of computers to create illustrations or designs.

computer language, *n* the vocabulary and syntax of a set of symbols that are used to instruct a computer what to do (for example, Java, Ada, C++).

computer literacy, *n* a functional knowledge of the use and application of computers, from word processing to data management.

computer output microfilm (COM), *n* a system that allows a computer user to produce microfilm copies of computer output. The COM unit operates independently of the CPU and is therefore called an *off-line* device. Output from computer processing is recorded on generic media and later recorded on microfilm.

computer simulation, *n* the use of computers to replicate a mechanical or biologic function.

computer-aided design, *n* the use of computers to assist a draftsman, architect, or artist in the creation of drawing, illustration, or visual art.

computer-controlled delivery (WAND), *n* a computer-driven arrangement of software, hardware, and dental implements used to administer anesthetic injections in which the amount of drug and injection speed are predetermined by a software-driven motor. The injection itself is manually applied.

concanavalin A, *n* a hemagglutinin, isolated from the meal of the jack bean, that reacts with polyglucosans in the blood of mammals, causing agglutination. It has been used to stimulate T-cell production.

conceal, *v* to hide; secrete; withhold from the knowledge of others.

concise, *n.pr* the brand name for diacrylate resin adhesives used in composite restorations and for bonding orthodontic appliances to the enamel.

concrescence (känkres′əns), *n* **1.** the union of two teeth after eruption, by the fusion of their cementum surfaces. **2.** the fusion of teeth after their roots have formed. The union is effected by cementum. See also fusion.

Concrescence. (Sapp/Eversole/Wysocki, 2004)

condensation (kän′densā′shən), *n* a commonly used term for the insertion and compression or compaction of dental materials into a prepared cavity. Compaction is a more accurate term than condensation. See also compaction.

condenser (kənden′sur), *n* (formerly called *plugger*), an instrument or device used to compact or condense a restorative material into a prepared cavity. Its working end is called the *nib,* or *point;* the end of the nib is termed the *face.* The face may be smooth or serrated.

condenser, amalgam **(amalgam plugger),** *n* an instrument used to condense plastic amalgam.

condenser, automatic, *n* See condenser, mechanical.

condenser, back-action, *n* a condenser with the shank bent into a U shape so that the condensing force is a pulling motion rather than the usual pushing force.

condenser, bayonet, n a condenser in which the offset of the nib and the approximately right-angled bends in the shank permit a better line of force for condensation of direct filling gold. There are many variations in angles, length, and diameter of the nib.

condenser, electromallet (**McShirley's electromallet**), n an electromechanical device for compacting direct filling gold. Frequency of blows may be varied from 200 to 3,600 strokes/min; the intensity of the blow is controlled electronically.

condenser, foil, n a condenser used to compact direct-filling gold.

condenser, foot, n a foil condenser with the nib shaped like a foot.

condenser, hand, n an instrument that compacts material, the force being applied by the muscular effort of the operator with or without supplementary force from a mallet in the hand of the assistant.

condenser, Hollenback, n.pr See condenser, pneumatic.

condenser, long-handled foil, n a hand condenser of varied design for compacting gold foil.

condenser, mechanical, n (automatic mallet), a device to supply an automatically controlled blow for condensing restorative material. It may be spring activated, pneumatic, or electronically controlled.

condenser, parallelogram, n a condenser the face of which is shaped like a rectangle or parallelogram.

condenser, pneumatic (**Hollenback condenser**), n a pneumatic mechanical device developed by George M. Hollenback to supply a compacting force. The force is delivered by controlled pneumatic pressure. Blows are variable in intensity, with speed variable up to 300 strokes/min.

condenser point, n See point, condenser.

condenser, round, n a condenser the face of which has a circular outline.

condenser, stepping, n the orderly movement of a condenser point over the surface of gold foil or amalgam during its placement and compaction.

condensing force, n See force, condensing.

condensing osteitis, n See osteitis, condensing.

condensor (spreader), n an instrument used in filling a root canal to compress the filling material in a lateral direction.

conditioner, n **1.** an additive substance used to increase the effectiveness of another substance. **2.** a substance added to enamel that improves a sealant's ability to adhere.

conditioning, n a form of learning based on the development of a response or set of responses to a stimulus or series of stimuli.

conduct, dishonorable, n conduct that mars the character and lessens the reputation; conduct that is shameful, disgraceful, base.

conduction, n the carrying of sound waves, heat, light, nerve impulses, and electricity.

conduction, air, n the process of transmitting sound waves to the cochlea by way of the outer and middle ear. In normal hearing, practically all sounds are transmitted in this way, except those of the hearer's own voice, which are transmitted partly by bone conduction.

conduction, bone, n the transmission of sound waves or vibrations to the cochlea by way of the bones of the cranium.

conduction, impulse, n the conduction of an impulse along the nerve fiber, accompanied by an alteration of the electrical potential of the fiber tissue and an exchange of electrolytes across the nerve fiber membrane.

conductivity, n the capacity for conduction; ability to convey.

conductivity, electrical, n the ability of a material to conduct electricity. Metals are usually good conductors, and nonmetals are poor conductors.

conductivity, thermal, n the ability of a material to transfer heat. Thermal conductivity is of great importance in dentistry, where a low thermal conductivity is desirable in restorative material and a high thermal conductivity is desirable when soft tissue is covered.

condylar (kän´dilur), adj pertaining to the mandibular condyle.

condylar axis, n See axis, condylar.

condylar guide, n See guide, condylar.

condylar guide inclination, n See guide, condylar, inclination.

condyle (kän´dīl), *n* the rounded surface at the articular end of a bone.

condyle head, n a redundant term—the word *condyle* means *head*. See also condyle.

condyle, lateral path, n the path of the condyle in the glenoid fossa when a lateral mandibular movement is made.

condyle, mandibular, n the articular process of the mandible; the condyloid process of the mandible.

condyle, neck of, n See process, condyloid, neck of.

condyle, orbiting, n See orbiting condyle.

condyle path, n the path traveled by the mandibular condyle in the temporomandibular joint during the various mandibular movements.

condyle, protrusive path, n the path of the condyle when the mandible is moved forward from its centric position.

condyle, rod, n See rod, condyle.

condyle, rotating, n the condyle on the side of the bolus formation, or the one that is braced and placed and rotated while the bolus is being chewed.

condylectomy (kän´dilek´tōmē), *n* the surgical removal of a condyle.

condyloid process, *n* See process, condyloid.

condyloplasty, *n* a surgical procedure to alter the shape of the condyle to remove the effects of degenerative disease.

condylotomy (kän´dilot´ōmē), *n* surgical division through, without removal of, a condyle; or removal of a portion, usually the articular surface, of a condyle.

cone, *n* **1.** a geometric shape with a circular base tapering evenly to an apex. **2.** a solid substance, usually guttapercha or silver, having a tapered form similar in length and diameter to a root canal; used to fill the space once occupied by the pulp in the root of the tooth. **3.** an accessory device on a dental x-ray machine, designed to indicate the direction of the central axis of its x-ray beam and to serve as a guide in establishing a desired source-to-film distance.

cone distance, n the distance between the focal spot and the outer end of the cone; usually expressed in inches or centimeters. Modern dental roentgen-ray units usually have cone distances of from 5 to 20 inches (12.5 to 50 cm).

cone, long, n a tubular "cone" designed to establish an extended anode-to-skin distance, usually within a range of from 12 to 20 inches (30 to 50 cm).

cone, sharpening, n a tapered or straight cylindrical stone that is used primarily to sharpen the curvature of dental instruments. See also stone, Arkansas and stone, Carborundum.

Sharpening cone. (Daniel/Harfst, 2002)

cone, short, n a conical or tubular "cone" having as one of its functions the establishment of an anode-to-skin distance of up to 9 inches (22.5 cm).

cone socket handles, *n.pl* the handheld parts of instruments which may be separated from the working ends in order to replace or exchange individual parts.

cone-cut, *n* a technical error in the x-ray taking process where the position-indicating device is improperly aligned, causing the film to be incompletely covered by the radiation beam.

Cone cutting. (Frommer, 2001)

confidence interval, *n* a statistical device used to determine the range within which an acceptable datum would fall. Confidence intervals are usually expressed in percentages, typically 95% or 99%.

confidential, *adj* pertaining to information that is only shared with those directly responsible for patient care.

confidentiality, *n* the nondisclosure of certain information except to another authorized person.

confusion, *n* a mental state characterized by disorientation regarding time, place, or person that causes bewilderment, perplexity, lack of orderly thought, and inability to act decisively or perform the activities associated with daily living.

congenital, *adj* present at birth and usually developed in utero.

congestion, *n* See hyperemia.

congestive heart failure, *n* an abnormal condition characterized by circulatory congestion (retention of fluids) caused by cardiac or kidney disorders. This condition usually develops chronically in association with the retention of sodium and water by the kidneys. Acute congestive heart failure may result from myocardial infarction of the left ventricle.

conjugate, *v* **1.** to unite. **2.** the product of conjugation.

conjugation, *n* in biochemistry, the union of a drug or toxic substance with a normal constituent of the body, such as glucuronic acid, to form an inactive product that is then eliminated.

conjunctiva, the mucous membrane lining the inner surfaces of the eyelids and anterior part of the sclera.

conjunctivitis, *n* an inflammation of the conjunctiva, caused by bacterial or viral infection, allergy, or environmental factors. Also called *pinkeye.*

connective tissue, *n* See tissue, connective.

connector, *n* the part of a partial denture that unites its components.

connector, anterior palatal major, n a major connector uniting bilateral units of a maxillary removable partial denture. It is a thin metal plate that is located in the anterior palatal region.

connector bar, n See bar, connector.

connector, cross-arch bar splint, n a removable cross-arch connector used to stabilize weakened abutments that support a fixed prosthesis by attachment to teeth on the opposite side of the dental arch. It can be removed by the dentist but not by the patient.

connector, lingual bar major, n a type of connector used to unite the right and left components of a mandibular removable partial denture and occupy a position lingual to the alveolar ridge.

connector, linguoplate major, n a major connector formed by the extension of a metal plate from the superior border of the regular lingual bar, across gingivae, and onto the cingulum of each anterior tooth.

connector, major, n a metal plate or bar (for example, lingual bar, linguoplate, palatal bar) used to join the units of one side of a removable partial denture to those located on the opposite side of the dental arch.

connector, minor, n the connecting link between the major connector or base of a removable partial denture and other units of the restoration, such as direct and indirect retainers and rests.

connector, nonrigid, n a connector used where retainers or pontics are united by a joint permitting limited movement. It may be a precision or a nonprecision type of connector.

connector, posterior palatal major, n (posterior palatal bar), a major transpalatal connector located in the posterior palatal region. It is used when the anterior palatal bar alone is insufficient to provide the necessary rigidity.

connector, rigid, n a connector used where retainers or pontics are united by a soldered, cast, or welded joint.

connector, saddle, n See connector, major.

connector, secondary lingual bar major **(Kennedy bar),** *n* often called a *continuous clasp* or *Kennedy bar.* It rests on the cingulum area of the lower anterior teeth and serves principally as an indirect retainer and/or stabilizer for weakened anterior lower teeth.

connector, subocclusal, n a nonrigid connector positioned gingival to the occlusal plane.

consanguinity, *n* a hereditary or "blood" relationship between persons, by virtue of having a common parent or ancestor.

conscious, *adj* pertaining to the state of mind in which an individual is able to breathe on his or her own and to respond to verbal commands and physical prompts.

conscious sedation, *n* a state of sedation in which the patient remains aware of his or her person, surroundings, and conditions but without experiencing pain or anxiety.

consciousness, *n* a state in which the individual is capable of rational response to questioning and has all protective reflexes intact, including the ability to maintain a patent airway.

consent, *n* the concurrence of wills; permission.

consent, express, *n* consent directly given by voice or in writing.

consent, implied, *n* consent made evident by signs, actions, or facts, or by inaction or silence.

consideration, *n* inducement to make a contract. It may be a benefit to the promisor or a loss or detriment to the promisee. Consideration must be regarded as by both parties.

Consolidated Omnibus Budget Reconciliation Act (COBRA), *n.pr* legislation relative to mandated benefits for all types of employee benefits plans. The most significant aspects within this context are the requirements for continued coverage for employees and their dependents for 18 months who would otherwise lose coverage (30 months for dependents in the event of an employee's death).

consonant, *n* a conventional speech sound produced, with or without laryngeal vibration, by certain successive contractions of the articulatory muscles that modify, interrupt, or obstruct the expired airstream to the extent that its pressure is raised.

consonant, semivowel, *n* consonants that are like vowels both perceptually and physiologically.

constipation, *n* difficulty passing stools or incomplete or infrequent passage of hard stools.

constituent (kənstich′yōō-ənt), *n* a part of the whole; component.

constitution, *n* the general makeup of the body as determined by genetic,

physiologic, and biochemical factors. An individual's constitution may be markedly influenced by environment.

constriction, *n* an abnormal closing or reduction in the size of an opening or passage of the body.

construction, single denture, *n* the making of one upper or lower denture as distinguished from a set of two complete dentures.

consultant, *n* a professional or nonprofessional person who, by virtue of special knowledge of professional or nonprofessional aspects of a dental practice, is sought out for advice and training.

consultation, *n* a meeting of persons to discuss or decide something.

consultation, patient, *n* a meeting between the dentist, patient, and other interested persons for the purpose of discussing the patient's dental needs, proposing treatment, and making business arrangements.

consultation, professional, *n* a joint deliberation by two or more dentists and/or physicians to determine the diagnosis, treatment, or prognosis for a particular patient.

consumer, *n* one who may receive or is receiving dental service; the term is also used in health legislation and programs as a reference to someone who is never a practitioner or is not associated in any direct or indirect way with the supplying or provision of dental services.

contact, *n* the act of touching or meeting.

contact, balancing, *n* the contact established between the upper and lower dentures at the side opposite the working side (anteroposteriorly or laterally) for the purpose of stabilizing the dentures.

contact, deflective occlusal, *n* (cuspal interference), a condition of tooth contacts that diverts the mandible from a normal path of closure to centric jaw relation or causes a denture to slide or rotate on its basal seat. See also contact, interceptive occlusal.

contact, faulty, *n* imperfections in the contact between adjacent teeth. Often leads to food impaction between the teeth, with subsequent initiation or perpetuation of periodontal lesions.

contact, initial, n the first meeting of opposing teeth on elevation of the mandible toward the maxillae.

contact, interceptive occlusal, n an initial contact of teeth that interferes with the normal movement of the mandible. See also contact, deflective occlusal.

contact, premature, n See deflective occlusal and contact, interceptive.

contact, working, n a contact of the teeth made on the side of the dental arch toward which the mandible has been moved.

contagious (kəntā′jus), *adj* capable of being transmitted from one person to another by direct or indirect contact.

contaminated, *v* made radioactive by the addition of minute quantities of radioactive material.

contamination, radioactive, n the deposition of radioactive material in any place where it is not desired, and particularly where its presence may be harmful or may constitute a radiation hazard.

contingent (kəntin′jənt), *adj* dependent for effect on something that may or may not occur.

continuant, n a speech sound in which the speech organs are held relatively fixed during the period of production.

continuing education, n postgraduate study offered either in an institution of higher learning by groups with an organized dental program or by individuals who are especially qualified in certain areas. Required by some state licensing boards for license renewal. Credit accumulates for special qualifications to join special interest groups.

continuing education unit (CEU), n educational classes or experiences for licensed professionals that extend, update, or renew their knowledge of practices in their field. Some classes may be required for relicensing. Usually, 1 CEU equals one clock hour of instruction.

continuous bar retainer, n See retainer, continuous bar.

continuous clasp, n See retainer, continuous bar.

continuous loop wiring, n See wiring, continuous loop.

contour, n the external shape, form, or surface configuration of an object.

contour, n height of, the greatest convexity of a tooth viewed from a predetermined position.

contour, anatomic height of, n a line encircling a tooth to designate its greatest convexity.

contour, buccal, n the shape of the buccal aspect of a posterior tooth. It normally has occlusocervical convexity, with its greatest prominence at the gingival third of the clinical buccal surface.

contour, gingival, n the shape of the natural or artificial gingiva as it approximates the natural or artificial tooth.

contour, proximal, n the form of the mesial or distal surface of a tooth.

contour, restoration, n the restoration of a proper contour where surfaces of teeth have been destroyed by disease processes or excessive wear.

contour, tooth, n a shape of a tooth that is essential to a healthy gingival unit because it enables the bolus of food to be deflected from gingival margins during mastication.

contouring, occlusal, n the correction, by grinding, of gross disharmonies of the occlusal tooth form (for example, uneven marginal ridges, plunger cusps, extruded teeth, malpositioned teeth) to establish a harmonious occlusion and protect the periodontium of the tooth.

contouring pliers, n See pliers, contouring.

contra-angle (kän′trə-ang′gəl), n more than one angle. An instrument having two or more offsetting angles such that the end of the instrument is kept within 3 mm of the axis of the shaft.

contraception, n a process or technique for the prevention of pregnancy by means of a medication, device, or method that blocks or alters one or more of the processes of reproduction in such a way that sexual union can occur without impregnation.

contract, n **1.** an agreement based on sufficient consideration between two or more competent parties to do or not to do something that is legal. **2.** a legally enforceable agreement between two or more individuals or entities that confers rights and duties on the parties. Common types of contracts include (1) those contracts between a dental benefits organization and an individual dentist to provide dental treatment to members of an alternative benefits plan. These contracts define the dentist's duties both to beneficiaries of the dental benefits plan and the dental benefits organization, and usually define the manner in which the dentist will be reimbursed; and (2) contracts between a dental benefits organization and a group plan sponsor. These contracts typically describe the benefits of the group plan and the rates to be charged for those benefits.

contract, breach of, n the failure, without legal excuse, to perform an obligation or duty in a contract.

contract dentist, n a practitioner who contractually agrees to provide services under special terms, conditions, and financial reimbursement arrangements.

contract dentistry, n 1. providing dental care under a specific set of guidelines and for a specific set of individuals under an accepted written agreement by the patient, dentist, and employer. 2. the practice of dentistry whereby the dentist enters into a written agreement with either patients or an employer to provide dental care for a set group of people.

contract, express, n a contract that is an actual agreement between the parties, with the terms declared at the time of making, being stated in explicit language either orally or in writing.

contract fee schedule plan, n a dental benefits plan in which participating dentists agree to accept a list of specific fees as the total fees for dental treatment provided.

contract, implied, n a contract not evidenced by explicit agreement of the parties but inferred by the law from the acts and circumstances surrounding the transactions.

contract, open-end, n 1. a contract that permits periodic reevaluation of the dental plan during the contract year. If indicated by the reevaluation, dental services may be deleted or added to achieve a balance between the premium and cost of service provided. 2. a contract that sets no dollar limits on the total services to be provided to beneficiaries but does list the particular services that will be included in the plan.

contract practice, n dental practice in which an employer or third-party administrator contracts directly with a dentist or group of dentists to provide dental services for beneficiaries of a plan. See also closed panel.

contract term, n the period of time, usually 12 months, for which a contract is written.

contraction, n 1. a shortening, shrinkage, or reduction in length or size. 2. a condition in which teeth or other maxillary and mandibular structures, such as the dental arch, are nearer than normal to the median plane.

contraction, concentric muscle, n an unresisted ordinary shortening of muscle.

contraction, eccentric muscle, n an increase in muscle tonus during lengthening of the muscle. Eccentric contraction occurs when muscles are used to oppose movement but not to stop it (for example, the action of the biceps in lowering the forearm gradually and in a controlled manner). Eccentric contractions are called *isotonic,* because the muscle changes length.

contraction, isometric muscle, n an increase in muscular tension without a change in muscle length, as in clenching the teeth.

contraction, isotonic muscle, n an increase in muscular tension during movement without resistance (either lengthening or shortening), as in free opening and closing of the jaws.

contraction, metal, n shrinkage associated with the congealing of a metal from its molten state to a solid after having been cast. See also expansion, thermal.

contraction, muscle, n the development of tension in a muscle in response to a nerve stimulus.

contraction, muscle, changes in striation bands, n.pl alterations in bands of striated muscle during contraction. Striated muscle is composed of a darker A band and a lighter I band. Both of these alternating bands develop tension during contraction but not to the same degree. In isometric contraction (clenched teeth), the sarcomere muscle unit remains unchanged in length, whereas the A band (the darker band) actually shortens and the I band (the lighter band) lengthens. When a muscle is passively stretched, such as when the mandible is opened by gravity, the A band lengthens relatively more than the I band, and during isotonic contraction, almost all the shortening is in the A segment. It is thus concluded that the contractile properties are not the same throughout the sarcomere, which is the unit of contractility. It is suggested that the darker A band has a greater concentration of contractile substance than the I band and that, in addition to contractile elements, the I band contains elastic noncontractile elements that constitute a series of elastic components throughout the fibril. Thus there is, throughout a fiber, an arrangement of dark, contractile components alternating with lighter, elastic components.

contraction, muscle, chemical factors in, *n.pl* the chemical constituents and action involved in the contraction of muscle fibers. Muscle is a structure with working units built up largely from two proteins, actin and myosin, which appear to be organized into separate filaments running longitudinally through the muscle fibers. Neither type of filament runs continuously along the length of the fiber, although the effect is that of a continuous structure. The filaments are organized into a succession of groupings of one type of fiber. Each group is arranged in a regular palisade to overlap the next group of fibers, which are similarly arranged in palisades. This gives a banded appearance to the fiber. The thicker filaments contain myosin and are restricted to the A bands, where they give rise to a higher density and double refraction. The thinner filaments contain actin and extend to either side of the Z band, which is at the center of the I band. When the muscle contracts or is stretched, the two groups of filaments slide past each other like the alternating units of a sliding gate. The controlled sliding motion is presumably brought about through the mediation of oblique cross links between the filaments. These cross links are the

structural expression of the biochemical interaction between actin and myosin. The chemical substance that initiates the interaction between these fibrils is adenosine triphosphate (ATP). The final effect of the interaction between ATP, myosin, and actin is to enable the two types of filaments to crawl past each other to create the shortened state of the muscle.

contraction, postural muscle, *n* maintenance of muscular tension (usually isometric muscular contraction) sufficient to maintain posture.

contraction, smooth muscle, mechanism of, *n* the mechanisms that regulate the functions of smooth muscle fibers. These regulatory mechanisms vary and are affected principally by two methods. First, the parasympathetic and sympathetic nerve fiber endings of the autonomic nervous system form a reticulum around the muscle cells before entering them. The action of these fibers is antagonistic; they act directly on the muscle cell, not on each other. Examples of the structures principally under the control of the autonomic nerve mechanism are the blood vessels and the pilomotor fibers. Second, the selection response to rhythmic activity associated with the automaticity of a viscus or other organ depends on local or hormonal factors. An example of this mechanism is the function of the uterus under the control of the estrogenic hormone.

contraction, static muscle, *n* contraction in which opposing muscles contract against each other and prevent movement. Fixation action of a muscle in a static contraction is termed *isometric,* because it develops tension without changing length.

contractor, independent, *n* one who, exercising an independent employment, contracts to do a piece of work according to the conditions of the contract and without being subject to control except as to the result of the work.

contracture, *n* a permanent shortening, or contraction, of a muscle.

contraindication (kon´trə-in´dikā´ shən), *n* any symptom or circumstance indicating the inappropriateness of a form of treatment otherwise advisable.

contralateral (kon'trəlat'ərəl), *adj* originating from or affecting the opposite side of a reference point.

contrast, radiographic (radiographic image), *n* the differences in photographic or film density produced on a radiograph by structural composition of the object radiographed or by varying amounts of radiation.

contrast, radiographic, long-scale, n an increased number of gradations of gray between the blacks and whites on a radiograph. Higher kilovoltages increase the scale of contrast.

contrast, radiographic, media, n a radiopaque substance injected into the body to facilitate radiographic imaging of internal structures that otherwise are difficult to visualize on x-ray films.

contrast, radiographic, short-scale, n a minimum number of gradations of gray between the blacks and whites on a radiograph. Lower kilovoltages decrease the scale of contrast.

contrast, subject, *n* See contrast, radiographic.

contributory negligence, *n* See negligence, contributory.

contributory plan, *n* a method of payment for group insurance coverage in which part of the premium is paid by the employee and part is paid by the employer or union.

contributory program, *n* a dental benefits program in which the enrollee shares in the monthly premium of the program with the program sponsor (usually the employer). Generally done through payroll deduction.

control group, *n* the group of participants in a clinical study who do not receive the drug or treatment being studied against which the reactions of individuals in the experimental group may be compared. See also controlled clinical trial.

control, stress, *n* any method used to diminish or remove the stress load generated by occlusal contact, whether the contact is functional in origin or the result of a habit cycle.

controlled clinical trial, *n* a research strategy that calls for two samples: an experimental sample of patients receiving a pharmaceutical, and a second sample of control patients receiving a placebo. Neither the patient nor the researcher knows which is receiving the pharmaceutical and which the placebo.

controlled substance, any drug as defined in the five categories of the federal Controlled Substances Act of 1970. The categories, or schedules, cover opium and its derivatives, hallucinogens, depressants, and stimulants.

controlled-release therapeutic systems, *n* a drug or hormone delivery system that releases predetermined amounts of drug or hormone into the body over a specified period of time.

contusion (kəntōō'zhən), *n* a bruise that is usually produced by impact from a blunt object and that does not cause a break in the skin.

convenience form, *n* See form, convenience.

convergence, cervical, *n* the angle formed between the cervicoaxial inclination of a tooth surface on one side and a diagnostic stylus of a dental cast surveyor in contact with the tooth at its height of contour.

conversion privilege, *n* the right of an individual covered by a group dental insurance policy to continue having coverage on a direct payment basis when association with the insured group is terminated.

converter, rotary, *n* a motor generator set or unit that, when operated by one type of current, produces another (for example, the conversion of alternating to direct current).

convertin, *n* See thromboplastin, extrinsic.

convulsion (kənvul'shən), *n* an intense seizure.

coolant (kōō'lənt), *n* air or liquid directed onto a tooth, tissue, or restoration to neutralize the heating effect of a rotary instrument.

Cooley's anemia, *n.pr* See thalassemia major.

Cooley's trait, *n.pr* See thalassemia minor.

Coolidge filament transformer, tube, *n.pr* See transformer, Coolidge.

coordination, *n* harmonious functioning of body systems.

coordination of benefits clause, n 1. a provision in an insurance contract that when a patient is covered under more than one group dental plan, benefits paid by all plans will be limited to 100% of the actual charges after each deductible has been satisfied. **2.** COB: a method of integrating benefits payable under more than one plan. Benefits from all sources should not exceed 100% of the total charges.

Copal resin, *n.pr* a mixed resin of diverse plant origin used in cavity varnishes. Its effectiveness in protecting the pulp from the phosphoric acid in dental cements is questioned.

copayment, *n* the beneficiary's share of the dentist's fee after the benefits plan has paid.

cope, *n* the upper half of a flask in the casting art; hence also the upper, or cavity, side of a denture flask.

coping (thimble), *n* a thin metal covering or cap over a prepared tooth.

coping, parallel, *n* a casting placed over an implant abutment to make it parallel to other natural or implant abutments.

coping, transfer, *n* a covering or cap, made of metal, acrylic resin, or other material used to position a die in an impression.

copolymer (kōpäl'imur), *n* polymerization of two or more monomers that have slightly different chemical formulas. Used in dentistry to impart certain desirable physical properties such as flow.

**copolymerization
(kōpäl'imərizā'shən),** *n* the formation of a copolymer.

copper, *n* a malleable, reddish brown metallic element. Copper is a component of several important enzymes in the body and is essential to good health. Copper deficiency is rare, because only 2 to 5 mg daily are necessary, and that amount is easily obtained in a normal diet.

coprolalia (kop'rōlā'lē-ə), *n* the uncontrollable vocalization of obscene or offensive words.

**coproporphyria
(kop'rōpôr'fir'ē-ə),** *n* the presence of an abnormal concentration of coproporphyrin in the urine. Normal values range from 70 mg to 250 mg/day. An increased amount of coproporphyrin III occurs in the urine in clinical lead poison-

ing, exposure to lead without clinically apparent symptoms, infections, malignant disease, alcoholic cirrhosis, after ingestion of small amounts of ethanol, and normally in some individuals.

coproporphyrin, *n* any of the nitrogenous organic substances normally excreted in the feces as a breakdown of bilirubin.

cord(s), *n* a long, rounded organ or body.

cord, spinal, *n* the central nervous system cord contained in the vertebral column. The spinal cord is essential to the regulation and administration of various motor, sensory, and autonomic nerve activities of the body. Through its pathways it conducts impulses from the extremities, trunk, and neck to and from the higher centers and to consciousness. It thus provides for simple reflexes, has control over visceral activities, and participates in the conscious activities of the body.

cord, vocal, the membranous structures in the throat that produce sound; the thyroarytenoid ligaments of the larynx. The inferior cords are called the *true vocal cords,* and the superior cords are called the *false vocal cords.*

core, *n* the central part. A section of a mold, usually of plaster, made over assembled parts of a dental restoration or construction to record and maintain the relationships of the parts so that the parts can be reassembled in their original positions. Synonym. *laboratory core.*

core, amalgam, *n* the foundational replacement of the badly mutilated crown of a tooth whose purpose is to provide a rigid base for retention of a cast crown restoration. The core may be retained by undercuts, slots, pins, or the pulp chamber of an endodontically treated tooth.

core, cast, *n* a metal casting, usually with a post in the canal or a root, designed to retain an artificial crown.

core, composite, *n* composite resin buildup to provide retention for a cast crown restoration.

core, laboratory, a section of a mold, usually of plaster, made over assembled parts of a dental restoration or construction to record and maintain the relationships of the parts so that the parts can be reassembled in their original positions.

core-vent implant system, *n* an endosseous implant system (provisionally accepted by the ADA) that uses the criteria of osseous integration constructed of medical grade titanium alloy after the design of Branemark, in which the apical portion that is able to be submerged is of a hollow-vented design. The superior part is machined to receive a variety of prosthodontic abutments.

corium, gingival (kō′rē-əm), *n* the most stable, inert, and mature phase of connective tissue elements of the gingiva lying between the periosteum and the lamina propria mucosae.

cornea, *n* the transparent anterior part of the eye.

cornification, *n* the conversion of epithelium to a hornlike substance. *Keratinization* is a more specific term implying the formation of true keratin.

cornu (kôr′nōō), *n* in anatomy, a bony projection shaped like a horn.

coronal, *adj* pertaining to the crown portion of teeth.

coronary angioplasty, percutaneous transluminal, *n* a surgical technique designed to improve circulation. It involves the insertion of a balloon-carrying catheter into a blood vessel of the heart that is clogged with plaque, then alternately inflating and deflating the balloon several times to flatten the plaque against the arterial walls and reestablish the free flow of blood. Also called *balloon angioplasty* or *coronary dilation.*

coronary artery bypass, *n* openheart surgery in which a section of a blood vessel is grafted onto one or more of the coronary arteries to improve the blood supply to the muscles of the heart.

Coronaviridae **(kôrō′nəvir′idā),** *n.pl* a family of enveloped, helical, airborne RNA viruses responsible for some respiratory and gastrointestinal diseases. It can also be contracted from unsanitary equipment or from human carriers.

coronoid notch, *n* See notch, coronoid.

coronoid process, *n* See process, coronoid.

coronoidectomy (kor′ōnoidek′tōmē), *n* the surgical removal of the coronoid process of the mandible.

corporate dentistry, *n* **1.** dental care provided for a specific group of employees within a single business under a contract arrangement or on a salaried basis, with costs borne by the corporation. **2.** a company-owned-and-operated dental care facility that provides services to employees and sometimes dependents.

corpus callosum, *n* the largest commissure of the brain connecting the cerebral hemispheres.

corpuscle(s), *n* any small body, mass, or organ.

corpuscle, blood, *n* a formed element in the blood. See also erythrocyte, leukocyte, lymphocyte, monocyte.

corpuscle, Golgi's, *n.pr* a small, spindle-shaped proprioceptive endorgan located in tendons and activated by stretch.

corpuscle, Krause's, *n.pr* bulboid encapsulated nerve endings located in mucous membranes and activated by cold.

corpuscle, Meissner's, *n.pr* medium encapsulated nerve endings found in the skin and activated by light touch.

corpuscle, Merkel's, *n.pr* specialized sensory nerve endings located in the submucosa of the mouth and activated by light touch.

corpuscle, Pacini's, *n.pr* large sensory nerve endings, scattered widely in subcutaneous tissues, joints, and tendons and activated by deep pressure.

corpuscle, Ruffini's, *n.pr* specialized sensory nerve organs in the skin and mucous membranes for perceiving heat. Temperature variations of less than 5° C are not readily received by these end organs.

corrected master cast, *n* See cast, master, corrected.

correction, occlusal, *n* correction of malocclusion, by whatever means is employed, including the elimination of disharmony of occlusal contacts.

corrective, *n* a prescription ingredient designed to compensate for or nullify specific undesirable effects of the principal pharmaceutical agent and the adjuvant.

correlation, *n* a statistical procedure

used to determine the degree to which two (or more) variables vary together. Correlation does not suggest a cause-effect relationship but only the degree of parallelism or concomitance between the variables, the cause of which may be unknown. The *Pearson product-moment correlation (r)* is the most frequently used, and this coefficient is used unless another is specified.

correlation, coefficient number, n the result of statistical computation that indicates the strength of the tendency of two or more variables to vary concomitantly. The coefficient is expressed in fractions (that is, r = 80), ranging from 21 to 11, and indicates the magnitude of the relationship between the variables. Perfect direct correspondence is expressed by 11; perfect inverse correspondence by 21; complete lack of correspondence by 0. Fractional values are not read as percents.

correlation, linear, n a correlation in which the regression line, the line that best describes the relationship between the two variables, is a straight line, so that for any increase in the magnitude of one variable there will be a proportional change in the magnitude of the other variable.

correlation, multiple, n a complex correlation procedure in which scores on two or more variables are combined to predict scores on another variable, called the *dependent variable.*

correspondence, n written or typed communication between two individuals or groups of individuals.

corrosion, n an electrolytic or chemical attack of a surface. Usually refers to the attack of a metal surface.

cortex, n the outer layer of an organ or other structure.

cortex, adrenal, n the outer layer of the adrenal gland, the site of secretion of the adrenocortical hormones.

cortex, cerebral, n the outer gray matter of cerebrum, where many of the higher functions, such as volition, consciousness, conceptualization, and sensation, are carried out.

corticalosteotomy (kôr′tikəlos′tē-ot′ōmē), n an osteotomy through the cortex at the base of the dentoalveolar segment, which serves to weaken the resis-

tance of the bone to the application of orthodontic forces.

corticoid, adrenal (kôr′tikoid), n an adrenal corticosteroid hormone (for example, 11-dehydrocorticosterone [compound A], corticosterone [compound B], 11-deoxycorticosterone [cortexone, DOC], cortisone [compound E], cortisol [compound F], 11-desoxycortisol [substance S], aldosterone, androgen, progesterone, estrogen, and many other inactive steroids). See also aldosterone, androgen, corticosterone, cortisone, estrogens, hydrocortisone, and progesterone.

corticosteroid (kôr′tikōstir′oid), n See steroid, adrenocortical.

corticosterone (Kendall's compound B) (kôr′tikōstir′ōn, kôr′tikos′tərōn), n an adrenal corticosteroid hormone necessary for the maintenance of life in adrenalectomized animals; protects against stress, influences muscular efficiency, and influences carbohydrate and electrolyte metabolism.

corticotropin (kôr′tikōtrō′pin), n a purified preparation of adrenocorticotropic hormone derived from the pituitary gland of animals. See also ACTH.

cortisol, n See hydrocortisone.

cortisone (17-hydroxy-11-dehydrocorticosterone, Kendall's compound E), n a hormone produced by the adrenal cortex; a glucocorticoid, 17-hydroxy-11-dehydrocorticosterone; useful in the treatment of rheumatoid arthritis, lupus erythematosus, and some allergic conditions. Has marked antiinflammatory properties. Excess production or administration produces signs of hyperadrenocorticalism (Cushing's syndrome) with hyperlipemia and obesity hyperglycemia and edema.

cortisone acetate, n trade name: Cortone; drug class: glucocorticoid, short acting; action: decreases inflammation by suppression of macrophage and leukocyte migration, reduces capillary permeability; uses: inflammation, severe allergy, adrenal insufficiency, collagen, and respiratory and dermatologic disorders.

corundum, n See emery.

Corynebacterium, n a common genus of rod-shaped, curved bacilli. The most common pathogenic species are *Corynebacterium acnes,* commonly found in acne lesions, and *C. diphtheriae,* the cause of diphtheria.

cosmetic orthodontics, *n* limited orthodontic therapy for the purpose of improving appearance, such as the closing of an unsightly diastema between central incisors that presents no other handicap.

cost containment, *n* the features of a dental benefits program or of the administration of the program designed to reduce or eliminate certain charges to the plan.

cost share, *n* the share of health expenses that a beneficiary must pay, including the deductibles, copayments, coinsurance, and charges over the amount reimbursed by the dental benefits plan.

cost-benefit analysis, *n* the comparative study of the service or production costs of a service or item and its value to the subject.

cost-effective, *n* the minimal expenditure of dollars, time, and other elements necessary to achieve the health care result deemed necessary and appropriate.

Costen's syndrome, *n.pr* See syndrome, Costen's.

cotherapist, *n* in oral health care, a designation for the relationships among patient, dental hygienist, and dentist in securing the patient's regular treatment.

cotinine (kō′tinēn), *n* substance that remains in body fluids after nicotine has been used. Presence of this chemical in body fluids is considered proof of recent nicotine use. It is currently being studied for its possible contribution to a range of oral diseases.

cotton, absorbent, *n* the fibers or hairs of the seed of cultivated varieties of *Gossypium herbaceum,* so prepared that the cotton readily absorbs liquid.

cotton pliers, *n* See pliers, cotton.

cough, *n* a sudden, noisy expulsion of air from the lungs.

cough, gander, *n* the characteristic clanging, brassy cough of tracheal obstruction.

Council on Dental Therapeutics, *n.pr* an appointed council within the Division of Scientific Affairs of the American Dental Association directed to study, evaluate, and disseminate information with regard to dental therapeutic agents, their adjuncts, and dental cosmetic agents that are offered to the public or profession.

counseling, *n* the act of providing advice and guidance to a patient or the patient's family.

count, blood, complete, *n* the determination of the number of red blood cells (erythrocytes), white blood cells, and platelets in an accurately measured volume of blood. It usually includes the quantity of hemoglobin per cubic millimeter of blood. A normal red blood count is 4 to 5.5 million cells/cubic mm of blood.

count, differential white blood cell, *n* the determination of the number of each type of white blood cell in the peripheral blood. The relative count is obtained by counting the number of each type of cell in every 100 cells. The results are expressed in percentages. The normal figure for neutrophils is 60% to 70%, lymphocytes 20% to 35%, monocytes 2% to 8%, basophils 0% to 1%, and eosinophils 2% to 4%.

count, platelet, *n* the determination of the number of platelets in a cubic millimeter of blood. The normal count is 200,000 to 500,000.

count, reticulocyte (rətik′yəlōsīt), *n* the number of reticulocytes in the circulating blood, giving some indication of bone marrow activity. The number is increased after acute blood loss and after recovery from anemia. The number is decreased in anemias associated with defective red cell or hemoglobin production (nutritional, endocrine, toxic, or displacement anemias). The normal range is 0.5% to 1.5% of the erythrocytes.

count, white blood cell, *n* the determination of the number of white blood cells in an accurately measured volume of blood. The normal value is from 4000 to 9000 per cubic millimeter of blood.

counter, *n* a device for enumerating ionizing events.

counter, Geiger-Muller **(G-M counter, Geiger counter),** *n.pr* a highly sensitive gas-filled device that measures radiation.

counter, proportional, n a gas-filled radiation detection tube in which the pulse produced is proportional to the number of ions formed in the gas by the primary ionizing particle.

counter, scintillation, n a combination of phosphor, photomultiplier tube, and associated circuits for counting the light emissions that are produced in the phosphor.

counterdie, n the reverse image of a die, usually made of a softer and lower-fusing metal than the die. It is used to swage metal, wax, or other material over a die. See also die.

counterirritant, n an irritant that blocks perception of pain by diverting attention to the sensation that it produces.

coverage, n **1.** benefits available to an individual covered under a dental benefits plan. **2.** See denture coverage.

coverage year, n the 12-month period over which deductibles and maximum benefits apply for each person.

covered charges, n.pl the charges for services rendered or supplies furnished by a dentist that qualify as covered services and are paid for in whole or in part by the dental benefits program. May be subject to deductibles, copayments, coinsurance, annual or lifetime maximums, or table of allowances, as specified by the terms of the contract.

covered person, n an individual who is eligible for benefits under a dental benefits program.

covered services, n.pl the services for which payment is provided under the terms of the dental benefits contract.

Coxiella, a genus of filterable bacteria of the order *Rickettsiales.*

Coxiella burnetii, a species of *Coxiella* that causes Q fever in man.

Coxsackie A disease, n See herpangina.

crack cocaine, n a street drug made by chemically converting cocaine hydrochloride to a form that can be smoked. Smoking crack is a faster, more direct way of getting cocaine into the brain. The narcotic effect of smoking crack cocaine is faster and more intense than it is when injected, inhaled, or ingested. No medical application exists for crack cocaine.

cracked tooth syndrome, n transient acute pain experienced occasionally while chewing. Difficult to locate and reproduce. Likely to occur among individuals who crack nuts and crush ice with their teeth, and among popcorn eaters. Usually a vertical crack or split in the tooth extends across a marginal ridge through the crown and into the root, involving the pulp. Visible by transilluminated light or with the use of disclosing dyes.

cranial base, n.pl the bones forming the base of the skull. In cephalometric analysis, defined by the angle formed by a line drawn basion to point S (sella turcica) and from point S to point N (frontonasal suture).

cranial nerves, n the twelve pairs of nerves that emerge from the cranial cavity through various openings in the base of the skull are the olfactory, optic, oculomotor, trochlear, trigeminal, abducens, facial, acoustic, glossopharyngeal, vagus, accessory, and hypoglossal.

cranial prosthesis, n an artificial replacement for a portion of the skull.

cranial sutures, n.pl the fibrous joints between the bones of the cranium, some of which are fused in adults.

craniofacial, adj pertaining to the portion of the skull that contains the face and brain.

craniofacial anomalies, n.pl congenital malformations of the skull and face, frequently associated with genetically transmitted syndromes.

craniofacial dysostosis (krā′nē-ōfā′shəl dis′ostō′sis), n See dysostosis, craniofacial.

craniofacial templates, n.pl a series of cephalometric tracings of normal faces by age, sex, and race by which variations in the facial form of a patient can be determined and a treatment objective arranged.

craniometry (krā′nē-om′ətrē), n the study of the measurements of the skull.

craniopharyngioma (krā′nē-ōfərin′jē-ō′mə), n a tumor histologically identical to ameloblastoma that arises from remnants of the craniopharyngeal duct.

craniosynostosis, n premature fusion of the cranial sutures resulting in a malformed head, which may lead to an increase in intracranial pressure and consequential brain damage.

craniotabes (kra′nē-ōtā′bēz), *n* a soft, yielding skull; shallow pitting and thinning of skull bones of infants as a result of congenital syphilis or rickets.

craniotomy, *n* any surgical opening into the skull, performed to relieve intracranial pressure, to control bleeding, or to remove a tumor.

crater formation, *n* the formation of interdental depressions in the gingival tissues or subjacent bone; often associated with the destructive effects of necrotizing ulcerative gingivitis.

crazing, *n* the formation of small cracks on the surface of structures induced by release of internal stress.

crazing of plastic teeth, *n* minute cracks appearing on the surface of plastic teeth.

creatine kinase, *n* an enzyme in muscle, brain, and other tissues that catalyzes the transfer of a phosphate group from adenosine triphosphate to creatine, producing adenosine diphosphate and phosphocreatine.

creatinine, *n* a substance formed from the metabolism of creatine, commonly found in blood, urine, and muscle tissue.

creative, *adj* describing the ability or talent to think or act in a new or original way.

credential, license by, *n* the establishment of a license to practice in one state or province based on licensing history from another state or province with comparable regulations and requirements. Also called *reciprocity.*

credit rating, *n* the evaluation of any person's responsibility toward meeting financial obligations.

creditor, *n* a person to whom a debt is owed.

crenation (krinā′shən), *n* a wrinkling of the surface of cells as a result of shrinkage in their volume.

crenation of tongue, *n* scalloping along the lingual periphery of the tongue caused by the tongue lying against the lingual surface of the mandibular teeth.

creosote, N.F. XI (wood creosote), *n* a mixture of phenols ob-

tained from wood tar and occasionally used to treat root canals.

crepitus (krep′itus), *n* a crackling sound such as that produced by the rubbing together of fragments of a fractured bone or by air moving in a tissue space.

crepitus, bony, *n* the crackling sound noted during auscultation; also the sensation noted during palpation when the fragments of a fractured bone are rubbed together.

crescent, sublingual, *n* the crescent-shaped area on the floor of the mouth formed by the lingual wall of the mandible and the adjacent part of the floor of the mouth.

crest, *n* a projecting ridge or structure.

crest, alveolar, *n* See bone crest.

crest, gingival, *n* the coronal margin of the gingival tissue.

crestal resorption, *n* bone resorption at the border or crest of the dental alveolus. This bone loss follows tooth extraction and may result from periodontal infection or through the use of heavy orthodontic forces.

cretin, *n* a thyroid-deficient dwarfed individual with mental subnormality.

cretinism (krē′tənizəm) (congenital hypothyroidism), *n* **1.** a marked retardation of physical and mental development caused by congenital lack of secretion of thyrotropic hormone by the pituitary gland. Slow tooth eruption is one of the results. **2.** a thyroid deficiency that results in retardation of physical and mental development.

crevice, *n* a narrow opening caused by a fissure or a crack.

crevice, gingival, *n* the fissure between the free gingiva and enamel.

crevicular fluid (krevik′yōōlur), *n* a clear, usually unnoticeable fluid that can serve as a defense mechanism against infection by carrying antibodies and other therapeutic substances between the connective tissue and sulcus or pocket. Also called *gingival sulcus fluid* or *sulcular fluid.*

crib, Jackson, *n.pr* a removable orthodontic appliance retained in position by crib-shaped wires.

crib, lingual, *n* an orthodontic appliance consisting of a wire framework suspended lingually to the maxillary incisor teeth; used to obstruct thumb and tongue habits.

crib splint, *n* See splint, crib.

cribriform, *adj* perforated (like a sieve).

cribriform plate, *n* the aveolar bone that forms the tooth socket and to which the periodontal ligament is attached (radiographically, the lamina dura).

cricoid cartilage (krī'koid), *n* See cartilage, cricoid.

cricoidynia (krī'koidī'nē-ə), *n* pain in the cricoid cartilage.

cricothyrotomy (krī'kōthīrot'ōmē), *n* an incision between the cricoid and thyroid cartilages for the purpose of maintaining a patent airway.

cri-du-chat syndrome (krē' dōōshä'), *n* See syndrome, cri-du-chat.

criminology, the study of crime, the people who commit crimes, and penal codes used to deter crime and punish criminals.

crisis, adrenal, an acute adrenocortical insufficiency, with clinical manifestations of headache, nausea, vomiting, diarrhea, confusion, costovertebral angle pain, circulatory collapse, and coma. May occur in relation to stress of dental or medical procedures in patients with latent adrenal disease or in patients who have undergone prior ACTH or cortisone therapy, especially without control or termination of therapy.

crisis, thyroid, *n* a complication occurring after thyroidectomy, or before or during other surgical procedures where even mild hyperthyroidism is present. It is characterized by tachycardia, a high temperature, nervousness, and occasionally delirium.

cristobalite (kristō'bəlīt), *n* a form of crystalline silica used in dental casting investments because of its relatively high capacity for thermal expansion and resistance to breaking down by heat.

criteria, *n.pl* predetermined rules or guidelines for dental care, developed by dentists relying on professional expertise, prior experience, and the professional literature, with which aspects of actual instances of dental care may be compared. *Explicit* criteria are predetermined, specific, and measurable; *implicit* criteria are im-

plied or understood but not directly expressed.

critical care, *n* See intensive care.

cromolyn sodium, *n* *trade names:* Intal, Nasalcrom, Rynacrom; *drug class:* antiasthmatic; *action:* stabilizes the membrane of the sensitized mast cell, preventing release of chemical mediators; *uses:* allergic rhinitis, severe perennial bronchial asthma, exercise-induced bronchospasm.

cross linkage, *n* See polymerization, cross.

cross-arch bar splint, *n* See connector.

cross-arch bar splint connector, *n* See connector, cross-arch bar splint.

cross-arch splinting, *n* See splinting, cross arch.

cross-bite, *n* an occlusion with the line of occlusion of the mandibular teeth anterior and/or buccal to the maxillary teeth. See also occlusion, cross-bite.

cross-bite, anterior, *n* primary or permanent maxillary incisors locked lingual to mandibular incisors.

cross-bite, posterior, *n* primary permanent maxillary posterior teeth in lingual position in relation to the mandibular teeth.

cross-contamination, *n* the transfer of an infection directly from one person to another or indirectly from one person to a second person via a fomite.

cross-examination, *n* questioning of a witness by the party against whom he or she has been called and examined.

cross-infection, *n* the transmission of a communicable disease from one person to another because of a poor barrier protection.

cross-resistance, *n* See resistance, cross-.

cross-section form, *n* See clasp, flexibility of.

cross-sectional study, *n* the scientific method for the analysis of data gathered from two or more samples at one point in time.

cross-tolerance, *n* See tolerance, cross-.

Crouzon's disease (krōōzonz'), See dysostosis, craniofacial.

Crouzon's syndrome, *n.pr* See dysostosis, craniofacial.

crowding, *n* **1.** more than filling the space provided or intended. In dentistry, when the dental arch length is less than the mesial distal width of the teeth intended to occupy it. **2.** malocclusion characterized by inadequate arch circumference to accommodate the teeth in proper alignment.

crown, *n* that portion of a human tooth covered by enamel.

crown, anatomic, n that portion of dentin covered by enamel.

crown and bridge prosthodontics, n the division of prosthodontics that deals with crown restorations and the fixed type of tooth-borne partial denture prosthesis. See also prosthodontics, fixed.

crown, artificial, n a dental prosthesis restoring the anatomy, function, and esthetics of part or all of the coronal portion of the natural tooth.

crown, clinical, n **1.** that portion of enamel visibly present in the oral cavity. **2.** the portion of a tooth that is occlusal to the deepest part of the gingival crevice.

crown, complete, n a restoration that reproduces the entire surface anatomy of the clinical crown and fits over a prepared tooth stump.

crown, crown veneer, n a restoration that reproduces the total clinical coronal surface contour of the tooth.

crown, dowel, n a restoration that replaces the entire coronal portion of a tooth and derives its retention from a dowel extending into a treated (filled) root canal.

crown, extraalveolar clinical, n the portion of a tooth that extends occlusally or incisally from the junction of the tooth root and the supporting bone.

crown, faced, n See crown, veneered metal.

crown, full, restoration, n an individual tooth prosthesis encompassing the entire prepared clinical crown. See also crown, complete veneer.

crown, jacket, n See crown, complete.

crown lengthening, n a surgical procedure to remove marginal gingival tissues to expose more of the crown of the tooth to facilitate a reconstructive or operative procedure.

crown, partial, n a restoration that covers three or more, but not all, surfaces of a tooth.

crown, porcelain-faced, n an artificial crown that makes use of porcelain inlayed in or veneered onto the labial or buccal surface.

crown, stainless steel, n a preformed steel crown used for the restoration of badly broken-down primary teeth and first permanent molars. Also used as a temporary restoration of fractured permanent incisors.

crown, three-quarter, n a term frequently used to designate a partial veneer crown.

crown, veneered metal, n a complete crown that has one or more surfaces prepared for and covered by a tooth-colored substance such as porcelain or resin.

crown-root ratio, *n* the relation of the clinical crown to the clinical roots of the teeth—an important consideration in diagnosis, prognosis, and treatment planning.

crown-rump length, *n* the length of an embryo, fetus, or newborn as measured from the crown of the head to the prominence of the buttocks.

Crozat appliance, *n.pr* See appliance, Crozat.

CRT, *n* the abbreviation for cathode-ray tube.

crucible (krōō′sibəl), *n* a vessel or container that will withstand high heat and is used for melting or holding material.

crucible crushing strength, n See strength, compressive.

crucible former (sprue base), n the stand or base into which a sprued pattern is placed. It establishes the shape or form of the hollowed-out end of the investment in the casting ring, which will receive the molten metal on its course through the sprue hole. See also sprue former.

crust, *n* a hard-coating surface layer composed of coagulated tissue fluid and blood products mixed with epithelial and inflammatory cells covering a lesion formed by the rupture of a bulla, vesicle, or pustule.

cryolite (krī′-ōlīt) (sodium aluminum fluoride [Na₃AlF₆]), *n* a fluoride often used as a flux in the manufacture of silicate cements.

cryosurgery, *n* the use of subfreezing temperature to destroy tissue. Cryosurgery is used to cause the edges of a detached retina to heal, to remove cataracts, and in the treatment of Parkinson's disease.

cryotherapy, *n* a use of cryosurgery in the treatment of cutaneous tags, warts, actinic keratosis, and dermatofibromas. The agent is usually liquid nitrogen, applied briefly with a sterile cotton-tipped applicator.

cryptococcosis (krip′tōkäkō′sis), *n* a fungal infection from the organism *Cryptococcosis neoformans*, found primarily in pigeon feces. It often affects individuals with weakened or compromised immune systems.

Cryptococcosis. (Neville/Damm/Allen/ Bouquot, 2002, Courtesy of Dr. Catherine Flaitz)

cryptogenic (krip′tōjen′ik), *n* a condition distinguished by an unknown cause.

crystal(s), *n* a naturally produced solid. The ultimate units of the substance from which it was formed are arranged systematically.

crystal gold, n See gold, mat.

crystal, silver halide, n silver compounds, usually silver bromide and silver iodide, that are impregnated in the photographic emulsion of film. These compounds, when acted on by actinic rays, are disintegrated, with the formation of metallic silver in a finely divided state. The photographic image results when the film is subjected to processing.

crystallization, *n* the production or formation of crystals, either by cooling a liquid or gas to a solid state or by cooling a solution until the solute precipitates as a crystalline deposit.

cubital (kyōō′bitəl), *adj* pertaining to the forearm.

cubitus (kyōō′bitus), *n* the forearm.

cuboid (kyōō′boid), *adj* (cuboidal), resembling a cube in form.

cuboidal, *adj* See cuboid.

cue, *n* a stimulus that determines or may prompt the nature of a person's response.

cultural characteristics, *n.pl* See culture 2.

cultural diversity, *n* a population consisting of two or more cultural groups.

culture, *n* **1.** the growth of microorganisms or other living cells on artificial media. **2.** a set of learned values, beliefs, customs, and behavior that is shared by a group of interacting individuals.

culture, bacterial, n bacterial growth on or in an artificial medium. The medium used may be selective for a given type or genus of organism (for example, tomato juice agar for lactobacilli).

culture, endodontic, n the growth of microorganisms obtained from root canals or periapical tissues.

culture, endodontic medium, n a specific medium used for endodontic cultures.

culture medium, n a substance, liquid or solid, used for cultivating bacteria.

cumulative, *adj* increasing in effect.

cup, chin, *n* **1.** an orthopedic device that directs a posterior and/or vertical force to the mandible, through the attachment of a cup fitting over the chin to a headcap. **2.** a drug used to cause muscle relaxation during anesthesia by blocking acetylcholine at the neuromuscular and synaptic junctions.

cure, *n* **1.** the successful treatment of a disease or wound. **2.** a procedure or reaction that changes a plastic material to a hard material (for example, vulcanization and polymerization). See also process.

curet, curette (kyōōret′), *n* a periodontal or surgical instrument having a sharp, spoon-shaped working blade; used for debridement. The periodontal curet, available in many sizes and shapes, is used for root and gingival curettage.

curet, area-specific, n any of a number of spoon-shaped scaling instruments designed for use on specific tooth surfaces. It may feature an elongated shank or shortened blade.

Mini-Five curet | After-Five curet | Standard Gracey curet | Vision curet

Comparison of area specific curets. (Daniel/Harfst, 2002)

curet, nonsurgical Gracey, n instrument used for removal of subgingival calculus and root debridement.

curet, nonsurgical Langer, n instrument that has combined features of the Gracey curet and universal curet for superior functioning.

curet, nonsurgical rigid, n instrument made with a rigid shank that is stronger and aids in removal of tenacious deposits of plaque.

curet, nonsurgical universal, n instrument designed to permit access to all surfaces of the tooth without the need to change instruments during debridement.

curet, universal, n a hand instrument used to treat subgingival sufaces. The universal curet has a blade with an unbroken cutting edge that curves around the toe and a flat face that is set at a 90° angle to the lower shank.

curettage (kyōō′rətäzh′), *n* scraping or cleaning with a curet.

curettage, angle for gingival, n an angle between 45° and 90° at which the curet should be held against the gingiva to clean out a pocket effectively. See also curettage, subgingival.

curettage, apical, n (apoxesis), curettement of diseased periapical tissue without excision of the root tip. See also curettage, subgingival.

curettage, gingival, n See curettage, subgingival.

curettage, gingival, closed, n See curettage, subgingival.

curettage, infrabony pocket, n enucleation, by means of suitable instrumentation, of the inflammatory soft tissue elements lying within and surrounding the crest of an infrabony resorptive defect; also includes the debridement and planing of the root surface of the pocket.

curettage, root, n debridement and planing to smoothness of the root surface of a tooth to eliminate accretions on the root and provide a suitable environment for the return of the gingival tissues to a state of health.

curettage, subgingival, n the process of debridement of the epithelial attachment, the ulcerated and entire (pocket) epithelium, and subjacent inflamed and altered gingival corium. The controversial procedure is thought to result in the resolution of the inflammatory process and desirable shrinkage and repair of the edematous tissue, but less invasive procedures have proven more effective. Some states still require hygienists to be tested on this procedure, while other states and programs have dropped testing and teaching the procedure altogether.

curette, *n* See curet.

curie (kyōō′rē), a measurement of radioactivity produced by the disintegration of unstable elements. The curie is that quantity of a radioactive nuclide in which the number of disintegrations per second is 3.700 times 10^{-10}. Since the curie is a relatively large unit, the millicurie (0.00 curie) and the microcurie (one-millionth of a curie) are more often used. The curie is based on the number of nuclear disintegrations and not on the number or amount of radiations emitted.

curing, *n* the act of polymerization.

curing, denture, *n* See denture curing.

current, *n* a measure of the number of electrons per second that pass a given point on a conductor.

current, alternating, *n* a current that alternately changes its direction of flow. It usually consists of 60 complete cycles/sec.

current, coagulating, *n* an electrical current, delivered by a needle, ball, or other variously shaped points, that coagulates tissue.

current dental terminology (CDT), *n* a listing of descriptive terms and identifying codes developed by the American Dental Association (ADA) for reporting dental services and procedures to dental benefits plans.

current, direct, *n* an electrical current in which the electron flow is in only one direction.

current, galvanic, *n* a direct current created by a battery.

current procedural terminology (CPT), *n* a listing of descriptive terms and identifying codes developed by the American Medical Association (AMA) for reporting practitioner services and procedures to medical plans and medicare.

current, saturation, *n* the maximum current in a roentgen-ray tube that fully uses all electrons that are available at the cathode for the production of roentgen rays.

curriculum, *n* a course of study; the linked series of academic courses leading to mastery of a discipline.

cursor, *n* the pointer on a PC monitor or other display that indicates where the next character will be entered.

curvature, occlusal, *n* See curve of occlusion.

curve, *n* a nonangular deviation from a straight line or surface.

curve, alignment, *n* See alignment.

curve, anti-Monson, *n.pr* See curve, reverse.

curve, compensating, *n* the curvature of alignment of the occlusal surfaces of the teeth that is developed to compensate for the paths of the condyles as the mandible moves from centric to eccentric positions. A means of maintaining posterior tooth contacts on the molar teeth and providing balancing contacts on dentures when the mandible is protruded. Corresponds to the curve of Spee of natural teeth.

curve, dose-effect, *n* a curve relating the dose of radiation with the effect produced.

curve, dose-response, *n* a graphical representation of the relationship between dosage (x-axis) and degree of response (y-axis); used to determine the effective dose of any given drug.

curve, milled-in, *n* See path, milled-in.

curve, Monson, *n.pr* the curve of occlusion, described by Monson, in which each cusp and incisal edge touch or conform to a segment of the surface of a sphere 8 inches (20 cm) in diameter, with its center in the region of the glabella. See also curve, compensating.

curve of occlusion (**occlusal curvature**), *n* **1.** a curved occlusal surface that makes simultaneous contact with the major portion of the incisal and occlusal prominences of the existing teeth. **2.** the curve of a dentition on which the occlusal surfaces of the teeth lie. See also curve, reverse.

curve of Spee, *n.pr* **1.** an anatomic curvature of the occlusal alignment of teeth, beginning at the tip of the mandibular canine, following the buccal cusps of the natural premolars and molars, and continuing to the anterior border of the ramus, as described by von Spee. **2.** the curve of the occlusal surfaces of the arches in vertical dimension, brought about by a dipping downward of the mandibular premolars, with a corresponding adjustment of the maxillary premolars.

curve of Wilson, *n.pr* by-product term of the thinking that supported the theory that occlusion should be spherical. The curve in the lower arch is concave, whereas the one in the upper arch is convex.

curve, reverse, *n* a curve of occlusion that is convex upward when viewed in the frontal plane.

curve, sine, *n* the wave form of an alternating current, characterized by a rise from zero to maximum positive potential, then descending below zero to its maximum negative value, and

C

then rising to its maximum positive potential, to fall to zero again.

curve, survival, n a curve obtained by plotting the number or percentage of organisms surviving at a given time against a given dose of radiation. A curve showing the percentage of individuals surviving at different intervals after a particular dosage of radiation.

Cushing's syndrome, *n.pr* See syndrome, Cushing's.

cusp, n a notably pointed or rounded eminence on or near the masticating surface of a tooth.

cusp, angle, n See angle, cusp.

cusp-fossa relations, n.pl organic relations between a stamp cusp and its fossa.

cusp height, n the shortest distance between the deepest part of the central fossa of a posterior tooth and a line connecting the points of the cusps of the tooth.

cusp, shoeing, n See restoration of cusps.

cuspal interference, n See contact, deflective occlusal.

cuspid, n See canine.

cuspidor, n a fixture provided on some dental operating units into which patients can expectorate. In current practice, most operating fields are kept clear of saliva by high-volume suction saliva ejectors.

customary fee, n the fee level determined by the administrator of a dental benefits plan from actual submitted fees for a specific dental procedure to establish the maximum benefit payable under a given plan for that specific procedure. See also fee, usual and fee, reasonable.

cutaneous (kyōōtā′nē-us), *adj* relating to the skin. Tests of cutaneous hypersensitivity may be indicators of malnutrition and are useful in determining a patient's readiness for surgery.

cuticle, n the outer layer of the skin. Also, a layer that covers the free surface of an epithelial cell.

cuticle, primary, n 1. the transitory remnants of the enamel organ and oral epithelium covering the enamel of a tooth after eruption. *Synonym:* Nasmyth's membrane. 2. believed to be the last substance formed by ameloblasts, mediating the attachment of ameloblasts to the enamel.

cuticle, secondary, n 1. the second cuticle formed when the ameloblasts are replaced by the oral epithelium. It then covers the primary cuticle on the enamel and is the only cuticle on the cementum. 2. a keratinized pedicle found between the gingival epithelium and the surface of a tooth.

cuticula dentis (kyōōtik′yōōlə den′tis), n See cuticle, primary.

cutting instrument, n See instrument, cutting.

CVA, n See accident, cerebrovascular.

cyanocobalamin, n (vitamin B_{12}), *trade names* (some): Alpha Redisol, Betalin-12, Cobex; *drug class:* Vitamin B_{12} water-soluble vitamin; *action:* needed for adequate nerve functioning, protein and carbohydrate metabolism, normal growth, red blood cell development, and cell reproduction; *uses:* vitamin B_{12} deficiency, pernicious anemia, hemolytic anemia, hemorrhage, and renal and hepatic diseases.

cyanosis (sīə-nō-sis), n a characteristic bluish tinge or color of the skin and mucous membranes associated with reduction in hemoglobin brought about by inadequate respiratory change (5 gm/100 ml are necessary for color to be perceptible).

cyclamate, n a noncaloric artificial sweetening agent used in conjunction with saccharin; presently banned by the FDA because of its carcinogenic potential.

cycle, n a succession of events.

cycle, chewing, n a complete course of movement of the mandible during a single masticatory stroke.

cycle, masticating, n three-dimensional patterns of mandibular movements formed during the chewing of food.

cyclic AMP cycloheximide, n a cyclic nucleotide formed from adenosine triphosphate by the action of adrenyl cyclase. Known as the "second messenger," it participates in the action of catecholamines, vasopressin, adrenocorticotropic hormone, and many other hormones.

cyclic neutropenia, n a hereditary disease primarily afflicting young children and infants; characterized by flu-like symptoms (weakness, tenderness in the throat, aching head, and fever) as well as stomatitis, periodontitis, and gingivitis; cycles every 3 to 4 weeks with painful lesions and damage to the alveolar bone; should be medicated with antibiotics prior to any oral surgery.

cyclizine HCl/cyclizine lactate, trade, *n trade name:* Marezine; *drug class:* antiemetic, antihistaminic, anticholinergic; *action:* may act centrally on vomiting center, also antagonizes histamine peripherally; *uses:* motion sickness, prevention of postoperative vomiting.

cyclobenzaprine HCl, *n trade name:* Cycoflex; *drug class:* skeletal muscle relaxant, centrally acting tricyclic; *action:* has actions similar to those of tricyclic antidepressants; *uses:* adjunct for relief of muscle spasm and pain in musculoskeletal conditions.

cyclophosphamide, *n trade names:* Cytoxan, Neosar, Procytox; *drug class:* antineoplastic alkylating agent; *action:* alkylates DNA, RNA, inhibits enzymes that allow synthesis of amino acids in proteins; *uses:* Hodgkin's disease; lymphomas; leukemia; cancer of female reproductive tract, lung, prostate; multiple myeloma; neuroblastoma; retinoblastoma; Ewing's sarcoma.

cycloserine, *n trade name:* Seromycin Pulvules; *drug class:* antitubercular; *action:* inhibits cell wall synthesis, analog of D-alanine; *uses:* pulmonary tuberculosis.

cyclosporine, *n trade name:* Sandimmune; *drug class:* immunosuppressant; *action:* produces immunosuppression by inhibiting lymphocytes; *uses:* to prevent rejection of tissues and/or organ transplants.

cyclothymia (sī′klōthī′mē-ə), *n* See psychosis, manic-depressive.

cyclotron (sī′kləträn), *n* a device for accelerating charged particles to high energies by means of an alternating electrical field between electrodes placed in a constant magnetic field.

cylindroma (sil′indrō′mə), *n* an adenocystic basal cell carcinoma of the salivary glands. A malignant tumor that may occur in the sublingual, submandibular, parotid, or labial salivary glands. See also carcinoma, adenocystic.

cyproheptadine HCl, *n trade name:* Periactin; *drug class:* antihistamine H_1-receptor antagonist; *action:* acts on blood vessels, gastrointestinal and respiratory systems by competing with histamine for H_1-receptor site; *uses:* allergy symptoms, rhinitis, pruritus, cold urticaria.

cyst (sist), *n* a pathologic space in bone or soft tissue containing fluid or semifluid material and, in the oral regions, almost always lined by epithelium.

cyst, aneurysmal bone, *n* a nonmalignant osteolytic lesion expanding a long bone or within a vertebra in which the space, filled with blood, is networked with fibrous tissue containing multinucleated giant cells.

cyst, branchial, *n* (branchial cleft cyst), soft-tissue cyst usually seen on the lateral side of the neck, arising from epithelial illusions within the cervical lymph nodes. Microscopic examination shows the epithelial lining of stratified squamous epithelium surrounded by lymphoid tissue.

Branchial cyst. (Regezi/Sciubba/Pogrel, 2000)

cyst, calcifying and keratinizing odontogenic, *n* a cyst arising from odontogenic epithelium, with abundant production of keratin-containing ghost cells and areas of dystrophic calcification. This lesion has no age or sex distribution.

cyst, dental, *n* See cyst, periodontal.

cyst, dentigerous, *n* an epithelium-lined sac filled with fluid or semifluid material that surrounds the crown of an unerupted tooth or odontoma.

cyst, dentoalveolar, *n* See cyst, periodontal.

cyst, dermoid, n an epithelium-lined sac with one or more skin appendages (hair follicles, sweat glands, sebaceous glands) in its wall. It may be found in the floor of the mouth. This lesion should not be confused with the teratomatous dermoid cyst of the ovary.

cyst, developmental, n a pathologic fluid sac which may be caused by infection or disease. See also cyst, dentigerous and cyst, odontogenic.

cyst, epidermoid, n an epithelium-lined sac containing fluid; possesses characteristics of the epidermis but does not have the skin appendages seen in dermoid cysts.

cyst, eruption, n a dentigerous cyst that causes a clinically evident bulging of the overlying alveolar ridge.

cyst, extravasation, n See cyst, traumatic.

cyst, fissural, n a cyst that arises from the enslaved epithelium in maxillary suture lines caused by fusion of the embryonic processes of the facial bones.

cyst, follicular, n an odontogenic cyst that arises from the epithelium of the tooth bud and dental lamina. Follicular cysts include dentigerous, primordial, and multilocular cysts.

cyst, globulomaxillary, n an epithelium-lined sac formed at the junction point of the globular (median nasal) and maxillary processes. It is seen as a pear-shaped radiolucency between the maxillary lateral incisor and canine, and it separates their roots.

cyst, hemorrhagic, n an extravasation cyst or lesion; traumatic bone cyst or lesion. This is not a true cyst but is probably a defect in the bone produced by trauma and repair. It appears as a definite radiolucent area with a sharply marked radiopaque border. It contains air and is lined by a thin endosteum. See also cyst, solitary bone.

cyst, incisive canal, n See cyst, nasopalatine.

cyst, indefinite bone, n See cyst, traumatic.

cyst, lateral, n See cyst, periodontal.

cyst, lateral follicular, n a follicular cyst occurring on the lateral surface of a tooth, usually near the cemento-dentinoenamel junction. See also cyst, follicular.

cyst, median palatal, n an epithelium-lined sac containing fluid; appears as a radiolucency in the midline of the palate. It is of developmental origin.

cyst, mucous (**mucocele**), n an epithelium-lined sac containing mucus. Mucous cysts in the sinus may appear as spherical, radiopaque areas.

cyst, multilocular, n a follicular cyst containing many loculi, or spaces, and not associated with a tooth.

cyst, nasoalveolar, n a fluid-containing sac lined by epithelium and located at the ala of the nose. A developmental cyst, it may simulate a nasal or periapical abscess.

cyst, nasopalatine (**nasopalatine duct**), n a cyst arising within the nasopalatine canal. Radiographically it may appear as a heart-shaped radiolucency between the maxillary central incisors. Histologically it may show mucous cells and nerve bundles in addition to a lining of stratified squamous or respiratory epithelium. The incisive canal cyst and the cyst of the papilla incisiva are the recognized subtypes.

cyst, odontogenic, n an epithelium-lined sac produced from the tooth-forming tissues (for example, primordial, dentigerous, and periodontal cysts).

cyst, periapical, n See cyst, radicular.

cyst, periodontal (**dental root cyst, dentoalveolar cyst, lateral cyst, periapical cyst**), n an epithelium-lined sac containing fluid usually found at the apex of a pulp-involved tooth. Lateral types occur less frequently along the side of the root.

cyst, primordial, n an epithelium-lined sac containing fluid and appearing as a radiolucency in the jaws. It is derived from an enamel organ before any hard tissue is formed.

cyst, radicular (**periapical cyst, root end cyst**), n a cyst that has a fibrous connective tissue wall and a lining of stratified squamous epithelium and that is attached to the apex of the root of a tooth with a nonvital pulp or a defective root canal filling.

cyst, residual, n an odontogenic cyst that remains within the jaw after the removal of the tooth with which it was associated. May be radicular or follicular.

cyst, root end, n See cyst, radicular.

cyst, soft tissue developmental, n a pathologic fluid sac which occurs in mucous membranes or other soft tissue of the body, as opposed to those occurring in bone or teeth. See also cyst, thyroglossal duct and cyst, lateral cervical.

cyst, solitary bone, n a pathologic bone space of disputed origin that may be either empty or filled with fluid. It may have a delicate connective tissue lining.

cyst, thyroglossal duct, n an epithelium-lined sac containing fluid formed in portions of the incompletely involuted thyroglossal duct, which connects the primitive pharynx with the tongue in embryonic life. These cysts may appear in the midline at any region from the subhyoid to the base of the tongue.

cyst, traumatic (**extravasation cyst, extravasation lesion, traumatic bone lesion**), n a radiolucent lesion appearing chiefly in the mandible as a well-defined area with a radiopaque border; clinically it appears as a cavity lined by extremely thin periosteum and filled with air. Assumed to be caused by injury to young spongy bone, hemorrhage resorption, and then walling off by cortical bone. See also cyst, solitary bone.

cysts, median mandibular, n a soft tissue sac which develops in the mouth near the middle of the lower jaw in conjunction with normal growth or as the result of an odontogenic cyst.

cysts, nonodontogenic, n a soft tissue abnormality that may develop in any number of locations within the mouth but is not directly associated with a tooth.

cysts, soft tissue, n a broad classification of oral abnormalities that may include blisterlike obstructions of salivary glands and growths in the thyroglossal tract, lymph nodes, and epithelial cells on the floor of the mouth.

cystadenoma (sist′adəno̅′mə), n an adenoma with the development of cystic spaces caused by dilation of acinar or ductal structures.

cystadenoma, papillary, lymphomatosum (**Warton's tumor**), n a benign salivary gland tumor that consists of numerous cystic spaces lined by a double layer of epithelium. A dense aggregate of lymphocytes containing germinal centers surrounds the cystic spaces.

cysteine, n a nonessential amino acid found in many proteins in the body.

cystic fibrosis, n an inherited disorder of the exocrine glands, causing those glands to produce abnormally thick secretions of mucus, elevation of sweat electrolytes, increased organic and enzymatic constituents of saliva, and overactivity of the autonomic nervous system.

cystinuria (sis′tinyo̅o̅′rē-ə), n a hereditary defect caused by the dysfunctional reabsorption of the amino acid cystine into the kidneys; it results in regular, abnormally high levels of cystine in urine.

cystostomy, n creating a surgical opening into the urinary bladder or gall bladder.

cytochrome, n one of a class of hemoproteins that act as electron transport. Cytochromes are classified as *a, b, c,* and *d.*

cytokine, n a nonantibody protein, such as lymphokine. Cytokines are released by a cell population on contact with a specific antigen. Cytokines act as intercellular mediators in the generation of immune response.

cytologic smear, n the product of a diagnostic technique where cells are scraped off the surface of a lesion found in the mouth. The gleaned cells are then examined under a microscope for indications of a variety of diseases. Considered a preliminary diagnostic test, it is not used to detect more serious conditions that require deeper tissue samples.

cytology (sītol'əjē), *n* the study of the anatomy, physiology, pathology, and chemistry of a cell.

cytology, exfoliative, n the study of desquamated cells.

cytomegalic inclusion disease, *n* See disease, salivary gland.

cytomegalovirus (CMV), *n* a visceral disease virus, a member of the group of herpetoviruses having special affinity for the salivary glands. Considered one of the indicator infections of AIDS.

cytoskeleton, *n* the intracellular filaments that serve to support or stiffen cells.

cytosol, *n* the totality of the intracellular substance exclusive of mitochondria and endoplasmic reticulum components.

cytozyme (sī'tōzīm), *n* See thromboplastin.

d-lysergic acid diethylamide (LSD) (lisur'jik as'id dī-eth'əlam'id), *n* a hallucinogenic street drug taken to induce a perceived state of euphoria, freedom, and control.

daily food requirements, *n* actively teaching patients proper nutrition, personal diet analysis, reasonable portion sizes, and how to choose foods from the Food Guide Pyramid to enjoy overall good health.

Dalton's law, *n* See law, Dalton's.

dam, a barrier to the passage of moisture or saliva.

dam, post-, n See seal, posterior palatal.

dam, rubber, n a thin sheet of latex rubber used to isolate a tooth or teeth and keep them dry during a dental procedure.

dam, rubber punch, n a hand-punch instrument with progressively larger openings, used to make a hole(s) in the rubber dam.

damages, *n.pl* compensation or indemnity that may be recovered in the courts by any person who has suffered loss, detriment, or injury to person, property, or rights through the unlawful act or negligence of another.

damages, compensatory, n.pl a sum that compensates the injured party for injury only.

damages, exemplary (punitive damages), n.pl damages awarded to the plaintiff over those that will barely compensate for property loss. Such compensation may be awarded when the wrong done to the plaintiff involves violence, malice, or fraud by the defendant. The object is to provide compensation for mental suffering or loss of pride. It may be employed as punishment for the defendant.

damages, nominal, n.pl a trifling sum awarded to a plaintiff in an action in which there is no substantial loss or injury to be compensated but in which the law still recognizes a technical invasion of rights or a breach of the defendant's duty. Also awarded in cases in which, although there has been a real injury, the plaintiff's evidence is not sufficient to show its amount.

damages, punitive, n.pl See damages, exemplary.

danazol, *n trade name:* Danocrine; *drug class:* androgen, alpha-ethinyl testosterone derivative; *action:* decreases FSH and LH output; *uses:* endometriosis, prevention of hereditary angioedema, fibrocystic breast disease.

dantrolene sodium, *n trade name:* Dantrium; *drug class:* skeletal muscle relaxant, direct acting; *action:* interferes with intracellular release of calcium necessary to initiate contraction; *uses:* spasticity in multiple sclerosis, stroke, spinal cord injury, cerebral palsy, malignant hyperthermia.

dapsone (DDS), *n trade name:* Avlosulfon; *drug class:* leprostatic, antibacterial; *action:* bactericidal and bacteriostatic against *M. leprae;* may also be immunosuppressant; *uses:* leprosy and dermatitis herpetiformis.

Darier's disease, *n.pr* See disease, Darier's.

darkroom, *n* a completely lightproof room or cubicle that is used in the processing of photographic, medical, and dental films. See also safe light.

darkroom, features of, *n* a dark-room for developing x-ray films, should be absolutely devoid of white light, as well as chemicals or dust that could damage the film while it is being processed; a filtered safe light of less than 15 watts should be the only light in the room.

Darvon, *n.pr* the brand name for pro-poxyphene hydrochloride, a mild, centrally acting narcotic analgesic agent.

data, *n.pl* facts and figures; data are processed and interpreted to yield information.

data aggregation, *n* a collection of protected health information used to conduct data analysis relating to the health care operations of the entity.

data base, *n* an organized collection of data. A medical data base is all the information that exists in the practice at any time.

data processing, *n* the collection of data, processing of the data to obtain usable information, and communica-tion of this usable information.

data set, *n* a hardware device that converts digital pulses (square wave-form) into modulated frequencies (si-nusoidal wave) for transmission, a process called modulation. It also converts modulated frequencies into voltage pulses, a process called de-modulation. Also called *modem.*

daughter (decay product), *n* a nu-clide formed from the radioactive decay of another nuclide called the parent.

day care, *n* **1.** a specialized program or facility that provides care for children from infants through pre-school age, usually within a group framework, either as a substitute for or an extension of home care. *n* **2.** a specialized program or facility that provides care for handicapped or dependent children or adults as a substitute for or an extension of home care.

day sheet, *n* a form that permits systematic record keeping of treat-ment of patients and of monies re-ceived and spent.

Day's syndrome, *n.pr* See syndrome, Riley-Day.

daylight loader method, *n* method for developing x-ray films without a darkroom, using a flexible apparatus that allows you to insert your hands into a dark space without admitting any light. Insert the exposed x-ray film in the daylight loader compart-ment and remove the protective packets. With ungloved hands, pro-cess the film, touching only the edges.

DDC, *n* the abbreviation for dideoxy-cytidine. See dideoxycytidine.

DDI, *n* the abbreviation for dideoxy-inosine. See dideoxyinosine.

dead, *adj* without life; destitute of life.

dead space, *n* See space; physiologic dead space, and anatomic dead space.

deaf, *adj* without usable hearing.

deafen, *v* to make deaf; to cause the loss of all usable hearing.

deafness (def'nes), *n* a condition characterized by a partial or complete loss of hearing.

deafness, central, *n* impaired hear-ing caused by interference with cere-bral auditory pathways or in the auditory centers in the brain (for example, cerebrovascular accidents and other degenerative brain dis-eases). Hearing aids are of little benefit.

deafness, conduction, *n* See deaf-ness, transmission.

deafness, nerve, *n* impaired hearing caused by pathologic conditions in the auditory nerve or the hair cells of the organ of Corti in the inner ear (for example, high-tone deafness, which comes with age; damage to the organ of Corti by noise; or a tumor of an auditory nerve). Hearing aids are usually of little benefit.

deafness, transmission (conduction deafness), *n* impaired hearing caused by interference with passage of sound waves through the external ear (for example, interference caused by wax) or middle ear (for example, interference caused by otitis media, aerotitis media, or otosclerosis). May be characterized by greater interfer-ence with hearing of low tones. Hearing aids that amplify may be helpful.

deaminated (dē-am'inātəd), *adj* pertaining to α-amino acids which have undergone the chemical alter-ation that removes ammonia (NH_3) from glutamate.

deamination (dē-am′inā′shun), *n* a chemical alteration of α-amino acids which removes ammonia (NH_3) from glutamate.

deanesthesiant (dē′-anəsthē′zē-ənt), *n* anything that will arouse a patient from a state of anesthesia.

death (deth), *n* **1.** cessation of life; the stoppage of life beyond the possibility of resuscitation. *n* **2.** the cause or occasion of loss of life. *n* **3.** the total absence of activity in the brain and central nervous system, the cardiovascular system, and the respiratory system as observed and declared by a physician or other legally authorized agent.

death, brain, n in addition to the generally accepted definition of death, some states, either by statute or court decision, have added a "brain death" definition to the law, applicable where there has been an irreversible cessation of brain function.

death certificate, n the signed affidavit that life has ceased, giving the time, place, and cause of death. Death certificates are required by law to be filed in the proper local or regional geopolitical office.

debility (dēbil′itē), *n* weakness; lack of strength; asthenia.

debonding, *n* a procedure by which brackets and bonding resin are removed and the surface of the tooth is restored to its previous condition.

debridement (dābrēd′mənt), *n* the removal of foreign material and/or devitalized tissue from the vicinity of a wound.

debridement, epithelial (deepithelization), n See curettage, subgingival.

debridement, nonsurgical periodontal, n removal of cellular debris and damaged tissue from areas surrounding the tooth by nonmechanical means.

debris (debrē′), *n* foreign material or particles loosely attached to a surface.

debris of Malassez (maləsə′), *n* the remnants of Hertwig's epithelial root sheath within the periodontal ligament.

debt, *n* a sum of money due by agreement; the contract may or may not be express and does not necessarily set the precise amount to be paid.

debug, *v* to locate and correct any errors in a computer program.

decalcification (dēkal′sifikā′shən), *n* loss or removal of calcium salts from calcified tissues.

decarboxylation, *n* a chemical reaction involving the removal of a molecule of carbon dioxide from carboxylic acid.

decay, *v* to deteriorate, putrefy.

decay, dental, n See caries, dental.

decay product, n See daughter.

decay, radioactive, n the disintegration of the nucleus of an unstable nuclide by the spontaneous emission of charged particles and/or photons.

decay, senile, n See caries, dental, senile.

decayed teeth, indices and scoring methods for, *n.pl* See index, DEF and index, DMF.

deceleration, *n* a decrease in the speed or velocity of an object or reaction.

decibel (des′ibel), *n* a logarithmic ratio unit that indicates by what proportion one intensity level differs from another.

deciduous (dēsid′yōō-əs), *adj* that which will be shed. Pertaining specifically to the first dentition of humans or animals. Preferred term is *primary*.

deciduous dentition, n teeth that will be shed.

deciduous teeth, n the teeth constituting the first dentition.

decision-making, *n* the process of coming to a conclusion or making a judgment.

decision-making, evidence-based, n a type of informal decision-making which combines clinical expertise, patient concerns, and evidence gathered from scientific literature to arrive at a diagnosis and treatment recommendations. See also evidence-based care.

decision-making, statistical, n a type of formal decision-making which proceeds from a hypothesis to a conclusion by incorporating such techniques as statistical inference and significance, probability analysis, literature review, sampling, and discussion.

decision tree, *n* an algorithm or a formal stepwise process used in coming to a conclusion or making a judgment.

declaration and provision for affairs, *n* a systematic statement of the affairs and estate of a person, in which all assets and property are listed.

decompensate, *n* development or worsening of a mental disorder.

decompression, *n* **1.** a technique used to readapt an individual to normal atmospheric pressure after exposure to higher pressures, as in diving. *n* **2.** the removal of pressure caused by gas or fluid in a body cavity such as the stomach or intestinal tract.

decompression, nerve, n the release of pressure on a nerve trunk by surgical widening of the bony canal.

decontamination, *n* the process of making a person, object, or environment free of microorganisms, radioactivity, or other contaminants.

deductible, *n* **1.** a stipulated sum the covered person must pay toward the cost of dental treatment before the benefits of the program go into effect. The deductible may be annual or payable only once and may vary in amount from program to program. *n* **2.** the amount of dental expense for which the beneficiary is responsible before a third party will assume any liability for payment of benefits. Deductible may be an annual or onetime charge and may vary in amount from program to program. See also family deductible.

deductible amount, n that portion of dental care expense the insured must pay before the plan's benefits begin.

deductible clause, n a provision in an insurance contract stipulating that the insurer will pay only that amount that is in excess of a specified amount.

deductive reasoning, *n* the ability to distill the pertinent facts and details of a situation from a wider body of evidence and generalizations.

deep bite, *n* See overbite.

deep sensibility, See sensibility, deep.

deepithelization (dē-ep′ithē′lizā′shən), *n* See debridement, epithelial.

DEF rate, See rate, DEF.

defamation (def′əmā′shən), *n* the act of detracting from the reputation of another. The offense of injuring a person's reputation by false and malicious statements.

default, *n* **1.** an omission of that which should be done. *v* **2.** to fail to fulfill an obligation or a promise.

defecation, *n* the elimination of feces from the digestive tract through the rectum.

defect, *n* **1.** the absence of some legal requisite. **2.** an imperfection.

defect, operative, n the incomplete repair of bone after root resection or periapical curettage.

defect, osseous, n a concavity in the bone surrounding one or more teeth, resulting from periodontal disease.

defect, speech, n any deviation of speech that is outside the range of acceptable variation in a given environment.

defective, mentally, *adj* a mentally subnormal individual. A person in whom a basic nervous system defect may be assumed because of social and intellectual deficiencies (for example, persons afflicted with microcephaly, hydrocephalus, or mongolism).

defendant, *n* the party against whom relief or recovery is sought in a lawsuit.

defense, *n* the reasons, in law or fact, offered by the defendant in a legal proceeding as to why the plaintiff should not prevail.

defense cell, n See cell, defense.

defense mechanism, n an unconscious, intrapsychic reaction that offers protection to the self from threatening or stressful situations. Defense mechanisms may be useful to diminish anxiety and facilitate coping behaviors, or may be harmful because of denying, displacing, isolating, or repressing anxiety and preventing useful coping responses.

defibrillation (dēfib′rilāshən), *n* the arrest of fibrillation, usually that of the cardiac ventricles. An intense alternating current is briefly passed through the heart muscle, throwing it into a refractory state.

defibrillator (dēfib′rilā′tur), *n* an apparatus for defibrillating the ventricles of the heart.

defibrillator, automatic external device, n an electric device attached to the abdomen or chest, which terminates erratic heartbeat by shock, thereby restoring the normal cardiac rhythm.

deficiency, *n* a lack or defect.

deficiency, ac-globulin, *n* See parahemophilia.

deficiency, dietary, *n* an inadequate amount of food intake or an insufficiency of any of the food elements necessary for proper nutrition.

deficiency, mineral, *n* a form of nutritional deficiency produced by the inadequate ingestion, absorption, use, and/or overexcretion of essential inorganic elements such as calcium, magnesium, and phosphorus.

deficiency, nicotinic acid, *n* a deficiency of nicotinic acid in the diet, resulting in acute erythematous stomatitis, papillary atrophy of the tongue, and ulcerative gingivitis.

deficiency, nutritional, *n* See deficiency, dietary.

deficiency, plasma thromboplastic antecedent, *n* See hemophilia C.

deficiency, protein, *n* a malnutritive state produced by inadequate ingestion, absorption, use, or overexcretion of essential protein elements. Degenerative lesions produced in the periodontium include osteoporosis of the alveolar and supporting bone and disappearance of fibroblasts and connective tissue fibers of the periodontal membrane.

deficiency, PTA, *n* See hemophilia C.

deficiency, vitamin A, gingival hyperplasia in, *n* hyperplastic and hyperkeratotic gingival changes occurring with decreased ingestion, diminished absorption, faulty use, or overexcretion of vitamin A. For example, in diabetes, the liver often cannot effectively convert carotene to vitamin A.

definition (image), *n* the property of projected images relating to their sharpness, distinctness, or clarity of outline. Penumbra width is a measure of definition. See also resolution.

definitive care, *n* refers to completion of recommended treatment.

deflective occlusal contact, *n* See contact, deflective occlusal.

deformation (dē′fôrmā′shən), *n* a distortion; a disfigurement.

deformation, elastic, *n* the term used to describe the change in shape of an object under an applied load from which the object can recover or

return to its original unloaded state when the load is removed.

deformation, inelastic, *n* a deformation occurring when a material is stressed beyond its elastic limit.

deformation, permanent, *n* a deformation occurring beyond the yield point so that the structure will not return to its original dimensions after removal of the applied force.

deformity, *n* a distortion or disfigurement of a portion of the body; may be congenital, familial, hereditary, acquired, pathologic, or surgical.

deformity, gingival, *n* a deviation from the normal gingival topographic and architectural pattern.

degeneration, ballooning, *n* a condition seen in vesicles of viral origin in which epithelial cells are washed from the vesicle wall. The cells swell and their nuclei undergo amitotic division, resulting in multinucleated giant cells that may be seen floating in vesicular fluid.

degeneration, basophilic granular, See basophilia.

degenerative joint disease, *n* a term to describe osteoarthritis. Osteoarthritis is a noninflammatory process as opposed to rheumatoid arthritis. Osteoarthritis occurs more frequently in women after the age of 40.

degloving, *n* an intraoral surgical exposure of the bony mandibular anterior region. This procedure can be performed in the posterior region if necessary.

Degloving injury. (Zitelli/Davis, 2002)

deglutition (dē′glōōtish′ən), *n* (swallowing), a succession of muscular contractions from above downward or from the front backward; propels food from the mouth toward the stomach. The action is generally initiated at the lips; it proceeds back through the oral cavity, and the food is moved automatically along the dorsum of the tongue. When the food is ready for swallowing, it is passed back through the fauces. Once the food is beyond the fauces and in the pharynx, the soft palate closes off the nasopharynx, and the hyoid bone and larynx are elevated upward and forward. This action keeps food out of the larynx and dilates the esophageal opening so that the food may be passed quickly toward the stomach by peristaltic contractions The separation between the voluntary and involuntary characteristics of this wave of contractions is not sharply defined. At birth the process is already well established as a highly coordinated activity, that is, the swallowing reflex.

degradation (deg′rədā′shən), *n* the reduction of a chemical compound to a less complex compound.

degrees of freedom (df), *n.pl* a statistic, based on the number of observations and groups in a study, that is necessary to determine statistical significance. One looks up the degrees of freedom and the significance level in a table of significance values to determine if the magnitude of the value obtained is significant. Used with the t-test, chi square, analysis of variance, and correlation.

dehiscence (dēhis′əns), *n* a fissural defect in the facial alveolar plate extending from the free margin apically.

dehiscent (dēhis′ənt), *adj* opened wide; fissured.
dehiscent mandibular canal, *n* a condition caused by bone resorption that leaves the mandibular canal without a covering or roof of bone.

dehydration (dē′hīdrā′shən), *n* **1.** the removal of water (for example, from the body or tissue). *n* **2.** a decrease in serum fluid coupled with the loss of interstitial fluid from the body. Dehydration is associated with disturbances in fluid and electrolyte balance.
dehydration of gingivae, *n* the drying of gingival tissue, leading to a lowered tissue resistance, which can result in gingival inflammation; seen in mouth breathing.

dehydrogenase, *n* an oxidoreductase class (EC 1) enzyme that induces the transportation of electrons or hydrogen from a donor, which usually indicates the dehydrogenase, to an acceptor compound.

delayed expansion, *n* See expansion, delayed.

delict (dilikt′), *n* a wrong or an injury; an offense; a violation of public or private obligation.

delinquent (deling′kwent), *n* pertaining to a debt or claim that is due and unpaid at the time due.

delirium (delir′ē-əm), *n* a condition of mental excitement, confusion, and clouded sensorium, usually accompanied by hallucinations, illusions, and delusions; precipitated by toxic factors in diseases or drugs.
delirium tremens, *n* a delirious state marked by distressing delusions, illusions, and hallucinations, constant tremor, fumbling movements of the hands, insomnia, and great exhaustion.

delivery, *n* a transfer of the possession of personal property from one person to another.

Delta Dental Plan, *n.pr* an active member organization of the Delta Dental Plans Association, formed and guided by state dental societies to provide prepaid dental care to the public on a group basis.

delusion, *n* a persistent, aberrant belief or perception held inviolable by a person despite evidence to the contrary.

demand, *n* in economics, refers to the buying of services or goods; in dental care, generally denotes the active request for and purchase of dental care services.

demeclocycline HCl, *n trade name:* Declomycin; *drug class:* tetracycline; *action:* inhibits protein synthesis, phosphorylation in microorganisms; *uses:* uncommon gram-positive or gram-negative bacteria or both, protozoa.

dementia, *n* a progressive, organic mental disorder characterized by chronic personality disintegration, confusion, disorientation, stupor, deterioration of intellectual capacity and function, and impairment or control of memory, judgment, and impulses (for example, senile psychosis, also associated with AIDS).

Demerol (dem′ərôl), *n.pr* the trade name for meperidine hydrochloride.

demineralization, *n* a measurable decrease in the level of inorganic salts or minerals in human tissue.

demography, *n* the study of human populations, particularly the size, distribution, and characteristics of members of population groups. Demographic techniques are employed in the long-term continuing study of the residents of Framingham, Massachusetts, by the National Institutes of Health.

demurrer (dēmur′ər), *n* an admission of the facts charged by the opponent while maintaining that those facts are legally insufficient to establish liability.

demyelinate (dēmī′-əlināt), *n* the process of removing or damaging the myelin sheath surrounding a nerve.

denasality (dēnəzal′itē), *n* the quality of the voice when the nasal passages are obstructed, preventing adequate nasal resonance during speech.

dendrite (den′drīt), *n* **1.** fingerlike projections formed during the solidification of crystalline materials. *n* **2.** a branched, treelike protoplasmic process of a neuron that carries nerve impulses toward the cell body. See also axon.

denervation (de′nurvā′shən), *n* the sectioning or removal of a nerve to interrupt the nerve supply to a part.

dens in dente (denz in den′tā), *n* (dens invaginatus, gestant odontoma), an anomaly of the tooth found chiefly in upper lateral incisors; characterized by invagination of the enamel, giving a radiographic appearance that suggests a "tooth within a tooth."

Dens in dente. (Bird/Robinson, 2002)

dens invaginatus (denz invajinä′təs), *n* See dens in dente.

Densite (den′sīt), *n.pr* the trade name for a form of alpha-hemihydrate with a low setting expansion and greater hardness; used for dies, models, and casts; sometimes referred to as a Class II stone.

densitometer (den′sitom′ətur), *n* an instrument for determining the degree of darkening of developed photographic or x-ray film, based on the use of a photoelectric cell to measure the light transmission through a given area of the film.

density, *n* the concentration of matter, measured by mass per unit volume.

density, radiographic, n the degree of darkening of exposed and processed photographic or x-ray film, expressed as the logarithm of the opacity of a given area of the film.

dental, *adj* relating to the teeth.

dental abutment, n See abutment.

dental alloy, n See alloy.

dental amalgam, n See amalgam.

dental ankylosis, n See tooth, ankylosed.

dental anxiety, n See anxiety.

dental arch, n See arch, dental.

dental articulator, n See articulator.

dental assistant, n See assistant, dental.

dental auxiliary, n See auxiliary personnel.

dental benefits organization, n any organization offering a dental benefits plan. Also known as dental plan organization.

dental benefits plan, n entitles covered individuals to specified dental services in return for a fixed, periodic payment made in advance of treatment. Such plans often include the use of deductibles, coinsurance, or maximums to control the cost of the program to the purchaser.

dental benefits program, n the specific dental benefits plan being offered to enrollees by the sponsor.

dental bonding, n See bonding.

dental calculus, n See calculus.

dental care, n the treatment of the teeth and their supporting structures.

dental care for children, n See pedodontics.

dental caries, n See caries, dental.

dental caries susceptible, n See susceptible.

dental cavity lining, n See cavity lining.

dental cement, n See cement, dental.

dental cementum, n See cementum.

dental chart, n See chart, dental.

dental clinic, n See clinic.

dental cooperative, n a dental facility organized to provide dental services for the benefit of subscribers and not for profit. There is no discrimination as to who may subscribe, and each subscriber has equal rights and voice in the control of the cooperative. The operation of the cooperative usually rests with a lay board of directors elected by subscribers.

dental deposit, n See calculus.

dental dysfunction, n See dysfunction, dental.

dental enamel, n See enamel.

dental enamel, hypoplastic, n See hypoplasia.

dental engine, n See engine, dental.

dental equipment, n See equipment.

dental fissure, n See fissure.

dental fistula, n See fistula.

dental floss, n waxed or plain thread of nylon or silk used to clean the interdental areas; an aid in oral physiotherapy.

dental floss, silk, n a particularly strong type of floss made from natural silk fibers loosely twisted into a strand, then waxed for maximum cleaning effectiveness between the teeth.

dental geriatrics, n See geriatrics.

dental granuloma, n See granuloma, dental.

dental handpiece, n See handpiece.

dental health services, n the sum of the diagnostic, preventive, consultative, supportive, and therapeutic dental care offered by the dental profession or that portion provided by a member of a dental health plan.

dental health surveys, n the use of questionnaires and oral examinations of a target population to determine the need or demand for dental care or the opinions or attitudes of patients or consumers.

dental history, n See history.

dental hygiene armamentarium, n See armamentarium.

dental hygiene diagnostic model, n one of four approaches to patient care. Its purpose is to arrive at a plan for recommended treatment by the systematic use of six steps that cover the major aspects of care, from initial inquiry to problem solving to patient education.

dental hygiene instrumentarium, n See instrumentarium.

dental hygiene process model, n one of four approaches to patient care, characterized by the documentation of a patient's expressed needs as they relate to a range of possible causes. Patient is questioned about various areas of concern, including overall health, gums, teeth, and brushing habits.

dental hygienist, n See hygienist, dental.

dental identification, n the process of establishing the unique characteristics of teeth and dental work of an individual, leading to the identification of an individual by comparison with the person's dental charts and records.

dental implant, n See implant.

dental impression material, n See impression.

dental instrument, n See instruments.

dental insurance, n a policy that insures against the expense of treatment and care of dental disease and accident to teeth.

dental jurisprudence, n the application of the principles of law as they relate to the practice of dentistry. See also jurisprudence, dental.

dental laboratory technician, n See technician, dental laboratory.

dental material, n See material, dental.

dental model, n See model.

dental neglect, n the purposeful denial of the minimum amount of oral health care or maintenance required to sustain functioning teeth and gums. The caretaker may exhibit a disregard for the patient's health, and may focus primarily on pain relief for the patient. Dental neglect is considered a warning sign of possible child or elder abuse.

D

Dental neglect. (Christensen, 2002)

dental occlusion, n See occlusion.

dental papilla, n See papilla.

dental pathology, n that branch of dentistry that deals with all aspects of dental disease. See also pathology.

dental pin, n See pin.

dental plan, n any organized method for the financing of dental care.

dental plaque, n See plaque.

dental porcelain, n See porcelain, dental.

dental prepayment, n a system for budgeting the cost of dental services in advance of their receipt.

dental prophylaxis, n See prophylaxis.

dental prosthesis, n See prosthesis.

dental prosthetic restoration, n See prosthesis, dental.

dental public health, n preferably called public health dentistry, this is a specialty of dentistry that deals with dental health on a community, regional, or national basis rather than on a provider-to-patient basis. However, some programs sponsored by public health dental agencies do provide for direct patient care for otherwise underserved populations. See also community dentistry.

dental pulp, n See pulp.

  dental pulp capping, n See capping, pulp.

  dental pulp cavity, n See cavity, pulp.

  dental pulp exposure, n See exposure.

dental record, n confidential documents containing the clinical and financial data of the dental patient, including the patient's identity, pertinent history, medical and dental conditions, services rendered, and charges and payments made.

dental research, n the formal scientific study of issues related to dentistry.

dental review committee, n a group of dentists and administrative personnel that reviews questionable dental claims and can suggest policy decisions regarding dental care.

dental sac, n connective tissue that envelops the developing tooth, and into which are implanted the enamel organ and dental papillae.

dental scaling, n See scaling.

dental sealant, n See sealant.

dental senescence, n See senescence, dental.

dental service corporation, n a legally constituted, not-for-profit organization that negotiates and administers contracts for dental care. Delta Dental and Blue Cross/Blue Shield corporations are two such organizations.

dental service, hospital, n **1.** the location of the dental facility within a hospital. *n* **2.** the array of dental procedures offered within a hospital setting.

dental splint, n See splint, dental.

dental staff, n the personnel employed or engaged by the dentist or the dentist's agent to conduct the assignable professional and management functions of the dental clinic, office, or practice.

dental stone, n See stone, dental.

dental tape, n See tape, dental.

dental technician, n See technician.

dental unit, n See unit, dental.

dentate (den′tāt), *adj* having teeth.

denticle (den′tikəl), *n* (endolith, pulp nodule, pulpstone), a calcified body found in the pulp chamber of a tooth; it may be composed either of irregular dentin (true denticle) or an ectopic calcification of pulp tissue (false denticle).

dentifrice, *n* a pharmaceutical compound used in conjunction with the toothbrush to clean and polish the teeth. Contains a mild abrasive, a detergent, a flavoring agent, a binder, and occasionally deodorants and various medicaments designed as caries preventives (for example, antiseptics).

dentifrice abrasion, n See abrasion, dentifrice.

dentifrice, anticalculus, n a commercially available toothpaste, gel, or powder formulated to inhibit the development of new calculus and which contains, among other ingredients, either pyrophosphate or zinc. It has no effect on existing calculus.

dentifrice, calculus-control, n See dentifrice, anticalculus.

dentifrice, flavoring agents, n any additive in liquid, powder, or paste oral hygiene products designed to enhance the product's taste. Flavors tend to be mint, and are derived primarily from essential oils.

dentifrice, foaming agents in, n also referred to as detergents or surfactants, these foam-generating ingredients are nontoxic, chemically compatible ingredients that also serve to remove unwanted matter from dental surfaces, make teeth feel smoother, and break down stains and deposits.

dentigerous cyst, *n* See cyst.

dentin (dun'tin), *n* (dentine), the portion of the tooth that lies subjacent to the enamel and cementum. Consists of an organic matrix on which mineral (calcific) salts are deposited; pierced by tubules containing filamentous protoplasmic processes of the odontoblasts that line the pulpal chamber and canal. It is of mesodermal origin.

dentin bonding agent, n a tissue compatible adhesive that adheres to dentin.

dentin, carious, n dentin that is involved in or affected by the carious process.

dentin dysplasia, n See dysplasia, dentinal.

dentin eburnation (ē'burnā'shən), n a change in carious teeth in which the softened and decalcified dentin assumes a hard, brown, polished appearance.

dentin, globular, n part of dentinal matrix consisting of completely fused and calcified globules of predentin.

dentin, hereditary opalescent, n See dentinogenesis imperfecta.

dentin, hyperesthesia of, n an excessive sensibility of dentin.

dentin, interglobular, n incompletely calcified dentinal matrix present between the calcified globules.

dentin, intertubular, n dentin present between the dentinal tubules.

dentin irritation (tertiary dentin, reparative dentin), n formed in response to an injury or irritant.

dentin, mantle, n outer portion of dentin bordering the enamel or cementum of the tooth.

dentin, residual carious, n See caries, dental, residual.

dentin, sclerotic, n See dentin, transparent.

dentin, secondary, n dentin formed or deposited on the walls of pulp chambers and canals subsequent to the complete formation of the tooth; caused by certain metabolic disturbances that result in irritation and stimulation of the odontoblasts to renewed activity.

dentin, transparent (sclerotic dentin), n dentin formed as a defense mechanism in reaction to various stimuli. Dental tubules are obliterated by deposits of calcium salts that are harder and denser than normal dentin. This dentin appears transparent in ground sections.

dentin wall, n the portion of the wall of a prepared cavity that consists of dentin.

dentinal, *adj* pertaining to the dentin.

dentinal fluid, n tissue fluid in the dentinal tubule that surrounds the odontoblasts which form the dentin tissue.

dentinal hypersensitivity, n condition caused by exposure of dentin due to caries, dental procedures, or attrition. May be painful in some cases.

dentinal permeability, n the degree to which fluids can pass through intact dentin.

dentine, *n* See dentin.

dentinocemental junction (dentin'ōsēmen'təl), *n* See junction, dentinocemental.

dentinoenamel junction, *n* See junction, dentinoenamel.

dentinogenesis imperfecta (den'tinōjen'əsis), *n* (hereditary opalescent dentin) **1.** a disturbance of the dentin of genetic origin; characterized by early calcification of the pulp chambers and root canals, marked attrition, and an opalescent hue to the teeth. *n* **2.** a localized form of mesodermal dysplasia affecting the dentin of the tooth. It may be hereditary and may be associated with osteogenesis imperfecta. *n* **3.** a hereditary condition associated with a defect in dentin formation; the enamel remains normal.

Dentinogenesis imperfecta. (Regezi/Sciubba/Jordan, 2003)

dentinoma (den'tinōmə), *n* an odontogenic tumor composed of regular or irregular dentin.

dentist, *n* one who is educated, trained, and licensed to treat diseases and injuries of the teeth and oral cavity and to construct and insert restorations of and for the teeth, jaws, and mouth.

dentistry, *n* the science and art of preventing, diagnosing, and treating diseases, injuries, and malformations of the teeth, jaws, and mouth and of replacing lost or absent teeth and associated structures.

dentistry, forensic, n See jurisprudence, dental.

dentistry, four-handed, n the technique of chairside operating in which four hands are kept busy working in the oral cavity simultaneously.

dentistry, operative, n the branch of oral health service concerned with operations to restore or reform the hard dental tissues (for example, operations necessitated by caries, trauma, and impaired function, and for improvement of appearance).

dentistry, prosthetic, n See prosthodontics.

dentistry, psychosomatic, n dentistry that concerns itself with the mind-body relationship.

dentistry, washed-field, n the constant flushing of the operative field with an irrigant (usually water) and the evacuation of the washing (debris) from the mouth by vacuum airstream. See also technique, hydroflow.

dentition (dentish'ən), *n* the natural teeth in position in the dental arches.

dentition, artificial, n artificial substitutes for the natural dentition. See also denture.

dentition, deciduous, n See dentition, primary.

dentition, mixed, n the complement of teeth in the jaws after the eruption of some of the permanent teeth but before all the primary teeth are absent.

dentition, permanent (secondary dentition, permanent teeth), n the 32 teeth of adulthood that either replace or are added to the complement of deciduous teeth.

dentition, primary, n the teeth that erupt first and are usually replaced by the permanent teeth. This term is currently preferred over *deciduous.*

dentition, prognosis of, n an evaluation by the dentist of the prospect of recovery from dental disease, combined with a forecast of the probability of maintaining the dentition and associated structures in function and health.

dentition, secondary, n See dentition, permanent.

dentition, transitional, n more commonly referred to as the *mixed dentition.* The transitional period usually begins with the eruption of the first permanent molars and ends with the exfoliation of the last primary tooth. In time span, about 6 years from age 6 to 12.

dentoalveolar surgery (den'tō-alvē'-əlur), *n* the category of oral surgery concerned with the extraction of teeth and the repair or restructuring of supporting bone. See also exodontics.

dentofacial deformity, *n* the malformation of the dentofacial complex with resultant disabling disharmony in size and form, as well as function. Includes malocclusion, cleft lip and palate, other skeletal deformities, and muscular dysfunctions.

dentofacial orthopedics, *n* a more descriptive synonym for orthodontics; the adjustment of relationships between and among teeth and facial bones by the application of outside forces and/or the stimulation and redirection of functional forces within the craniofacial complex.

dentoform, *n* a mock-up of the dentition and alveolar structures; used as a teaching aid or for display purposes.

dentogenesis (den'tōjen'əsis), *n* formation of the connective tissue, dentin, from odontoblasts during the development of the tooth. See also dentin.

dentogingival junction (den′tōjin′jivəl), *n* formed from the reduced enamel epithelium which is made up of the enamel organ remnants.

dentulous (dent′yōōləs), *adj* (dentulism), having the natural teeth present in the mouth.

denture, *n* an artificial substitute for missing natural teeth and adjacent tissues.

denture, acrylic resin, n a denture made of acrylic resin.

denture adhesive, n a pliable, self-adjusting product used to hold a dental prosthesis in position. Also referred to as an *adherent.*

denture, artificial, n See denture.

denture, basal surface of (impression surface of denture, foundation surface of denture), n the part of a denture base that is shaped to conform to the basal seat for the denture.

denture-bearing area, n See area, basal seat.

denture, bilateral partial, n a dental prosthesis that supplies teeth and associated structures on both sides of a semiedentulous arch.

denture brush, n a brush designed especially for cleaning dentures.

denture characterization, n a modification of the form and color of the denture base and teeth to produce a more lifelike appearance.

denture, complete (complete dental prosthesis), n a dental prosthesis that replaces all of the natural dentition and associated structures of the maxillae or mandible. It may be supported solely by the mucosa, or attached to implants in the alveolar process.

   denture, complete, lower, n a prosthetic replacement of all the teeth in the mandibular dental arch.

   denture, complete, upper, n a prosthetic replacement of all the teeth in the maxillary dental arch.

denture, coping, n See overdenture.

denture coverage, n the extent to which the oral tissue is covered by the denture base.

denture curing, n the process by which the denture base materials are hardened in a denture mold to the form of a denture. See also process.

denture delivery, n See denture placement.

denture deposits, n ranging in degree of severity and ease of removal, these first appear as easily dissolved food matter or mucin, can progress to dental plaque or yeast infection, and in severe cases can result in the formation of calculus, a deposit that requires professional intervention to remove.

denture design, n a planned visualization of the form and extent of a denture.

denture dislodging force, n See force, denture dislodging.

denture, duplicate, n a second denture intended to be a copy of the first denture.

denture edge, n See border, denture.

denture engraving tool, n a tool used to permanently inscribe the patient's name on the flange of his or her dental prosthesis for identification purposes.

denture esthetics, n See esthetics, denture.

denture, finish of, n the final perfection of the form of the polished surfaces of a denture.

denture flange, n See flange.

denture foundation, n the portion of the oral structures that supports the complete or partial denture base under occlusal load. See also area, basal seat.

   denture foundation, surface of, n See denture, basal surface of.

denture, full, n improper term. See denture, complete.

denture, heel of, n See distal end.

denture, immediate (immediate-insertion denture), n a removable dental prothesis constructed for placement immediately after removal of the remaining natural teeth.

denture, implant, n a denture that gains its support, stability, and retention from a substructure that is implanted under the soft tissues of the basal seat of the denture and is in contact with bone.

   denture, implant, substructure, n See substructure, implant.

   denture, implant, superstructure, n See superstructure, implant.

denture, impression surface of, n See denture, basal surface of.

denture, inclusion markers, n temporary labels affixed to the impression surface of the denture for identification during processing.

denture, insertion, *n* See denture, placement.

denture, interim, *n* a dental prosthesis that is to be used for a short interval of time.

denture liner, *n* a resin used to coat the tissue surface of a dental prosthesis to restore or improve the conformation of the prosthesis to the tissue; generally used to improve the retention of the denture.

denture, maintenance of, *n* an important part of prosthodontic treatment and a major factor in the longevity of the service that the restoration can be expected to give.

denture, metal base, *n* a denture with a base of gold, chrome-cobalt alloy, aluminum, or other metal.

denture, model, wax, *n* See denture, trial.

denture overlay, *n* a complete denture that is supported by both tooth and mucosa. Remaining teeth are used to provide additional stability to the denture.

denture packing, *n* See packing, denture.

denture, partial (partial dental prosthesis), *n* a prosthesis that replaces one or more, but less than all, of the natural teeth and associated structures.

   denture, partial, cantilever, *n* See denture, partial, cantilever fixed.

   denture, partial, cantilever fixed, *n* a fixed dental prosthesis that has one or more abutments at one end of the denture supporting pontic(s) at its other end.

   denture, partial, components of, *n* the units that compose a removable partial denture (for example, the base, the artificial teeth, direct and indirect retainers, major and minor connectors).

   denture, partial, construction of, *n* the science and technique of designing and constructing partial dentures.

   denture, partial, extension, *n* a removable partial denture that is retained by natural teeth at one end of the denture base segments only; a portion of the functional load is carried by the residual ridge.

denture, partial, fixed, *n* a tooth-borne partial denture that is intended to be permanently attached to the teeth or roots that furnish support to the restoration.

denture, partial, removable, *n* a partial denture that can be readily placed in the mouth and removed by the wearer.

denture, partial, temporary, *n* See denture, partial, treatment.

denture, partial, tissue-borne, *n* a removable partial denture that is not supported entirely by the natural teeth.

denture, partial, tooth-borne, *n* a partial denture that is supported entirely by the teeth that bound the edentulous area covered by the base.

denture, partial, tooth-borne/tissue-borne, *n* a partial denture that gains support from both an abutment tooth or teeth and from the structures of the edentulous area covered by the base.

denture, partial, treatment (temporary partial denture), *n* a dental prosthesis used for the purpose of treating or conditioning the tissues that are needed to support and retain a denture base.

denture, partial, unilateral, *n* a dental prosthesis that restores lost or missing teeth on one side of the arch only.

denture periphery, *n* See border, denture.

denture placement, *n* the act of inserting a dental prosthesis into the place in a patient's mouth for which it was designed. Also called *denture delivery* or *denture insertion.*

denture, polished surface of, *n* the portion of the surface of a denture that extends in an occlusal direction from the border of the denture and includes the palatal surface. It is the part of the denture base that is usually polished and includes the buccal and lingual surfaces of the teeth.

denture processing, *n* See processing, denture.

denture, provisional, *n* a prosthetic appliance to be used for a short period of time for reasons of esthetics, function, or occlusal support; more commonly referred to as a temporary, interim, or transitional denture. A provisional denture is usually an immediate denture and is most often employed in the maxillary arch.

denture repair, n the restoration of a broken or damaged dental prosthesis.

denture retention, n See retention, denture.

denture sore mouth, n See mouth, denture-sore.

denture space, n the space between the residual ridges and the cheeks and tongue that is available for dentures. See also distance, interarch.

denture stability, n See stability, denture.

denture, stomatitis, n See mouth, denture sore

denture supporting area, n See area, basal seat.

denture supporting structure, n See structure, denture supporting

denture, temporary, n a denture intended to serve for a very short time in a temporary or emergency situation.

denture, tooth-mucosa-supported, n See denture.

denture, transitional, n a removable partial denture that serves as a temporary prosthesis to which teeth will be added as more teeth are lost and that will be replaced after postextraction tissue changes have occurred. A transitional denture may become an interim denture when all the teeth have been removed from the dental arch.

denture, trial (wax model denture), n a temporary denture, usually made of wax on a baseplate, that is used for checking jaw relation records, occlusion, and the arrangement and observation of teeth for esthetics.

denture cleanser, n any of a variety of products designed to safely remove stains, deposits, and debris from the surfaces of dental prostheses, by means of immersion or brushing with a denture brush and paste, toothpaste, or powder.

denture cleanser, alkaline hypochlorite (hī′pōklôr′īt), n chemical ingredient used in some solutions to clean removable oral prostheses. The active ingredient is dilute sodium hypochlorite. It effectively removes food, stains, and plaque, and is read-

ily available in household bleach; it has a strong lingering scent and may damage prostheses.

denture cleanser, alkaline peroxide, n considered a light-duty denture cleaner; active ingredient is typically sodium perborate or sodium percarbonate. Comes in tablet or powder form; when combined with water, it creates bubbles. Does not effectively deal with calculus or darker staining.

denture cleanser, dilute acid, n chemical containing inorganic acids as its active ingredient; used to clean prosthetic dental appliances in an immersion regimen. Solutions range from 3% to 5% hydrochloric acid, a combination of phosphoric and hydrochloric acids, and vinegar (acetic acid), which is very mild and has limited effectiveness. Regular use of dilute acids can damage any metal on the prosthetic device.

denture cleanser, enzyme, n an agent that is sometimes added to immersion cleaning solutions, which works by weakening polysaccharides and plaque proteins.

denturist, n a person other than a dentist (usually a technician) who engages in the practice of dentistry that is usually limited to making and fitting complete or partial dentures. Such activity is outside the dental practice act of most states.

denudation (den′yōōdā′shən), n stripping bare; the process of removing the outer (epithelial) layer by surgery or disease.

deoxyribonucleic acid probes, n a nucleic acid fragment labeled with a radioisotope that is complementary to a sequence in another nucleic acid fragment that will bind to it and thus identify it. It is used as a diagnostic tool to identify the species of microbe involved in an infectious process such as refractory periodontal disease.

dependence, physical, n the level of substance abuse at which disagreeable or severe physiologic symptoms will occur if use of the substance is suddenly terminated.

dependency, n the state of being dependent.

dependency, drug, n a psychologic craving for, habituation to, or addiction to a chemical substance; the term replaces drug addiction, which emphasizes physiologic craving.

dependency, emotional, n an emotional need manifested by a marked and habitual inclination to rely on another for comfort, support, guidance, and decision making; the tendency to seek help from others in making decisions or in carrying out difficult actions; the need to be mothered, loved, taken care of, emotionally supported. In extreme cases such persons lose their ability to function independently.

dependents, *n.pl* generally the spouse and children of a subscriber, as defined in a contract. Under some contracts, parents or other members of the family may be beneficiaries.

depletion, salt (dēplē'shən), *n* a condition resulting from inadequate water intake, low intake of sodium and chlorides in the alimentary tract, and secretion of sweat and urine. The most significant of these losses are the gastrointestinal fluid losses resulting from vomiting, diarrhea, and fistulas.

depolarization (dēpō'lərizā'shən), *n* a neutralization of polarity; the breaking down of polarized semipermeable membranes, as in nerve or muscle cells in the induction of impulses.

deponent, *n* one who gives under oath testimony reduced to writing.

deposit, bismuth, *n* See stomatitis, bismuth.

deposit, calcareous, *n* See calculus.

deposition (dep'ōzish'ən), *n* evidence given by a witness under interrogation, oral or written, and usually written down by an official person and intended to be used in the trial of an action in court.

deposits, assessment of, *n* the examination of the teeth for evidence of food particles, calculus, bacterial plaque, and miscellaneous debris which, if not removed, may lead to tooth decay and periodontal infection.

deposits, nonmineralized (soft), *n.pl* soft deposits, consisting of acquired pellicle, bacterial plaque, materia alba, and food debris, which accumulate on tooth surfaces and within periodontal pockets. If left unattended, will harden into calculus

and may cause tooth decay and/or periodontal infections.

depot (dē'pō), *n* in physiology, the site of accumulation, deposit, or storage of body products not immediately or actively involved in metabolic processes (for example, a fat depot).

depreciation, *n* normally, charges against earnings to write off the cost, less salvage value, of an asset over its estimated useful life. It is a bookkeeping entry and does not represent any cash outlay, nor are any funds earmarked for the purpose. Following are three classic methods of applying depreciation: straight line, sum of the year's digits, and double declining balance.

depressant (dēpres'ənt), *n* a medicine that diminishes functional activity.

depressed oral lesions, *n.pl* abnormalities found in the mouth, characterized by their subsurface occurrence and nonuniform shape. They may be classified as either erosions, which are considered superficial (that is, having a depth of less than 3 mm), or the more frequently occurring ulcers, which may be up to 3 mm in depth. Ulcers may be the result of elevated lesions that have burst, and vary in appearance, with centers being yellow to gray, while the borders are typically red.

depression (dēpresh'ən), *n* **1.** a decrease of functional activity. *n* **2.** a pitted area on a tooth or other anatomical surface.

depression, developmental, n depression seen in a defined region on a tooth.

depression, mandible, n lowering of the mandible caused by rotational movement of the temporomandibular joint.

depression, postpartum, n a moderate to severe form of depression which occurs in women beginning approximately 2 to 3 weeks after childbirth as a result of physical and psychological factors. Symptoms include fatigue, loss of appetite, and lack of enthusiasm for everyday activities.

depression, psychologic, n a clinical syndrome of neurotic or psychotic proportions, consisting of lowering of mood tone (feelings of painful dejection), difficulty in thinking, and psychomotor retardation. As used by the layman, depression ordinarily refers only to the mood element, which would be more appropriately labeled dejection, sadness, gloominess, despair, or despondency. Many such patients lack motivation and concern for their oral health or dental needs.

derivative (dēriv′ətiv), *n* a chemical substance that is the result of a chemical reaction.

dermal undergloves, *n* an additional pair of protective hand coverings, worn to protect sensitive skin from the latex or nonlatex material of the outer glove.

dermatalgia (durmətal′jē-ə), *n* pain, burning, and other sensations of the skin unaccompanied by any structural change; probably caused by some nervous disease or reflex influence.

dermataneuria (dur′matənŏŏrē-ə), *n* a derangement of the nerve supply of the skin, causing disturbance of sensation.

dermatitis (durmətī′tis), *n* an inflammation of the skin.

dermatitis, allergic contact, n the reaction of the skin to direct contact with a specific antigen. Poison ivy rash is a common example of an allergic contact dermatitis.

dermatitis, atopic, n atopic eczema characterized by the distinctive phenomenon of atopy, a familial related allergic response associated with IgE antibody.

dermatitis, contact, n a delayed type of induced sensitivity (allergy) of the skin with varying degrees of erythema, edema, and vesiculation, resulting from cutaneous contact with a specific allergen. Contact dermatitis is an occupational hazard in dentistry.

dermatitis herpetiformis, n dermatitis characterized by grouped, erythematous, papular, vesicular, pustular, or bullous lesions occurring in various combinations, often accompanied by vesicobullous and ulcerative lesions of the oral mucous membranes.

dermatitis infectiosa eczematoides (Engman's disease), n a pustular eczematous eruption that frequently follows or occurs coincidentally with some pyogenic process.

dermatitis, occupational, n generally a contact dermatitis associated with allergens found in the workplace.

dermatitis, radiation, n an inflammation of the skin resulting from a high dose of radiation. The reaction varies with the quality and quantity of radiation used and is usually transitory.

dermatitis, seborrheic, n a chronic inflammatory skin disease that can affect the scalp, face, ears, armpits, breasts, and groin. Its symptoms include moist, greasy, or dry scaling and patches of yellowish crust. Although the cause of seborrheic dermatitis is unknown, it can be treated with selenium sulfide shampoos, topical antibiotics, and topical and oral corticosteroids.

dermatoglyphics, *n* the study of the skin ridge patterns on fingers, toes, palms of hands, and soles of feet. The patterns are used as a basis of identification (fingerprinting).

dermatology, *n* the study of the skin, including the anatomy, physiology, and pathology of the skin and the diagnosis and treatment of skin disorders.

dermatoma, *n* a circumscribed thickening or hypertrophy of the skin.

dermatome, *n* an instrument for cutting thin slices or layers of skin for grafting or for sequentially removing small lesions.

dermatomyositis (dur′mətōmī′-ōsī′tis), *n* (polymyositis, dermatomucosomyositis) a form of collagen disease related to scleroderma and lupus erythematosus. The skin lesions are diffuse erythematous desquamations or rashlike lesions. The skin symptoms are related to a variety of patterns of myositis.

dermatophyte, *n* any of several fungi that cause parasitic skin disease in humans.

dermatosclerosis (dur′mətōsklərō′sis), *n* See scleroderma.

dermatosis (dur′mətō′sis), *n* any disease of the skin.

dermis (dur′mis), *n* the layer of skin just below the epidermis consisting of vascular connective tissue.

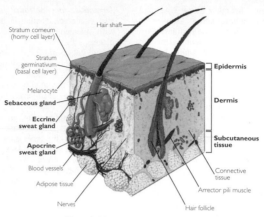

Labels on figure:
Stratum corneum (horny cell layer)
Stratum germinativum (basal cell layer)
Melanocyte
Sebaceous gland
Eccrine sweat gland
Apocrine sweat gland
Blood vessels
Adipose tissue
Nerves
Hair shaft
Epidermis
Dermis
Subcutaneous tissue
Connective tissue
Arrector pili muscle
Hair follicle

Normal skin anatomy. (Jarvis, 2000)

dermoid cyst, *n* See cyst, dermoid.

desaturation (dēsat′yərā′shən), *n* the conversion of a saturated compound such as stearin into an unsaturated compound such as olein by the removal of hydrogen.

desensitization (dēsen′sitizā′shən), *n* **1.** a condition of insusceptibility to infection or an allergen; established in experimental animals by the injection of an antigen that produces sensitization or an anaphylactic reaction. After recovery, a second injection of the antigen is made, bringing about no reaction and thus producing desensitization. *n* **2.** reduction in dentinal hypersensitivity by the addition of medicaments to the exposed dentin surface.

desensitization, psychological, *n* the deliberate exposure of an individual to imagined or actual emotionally stressful experiences to treat phobias and other related conditions.

desiccate (des′ikāt), *n* to dry by chemical or physical means; for example, electrocoagulation can produce desiccation in tissues.

desiccation (des′ikā′shən), *n* excessive loss of moisture; the process of drying up. See also electrocoagulation.

design, *v* **1.** to plan or delineate by drawing the outline of a proposed prosthesis. *n* **2.** the graphical and artistic representation of a plan.

designer drugs, *n.pl* synthetic organic compounds that are designed as analogs of illicit drugs and have the same narcotic or other dangerous effects.

desipramine HCl, *n trade names:* Norpramin, Petrofrane; *drug class:* antidepressant, tricyclic; *action:* inhibits both norepinephrine and serotonin (5-HT) uptake in the brain; *use:* depression.

desmins, *n.pl* α-amino acids, usually lysine and norleucine, condensed through their sidechains rather than through the α-amino and carboxyl groups. They copolymerize with vimentin to form constituents of connective tissue.

desmolysis (desmol′isis), *n* the destruction and disintegration of connective tissue. Some authorities associate this desmolytic process with the destruction of connective tissue lying between the enamel and oral epithelium, which thus permits proliferation of the oral epithelium and fusion of enamel and oral epithelium.

desmopressin acetate, *n trade name:* Stimate; *drug class:* synthetic antidiuretic hormone; *action:* promotes reabsorption of water by action on renal tubular epithelium; *uses:* primary nocturnal enuresis, hemophilia A with factor VIII levels of less than 5%, von Willebrand's disease, and neurogenic diabetes insipidus.

desmosomes, *n.pl* See epithelium, desmosomes of.

desonide, *trade names:* DesOwen, Tridesilon; *drug class:* topical corticosteroid, group IV low potency; *action:* possesses antipruritic, antiinflammatory actions; *uses:* psoriasis, eczema, contact dermatitis, pruritus.

desoximetasone, *n* *trade names:* Topicort, Topicort LP; *drug class:* topical corticosteroid, group II potency (0.25%), group III potency (0.05%); *action:* interacts with steroid cytoplasmic receptors to induce antiinflammatory effects; *uses:* psoriasis, eczema, contact dermatitis, pruritus.

desquamation (des'kwəmā'shən), *n* a naturally occurring process in which the outer layer of skin or mucosa cells is sloughed off.

detector, radiation, *n* See radiation detector.

detention, *n* restraint; custody; confinement.

detergent (dētur'jənt), *n* a cleanser. Also applied in a more specific sense to chemicals that possess surface-active properties in water and whose solutions are therefore able to wet surfaces that are normally water repellent, thereby assisting in the mechanical dispersion and emulsification of fatty or oily material and other substances that soil the surface.

detergent, **anionic,** *n* a detergent in which the cleansing action resides in the anion. Soaps and many synthetic detergents are anionic.

detergent, **cationic,** *n* a detergent in which the cleansing action resides in the cation. Many such detergents are strong germicides (for example, those that contain quaternary ammonium compounds).

detergent, **nonionic,** *n* a cleanser that acts by depressing the surface tension of water but does not ionize.

detergent, **synthetic,** *n* a cleanser, other than soap, that exerts its effect by lowering the surface tension of an aqueous cleansing mixture.

detoxicate (dētok'sikāt), *v* See detoxify.

detoxify, *v* (detoxicate), to remove the toxic quality of a substance.

detritus (det'ritus), *n* fragments or scraps that cling to teeth, gums, or other oral surfaces.

deuterium, a stable isotope of the hydrogen atom, used as a tracer. Also called *heavy hydrogen.*

deuterium oxide, *n* heavy water, so named because it is formed from an isotope of hydrogen, which has twice the weight of ordinary hydrogen.

developed countries, *n.pl* countries with an economic base built largely on manufacturing and technology rather than agriculture. Although the need for medical and dental care may not differ from undeveloped to developed countries, the effective demand does vary. Developed countries have the available health professionals, the economic base to support the purchase of health care, and an informed public.

developer, *n* a chemical solution that converts the invisible (latent) image on a film into a visible one composed of minute grains of metallic silver.

developer stain, *n* See film fault, black spots.

developing countries, *n.pl* countries in transition from an agrarian economy to a manufacturing- and technology-based economy.

developing, time-temperature method, *n* the procedure of developing dental films; a solution of fixed temperature is used, and the films are immersed in the solution for a specific length of time.

developing, visual method, *n* the procedure of developing dental films by placing the films in the developing solution and holding them from time to time before a safelight. Correct development has occurred when the film becomes so dark that it is difficult to distinguish between tooth and bone structure.

development, *n* the process by which an individual reaches maturity.

development hyperactivity, *n* a condition distinguished by continuous movement, restlessness, impetuosity, excitability, and a short span of attention. Also called *hyperkinesis.*

developmental biology, *n* the study of life processes occurring during growth and maturation.

developmental disabilities (DD), *n.pl* pathologic conditions that have their origin in the embryology and growth and development of an individual. DDs usually appear clinically

D

before 18 years of age. The limitations of physiologic or mental function usually persist throughout life.

deviation (dē′vē-ā′shən), *n* turning from a regular course; deflection.

device, scavenging, *n* a device which collects and removes exhaled nitrous oxide during the administration of nitrous oxide and oxygen for sedation. The device is recommended by the American Dental Association to avoid occupational exposure to the gas.

devital tooth, See tooth, pulpless.

dexamethasone/dexamethasone acetate/dexamethasone sodium phosphate, *n trade names:* Decadron, Hexadrol, Oradexan; *drug class:* glucocorticoid, long-acting; *action:* decreases inflammation by suppression of macrophage and leukocyte migration, reduces capillary permeability; *uses:* inflammation, allergies, neoplasm, cerebral edema, shock, collagen disorders.

dexamethasone/dexamethasone sodium phosphate, *n trade name:* Decaderm; *drug class:* synthetic topical corticosteroid; *action:* interacts with steroid cytoplasmic receptors to induce antiinflammatory effects; *uses:* corticosteroid-responsive dermatoses; oral ulcerative inflammatory lesions.

dexchlorpheniramine maleate, *n trade names:* Dexchlor, Poladex TD; *drug class:* antihistamine; *action:* acts on blood vessels, gastrointestinal system, respiratory system by competing with histamine for H_1-receptor sites; decreases allergic response by blocking histamine; *uses:* allergy symptoms, rhinitis, pruritus, contact dermatitis.

dextran (dek′stran), *n* ($C_6H_{10}O_5$) a water-soluble polymer of glucose of high molecular weight. A purified form, having an average molecular weight of 75,000, is used in a 6% concentration in isotonic sodium chloride solution to expand plasma volume and maintain blood pressure in emergency treatment of hemorrhagic and traumatic shock.

dextro-, *adj/comb* the prefix designating that an aqueous solution of a substance rotates the plane of polarized light to the right. See also isomers, optical.

dextroamphetamine sulfate, *n trade names:* Dexedrine, Oxydess II; *drug class:* amphetamine, Controlled Substance Schedule II; *action:* increases release of norepinephrine and dopamine in the cerebral cortex to the reticular activating system; *uses:* narcolepsy, attention deficit disorder with hyperactivity.

dextromethorphan hydrobromide, *n trade names:* Benylin DM, Robitussin Pediatric, Vicks Formula 44; *drug class:* antitussive, nonnarcotic; *action:* depresses cough center in medulla; *use:* nonproductive cough.

dextrorotatory (dek′strōrō′tətôrē), *adj* turning the plane of polarization, or rays of polarized light, to the right.

dextrose (dek′strōs), *n* dextrorotatory glucose, a monosaccharide occurring as a white, crystalline powder; colorless and sweet.

diabetes (dī-əbē′tēz), *n* a deficiency condition involving carbohydrate metabolism and characterized by the habitual discharge of an excessive amount of urine.

diabetes, bronzed, *n* the combination of hemochromatosis and diabetes mellitus. The skin takes on a bronzed appearance as a result of the deposition of an iron-containing pigment in the skin.

diabetes, gestational, *n* the term describing patients who acquire glucose intolerance when pregnant.

diabetes insipidus, *n* **1.** a metabolic disturbance characterized by marked urinary excretion and great thirst but no elevation of sugar in the blood or urine. *n* **2.** a pituitary dysfunction characterized by an insufficient output of antidiuretic hormone, leading to polyuria and polydipsia.

diabetes, juvenile, *n* diabetes mellitus occurring in children and adolescents, usually of a more severe and rampant nature than diabetes mellitus in adults, with consequent difficulty of regulation.

diabetes mellitus, *n* a metabolic disorder caused primarily by a defect in the production of insulin by the islet cells of the pancreas resulting in an inability to use carbohydrates. Characterized by hyperglycemia, glycosuria, polyuria, hyperlipemia (caused by imperfect catabolism of fats), acidosis, ketonuria, and a lowered resistance to infection. Periodontal manifestations may include recurrent and multiple periodontal abscesses, osteoporotic changes in alveolar bone, fungating masses of granulation tissue protruding from periodontal pockets, a lowered resistance to infection, and delay in healing after periodontal therapy.

diabetes mellitus, amputation, n a great number of limb amputations are caused by diabetes, especially amputations of the feet; blood infections in the feet can go unnoticed by the patient because of a lack of feeling caused by diabetic neuropathy.

diabetes mellitus, insulin-dependent (IDDM), n a type 1 diabetes that includes patients requiring the administration of insulin to prevent ketosis. Previously called *juvenile-onset diabetes, brittle diabetes,* and *ketosis-prone diabetes.*

diabetes mellitus, non-insulin-dependent (NIDDM), n a type 2 diabetes that includes patients who can maintain proper blood sugar levels within the administration of insulin. Previously called *maturity-onset diabetes, adult-onset diabetes, ketosis-resistant diabetes,* and *stable diabetes.*

diabetes, phlorizin, n a condition of glycosuria caused by inhibition of phosphorylation of phlorizin. It is not related to an endocrine disturbance.

diabetic, *adj* of or pertaining to diabetes.

diabetic ketoacidosis (DKA), n diabetic coma, an acute, life-threatening complication of uncontrolled diabetes mellitus in which urinary loss of water, potassium, ammonium, and sodium results in hypovolemia, electrolyte imbalance, extremely high blood glucose levels, and the breakdown of free fatty acids causing acidosis.

diabetic nephropathy, n the negative effects on the kidneys or renal system caused by diabetes mellitus. The condition may necessitate dialysis or kidney transplant.

diabetic neuropathy, n the negative effects on the nervous system that can be caused by diabetes mellitus, some of which may necessitate amputation or result in oral or facial symptoms.

diabetic retinopathy **(ret′inop′əthē),** *n* the negative effects on the eye that can be caused by diabetes mellitus, some of which may result in blindness.

diadochokinesia (dī-ad′əkōkīnē′zē-ə, -zhə), *n* the act or process of repeating at maximum speed a simple cyclical, reciprocating movement such as raising and lowering of the mandible or protrusion and retracting the tongue.

diagnose, *v* to distinguish irregularities and other issues of concern based upon a patient's examination and interview.

diagnosis, *n* the translation of data gathered by clinical and radiographic examination into an organized, classified definition of the conditions present.

diagnosis, clinical, n the determination of the specific disease or diseases involved in producing symptoms and signs by examination of the patient and use of analogy.

diagnosis, differential, n the process of identifying a condition by differentiating all pathologic processes that may produce similar lesions.

diagnosis, final, n the diagnosis arrived at after all the data have been collected, analyzed, and subjected to logical thought. Treatment may be necessary in some instances before the final diagnosis is made.

diagnosis, laboratory, n a diagnosis made from chemical, microscopic, microbiologic, immunologic, or pathologic study of secretions, discharges, blood, or tissue sections.

diagnosis, oral, n the identification of the cause of a dental disease or abnormality.

diagnosis, radiographic, n a limited term used to indicate those radiologic interpretations that cannot be verified or disproved by clinical examination.

diagnosis-related group (DRG), n a system of classifying hospital patients on the basis of diagnosis consisting of distinct groupings. A DRG assignment to a case is based on the patient's principal diagnosis, treat-

D

ment procedures performed, age, gender, and discharge status.

diagnosis, surgical, *n* a surgical incision into a body part or the excision of a lesion for the purpose of determining the cause or nature of an illness.

diagnostic cast, *n* See cast, diagnostic.

diagnostic equilibration, a measuring method of determining and recording on dentodes the amount and direction that interfering cusps deflect the closure direction of the mandible, as can be seen in mountings.

diagnostic error, *n* a mistake in judgment regarding the cause of an illness.

diagnostic imaging, *n* the use of radiographic, sonographic, and other technologies to create a graphic depiction of the body part(s) in question.

diagnostic services, *n.pl* those imaging and laboratory capabilities available for determining the cause of an illness.

dialysis (dī-al′isis), *n* a type of filtration used to separate smaller molecules from larger ones contained in a solution. The molecular solution is placed on one side of a semipermeable membrane and water on the other side. The smaller molecules pass through the membrane into the water; the larger molecules are retained in the solution.

diamond, *n* a crystalline carbon substance, the hardest natural substance known, used industrially and in dentistry for cutting and grinding.

diamond particles, *n.pl* elements of a diamond polishing paste which are used to bring out the natural luster of porcelain surfaces.

diaphragm (dī′-əfram), *n* **1.** a musculotendinous partition that separates the thorax and abdomen. *n* **2.** a metal barrier plate, often of lead, pierced with a central aperture so arranged as to limit the emerging, or useful, beam of roentgen rays to the smallest practical diameter for making radiographic exposures. See also collimation; collimator; distance, cone.

diaphragm, lead, *n* a collimating device with a small opening, designed to limit the size of the outgoing x-ray

beam. It is usually made of lead one-eighth of an inch thick and located between the position-indicating device and the x-ray tube itself.

diaphragm, Potter-Bucky, See grid, Potter-Bucky.

diaphysis (di-af′isis), *n* the shaft of a long bone.

diarrhea, *n* the frequent passage of loose, watery stools. The stool may also contain mucus, pus, blood, or excessive amounts of fat. Diarrhea is usually a symptom of some underlying disorder. See antidiarrheals

diarthrosis (dī′-ärthrō′sis), *n* See synovial joint.

diastema (dī′-əstē′mə), *n* an abnormal space between two adjacent teeth in the same dental arch.

Diastema. (Zitelli/Davis, 2002)

diastole (dī-as′təlē) *n* **1.** the rhythmic period of relaxation and dilation of a chamber of the heart during which it fills with blood. *n* **2.** the period after the contraction of the heart muscle, during which the aorta releases the potential energy stored in its elastic tissue. The energy is converted into kinetic energy and sustains the pressure necessary for steady flow of blood in the vessels. The pressure measured at this period is the lowest attained during the cardiac pumping cycle and is called the *diastolic pressure.* The normal pressure in the adult is approximately 120/80 mm Hg (systolic/diastolic) and increases with age from 128/85 at 45 years of age to 135/89 at 60 years of age.

diathermy (di′əthur′mē), *n* a generalized rise in tissue temperature produced by a high-frequency alternating current between two electrodes. The temperature rise is produced without causing tissue damage.

diathesis (dī-ath´əsis), *n* a tendency, based on body makeup or constitutional, hereditary, or acquired states of the body, that causes a predisposition or susceptibility to disease.

diathesis, hemorrhagic, n a condition that may be caused by defects in the coagulation mechanism, blood vessel wall, or both.

diazepam, *n trade name:* Valium; *drug class:* benzodiazepine, anxiolytic Controlled Substance Schedule IV; *action:* produces CNS depression by acting on parts of the limbic system and the thalamus and hypothalamus, inducing a calming effect; *uses:* management of short-term anxicty disorders and relief of symptoms of anxiety, short-term relief of skeletal muscle spasm, acute alcohol withdrawal.

Dick's test, *n* See test, Dick's.

diclofenac, *n trade names:* Cataflam, Voltaren; *drug class:* nonsteroidal antiinflammatory; *action:* inhibits prostaglandin synthesis; *uses:* acute and chronic rheumatoid arthritis, osteoarthritis, ankylosing spondylitis.

dicloxacillin sodium, *n trade names:* Dycill, Dynapen, Pathocil; *drug class:* penicillinase-resistant penicillin; *action:* interferes with cell wall replication of susceptible organisms; *uses:* infections caused by penicillinase-producing *Staphylococcus.*

dicyclomine HCl, *n trade names:* Antispas, Dibent; *drug class:* GI anticholinergic; *action:* inhibits muscarinic actions of acetylcholine at postganglionic parasympathetic neuroeffector sites; *uses:* peptic ulcer disease in combination with other drugs; infant colic.

didanosine, *n trade name:* Videx; *drug class:* synthetic antiviral; *action:* converted by cellular enzymes that act as antimetabolites to inhibit HIV replication; *uses:* advanced HIV infections in adults and children who have been unable to use zidovudine or who have not responded to treatment with zidovudine.

dideoxycytidine, *n* a dideoxynucleoside under study as an antiviral in the treatment of AIDS. See also Zalcitabine.

dideoxyinosine, *n* a dideoxynucleoside under study as an antiviral in the treatment of AIDS. See also didanosine.

die, *n* the positive reproduction of the form of a prepared tooth in any suitable hard substance, usually in metal or specially prepared (improved) artificial stone.

die, lubricant, n a material applied to a die to serve as a separating medium so that the wax pattern will not adhere to the die but may be withdrawn from it without sticking.

die, stone, n a positive likeness in artificial (dental) stone; used in the fabrication of a dental restoration.

die, waxing, n a mold into which wax is forced for the production of standardized wax patterns.

dienestrol, *n trade name:* Ortho Dienestrol; *drug class:* nonsteroidal synthetic estrogen; *action:* needed for adequate functioning of female reproductive system; affects release of pituitary gonadotropins, inhibits ovulation; *uses:* atrophic vaginitis, kraurosis vulvae.

diet, *n* **1.** the food and drink consumed by a given person from day to day. Not all the diet is necessarily used by the body. For this reason, diet and nutrition must be differentiated. *v* **2.** to eat according to a plan.

diet, alkaline, n a diet that is basic in reaction; produced by the addition of alkaline salts, including sodium bicarbonate.

diet, cariogenic, n the intake of food that is heavy in refined carbohydrates and other food stuffs that support the growth of caries-producing bacteria.

diet, lysine-poor, n a diet deficient in lysine, an essential amino acid. All the essential amino acids must be present in the diet; should one or more be absent, proper use of the others cannot occur. Periodontal changes described in experimental animals with lysine deficiency include osteoporosis of supporting bone and disintegration and failure of replacement of periodontal fibers.

dietary carbohydrates, *n* the amount of simple and complex sugars consumed; the physical character of the diet. It may tend to produce or modify periodontal disease.

dietary fiber, *n* a generic term for nondigestible chemical substances found in plant cell walls. Foods high in dietary fiber are fruits, green leafy vegetables, root vegetables, and whole grain cereals and bread.

dietary history, *n* See analysis, dietary.

dietary reference intakes (DRIs), *n.pl* a set of nutritional guidelines concerning the intake of vitamins and minerals from food rather than supplements.

dietetics, *n* the science of applying nutritional principles to the planning and preparation of foods and the regulation of the diet in relation to both health and disease.

diethylpropion HCl, *n trade names:* Tenuate Dospan, Ten-Tab; *drug class:* anorexant, amphetamine-like analog Controlled Substance Schedule IV; *action:* exact mechanism of appetite suppression is unknown, may have an effect on the satiety center of the hypothalamus; *use:* exogenous obesity.

diethylstilbestrol (dī-eth′ilstilbes′ trôl), *n* an estrogenic substance, $C_{18}H_{20}O_2$, that has an estrogenic activity considered to be greater than that of estrone. Useful in treating menopausal symptoms and occasionally used in the therapy of chronic desquamative gingivitis associated with artificial or natural menopause.

dietitian, registered (dī-ətish′ən), *n* an individual who meets the requirements of the American Dietetic Association (ADA) including possession of a bachelor's degree in dietetics or nutrition, a passing grade on the registration exam, and a demonstrated commitment to continuing education through updated courses taken annually.

difenoxin HCl with atropine sulfate, *n trade name:* Motofen; *drug class:* antidiarrheal Controlled Substance Schedule IV; *action:* inhibits gastric motility by acting on mucosal receptors responsible for peristalsis; *uses:* acute nonspecific diarrhea and acute exacerbations of chronic functional diarrhea.

differential force, *n* a term sometimes used to describe the design and application of an orthodontic appliance to distribute the reciprocal forces of the appliance over significantly different root areas with the objective of eliciting a differential response.

difficult eruption, See teething.

diffusibility (difyōōz′ibil′itē), *n* capable of being diffused.

diffusion (difyōō′zhən), *n* a property of ions or molecules of a solute that permits them to pass through a membrane or to intermingle by rapid or gradual permeation with the molecules of a solvent.

diffusion, facilitated, *n* an absorption process during which only certain recognized molecules are allowed to pass into the receiving area.

diflorasone diacetate, *n trade names:* Florone, Maxiflor, Psorcon; *drug class:* topical corticosteroid, group II high potency; *action:* possesses antipruritic, antiinflammatory actions; *uses:* psoriasis, eczema, contact dermatitis, pruritus.

diflunisal, *n trade name:* Dolobid; *drug class:* salicylate derivative, nonsteroidal antiinflammatory; *action:* inhibits prostaglandin synthesis; *uses:* mild-to-moderate pain, symptoms of rheumatoid arthritis and osteoarthritis.

digestion, *n* the conversion of food into absorbable substances in the GI tract.

digit, *n* **1.** a single symbol or character representing a quantity. *n* **2.** a finger or toe.

digit sucking, *n* an oral habit, usually referred to as *finger* or *thumb sucking,* that is not unusual in preschool children. Prolonged, persistent, or vigorous sucking into the transition dentition period can cause tooth displacement malocclusions.

digital, *adj* **1.** involving the use of the fingers. *adj* **2.** a means of data storage in which information is converted to numeric strings. *adj* **3.** using alphanumeric characters to display data, as opposed to analog, which uses the relative position of needles or "hands" (as with a clock) against a background scale.

digital massage, *n* a manual technique developed to increase blood flow to the area of the mouth where dentures are worn. The technique involves a moderate, pulse-squeeze movement with the index finger and the thumb over the affected region. The roof of the mouth is gently pressed with the thumb pad.

digitalization (dij′italizā′shən), *n* the administration of digitalis in sufficient amount by any of several types of dosage schedules to build up the concentration of digitalis glycosides in the body of a patient.

digitoxin, *n trade names:* Crystodigin, Digitaline; *drug class:* cardia glycoside; *action:* inhibits the formation of sodium-potassium ATPase, which makes more calcium available for contractile proteins; *uses:* congestive heart failure (CHF), atrial fibrillation, paroxysmal atrial flutter, atrial tachycardia.

digoxin, *n trade names:* Lanoxicaps, Lanoxin, Novadigoxin; *drug class:* cardiac glycoside; *action:* acts by inhibiting the sodium-potassium ATPase, which makes more calcium available for contractile proteins; *uses:* CHF, atrial fibrillation, atrial flutter, paroxysmal atrial tachycardia.

dihydrotachysterol (DHT), *n trade names:* DHT Intensol, Hytakerol; *drug class:* vitamin D analog; *action:* increases intestinal absorption of calcium, increases renal tubular absorption of phosphate; *uses:* nutritional supplement, rickets, hypoparathyroidism, postoperative tetany.

dihydroxyaluminum sodium carbonate, *n trade name:* Rolaids; *drug class:* antacid; *action:* neutralizes gastric acidity; *use:* antacid.

dilaceration (dīlas′ərā′shən), *n* a severe angular distortion in the root of a tooth or at the junction of the root and crown. Dilaceration results from trauma during tooth development.

Dilaceration. (Sapp/Eversole/Wysocki, 2004)

Dilantin enlargement, *n.pr* See hyperplasia, gingival, Dilantin.

Dilantin gingival hyperplasia, *n.pr* See hyperplasia, gingival, Dilantin.

Dilantin sodium (dīlan′tin sō′dē-əm), *n.pr* the trade name for diphenylhydantoin sodium.

dilation (dīlā′shən), *n* the act of stretching or dilating.

diltiazem HCl, *n trade names:* Cardizem, Cardizem SR, Cardizem CD; *drug class:* calcium channel blocker; *action:* inhibits calcium ion influx across cell membrane during cardiac depolarization; produces relaxation of coronary vascular smooth muscle, dilates coronary arteries, slows SA/AV node conduction; *uses:* chronic stable angina pectoris, coronary artery spasm, hypertension.

diluent (dil′yōō-ənt), *n* an agent that dilutes the strength of a solution or mixture; medication that dilutes any one of the body fluids.

dilute (dilōōt′, dīlōōt′), *v* to make weaker the strength of a solution or mixture.

dimenhydrinate, *n trade names:* Calm-X, Dimentabs, Dinate, Dramamine; *drug class:* antihistamine, H_1-receptor antagonist; *actions:* acts on blood vessels and gastrointestinal and respiratory systems by competing with histamine for H_1-receptor sites; decreases allergic response by blocking histamine; *uses:* motion sickness, nausea, vomiting.

dimension, vertical, *n* **1.** a vertical measurement of the face between any two arbitrarily selected points that are conveniently located one above and one below the mouth, usually in the midline. *n* **2.** the vertical height of the face with the teeth in occlusion or acting as stops. See also relation, vertical.

dimension, vertical, decrease, *n* a decrease of the vertical distance between the mandible and the maxillae by modifications of teeth or the positions of teeth or occlusion rims, or through alveolar or residual ridge resorption.

dimension, vertical, increase, *n* an increase of the vertical distance between the mandible and the maxillae by modifications of teeth or the positions of teeth or occlusion rims.

dimension, vertical, occlusal, *n* the

vertical dimension of the face when the teeth or occlusion rims are in contact in centric occlusion.

dimension, vertical, rest, *n* the vertical dimension of the face with the jaws in the rest relation.

dimension, vertical, rest, decrease, *n* may or may not accompany a decrease in occlusal vertical dimension. It may occur without a decrease in occlusal vertical dimension in patients with a preponderant activity of the jaw-closing musculature, as in chronic gum chewers or patients with muscular hypertension.

dimension, vertical, rest, increase, *n* may or may not accompany an increase in occlusal dimension. It sometimes occurs after the removal of remaining occlusal contacts, perhaps as a result of the removal of noxious reflex stimuli.

dimensional stability, *n* See stability, dimensional.

dimethyl sulfoxide, *n* an antiinflammatory agent and organic solvent.

dimethylbenzene (dīmeth′ilben′zēn), *n* See xylene.

Dimitri's disease (dimē′trēz), *n.pr* See disease, Sturge-Weber-Dimitri.

diphenhydramine HCl, *n* *trade names:* Benadryl, Sominex Formula 3; *drug class:* antihistamine, H_1-receptor antagonist; action: acts on blood vessels and gastrointestinal and respiratory systems by competing with histamine for H_1-receptor sites; decreases allergic response by blocking histamine; *uses:* allergy symptoms, rhinitis, motion sickness, antiparkinsonism, nighttime sedation, infant colic, nonproductive cough.

diphenoxylate HCl with atropine sulfate, *n trade names:* Lofrol, Logene, Lomotil, Lonox; *drug class:* antidiarrheal (opioid with atropine) Controlled Substance Schedule V; *action:* inhibits gastric motility by acting on muscosal receptors responsible for peristalsis; *use:* simple diarrhea.

diphenylhydantoin sodium (dīfen′ilhīdan′tō-in), *n* (Dilantin sodium), a drug used for the control of convulsive grand mal and petit mal epileptic seizures; often associated with the production of a profuse gingival hyperplasia. See also phenytoin sodium.

diphtheria (difthir′ē-ə), *n* an acute disease caused by *Corynebacterium diphtheriae* resulting in swelling of the pharynx and larynx with fever.

dipivefrin HCl, *n trade name:* Propine; *drug class:* adrenergic agonist; *action:* converted to epinephrine with decreased aqueous production and increased outflow; *use:* open-angle glaucoma.

diplococci, morphologic form of, *n.pl* the uniformly scattered pairs of half ovals, resembling shoeprints, which are characteristic of the diplococci bacteria.

diplomate, *n* a dental specialist who has achieved certification by the recognized certification board in that specialty, as attested by a diploma from the board.

diplopia (diplō′pē-ə), *n* seeing a single object as two images. May occur after fracture of the bony orbital cavity as a result of displacement of the globe of the eye inferiorly.

dipyridamole, *n trade name:* Persantine; *drug class:* platelet aggregation inhibitor; *action:* specific action unclear, inhibits ability of platelets to aggregate; *uses:* prevention of transient ischemic attacks (TIA), inhibition of platelet aggregation to prevent myocardial reinfarction, prevention of coronary bypass graft occlusion with aspirin.

dipyrone, *n* an analgesic, antiinflammatory, and antipyretic agent that is rarely used because of a high incidence of agranulocytosis.

direct (dīrekt′), *adj* relating to any restorative procedure performed directly on a tooth without the use of a die (for example, a wax pattern formed in the prepared cavity), silver amalgam, or one of the powdered, granular, or foil golds compacted into a prepared cavity.

direct access storage device, *n* a device used for storage of direct access files. It could be a magnetic disk or diskette units.

direct billing, *n* a process whereby the dentist bills a patient directly for his or her fees.

direct gold, *n* any of the forms of pure gold that may be compacted directly into a prepared cavity to form a restoration.

direct pulp capping, n See capping, pulp, direct.

direct reimbursement, n a self-funded program in which the individual is reimbursed based on a percentage of dollars spent for dental care provided, allowing the beneficiary to seek treatment from the dentist of his or her choice.

direct retainer, n See retainer, direct.

direct retention, n See retention, direct.

direct supervision, n a circumstance of treatment in which the dentist must be present on the premises to diagnose, authorize, and approve all work performed on the patient by the dental hygienist.

director, n a person elected by shareholders at the annual meeting to establish company policies. The directors appoint the president, vice presidents, and all other operating officers. Directors decide, among other matters, if and when dividends shall be paid.

directory, n **1.** an organized list of names, organizations, or other data bases for ease of retrieval or reference. n **2.** the listing of files in a computer storage system.

dirithromycin, n *trade name:* Dynabac; *drug class:* macrolide antibiotic; *action:* binds to 50S ribosomal subunits of susceptible bacteria to inhibit bacterial growth; *uses:* treatment of secondary bacterial infection of acute bronchitis, community-acquired pneumonia, streptococcal pharyngitis, and uncomplicated skin and skin structure infections.

disability, n **1.** the lack of legal qualification to do a thing; legal incompetency. n **2.** the inability to function in the normal or usual manner; examples of an outcome measure are days missing from work or lessened productivity.

disability, denial of, n a symptom in which patients deny the existence of a disease or disability. A patient who is edentulous may insist he eats better, looks better, and speaks better than if he had teeth. Another may insist that filthy, carious, periodontally involved teeth are beautiful and healthy and enhance his appearance.

Denial by these patients is a nonrealistic attempt to maintain their predisease status. These patients regard ill health and disability as an imperfection, a weakness, and even a disgrace.

disaccharide, n a general term for simple carbohydrates (sugars) formed by the union of two monosaccharide molecules. Sucrose is the most common disaccharide sugar.

disarticulation
(dis'ärtik'yōōlā'shən), n the amputation or separation of joint parts, as in hemimandibulectomy, with inclusion of the condyloid process of the mandible.

disc, n See disk.

discharge, v **1.** to release; liberate; annul; unburden. To cancel a contract; to make an agreement or contract null and void. n **2.** Any substance which exudes from an opening.

discharge, purulent, n See pus.

discharge summary, n the clinical notes written by the discharging physician or dentist at the time of releasing a patient from the hospital or clinic, outlining the course of treatment, the status at release, and the postdischarge expectations and instructions.

disclosing solution, n a material, usually some form of dye, applied to the teeth to stain bacterial and mucinous plaque on the tooth surface.

disclosing solution, aniline (an'ilin), n a dye used to reveal deposits on the teeth by temporarily coloring them. Its use is not recommended due to properties that pose cancer risks to patients. Found in basic fuchsin and beta rose.

disclosing solution, two-tone, n a staining substance used to help patients identify plaque in their own mouths. It stains older plaque blue and newer plaque red.

disclosure, n a release of information.

disclusion (disklōō'zhən), n a separation of the occlusal surfaces of the teeth directly and simply by opening the jaws, or indirectly in excursions by the anterior teeth.

discoid (dis'koid), n a carving instrument with a blade of circular form that has a cutting edge around the entire periphery.

Discoid blade carving amalgam.
(Roberson/Heymann/Swift, 2002)

discoloration, enamel, n See tetracycline.

discoloration, gingival, n See gingival discoloration.

discoplasty, n the surgical shaping or contouring of the meniscus of the temporomandibular joint.

discount, n **1.** an allowance or deduction made from a gross sum. v **2.** to reduce the amount of a professional fee.

discrimination, legal, n to treat unequally or unfairly on the basis of race, gender, national origin, religion, or handicap.

discrimination, tactile, n the ability to perceive two simultaneous touch stimuli; two-point discrimination. When the distance between the two stimuli is diminished to the point where only one stimulus is perceived, a value is determined for the two-point discrimination capacity of a special part. When patients are anesthetized by local agents, they have diminished tactile sense and frequently bite their lips rather severely without being aware of it. Thus patients should be instructed not to eat or chew until the "numbness" has completely gone and full tactile sense has returned.

disease(s) (dizēz'), n a definite deviation from the normal state characterized by a series of symptoms. Disease may be caused by developmental disturbances, genetic factors, metabolic factors, living agents, or physical, chemical, or radiant energy, or the cause may be unknown.

disease activity, n the ongoing and ever-worsening condition in which gingival tissues continue to pull away from the tooth structures and the supporting bones shrink to the point where they are no longer able to hold the teeth in place. Also called *aggressive periodontal disease.*

disease, Adams-Stokes (Adams-Stokes syndrome), n.pr a disease characterized by a slow and perhaps irregular pulse, vertigo, syncope, occasional pseudoepileptic convulsions, and Cheyne-Stokes respirations.

disease, adaptation (adaptation syndrome), n metabolic disorders occurring as a result of adaptation or resistance to severe physical or psychologic stress. See also syndrome, general adaptation.

disease, Addison's, n.pr chronic adrenocortical insufficiency caused by bilateral tuberculosis, aplasia, atrophy, or degeneration of the adrenal glands. Symptoms include severe weakness, weight loss, low blood pressure, digestive disturbances, hypoglycemia, lowered resistance to infection, and abnormal pigmentation (bronze color of the skin, with associated melanotic pigmentation of the oral mucous membranes, particularly of the gingival tissues).

disease, adrenocortical, n disorders of adrenocortical function, giving rise to Addison's disease, Cushing's syndrome, adrenogenital syndrome, and primary aldosteronism.

disease, Albers-Schönberg, n.pr See osteopetrosis.

disease, autoallergic, n See disease, autoimmune.

disease, autoimmune (autoallergic disease, autoimmunization syndrome, chronic hypersensitivity), n any one of the diseases that are believed to be caused in part by reactions of hypersensitivity of the host tissue (antigens). Includes various hemolytic anemias, idiopathic thrombocytopenias, rheumatoid arthritis, systemic lupus erythematosus, glomerulonephritis, scleroderma, Hashimoto's thyroiditis, and Sjögren's syndrome.

disease, Barlow's, n.pr See scurvy, infantile.

disease, Basedow's, n.pr See goiter, exophthalmic.

disease, Behçet's, n.pr See syndrome, Behçet's.

disease, Besnier-Boeck-Schaumann, *n.pr* See sarcoidosis.

disease, bleeder's, *n* See hemophilia.

disease, blood, *n* a disease affecting the hematologic system (e.g., anemia, leukemia, agranulocytosis purpura, infectious mononucleosis). Such a disease often results in lesions of the oral structures, particularly the mucosal surfaces.

disease, Bowen's, *n.pr* See carcinoma in situ.

disease, Brill-Symmers, *n.pr* See lymphoblastoma, giant follicular.

disease, brittle bone, *n* See osteogenesis imperfecta.

disease, Caffey's, *n.pr* See hyperostosis, infantile cortical.

disease, Cannon's, *n.pr* See nevus spongiosus albus mucosa.

disease, cardiac, *n* a disease affecting the heart

disease, cat-scratch, *n* See fever, cat-scratch.

disease, Cheadle's, *n.pr* See scurvy, infantile.

disease, Christmas, *n.pr* See hemophilia B.

disease, chronic hypersensitivity, *n* See disease, autoimmune.

disease, chronic obstructive pulmonary, *n* disease marked by decreased expiratory flow rates resulting in increased total lung capacity. Patients with this condition are prone to acute respiratory failure from infections or general anesthesia.

disease, collagen (group disease, visceral angiitis), *n* collectively, a group of diseases affecting the collagenous connective tissue of several organs and systems. These diseases have similar biochemical structural alterations and include rheumatic fever, scleroderma, rheumatoid arthritis, systemic lupus erythematosus, periarteritis, and serum sickness.

disease, combined system, *n* pernicious anemia in which there is central nervous system damage associated with the hematologic findings.

diseases, communicable, *n* any disease that may be transmitted directly or indirectly to a well person or animal from an infected person or animal. Any disease with the capacity for maintenance by natural modes of spread (for example, by contact, by airborne routes, through drinking water or food, by arthropod vectors).

disease, congenital, *n* any disease present at birth, or, more specifically, one that is acquired in utero.

disease, Coxsackie A, *n.pr* See herpangina.

disease, Crouzon's, *n.pr* See dysostosis, craniofacial.

disease, Cushing's, *n.pr* See syndrome, Cushing's.

disease, cytomegalic inclusion, generalized, *n* See disease, salivary gland.

disease, Darier's (keratosis follicularis), *n.pr* an apparently genetic dermatologic disease that also involves mucous membranes. The oral lesions are whitish papules of the gingiva, tongue, or palate. Darier's disease is characterized histologically by the presence of corps ronds.

disease, deficiency, *n* a disturbance produced by lack of nutritional or metabolic factors. Used chiefly in reference to avitaminosis.

disease, degenerative joint, *n* See osteoarthritis.

disease, dermatologic, *n* any one of the diseases affecting the skin; often accompanied by pathologic manifestations of various mucosal surfaces of the body (for example, the oral mucosa, genital mucosa, conjunctiva).

disease, Engman's, *n.pr* See dermatitis infectiosa eczematoides.

disease, exanthematous, *n* any one of a group of diseases caused by a number of viruses but having as a prominent feature a skin rash (for example, smallpox, chickenpox, cowpox, measles, rubella).

disease, familial, *n* a disease occurring in several members of the same family. Often used to mean members of the same generation and occasionally used synonymously with hereditary disease.

disease, Feer's, *n.pr* See erythredema polyneuropathy and acrodynia.

disease, fibrocystic (mucoviscidosis), *n* a hereditary defect of most of the exocrine glands in the body, including the salivary glands. The secretion of the affected mucous glands is abnormally viscous.

disease, fifth, *n* a viral infection caused by the human parvovirus B19; spread via the upper respiratory tract, this virus impacts on children

D

more strongly than adults. Also called *erythema infectiosum*.

disease, Fordyce's, n.pr See spots, Fordyce's.

disease, functional, n a disease that has no observable or demonstrable cause.

disease, Gaucher's, n.pr a constitutional defect in the metabolism of the cerebroside kerasin. This glycoprotein accumulates in the reticuloendothelial system and leads to splenomegaly, hepatomegaly, lymph node enlargement, and bone defects.

disease, Graves', n.pr See goiter, exophthalmic.

disease, hand-foot-and-mouth (aphthous fever, epidemic stomatitis, epizootic stomatitis), n primarily a disease of animals caused by a filterable virus that may be transmitted to humans and that occasionally produces symptoms. The human form is characterized by fever, nausea, vomiting, malaise, and ulcerative stomatitis. Skin lesions consisting of vesicles may appear, usually on the palms of the hands and soles of the feet. Spontaneous regression usually occurs within 2 weeks.

Hand, foot, and mouth disease.
(Regezi/Sciubba/Pogrel, 2000)

disease, Hand-Schüller-Christian (chronic disseminated histiocytosis X), n.pr a type of cholesterol lipoidosis characterized clinically by defects in membranous bones, exophthalmos, and diabetes insipidus.

disease, Hansen's, n.pr See leprosy.

disease, heart, n any abnormal condition of the heart (organic, mechanical, or functional) that causes difficulty.

disease, heart, arteriosclerotic, n a variety of functional changes of the myocardium that result from arteriosclerosis.

disease, heart, congenital, n a defective formation of the heart or of the major vessels of the heart.

disease, heart, rheumatic, n scarring of the endocardium resulting from involvement in acute rheumatic fever. The process most often involves the mitral valve.

disease, heart, thyrotoxic, n cardiac failure occurring as the result of hyperthyroidism or its superimposition on existing organic heart disease. Thyrotoxicosis is an important cause of auricular fibrillation.

disease, hemoglobin C, n a disease resulting from an abnormal hemoglobin (hemoglobin C); occurs primarily in African Americans and causes a mild normochromic anemia, target cells, and vague, intermittent arthralgia.

disease, hemolytic, of newborn, n hemolysis caused by isoimmune reactions associated with Rh incompatibility or with blood transfusions in which there is an incompatibility of the ABO blood system. Several forms of the disease occur: erythroblastosis fetalis, congenital hemolytic disease, icterus gravis neonatorum, and hydrops fetalis.

disease, hemophilioid, n hemophilic states (conditions) that clinically resemble hemophilia (for example, parahemophila, hemophilia B [Christmas disease]).

disease, hemorrhagic, of newborn, n a hemorrhagic tendency in newborn infants occurring usually on the third or fourth day of life; believed to be caused by defects of prothrombin and factor VII, resulting from a deficiency of vitamin K.

disease, hereditary, n a disease transmitted from parent to offspring through genes. Three main types of mendelian heredity are recognized: dominant, recessive, and sex-linked.

disease, hidebound, n See scleroderma.

disease, Hodgkin's, n.pr a generally fatal lymphomatous disorder of unknown etiology that has neoplastic and granulomatous characteristics. Chiefly involves the lymph nodes, but sometimes the spleen, liver, bone marrow, and other organs are involved as well. Three variants include Hodgkin's paragranuloma, Hodgkin's granuloma (classical or common type), and Hodgkin's sarcoma. All have in common the presence of Sternberg-Reed, or Dorothy Reed, cells and lymph node enlargement. Cervical lymph nodes are often the first to be affected. See also cell, Sternberg-Reed.

Hodgkin's disease. (Seidel/Ball/Dains/Benedict, 2003)

disease, hypersensitivity, n See disease, autoimmune.

disease, iatrogenic, n a disease arising as a result of the actions or words of a physician or dentist (for example, an obsession of having heart disease or bruxism as a result of a misunderstanding on the part of a patient).

disease, idiopathic (id′ē-ōpath′ik), *n* a disease in which the cause is not recognized or determined.

disease, infectious, n pathologic alterations induced in the tissues by the action of microorganisms and/or their toxins. Some infectious diseases involving the oral tissues are herpes zoster, herpetic gingivostomatitis, moniliasis, syphilis, and tuberculosis.

disease, inflammatory neoplastic, n See granuloma; tumor, inflammatory.

disease, kissing, n See mononucleosis, infectious.

disease, Langerhans' cell, n a group of three diseases identified by an abundance of Langerhans' cells-eosinophils combined with histiocytic cells. See also disease, Letterer-Siwe; disease, Hand-Schüller-Christian; and granuloma, eosinophili.

disease, Letterer-Siwe (sē′vā), *n.pr* (acute disseminated histiocytosis X, nonlipid histiocytosis, nonlipid reticuloendotheliosis), a fatal febrile disease of unknown cause occurring in infants and children; characterized by focal granulomatous lesions of the lymph nodes, spleen, and bone marrow. Results in enlargement of the lymph nodes, spleen, and liver, defects of the flat and long bones, anemia, and sometimes purpura.

disease, lipoid storage (lipoidosis, reticuloendothelial granuloma), n any one of a group of diseases in which lipid substances accumulate in the fixed cells of the reticuloendothelial system. Included are Gaucher's disease, Niemann-Pick disease, and the Hand-Schüller Christian disease complex. Other storage diseases include lipochondrodystrophy (gargoylism) and cerebral sphingolipidosis.

disease, Lobstein's, n.pr See osteogenesis imperfecta.

disease, Marie's, n.pr See acromegaly.

disease, Mediterranean, n.pr See thalassemia major.

disease, metabolic bone, n.pl diseases of the bone which may be attributed to cellular changes or to nutritional deficiencies/excesses brought on by dietary imbalances. Diseases include hyperparathyroidism, osteoporosis, osteomalacia, rickets, and the many diseases associated with an abnormal abundance of Langerhans' cells.

disease, Mikulicz' (mlk′yōōlich′əz), *n.pr* a benign hyperplasia of the lymph nodes of the parotid or other salivary glands and/or the lacrimal glands.

disease, Moeller's, n.pr See scurvy, infantile.

disease, molecule, n a disease associated with genetically determined abnormalities of protein synthesis at the molecular level.

disease, muscle, n pathologic muscle tissue changes. Such changes reveal few structural alterations, and the highly differentiated contents of muscle fibers tend to react as a whole. The pathologic features that distinguish one muscle disease from another are the age and character of changes within a muscle, distribution of those changes within one or several muscles, presence of inflammatory cells and parasites, and coexistence of pathologic changes in other organs. Muscles undergo a number of degenerative changes. There are alterations in the striation in certain pathologic states caused by cloudy swelling, granular degeneration, waxy or hyaline degeneration, and other cellular modifications such as multiplication of the sarcolemmic nuclei and phagocytosis of muscle fibers.

disease, necrotizing periodontal, *n.pl* bacterial disease of the teeth and gums that leads to tissue degeneration and death if not properly treated. It can comprise symptoms or side effects of other illnesses and treatments.

disease, neuromuscular, *n* a condition in which various areas of the central nervous system are affected; results in dysfunction or degeneration of the musculature and disabilities of the organ.

disease, Niemann-Pick (nē′män), *n.pr* a congenital, familial disorder occurring chiefly in Jewish female infants that terminates fatally before the third year and is characterized by the accumulation of the phospholipid sphingomyelin in the cells of the reticuloendothelial system.

disease, oral, hereditary, *n* heritable defects of oral and paraoral structures (excluding the dentition) without generalized defects; includes ankyloglossia, hereditary gingivofibromatosis, and possibly cleft lip and cleft palate. Many oral and paraoral defects are associated with generalized defects (for example, Peutz-Jeghers, Franceschetti, Ehlers-Danlos, Pierre Robin, and Sturge-Weber syndromes; hemorrhagic telangiectasia; Crouzon's disease; sickle cell disease; acatalasemia; white spongy nevus; xeroderma pigmentosum; gargoylism; neurofibromatosis; familial amyloidosis; and achondroplasia).

disease, oral manifestations of systemic, *n* the lesions occurring within the stomatologic system in association with systemic disease, often influenced by the local environmental factors within the oral cavity.

disease, organic, *n* a disease in which actual structural changes have occurred in the organs or tissues.

disease, Osler's, *n.pr* See erythremia.

disease, Owren's, *n.pr* See parahemophilia.

disease, Paget's, *n.pr* See osteitis deformans.

disease, Parkinson's, *n.pr* a progressive neurologic disorder for which there is no known cure that is thought to be the result of neuron degeneration in the section of the brain controlling spontaneous movement and balance. The disease causes postural changes, tremors, muscle rigidity, and weakness. Oral manifestations include difficulty in swallowing and excess salivation.

disease, periodic, *n* See disorder(s), periodic.

disease, periodontal, *n* any disturbance of the periodontium or supporting structures of the teeth. Diseases affecting the periodontium include periodontitis, periodontosis, gingivitis, gingival enlargement, atrophy, and traumatism and may be loosely divided into two types: inflammatory and dystrophic. Etiologic factors may be local or systemic or may involve an interplay between the two.

　disease, periodontal, etiologic factors of, *n.pl* the local and systemic factors, singly or in combination, that initiate periodontal lesions.

　disease, periodontal, local factors of, *n.pl* the environmental conditions within the oral cavity that initiate, perpetuate, or alter the course of diseases of the periodontium (for example, calculus, diastemata between teeth, food impaction, prematurities in the centric path of closure, and tongue habits).

disease, peripheral vascular, *n* a disease of arteries, veins, and/or lymphatic vessels.

disease, pink, *n* See acrodynia.

disease, Pott's, *n.pr* a spinal curvature (kyphosis) resulting from tuberculosis.

disease progression, *n* the course of the disease within a patient/host from onset to resolution.

disease, psychosomatic, *n* a disease that appears to have been precipitated or prolonged by emotional stress; manifested largely through the autonomic nervous system. Various conditions may be included (for example, certain forms of asthma, dermatosis, migraine headache, hypertension, peptic ulcer, rheumatoid arthritis, and ulcerative colitis). Occlusal trauma associated with bruxism is often considered a disease of this type. See also disorder, psychophysiologic, autonomic, and visceral.

disease, Quincke's, *n.pr* See edema, angioneurotic.

disease, Rendu-Osler-Weber **(ron′dōō),** *n.pr* See telangiectasia, hereditary hemorrhagic.

disease, rheumatic, *n* See rheumatism.

disease, rickettsial, *n* a disease caused by microorganisms of the order Rickettsiales (for example, Rocky Mountain spotted fever, rickettsialpox, typhus, and Q fever).

disease, Riga-Fede **(rē′gə-fā′də),** an ulceration of the lingual frenum of infants caused by abrasion by natal or neonatal teeth.

disease, Sainton's, *n.pr* See dysostosis, cleidocranial.

disease, salivary gland (generalized cytomegalic inclusion), *n* a generalized infection in infants caused by intrauterine or postnatal infection with a cytomegalovirus of the group of herpesviruses. Manifestations include jaundice, purpura, hemolytic anemia, vomiting, diarrhea, chronic eczema, and failure to gain weight.

disease, Schüller's **(shü′lerz),** *n.pr* See osteoporosis.

disease, Selter's, *n.pr* See acrodynia.

disease, sex-linked, *n* a hereditary disorder transmitted by the gene that also determines sex (for example, hemophilia).

disease, sickle cell, *n* a hematologic disorder caused by the presence of an abnormal hemoglobin (hemoglobin S) that permits the formation or results in the formation of sickle-shaped red blood cells. Two forms of the disease occur: sickle cell trait and sickle cell anemia. See also anemia, sickle cell; trait, sickle cell.

disease, Simmonds' (pituitary cachexia, hypophyseal cachexia, hypopituitary cachexia), *n.pr* panhypopituitarism resulting from destruction of the pituitary gland, usually from hemorrhage or infarction.

disease, skin, *n* disease characterized by various types of ulcerative eruptions and/or lesions that may appear in or affect the oral cavity.

Types include erythema multiforme, Stevens-Johnson syndrome, Behçet's syndrome, and pemphigus vulgaris.

disease, students', *n* See mononucleosis, infectious.

disease, Sturge-Weber-Dimitri (encephalotrigeminal angiomatosis), *n.pr* a congenital condition characterized by venous angioma of the meninges and cerebral cortex and ipsilateral angiomatous lesions of the face and jaws.

disease, subclinical, *n* a latent, incipient, or mild form of a disease that does not produce known, clinically detectable manifestations. Abuse of the term occurs by including diseases deduced to be present only on the basis of borderline laboratory values.

disease susceptibility, *n* the degree to which a patient or host is vulnerable to a disease.

disease, Sutton's, *n.pr* See periadenitis mucosa necrotica recurrens.

disease, Swift's, *n.pr* See acrodynia.

disease, systemic, *n* any disease involving the whole body.

disease, Takahara's **(tä′kəhä′rəz),** *n.pr* a form of rare progressive oral gangrene occurring in childhood and seen only in Japan. Apparently related to a congenital lack of the enzyme catalase (acatalasemia). Characterized by a mild to severe form of a peculiar type of oral gangrene that may develop at the roots of the teeth or the tonsils. Loss of teeth occurs, with necrosis of the alveolar bone. Patients become symptom free after puberty.

disease, transmissible, *n* any disease capable of being transmitted from one individual to another; any disease capable of being maintained in successive passages through a susceptible host, usually under experimental conditions such as by injection. See also disease, communicable.

disease transmission, *n* the method by which a disease is passed from one patient or host to another. The three most common methods of transmission are direct contact, aerosols, and vectors, such as insects.

disease, Vaquez' **(väkēz′),** *n.pr* See erythremia.

disease vectors, *n.pl* intermediary hosts that carry the disease from one species to another, such as mosquitoes, ticks, and rabid animals.

disease, von Recklinghausen's (von Recklinghausen's disease), n.pr See hyperparathyroidism; osteitis; generalized fibrosa cystica; and neurofibromatosis.

disease, von Recklinghausen's, of bone, n.pr See hyperparathyroidism; osteitis fibrosa cystica,

disease, von Recklinghausen's, of skin, n.pr See neurofibromatosis.

disease, von Willebrand's, n.pr an inherited blood coagulation disorder attributed to a deficiency or malfunction of factor VIII. It may cause prolonged or excessive gingival bleeding.

disease, Weil's (epidemic jaundice) (vīlz), n.pr an acute febrile disease caused by *Leptospira icterohaemorrhagiae* or *L. canicola.* Manifestations include fever, petechial hemorrhage, myalgia, renal insufficiency, hepatic failure, and jaundice.

disease, Werlhof's (verl'hôfs), n.pr See purpura, thrombocytopenic.

diseases, demyelinating, n the diseases that have in common a loss of myelin sheath, with preservation of the axis cylinders (for example, multiple sclerosis, Schilder's disease).

diseases, dental, hereditary, n.pl heritable defects of the dentition without generalized disease include amelogenesis imperfecta, dentinogenesis imperfecta, dentinal dysplasia, localized and generalized hypoplasia of enamel, peg-shaped lateral incisors, familial dentigerous cysts, missing teeth, giantism, and fused primary mandibular incisors. Dental defects occurring with generalized disease include dentinogenesis imperfecta with osteogenesis imperfecta, missing teeth with ectodermal dysplasia, enamel hypoplasia with epidermolysis bullosa dystrophica, retarded eruption with cleidocranial dysostosis, missing lateral incisors with ptosis of the eyelids, missing premolars with premature whitening of the hair, and enamel hypoplasia in vitamin D-resistant rickets.

diseases, group, n See disease, collagen.

disharmony, occlusal, n a phenomenon in which contacts of opposing occlusal surfaces of teeth are not in harmony with other tooth contacts

and with the anatomic and physiologic controls of the mandible. See also contact, deflective occlusal; contact, interceptive occlusal; and malocclusion.

disinfect (dis'infekt'), v to destroy pathogenic microorganisms.

disinfectant (dis'infek'tənt), n a chemical intended especially for use on instruments to destroy most pathogenic microorganisms.

disinfectant, alcohol, n an unaccepted method of sterilization. While ethanol and isopropanol both have cleansing properties when used on the skin, they are insufficient as sterilizers.

disinfectant, chlorine dioxide, n a chemical disinfectant which can be used for 24 hours once it is activated. It can corrode some steel tools.

disinfectant holding solution, n an antimicrobial liquid into which an object can be temporarily placed while awaiting sterilization.

disinfection, n the process of destroying pathogenic organisms or rendering them inert.

disinfection, full mouth, n procedure used to reduce active periodontal disease, usually completed within 24 hours.

disintegration, induced nuclear, n disintegration resulting from artificial bombardment of a material with high-energy particles such as alpha particles, deuterons, protons, neutrons, or gamma rays.

disintegration, nuclear, n a spontaneous nuclear transformation (radioactivity) characterized by the emission of energy or mass from the nucleus. When numbers of nuclei are involved, the process is characterized by a definite half-life.

disk, n a thin, flat, circular object.

disk, abrasive, n a disk with abrasive particles attached to one or both of its surfaces or its edge.

disk, diamond, n a disk of steel with diamond chips bonded to its surface.

disk, garnet, n a disk with particles of garnet as the abrading medium.

disk, Joe Dandy, n.pr the trade name for a separating disk. See also disk, separating.

disk, lightning, a steel separating disk.

disk, Merkel's, n.pr See corpuscle, Merkel's.

disk, pack, n a set of circular magnetic surfaces mounted coaxially on a shaft for computer storage of files. Can be used for storage of serial or direct access files.

disk, polishing, n a disk with an extremely fine abrasive; used to finish and polish a surface.

disk, safe-side, n a separating disk with abrasive on one side only; the other side is smooth.

disk, sandpaper, n an abrasive disk with sandpaper as the abrading medium.

disk, separating, n a disk of steel or hard rubber.

disk, storage, n a storage device that uses magnetic recording on flat, rotating disks.

disk, temporomandibular joint, n a plate of fibrous tissue that divides the temporomandibular joint into an upper and lower cavity. The disk is attached to the articular capsule and moves forward with the condyle in free opening and protrusion. See also articulation, temporomandibular.

dislocation, n the displacement of any part, especially a bone or bony articulation.

dislodgment, n movement or removal of a prosthesis from its established position.

disopyramide, n *trade name:* Norpace CR; *drug class:* antidysrhythmic (Class IA); *action:* prolongs action potential duration and effective refractory period; *uses:* PVCs, ventricular tachycardia, atrial flutter, atrial fibrillation.

disorder(s), n derangement of function.

disorder, bipolar, n a major mood disorder characterized by alternating periods of mania or elation and depression. Formerly called *manic-depressive disorder.*

disorder, body dysmorphic (dismôr′fik), WEB:(dismôr′fik), n a mental disorder in which an otherwise physiologically healthy person obsesses about an imaginary physical defect.

disorder(s), coagulation, n any one of the hemorrhagic diseases caused by a deficiency of plasma thromboplastin formation (deficiency of antihemophilic factor, plasma thromboplastic antecedent, Hageman factor, Stuart factor), deficiency of thrombin

formation (deficiency of prothrombin, factor V, factor VII, Stuart factor), and deficiency of fibrin formation (afibrinogenemia, fibrinogenopenia).

disorder, conversion, n uncontrolled change or loss of control of physical function due to a mental, not physical, need or conflict.

disorder, panic, n disorder marked by repeated panic attacks and fear, which interrupts normal functioning.

disorder(s), periodic, n.pl a variety of disorders of unknown cause that have in common periodic recurrence of manifestations. Such disorders are usually benign, resist treatment, often begin in infancy, and occasionally have a hereditary pattern. Included are periodic sialorrhea, neutropenia, arthralgia, fever, purpura (anaphylactoid purpura), edema (angioneurotic edema), abdominalgia, and periodic parotitis (recurrent parotitis).

disorder, pervasive developmental, n a disorder of behavioral and sensory impairment which generally appears during infancy or early childhood and continues to affect the individual's ability to communicate and interact with others throughout his or her life. See also autism.

disorder(s), platelet, n.pl hemorrhagic disease caused by an abnormality of the blood platelets (for example, thrombocytopenia, thrombasthenia).

disorder, posttraumatic stress, n a condition characterized by acute or recurring anxiety which has been brought about as the result of experiencing a traumatic event, such as a natural disaster, automobile accident, terrorist attack, military combat, rape, physical torture, or childhood sexual abuse. Symptoms may include flashbacks, nightmares, mild to severe depression, and panic attacks.

disorder(s), psychophysiologic, autonomic, and visceral, n standard psychiatric nomenclature for what are commonly known as psychomotor disorders. The disorders are disturbances of visceral function, secondary to chronic attitude and long-continued reaction to stress. These disorders may occur in any organ innervated by the autonomic nervous system, since overactivity or underactivity of that system as a result of stress appears to trigger the disorder. See also disease, psychosomatic.

disorder(s), visual, n.pl disorders that may result from injury or disease to the eyeball and its adnexa, the retina, or the cornea (for example, contusions of the orbit and eyelids, opacities of the lens, corneal scars, vascular changes to the retina). These peripheral disorders are effective in causing partial or total loss of vision in one or both eyes. They are simple, concrete, and fundamental. One sees or one does not see, and gray visions are generally quantitative differences that affect the perception of light and shadow and color and form. Visual disorders may also result from injury or disease to the optic tract fibers, optic chiasma, cerebral pathways, and visual cortex in the occipital region of the cerebrum. These disorders are qualitative deviations from normal, and the symptoms include visual field defects such as tubular vision found in hysteria, complete blindness in one or both eyes as a result of optic nerve injury, and hemianopsia, in which vision may be lost in one half of the visual field of one or both eyes. Other visual disorders include night and day blindness, color blindness, and the serious visual agnosia that results from trauma, tumor, or vascular disorders in the visual cortex of the cerebrum.

disorders, cognitive impairment, n.pl mental disorders distinguished by a limitation of mental functions (e.g., memory, comprehension, and judgment).

disorders, dissociative, n.pl mental disorders distinguished by the psychologically induced, distinct partition of separate mental functions from normal behavior or consciousness (e.g., dissociative amnesia and depersonalization disorder).

disorders, factitious, n.pl mental disorders distinguished by the self-induced creation of artificial physical or mental symptoms to assume the role of a sick individual.

disorders, feeding, n.pl conditions distinguished by an inability to eat sufficiently, a continual need to consume abnormal items of food or substances lacking nutrients, or frequent vomiting episodes without any indications of a gastrointestinal infection.

disorders, impulse control, n.pl mental disorders distinguished by an uncontrollable tendency to commit an unplanned behavior (e.g., pathologic gambling, kleptomania, and pyromania).

disorders, sexual, n.pl disorders of sexual performance or desire, which may include sexual dysfunction, feelings of discomfort about one's gender, and perverse sexual urges or activities. Also called paraphilia.

disorders, sleep, n.pl conditions characterized by a disruption in normal sleeping patterns which may be the result of serious medical conditions, including breathing difficulties or thyroid disorders, or external factors such as stress or substance abuse. Manifestations include insomnia, sleep apnea, and narcolepsy.

disorders, somatoform, n.pl disorders characterized by symptoms which seem to suggest the presence of an illness, but for which there is no physical proof. Often may be attributed to unresolved emotional conflicts. Types include conversion disorder, hypochondriasis, body dysmorphic disorder, and pain disorder.

disorders, substance-related, n.pl conditions or illnesses which may be directly attributed to overuse of drugs, alcohol, nicotine, or caffeine and may also include nutritional deficiencies, cardiovascular disease, oral lesions, liver disease, and sleep disorders.

disorders, tic, n.pl conditions characterized by involuntary and sometimes violent muscle spasms, including Tourette's syndrome and chronic motor or vocal tic disorders.

disprove, *v* to refute or to prove false by affirmative evidence to the contrary.

dissection, neck, *n* the removal of the lymph nodes and contiguous tissues from a primary site in the mandibular or maxillofacial area as treatment of neoplastic cells that have involved the regional cervical lymphatic system.

disseminated intravascular coagulation (DIC), *n* a grave coagulopathy resulting from the overstimulation of clotting and anticlotting processes in response to disease or injury, such as septicemia, acute hypotension, poisonous snake bites, neoplasms, and severe trauma.

dissociation, *n* the psychologically induced, distinct partition of separate mental functions (e.g., identity, memory, and awareness) from normal behavior or consciousness.

dissociative fugue (fȳoog), *n* a sudden departure from a home or workplace without any ability to recall personal history or identity.

dissolve, *v* to terminate, cancel, annul, disintegrate. To release the obligation of anything, as to dissolve a partnership.

distal, *adj* away from the median sagittal plane of the face and following the curvature of the dental arch.

distal end, adj the most posterior part of a removable dental restoration or denture flange.

distance, *n* the measure of space intervening between two objects or two points of reference.

distance, cone, n the distance between the focal spot and the outer end of the cone; usually expressed in inches or centimeters. Modern dental roentgen-ray units usually have cone distances of from 5 to 20 inches (12.5 to 50 cm).

distance, interarch (interridge distance), n the vertical distance between the maxillary and mandibular arches under conditions of vertical relations that must be specified.

distance, interocclusal (interocclusal gap, free-way space), n the distance between the occluding surfaces of the maxillary and mandibular teeth when the mandible is in its physiologic rest position. This can be determined by calculating the difference between the rest vertical dimension and the occlusal vertical dimension of the face.

distance, interridge, n See distance, interarch.

distance, large interarch, n a large distance between the maxillary and mandibular arches.

distance, long cone, n long (extended) cone distance is usually 14 to 20 inches (35 to 50 cm). See also cone, long.

distance, object-film, n the distance, usually expressed in centimeters or inches, between the object being radiographed and the cassette or film.

distance, operator, n See positions at the chair.

distance, short cone, n a focal-skin distance of 9 inches (22.5 cm) or less; usually refers to the distance as determined by the cone supplied by the manufacturer of the basic x-ray unit.

distance, small interarch, n a small distance between the maxillary and mandibular arches.

distance, target-film (anode-film distance, focal-film distance), n the distance between the focal spot of the tube and the film; usually expressed in inches or centimeters.

distention, *n* a state of dilation.

distoclusion, *n* mandibular teeth occluding distal to their normal relationship to the maxillary teeth, as in an Angle Class II malocclusion.

distoclusion, bilateral, n distoclusion on both sides.

distoclusion, unilateral, n distoclusion on one side.

distomolar, *n* a supernumerary (fourth) molar located posterior to the third molar.

distortion, *n* **1.** a deviation from the normal shape or condition. *n* **2.** a modification of the speech sound in some way so that the acoustic result only approximates the standard sound and is not accurate. *n* **3.** a twisting or deformation. A loss of accuracy in reproduction of cavity form.

distortion, film-fault, n an imperfection in the size or shape of a film image by either magnification, elongation, or foreshortening.

distortion, horizontal, n a disproportional change in size and shape of the image in the horizontal plane as a result of oblique horizontal angulation of the x-ray beam.

distortion, magnification, n a proportional enlargement of a radiographic image. It is always present to some degree in oral radiography but is minimized with extended focal-film distances.

distortion, vertical (foreshortening), n a disproportional change in size, either elongation or foreshortening, caused by incorrect vertical angulation or improper film placement.

distoversion, *n* the placement of a tooth farther than normal from the median plane or midline.

distraction, *n* the placement of teeth or other maxillary or mandibular structures farther than normal from the median plane.

disturbances, occlusal, *n.pl* derangements in the patterns of occlusion.

disulfiram, *n trade name:* Antabuse; *drug class:* aldehyde dehydrogenase inhibitor; *action:* blocks oxidation of alcohol at acetaldehyde stage; *uses:* chronic alcoholism (as adjunct).

ditch (ditching), *n* the undesirable loss of tooth substance in the region of a restoration margin (usually gingival).

ditching, *n* See ditch.

diuretic (dī'yōōret'ik), *n* **1.** a drug that increases the formation of urine. *adj* **2.** pertaining to the increased formation of urine.

diuretic, loop, *n* a high-potency therapeutic agent used to control hypertension by exerting influence on the loop of Henle in order to facilitate the removal of surplus water and sodium from the body. See furosemide.

diurnal (dī-ur'nəl), *adj* relating to or happening in the daytime or portion of the day which is light.

diverticulitis, *n* an inflammatory pouching of the intestinal wall.

dizziness, *n* a sensation of faintness or an inability to maintain normal balance in a standing or seated position. A patient who experiences dizziness should be carefully lowered to a safe position on a bed, chair, or floor because of the danger of injury from falling. See also syncope.

DMF index rate, *n* See rate, DMF index.

DNA, bacterial, *n* the DNA specific to a bacterial strain.

DNA fingerprinting, *n* the use of DNA analysis to identify a subject from blood or other suitable tissue.

DNA probe, *n* See deoxyribonucleic acid probes.

DO cavity, *n* a cavity on the distal and occlusal surfaces of a tooth. See also cavity, Class 2.

doctor, *n* a learned person; one qualified in a science or art; one who has received the highest academic degree in a particular field.

documentation, *n* the permanent recording of information properly identified as to time, place, circumstances, and attribution.

docusate calcium/docusate potassium/docusate sodium, *n trade names:* Colace, Correctol Extra Gentle, Sulfalax; *drug class:* laxative; *action:* increases water, fat penetration in intestine; allows for easier passage of stool; *uses:* stool softener.

dolichocephalic (dol'ikōsəfəl'ik), *adj* pertaining to a long and narrow head (with a cephalic index below 75).

dolor (dō'lôr), *n* any kind of pain.

donor site, *n* the portion of the body from which an organ or tissue is removed for transplant or grafting.

donor tissue, *n* tissue contributed by a donor to be used in tissue or organ transplant.

dopa, *n* an amino acid derived from tyrosine that occurs naturally in plants and animals. It is a precursor of dopamine, epinephrine, and norepinephrine.

dopamine, *n* a sympathomimetic catecholamine used in the treatment of shock, hypotension, and low cardiac output.

dope, *n* a slang term denoting any drug taken temporarily or habitually without medical cause and that is intended to alter mood.

dornase alfa, *n trade name:* Pulmozyme; *drug class:* recombinant human deoxyribonuclease (DNase); *action:* reduces sputum viscosity; *uses:* cystic fibrosis, reduces incidence of pulmonary infection, improves pulmonary function.

dorsal (dôr'səl), *adj* pertaining to the back or to the posterior part of an organ.

dorsum sellae (dôr'səm sel'ē), *n* the most posterior point on the internal contour of the sella turcica.

dosage (dō'səj), *n* the amount of a medicine or other agent administered for a given case or condition.

dose, *n* **1.** the quantity of drug necessary to produce a desired effect. *n* **2.** the total radiation delivered to a specified area or volume or to the whole body. See also dose, radiation-absorbed.

dose, absorbed (D), n the amount of energy imparted by ionizing particles to unit mass of irradiated material at a place of interest. The unit of absorbed dose is the rad (100 ergs/Gm).

dose, air, n an x-ray dose delivered at a point in free air; expressed in roentgens. It consists only of the radiation of the primary beam and the radiation scattered from surrounding air; does not include backscatter from radiated matter (for example, tissue).

dose, booster, n the portion of an immunizing agent given at a later time to stimulate the effects of a previous dose of the same agent.

dose, cumulative, n the total accumulated dose resulting from a single or repeated exposure to radiation of the same region or of the whole body. If used in area monitoring, it represents the accumulated radiation exposure over a given period of time.

dose, depth, n the absorbed dose of radiation imparted to matter at a particular depth below the surface, usually expressed as "percentage depth dose." See also dose, percentage depth.

dose, distribution, n a representation of the variation of dose with position in any region of an irradiated object. The dose distribution may be measured using detectors small enough to avoid disturbing the distribution, or it may be calculated and expressed in mathematical form.

dose, doubling, n the amount of ionizing radiation, absorbed by the gonads of the average person in a population over a period of several generations, that will result in a doubling of the current rate of spontaneous mutations.

dose, effect curve, n See curve, dose effect.

dose, equivalent (DE), n the product of absorbed dose and modifying factors, namely the quality factor (QF), distribution factor (DF), and any other necessary factors. The unit of dose equivalent is the rem (rads times qualifying factors).

dose, erythema, n the dose of radiation necessary to produce a temporary redness of the skin. This dose varies with the quality of radiation.

dose, exit, n the absorbed dose delivered by a beam of radiation at the surface through which the beam emerges from a phantom or patient.

dose, exposure, n See exposure.

dose, fractionation, n a dose given by a number of shorter exposures over a longer period than would be required if the dose was given by a continuous exposure in one session at the same dose rate.

dose, gonadal, n the dose of radiation absorbed by the gonads.

dose, integral (integral absorbed dose, volume dose), n the total energy absorbed by a part or object during exposure to radiation. The unit of integral dose is the gram rad (100 ergs/gm).

dose, lethal, n **1.** the amount of a drug that would prove fatal to the majority of persons. n **2.** the amount of radiation that will be or may be sufficient to cause the death of an organism.

dose, maintenance, n the quantity of drug necessary to sustain a normal physiologic state or a desired blood or tissue level of drug.

dose, maximum permissible (MPD), n the maximum relative biologic effect dose that the body of a person or specific parts thereof shall be permitted to receive in a stated period of time. In most instances, for the roentgen rays used in dental radiography, it is satisfactory to consider the RBE dose in rems numerically equal to the absorbed dose in rads and the absorbed dose in rads numerically equal to the exposure dose in roentgens. See also dose, weekly permissible.

dose, median effective (ED50), n a dose that, under standard conditions, is effective in 50% of a randomly selected group of subjects.

dose, median lethal (LD50), n the amount of ionizing radiation required to kill, within a specified period, 50% of the individuals in a large group or population of animals or organisms.

dose, minimum lethal (MLD), n the minimal amount of a drug that will kill an experimental animal.

dose, percentage depth, n the ratio (expressed as a percentage) of the absorbed dose at a given depth in an irradiated body, to the absorbed dose at a fixed reference point on the central ray, usually the surface-absorbed dose.

dose, priming, n a quantity several times larger than the maintenance dose; used at the initiation of therapy to rapidly establish the desired blood and tissue levels of the drug.

dose, protraction, n a method of radiation administration delivered continuously over a relatively long period at a relatively low dosage rate.

dose, radiation, n the amount of energy absorbed per unit mass of tissue at a site of interest. Note: This definition limits the use of "dose" to conform with the 1962 recommendations of the International Commission on Radiological Units and Measurements (ICRUM). The following terms therefore become obsolete but will be found in this dictionary under the general heading of exposure: air dose, cumulative dose, exposure dose, and threshold dose.

dose, radiation-absorbed (rad), n the unit of absorbed dose, with a value of 100 ergs per gram.

dose, rate, n the time rate at which radiation dose is applied, expressed in either roentgens per unit time or rads per unit time.

dose, skin, n See dose, surface-absorbed.

dose, surface-absorbed, n the absorbed dose delivered by a radiation beam at the point where the central ray passes through the superficial layer of the phantom or patient.

dose, therapeutic, n a quantity several times larger than the maintenance dose; used in vitamin therapy in which a marked deficiency exists.

dose, threshold, n the minimum dose that will produce a detectable degree of any given effect.

dose, tissue, n the dose absorbed by a tissue or tissues in a region of interest.

dose, tolerance, n See dose, maximum permissible.

dose, toxic, n the amount of a drug that causes untoward symptoms in the majority of persons.

dose, transit, n a measure of the primary radiation transmitted through the patient and measured at a point on the central ray at some point beyond the patient.

dose, U.S.P, n See dose, median effective (ED50); dose, lethal.

dose, volume, n See dose, integral.

dose, weekly permissible, n a dose of ionizing radiation accumulated in 1 week and of such magnitude that, in view of present knowledge, exposure at this weekly rate for an indefinite period of time is not expected to cause appreciable bodily injury during a person's lifetime.

dosimetry (dōsim′etrē), n the accurate and systematic determination of the amount of radiation to which an animal or person has been exposed during a given period of time.

dovetail, n a widened or fanned-out portion of a prepared cavity, usually established deliberately to increase the retention and resistance form.

dovetail, lingual, n a dovetail established as a step portion, with lingual approach, in some Class 3 and Class 4 preparations; used to supplement the retentions and resistance form.

dovetail, occlusal, n a dovetail established at the terminal of the occlusal step of a proximal cavity.

dowel, n a post or pin, usually made of metal, fitted into a prepared root canal of a natural tooth to improve retention of a restoration.

Down syndrome, n a congenital condition characterized by varying degrees of mental retardation and multiple developmental defects. It is most commonly caused by the presence of an extra chromosome 21. It is also called *trisomy 21* and *trisomy G syndrome.* Mongolism is an archaic and discredited term.

downcoding, n a practice of third-party payers in which the benefits code has been changed to a less complex or lower cost procedure than was reported.

downtime, n the time interval during which a device is malfunctioning or inoperative.

doxazosin mesylate, n *trade name:* Cardura; *drug class:* peripheral α-adrenergic blocker; *action:* peripheral blood vessels are dilated, peripheral resistance lowered, reduction in blood pressure reduced; *uses:* hypertension.

doxepin (topical), n *trade name:* Zonolon; *drug class:* topical antipruritic (tricyclic antidepressant); *action:*

antipruritic mechanism unknown; has antihistaminic activity; also produces drowsiness; *uses:* pruritus associated with eczema, atopic dermatitis, lichen simplex chronicus.

doxepin HCl, *n trade name:* Sinequan; *drug class:* antidepressant, tricyclic; *action:* inhibits both norepinephrine and serotonin (5-HT) reuptake in synapses in brain; *uses:* major depression, anxiety.

doxycycline hyclate, *n trade names:* Doryx, Doxy-Caps, Vibra-Tabs; *drug class:* tetracycline, broad-spectrum antiinfective; *action:* inhibits protein synthesis, phosphorylation in microorganisms; *uses:* syphilis, chlamydia trachomatis, gonorrhea, lymphogranuloma venereum, uncommon gram-negative and gram-positive organisms, necrotizing ulcerative gingivostomatitis.

drachm (dram), *n* See dram.

draft, *n* See draw.

drag, *n* the lower, or cast, side of a denture mold or flask, to which the cope is fitted. The base of the cast is embedded in plaster or stone, with the remainder of the denture pattern exposed to be engaged by the plaster or stone in the cope (the upper part of the flask).

drain, *n* **1.** any substance that provides a channel for release or discharge from a wound. *v* to release or remove a fluid substance.

drain, cigarette, n See drain, Penrose.

drain, Penrose (cigarette), n.pr a thin-walled rubber tube through which a piece of gauze has been pulled.

drainage, *n* the placement or creation of a pathway from a deep lesion to the surface of the body to provide an avenue for the body to expel the byproducts of an infection or inflammation.

dram (drachm), *n* a unit of weight that equals the eighth part of the apothecaries' ounce. Symbol ʒ.

draught (draft), *n* See draw.

draw (draft, draught), *n* the taper or divergence of the walls of a preparation for insertion of a cemented restoration.

dressing, chemically cured, *n* a protective covering which contains the ingredients and accelerator necessary to initiate a chemical process upon application to a wound.

dressing, Coe-pak, *n.pr* the brand name of a commonly used chemical-cured dressing that is easy to place and remove. It is available as a pliable paste.

dressing, collagen, *n* protective coverings made of natural materials that are particularly suited for application over moist or bleeding wounds.

dressing, Kirkland cement, *n.pr* a surgical dressing applied to the tissues after periodontal surgery; consists of zinc oxide, tannic acid, and powdered rosin, admixed with a liquid composed of lump rosin, sweet almond oil, and eugenol.

dressing, PerioCare, *n.pr* the brand name of a commonly used chemical-cured dressing that provides comfortable protection and is easy to apply and remove; available as a pliable paste-gel.

dressing, postoperative surgical, *n* a surgical cement dressing applied to the teeth and tissues after surgical periodontal therapy. Possesses supportive, protective, hemostatic, analgesic, and other properties.

dressing, pressure, *n* a protective covering applied with pressure on top of a wound in order to stop bleeding or to hold a tissue flap or graft in place.

dressing, Ward's, *n.pr* See Ward's Wonderpack.

DRG, *n* the abbreviation for diagnosis-related group.

drift, *n* See tooth, drifting.

drill, *n* a cutting instrument for boring holes by rotary motion.

drill, bibevel, n a drill with two flattened sides and the end cut in two beveled planes.

drill, spear-point, n a drill with a tri-beveled, or threeplaned, point.

drill, twist, n a drill with one or more deep spiral grooves that extend from the point to the smooth part of the shaft.

drilling, *n* boring a hole with a rotary cutting instrument; used in reference to pinholes. (Objectionable as a term describing the general preparation of cavities with rotary instruments.)

drip, *n* the continuous slow intravenous introduction of fluid containing nutrients or drugs.

droperidol, *n* a butyrophenone drug used in neuroleptanalgesia and preanesthetic medication.

droplet spread, *n* transmission of an infection through the projection of oral and nasal secretions by coughing, sneezing, or talking.

dropsy (drop′sē), *n* See anasarca.

drowning, *n* asphyxiation because of submersion in a liquid.

drug(s), *n* a substance used in the prevention, cure, or alleviation of disease or pain or as an aid in some diagnostic procedures.

drug absorption, *n* See absorption, drug.

drug abuse, *n* an excessive or improper use of drugs, especially through self-administration for non-medical purposes. This term has increased significance because of the enactment of the Comprehensive Drug Abuse Prevention and Control Act of 1970, which replaces the Harrison Narcotic Act.

drug combinations, *n.pl* the use of drugs together to enhance the properties of both to the benefit of the patient.

drug dependence, *n* a physical or psychological state in which a person displays withdrawal symptoms if drug use is halted suddenly; can lead to addiction.

Drug Enforcement Administration (DEA), *n.pr* the federal agency charged with monitoring use and abuse of narcotics. It provides the drug schedules used to determine the addiction potential of dental drugs.

drug interaction, *n* a modification of the effect of a drug when administered with another drug. The effect may be an increase or a decrease in the action of either substance, or it may be an adverse effect that is not normally associated with either drug.

drug resistance, *n* the capacity of a microorganism to build a tolerance to a drug.

drug stability, *n* the length of time a drug retains its properties without loss of potency; usually referred to as shelf life.

drug therapy, *n* the use of a drug in the treatment of a patient with a specific disease or illness.

drug tolerance, *n* the body's ability to increasingly withstand the effects of the substance being used, thereby requiring larger quantities of said substance in order to bring about the desired result.

drugs, antibiotic, *n.pl* chemical compounds obtained from certain living cells of lower plant forms, such as bacteria, yeasts, and molds, and from synthesis. They are antagonistic to certain pathogenic organisms and have a lethal effect on them.

drugs, antimicrobial, *n.pl* any number of drugs, the chief of which are penicillin and its derivatives, used to combat viral, fungal, and parasitic infections.

drugs, antiseptic, *n.pl* chemical compounds used to reduce the number of microorganisms in the oral cavity.

drugs, autonomic, *n.pl* drugs that mimic or block the effects of stimulation of the autonomic nervous system.

drugs, desensitizing, *n.pl* pharmaceuticals used to diminish or eliminate sensitivity of teeth to physical, chemical, thermal, or other irritants (for example, strontium chloride, silver nitrate [ammoniacal], sodium fluoride, formalin, zinc chloride).

drugs, endodontic, *n.pl* any of the drugs used in treating the dental pulp and dental periapical tissues.

drugs, nonofficial, *n.pl* drugs that are not listed in the United States Pharmacopeia (U.S.P.) or the National Formulary (N.F.).

drugs, official, *n.pl* drugs listed in the U.S.P. or N.F.

drugs, officinal **(ōfis′inəl),** *n.pl* drugs that may be purchased without a prescription. More commonly called *over-the-counter (OTC) drugs.*

drugs, over-the-counter (OTC), *n.pl* drugs that may be purchased without a prescription. Sometimes called nonlegend drugs because the label does not bear the prescription legend required on all drugs that may be dispensed only on prescription.

drugs, parasympathetic, *n.pl* belladonna alkaloids that inhibit glandular secretions of the nose, mouth, pharynx, and bronchi. This is the chief reason for using atropine and scopolamine for preanesthetic medication.

drugs, parasympatholytic **(per′əsim′pəthōlit′ik),** *n.pl* drugs that block nerve impulses passing from parasympathetic nerve fibers to postganglionic neuroeffectors.

drugs, parasympathomimetic **(per´əsim´pəthōmimet´ik),** *n.pl* drugs that have an effect similar to that produced when the parasympathetic nerves are stimulated.

drugs, proprietary, *n.pl* drugs that are patented or controlled by a private organization or manufacturer.

drugs, psychoactive, *n.pl* drugs or other agents which have the capacity to become habit forming because of their influence on mood, behavior, or conscious thought; may be therapeutic or recreational.

drugs, sympathetic, *n.pl* agents that imitate the sympathetic autonomic nervous system actions. They usually causes raised levels of alertness and anxiety. Some types are used in dentistry as vasoconstricters in conjunction with local anesthetics. See also adrenergic agents.

dry field, *n* the isolation of a surgical or operating field from body fluids such as saliva and blood. A dry field is essential in the placement of some sealants and restorative fillings.

Dry-foil, *n.pr* the trade name for tinfoil that is supplied with an adhesive powder or coating on one side.

dry heat, *n* a method of sterilization of suitable instruments using a well-calibrated and time-controlled convection oven.

dry ice, *n* solid carbon dioxide, with a temperature of about −140° F.

dry socket, *n* See socket, dry.

drying, for sealant application, *n* the removal of moisture from the affected area prior to applying a sealant.

DSM-IV (Diagnostic and Statistical Manual of Mental Disorders), *n* a publication of the American Psychiatric Association that classifies more than 200 mental conditions.

dual choice (dual option), *n* federal legislation that requires employers to give their employees the option to enroll in a local health maintenance organization rather than in the conventional employer-sponsored health program.

dual impression technique, *n* See technique, impression, dual.

duct, *n* a small passage.

duct, intercalated, *n* duct that is connected to an acinus of the salivary glands. See also acinus.

duct, nasopalatine, *n* See cyst, nasopalatine.

duct, Stensen's, *n.pr* the excretory duct of the parotid gland; it passes lateral to the masseter muscle and enters the oral cavity through the buccal tissues adjacent to the maxillary first and second molars.

duct, striated, *n* part of the ductal system to which the intercalated ducts are connected in the lobules of the salivary gland.

duct, Wharton's, *n.pr* the excretory duct of the submaxillary glands; opens into the oral cavity at the sublingual papillae of the mucous membrane of the floor of the mouth posterior to the mandibular incisor teeth.

ductility (duktil´itē), *n* the property of a material that allows permanent deformation under tension without rupture. It is measured as a percentage increase in length on rupture compared with original length and is termed percentage elongation, or elongation.

due process, *n* the rules governing the fair practice of law. Due process dictates that everyone is equal in the eyes of the law, and it also states that the law must be fair and clearly stated to prevent arbitrary actions by the state.

Duke's test, *n.pr* See test, Duke's.

duodenal ulcer, *n* a peptic ulcer located in the duodenum.

duodenum, *n* the first, shortest, and most fixed portion of the small intestine. The duodenum courses from the pyloric valve of the stomach and terminates in a junction with the jejunum at the duodenojejunal flexure.

duplication, *n* the procedure of accurately reproducing a cast or other object.

duplication impression, *n* See duplication.

dust-borne organisms, *n.pl* organisms, including pathogens, which enter an inhabited space attached to dust particles and contaminate the contents of the inhabited space or the respiratory tracts of the inhabitants.

duty, *n* that which is due from a person; that which a person owes to another; an obligation.

dwarf, pituitary (pitōō′iterē), *n* an individual who is of small stature as a result of a deficiency of growth hormones. Such dwarfs usually are well proportioned.

dwarfism, *n* deficient growth and development leading to small stature and often skeletal deformity. It may be associated with ovarian agenesis, pituitary insufficiency, mongolism, progeria, rickets, renal disease, dietary deficiency, achondroplasia, cleidocranial dysostosis, osteogenesis imperfecta, microcephaly, hydrocephaly, sexual precocity, and delayed adolescence.

dyclonine hydrochloride (dī′klənēn), *n* a ketone-type liquid topical anesthetic agent which may be applied with a cotton swab or used as a mouthrinse.

dye, occlusal registration, *n* a water-soluble dye used as an aid in locating occlusal contacts. A valuable aid in effecting fine adjustments in the final phases of the selective grinding procedure.

dyes, plaque detection, *n.pl* See disclosing solution.

dyes, treatment, *n.pl* the dyes used in medicine and dentistry in the treatment of diseased states, the most useful of which are the rosaniline dyes (for example, gentian violet, crystal violet) and the fluorescein dyes (for example, Mercurochrome), which possess antiseptic and protective properties.

dynamic relation, *n* See relation, dynamic.

dyphylline, *n trade names:* Dilor, Dyflex, Lufyllin; *drug class:* Xanthine derivative; *action:* relaxes smooth muscle of respiratory system by blocking phosphodiesterase; *uses:* bronchial asthma, bronchospasm in chronic bronchitis, COPD, emphysema.

dysarthria (disärth′rē-ə), *n* a speech impediment brought on by emotional distress, paralysis, or muscle spasticity.

dysautonomia, familial (dis′ôtōnō′mē-ə), *n* See syndrome, Riley-Day.

dyscrasia (diskrā′zhə, -zē-ə), *n* I. a morbid condition, especially one that involves an imbalance of component elements. *n* 2. an abnormal composition of the blood, such as that found in leukemia and anemia.

dysdiadochokinesia (dis′dī-ad′ōkōkinē′zhə, zē-ə), *n* a disturbance of musculoskeletal function. There is a disorganization in the reciprocal innervation of agonists and antagonists and a loss of the ability to stop one act in terms of rate, magnitude, and the direction of movement and immediately to follow it with another act diametrically opposite (for example, alternately elevating and depressing the mandible). Another example is observed in the inappropriate use of the tongue during mastication when it is necessary to change, reverse, and modify the energy and direction of movement.

dysentery, *n* an inflammation of the intestine, especially of the colon, that may be caused by chemical irritants, bacteria, protozoa, or parasites. It is characterized by frequent and bloody stools and severe abdominal pain.

dysesthesia (dis′esthē′zhə, -zē-ə), *n* an impairment of the senses, especially the sense of touch. No sensation is painful with dysesthesia.

dysfunction (disfunk′shən), *n* (malfunction), any abnormality or impairment of function or the inability of a body, organ, or organ system to perform normally.

dysfunction, dental, *n* an abnormal functioning or impairment of the functioning of the dental organ.

dysfunction, endocrine, *n* an abnormality in the function of an endocrine gland, either by hypofunction or hyperfunction of the secretory elements of the gland.

dysgeusia, *n* an abnormal or impaired sense of taste.

dysgnathia (disnā′thē-ə), *n* those abnormalities that extend beyond the teeth and include the maxilla, the mandible, or both. See also anomaly, dysgnathic.

dyskeratosis (dis′kerətō′sis), *n* an irreversible alteration in the maturation of stratified squamous epithelium. Refers to an increase of abnormal mitosis, individual cell keratinization, epithelial pearls within the spinous layer, loss of polarity of the cells, hyperchromatism, nuclear atypia, and basilar hyperplasia.

Dyskeratosis. (Neville/Damm/Allen/Bouquot, 2002)

dyslexia, *n* an impairment of the ability to read. Dyslexic persons often reverse letters and words, cannot adequately distinguish the letter sequences in written words, and have difficulty determining left from right.

dysmenorrhea (dis′menərē′-ə), *n* painful menstruation.

dysmetria (dismē′trē-ə), *n* the loss of ability to gauge distance, speed, or power of movement associated with muscle function; for example, the patient is unable to control the force of closure and strikes the opposite occluding teeth with greater vigor than necessary.

dysmorphism (dismôr′fizəm), *n* an aberration of form.

dysostosis (disostō′sis), *n* defective ossification.

dysostosis, cleidocranial **(klī′dōkrā′nē-əl),** *n* (Sainton's disease), a familial disease or congenital disorder characterized by failure to form, or retarded formation of, the clavicles; delayed closure of the sutures and fontanels; and delayed eruption of teeth, with formation of supernumerary teeth. Cleidocranial dysostosis is characterized by underdevelopment of the maxillae, agenesis or aplasia of the clavicle, abnormalities in other skeletal bones and muscles, and irregularities of the dentition. The syndrome may be mutational or transmitted on an autosomal dominant basis.

dysostosis, craniofacial (Crouzon's disease, Crouzon's syndrome), *n* a condition of unknown etiology that is similar to cleidocranial dysostosis but differs in that the clavicles are not affected. See also dysostosis, cleidocranial.

dysostosis, faciomandibular, *n* a developmental disturbance of the cranial bones and hypoplasias of the upper part of the face. The mandibular body is underdeveloped, but the ramus is hyperplastic. The teeth are crowded and malposed.

dysostosis multiplex, *n* See syndrome, Hurler's.

dyspepsia, *n* a vague feeling of epigastric discomfort, felt after eating. Dyspepsia is not a distinct condition but may be a sign of underlying intestinal disorder, such as peptic ulcer, gallbladder disease, or chronic appendicitis. The symptoms usually increase during periods of stress.

dysphagia (disfā′jē-ə), *n* difficulty in swallowing. It may be caused by lesions in the mouth, pharynx, or larynx; neuromuscular disturbances; or mechanical obstruction of the esophagus (for example, dysphagia of Plummer-Vinson syndrome [sideropenic dysphagia], peritonsillar abscess, Ludwig's angina, and carcinoma of the tongue, pharynx, larynx).

dysphoria (disfôr′ē-ə), *n* a feeling of discomfort or restlessness. See also euphoria.

dysplasia (displā′zhə), *n* **1.** developmental abnormality. See also dysplasia, dentinal. *n* **2.** reversible, regressive alteration in adult cells, seen as alterations in their size, shape, orientation, and functions; leads to change in tissue architecture and is related to chronic inflammation or protracted irritation. Abnormality of development. *n* **3.** disharmony between component parts.

dysplasia, anteroposterior (anteroposterior facial dysplasia), *n* an abnormal anteroposterior relationship of the maxillae and mandible to each other or to the cranial base.

dysplasia, craniofacial, *n* a disharmony between the cranium and the face.

dysplasia, dentinal, *n* a genetic disturbance of the dentin characterized by early calcification of the pulp chambers and root canals and by root resorption. It is differentiated from dentinogenesis imperfecta by the latter's characteristics of attrition and relative freedom from root resorption.

dysplasia, dentofacial, n a disharmony between teeth and bones of the face (for example, crowding and spacing).

dysplasia, ectodermal, n a disease of genetic origin characterized by failure to form ectodermal derivatives. Sweat glands and teeth may be missing (anhidrosis and anodontia, respectively), and there may be scant hair, faulty fingernails, and malformation of the iris.

dysplasia, enamel, n a development abnormality of enamel tissue.

dysplasia, fibroosseous, n See dysplasia, fibrous.

dysplasia, fibrous (fibroosseous dysplasia), n a metabolic disturbance characterized by replacement of the bone marrow with fibrous tissue and slow, progressive remolding and enlargement of the bone. It may be monostotic (limited to one bone) or polyostotic (present in many bones). Albright's syndrome shows polyostotic fibrous dysplasia and other symptoms. The monostotic lesions may be identical with ossifying fibroma or with osseous dysplasia. See also osteofibroma and syndrome, Albright's.

dysplasia, focal osseous, n See fibroma, periapical.

dysplasia, maxillomandibular, n a disharmony between one jaw and the other.

dysplasia, osseous, n a chronic reaction of the bone to injury characterized by replacement of the bone marrow with fibrous connective tissue, unilateral enlargement of the maxillae or mandible, and characteristic radiographic findings. It is similar to or identical with monostotic fibrous dysplasia and ossifying fibroma.

dysplasia, periapical cementoosseous, n See cementoma.

dysplasia, polyostotic fibrous, n fibrous dysplasia occurring in more than one bone. See also dysplasia, fibrous; osteofibroma; and syndrome, Albright's.

dyspnea (dispnē′-ə), n difficult, labored, or gasping breathing; inspiration, expiration, or both may be involved.

dystonia (distō′nē-ə), n a disorder or lack of tonicity.

dystrophy (dis′trōfē), n faulty nutrition. Often used to refer to the results of faulty nutrition, that is, wasting away.

E space, n the net difference between the combined mesiodistal width of the primary canine, primary first molar, and the primary second molar and that of the permanent canine, first premolar, and second premolar. In the mandible the mean leeway space is 3.4 mm, and in the maxilla it is 1.9 mm. Also called *leeway space.*

Eames' technique (ēmz), n See technique, Eames'.

earnings report, n a statement issued by a company showing its earnings or losses over a given period. The earnings report lists the income earned, expenses, and net result. Also called *income statement.*

Eastman Interdental Bleeding Index (EIBI), n.pr an assessment tool used to determine the extent of interdental inflammation based on bleeding that occurs within 15 seconds after a wooden cleaning stick is inserted between the teeth.

eating disorders, n.pl a group of dysfunctional behaviors of nutrition, including anorexia, bulimia, or cravings for such nonfood items as ice, clay, or starch.

EBIT, n the abbreviation for **earnings before interest and taxes.**

eburnation (ē′bur-nā′shən), n an increase in bony density into an ivory-like mass. See also *osteitis, condensing* and *dentin eburnation.*

eccentric (ek-sen′trik), n **1.** a deviation from the normal or conventional. adj **2.** away from the central or reference position.

eccentric checkbite, n See record, interocclusal, eccentric.

eccentric jaw relation, n See relation, jaw, eccentric.

eccentric occlusion, n See occlusion, eccentric.

eccentric position, n See *position, eccentric.*

ecchymosis (ek′i-mō′sis), n a discoloration of mucous membranes caused by a diffuse extravasation of blood. Frequently called a *bruise.*

Ecchymosis. (Regezi/Sciubba/Jordan, 2003)

echocardiography, n a diagnostic procedure for studying the structure and motion of the heart using ultrasonic waves that pass through the heart and are reflected backward, or echoed, when they pass from one type of tissue to another.

echolalia (ek″o-la′le-ə), n an uncontrollable reiteration of a word or phrase recently stated by another individual.

echoviruses (ECHO virus), n.pl an enteric pathogen associated with fever and mild respiratory disease; sometimes may produce an aseptic meningitis.

ecology, n the study of the interaction between living organisms and their environment.

econazole nitrate (topical), n *trade name:* Ecostatin; *drug class:* local antifungal; *action:* interferes with fungal cell membrane, which increases permeability, leaking of cell nutrients; *uses:* tinea pedis, tinea cruris, tinea corporis, tinea versicolor, cutaneous candidiasis.

economics, n in dentistry, a broad term that covers all the business aspects of dental practice.

ecosystem, n the sum total of all living and nonliving things that support the chain of life events within a particular area.

ectoderm, n the outermost of the three primary cell layers of an embryo. The ectoderm gives rise to the nervous system, the organs of special sense, the epidermis, and epidermal tissues such as fingernails, hair, and skin glands.

ectodermal dysplasia, n a developmental disturbance of tissues derived from the ectoderm (for example, hair, nails, sweat glands, and teeth). Dental findings are partial anodontia and microdontia.

ectomorph (ek′tōmôrf), n a constitutional body type (Sheldon's classification) characterized by long, fragile bones and a highly developed nervous system.

ectopia lentis, n a displacement of the lens of the eye.

ectopic (ek-top′ik), adj occurring outside of the expected or usual location; displaced.

ectopic eruption, n See *eruption, ectopic.*

ectropion (ek-trō′pē-on), n eversion, or rolling outward, of the eyelid margin.

eczema (ek′zē-mə), n an inflammatory skin disease characterized by vesiculation, inflammation, watery discharge, and the development of scales and crusts. The large variety of types can be distinguished according to location and causal agent.

Eczema. (Zitelli/Davis, 2002)

ED50, n See *dose, median effective.*

edema (e-dē′mə), n the accumulation of fluid in the tissues or in the peritoneal or pleural cavities. Primary factors favoring edema are increased capillary hydrostatic pressure (increased venous pressure), decreased osmotic pressure of plasma (hypoproteinemia), decreased tissue tension and lymphatic drainage, increased osmotic pressure of tissue fluids, and increased capillary permeability. Additional renal and hormonal factors are important. Clinical manifestations may consist of a steady weight gain or localized or generalized swelling.

edema, angioneurotic, n (angioedema, giant urticaria, Quincke's disease) the spontaneous swelling of the lips, cheeks, eyelids, tongue, soft palate, pharynx, and glottis, frequently associated with allergy to foods or drugs and lasting from several hours to several days. Involvement of the glottis results in obstruction of the airway.

Angioneurotic edema. (Regezi/Sciubba/Pogrel, 2000)

edema, cardiac, n edema caused by venous congestion in association with congestive heart failure; tends to appear first in such dependent parts as the legs.

edema, dependent, n edema that changes its position with the posture of dependent parts (for example, edema of the legs in progressive heart failure).

edema of glottis, n a swelling caused by fluid accumulation in the soft tissues of the larynx. The condition, usually inflammatory, may result from an infection, injury, allergy, or inhalation of toxic substances.

edema, periorbital, n edematous swelling of the eyelids in association with local injury, allergic reactions, hypoproteinemia, trichinosis, and myxedema.

edema, pitting, n a persistent indentation of the skin when pressure is applied to an edematous area.

edentulism (ē-den′tyōō-liz-əm), *n* the condition of being edentulous, without teeth.

edentulous (ē-den′tyōō-ləs), *adj* without teeth; lacking teeth.

edge strength, *n* See *strength, edge.*

edge-to-edge bite, *n* See *occlusion, edge-to-edge.*

edge-to-edge occlusion, *n* See *occlusion, edge-to-edge.*

edgewise appliance, *n* See *appliance, edgewise.*

EDP, *n* the abbreviation for **electronic data processing.**

Edtac, *n* the trade name for a chelating agent used to soften calcified tissue.

education, *n* the act or process of imparting or acquiring knowledge, skill, or judgment.

education, continuing, n education that occurs after the completion of a course of study leading to a degree. Usually taken in short (1- to 2-day) courses covering a specific topic or procedure.

education dental, n the formal education necessary to become qualified to practice dentistry; typically 4 years of full-time study in an accredited school of dentistry.

education of patient, n effective communication between the dentist (and/or auxiliaries) and the patient concerning dentistry and the principles of treatment and prevention. The procedure of increasing the patient's knowledge of the oral cavity and its care to the point where the reasons for proposed dental services are understood.

education, predental, n the formal education necessary to qualify for placement in a dental curriculum, typically 4 years of full-time study at the baccalaureate level.

educational status, *n* the level of education and skill obtained within a discipline or profession, usually referred to as a generalist or specialist in a discipline.

effect, *n* the result of an action.

effect, heel, (anode heel effect), n the variation of intensity over the cross section of a useful x-ray beam, caused by the angle at which x-rays emerge from beneath the surface of the focal spot, which causes a differential attenuation of photons composing the useful beam.

effect of external radiation on bone, n See *osteoradionecrosis.*

effect of function on bone, n See *law, Wolff's.*

effect, photoelectric, n the process

by which x-ray images are produced when the energy of an incident photon is absorbed as the result of bound electron ejection.

effect, wedging, *n* an effect produced by food impaction that forces the teeth apart.

effective half-life, *n* See *life, radioactive.*

effectiveness, *n* the degree to which action(s) achieves the intended health result under normal or usual circumstances.

effector (ēfek'tur), *n* **1.** a motor or secretory nerve ending in an organ, gland, or muscle; consequently called an *effector organ. n* **2.** an on-the-job organ of the body that responds to stimulations asking for corrections. Antonym: receptor.

efferent (ef'ər-ənt), *adj* conveying away from a center toward the periphery.

efferent neurons, *n.pl* See *neuron, efferent.*

efficacy, *n* the ability to provide a clinically measurable effect, preferably beneficial.

efficiency, *n* the operation of a dental practice in such a way that both business and professional services are performed in a minimal amount of time without sacrificing quality of work, sympathetic attitude, and kindliness.

eH, *n* the symbol for oxidation-reduction potential, which is regarded as a significant factor in the protection of the body against anaerobic bacteria. The eH of living tissue of pH level 7.4 is about 0.12 volt.

Ehlers-Danlos syndrome (ā'lurz-dan'lus), *n.pr* a hereditary disorder of connective tissue, marked by hyperplasticity of skin, tissue fragility, and hypermotility of joints. Minor trauma may cause a gaping wound with little bleeding. Sprains, dislocations, and synovial effusions are common. See also *syndrome, Ehlers-Danlos.*

EIA, *n* the abbreviation for **enzyme immunoassay;** better known as ELISA for enzyme-linked immunosorbent assay, used to detect the presence of HIV antibody to HIV in the blood.

Eikenella corrodens, *n.pr* a gram-negative, rod-shaped, facultatively anaerobic bacteria that is part of the normal flora of the oral cavity but may become an opportunistic pathogen in immunocompromised patients.

ejector, *n* by common usage, a device used to remove debris and fluids by negative pressure. The correct term for such a device, however, is *aspirator.* See also *aspirator.*

ejector, saliva, *n* a device (containing a removable tip) that is attached to a vacuum supply to remove saliva from a dental field of operation.

ejector, saliva, tip, *n* a removable tip, made of metal, glass, rubber, plastic, or a combination of these, that is attached to a saliva ejector and bent to fit over lower teeth and reach the floor of the oral cavity.

elastic, *adj* referring to property of a solid substance that permits recovery of its shape after a deformation resulting from force application.

elastic deformation, *n* See *deformation, elastic.*

elastic impression, *n* See *impression, elastic.*

elastic, intermaxillary, *n* See *elastic, maxillomandibular.*

elastic, intramaxillary, *n* an elastic band used within either the maxillary or mandibular arch.

elastic limit, *n* See *limit, elastic.*

elastic, maxillomandibular, *n* an elastic band used between the maxillary and mandibular dentitions.

elastic memory, *n* **1.** the property of a material such as wax that enables it, after being warmed, bent, and cooled, to return to its original form upon rewarming. *n* **2.** a rubber plastic band used to apply force to the teeth.

elasticity, *n* the quality or condition of being elastic.

elasticity, modulus of, *n* (Young's modulus) a measurement of elasticity obtained by dividing stress below the proportional limit by its corresponding strain value. A measure of stiffness.

elastomer (ē-las'tō-mur), *n* a soft, rubberlike material; synthetic rubber. A rubber base impression material (for example, silicone, mercaptan).

elastosis (ē'las-tō'sis), *n* a degeneration of the elastic tissues; found particularly in the lips and associated with senile or actinic cheilitis.

elastosis, senile, *n* a dermatologic

disease that results from degeneration of the elastic connective tissue.

elder abuse, *n* the infliction of physical, sexual, or emotional trauma on a senior citizen.

elderly, *adj* an adjective used to describe a person who is beyond middle age and approaching old age. It is politically correct to refer to those older than 65 as *senior citizens.* See also *geriatric dentistry.*

electroanesthesia (i-lek′trō-an-es-thē′zē-ə, -zhə), *n* local or general anesthesia induced by electric current.

electrocardiography, *n* a method of recording electrical activity generated by the heart muscle.

electrochemistry, *n* chemical reactions that elicit electrical potentials, and electrical potentials that initiate chemical reactions.

electrocoagulation (ē-lek′trō-kō-ag′yōō-la′shən), *n* the use of electrically generated heat to destroy tissue by coagulation necrosis. Usually a platinum wire electrode or loop is used.

electroconvulsive therapy, *n* the induction of a brief convulsion by passing an electric current through the brain for the treatment of affective disorders, especially in patients resistant to psychoactive drug therapy.

electrode (ē-lek′trōd), *n* an instrument with a point or a surface from which a current can be discharged into or received from the body of a patient or a solution.

electrodiagnosis, *n* the diagnosis of disease or injury by applying electric stimulation to various nerves and muscles.

electroencephalograph (EEG) (ē-lek′trō-en-sef′ə-lō-graf), *n* an instrument for recording the electrical activity of the brain.

electrogalvanism (galvanism) (ē-lek-trō-gal′vən-iz-əm), *n* the flow of electric current between two different metals in an electrolyte solution. Dissimilar metals used in different intraoral restorations.

electrolyte (ē-lek′trō-līt), *n* a solution that conducts electricity by means of its ions.

electrolyte affinity, *n* the attraction of the electrolytes in the body to the

different fluid compartments of the intracellular and extracellular environments. Sodium is the predominant cation in the extracellular fluid; potassium is the predominant cation within the cells; chlorine and bicarbonate are the predominant anions in the plasma and interstitial fluids; and phosphates and proteins are the chief anions in the cells.

electrolyte balance, fluid and, *n* See *fluid and electrolyte balance.*

electrolyzer (ionizer) (ē-lek′trō-līz-ur), *n* an electric apparatus designed for use in a root canal to break down a treatment chemical into its various ions by direct current. See also *electrosterilizer.*

electromallet, McShirley's, *n* See *condenser, electromallet.*

electrometer (ē-lek-trom′ə-tur), *n* an electrostatic instrument for measuring the potential difference between two points. In radiology, electrometers are used to measure changes in the potential of charged electrodes resulting from ionization occasioned by radiation.

electromyography (ē-lek′trō-mī-og′rə-fē), *n* the detection, recording, and interpretation of electric voltage generated by the skeletal muscles.

electron (e) (ē-lek′tron), *n* a negatively charged elementary particle constituent in every neutral atom, with a mass of 0.000549. (Particles with an equal but opposite charge are called *positrons.*)

electron beam, *n* See *electron stream.*

electron stream, *n (electron beam, cathode ray, cathode stream),* a stream of electrons emitted from the negative electrode (cathode) in a roentgen-ray tube; their bombardment of the anode gives rise to the roentgen rays.

electronic, *adj* pertaining to the application of that branch of science that deals with the motion, emission, and behavior of currents of free electrons, especially in vacuum, gas, or phototubes and special conductors or semiconductors. Contrasted with *electric,* which pertains to the flow of large currents in wires only.

electronic knife, *n* See *knife, electronic.*

electrophoresis, *n* the movement of

charged suspended particles through a liquid medium in response to changes in an electric field.

electroplating, *n* plating by electrolysis. Impressions are plated in dentistry to form metalized working dies.

electropolishing, *n* the removal of a minute layer of metal by electrolysis to produce a bright surface.

electrosection, *n* an incision created by electrosurgery, ideally by using a fully rectified, alternating highfrequency current and producing minimal cellular injury.

electrosterilization, *n* medication of a prepared root canal by use of electrolysis of the medicament.

electrosterilizer, *n* an electric apparatus designed for use in root canal treatment for the electrolysis of a halide, such as sodium iodide, to release iodine in the cleaned root canal for the purpose of destroying residual organisms. See also *electrolyzer.*

electrosurgery, *n* the use of electrically generated energy from highfrequency alternating currents to cut or alter tissue within definite limits.

element, *n* a simple substance that cannot be decomposed by chemical means and is made up of atoms that are alike in their peripheral electronic configuration and chemical properties but differ in their nuclei, atomic weights, and radioactive properties.

elephantiasis (el′ə-fən-tī′-ə-sis), *n* a chronic disease caused by filariasis of the lymph channels with resultant inflammation and blockage. The term is also used for hypertrophy of tissues from other causes (for example, gingival elephantiasis).

elephantiasis gingivae, n See *fibromatosis gingivae.*

elevated oral lesions, *n.pl* abnormalities occurring above the surface of the interior of the mouth, categorized as either blisterform (bulla, pustule, or vesicle) or nonblisterform (nodules, tumors, plaques, or papules).

elevator, *n* an instrument used to raise or lift something.

elevator, dental, n one of a variety of blades used for engaging teeth and roots to remove them from their alveoli.

elevator, malar, n an instrument

used to elevate or reposition the zygomatic bone.

elevator, periosteal, n a thin blade used to lift periosteum from bone.

eligibility date, *n* the date an individual and dependents become eligible for benefits under a dental benefits contract. Often referred to as *effective date.*

eligibility rules, *n.pl* conditions that define who may be entitled to dental benefits, when persons first become entitled to such benefits, and any provisions that determine how long an individual remains entitled to benefits.

eligible person, *n* See *beneficiary.*

ELISA, *n* the abbreviation for **enzyme-linked immunosorbent assay** used to detect the presence of HIV antibody to HIV in the blood.

elixir (ē-lik′sur), *n* a pleasantly flavored, sweetened hydroalcoholic solution of a drug intended for oral administration.

elliptocytosis (ē-lip′tō-sĭ-tō′sis), *n* (ovalcytosis, oval cell anemia), a hereditary anomaly in which the red blood cells are elliptical, or oval shaped, and are predisposed to hemolysis.

elongation (ē′lông-gā′shən), *n* the process or condition of increasing in length before breaking; indicates ductility (for example, of a metal).

elongation, percent, n **1.** the increase in length of a material after fracture in tension. *n* **2.** a mechanical test usually employed to measure ductility.

emaciation, *n* excessive leanness caused by disease or lack of nutrition.

embedded, *adj* referring to a tooth, root tip, or foreign body that is covered in bone.

embolism (em′bə-liz-əm), *n* the clogging of a vessel by matter, such as a clot, air, or oil, that is carried by the bloodstream to some point where the lumen of the vessel narrows. This is the opposite of thrombosis, in which the clotting mechanism is organized in situ.

embolism, air, n See *aeroembolism.*

embolus (em′bə-lus), *n* a blood clot or other material that travels in the bloodstream and then lodges in a vessel and obstructs circulation.

E

embrasure, *n* an opening, as in a wall. The space between the curved proximal surfaces of the teeth.

embrasure, buccal, *n* an embrasure that opens toward the cheeks.

embrasure clasp, *n* See *clasp, embrasure.*

embrasure hook, *n* an extension of a removable partial denture into the embrasure above the contact area between two adjacent teeth, which resists movement in a cervical direction.

embrasure, interdental, *n* the spaces formed by the interproximal contours of adjoining teeth, beginning at the contact area and extending lingually, facially, occlusally, and apically.

embrasure, labial, *n* an embrasure that opens toward the lips.

embrasure, lingual, *n* an embrasure that opens toward the tongue.

embrasure, occlusal, *n* an embrasure that opens toward the occlusal surface or plane.

embryo, *n* an organism in the earliest stages of development; in humans, the stage between the time of implantation of the fertilized ovum until the end of the seventh or eighth week of gestation.

embryoblast (em′bre-o-blast″), *n* a group of cells near the embryonic axis of the blastocyst that develop into the embryo.

embryology, *n* the study of the origin, growth, development, and function of an organism from fertilization to birth.

embryonic period (em″bre-on′ik pe′re-od), *n* in humans, the stage between the second and eighth week of embryonic development, during which differentiation of organs and organ systems occurs.

emergency, *n* an unforeseen occurrence or combination of circumstances that calls for immediate action or remedy; pressing necessity; exigency.

emergency cart/kit, *n* a portable container holding all of the equipment and medicines that one would need to assist a patient in case of a medical crisis.

emergency medicine, *n* a branch of medicine concerned with the diagnosis and treatment of conditions resulting from trauma or sudden illness.

emergency prevention, *n* the procedures necessary to avoid creating a life-threatening crisis for a patient.

emergency training, *n* the system of imparting knowledge and skills to be used in case of an accident or an unforeseen occurrence.

emergency treatment, *n* treatment that must be rendered to the patient immediately because of acute infection or pain.

emergency treatment, burns, *n* the immediate, urgent care given to a burn victim to stabilize the individual until further medical assistance can be found.

emergency treatment, cortical deficiency, *n* the immediate, urgent care given to an individual experiencing adrenal crisis to stabilize that individual until further medical assistance can be found.

emergency treatment, facial fractures, *n* the immediate, urgent care given to a patient with facial fractures to stabilize the individual until further medical assistance can be found.

emergency treatment, heart failure, *n* the immediate, urgent care given to a patient experiencing heart failure to stabilize the individual until further medical assistance can be found.

emery, *n* an aluminum-based abrasive agent. Two types are aluminum oxide and levigated alumina. Emery is not suitable for polishing dental enamel. Also called *corundum.*

emesis (em′ə-sis), *n* the sudden expulsion of gastric contents through the esophagus into the pharynx. The act is partly voluntary and partly involuntary. See also *vomiting.*

emesis basin (em′ə-sis, əmē′sis), *n* a bowl that catches fluids and solids spewed from the mouth.

emetic (ə-met′ik), *n* a drug that induces vomiting.

emetine hydrochloride (em′ə-tēn), *n* an alkaloid, $C_{29}H_{40}N_2O_4$ 2HCl, regarded as a protozoacide and formerly used in the treatment of periodontitis and amebic dysentery.

EMF, *n* the abbreviation for **erythrocyte-maturing factor.**

emigration, *n* movement of erythrocytes or leukocytes through the walls of the vessels that carry them.

eminence, retromylohyoid (em′in-əns, ret′rō-mī′lō-hī′-oid), *n* the distal end of the lingual flange of a lower denture. It occupies the retromylohyoid space.

eminenectomy (em'inenek'tōmē), *n* the operative removal of the anterior articular surface of the glenoid fossa.

emollient (ē-mï'lē-ənt), *n* an agent that is soothing to the skin or mucous membrane; makes the skin softer or smoother.

emotion, *n* a complex feeling or state (affect) accompanied by characteristic motor and glandular activities; feelings; mood.

emotional, *adj* describing of a person experiencing an emotion; manifesting emotional behavior, rather than logical, rational behavior; describing a person who is easily or excessively given to emotion.

empathy, *n* putting oneself into the psychologic frame of reference of another, so that the other person's feeling, thinking, and acting are understood and to some extent predictable. A desirable trust-building characteristic of a helping profession. It is embodied in the sincere statement, "I understand how you feel." Empathy is different from sympathy in that to be empathetic one understands how the person feels rather than actually experiencing those feelings, as in sympathy.

emphysema (em'fi-zē'mə), *n* **I.** a swelling caused by air in the tissue spaces. In the oral and facial regions it may be caused either by air introduced into a tooth socket or gingival crevice with the air syringe, or by blowing of the nose. *n* **2.** a permanent dilation of the respiratory alveoli.

employee, *n* a person who, under the direction and control of the employer, performs services for remuneration.

Employee Retirement Income Security Act (ERISA), *n.pr* a federal act, passed in 1974, that established new standards and reporting and disclosure requirements for employer-funded pension and health benefits programs. To date, self-funded health benefit plans operating under ERISA have been held to be exempt from state insurance laws. This exemption is currently under review.

employer-sponsored plan, *n* a program supported totally or in part by an employer or group of employers to provide dental benefits for employees. The plan may be administered directly by the employer or another person or group under a contractual arrangement. Part of the cost may be borne by the employee.

employment, *n* **I.** to be engaged in work for hire. *n* **2.** use of a specific tool or technique in the accomplishment of a task.

empyema (em'pī-ē'mə, em'pē-ē'mə), *n* the presence of pus in a cavity, hollow organ, or space (for example, the pleural cavity).

emulsifier, *n* an agent such as gum arabic or egg yolk used to suspend droplets of oil in a water-based solution. An agent to maintain any element or particle in suspension within a fluid medium.

emulsion (ē-mul'shən), *n* a colloidal dispersion of one liquid in another. See also *suspension.*

emulsion, digestive, *n* the suspension of fat globules, usually in the bile acid of the small intestine, and their resulting breakdown into smaller particles as part of the digestive process. See also *emulsifiers.*

emulsion, double, *n* a suspension of sensitive silver halide salts impregnated in gelatin and coated on both sides of a radiographic film base.

emulsion, silver, *n* a suspension of sensitive silver halide salts impregnated in gelatin and used for coating photographic plates and radiographic films.

emulsion, single, *n* a suspension of sensitive silver halide salts impregnated in gelatin and coated on only one side of a radiographic film base.

enalapril maleate, *n trade names:* Vasotec, Vasotec IV; *drug class:* angiotensin-converting enzyme (ACE) inhibitor; *action:* selectively suppresses renin-angiotensin-aldosterone system; inhibits ACE; prevents conversion of angiotensin I to angiotensin II leading to dilation of arterial and venous vessels; *uses:* hypertension, heart failure adjunct.

enamel, *n* **I.** the hard, glistening tissue covering the anatomic crown of the tooth. It is composed chiefly of hexagonal rods of hydroxyapatite, sheathed in an organic matrix (approximately 0.15%) and oriented with their long axes approximately at right angles to the surface. *n* **2.** the outermost layer or covering of the coronal portion of the tooth that overlies and protects the dentin.

enamel, junction of cementum, *n* association of enamel with cementum by edge-to-edge contact or by overlapping. In some cases, the two do not form a junction, thereby exposing dentin.

enamel lamellae, *n.pl* incompletely calcified, microscopic structures present in the enamel. They may extend to the dentinoenamel junction and beyond.

enamel matrix, *n* the mineral structure of enamel, secreted by ameloblasts.

enamel, mottled, *n* See *fluorosis, chronic endemic dental.*

enamel, opacity, (white spot), *n* a visibly lighter area on a tooth's surface; may be caused by fluorosis, or demineralization.

enamel organ, *n* the part of a developing tooth that is destined to produce the enamel.

enamel pearl, *n* See *pearl, enamel.*

enamel spindles, *n.pl* tubular projections from the dentinoenamel junction into the enamel, caused by penetration by odontoblasts before the junction is formed.

enamel tufts, *n.pl* brush-shaped projections from the dentinoenamel junction into the enamel, caused by crystallization defects.

enamel epithelium, *n* See *epithelium, enamel.*

enameloma, *n* See *pearl, enamel.*

enanthem (e-nan´thəm), *n* See *enanthema.*

enanthema (enanthem) (en´an-thē´mə), *n.pl* lesions involving the mucous membrane.

encephalitis, *n* an inflammatory condition of the brain.

encounter form, *n* a document or record used to collect data about given elements of a patient visit to a dental office or similar site that can become part of a patient record or be used for management purposes or for quality review activities.

end organ, *n* the expanded termination of a nerve fiber in muscle, skin, mucous membrane, or other structure.

end organ, proprioceptor, *n.pl* sensory end organs, located chiefly in the muscles, tendons, and labyrinth, that provide information on the movements and position of the body. Four specific end organs are the muscle spindles; Golgi corpuscles, stimulated by tension; Pacini's corpuscles, stimulated by pressure; and bare nerve endings, stimulated by pain.

end organ, sensory, *n* sensory nerve fibers that end peripherally as either unmyelinated fibers or special structures called receptors. Receptors are situated in the skin, mucous membranes, muscles, tendons, joints, and other structures and also in such special sense organs as those for vision, hearing, smell, and taste. The receptors are organized into a system that relates them to the environment: exteroceptors, interoceptors, and proprioceptors.

end points, *n.pl* **1.** preestablished steps that, when completed, mark the achievement of a treatment goal. *n.pl* **2.** clinical indications that a specific infectious condition has been lessened or eliminated altogether.

end section, *n* the distal portion of a twin-wire labial arch wire, consisting of a tube in which the anterior section of the labial arch is engaged.

end-bulb, *n* See *end-feet.*

end-feet (boutons terminaux, end-bulb), *n.pl* small, terminal enlargements of nerve fibers that are in contact with the dendrites or cell bodies of other nerve cells; the synaptic endings of nerve fibers.

end-plate, *n* the terminal fibers of the motor nerves to the voluntary muscles. The nerve endings lose their myelin sheaths as they enter the sheaths of striated muscle fibers, at which point they ramify across the muscle fiber like the roots of a tree.

end-plate, motor, *n* the end-plate by which impulses from nerves are transmitted to the muscle fibers. It is a modification of the sarcolemma and is continuous with it. The end-plate potential generated by the nerve impulse activates the muscle impulse.

end-to-end bite, *n* See *occlusion, edge-to-edge.*

end-to-end occlusion, *n* See *occlusion, edge-to-edge.*

endemic, *adj* peculiar to a specific location or region, or within a specific group of people.

ending, *n* a termination; the point at which something is concluded.

ending, annulospiral, *n* a nerve ending, associated with an intrafusal muscle fiber, that is stimulated by a stretch impulse resulting from the extension of a muscle. The ending is in the form of a gradual spiral around the length of the intrafusal muscle fiber in the muscle spindle and is connected to the coarse myelinated fibers.

ending, flower spray, *n* a sensory nerve ending that is attached to the distal end of an intrafusal muscle fiber and that is stimulated when the muscle fiber contracts, pulling on the nerve ending.

ending, free nerve, *n* the peripheral terminal of the sensory nerve.

endocarditis and rheumatic fever, *n* a history of rheumatic fever should be a warning sign to the dental professional that the patient may have a risk of infective endocarditis. See *rheumatic heart disease.*

endocarditis, bacterial (en'dō-kar-dī'tis), *n* an inflammation of the heart valves and lining of the heart as a result of a bacterial infection.

endocarditis, infective, *n* bacterial infection of the heart valves. It may occur in normal or compromised valves. An increasing occurrence of the disease has been documented in those with prosthetic valve replacements, known as *prosthetic valve endocarditis (PVE).*

endocarditis, subacute bacterial (SBE), *n* a bacterial infection involving the endocardium that occurs primarily after bacteremia and the establishment of bacterial vegetation on an area of defective endocardium such as is found in patients with rheumatic or congenital heart disease.

endochondral bone, *n* See *bone, endochondral.*

endocrine, *adj* refers to either the gland that secretes directly into the systemic circulation or the substance secreted.

endocrine disease, *n* an abnormal condition caused by some malfunction of an endocrine gland.

endocrine system, *n* the interrelated nature of the physiologic function of endocrine glands.

endocrinology, *n* the study of the anatomy, physiology, biochemistry, and pathology of the endocrine system and the treatment of endocrine problems.

endodontally involved (en'dō-don'təl-ē), *adj* pertaining to disease of the dental pulp and dental periapical tissues.

endodontic implant, *n* a metallic implant extending through the root canal into the periapical bone structure to increase support and retention of the tooth.

endodontic techniques, *n.pl* procedures used in pulpless teeth or teeth that are to be made pulpless.

endodontics (en'dō-don'tiks), *n* the branch of dental practice that applies the knowledge of endodontology.

endodontist (en'dō-don'tist), *n* a dentist who practices endodontics as a specialty.

endodontology (en'dō-don-tol'ō-jē), *n* (endodontia, pulp canal therapy, root canal therapy), the division of dental science that deals with the causes, diagnosis, prevention, and treatment of diseases of the dental pulp and their sequelae.

endogenous (en-doj'ə-nəs), *adj* originating within.

endolith (en'dōlith), See *denticle.*

endometrium, *n* the uterine mucous membrane lining.

endonuclease, *n* an enzyme (nuclease) that cleaves polynucleotides at interior bonds, producing polynucleotide or oligonucleotide fragments.

endophthalmitis, *n* an inflammation of the tissues of the eyeball.

endophytic (en"do-fit'ik), *adj* growing inward or on the inner surface of a structure.

endoplasmic reticulum, *n* an extensive network of membrane-enclosed tubules in the cytoplasm of a cell.

endorphins (en'dor-fins), *n.pl* substances produced in the brain and pituitary gland that reduce pain sensations by binding to receptors in the nervous system. The three endorphins, called alpha-, beta-, and gamma-endorphin, are subsequences of the 91-amino-acid peptide hormone, beta-lipotropin.

endoscopy, *n* the visualization of the interior of organs and cavities of the body with an illuminated, flexible optical tube.

endoscopy, gastrointestinal, n the visualization of the interior of the stomach and intestines with an illuminated, flexible optical tube.

endoscopy, periodontal, n use of a small fiber optic endoscope attached to a specially designed dental instrument, such as an explorer, showing subgingival deposits in a magnified view.

endosteal implants, n.pl See *implants, endosteal.*

endosteum (en-dos′tē-əm), n a thin layer of connective tissue that lines the walls of the bone marrow cavities and haversian canals of compact bone and covers the trabeculae of cancellous bone. Endosteum has both osteogenic and hematopoietic potencies and, like the periosteum, takes an active part in the healing of fractures.

endothelioma (en′dō-thē′lē-ō′mə), n See *tumor, Ewing's.*

endothelium, n the layer of simple squamous epithelial cells that line the heart, the blood and lymph vessels, and the serous cavities of the body.

endotoxin (en′dō-tok′sin), n a non-diffusible lipid polysaccharide-polypeptide complex formed within bacteria (some gram-negative bacilli and others); when released from the destroyed bacterial cells, endotoxin is capable of producing a toxic manifestation within the host.

Endur, n.pr the brand name for a two-paste diacrylate resin adhesive used as a bonding agent in orthodontics.

enema, n a procedure in which a solution is introduced into the rectum for cleansing or therapeutic purposes.

energy, n the capacity for doing work.

energy, atomic, n energy that can be liberated by changes in the nucleus of an atom.

energy binding, n energy represented by the difference in mass between the sum of the component parts and the actual mass of the nucleus of an atom.

energy dependence, n the characteristic response of a radiation detector to a given range of radiation energies or wavelengths as compared with the response of a standard free-air chamber. Emulsions also show energy dependence.

energy excitation, n energy required to change a system from its ground state to an excited state. With each excited state there is associated a different excitation energy. See also *excitation.*

energy ionizing, n the average energy lost by ionizing radiation in producing an ion pair in a gas. (For air, ionizing energy is approximately 33 V.)

energy kinetic, n energy possessed by a mass because of its motion.

energy nuclear, n See *energy, atomic.*

energy photon (hv), n electromagnetic energy in the form of photons, with a value in ergs equal to the product of their frequency in cycles per second and Planck's constant (E-hv).

energy potential, n energy inherent in a mass because of its position with reference to other masses.

energy radiant, n the energy of electromagnetic waves, such as radio waves, visible light, x-rays, and gamma rays.

enflurane, n a nonflammable anesthetic gas belonging to the ether family, used for induction and maintenance of general anesthesia.

engine, dental, n an electric motor that, by means of a continuous-cord drive over pulleys, activates a handpiece that holds a rotary instrument.

engineering, n the organized application of the sciences of mathematics, physics, chemistry, and biology to the solving of problems.

engineering, dental, n the application of physical, mechanical, and mathematical principles to dentistry.

Engman's disease See *dermatitis, infectiosa eczematoides.*

enkephalin, n one of two pain-relieving pentapeptides produced in the body.

enlargement, n an increase in size.

enlargement, Dilantin, n.pr See *hyperplasia, gingival, Dilantin.*

enlargement, idiopathic, n gingival enlargement, of unknown causation, clinically characterized by a firm, rounded thickening of the gingival tissues and histologically characterized by connective tissue hyperplasia of the gingival corium.

enolase (e´no-lās), *n* enzyme characterized by its crystalline structure and role in carbohydrate utilization.

enostosis (en´os-tō´sis), *n* a bony growth located within a bone cavity or centrally from the cortical plate. See also *osteoma.*

enoxacin, *n trade name:* Penetrex; *drug class:* fluoroquinolone antiinfective; *action:* a broad-spectrum bactericidal agent that inhibits the enzyme deoxyritonucleic acid (DNA) gyrase, needed for replication of DNA; *uses:* uncomplicated urethral or cervical gonorrhea, uncomplicated and complicated urinary tract infections.

enrollee, *n* an individual covered by a benefit plan. See also *beneficiary.*

***Entamoeba gingivalis* (en´tə-mē´bə),** *n* a genus of protozoan found in the mouth; repeatedly, but not conclusively, associated with the initiation and perpetuation of periodontitis.

enteral (en´tər-əl), *adj* directly into the gastrointestinal tract; pertains to tube feedings that may be necessary when a patient cannot ingest food orally.

enteric coating (en-ter´ik), *n* See *coating, enteric.*

enteritis, *n* an inflammation of the mucosal lining of the small intestine.

***Enterobacter cloacae,* n.pr** a common species of bacteria found in human and animal feces, dairy products, sewage, soil, and water. It is rarely the cause of disease.

***Enterobacteriaceae,* n.pr** a family of aerobic and anaerobic bacteria that includes both normal and pathogenic enteric microorganisms such as *Escherichia, Klebsiella, Proteus,* and *Salmonella.*

***Enterobius vermicularis* (en˝tər-o´be-əs),** *n* a parasitic worm that resides in the large intestine, more commonly found in children, which may cause pruritis in the anal region. It can be contracted from contact with fomites or by ingesting or inhaling immature forms of the worm. Also called *pinworm.*

enterococcus, *n* any *Streptococcus* bacterium that inhabits the intestinal tract.

entropion (en-trō´pē-on), *n* the inversion, or infolding, of the eyelid margin.

entry, port of, *n* the point on the body through which infectious microorganisms may enter, such as the eyes, nose, respiratory tract, or open wound.

enucleate (e-nōō´klē-āt), *v* to remove a lesion in its entirety.

enunciation, *n* an auxiliary function of teeth, particularly those in the anterior sector of the dental arch; the formation of sounds as in speech.

enuresis (en-yōō-rē´sis), *n* involuntary urination (for example, during general anesthesia, at night).

environment (en-vī´rən-ment, en-vī´urn-ment), *n* the aggregate of all the external conditions and influences affecting the life and development of an organism.

environment, extracellular, *n* the external, or interstitial, environment provided and maintained for the tissue cells.

environment, oral, the aggregate of all oral conditions and influences.

environmental health, *n* the total of various aspects of substances, forces, and conditions in and about a community that affect the health and well-being of the population.

environmental pollutants, *n.pl* substances and conditions, including noise, that adversely affect the health and well-being of the people within a community.

environmental pollution, *n* the presence of substances and conditions that adversely affect the health and well-being of people within a community; usually substances in the air and water supply.

Environmental Protection Agency (EPA), *n.pr* a federal agency charged with the approval and overseeing of the use and disposal of hazardous materials. Workplace management of hazardous materials falls under the jurisdiction of the Occupational Safety and Health Administration (OSHA).

EPA registered, *adj* indicates that an object or substance has been approved by the Environmental Protection Agency.

environmental tobacco smoke (ETS/passive smoke), *n* gaseous by-product of burning tobacco products, including but not limited to commercially manufactured cigarettes and cigars; contains toxic elements harmful to the health of adults and children exposed to it. Also called *second-hand smoke.*

enzyme (en′zīm), *n* a protein substance that acts as a catalyst to speed up metabolic and other processes involving organic materials. Some enzymes function within cells; others function in the extracellular fluids and tissue spaces and organs. They are active in all major tissue functions, such as cellular respiration, muscle contraction, digestive processes, and energy consumption, and are produced intracellularly.

enzyme-linked immunosorbent assay, *n* a species-specific serologic laboratory procedure used to identify microorganisms infecting or inhabiting a tissue or organ system. Its dental use is in the identification of pathogens involved in periodontal disease.

eosin (e′o-sin), *n* one of a pair of dyes used to color tissue samples to augment visibility under a microscope. The dyes are rose-colored, causing the cytoplasm to appear pink.

eosinophil (ē′-ə-sin′ə-fil), *n* See *leukocyte, eosinophilic.*

eosinophilia (ē′-ə-sin′ə-fil′ē-ə), *n* an absolute or relative increase in the normal number of eosinophils in the circulating blood. Various limits are given (for example, absolute eosinophilia if the total number exceeds 500 mm^3) and relative if greater than 3% but total less than 500 mm^3. It may be associated with skin diseases, infestations, hay fever, asthma, angioneurotic edema, adrenocortical insufficiency, and Hodgkin's disease.

eosinophilic granuloma, *n* See *granuloma, eosinophilic.*

EPA, *n.pr* See *Environmental Protection Agency.*

ephebodontics (ə-fe″bo-don′tiks), *n* adolescent dentistry. See also *pedodontics.*

ephedrine sulfate, *n trade name:* generic; *drug class:* adrenergic, mixed direct and indirect effects; *action:* causes increased contractility and heart rate by acting on β-receptors in heart; also acts on α-receptors, causing vasoconstriction in blood vessels; *uses:* shock, increased perfusion, hypotension, bronchodilation.

ephelis (ə-fe′lis), *n* (freckle) a circumscribed macular collection of pigment in the epidermis or oral mucosa. An increased amount of melanin pigment is seen in the region of the basal layer of cells.

epicanthic fold, *n* a characteristic crease in the eyelid; seen in persons with Down syndrome.

epidemic, *adj* spreading rapidly and widely among many individuals in a single location or region; illnesses labeled epidemic are those that occur beyond normal expectations and are usually traceable to a single source.

epidemiologic survey, *n* See *research, epidemiologic survey.*

epidemiology (ep′i-dē′mē-ol′ə-jē), *n* the science of epidemics and epidemic diseases, which involve the total population rather than the individual. The aim of epidemiology is to determine those factors in the group environment that make the group more or less susceptible to disease.

epidemiology, indices in, *n.pl* data collection tools that aid in the measurement and evaluation of disease indicators and conditions; classification systems featuring numbered scales against which a specific population may be compared.

epidermal cyst, *n* a common, benign, variable, subcutaneous swelling lined by keratinizing epithelium and filled with a cheesy material composed of sebum and epithelial debris.

epidermis, *n* the superficial, avascular layers of the skin.

epidermolysis bullosa (ep′i-dur-mol′i-sis), *n* a disease of the skin characterized by bullae, vesicles, cysts, and, often, associated mandibular enlargement. See also *syndrome, Goldscheider's* and *syndrome, Weber-Cockayne.*

Epidermolysis bullosa. (Regezi/Sciubba/Jordan, 2003)

epiglottis (ep′i-glot′is), *n* an elastic cartilage, covered by mucous membrane, that forms the superior part of the larynx and guards the glottis during swallowing.

epilepsy (ep′i-lep′sē), *n* a group of neurologic disorders characterized by recurrent episodes of convulsive seizures, sensory disturbances, abnormal behavior, and loss of consciousness. Most epilepsy is of an unknown cause but may be associated with cerebral trauma, brain tumors, vascular disturbances, or chemical imbalance. Drugs used in the treatment of symptoms (for example, hydantoin sodium, diphenylhydantoin sodium) promote gingival hyperplasia.

epiloia (ep-i-loi′-ə), *n* See *syndrome, Bourneville Pringle.*

epinephrine (ep′i-nef′rin), *n* a hormone secreted by the adrenal medulla that stimulates hepatic glycogenolysis, causing an elevation in the blood sugar, vasodilation of blood vessels of the skeletal muscles, vasoconstriction of the arterioles of the skin and mucous membranes, relaxation of bronchiolar smooth muscles, and stimulation of heart action. Used in local anesthetics for its vasoconstrictive action.

epinephrine/epinephrine bitartrate/ epinephrine HCl, n trade names. EpiPen Jr., Bronkaid Mist, Primatene Mist; *drug class:* adrenergic agonist, catecholamine; *action:* β1- and β2- agonist, causing increased levels of cAMP, producing bronchodilation and cardiac stimulation; *uses:* acute asthmatic attacks, hemostasis, bronchospasm, anaphylaxis, allergic reactions, cardiac arrest, vasopressor.

epiphysis (e-pif′i-sis), *n* the terminal portion of a long bone. The epiphysis is separated from the diaphysis during growth by a cartilaginous zone that serves as a growth center. Once ossification unites the epiphysis with the diaphysis, growth is completed.

epispinal (ep-i-spī′nəl), *adj* located on the spinal column.

epistaxis (ep′is-tak′sis), *n* (nosebleed) bleeding from the nose.

epithelial (ep′i-thē′lē-əl), *adj* pertaining to the epithelium.

epithelial attachment, n See *attachment, epithelial.*

epithelial cells, n.pl form the epithelial tissue that lines both the inner and outer surfaces of the body; serve a protective function and also aid in absorption and secretion.

epithelial cuff, attached, n the attachment of the gingival epithelium to the enamel, including the close approximation of the free gingiva to the tooth.

epithelial cuff, implant, n the band of tissue that is constricted around an implant abutment post.

epithelial desquamation, anesthetic, n the shedding of oral epithelial tissue that occurs as the result of prolonged exposure to topical anesthesia.

epithelial inclusion, n bits of epithelial tissue introduced into bone crypts during perforation osteotomies. See also *osteotomy, perforation.*

epithelioma (ep′i-thē′lē-ō′mə), *n* an epithelial cancer.

epithelioma adenoides cysticum, n (*Brooke's tumor, trichoepithelioma*) a form of basal cell carcinoma believed to arise from the epithelium of hair follicles. Regarded as a less invasive form of basal cell carcinoma.

epithelioma, basal cell, n See *carcinoma, basal cell.*

epithelium (ep′i-thē′lē-əm), *n* the structural arrangement of the various cellular components of epithelium, characterized by two basic forms: medium suprapapillary width with medium-length rete pegs, and narrow suprapapillary width with long rete pegs.

epithelium, basement membrane of, n See *membrane, basement.*

epithelium, desmosomes of, n an electronmicroscopic finding of intercellular bridges that serve to attach adjacent epithelial cells to each other.

epithelium, enamel, inner, n the innermost layer of cells (ameloblasts) of the enamel organ that deposit the organic matrix of the enamel on the crown of the developing tooth. Also the innermost layer of Hertwig's epithelial root sheath.

epithelium, enamel, outer, n the outermost layer of cells of the enamel organ. It is separated from the inner enamel epithelium in the area of the developing crown by the stratum intermedium and stellate reticulum and lies immediately adja-

E

cent to the inner enamel epithelium in the area of the developing root.

epithelium, enamel, reduced, n combined enamel epithelium; the remains of the enamel organ after enamel formation is complete. After eruption of the tip of the crown, that part of the combined epithelium remaining on the enamel surface is called the *epithelial attachment.*

epithelium, gingival, n a stratified squamous epithelium consisting of a basal layer; it is keratinized or parakeratinized when comprising the attached gingiva.

epithelium, hyperplastic, n an increase in thickness, with alterations in structure, produced by proliferation of cellular elements of epithelium. The stratum spinosum epidermidis is usually the layer of cells that become thickened, resulting in acanthosis.

epithelium, oral, n the epithelial covering of the oral mucous membranes. Composed of stratified squamous epithelium of varying thickness and varying degrees of keratinization.

epithelium, pocket, n the epithelium that lines the gingival or periodontal pocket. Its most prominent characteristics are the presence of hyperplasia and ulceration, with exposure to the corium of the gingiva.

epithelium, squamous, n epithelium consisting of flat, scalelike cells.

epithelium, stratified squamous, n the variety of epithelium prevalent as the covering of the oral mucous membrane and of dermal surfaces; composed of layers of cells oriented parallel to the surface. The various layers of cells in order of ascent from basement membrane to surface are stratum germinativum, stratum spongiosum, stratum granulosum, stratum lucidum (in dermal epithelium), and stratum corneum. The gingival epithelium generally exhibits some degree of keratinization, variable from parakeratosis to hyperkeratosis.

epithelium, sulcal, n the stratified squamous epithelium forming the covering of the soft tissue wall of the gingival sulcus, or crevice. Extends from the gingival margin to the line of attachment of the epithelium to the tooth surface.

epithelization (ep′i-thē′li-zā′shən), *n* the natural act of healing by secondary intention; the proliferation of new epithelium into an area devoid of it but that naturally is covered by it.

epizootic fever, *n* another name for foot and mouth disease in clovenfoot animals; also known as aphthous fever; caused by a type of coxsackievirus, uncommon in the United States. The disease in man is characterized by malaise, fever, headache, itchy skin, and a sensation of dry mouth despite heavy salivation. Vesicles appear in the mouth, around the lips, and on the hands and feet. Vesicles and ulcers of the mouth disappear within approximately 10 days.

epoxy resin (ē-pok′sē, ə-pok′sē), *n* See *resin, epoxy.*

Epstein's pearls, *n.pr* See *nodules, Bohn's.*

Epstein-Barr virus, *n.pr* a herpesvirus associated with Burkitt's lymphoma and reported in cases of infectious mononucleosis; more recently reported associated with acquired immune deficiency syndrome.

epulis (e-pyōō′lis), *n* a tumor (tumescence) of the gingiva.

epulis, congenital of newborn, n a raised or pedunculated lesion located on the anterior gingivae of the newborn. It is histologically similar to granular cell myoblastoma. See also *myoblastoma, granular cell.*

epulis fissuratum, n a curtainlike fold of excess tissue associated with the flange of a denture *(inflammatory fibrous hyperplasia, redundant tissue).*

Epulis fissuratum. (Neville/Damm/Allen/Bouquot, 2002)

epulis, giant cell, n See *granuloma, giant cell reparative, peripheral.*

epulis granulomatosa, n a tumorlike mass of red, easily bleeding, infected granulation tissue that occurs as a result of exuberant reparative phenomena. Seen arising from tooth sockets or is associated with exfoliating necrotic bone.

equal protection, *n* clause set out in the Fourteenth Amendment of the Constitution that dictates that state governments cannot pass or enforce any laws based solely on a specific classification of person by race, gender, religion, ethnicity, or age.

equilibration (ē-kwil'i-brā'shən), *n* the act of placing a body in a state of equilibrium.

equilibration diagnostic, n See *diagnostic equilibration.*

equilibration, mandibular, n the act or acts performed to place the mandible in a state of equilibrium.

equilibration, occlusal, n the modification of occlusal forms of teeth by grinding, with the intent of equalizing occlusal stress and of harmonizing cuspal relations in function.

equilibration of mounted casts, n equilibration of the occlusion of mounted casts made of a patient for the purpose of observing and recording what must be done to adjust the natural occlusion.

equilibrator (ē-kwil'i-brā-tur), *n* an instrument or device used in achieving or maintaining a state of equilibrium.

equilibrium (ē'kwil-ib'rē-əm), *n* a state of balance between two opposing forces or processes.

equilibrium, functional, n the state of homeostasis within the oral cavity existing when biologic processes and local environmental factors, including the forces of mastication, are in a state of balance.

equipment, *n* the nonexpendable items used by the dentist in the performance of professional duties.

equity, *n* a free and reasonable claim or right; fairness; impartiality. The money value of a property or of an interest in a property in excess of claims or liens against it; a risk interest or ownership right in property.

equivalent, *n* equal in force, value, measure, or effect; corresponding in function.

equivalent, aluminum, n the thickness of pure aluminum affording the same radiation attenuation, under specified conditions, as the material or materials being considered.

equivalent, concrete, n the thickness of concrete having a density of 2.35 g/cm³ that would afford the same radiation attenuation, under specified conditions, as the material or materials being considered.

equivalent, lead, n the thickness of pure lead that would afford the same radiation attenuation, under specified conditions, as the material or materials being considered.

erbium, *n* a rare earth, metallic element with an atomic number of 68 and an atomic weight of 167.26.

erg, *n* a unit of energy equal to the energy consumed by 1 dyne acting through 1 cm, which is equal to 10^{-7} joule.

ergoloid mesylate, *n trade names:* Hydergine LC, Gerimal; *drug class:* ergot alkaloids; *action:* may increase cerebral metabolism and blood flow; *uses:* senile dementia, Alzheimer's dementia, primary progressive dementia.

ergonomics, *n* the field of science including all aspects pertaining to a comparison of the mental and physical exhaustion produced to the quantity and quality of the deliverable care.

ergotamine tartrate, *n trade names:* Ergomar, Ergostat; *drug class:* α-adrenergic blocker; *action:* constricts by direct action vascular smooth muscle in peripheral and cranial blood vessels, relaxes uterine muscle; *uses:* vascular headache (migraine or histamine), cluster headache.

ergotoxine (ur'gō-tox'in), *n* a potent alkaloid that paralyzes the motor and secretory nerves of the sympathetic system but has no effect on the inhibitory or parasympathetic nerves.

ERISA, *n.pr* the acronym for the **Employee Retirement Income Security Act of 1974.** See also *Employee Retirement Income Security Act.*

erosion (ē-rō'zhən), *n* the chemical or mechanicochemical destruction of tooth substance, the mechanism of which is incompletely known, which leads to the creation of concavities of many shapes at the cementoenamel junction of teeth. The surface of the cavity, unlike dental caries, is hard and smooth.

Erosion. (Sapp/Eversole/Wysocki, 2004)

error, *n* a violation of duty; a fault; a mistake in the proceedings of a court in matters of law or of fact.

error, legal, *n* a mistaken judgment or incorrect belief as to the existence or effect of matters of fact, or a false or mistaken conception or application of the law.

error, numerical, *n* the amount of loss or precision in a quantity; the difference between an accurate quantity and its calculated approximation. Errors occur in numerical methods; mistakes occur in programming, coding, data transcription, and operating; malfunctions occur in computers and are caused by physical limitations of the properties of materials.

error of measurement, *n* the deviation of an individual score or observation from its true value, caused by the unreliability of the instrument and the individual who is measuring.

error, sampling, *n* any mistake in drawing a sample that keeps it from being unrepresentative; selection procedures that are biased; error introduced when a group is described on the basis of an unrepresentative sample.

error, variance, *n* that part of the total variance caused by anything irrelevant to a study that cannot be experimentally controlled.

eruption (ē-rup′shən), *n* the migration of a tooth from within its follicle in the alveolar process of the maxilla or mandible into the oral cavity.

eruption, continuous, *n* the normal occlusal progression of teeth noted throughout a lifetime.

eruption cyst, *n* a dentigerous cyst that causes a clinically evident bulging of the overlying alveolar ridge. See also *cysts, eruption.*

eruption, ectopic, *n* the abnormal direction of tooth eruption, most common to mandibular first and third molars, which sometimes leads to abnormal resorption of the adjacent tooth.

eruption hematoma, *n* an eruption cyst that is blood-filled, visualized as a bluish purple area of elevated tissue of the overlying alveolar ridge.

eruption, passive, *n* an increasing length of the clinical crown often seen with aging and in the absence of clinical evidence of inflammation. The stages of passive eruption are as follows: (1) the most apical limit of the epithelial attachment is at the cementoenamel junction; (2) the most apical limit of the attachment is on the cementum, with the base of the gingival sulcus still on the enamel surface; (3) the most apical limit of the epithelial attachment is on the cementum, with the base of the sulcus at the cementoenamel junction; and (4) both the base of the sulcus and the epithelial attachment are on the surface of the cementum.

eruption, surgical, *n* the surgical removal of tissues covering an abnormally unerupted tooth to allow its natural progress into position.

eruptive gingivitis, *n* See *gingivitis, eruptive.*

erysipelas, *n* an infectious skin disease characterized by redness, swelling, vesicles, bullae, fever, pain, and lymphadenopathy. It is caused by a species of group A β-hemolytic streptococci.

Erysipelothrix (er″ə-sip′ə-lo-thriks″), *n* gram-positive bacterium that does not produce spores and has cell walls.

erythema (er′i-thē′mə), *n* a patchy, circumscribed, or marginated macular redness of the skin or mucous membranes caused by hyperemia or inflammation.

erythema multiforme complex, *n* an acute, inflammatory dermatologic disease of uncertain cause (although occasionally related to drug administration), characterized by erythematous macules, papules, vesicles, and bullae that appear on the skin and not infrequently on the oral mucosa. See also *syndrome, Stevens-Johnson.*

Erythema multiforme. (Daniel/Harfst, 2002)

erythredema polyneuropathy (ər-ith′re-dē′mə pol′ē-nyōōr-op′ə-thē), *n* (acrodynia, Feer's disease, pink disease, Selter's disease, Swift's disease) a disease of infancy believed to be caused by mercury poisoning. It is manifested by itching of the hands and feet, profuse sweating, hypertension, vasomotor disturbances, bruxism, and precocious shedding of the teeth.

erythremia (er′ith-rē′mē-ə), *n* (Osler's disease, polycythemia rubra, polycythemia vera, primary polycythemia, Vaquez' disease) a myeloproliferative disease characterized by a marked increase in the circulating red blood cell mass. Erythremia may represent a neoplastic growth of erythropoietic tissue. Neutrophilia, thrombocytopenia, and splenomegaly are common. Manifestations include plethora, vertigo, headache, and thrombosis.

erythrityl tetranitrate, *n trade name:* Cardilate; *drug class:* organic nitrate; *action:* causes relaxation of vascular smooth muscle; decreases preload/afterload, which is responsible for decreasing left ventricular end diastolic pressure; systemic vascular resistance; improved exercise tolerance; *uses:* chronic stable angina pectoris, prophylaxis of angina pain.

erythroblastosis fetalis (ər-ith′rō-blas-tō′sis fē-tal′is), *n* an excessive destruction of red blood cells begun before or shortly after birth. It may be caused by an Rh factor reaction. The skin is yellow, and the teeth may be markedly discolored.

Erythrocin, *n.pr* the brand name for erythromycin.

erythrocyte (ər-ith′rō-sīt), *n* red blood cell; a nonnucleated, circular, biconcave, discoid, hemoglobin-containing, oxygen-carrying formed element circulating in the blood.
erythrocyte count, *n* the number of red blood cells per cubic millimeter of blood.
erythrocyte indices, *n.pr* the standard values of red blood cell numbers, morphologic characteristics, and behavior in comprehensive hematologic laboratory testing.
erythrocyte sedimentation rate (ESR), *n* the rate at which red blood cells settle in a pipette of unclotted blood, measured in millimeters per hour. It is used as an index of inflammation.

erythrocytosis (ər-ith′rō-sī-tō′sis), *n* (secondary polycythemia) an increased circulating red blood cell mass resulting from compensatory effort to meet reduced oxygen content. May be seen in persons living at high altitudes, as well as in persons with emphysema, pulmonary insufficiency, and heart failure.

erythromycin, *n* an antibiotic produced by a strain of *Streptomyces erythroeus,* only slightly effective against β-hemolytic streptococci (viridans group), and upper and lower respiratory tract, skin, and soft tissue infections of mild to moderate severity. It is no longer recommended by the American Heart Association and the American Dental Association for treatment of bacterial endocarditis in patients hypersensitive to penicillin.
erythromycin base (et al.), *n trade names:* E-mycin, Ery-Tab (et al.); *drug class:* macrolide antibiotic; *action:* binds to 50S ribosomal subunits of susceptible bacteria and suppresses protein synthesis; *uses:* infections caused by *Neisseria gonorrhoeae;* mild-to-moderate respiratory tract, skin, soft tissue infections caused by *Streptococcus pneumoniae, Corynebacterium diphtheriae, Bordetella pertussis;* syphilis; Legionnaire's disease; *Haemophilus influenzae;* endocarditis prophylaxis.

erythroplakia (ə-rith″ro-pla′ke-ə), *n* a distinct disease of the oral mucosa distinguished by red patchy lesions.

E

Erythroplakia. (Regezi/Sciubba/Jordan, 2003)

erythroplasia of Queyrat (ər-ith'rō-plā'zhə əv kə-rat', kā-rĭ'), *n.pr* a form of intraepithelial carcinoma. The oral lesions are usually seen as plaques with a bright, velvety surface.

erythropoiesis, *n* the process in which red blood cells are formed.

erythrosin (ə-rith'ro-sēn), *n* a red dye used to reveal plaque deposits on teeth; administered in both tablet and liquid form.

escharotic (es'kĭr-ot'ik), *n* a caustic or corrosive agent that has the strength to burn tissue.

Escherichia coli, *n.pr* a species of coliform bacteria normally present in the intestines and common in water, milk, and soil.

esculin, *n* a glucoside from horsechestnut bark; used as a sunburn protective.

esophageal atresia, *n* an abnormal esophagus that ends in a blind pouch or narrows to a thin cord and thus fails to provide a continuous passage to the stomach. It is usually a congenital anomaly.

esophageal stenosis, *n* a narrowing or restriction of the lumen of the esophagus that slows or impedes the passage of fluid and foods from the mouth to the stomach.

esophagitis, *n* an inflammation of the mucosal lining of the esophagus caused by infection or irritation of the mucosa by reflux of gastric juice from the stomach.

esophagus, *n* the muscular canal, about 25 cm long, extending from the pharynx to the stomach.

essence (es'ens), *n* an alcoholic solution of an essential oil.

essential oil, *n* See *oil, essential.*

essentials oils mouthrinses, *n.pl* mouthwashes made from thymol, menthol, eucalyptol, and methylsalicylate in combination with alcohol that are available over the counter for use in controlling plaque and gingivitis. See also *mouthwash.*

estate, *n* one's interest in land or other property.

estate planning, *n* a detailed, written-out plan (usually arrived at with the advice of estate counselors) in which all the financial affairs of the dentist are clearly stated and provisions are made for alterations when changing conditions warrant it.

estazolam, *n trade name:* ProSom; *drug class:* benzodiazepine, sedative-hypnotic, Controlled Substance Schedule IV in United States; *action:* produces central nervous system depression by interaction with benzodiazepine receptor; *use:* insomnia.

ester (es'tur), *n* any compound formed from alcohol and an acid.

ester linkage, *n* the bonding between fatty acids and glycerol that characterizes true fats.

esterase (es'tər-ās), *n* an enzyme that catalyzes the hydrolysis of an ester into its alcohol and acid.

esterified estrogens, *n.pl trade names:* Estabs, Estratab, Menest; *drug class:* synthetic estrogen; *action:* required for development, maintenance, and adequate function of female reproductive system by increasing synthesis of deoxyribonucleic acid, ribonucleic acid, and selected proteins; decreases release of gonadotropine-releasing hormone; inhibits ovulation and helps maintain bone structure; *uses:* menopause, breast cancer, prostatic cancer, hypogonadism, ovariectomy, primary ovarian failure.

esthetics (es-thet'iks), *n* (aesthetics) the branch of philosophy dealing with beauty, especially with the components thereof; that is, color and form.

esthetics, dentistry, *n* refers to those skills and techniques used to improve the art and symmetry of the teeth and face to improve the appearance as well as the function of the teeth, mouth, and face.

esthetics, denture, *n* the cosmetic effect, produced by a denture, that affects the desirable beauty, charm, character, and dignity of the individual.

esthetics, denture base, *n* the esthetically proper tinting, contouring, and festooning of the gingival tissue portion of a denture base.

esthetics, gingival tissue (gingival tissue esthetics), n See *esthetics, denture base.*

estimate, n the anticipated fee for dental services to be performed.

estimated average requirement (E.A.R.), n the accepted standard level of nutrients that an average person requires. The basis for the Recommended Daily Allowance is established by the U.S. government.

estoppel (es-top'əl), n a preclusion, in law, that prevents a person from alleging or denying a fact because of his or her own previous act or allegation.

estradiol benzoate (es'trə-dī'ōl ben'zō-āt), n a topical steroid (β-estradiol-3-benzoate) with estrogenic activity, useful in the treatment of lesions produced by diminution of bodily production of estrogens. Experimental administration to aged laboratory mice has resulted in an increased downgrowth of epithelial attachment along the root surface of teeth and subsequent production of periodontal disease.

estradiol/estradiol cypionate/estradiol valerate, n *trade names:* Deladiol, Depogen, Estro-Cyp, Estra-LA; *drug class:* estrogen; *action:* increases synthesis of deoxyribonucleic acid, ribonucleic acid, and selected proteins, decreases release of gonadotropin-releasing hormone, inhibits ovulation, and helps maintain bone structure; *uses:* menopause, prostatic cancer, atrophic vaginitis, kraurosis vulvae, hypogonadism, ovariectomy, primary ovarian failure.

estradiol transdermal system, n *trade names:* Estraderm, Climera; *drug class:* estrogen; *action:* increases synthesis of deoxyribonucleic acid, ribonucleic acid, and selected proteins; decreases release of gonadotropin-releasing hormone; inhibits ovulation and helps maintain bone structure; *uses:* menopause, prostatic cancer, abnormal uterine bleeding, hypogonadism, ovariectomy, osteoporosis.

estrin (es'trin), n the generic term for the ovarian estrogens estriol, estrone, and estradiol.

estrogens (es'trō-jenz), n.pl the collective term for substances capable of producing estrus. The term also applies to the estrogenic hormones in

women. Estriol is the principal estrogen found in the urine of pregnant women and in the placenta. Synthetic estrogens include diethylstilbestrol, hexestrol, and ethinyl estradiol.

etch, acid, v See *acid etching.*

etching, n a process used to decalcify the superficial layers of enamel as a step in the application of sealants or bonding agents in preventive dentistry and orthodontics. The agent of choice is phosphoric acid in concentrations of 30% to 40%.

ethacrynate sodium/ethacrynic acid, n *trade name:* Edecrin Sodium; *drug class:* loop diuretic; *action:* acts on loop of Henle by increasing excretion of chloride, sodium; *uses:* pulmonary edema, edema in congestive heart failure, liver disease, nephrotic syndrome, ascites, hypertension.

ethambutal HCl, n *trade name:* Myambutol; *drug class:* antitubercular; *action:* inhibits ribonucleic acid synthesis, decreases tubercle bacilli replication; *uses:* pulmonary tuberculosis, as adjunct.

ethane, n a constituent of natural and "bottled" gases.

ether, diethyl (e'thər, dī-eth'il), n (ethyl ether, ether [C_2H_5]2O) a volatile ether used as an anesthetic that causes excellent muscle relaxation with minimal effect on blood pressure, pulse rate, and respiration. It is irritating to the respiratory passages and produces nausea.

ether, divinyl (e'thər, dīv-ī'nəl), n (divinyl oxide [CH_2:CH]2O) a highly volatile, unsaturated ether that is a rapid-acting anesthetic without the aftereffect of nausea produced by diethyl ether.

etherization (e'ther-i-zā'shən), n administration of ether to produce anesthesia.

ethics (eth'iks), n **1.** the science of moral obligation; a system of moral principles, quality, or practice. n **2.** the moral obligation to render to the patient the best possible quality of dental service and to maintain an honest relationship with other members of the profession and mankind in general.

ethics, dental, n See *ethics, professional.*

ethics, professional, n the principles and norms of proper professional conduct concerning the rights and duties of health professionals themselves and their conduct toward patients and fellow practitioners, including the actions taken in the care of patients and family members.

ethinyl estradiol, *n trade names:* Estinyl; *drug class:* nonsteroidal synthetic estrogen; *action:* affects release of pituitary gonadotropins, inhibits ovulation, promotes adequate calcium use in bone structure; *uses:* menopause, prostatic cancer, breast cancer, postmenopausal osteoporosis.

ethionamide, *n trade name:* Trecator-SC; *drug class:* antitubercular; *action:* bacteriostatic against Mycobacterium tuberculosis; may inhibit protein synthesis; *uses:* pulmonary, extrapulmonary tuberculosis when other antitubercular drugs have failed.

ethnic group, *n* a population of individuals organized around an assumption of common cultural origin.

ethosuximide, *n trade name:* Zarontin; *drug class:* anticonvulsant; *action:* suppresses spike wave formation in absence seizures (petit mal); decreases amplitude, frequency, duration, spread of discharge in minor motor seizures; *uses:* absence seizures (PM).

ethotoin, *n* trade name: Peganone; drug class: hydantoin derivative anticonvulsant; action: inhibits spread of seizure activity in motor cortex; uses: generalized tonic-clonic or complex-partial seizures.

ethyl acetate, abuse of (eth′əl as′ə-tāt), *n* recreational, often compulsive inhaling of the fumes of a liquid solvent, especially those found in paint thinners.

ethyl aminobenzoate (eth′əl ə-me″no-ben′zo-āt), *n* an ester-type anesthetic agent formulated for surface application as a liquid, gel, ointment, or spray; the most widely used topical numbing agent.

ethyl chloride (eth′il klôr′īd), *n* (C_2H_5Cl) a colorless liquid that boils between 12° and 13° C. It acts as a local, topical anesthetic of short duration through the superficial freezing produced by its rapid vaporization from the skin. Ethyl chloride is used occasionally in inhalation therapy as a rapid, fleeting general anesthetic, comparable to nitrous oxide but somewhat more dangerous.

ethylene (eth′il-ēn), *n* (olefiant gas, CH_2CH_2) a colorless gas of slightly sweet odor and taste; used as an inhalation anesthetic.

ethylene oxide sterilization, *n* a process that uses gas to sterilize instruments, equipment, and materials that would otherwise be damaged by heat or liquid chemicals. Effective at room temperature. Requires between 10 and 16 hours to be effective. Gas must penetrate the material. The gas is highly toxic and must be vented before opening the sealed sterilizing unit. Sterilized materials must also be well aerated before using.

etidocaine HCl (local), *n trade names:* Duranest, Duranest MPF; *drug class:* amide, local anesthetic; *action:* inhibits ion fluxes across membranes, particularly sodium transport across cell membrane; decreases rise of depolarization phase of action potential; blocks nerve action potential; *uses:* local dental anesthetic, peripheral nerve block, caudal anesthetic, central neural block, vaginal block.

etidronate disodium, *n trade name:* Didronel IV; *drug class:* antihypercalcemic; *action:* decreases bone resorption and new bone development (accretion); *uses:* Paget's disease, heterotopic ossification, hypercalcemia of malignancy.

etiology (ē′tē-ol′ə-jē), *n* **1.** causative factors. *n* **2.** the factors implicated in the causation of disease. *n* **3.** the study of the factors causing disease.

etiology, local factors, the environmental influences that may be implicated in the causation or perpetuation of a disease process.

etiology, systemic factors, *n* generalized biologic factors that are implicated in the causation, modification, or perpetuation of a disease entity. Within the oral cavity, the actions of the systemic factors are modified by interaction with local factors.

etodolac, *n trade name:* Lodine; *drug class:* nonsteroidal antiinflammatory; *action:* inhibits prostaglandin synthesis by interfering with cyclooxygenase, which is needed for biosynthesis; *uses:* mild-to-moderate pain, osteoarthritis.

Eubacterium, *n.pr* a genus of anaerobic, non-spore-forming, nonmotile bacteria containing straight or curved gram-positive rods that usually occur singly, in pairs, or in short chains. They usually metabolize carbohydrates and may be pathogenic.

eugenol (yōō´jən-ol), n **1.** an allyl guaiacol obtainable from oil of cloves. Used with zinc oxide in a paste for temporary restorations, bases under restorations, and impression materials. Believed to have a palliative effect on dental pulp and possibly a limited germicidal effect. n **2.** a colorless or pale yellow liquid obtained from clove oil; has a clove odor and pungent, spicy taste. Used as the liquid portion of zinc oxide and eugenol cements and in toothache medications.

eugnathia (yōō-nā´thē-ə), n the normal or proper relationship of the jaws to each other.

euphoria (yōō-fôr´ē-ə), n a sense of well-being or normalcy. Pleasantly mild excitement.

euphoric (yōō-fôr´ik), n a substance that produces an exaggerated sense of well being.

eupnea (yōōp-nē´-ə), n easy or normal respiration.

europium, n a rare earth metallic element with an atomic number of 63 and an atomic weight of 151.96.

eustachian tube, n a tube, lined with mucous membrane, that joins the nasopharynx and the middle ear cavity, allowing equalization of the air pressure in the middle ear with atmospheric pressure. Also called the *auditory tube.*

Eutectic Mixture of Local Anesthetics (EMLA) (u-tek´tik), n a topical anesthetic made from equal parts of lidocaine and prilocaine that is applied as a cream on unbroken skin, then covered with an occlusive dressing, to kill pain prior to venipuncture, intramuscular injections, intravenous cannulation, or minor skin procedures. See lidocaine HCl (topical), prilocaine hydrochloride.

euthanasia, n deliberately bringing about the death of a person who is suffering from an incurable disease or condition; also called *mercy killing.* Active euthanasia is illegal in most jurisdictions; passive euthanasia, or the withholding of some life support systems, has legal standing in some jurisdictions.

euthyroidism (yōō-thī´roid-īz-əm), n a state of normal thyroid function.

evacuation system, n a centralized vacuum system connected to each dental operating unit, used to keep the oral cavity clear of water, saliva, blood, and debris, generally operating at a high volume, high velocity, and low pressure.

evaluation, n to make a judgment or appraisal of a condition or situation. In dentistry, used to describe the clinical judgment of a patient's dental health or an appraisal of staff performance.

evaluation studies, n.pl the control study of the comparative value of different treatment modalities or medications.

Evans blue, n.pr a diazo dye used for the determination of the blood volume on the basis of the dilution of a standard solution of the dye in the plasma after its intravenous injection.

evidence, n proof presented at a trial by the parties through witnesses, records, documents, and concrete objects for the purpose of inducing the court or jury to believe their contentions.

evidence, radiographic, n the shadow images depicted in radiographs.

evidence-based care, n a philosophy of treatment that relies on up-to-date, germane research as its foundation.

Evipal (ē´vi-pil), n.pr the trade name for **hexobarbital,** a rapid-acting barbiturate.

Evipal sodium, n the trade name for **hexobarbital sodium.** An ultrashort-acting barbiturate of the N-methyl type whose pharmacologic actions, from a clinical standpoint, are essentially similar to thiopental (Pentothal).

evoked potential, n an electrical response in the brainstem or cerebral cortex that is elicited by a specific stimulus. This property of the brain may be used to monitor brain function during surgery.

evulsed tooth, n See *tooth, evulsed.*

(avulsion), n the sudden tearing out, or away, of tissue as a result of a traumatic episode.

evulsion, nerve, n the operation of tearing a nerve from its central origin by traction.

evulsion, tooth, n the displacement of a tooth from its alveolar housing; may be partial or complete.

E

Ewing's sarcoma, *n.pr* See *tumor, Ewing's.*

Ewing's tumor, *n.pr* See *tumor, Ewing's.*

examination, *n* **1.** inspection; search; investigation; inquiry; scrutiny; testing. *n* **2.** inspection or investigation of part or all of the body to measure and evaluate the state of health or disease. The examination may include visual inspection, percussion, palpation, auscultation, and measurement of mobility as well as various laboratory and radiographic procedures.

examination, anteroposterior extraoral radiographic, n an examination in which the film is placed at the posterior direction with the rays passing from the anterior to the posterior direction to record images.

examination, bite-wing intraoral radiographic, n radiography in which an intraoral radiograph records on a single film the shadow images of the outline, position, and mesiodistal extent of the crowns, necks, and coronal third of the roots of both the maxillary and mandibular teeth and alveolar crests.

examination, body section extraoral radiographic, n (tomogram), a radiographic procedure of various internal layers of the head and body accomplished by the synchronized movement of the roentgen-ray tube and film in parallel planes but in opposite directions from each other. Also known as *tomography, laminagraphy, planigraphy,* and *stratigraphy.*

examination, bregmamentum extraoral radiographic, n radiography in which the film is placed beneath the chin, with the rays directed downward through the junction of the coronal and sagittal sutures (bregma) to the chin (mentum).

examination, cephalometric extraoral radiographic, n See *cephalometric radiography.*

examination, clinical, n **1.** the visual and tactile scrutiny of the tissues of and surrounding the oral cavity. *n* **2.** The formal testing of the dental hygienist student to determine whether his or her skills meet or exceed established standards.

examination, complete, n a methodical, complete assessment of an individual involving basic and supplementary procedures as well as evaluation of the plan for preventive care.

examination, extradental intraoral radiographic, n an examination in which the film is placed between the teeth and the tissue of the cheek or lip for the exploration or localization of the internal structures of these tissues.

examination, extraoral radiographic, n an examination of the oral and paraoral structures by exposing films placed extraorally, in contrast to intraorally.

examination, gingival, n the observation of the primary visual symptoms of periodontal disease, including color changes; changes in surface texture; deviations from normal contour and structure, tissue tone, and vitality; presence or absence of clefts; and the position of attachment.

examination, intraoral, n an examination of all the structures contained within the oral cavity.

examination, intraoral radiographic, n the examination of the oral and paraoral structures by exposing films placed within the oral cavity.

examination, lateral facial extraoral radiographic, n an examination by means of a lateral head film.

examination, lateral head extraoral radiographic, n an examination in which the film is placed parallel to the sagittal plane of the head.

examination, lateral jaw extraoral radiographic, n an examination in which the film is placed adjacent to the mandible.

examination, limited, n an assessment typically conducted during an emergency situation for the management of a critical medical condition.

examination, mental extraoral radiographic, n an examination in which the film is placed beneath the chin, and the radiation is directed through the long axis of the lower central incisors while the mouth is open.

examination, oblique occlusal intraoral radiographic, n an exploratory examination of the maxillae or mandible using an occlusal type of film placed between the teeth. The rays are directed obliquely downward or upward (usually 60 degrees to 75 degrees in the vertical plane) and parallel to the sagittal plane.

examination, panoramic extraoral radiographic, n curved, single-film radiography in which the beam source and film rotate in a synchronized manner about the head, exposing oral structures sequentially with simultaneous exposure of corresponding areas of the film.

examination, periapical intraoral radiographic, n the basic intraoral examination, showing all of a tooth and the surrounding periodontium.

examination, posteroanterior extraoral radiographic, n an examination in which the film is placed anteriorly, with the rays passing from the posterior to the anterior direction.

examination, profile extraoral radiographic, n a lateral head examination to show the profile of bone and soft tissue outline. It uses a decrease in milliampere seconds or an increase in target-film distance for recording the soft tissue image.

examination, radiographic, n 1. the production of the number of radiographs necessary for the radiologic interpretation of the part or parts in question. n 2. the study and interpretation of radiographs of the mouth and associated structures.

examination, stereoscopic extraoral radiographic, n a radiographic examination used in conjunction with a stereoscope for localization. Exposures of two films are made, with identical placement of each film adjacent to the part in question and with a different angulation for each exposure.

examination, temporomandibular extraoral radiographic, n an examination in which the film is placed adjacent to the area to be examined, with the rays directed through a point that is 2.5 inches (6.25 cm) above the tragus of the opposite external ear, with a vertical angulation of 15 degrees and a horizontal angulation of 5 degrees downward. Various other techniques and angulations are used, including laminagraphy, in examining this area.

examination, true occlusal topographic intraoral radiographic, n the radiography of the maxillae or mandible using an occlusal type of film placed between the teeth, with the rays directed at right angles to the

plane of the film or through the long axis of the teeth adjacent to the part in question.

examination, Waters extraoral radiographic, n.pr posteroanterior examination of the paranasal sinuses. The film is placed in contact with the nose and chin, with the rays directed at right angles to the plane of the film.

excavator, spoon (eks′kə-vā-tur), n a paired hand instrument intended primarily to remove carious material from a cavity.

excess, n more than is necessary, useful, or specified.

excess, marginal, n a condition in which the restorative material extends beyond the prepared cavity margin.

excess overhang, n gingival margin excess.

excipient (ek-sip′ē-ənt), n an ingredient included in a pharmaceutical preparation for the purpose of improving its physical qualities. See also *binder; filler;* and *vehicle.*

excision (ek-sizh′ən), n the act of cutting away or taking out.

excision, local, n an excision limited to the immediate area of the lesion in question.

excision, radical, n an excision involving not only the lesion in question but also anatomic parts remote from the site.

excision, wide, n an excision involving the lesion in question and immediately adjacent anatomic structures.

excitant (ek-sīt′ənt), n an agent that stimulates the activity of an organ.

excitation (ek-sī-tā′shən), n the addition of energy to a system, thereby transferring it from its ground state to an excited state.

exclusions, n.pl dental services not covered under a dental benefits program.

exclusive provider organization (EPO), n a dental benefits plan that provides benefits only if care is rendered by institutional and professional providers with whom the plan contracts (with some exceptions for emergency and out-of-area services).

excursion, n a trip; movement from a mean position.

excursion, lateral, n the movement of the mandible from the centric position to a lateral or protusive position.

execute, *v* to finish; accomplish; fulfill. To carry out according to certain terms.

exercise, *n* the performance of any physical activity for the purpose of conditioning the body, improving health, or maintaining fitness or as a means of therapy for correcting a deformity or restoring the organs and bodily function to a state of health.

exercise, myotherapeutic, *n* See *therapy, myofunctional.*

exercise prosthesis, *n* See *prosthesis, exercise.*

exertion, *n* vigorous action, a great effort, a strong influence.

exfoliation **(eks-fō'lē-ā'shən),** *n* (shedding) the physiologic loss of the primary dentition.

exhalation (eks-həl-ā'shən), *n* giving off or sending forth in the form of vapor; expiration.

exhaustion **(eg-zôs'chən),** *n* the loss of vital and nervous power from fatigue or protracted disease.

exhibit (eg-zib'it), *n* a paper, document, or object presented to a court during a trial or hearing as proof of facts, or as otherwise connected with the subject matter, and which, on being accepted, is marked for identification and considered a part of the case.

exit, port of, *n* the means by which infectious microorganisms may leave the body, such as secretions of mucus, blood, saliva, or other fluids.

exocrine (ek'so-krin), *adj* exuding outside the body, from a duct.

exocytosis, *n* the appearance of migrating inflammatory cells in the epidermis.

exodontics (ek'sō-don'tiks), *n* the science and practice of removing teeth from the oral cavity as performed by dentists.

exogenous (ek-soj'ə-nəs), *adj* originating or caused by aspects external to a body.

exophthalmos (ek'sof-thal'mōs), *n* an abnormal protrusion of the eyeball. It is characteristic of toxic (exophthalmic) goiter.

exophytic (ek''so-fit'ik), *adj* developing externally.

exostosis (ek'sos-tō'sis), *n* (hyperostosis) a bony growth projecting from a bony surface.

exotoxin (ek'sō-tok-sin), *n* the toxic material formed by microorganisms and subsequently released into their surrounding environments.

expanded duty auxiliary, *n* a person trained to carry out dental procedures more complex than the responsibilities usually delegated to dental auxiliaries.

expansile infrastructure endosteal implant, *n* an intraosseous implant device designed to enlarge or open after its insertion into the bone to provide retention.

expansion, *n* an increase in extent, size, volume, or scope.

expansion, delayed (secondary expansion), *n* **1.** an expansion occurring in amalgam restorations as a result of moisture contamination. *n* **2.** an expansion exhibited by amalgam that has been contaminated by moisture during trituration or insertion.

expansion, dental arch, *n* the therapeutic increase in circumference of the dental arch by buccal or labial movement of the teeth.

expansion, hygroscopic, *n* an expansion, caused by absorption of water during setting of an investment, used to compensate for the shrinkage of metal from the molten to the solid state.

expansion, secondary, *n* See *expansion, delayed.*

expansion, setting, *n* an expansion that occurs during the setting or hardening of materials such as amalgam and gypsum products.

expansion, thermal, *n* an expansion caused by heat. Thermal expansion of the mold is one of the important factors in achieving adequate compensation for the contraction of cast metal when it solidifies.

expansion, thermal coefficient, *n* a number indicating the amount of expansion caused by each degree of temperature change. The rate of change in restorative materials and tooth substance should be relatively the same.

experience rating, *n* a determination of the premium rate for a particular group partially or wholly on the basis of that group's own experience. Age, sex, use, and costs of services provided determine the premium.

experiment, *n* a trial or special observation made to confirm or disprove something doubtful; an act or operation undertaken to discover some unknown principle or effect or to test, establish, or illustrate some suggested or known truth.

experimental group, *n* the group of participants in a clinical study who receive the actual drug or treatment being studied. See also *controlled clinical trial.*

expert, *n* one who has special skill or knowledge in a particular subject, such as a science or art, whether acquired by experience or study; a specialist.

expert system, n a computer program that follows a logical pathway or algorithm to a conclusion in a manner that mimics what an expert in the field would follow.

expert testimony, n the sworn statements of a person with special knowledge about a subject under consideration by a court of law.

expert witness, n a person who has special knowledge of a subject about which a court requests testimony to educate the court and the jury in the subject under consideration.

expiration, *n* **1.** the act of breathing forth or expelling air from the lungs.

n **2.** a cessation; a termination; the expiration of a lease.

expiration date, n **1.** the date on which a dental benefits contract expires. *n* **2.** the date an individual ceases to be eligible for benefits.

explanation of benefits, *n* a written statement to a beneficiary, from a third-party payer, after a claim has been reported, indicating the benefits and charges covered or not covered by the dental benefits plan.

exploration, *n* **1.** an examination by touch, either with or without instruments. For example, a carious lesion is explored with a special explorer, but the mucobuccal fold may be explored with the finger. *n* **2.** the process of examination of a surface, with or without the use of instruments, to determine the condition or the surface depth of a defect or other similar diagnostic parameters.

explore, *v* to investigate.

explorer, *n* a dental instrument with a slender head that is honed to a fine point, used to conduct a tactile examination and appraisal of pits and fissures, carious lesions, root surfaces, and margins of restoration.

3A
6L
9 mm
17
20F
Orban

3
6
6XL
12 mm

TU17
Wilkins/
Tufts

23
Shepherd's
hook

Explorers. (Daniel/Harfst, 2002)

explorer, 11/12-type, n a hand-activated assessment tool with a paired working end and long lower shank whose specially-angled tip design makes it suited for use in either shallow depressions or deep pockets.

explorer, cowhorn, n a hand-activated assessment tool so named because of the shape of its shank that is used to examine teeth for calculus, caries, and restoration margins. Also called *pigtail explorer.*

explorer, curved shank, n a design adaptation to the instrument used to examine proximal tooth surfaces for calculus and caries which, because of its arc, allows easier access to back teeth.

explorer, Orban No. 20, n.pr the name given to a specific explorer that is used to detect calculus, caries, lesions, and cemental changes on the subgingival surfaces of a tooth.

explorer, pigtail, n See *explorer, cowhorn.*

explorer, pocket, n See *explorer, Orban No. 20.*

explorer, sickle, n a hand-activated assessment tool, so named because of the distinctive shape of its shank, that is used to examine fissures and the surfaces of natural teeth, restorations, and sealants; not suited for exploration inferior to the gingival margin.

explorer, straight, n a hand-activated, sharply pointed tool with an unpaired working end and short lower shank that is used to examine caries inferior to the gingival margin and in restorations with irregular margins; not suited to detecting calculus inferior to the gingival margin.

explorer, TU-17, n.pr the name given to a specific explorer that is used to detect calculus, caries, lesions, and cemental changes on the subgingival surfaces of a tooth; may be adapted for use on selected supragingival surfaces.

explorers, paired, n.pl two identical instruments with contralateral curves that are used to examine opposite tooth surfaces superior to the gingival margin; mirrored-image explorers.

explosion, n a violent, noisy outbreak caused by a sudden release of energy.

exposure, n uncovering: subjection to viewing or radiation.

exposure, accidental pulp, n pulp exposure unintentionally created during instrumentation.

exposure, air, n radiation exposure measured in a small mass of air under conditions of electronic equilibrium with the surrounding air, that is, excluding backscatter from irradiated parts or objects.

exposure, cariogenic, n refers to an incident in which teeth come into contact with foods that tend to create a favorable environment for development of dental caries.

exposure, carious pulp, n pulp exposure occasioned by extension of the carious process to the pulp chamber wall.

exposure, chronic, n radiation exposure of long duration, either continuous (protraction exposure) or intermittent (fractionation exposure); usually referring to exposure of relatively low intensity.

exposure, cumulative, n the total accumulated exposure resulting from repeated radiation exposures of the whole body or of a particular region.

exposure, double, n two superimposed exposures on the same radiographic or photographic film.

exposure, entrance, n exposure measured at the surface of an irradiated body, part, or object. It includes both primary radiation and backscatter from the irradiated underlying tissue or material.

exposure, erythema, n the radiation exposure necessary to produce a temporary redness of the skin. The exposure required varies with the quality of the radiation to which the skin is exposed.

exposure incident, n an event in which a health care professional's potential for infection is heightened after coming into contact with a patient's blood, body fluids, mucous membranes, or broken skin.

exposure, mechanical pulp, n See *exposure, pulp, surgical.*

exposure, protraction, n continuous exposure to radiation over a relatively long period at a low exposure rate.

exposure, pulp, n an opening through the wall of the pulp chamber uncovering the dental pulp.

exposure, radiographic, n a measure of the x or gamma radiation to which a person or object, or part of either, is exposed at a certain place, this measure being based on its ability to produce ionization. The unit of x- or γ-radiation exposure is the roentgen (R).

exposure, radiographic, entrance (surface), *n* radiation exposure measured at the external surface of a person or thing that has been irradiated. Measurement includes both backscatter radiation from the exposed tissues and primary radiation.

exposure rate, output, *n* exposure to radiation at a specified point per unit of time, usually expressed in roentgens per minute.

exposure, surface, *n* See *exposure, entrance.*

exposure, surgical pulp, *n* (mechanical pulp exposure) pulp exposure created intentionally or unintentionally during instrumentation.

exposure, threshold, *n* the minimum exposure that will produce a detectable degree of any given effect.

exposure time, *n* the time during which a person or object is exposed to radiation, expressed in one of the conventional units of time.

express, *v* to state distinctly and explicitly and not leave to inference; to set forth in words.

exsufflation (ek′su-flā′shən), *n* forced discharge of the breath.

extension, *n* **1.** an enlargement in boundary, breadth, or depth. *n* **2.** the process of increasing the angle between two skeletal levers having end-to-end articulation with each other; the opposite of flexion.

extension base, *n* See *base, extension.*

extension base for prevention, *n* a principle of cavity preparation enunciated by G.V. Black in 1891. To prevent the recurrence of decay, he advocated extension of the preparation subgingivally, axially, and occlusally into an area that is readily polished and cleaned.

extension base, gingiva, attached, *n* a gingival extension operation; a surgical technique designed to broaden the zone of attached gingiva by repositioning the mucogingival junction apically.

extension base, groove, *n* the enlargement of a cavity preparation outline to include a developmental groove.

extension base of benefits, *n* an extension of eligibility for benefits for covered services, usually designed to ensure completion of treatment commenced before the expiration date. Duration is generally expressed in terms of days.

extension base, ridge, *n* an intraoral surgical operation for deepening the labial, buccal, or lingual sulci.

extenuate, *v* to lessen; to mitigate.

external oblique line (ōb-lēk′), *n* See *line, external oblique.*

external pin fixation, *n* See *appliance, fracture.*

external traction, *n* See *traction, external.*

exteroceptors (ek′stər-ō-sep′turz), *n.pl* sensory nerve end receptors that respond to external stimuli; located in the skin, mouth, eyes, ears, and nose.

extirpation, pulp (ek′stur-pā′shən), *n* See *pulpectomy.*

extracellular (eks″trə-sel′u-lər), *adj* taking place outside of a cell.

extracellular matrix, *n* an amorphous or structured substance produced by cellular activity that lies within the tissue but outside of the cell.

extracoronal (ek′strə-kôr′ōn-əl), *adj* pertaining to that which is outside, or external to, the body of the coronal portion of a natural tooth.

extracoronal retainer, *n* See *retainer, extracoronal.*

extract, *n* a concentrate obtained by treating a crude material, such as plant or animal tissue, with a solvent, evaporating part or all of the solvent from the resulting solution, and standardizing the resulting product.

extraction, *n* the removal of a tooth from the oral cavity by means of elevators and/or forceps.

extraction, serial, *n* the extraction of selected primary teeth over a period of years (often ending with removal of the first premolar teeth) to relieve crowding of the dental arches during eruption of the lateral incisors, canines, and premolars.

extraoral, *adj* literally, outside of the mouth. Generally refers to an orthodontic appliance that extends outside the mouth to secure a firm base for force application within the mouth. See also *anchorage, extraoral.*

extraoral anchorage, *n* orthodontic force applied from a base outside the mouth. See also *anchorage.*

extrapolate (ek-strap′ō-lāt), *v* to infer values beyond the observable range from an observed trend of variables; to project by inference into the unexplored.

extrasystole (ek′strə-sis′tōlē), *n* a heartbeat occurring before its normal time in the rhythm of the heart and followed by a compensatory pause.

extravasation (ek-strav′ə-zā′shən), *n* the escape of a body fluid out of its proper place (for example, blood into surrounding tissues after rupture of a vessel, urine into surrounding tissues after rupture of the bladder).

extremity, *n* an arm or a leg; the arm may be identified as an upper extremity, and the leg as a lower extremity.

extrinsic, *adj* originating outside; not inherent or essential.

extroversion, *n* a tendency of the teeth or other maxillary structures to become situated too far from the median plane.

extrude, *v* to elevate; to move a tooth coronally.

extrusion, *n* the movement of teeth beyond the natural occlusal plane that may be accompanied by a similar movement of investing tissues. See also *eruption, continuous.*

extubate (eks′tōō-bāt), *v* to remove a tube, usually an endotracheal anesthesia tube or a Levin gastric suction tube.

extubation (eks′tōō-bā′shən), *n* the removal of a tube used for intubation.

exudate (eks′ōō-dāt), *n* the outpouring of a fluid substance, such as exudated pus or tissue fluid.

exudates, gingival, *n* the outpouring of an inflammatory exudate from the gingival tissues.

exudation (eks′ōō-dā′shən), *n* See *exudate.*

eye, *n* one of a pair of organs of sight, contained in a bony orbit at the front of the skull.

eye, assessment of, *n* an examination of the eyes—which includes an observation of pupil size, sclera color, the relative location of the eyeball,

and use of corrective eyeware—to determine the presence of disease.

eye-ear plane, *n* See *plane, Frankfort horizontal.*

eye wash station, *n* a cleansing receptacle set apart for the purpose of emergencies in which the eyes must be quickly flushed with water.

Eye wash station. (Hatrick/Eakle/Bird, 2003, Courtesy Lab Safety Supply Inc., Janesville, WI)

eyeglass, postmydriatic (pōst″ mid″re-at′ik), *n* disposable protective eyewear made of pliable plastic material, handed out by ophthalmologists to patients whose pupils have been dilated during a mydriatic examination.

eyeglasses, *n* transparent devices held in metal or plastic frames in front of the eyes to correct refractive errors or to protect the eyes from harmful electromagnetic waves or flying objects.

eyelids, *n.pl* a moveable fold of thin skin over the eye. The orbicularis oculi muscle and the oculomotor nerve control the opening and closing of the eyelid.

eyewear, protective, *n* **1.** goggles or safety glasses that are worn to protect the eyes from dust and debris while using dental powders or trimmers in the preparation of a study cast. *n* **2.** goggles or safety glasses worn to protect the dental care worker or the patient from accidental eye exposure to blood or other body fluids, or to prevent accidental injury from dental instruments. Pediatric patients or patients with sensitive eyes may be given shaded glasses or goggles to protect the eyes from the brightness of the examination lamp.

eythema infectiosum, *n* See *disease, fifth.*

fabrication
(fab'rikā'shən), *n* the construction or making of a restoration.

face, *n* the front of the head from the chin to the brow, including the skin and muscles and structures of the forehead, eyes, nose, mouth, cheeks, and jaw.

face, changeable area of, *n* the part of the face from the nose to the chin.

face form, *n* See form, face.

face, instrument blade, *n* See instrument blade face.

face shield, *n.pl* a type of protective eyewear sometimes used by oral healthcare workers in place of safety glasses. Although intended to cover the face completely for high-spatter treatments such as polishing and scaling, they may have limited impact resistance and should not be considered a replacement for protective breathing masks.

face-bow, *n* a caliper-like device that is used to record the relationship of the maxillae to the temporomandibular joints (or opening axis of the mandible) and to orient the casts in this same relationship to the opening axis of an articulator.

face-bow adjustable axis, *n* See face-bow, kinematic.

face-bow, kinematic (hinge-bow), *n* a face-bow attached to the mandible with caliper ends (condyle rods) that can be adjusted to permit the accurate location of the axis of rotation of the mandible.

Face shield. (Bird/Robinson, 2002)

facet (fas'et), *n* a flattened, highly polished wear pattern, as noted on a tooth.

facial angle, *n* an anthropomorphic expression of the degree of protrusion of the lower face, assessed by the measured inclination of the facial plane in relation to the Frankfort horizontal reference plane.

facial artery, *n* one of a pair of tortuous arteries that arise from the external carotid arteries, divide into four cervical and five facial branches, and supply various organs and tissues in the head. The cervical branches of the facial artery are the ascending palatine, tonsillar, glandular, and submental. The facial branches are the inferior labial, superior labial, lateral nasal, angular, and muscular.

facial asymmetry, *n* the variation in the configuration of one side of the face from the other when viewed in relation to a projected midsagittal line.

facial bones, *n.pl* the bones of the face, which include the frontal, nasal, maxillary, zygomatic, and mandibular bones.

facial cleft, *n* See cleft, facial.

facial expression, *n* the use of the facial muscles to communicate or to convey mood.

facial injuries, *n.pl* trauma to the face and its associated structures, most frequently from traffic accidents, contact sports, and domestic conflicts.

facial muscle, *n* one of numerous muscles of the face, seldom remaining distinct over its entire length because of a tendency to merge with neighboring muscles at its termination or attachment. The five groups of facial muscles include the muscles of the scalp, the extrinsic muscles of the ear, the muscles of the nose, the muscles of the eyelid, and the muscles of the mouth. The platysma is one muscle of the facial group but is described with the muscles of the neck. Also called *muscles of facial expression.*

facial nerve, *n* either of a pair of mixed sensory and motor cranial nerves that arise from the brainstem at the base of the pons and divide just in front of the ear into six branches, innervating the scalp, forehead, eyelids, muscles of facial expression, cheeks, and jaw. Also called the *seventh cranial nerve.*

facial neuralgia, *n* See neuralgia, trigeminal.

facial pain, *n* See pain, facial.

facial profile, *n* See profile, facial.

facial tic, *n* any repetitive spasmodic and involuntary contraction of groups of facial muscles.

facies (fā'shē-ēs), *n.pl* the features, general appearance, and expression of a face.

facilitation, *n* the reinforcement of a lower level nerve stimulus by a higher level nerve stimulus. Thus a reflex that cannot be elicited by a subliminal impulse may be reinforced by an additional stimulus from a higher center. The combined effect of the two stimuli may cause a reflex response.

facsimile (faksim'ilē), *n* a true copy that preserves all the markings and contents of the original.

fact, *n* a thing done; an event or a circumstance; an actual occurrence.

factitious (faktish'us), *adj* false or self-manufactured.

factor(s), *n* a constituent, element, cause, or agent that influences a process or system; a gene; a dietary substance.

factor I (fibrinogen, profibrin), *n* See fibrinogen.

factor II (prothrombin, component A, prothrombase, prothrombin B, thrombogen, thrombozyme), *n* considered the only essential precursor of thrombin.

factor III (thromboplastin [tissue], thrombokinase, cytozyme [platelet], thrombokinin [blood], thromboplastic protein), *n* See thromboplastin.

factor IV (calcium, Ca^{++}), *n* ionized and/or bound calcium, generally required for the coagulation of blood, although some early phases of coagulation and the thrombin-fibrinogen reaction can take place without calcium.

factor V (labile factor, proaccelerin, accelerin, acceleration factor, cofactor of thromboplastin, component A of prothrombin, plasma ac-globulin, plasma prothrombin conversion factor [PPCF], prothrombinase, prothrombin accelerator, prothrombin conversion accelerator I, thrombo-

gen, thrombogene, proaccelerinaccelerin system), *n* a factor apparently necessary for the formation of a prothrombin-converting substance in blood and tissue extracts—that is, intrinsic and extrinsic prothrombin activators. A deficiency results in parahemophilia (hypoproaccelerinemia).

factor VI, *n* term formerly used to indicate an intermediate product in the formation of thromboplastin and also used synonymously with accelerin and activated factor V. It has no designation at present.

factor VII (stable factor, serum prothrombin conversion accelerator [SPCA], proconvertin, autoprothrombin I, cofactor V, component B of prothrombin, cothromboplastin, kappa factor, precusor of serum prothrombin conversion accelerator [pro-SPCA], prothrombin conversion factor, prothrombin converting factor, prothrombin conversion accelerator II, proconvertinconvertin system, prothrombinogen, serozyme, stable factor), *n* a factor that accelerates the conversion of prothrombin to thrombin in the presence of factors III, IV, and V; a serum factor necessary for the formation of extrinsic prothrombin activator.

factor VII deficiency, *n* a deficiency associated with a lack of vitamin K. A deficiency may be congenital, or it may be acquired in liver disease, or from prothrombinopenic agents used in anticoagulation therapy; it results in a prolonged (quantitative) one-stage prothrombin time test.

factor VIII (antihemophilic factor [AHF], antihemophilic globulin, antihemophilic globulin A, antihemophilic factor A, plasma thromboplastin factor [PTF], plasmokinin, platelet cofactor I, prothrombokinase, thrombocatalysin, thrombocytolysin, thrombokatilysin, thromboplastic plasma component [TPC], thromboplastinogen), *n* a factor essential for the formation of blood thromboplastin. A deficiency results in classic hemophilia (hemophilia A); the clotting time is prolonged, and thromboplastin and prothrombin conversion is diminished.

factor IX (Christmas factor, plasma

thromboplastin component [PTC], antihemophilic factor B, antihemophilic globulin B, autoprothrombin II, beta prothromboplastin, plasma factor X, plasma thromboplastin factor B [PTF-B], platelet cofactor II), n a factor that is active in the formation of intrinsic blood thromboplastin. A deficiency results in Christmas disease (hemophilia B), which is caused by a decrease in the amount of thromboplastin formed.

factor X (Stuart-Prower factor, Stuart factor, Prower factor), n a factor influencing the yield of intrinsic (plasma) thromboplastin. A deficiency results in a prolonged one-stage prothrombin time. Brain tissue or Russell's viper venom are used to test for thromboplastin deficiency.

factor XI (plasma thromboplastin antecedent [PTA], antihemophilic factor C, PTA factor, plasma thromboplastin factor C [PTF-C]), n a factor related to intrinsic (plasma) thromboplastin activation, which occurs when blood is exposed to a foreign surface.

factor XI deficiency, n a deficiency caused by an autosomal recessive gene resulting in a hemorrhagic tendency. See also hemophilia C.

factor XII (Hageman factor, antihemophilic factor D, clot-promoting factor, fifth plasma thromboplastin precursor, glass factor), n a factor the absence of which results in a long clotting time and abnormal prothrombin consumption and thromboplastin generation tests when tests are carried out in glass tubes. No abnormal bleeding tendency occurs with a deficiency of the factor.

factor XIII, n a coagulation factor present in normal plasma that acts with calcium to produce an insoluble fibrin clot. Also called *fibrinase* or *fibrin stabilizing factor.*

factor XIII deficiency, n a deficiency caused by a deficiency of vitamin E.

factor, acceleration, n See factor V.

factor, antihemophilic (AHF), n See factor VIII.

factor, antihemophilic A, n See factor VIII.

factor, antihemophilic B, n See factor IX.

factor, antihemophilic C, n See factor XI.

factor, antihemophilic D, n See factor XII.

factor, antipernicious, n See vitamin B_{12}.

factor, C (contact factor, contact activation product, third thromboplastic factor), n a coagulation accelerator product formed by the interaction of active factor XII and factor XI.

factor, Castle's intrinsic (intrinsic factor), n.pr a factor produced by the gastric mucosa and possibly the duodenal mucosa, and considered to be responsible for the absorption of vitamin B_{12}. See also anemia, pernicious.

factor, Christmas, n See factor IX.

factor, clot-promoting, n See factor XII.

factor, clotting, n "trace" proteins (excluding calcium) present in normal blood in such small amounts (except fibrinogen) that their presence is usually established by deductive reasoning and by genetic and biochemical characteristics. They are associated with thromboplastic activity and the conversion of prothrombin to thrombin.

factor, contact, n See factor C.

factor, environmental, n local conditions that modify tissue response (for example, narrow interdental spaces, saddle areas, attachment of frenula, oblique ridges).

factor, erythrocyte-maturation (EMF), n See vitamin B complex.

factor, etiologic, n the element or influence that can be assigned as the cause or reason for a disease or lesion.

factor, extrinsic, n See vitamin B complex.

factor, familial, n a characteristic derived through heredity.

factor, glass, n See factor XII.

factor, glucocorticoid, n See hormone, "S."

factor, Hageman, n See factor XII.

factor, Hr, n blood factors that are reciprocally related to the Rh factors. They are present in agglutinogens when the corresponding Rh factor is absent from the gene.

factor, hyperglycemic, n See glucagon.

factor, hyperglycemic-glycogenolytic, n See glucagon.

factor, intrinsic, n See factor, Castle's intrinsic.

factor, kappa, n See factor VII.

factor, labile, n See factor V.

factor, local, n includes dental and bacterial plaques, bacterial toxins and irritants, calculus, food impaction, and other surface and locally placed irritants that are capable of injuring the periodontium.

factor, pellagra-preventive, n See acid, nicotinic.

factor, plasma prothrombin conversion (PPCF), n See factor V.

factor, plasma thromboplastin (PTF), n substances with thromboplastic activity contributed by the plasma. Included are the antihemophilic factor, Christmas factor, plasma thromboplastin antecedent, and Hageman factor. See also factor VIII.

factor, plasma thromboplastin, A (PTF-A), n See factor VIII.

factor, plasma thromboplastin, B (PTF-B), n See factor IX.

factor, plasma thromboplastin, C (PTF-C), n See factor XI.

factor, plasma thromboplastin, D (PTF-D), n considered by some to be a fourth plasma substance with thromboplastic activity; not well characterized.

factor, plasma, X, n See factor IX.

factor, platelet, n a substance on or in the surface of blood platelet necessary for coagulation in the absence of extravascular thromboplastic substances.

factor, platelet, 1, n either factor V or a factor with factor V activity; absorbed on platelets and accelerates conversion of prothrombin to thrombin.

factor, platelet, 2, n a substance that accelerates the conversion of fibrinogen to fibrin.

factor, platelet, 3, n a substance associated with thromboplastin generation activity.

factor, platelet, 4, n an antiheparin factor.

factor, prothrombin conversion, n See factor VII.

factor, prothrombin-converting, n See factor VII.

factor, Prower, n.pr See factor X.

factor, psychosomatic, n psychic, mental, or emotional factors that play a role in determining the initiation, course, and extent of a physical process, either directly or indirectly. Psychosomatic factors have been implicated in necrotizing ulcerative gingivitis (NUG), bruxism, clenching, and other oral habits.

factor, PTA (plasma thromboplastin antecedent factor), n See factor XI.

factor, reparative, n the ability of the tissues to heal or regenerate when they have been subjected to injury or disease.

factor, Rh, n agglutinogens of red blood cells responsible for isoimmune reactions such as occur in erythroblastosis fetalis and incompatible blood transfusions.

factor, spreading, n an enzyme that increases the permeability of ground substance.

factor, stable, n See factor VII.

factor, Stuart, n.pr See factor X.

factor, Stuart-Prower, n.pr See factor X.

factor, third thromboplastic, n See factor C.

facultative (fak′əltātiv), adj pertaining to an organism's ability to survive under different or varying environmental conditions.

faculty, n **1.** any normal physiologic function or natural ability of a living organism. **2.** an ability to do something specific, such as learn languages or to perceive and distinguish sensory stimuli. **3.** any mental ability or power. **4.** the group of people who teach within an institution of learning.

FAD, n abbreviation for *flavinadenine dinucleotide.*

failure, n a deficiency; an inefficiency as measured by some legal standard; an unsuccessful attempt.

failure to thrive, n the abnormal retardation of the growth and development of an infant resulting from conditions that interfere with normal metabolism, appetite, and activity.

faint, n a state of syncope, or swooning.

false light, n a misleading fashion in which a person is depicted before the public that a reasonable person finds offensive and damaging.

falsify, v to forge; to give a false

appearance to anything, as to falsify a record.

famciclovir, *n* *trade name:* Famvir; *drug class:* antiviral; *action:* converted to active metabolite, penciclovir triphosphate, which inhibits viral DNA synthesis and replication; *uses:* acute herpes zoster (shingles) infection.

family, *n* **1.** a body of persons who live in one house and under one head; a father, a mother, and a child or some children; a husband and wife living together. **2.** a group of people related by heredity, such as parents, children, and siblings. The term is sometimes broadened to include related by marriage or those living in the same household, who are emotionally attached, interact regularly, and share concerns for the growth and development of the group and its individual members. **3.** a group of persons who have a common surname, such as the Anderson family. **4.** a category of animals or plants situated on a taxonomic scale between order and genus. **5.** the legal definition varies, depending on the jurisdiction and purpose for which the term is defined.

family counseling, *n* a program that consists of providing information and professional guidance to members of a family concerning specific health matters.

family deductible, *n* a deductible that is satisfied by combined expenses of all covered family members. A plan with a $25 deductible may limit its application to a maximum of three deductibles, or $75, for the family, regardless of the number of family members.

family dentistry, *n* the branch of dentistry that is concerned with the diagnosis and treatment of dental problems in people of either sex and at any age. Family dentists were formerly known as *general practitioners,* and therefore family dentistry does not constitute one of the specialty areas of dentistry.

family history, *n* part of the medical history process; practitioner should ask patient about history of diseases or serious illness in family to determine if the patient might be predisposed to certain illnesses.

family membership, *n* a membership that includes spouses and/or dependents.

family unit, *n* an insured group member and dependents who are eligible for benefits under a dental care contract; an accounting unit.

famotidine, *n* *trade names:* Pepcid, Pepcid IV; *drug class:* H_2 histamine receptor antagonist; *action:* inhibits histamine at H_2 receptor site in parietal cells, which inhibits gastric acid secretion; *uses:* short-term treatment of active duodenal ulcer, gastric ulcer, and heartburn.

fascia, *n* the fibrous connective tissue of the body that may be separated from other specifically organized fibrous structures such as the tendons, the aponeuroses, and the ligaments. Fascia generally covers and separates muscles and muscle groups.

fascia lata, *n* the strong fascia that envelopes the muscles of the thigh.

fasciitis (fəsī'tis), *n* a tumorlike growth occurring in subcutaneous tissues in the mouth, usually in the cheek. A benign lesion sometimes mistaken for fibrosarcoma, fasciitis consists of young fibroblasts and numerous capillaries. It grows rapidly and may regress spontaneously.

fast, *v* to abstain from ingesting food for a specific period of time, usually for diagnostic, therapeutic, or religious purposes.

fast green, *n* a green dye used to reveal plaque deposits on teeth; consists of F.D. & C. Green No. 3 in concentrations of either 5% or 2.5%.

fat, *n* **1.** a substance composed of lipids or fatty acids and occurring in various forms or consistencies ranging from oil to tallow. **2.** a type of connective tissue containing stored lipids.

fat embolism, *n* a circulatory condition characterized by the blocking of an artery by an embolus of fat that enters the circulatory system after the fracture of a long bone, or less commonly, after traumatic injury to fatty tissue or to a fatty liver.

fatal outcome, *n* a consequence that results in death. The course of a disease that results in the death of the patient.

fate, *n* a synonym for the more modern term *biotransformation.* See also biotransformation.

fatigue, *n* a condition of cells or organs under stress resulting in a diminution or loss of an individual's capacity to respond to stimulation.

fatigue, dental materials, *n* dysfunction due to damage caused by recurring use or stress.

fatigue, muscle, *n* a peripheral phenomenon caused by the failure of the muscle to contract when stimuli from the nervous system reach it. Occurs when muscle activity exceeds tissue substrate and oxygenation capacity.

fatty acid, *n* any of several organic acids produced by the hydrolysis of neutral fats.

fauces (fô'sēz), *n* the archway between the pharyngeal and oral cavities; formed by the tongue, anterior and posterior tonsillar pillars, and soft palate.

faucial pillars, *n.pl* two pairs of vertical folds of tissue created by muscles that create the fauces, which surround the palatine tonsils.

FDA, *n.pr* the abbreviation for the Food and Drug Administration. See also Food and Drug Administration.

F. D. & C., *n* See Food, Drug, and Cosmetic Act.

fear, *n* an emotion, generally considered negative and unpleasant, that is a reaction to a real or threatened danger; fright. Fear is distinguished from anxiety, which is a reaction to an unreal or imagined danger.

febrile, *adj* pertaining to or characterized by an elevated body temperature. A body temperature of over 100° F is commonly regarded as febrile.

feces, *n* waste or excrement from the digestive tract that is formed in the intestine and expelled through the rectum. Feces consist of water, food residue, bacteria, and secretions of the intestines and liver.

Fede's disease, See disease, Riga-Fede.

Federal Tort Claims Act, *n.pr* a statute passed in 1946 that allows the federal government to be sued for the wrongful action or negligence of its employees. The act, for most purposes, eliminates the doctrine of governmental immunity, which formerly prohibited or limited the bringing of suit against the federal government.

Fédération Dentaire Internationale (F. D. I) Two-Digit System (fā'därä syōN dôNter' eN'ternäs'yōnäl'), *n.pr* a recognized method used to identify and designate permanent and primary and deciduous teeth within the oral cavity. The first digit represents the quadrant number (1–4) starting with the maxillary right quadrant, moving around the maxillary arch to the left, then down and back to the right, and ending with the mandibular right quadrant. The second digit represents each tooth in the quadrant, numbered distally from the midline. Also called the *International System.*

fee, *n* compensation for services rendered or to be rendered; payment for professional services.

fee, customary, *n* a fee is customary if it is in the range of the usual fees charged by dentists of similar training and experience for the same service within the specific and limited geographic area (that is, the socioeconomic area of a metropolitan area or of a county).

fee-for-service plan, *n* a plan providing for payment to the dentist for each service performed rather than on the basis of salary or capitation fee.

fee, reasonable, *n* a fee is considered reasonable if, in the opinion of a responsible dental association's review committee, it is the usual and customary fee charged for services rendered, considering the special circumstances of the case in question.

fee schedule, *n* **l.** a list of maximum dollar allowances for dental procedures that apply under a specific contract. **2.** a list of the charges established or agreed to by a dentist for specific dental services.

fee, usual, *n* the fee customarily charged for a given service by an individual dentist to a private patient.

feedback, *n* the constant flow of sensory information back to the brain. When feedback mechanisms are deficient because of sensory deprivation, motor function becomes distorted, aberrant, and uncoordinated.

Feer's disease (fārz), *n.pr* See erythredema polyneuropathy.

felbamate, *n* *trade name:* Felbatol; *drug class:* anticonvulsant; *action:* anticonvulsant action is unclear;

uses: alone or as an adjunct therapy in partial seizures.

feldspar (feld'spär), *n* a crystalline mineral of aluminum silicate with potassium, sodium, barium, or calcium—$NaAlSi_3O_8$ or $KA_lSi_3O_8$. Feldspar melts over a range of 1,100° to 2,000° F (593.5° to 1093.5° C). An important constituent of dental porcelain.

feldspar, orthoclase ceramic, n a clay found in large quantity in the solid crust of the earth. It acts as a filler and imparts body to the fused dental porcelain.

felodipine, *n trade names.* Plendil, Renedil; *drug class:* calcium channel blocker; *action:* inhibits calcium ion influx across cell membrane during cardiac depolarization; produces relaxation of coronary vascular smooth muscle; dilates coronary arteries; decreases SA/AV node conduction; *uses:* essential hypertension, alone or with other antihypertensives, chronic angina pectoris.

felony, *n* a crime declared by statute to be more serious than a misdemeanor and deserving of a more severe penalty. Conviction usually requires imprisonment in a penitentiary for longer than one year.

felypressin (fel'ipres'in), *n* an ingredient that may be added to a local anesthetic for the purpose of constricting blood vessels. It helps to contain the anesthetic in a specific area by reducing systemic absorption, decreasing blood flow, and prolonging effectiveness. *Trade name:* Octapressin. It is not available in the United States.

Fen-Phen, *n* a combination of fenfluramine hydrochloride and phentermine hydrochloride, two stimulants, which promotes weight loss by reducing appetite. See also fenfluramine hydrochloride and phentermine hydrochloride.

fenestration (fenestrā'shən), *n* an opening, a window, an interstice.

fenestration, in alveolar plate, n a round or oval defect or opening in the alveolar cortical plate of bone over the root surface.

fenfluramine HCl, *n trade name:* Pondimin; *drug class:* nonamphetamine anorexiant, Controlled Substance Schedule IV; *action:* influences serotonin pathways in the central nervous system; anorexic mechanisms unknown; *use:* exogenous obesity.

fenoprofen calcium, *n trade name:* Nalfon; *drug class:* nonsteroidal antiinflammatory; *action:* inhibits prostaglandin synthesis by interfering with cyclooxygenase needed for biosynthesis; *uses:* mild-to-moderate pain, osteoarthritis, rheumatoid arthritis, acute gout, dysmenorrhea.

fentanyl transdermal system, *n trade name:* Duragesic 25, 50, 75, 100 Transdermal Patches; *drug class:* narcotic analgesic, Controlled Substance Schedule II; *action:* interacts with opioid receptors in the central nervous system to alter pain perception; *uses:* management of chronic pain when opioids are necessary.

fermentable, *adj* the ability to undergo a chemical reaction in the presence of an enzyme that results in the creation of either acid or alcohol; in the mouth, the ability to create acid in plaque.

fermentation, *n* a chemical change that is brought about in a substance by the action of an enzyme or microorganism, especially the anaerobic conversion of foodstuffs to certain products such as acetic fermentation, alcoholic fermentation.

Ferrier's separator (fer'ē-urz), *n.pr* See separator, Ferrier's.

ferritin (fer'itin), *n* the compound iron-appoferritin, which is produced in the intestine and stored primarily in the liver, spleen, and bone marrow. It eventually becomes a component of hemoglobin, and can be measured to estimate the body's iron levels.

ferromagnetic (fer'ōmagnet'ik), *adj* pertaining to substances that exhibit unusually strong magnetic properties; iron-like substances.

ferrous fumarate/ferrous gluconate/ferrous sulfate, *n trade names:* Femiron, Feostat; *drug class:* hematinic, iron preparation; *action:* replaces iron stores needed for red blood cell development; *uses:* irondeficiency anemia, prophylaxis for iron deficiency in pregnancy.

fertility, *n* the ability to reproduce.

festoon(s) (festōōn'), *n* a carving in the base material of a denture that simulates the contours of the natural tissues being replaced by the denture.

festoon, gingival, n the distinct

rounding and enlargement of the margins of the gingival tissue found in early gingival involvement.

festoons, McCall's, n.pr enlargements of the gingival margins that may be associated with occlusal trauma.

festooning (festōōn´ing), *n* the process of carving the base material of a denture or denture pattern to simulate the contours of the natural tissues to be replaced by the denture.

fetal alcohol syndrome, *n* a set of congenital psychologic, behavioral, cognitive, and physical abnormalities that tend to appear in infants whose mothers consumed alcoholic beverages during pregnancy. It is characterized by typical craniofacial and limb defects, cardiovascular defects, and retarded development.

Fetal alcohol syndrome. (Zitelli/Davis, 2002)

fetal period, *n* the stage between the third and ninth months of in utero human development, during which there is growth of preformed structures.

fetor ex ore (fē´tôr eks ō´rē), *n* See halitosis.

fetor oris (fē´tôr ō´ris), *n* bad breath. See also halitosis.

fetus, *n* the unborn offspring of any viviparous animal after it has attained the particular form of the species, more specifically, the human being in utero after the embryonic period and the beginning of the development of the major structural features, usually from the eighth week after fertilization until birth.

fever (pyrexia), *n* elevation of the body temperature.

fever, acute necrotizing ulcerative gingivitis (ANUG) and acute primary keratotic gingivostomatitis, n a moderate-to-high elevation of temperature is not a symptom of ANUG; however, the presence of a significantly elevated temperature might suggest the presence of APKG, a viral disease accompanied by a bleeding and tender gingiva, marked halitosis, and lymphadenopathy.

fever, aphthous, n See disease, hand, foot, and mouth.

fever, cat-scratch (benign inoculation lymphoreticulosis, cat-scratch disease), n a granulomatous process that occurs at the site of a scratch or bite of a house cat. Local lesions occur at the site of injury, with a regional adenitis that is out of proportion to the primary lesion occurring within 1 to 3 weeks. Systemic symptoms of infection may occur. Diagnosis is confirmed by reaction to cat-scratch antigen or the antigen of lymphogranuloma venereum, which is a related form of disease.

Cat-scratch fever. (Zitelli/Davis, 2002)

fever, hay, n rhinitis and conjunctivitis resulting from allergy; frequently caused by allergy to pollens.

fever, of unknown origin, n the persistent elevation of body temperature without an identifiable cause.

fever, rheumatic (rōōmat´ik), n a severe, apparently infectious disease produced by hemolytic streptococci organisms or associated with their presence in the body; characterized by upper respiratory tract inflammation, cervical lymphadenopathy and lymphadenitis, polyarthritis, cardiac involvement, and subcutaneous nodules. The disease may be produced by an autoantibody reaction.

fever, scarlet (scarlatina), *n* an acute disease caused by a specific type of Streptococcus organism and characterized by a rash and strawberry tongue.

fever, uveoparotid (Heerfordt's syndrome, uveoparotitis), *n* **1.** a disease characterized by inflammation of the parotid gland and of the uveal regions of the eye. **2.** firm, nodular enlargement of the parotid glands, uveitis, and cutaneous lesions may be present. Considered to be a form of sarcoidosis. **3.** a syndrome consisting of sarcoidosis affecting the parotid glands, inflammation of the lacrimal glands, and inflammation of the uveal tract of the eye.

fever blister, *n* See herpes labialis.

fiber(s), *n* an elongated, threadlike structure of organic tissue.

fibers, A-alpha nerve, *n.pl* large-diameter nerve fibers that connect into the substantia gelatinosa of the dorsal horns of the spinal cord before synapsing with the central transmission of the dorsal horn. A-alpha fibers are associated with the "gate-control" theory of pain.

fibers, A-beta nerve, *n.pl* large-diameter nerve fibers that are mechanoreceptors for pressure occurring in both the pulp and periodontal ligament, necessary to operate the gate mechanism.

fibers, A-delta nerve, *n.pl* small-diameter nerve fibers that are mechanoreceptors for pain occurring in both the pulp and the periodontal ligament, necessary to operate the gate mechanism.

fibers, adrenergic, *n.pl* those nerve fibers, including most of the postganglionic sympathetic fibers, that transmit their impulses across synapses or neuroeffector junctions through the local release of the neurohormone, more recently identified as *norepinephrine* and formerly designated *sympathin.*

fibers, alveolar, *n.pl* white collagenous fibers of the periodontal membrane (ligament) that extend from the alveolar bone to the intermediate plexus, where their terminations are interspersed with the terminations of the cemental group of fibers.

fibers, alveolar crest, *n.pl* collagenous fibers of the periodontal membrane that extend from the cervical area of the tooth to the alveolar crest.

fibers, alveolgingival, *n.pl* supportive fibers that extend from the alveolar crest into the gingiva.

fibers, apical, *n.pl* the fibers of the periodontal ligament radiating apically from tooth to bone.

fibers, association, *n.pl* extensions of nerve cells that are neither efferent nor afferent neurons but furnish a pathway of connection between them.

fibers, bundle, *n.pl* the gathering together of collagen fibers in a group, particularly the collagen fiber bundles of the periodontal membrane.

fibers, C nerve, *n.pl* small-diameter nerve fibers that are mechanoreceptors for pain occurring in both the pulp and the periodontal ligament, necessary to operate the gate mechanism.

fibers, cemental, *n.pl* the fibers of the periodontal membrane extending from the cementum to the zone of the intermediate plexus, where their terminations are interspersed with the terminations of the alveolar group of periodontal fibers.

fibers, circular, *n.pl* the fibers in the free gingiva that encircle the tooth in a ringlike fashion.

fibers, collagen, *n.pl* white fibers composed of collagen. The most conspicuous part of connective tissue, including the gingivae and periodontal membrane. Some fibers are distributed haphazardly throughout the connective tissue ground substance, and others are arranged in coarse bundles that exhibit a distinct orientation. Characterized by its hydroxyproline and hydroxylysine content.

fiber, crestal, *n* one group of periodontal ligament fibers extending from the cervical area of the tooth to the alveolar crest.

fibers, dentogingival, *n.pl* the part of a fan-shaped fiber system that emerges from the supraalveolar connective tissue; composed of circular, dentogingival, dentoperiosteal, and transseptal fiber groups.

fibers, dentoperiosteal, *n* a fiber system emerging from the supraalveolar part of the cementum of the tooth and passing outward beyond the alveolar crest in an apical direction into the mucoperiosteum of the attached gingiva.

F

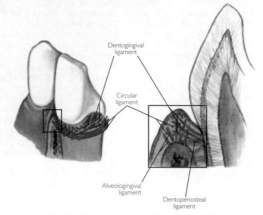

Gingival fibers. (Bath-Balogh/Fehrenbach, 1997)

fibers, gingival, *n* the group of fiber systems belonging to the gingival and supraalveolar connective tissue; composed of circular, dentogingival, dentoperiosteal, and transseptal fiber groups.

fibers, horizontal, *n.pl* collagen fibers of the periodontal membrane that extend horizontally from the cementum to the alveolar bone.

fibers, interradicular, *n.pl* fibers peculiar to multirooted teeth that extend from the cementum to the bone between the roots. The fibers help keep the tooth from shifting position.

fiber, myelinated nerve, *n* a nerve fiber inside or outside the brain that is covered with an insulating medullary sheath along which are located nodes of Ranvier that facilitate as relay points the speed of nerve impulses over that of an equivalent nonmedullated fiber.

fibers, nerve, *n.pl* See fiber, myelinated nerve, and fiber, nonmedullated nerve.

fibers, nonmedullated nerve, *n* a nerve fiber not covered by an insulating medullary sheath that is thus exposed to other tissue fluids and

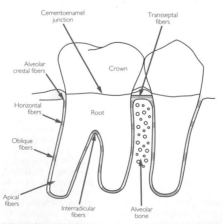

Tissues and fibers of the gingiva and attachment apparatus. (Daniel/Harfst, 2002)

their respective electric potentials. In nonmedullated fibers, the impulse is relayed from point to contiguous point. Most of the nonmedullated fibers are within the substance of the central nervous system, and the distances between the cells are short.

fibers, oblique, n the group of collagen fibers in bundle arrangement in the periodontal ligament that are obliquely situated, with insertions in the cementum, and that extend more occlusally in the alveolus (approximately two-thirds of the periodontal fibers fall into this group).

fibers, periodontal, n See ligament, periodontal.

fibers, principal, n.pl the numerous bundles of collagenous tissue fibers arranged in groups that function as the mode of attachment of the tooth to the alveolus.

fibers, Sharpey's, n.pr collagenous fibers that become incorporated into the cementum.

fibers, transseptal, n.pl a part of the gingival fiber system that extends from the supraalveolar cementum of one tooth horizontally through the interdental attached gingiva above the septum of the alveolar bone to the cementum of the adjacent tooth.

fiberoptic light, n a miniaturized light source that uses the property of flexible fiberglass strands to conduct light over long distances with little or no distortion; used in intraoral application, such as a light attached directly to the dental handpiece.

fiberoptics, n the technical process by which an internal organ or cavity can be viewed, using glass or plastic fibers to transmit light through a special tube designed to magnify and reflect an image of the surface of the internal region under observation.

fibrillation (fib′rilā′shən), n a local quivering of muscle fibers.

fibrillation, atrial, n a cardiac arrhythmia caused by disturbed spread of excitation through atrial musculature.

fibrillation, auricular **(ôrik′yōōlur),** n an uncoordinated, independent contraction of the heart that results in marked irregularity of heart action.

fibrillation, ventricular, n an uncoordinated, independent contraction of the ventricular musculature resulting in cessation of cardiac output.

fibrinogen (fībrin′əjən) (factor I, profibrin), n a soluble plasma protein (globulin) that is acted on by thrombin to form fibrin. The normal level is 200 to 400 mg/100 ml in plasma. Coagulation is impaired if the concentration is less than 100 mg/100 ml. Another form of fibrinogen called *tissue fibrinogen,* which has the power of clotting the blood without the presence of thrombin, occurs in body tissues.

fibrinokinase (fī′brinōkī′nās) (fibrinolysokinase, lysokinase), n an activator of plasminogen found in many animal tissues.

fibrinolysin (fī′brinol′isin), n See plasmin.

fibrinolysis, n the continual process of fibrin decomposition during the removal of small fibrin clots by the action of enzyme fibrinolysin.

fibrinolysokinase, n See fibrinokinase.

fibrinolytic agents, n.pl agents that decrease the breakdown of fibrin.

fibroblast (fī′brōblast), n a cell found within fibrous connective tissue, varying in shape from stellate (young) to fusiform and spindle shaped. Associated with the formation of collagen fibers and ground substance of connective tissue.

fibroblast, of periodontal ligament, n cells that play an important role in formation and remodeling of fibrous matrix and ground substance.

fibroblastoma (fī′brōblastō′mə), n a tumor arising from an ordinary connective tissue cell or fibroblast. The tumor may be a fibroma or a fibrosarcoma.

fibroblastoma, neurogenic, n See neurofibroma.

fibroblastoma, perineural, n See neurilemoma and neurofibroma.

fibrocystic disease, n See disease, fibrocystic.

fibroma (fībrō′mə), n a benign mesenchymal tumor composed primarily of fibrous connective tissue.

fibroma, ameloblastic, n a mixed tumor of odontogenic origin characterized by the simultaneous proliferation of both the epithelial and mesenchymal components of the tooth germ without the production of hard structure.

fibroma, calcifying, n See osteofibroma.

fibroma, cementifying, n an intrabony lesion not associated with teeth, composed of a fibrous connective tissue stroma containing foci of calcified material resembling cementum; a rare odontogenic tumor composed of varying amounts of fibrous connective tissue with calcified material resembling cementum. Central lesion of the jaws.

fibroma, irritation, n a localized peripheral, tumorlike enlargement of connective tissue caused by prolonged local irritation and usually seen on the gingiva or buccal mucosa.

fibroma, neurogenic, n See neurilemoma; neurofibroma.

fibroma, odontogenic, n a central odontogenic tumor of the jaws, consisting of connective tissue in which small islands and strands of odontogenic epithelium are dispersed. A mesodermal odontogenic tumor composed of active dense or loose fibrous connective tissue; contains inactive islands of epithelium.

fibroma, ossifying, n See osteofibroma.

fibroma, periapical (benign periapical fibroma, fibrous dysplasia, first-state cementoma, focal osseous dysplasia, traumatic osteoclasia), n a benign connective tissue mass formed at the apex of a tooth with a normal pulp.

fibroma, peripheral odontogenic, n a fibrous connective tissue tumor associated with the gingival margin and believed to originate from the periodontium. Often contains areas of calcification. Localized form of fibromatosis gingivae.

fibroma, with myxomatous degeneration, n See fibromyxoma.

fibromatosis (fī′brōmətō′sis), n a gingival enlargement believed to be a hereditary condition that is manifested in the permanent dentition and characterized by a firm hyperplastic tissue that covers the teeth. Differentiation between this and diphenylhydantoin (Dilantin) hyperplasia is based on a history of drug ingestion.

Fibromatosis. (Neville/Damm/Allen/Bouquot, 2002)

fibromatosis gingivae (elephantiasis gingivae, idiopathic fibromatosis, idiopathic gingival hyperplasia), n a generalized enlargement of the gingivae caused by fibrous hyperplasia. Idiopathic in nature and similar in appearance to Dilantin hyperplasia.

fibromatosis, hereditary gingival, n a condition possessing a familial attribute of distribution, in which there is gingival enlargement resulting from marked fibroplasia.

fibromatosis, idiopathic, n See fibromatosis gingivae.

fibromyalgia, n a form of nonarticular rheumatism characterized by musculoskeletal aching and stiffness, fatigue, and poor sleep, as well as tenderness on palpation at various sites. Common sites of pain or stiffness are the lower back, neck, shoulder region, arms, hands, knees, hips, thighs, legs, and feet.

fibromyxoma (fī′brōmiksō′mə) (fibroma with myxomatous degeneration), n a fibroma that has certain characteristics of a myxoma; a fibroma that has undergone myxomatous degeneration. Combination of both fibrous and myxomatous elements.

fibroosteoma (fī′brō-äs′tē-ō′mə), n See osteofibroma.

fibropapilloma (fī′brōpap′ilō-mə), n a lesion that resembles a benign neoplasm and shows fibroblastic and epithelial proliferation. Such lesions occur in regions of cheek chewing or other trauma. Because they are not true neoplasms, they may be better designated as *irritation fibroses* or *fibrous hyperplasias.*

fibrosarcoma (fī'brōsärkō'mə), *n* a malignant mesenchymal tumor, the basic cell type being a fibroblast. Most fibrosarcomas are locally infiltrative and persistent but do not metastasize.

Fibrosarcoma. (Regezi/Sciubba/Jordan, 2003)

fibrosarcoma, odontogenic, *n* an extremely rare malignant form of odontogenic fibroma.

fibrosis (fībrō'sis), *n* **1.** the process of forming fibrous tissue, usually by degeneration (for example, fibrosis of the pulp). The process occurs normally in the formation of scar tissue to replace normal tissue lost through injury or infection. **2.** an abnormal condition in which fibrous connective tissue spreads over or replaces normal smooth muscle or other normal organ tissue. Fibrosis is most common in the heart, lung, peritoneum, and kidney.

fibrosis, diffuse hereditary gingival, *n* an uncommon form of severe gingival hyperplasia considered to be of genetic origin. The tissue is pink, firm, dense, and insensitive and has little tendency to bleed.

fibrosis, hereditary gingival, *n* an uncommon form of severe gingival hyperplasia that may begin with the eruption of the deciduous or permanent teeth and is characterized by a firm, dense, pink gingival tissue with little tendency toward bleeding.

fibrous diseases, *n.pl* See dysplasia, fibrous.

fiduciary (fidōō'shē-erē), *n* a person who has a duty to act primarily for another's benefit, as a trustee. Also, pertaining to the good faith and confidence involved in such a relationship.

field, *n* an area, region, or space.

field block, *n* See block, field.

field, operating, *n* the area immediately surrounding and directly involved in a treatment procedure (for example, all the teeth included in a rubber dam application for the restoration of a single tooth or portions thereof).

field, radiation, *n* the region in which radiant energy is being propagated.

fifth disease, *n* an infectious disease primarily found in children that is caused by transmission of the human parvovirus B19 through the upper respiratory tract. Symptoms include fever and a skin rash that begins on the cheeks and spreads to other body surfaces. Also called *erythema infectiosum.*

filament, *n* an individual manufactured toothbrush bristle.

filament, curved, *n* refers to a single toothbrush bristle, manufactured to bend with the curve of the dental surface, designed to assist contact with the gum line when used at a 45° angle.

filament, end rounded, *n* refers to the manufactured shaping of an individual toothbrush bristle with an exceptionally rounded tip designed to protect teeth and gums during brushing.

filamentous bacilli, morphologic form of, *n* the clustered strands of narrow filaments, rounded at one end and tapered at the other, which are characteristic of the filamentous bacilli.

file, *n* **1.** a metal tool of varying size and form with numerous ridges or teeth on its cutting surfaces; may be push-cut or pull-cut; used for smoothing or dressing down metals and other substances. **2.** a collection of records; an organized collection of information directed toward some purpose such as patient demographic data. The records in a file may or may not be sequenced according to a key contained in each record. *v* **3.** to reduce by means of a file.

file, gold, *n* a file designed for removing surplus gold from gold restorations; may be pull-cut or push-cut.

file, Hirschfeld-Dunlop, n.pr a kind of periodontal file used with a pull stroke for the removal of calculus; available in various angulations for approach to different surfaces of teeth.

file, periodontal, *n* an instrument with multiple, angled cutting edges used to roughen the surface of a smooth calculus deposit before removal with a curet.

file, root canal, *n* a small metal hand instrument with tightly spiraled blades used to clean and shape the canal.

file, sharpening, *n* a difficult honing procedure requiring special tools designed to address the file's numerous parallel ridges; best left to a professional sharpener or the manufacturer.

file-access safeguards, *n.pl* methods of limiting certain users' access to particular data.

filing, *n* the act of using a file to shape or smooth an object, usually metal.

filled resin, *n* See resin, composite.

filled sealant, *n* See resin, composite and resin-filled.

filled teeth, indices and scoring methods for, *n.pl* See index, DEF and index, DMF.

filling, *n* a material used to fill a space. (Objectionable as a synonym for restoration.) See also restoration.

filling, dental, *n* a lay term for restoration.

filling, "ditched," *n* the marginal failure of amalgam restorations caused by fracture of either the material or the tooth structure itself in that area.

filling, material, *n* See material, filling.

filling, postresection, *n* See filling, retrograde.

filling, retrograde (postresection filling, retrograde obturation), *n* a filling placed in the apical portion of a tooth root to seal the apical portion of the root canal.

filling, root canal, *n* material placed in the root canal system to seal the space previously occupied by the dental pulp.

filling, technique, *n* See technique, filling.

filling, treatment, *n* a temporary filling, usually of a sedative nature, used to allay sensitive dentin before the final restoration of the cavity.

film, *n* a thin, flexible, transparent sheet of cellulose acetate or similar material coated with a light-sensitive emulsion.

film badge, *n* a pack of x-ray-sensitive film used for the detection and approximate measurement of radiation exposure for personnel-monitoring purposes; the badge may contain two or three films of differing sensitivity, and it may contain a filter that shields part of the film from certain types of radiation.

film base, *n* See base, film.

film, bite-wing (interproximal film), *n* a type of dental x-ray film that has a central tab or wing on which the teeth close to hold the film in position. See also examination, bite-wing radiographic.

film emulsion, *n* See emulsion, silver.

film fault, *n* a defective result in a radiograph; usually caused by a chemical, physical, or electrical error in its production.

film fault, black spots, n.pl spots caused by dust particles or developer on the films before development; also caused by outdated (expired) film.

film fault, blurred, *n* a fault caused by film movement during exposure, bent film during exposure, double exposures, or flowing of emulsion during processing in excessively warm solution.

film fault, clear radiographic, *n* the result of treating the film with fixer before developing or by excessive washing. The problem can be prevented by following appropriate procedures.

film fault, dark, *n* a fault caused by overexposure of the film to radiation, film fog from extended development, accidental exposure to light (light leaks in film packet or dark room), or an unsafe darkroom light.

film fault, distorted, n See distortion, film-fault.

film fault, dyschroic fog, n a fogging of the radiograph, characterized by the appearance of a pink surface when the film is viewed by transmitted light and a green surface when the film is seen by reflected light. It usually is caused by an exhaustion of the acid content of the fixing solution (incomplete fixation).

film fault, fogged, n a fault caused by stray radiation, use of expired film, or an unsafe darkroom light.

film fault, light, n a fault caused by underexposure, underdevelopment (expired or diluted developing solution), development in temperatures that are too cold, or accidental use of a wrong film speed.

film fault, reticulation, n a network of corrugations produced because of an excessive difference in temperature between any two of the three darkroom solutions.

film fault, roller marks on, n.pl dark lines on films caused by contaminated chemicals in automatic film processing units. Prevented by cleaning and replenishing the developer and fixer solutions regularly.

film fault, stained, n a fault caused by contaminated solutions, improper rinsing, exhausted solutions, improper washing, contamination by improper handling of the emulsions during or after processing, or film hangers containing dried fixer on the clips.

Stain on film from fixer. (Frommer, 2001)

film fault, static electricity, n an image in the emulsion that has the appearance of lightning. Caused by rapid opening of the film pocket or transfer of static electricity from the technician to the film.

film fault, white spots, n a fault caused by air bubbles clinging to the emulsion during development or by fixing solution spotted on the emulsion before development.

film hanger, n an instrument or device for holding x-ray film during processing procedures.

film holder, cardboard, n See cassette, cardboard.

film image, n the shadow of a structure as depicted on a radiographic or photographic emulsion.

film immersion method, n a procedure for processing x-ray films involving submerging the films in a sodium hypochlorite solution for anywhere between 30 seconds and 5 minutes. The solution should be 5.25% sodium hypochlorite.

film, interproximal, n See film, bitewing.

film mounting, n the placement of radiographs in an orderly sequence on a suitable carrier for illumination and study.

film on teeth, n mucinous deposits on teeth, containing microorganisms, desquamated tissue elements, and blood cellular elements; usually thin and adherent.

film packet, n a small, lightproof, moisture-resistant, sealed paper or plastic envelope containing an x-ray film (or two x-ray films) and a lead-foil backing designed for use in making intraoral radiographs.

film placement, n the positioning of the x-ray film to receive the image cast by the roentgen rays.

film processing, n a chemical transformation of the latent image, produced in a film emulsion by exposure to radiation, into a stable image visible by transmitted light. The usual procedure is basically a selective reduction of affected silver halide salts to metallic silver grains (development), followed by the selective removal of unaffected silver halide (fixation), washing to remove the processing chemicals, and drying.

film, processing, acids in, n chemicals that arrest the process of film development and also neutralize leftover developer.

film processing, automatic, n fast and efficient method of processing in which the film is mechanically transferred from the developer to the fixer, is washed and finally dried.

film processing, rapid, n the use of high-speed chemicals or elevated temperatures to reduce processing time.

film speed (film sensitivity), n the amount of exposure to light or roentgen rays required to produce a given image density. It is expressed as the reciprocal of the exposure in roentgens necessary to produce a density of 1 above base and fog; films are classified on this basis in six speed groups, between each of which is a twofold increase in film speed.

film thickness, n refers to the thickness of a layer of material, particularly in reference to dental cements. In standardization tests, film thickness is the minimal thickness or layer obtained under a specific load.

film, x-ray, n See survey, radiographic.

Filoviridae (fī'lōvir'idā), n one of the major virus families, to which both the Marburg and Ebola viruses belong. Viruses in this family have a single-stranded RNA molecular structure with complex symmetry.

filter, n a material placed in the useful beam to absorb preferentially the less energetic (less penetrating) radiations. See also filtration.

filter, added, n a filter added to the inherent filter.

filter, compensating, n a filter designed to shield less dense areas so that a more uniform image quality will be produced.

filter, inherent, n filtration introduced by the glass wall of the x-ray tube, any oil used for tube immersion, or any permanent tube enclosure in the path of useful beam.

filter, orange, n the recommended safelight filter for darkroom illumination when processing intraoral film only. Also called *filter type ML-2.*

filter, red, n the recommended safelight filter for darkroom illumination when processing either intraoral or extraoral film. Also called filter type GBX-2.

filter, total, n the sum of inherent and added filters.

filtration, n the use of absorbers for the selective attenuation of radiation of certain wavelengths from a useful primary beam of x-radiation.

filtration, built-in, n filtration put into effect by nonremovable absorbers deliberately built into the tubehead assembly to increase the inherent beam filtration.

filtration, external, n the action of absorbers external to the tube-head assembly, consisting of added filtration plus the attenuating effect of materials of which any closed-end cone such as a pointer cone may be made. See also filter, added.

financial management, n the management or control of the money or cash flow of a business or enterprise.

financial support, n the funding of a project to assist in its accomplishment.

finasteride, n *trade name:* Proscar; *drug class:* synthetic steroid; *action:* competitive inhibitor of 5-α-reductase, which converts testosterone to 5-α-dihydrotestosterone; *use:* symptomatic benign prostatic hyperplasia.

findings, radiographic (roentgenographic findings), n the recorded radiographic evidence of normal and deviated anatomic structures.

fineness, n a means of grading alloys with regard to gold content. The fineness of an alloy is designated in parts per thousand of pure gold, pure gold being 1,000 fine.

finger, n any one of the five digits of the hand.

finger, clubbed, n a condition seen in hypertrophic osteoarthropathy where the base angle between the base of the fingernail and adjacent dorsal surface of the terminal phalanx is obliterated and becomes 180 degrees or greater. The base of the nail projects downward, and the area of nail is increased.

finger positions, n.pl the positions of the fingers when operating; refers not only to the fingers grasping the instrument but also to the fingers used for rests, support, and holding the tissues out of the way.

finger rest, n an integral part of instrumentation, in which the fingers of the working hand rest on the teeth, adjacent tissues, and fingers of the opposing hand to improve control of the working stroke of an instrument by providing a fulcrum for movement of the working fingers and instruments.

finger rest, reinforced, n provides additional force to the instrument by allowing the thumb of the nondominant hand to be placed on the handle or shank of the instrument while the index (first) finger of the nondominant hand is placed on the adjacent tooth.

finger rest, substitute, n when the customary resting point on an adjacent tooth is inhibited by a missing or inadequately supported tooth, the substitute finger rest may be the dental arch or a gauze sponge or cotton roll packed into the appropriate area.

finger rest, supplementary, n provides additional support by allowing the index (first) finger of the dominant or instrument hand to rest on the index finger of the nondominant hand when it is placed on the occlusal surface of the adjacent teeth.

finger strut, n a bar or similar component of the infrastructure of a subperiosteal or endosteal implant that projects from it, being attached at only one side.

finger sucking, n the habit of sucking the finger (or thumb) for oral gratification. It is normal in infants and young children as a comforting device, especially when tired or hungry. If the habit persists beyond the eruption of the permanent teeth, it may cause a malocclusion of the anterior teeth.

finger sweep, n a method whereby one uses fingers to remove a foreign object from the mouth of an unconscious individual. Finger sweeps should not be performed on small children unless one can clearly see the object.

fingerspelling, *n* the manipulation of fingers into different positions, usually based on the manual alphabet, to represent letters of the alphabet.

finish line, *n* See line, finish.

finish, satin, *n* the degree of finish of a polished surface that has been made very smooth but without a high sheen.

finishing and polishing, *n* the removal of excess restoration material from the margins and contours of a restoration, and polishing of the restoration.

finishing stones, *n.pl* abrasive stones of varying shapes (flame, round, or pear) used to smooth the surfaces of a restoration.

finishing strip, *n* See strip, abrasive.

firmicutes (fur′mikyōōts), *n.pl* one of four major categories of disease-causing bacteria with many subgroups, to which the *Streptococcus* and *Staphylococcus* varieties belong. A gram-positive type of bacteria that has cell walls.

firmness, *n* term used to describe the relative flexibility of toothbrush bristles; determined by bristle thickness and height. See also stiffness.

firmware, *n* a special type of permanent program that takes the place of or accomplishes the function of traditional hardware components. Firmware is loaded into the equipment, either at the time it is manufactured or later, by the person installing the equipment or the person using it.

first aid, *n* the immediate care that is given to an injured or ill person before treatment by medically trained personnel.

first surgical stage (subperiosteal), *n* the operation performed to obtain a direct bone impression.

fission (fish′ən), *n* the splitting of a nucleus into two fragments. Fission may occur spontaneously or may be induced artificially. In addition to the fission fragments, particulate radiation energy and gamma rays are usually produced during fission.

fission, nuclear, products, n.pl elements (nuclides) or compounds resulting from nuclear fission.

fission products, n.pl the nuclides produced by the fission of a heavy-element nuclide.

F

fissure, *n* a deep groove or cleft; commonly the result of the imperfect fusion of the enamel or adjoining dental lobes.

fissure, gingival, *n* See cleft, gingival.

fissure, pterygomaxillary, *n* the most posterior point in the anterior contour of the maxillary tuberosity.

fissured tongue, *n* See tongue, fissured.

fistula (fis′tyōōlə), *n* an abnormal tract connecting two body surfaces or organs or leading from a pathologic or natural internal cavity to the surface. The tract may be lined with epithelium.

fistula, alveolar, *n* a fistula communicating with the cavity of an alveolar abscess. More properly called *alveolar sinus.* See also sinus, alveolar.

fistula, arteriovenous, *n* See shunt, arteriovenous.

fistula, branchial, *n* a fistula associated with a branchial cyst; usually seen on the lateral surface of the neck.

fistula, dental, *n* See fistula, alveolar.

fistula, of lip, *n* a congenital malformation in which there is a deep pit or fistula on the mucosa of the lip; often bilateral and usually found on the lower lip.

fistula, oroantral, *n* an opening between the maxillary sinus and the oral cavity, most often through a tooth socket. See also fistula.

fistula, orofacial, *n* an opening between the cutaneous surface of the face and the oral cavity.

fistula, oronasal, *n* an opening between the nasal cavity and the oral cavity.

fistula, salivary, *n* an opening between a salivary duct and/or gland and the cutaneous surface or into the oral cavity through other than the normal anatomic pathway.

fit, *n* an adaptation of any dental restoration. An adaptation of a denture to its basal seat, a clasp to a tooth, an inlay to a cavity preparation.

fix, *v* to make firm, stable, immovable; to place in a desired position and hold there. In dentistry, to secure in

position, usually by means of cementation, a prosthesis such as a crown or a fixed partial denture.

fixation, *n* the act or result of fixing, such as being bound or limited in position or relationship.

fixation, biphase pin, *n* See appliance, fracture.

fixation, elastic band, *n* the stabilization of fractured segments of the jaws by means of intermaxillary or maxillomandibular elastic bands applied to splints or appliances.

fixation, external pin, *n* See appliance, fracture.

fixation, intermaxillary, *n* See fixation, maxillomandibular.

fixation, intraosseous, *n* the reduction and stabilization of fractured bony parts by direct fixation to one another with surgical wires, screws, pins, and/or plates.

fixation, mandibulomaxillary, *n* See fixation, maxillomandibular.

fixation, maxillomandibular (mandibulomaxillary fixation), *n* a retention of fractures of the maxillae or mandible in the functional relations with the opposing dental arch through the use of elastic wire ligatures and interdental wiring and/or splints.

fixation, nasomandibular, *n* mandibular immobilization, especially for edentulous jaws, using mandibulomaxillary splints, circummandibular wiring, and intraoral interosseous wiring through the nasal process of the maxillae.

fixation, of elements by the skeleton, *n* the fixation of many elements for long periods of time in the bone matrix as a result of a special affinity of the elements for the matrix. Recent work with radioactive isotopes has firmly established the concept of the skeleton as a dynamic system. In addition to the changes in structure and distribution of the bone mineral mediated by cellular activity, every ionic grouping in the mineral is capable of replacement.

fixation, osseous, *n* the immobilization of fractured bony segments.

fixation, radiographic, *n* in film processing, the chemical removal of all the undeveloped salts of the film emulsion, so that only the developed (reduced) silver will remain as a permanent image.

fixation, restorative, *n* the act of securing in position, usually by means of cementation, some treatment appliance such as a crown or fixed partial denture when willful removal of the restoration by the patient is not intended.

fixation, Roger-Anderson pin, *n.pr* an appliance used in extraoral fixation of mandibular fractures and prognathisms. See also appliance, fracture.

fixative, *n* **1.** any substance used to bind, glue, or stabilize. **2.** any substance used to preserve gross or histologic specimens of tissue for later examination.

fixed appliance system, *n* See prosthesis, fixed expansion and prosthodontics, fixed.

fixed costs, *n.pl* costs that do not change to meet fluctuations in enrollment or in use of services (for example, salaries, rent, business license fees, and depreciation).

fixed fee schedule, *n* a list of specified fees for services that will be paid to dentists participating in a dental plan.

fixed partial denture, *n* See denture, partial, fixed.

fixed premium, *n* a specified amount charged for insurance that is not changed by such factors as family size or initial year versus maintenance year of dental care coverage. Also called *set premium.*

fixer, *n* the chemicals used in the final step of film processing that remove the unaffected silver halide particles from the developed film.

fixer stains on film, *n.pl* See film fault, stained.

flabby tissue, *n* See tissue, hyperplastic.

flaccid (flas′id, flak′sid), *adj* being in a relaxed or flabby state, as in a flail-like condition or paralysis of a muscle.

flag, *n* **1.** any of various types of indicators used for identification. **2.** a character that signals the occurrence of some condition, such as the end of a word.

flagella, *n.pl* hairlike projections that extend from some unicellular organisms and aid in their movement.

flagellates (flaj′əlāts), *n.pl* one of four phyla of parasitic protozoa, also called *Mastigophora.* They can cause diseases such as enteritis, urethritis, vaginitis, and Chagas' disease by means of drinking water contamination, vaginal discharge, and bug bite.

flange (flanj), *n* the part of the denture base that extends from the cervical ends of the teeth to the border of the denture.

flange, buccal, *n* the portion of the flange of a denture that occupies the buccal vestibule of the mouth and that extends distally from the buccal notch.

flange, contour of, *n* the topographic design of the flange of a denture.

flange, labial, *n* the portion of the flange of a denture that occupies the labial vestibule of the mouth.

flange, lingual, *n* the portion of the flange of a mandibular denture that occupies the space adjacent to the residual ridge and next to the tongue.

flange-guide appliance, *n* an appliance (prosthesis) with a lateral vertical extension designed to direct a resected mandible into centric occlusion.

flap(s), *n* a sheet (or sheets) of soft tissue partially or totally detached to gain access to structures underneath or to be used in repairing defects in an adjacent or a remote part of the body.

flap, envelope, *n* mucoperiosteal tissue retracted from a horizontal linear incision (as along the free gingival margin), with no vertical component of the incision.

flap, lingual tongue, *n* a flap used to repair a fistula of the hard palate, which combines the raising of a palatal flap to form the floor of the nose with a flap taken from the back or edge of the tongue to form the palatal surface.

flap, mucoperiosteal, *n* a flap of mucosal tissue, including the periosteum, reflected from a bone.

flap, pedicle, *n* a stalk-shaped attachment to a flap.

flaps, periodontal, *n* a portion of periodontal tissue partially removed for curettage or for removing a pocket by rearranging the soft tissue;

also useful for gaining access to the alveolar bone.

flap, sliding, n a flap that is advanced from its original location in a direction away from its base, to close a defect.

flap, V-Y, n a flap in which the incision is shaped like a V and after closure like a Y, to lengthen a localized area of tissue. See also flap, Y-V.

flap, Y-V, n a flap in which the incision is shaped like a Y and after closure like a V, to shorten a localized area of tissue. See also flap, V-Y.

flash, *n* excess material that is squeezed out of the mold (for example, during packing of a denture by compression technique).

flash, proximal-gingival, n an overhang that may occur inside the matrix band when a proximal wedge is positioned improperly or not used at all; more likely to occur on concave proximal surfaces.

flask, *n* a metal case or tube used in investing procedures.

flask, casting, n See flask, refractory.

flask, closure, n the procedure of bringing the parts of a flask together to form a complete mold.

flask, crown, n a small, sectional, metal, boxlike case in which a sectional mold of plaster of paris or artificial stone is made for the purpose of compressing and curing plastics on small dental restorations.

flask, denture, n a sectional, metal, boxlike case in which a sectional mold of plaster of paris or artificial stone is made for the purpose of compressing and curing dentures or other resinous restorations.

flask, final, closure, n the last closure of a flask before curing and after trial packing the mold with a denture base material.

flask, injection, n a special flask designed to permit the filling of the mold after the flask is closed or to permit the addition of denture base material to that in the flask after the flask is closed.

flask, refractory (casting flask, casting ring), n a metal tube in which a refractory mold is made for casting metal dental restorations or appliances.

flask, trial, closure, n a preliminary closure made for the purposes of

eliminating excess denture base or other plastic material and of ensuring that the mold is completely filled.

flasking, *n* the act of investing a pattern in a flask. The process of investing the cast and a wax denture in a flask preparatory to molding the denture base material into the form of the denture.

Flavobacterium, n a genus of aerobic to facultatively anaerobic, nonsporeforming, motile, and nonmotile bacteria. These organisms characteristically produce yellow, orange, red, or yellow-brown pigments. They are found in soil and fresh and salt water. Some species are pathogenic.

flavonoids, *n.pl* a group of substances containing the plant pigment flavone. There is no known human requirement for them. They have a constrictor effect on the capillary bed and decrease permeability of blood vessels. Some beneficial effects of flavonoids have been described in the treatment of bruises, contusions, and sprains. Also known as *bioflavonoid.*

flavoxate HCl, *n trade name:* Urispas; *drug class:* antispasmodic; *action:* relaxes smooth muscles in urinary tract; *uses:* relief of nocturia, incontinence, suprapubic pain, dysuria.

flecainide acetate, *n trade name:* Tambocor; *drug class:* antidysrhythmic (Class IC); *action:* decreases conduction in all parts of the heart with greatest effect on His-Purkinje system; *uses:* life-threatening ventricular dysrhythmias, sustained supraventricular tachycardia.

flexibility, *n* the property of elastic deformation under loading.

flexible benefits, *n.pl* a benefits program in which an employee has a choice of credits or dollars for distribution among various benefit options (for example, health and disability insurance, dental benefits, child care, pension benefits). See also cafeteria plans and flexible spending account.

flexible spending account, *n* an employee reimbursement account primarily funded with employee-designated salary reductions. Funds are reimbursed to the employee for health care (medical and/or dental), dependent care, and/or legal expenses and are considered a nontaxable benefit.

flexion (flek′shən), *n* the bending of a joint between two skeletal members to decrease the angle between the members; opposite of extension.

flexion-extension reflex, *n* See reflex, flexion-extension.

flexure (flek′shur), *n* the quality or state of being flexed.

flexure, clasp, *n* the flexure of a retentive clasp arm to permit passage over the surveyed height of contour, thus permitting the seating or removal of the clasp.

floater, *n* one or more spots that appear to drift in front of the eye, caused by a shadow cast on the retina by vitreous debris.

floor of cavity, *n* See cavity floor.

floppy disk, *n* a lightweight computer disk platter that is kept in a protective envelope and can be used for file information (storage). Also called *diskette* and *flexible disk.*

flora (flôr′ə), *n.pl* the bacteria living in various parts of the alimentary canal.

flora, fusospirochetal, *n.pl* the microorganisms *Fusobacterium fusiforme* and *Borrelia vincentii.* Present in most individuals as normal inhabitants of the oral cavity. Believed by some to be the primary and by others the secondary cause of acute necrotizing ulcerative gingivitis (ANUG).

flora, normal oral, *n.pl* the varying types of bacteria that are usually present in the mouth.

flora, oral, *n.pl* the microorganisms inhabiting the oral cavity of an individual. They are usually saprophytic in nature and live together in a symbiotic relationship. Some are potentially pathogenic, assuming a pathologic role when adverse local or systemic factors such as increased body temperature influence the symbiotic balance of the microorganic flora.

floss, *n* a waxed or unwaxed string or tape used to remove plaque from the interproximal and contact areas of the teeth. Its regular and proper use is essential to good oral hygiene and prevention of both dental caries and periodontal disease.

floss cleft, *n* a narrow gap created in the gum between the teeth by floss

that is repeatedly positioned incorrectly so that it presses against the gingiva.

floss cuts, prevention of, *n* patient care information centered around the protection of injury to the gums, particularly the col. Instruction includes careful attention to the angle and thickness of floss used, as well as proper flossing technique.

floss, expanded PTFE dental, *n* one of three varieties of filament-based dental hygiene tools; consists of a waxy man-made chemical called polytetrafluoroetilene; tends to resist shredding and breaking.

floss, tape, *n* a silk tape often incorporated with pumice and used to polish the proximal surfaces of teeth.

floss, tufted dental, *n* floss made from alternating sections of traditional thin fiber and thicker tufted fiber which is especially suited to removing plaque from teeth separated by wide spaces.

flossing, *n* the mechanical cleansing of interproximal tooth surfaces with stringlike, waxed or unwaxed dental floss or tape.

flossing aids, *n.pl* commercially available devices designed to make flossing easier and more effective, particularly in places that are tight or difficult to reach. These include plastic holders and threaders.

Flossing aids. (Daniel/Harfst, 2002)

flow, *n* to move in a manner similar to a liquid stream.

flow, dental material, *n* the continued deformation or change in shape under a static load, as with waxes and amalgam.

flow, traffic, *n* the pattern of office personnel and patient movement from one area within the office to another.

flowchart, *n* a graphic representation of a sequence of operations using symbols to represent the operations. Flowcharts often symbolize the most important steps of the process without detailing the algorithm of the way the work is to be performed.

flowmeter, *n* a physical device for measuring the rate of flow of a gas or liquid.

fluconazole, *n trade name:* Diflucan; *drug class:* antifungal; *action:* inhibits ergosterol biosynthesis; *uses:* oropharyngeal candidiasis, urinary candidiasis, cryptococcal meningitis, vaginal candidiasis.

fluctuation, *n* a wavelike motion produced in soft tissues in response to palpation or percussion. Fluctuation is caused by a collection of fluids or exudates in the tissues.

flucytosine, *n trade name:* Ancobon; *drug class:* antifungal; *action:* converted to fluorouracil after entering fungi, which inhibits DNA and RNA synthesis; *uses: Candida* infections.

fludrocortisone acetate, *n trade name:* Florinef Acetate; *drug class:* glucocorticoid, mineralocorticoid; *action:* promotes increased reabsorption of sodium and loss of potassium from renal tubules; *uses:* adrenal insufficiency, salt-losing adrenogenital syndrome.

fluid (flōō′id), *n* a liquid or gaseous substance.

fluid, crevicular, *n* a clear, usually unnoticeable fluid that can serve as a defense mechanism against infection by carrying antibodies and other therapeutic substances between the connective tissue and sulcus or pocket. Also called *gingival sulcus fluid* or *sulcular fluid.*

fluid delivery, *n* the continual fluid stream of an ultrasonic instrument, either over or through the vibrating tip, which is necessary to maintain a stable instrument temperature throughout a procedure.

fluid, synovial, *n* the small amount of fluid occurring in normal joints. Its principal function is to lubricate the joint surfaces and nourish the articular cartilage. Its content is approximately 95% water, with only 1% to 2% protein concentration.

fluid, total body, *n* all the fluids contained in the body. There are two main types: the intracellular fluid, which is contained totally within the cells, and the extracellular fluid, which is contained entirely outside the cells.

fluid wax, *n* See wax, fluid.

flumazenil, *n trade name:* Romazicon; *drug class:* benzodiazepine receptor antagonist; *action:* antagonizes actions of benziodiazepines on the central nervous system; *use:* reversal of sedative effects of benzodiazepines.

flunisolide, *n trade name:* Oral INH aerosol, AeroBid; *drug class:* synthetic glucocorticoid; *action:* long-acting synthetic adrenocorticoid with antiinflammatory activity; *use:* rhinitis (seasonal or perennial).

fluocinonide, *n trade names:* Licon, Lidex, Lidex-E; *drug class:* topical corticosteroid; *action:* interacts with steroid cytoplasmic receptors to induce antiinflammatory effects; possesses antipruritic, antiinflammatory actions; *uses:* psoriasis, eczema, contact dermatitis, pruritus, oral lichen planus lesions.

fluorapatite (flôrap′ətīt), *n* a member of the family of minerals that make up the basic structure of bones and teeth; basically a hydroxapatite form in which fluoride ions replace hydroxyl ions.

fluorescein (flôres′ē-in), *n* a dye applied to teeth to reveal plaque. In ophthalmology, it is used to discover corneal lesions.

fluorescence (fləres′əns), *n* the emission of radiation of a particular wavelength by certain substances as the result of absorption of radiation of a shorter wavelength.

fluorescent screen, *n* See screen, intensifying.

fluorhydroxyapatite (flôr′hīdrok′sē-ap′ətīt), *n* a member of the family of minerals that make up the basic structure of bones and teeth. It is formed when small amounts of fluoride and teeth mineral react. When higher concentrations of fluoride are involved, the result is the formation of calcium fluoride.

fluoridate (flôr′idāt), v to add fluoride to a water supply.

fluoridated salt, n sodium chloride with fluoride added; not considered as effective as fluoridated water.

fluoridation, n 1. the process of adding fluoride to a public water supply to reduce tooth decay. 2. the use of a fluoride to reduce caries activity; may be by means of communal water supplies; oral hygiene preparations for home use; or topical applications for the purpose of prophylaxis.

fluoride(s), n a salt of hydrofluoric acid, commonly sodium or stannous (tin).

fluoride dietary supplements, n.pl orally administered nutritional additives of the chemical fluoride; often taken by individuals without regular access to a fluoridated water supply; available as a mouthrinse, chewable tablet, drops, lozenge, pill, and in combination with vitamin supplements.

fluoride drops, n a supplemental liquid form of the chemical fluoride. They are primarily administered to children from six months to three years of age.

fluoride tablets/lozenges, n.pl supplemental forms of the chemical fluoride. Tablets must be chewed, and lozenges must be held in the mouth until dissolved in order to benefit from the fluoride's contact with the teeth.

fluorides, topical, n.pl salts of hydrofluoric acid (usually sodium or tin salts) that may be applied in solution to the enamel surface of the teeth to prevent dental decay.

fluorides, topical, paint-on technique, n a professionally administered procedure in which the dental surfaces are coated with a fluoride solution or gel to discourage caries and encourage remineralization.

fluoridization (flôr′idizā′shən), n the topical application of a solution of a fluoride to teeth. See also fluorides, topical.

fluorine, n an element of the halogen family and the most reactive of the nonmetals. Its atomic number is 9, and its atomic weight is 19. Small amounts of sodium fluoride added to

the public water supply will reduce the incidence of dental caries, particularly among children. Excessive amounts of fluoride can mottle tooth enamel and cause osteosclerosis. Acute fluoride poisoning can cause death.

fluoroscope (flôr′əscōp), n a device consisting of a fluorescent screen mounted in a metal frame covered with lead glass. In the presence of a roentgen ray, the screen glows in direct proportion to the intensity of the remnant x-radiation, producing visual impressions of the densities traversed.

fluorosis (flərō′sis), n enamel hypoplasia caused by the ingestion of water containing excess fluoride during the time of enamel formation. General term for chronic fluoride poisoning.

Fluorosis. (Bird/Robinson, 2002)

fluorosis, chronic endemic dental (mottled enamel), n an enamel defect caused by excessive ingestion of fluoride in the water supply (usually 2 to 8 ppm) during the period of tooth calcification. Affected teeth appear chalky white on eruption and later turn brown.

fluorosis, index of dental, n a classification system for determining the presence and severity of chronic fluoride poisoning in which the enamel on individual teeth is rated against a 0 to 4 scale with 0 representing normal enamel and 4 severely damaged enamel. This index may be used by communities to adjust the levels of fluoride in their water systems.

fluorouracil (topical), n *trade names:* Efudex, Fluoroplex; *drug class:* topical antineoplastic; *action:*

inhibits synthesis of DNA and RNA in susceptible cells; *uses:* keratosis, basal cell carcinoma.

Fluothane, *n.pr* the trade name for halothane.

fluoxetine, *n* *trade name:* Prozac; *drug class:* antidepressant; *action:* inhibits CNS neuron uptake of serotonin but not norepinephrine; *use:* depressive disorders.

fluoxymesterone, *n* *trade names:* Android-F, Halotestin; *drug class:* androgenic anabolic steroid, Controlled Substance Schedule III; *action:* increases weight by building body tissue; increases potassium, phosphorus, chloride, nitrogen levels; increases bone development; *uses:* impotence from testicular deficiency, hypogonadism, breast engorgement, palliative treatment of female breast cancer.

fluphenazine decanoate/fluphenazine enanthate/fluphenazine HCl, *n* *trade names:* Decanoate, Moditen, Prolixin Enanthate; *drug class:* phenothiazine antipsychotic; *action:* blocks neurotransmission at dopaminergic synapses in the cerebral cortex, hypothalamus, and limbic system; *uses:* psychotic disorders, schizophrenia.

flurandrenolide, *n* *trade names:* Cordran, Cordran SP; *drug class:* topical corticosteroid, group III medium potency; *action:* possesses antipruritic, anti-inflammatory actions; *uses:* corticosteroid-responsive dermatoses, pruritus.

flurazepam HCl, *n* *trade name:* Dalmane; *drug class:* benzodiazepine, sedative-hypnotic, Controlled Substance Schedule IV; *action:* produces central nervous system depression by interaction with benzodiazepine receptor to facilitate action of inhibitory neurotransmitter γ-aminobutyric acid (GABA); *uses:* insomnia.

flurbiprofen, *n* *trade name:* Ansaid; *drug class:* nonsteroidal antiinflammatory; *action:* inhibits prostaglandin synthesis by interfering with cyclooxygenase needed for biosynthesis; possesses analgesic, antiinflammatory, antipyretic properties; *uses:* acute, long-term treatment of rheumatoid arthritis, osteoarthritis.

flurbiprofen sodium, *n* *trade name:* Ocufen; *drug class:* nonsteroidal an-

tiinflammatory ophthalmic; *action:* inhibits enzyme system necessary for biosynthesis of prostaglandins, inhibits miosis; *uses:* inhibition of intraoperative miosis, corneal edema.

flush, *n* **1.** a blush or sudden reddening of the face and neck caused by vasodilation of small arteries and arterioles. **2.** a sudden, subjective feeling of heat. **3.** a sudden, rapid flow of water or other liquid.

flutamide, *n* *trade name:* Eulexin; *drug class:* antineoplastic; *action:* interferes with testosterone at cellular level, inhibits androgen uptake; *uses:* metastatic prostatic carcinoma, stage D2 in combination with LHRH agonistic analogs (leuprolide).

fluticasone propionate, *n* *trade name:* Cutivate (topical), Flonase (nasal spray); *drug class:* synthetic corticosteroid, medium potency; *action:* interacts with steroid cytoplasmic receptors to induce antiinflammatory effects; possesses antipruritic, antiinflammatory actions; *uses:* topical for inflammation of corticosteroid-responsive skin disorders; spray for seasonal and perennial allergic rhinitis.

fluting, *n* depressions along tooth root surfaces, formed during development.

flutter, *n* a quick, irregular motion.

fluvastatin sodium, *n* *trade name:* Lescol; *drug class:* cholesterol-lowering agent; *action:* inhibits HMG-CoA reductase enzyme, which reduces cholesterol synthesis; *uses:* adjunct in primary hypocholesterolemia (types IIa and IIb).

fluvoxamine maleate, *n* *trade name:* Luvox; *drug class:* antidepressant; *action:* selectively inhibits reuptake of serotonin in central nervous system neurons; *uses:* obsessive-compulsive disorder.

flux, *n* any substance or mixture used to promote fusion, especially the fusion of metals or minerals. Used principally in dentistry as an inclusion in ceramic materials and in soldering and casting metals.

flux, casting, *n* a flux that increases fluidity of the metal and helps to prevent oxidation.

flux, ceramic, *n* a flux used in the manufacture of porcelain and silicate powders.

flux, reducing, *n* a flux that contains powdered charcoal to remove oxides.

flux, soldering, *n* a ceramic material such as borax, boric acid, or a combination, in paste, liquid, or granular form; used to keep metallic parts clean while they are being heated during a soldering procedure. It is a solvent for metallic oxides and will flow over the parts to be soldered at temperatures well below the fusion temperature of solder, but it becomes separated from the solid metal by the molten solder.

FMIA, *n pr* See angle, Frankfort-mandibular incisor.

focal infection, *n* the site or origin of an infectious process. Endodontically treated teeth have frequently been accused of being the source of septicemias, often without justification. See also infection, focal.

focal spot, *n* See spot, focal.

focal-film distance, *n* See distance, target-film.

focus group, *n* a demographic target group of people used to gather opinions or data descriptive of the population represented by the sample selected.

fog (fogging), *n* See film fault, fogged.

fog, chemical, *n* See film fault.

fog, dyschroic, *n* See film fault, dyschroic fog.

fog, light, *n* See film fault.

fog, radiation, *n* film darkening caused by radiation from sources other than intentional exposure to the primary beam; for example, film may be exposed to scatter radiation, or accidental exposure may occur if stored film is not protected from radiation.

foil, *n* a very thin, flexible sheet of metal, usually gold, platinum, or tin.

foil, adhesive, *n* tin foil that is covered on one side with powdered gum arabic or karaya gum.

foil assistant, *n* See foil holder.

foil, cohesive gold, *n* a gold foil that has been annealed or had a surface so completely pure so that it will cohere or weld at room temperature.

foil, corrugated gold, *n* a gold foil made by burning gold foil sheets between paper in the absence of air.

foil cylinder, *n* a cylinder of gold foil formed by repeatedly folding a sheet of foil into a narrow ribbon, which is then rolled into cylindrical form.

foil, gold (fibrous gold), *n* pure gold that has been rolled and beaten from ingots into a very thin sheet. Thickness usually varies from 1/40,000 inch (No. 2 foil) to 1/20,000 inch (No. 4 foil). Classified as cohesive, semicohesive, or noncohesive. One of the oldest restorative materials, the most permanent if used properly, and the yardstick by which all others are measured. It is compacted or condensed into a retentive cavity form piece by piece, using this metal's property of cold welding.

foil holder (foil assistant), *n* an instrument used to retain a foil pellet in place while it is being condensed or to retain a bulk of gold while additions to it are made.

foil, noncohesive gold, *n* a gold foil that will not cohere at room temperature because of the presence on its surface of a protecting or contaminating coating. If the coating is a volatile substance, such as ammonia, the foil may be rendered cohesive by heating or annealing it to remove the protection.

foil passer (foil carrier), *n* a pointed or forked instrument used to carry pellets of gold foil through an annealing flame or from the annealing tray to the prepared cavity for compaction.

foil pellet, *n* See pellet, foil.

foil, platinized gold, *n* a form rolled or hammered from a "sandwich" made of platinum placed between two sheets of gold; used in portions of foil restorations where greater hardness is desired.

foil, platinum, *n* pure platinum rolled into extremely thin sheets. A precious-metal foil whose high fusing point makes it suitable as a matrix for various soldering procedures; also suitable for providing the internal form of porcelain restorations during fabrication.

foil, tin, *n* a base-metal foil used as a separating material, or protective covering (for example, between the cast and denture base material during flasking and curing procedures).

folate (fō'lāt), *n* a form of folic acid that helps transport single carbon units between molecules.

fold, *n* a doubling back of a tissue surface.

fold, mucobuccal (mucobuccal reflection), *n* the line of flexure of the oral mucous membrane as it passes from the mandible or maxillae to the cheek.

fold, mucolabial, *n* the line of flexure of the oral mucous membrane as it passes from the mandible or maxillae to the lip.

fold, sublingual, *n* the crescent-shaped area on the floor of the mouth following the medial wall of the mandible and tapering toward the molar regions. It is formed by the sublingual gland and the submandibular duct inferior to the mucous membrane of the alveololingual sulcus.

folder, *n* usually a heavy paper envelope in which the patient's records are kept.

folic acid, *n* vitamin B$_9$, a water-soluble B vitamin needed for erythropoiesis, increases red blood cell, white blood cell, and platelet formation in megaloblastic anemias. Folic acid functions as a coenzyme with vitamin B$_{12}$ and C in the breakdown and utilization of proteins and in the formation of nucleic acids. It is prescribed for use during pregnancy, megaloblastic or macrocytic anemia caused by folic acid deficiency, liver disease, alcoholism, hemolysis, and intestinal obstruction.

folic acid analog, *n* an antimetabolite drug used as an antineoplastic agent in the treatment of malignant cell growths.

follicle (dental), *n* the small sac that contains and protects a developing tooth prior to its emergence from the gingiva.

follicular cyst, *n* an odontogenic cyst that arises from the epithelium of a tooth bud and dental lamina.

follow-up, *n* the process of monitoring the progress of a patient after a period of active treatment.

fomite (fomes) (fō'mīt, fō'mēz), *n* a nonliving object that may carry germs. An inanimate source of disease, such as a drinking glass used by an infected person.

Fones's method, *n.pr* See method, Fones's.

food, *n* ingested solids and liquids that supply the body with nutrients and energy.

food additives, *n.pl* substances that are added to foods to prevent spoilage, improve appearance, enhance the flavor or texture, or increase the nutritional value.

Food and Drug Administration (FDA), *n.pr* an agency of the Department of Health and Human Services responsible for the enforcement of the Federal Food, Drug, and Cosmetic Act and other statutes as assigned.

food, comminution of (kom'inōō' shən), *n* the reduction of food into small parts.

food debris, *n* particles of food remaining in the mouth after eating which collect in tooth crevices and between the teeth and may contribute to the formation of dental caries.

Food Drug and Cosmetic Act (FD & C), *n.pr* legislation passed in 1906 dealing with import and export activity as well as the enforcement of packaging and labeling requirements of all food, drug, and cosmetic commerce within the United States.

food frequency checklist, *n* a tool used by individuals to determine how often they are ingesting certain types of foods. Consists of a list of various foods from all food groups, and a grid allowing for a range of answers, from never to five or more times per day.

food gorging, *n* rapidly ingesting large amounts of food; stuffing; in bulimia, gorging is alternated with purging as a weight-maintenance regimen.

Food Guide Pyramid, *n.pr* a graphic list issued and endorsed by the US Departments of Agriculture and Health and Human Services; outlines recommendations for a healthy, balanced diet. Through the illustration of a three-dimensional triangle, it divides daily diet choices according to recommended frequency of ingestion.

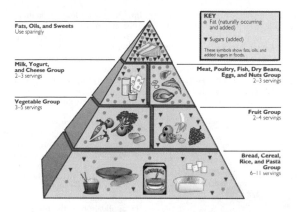

Food guide pyramid. (US Department of Agriculture)

food impaction, *n* See impaction, food.

food, physical character of, *n* the consistency, as the firmness, viscosity, or density, of food substances. Soft, adhesive, and nonabrasive foods tend to cling to the teeth, which may lead to calculus formation, whereas coarse foods leave little debris and create a frictional effect on the tissues, thus cleansing them.

food record, *n* a manually recorded history of an individual's dietary intake over a twenty-four hour period; subsequently analyzed by a dental hygienist in order to help correct any nutritional imbalances.

Food	Veg	Fruit	Meat	Milk	Bread	Other
Patient's name _____ Date _____						
Orange juice		1				
Coffee						1
Toast					1	
Butter						1
Jam						1
Pizza	1			1	1	
Diet soda						1
Candy bar						1
Chicken, roasted			1			
Baked potato	1					
Butter						1
Sour cream						1
Broccoli	1					
Cheese sauce				1		
Ice cream				1		
Totals	3	1	1	3	2	7

Food record. (Bird/Robinson, 2002)

football, *n* a popular American high school, collegiate, and professional team contact sport that may result in facial and dental injuries despite the use of protective headgear.

foramen (fôrā′mən), *n* **1.** a natural opening in a bone or other structure. **2.** a natural opening in the root, usually at or near the apical end.

Sphenopalatine foramen

Foramen. (Liebgott, 2001)

foramen cecum **(fôrā′men sē′kum),** *n* a small depression in the dorsal surface of the tongue where the median lingual sulcus meets the lingual tonsil.

foramen, incisive **(insī′siv),** *n* (nasopalatine foramen), **1.** the opening of the nasopalatine canal. **2.** the foramen, or opening, in the midline of the palate in the region where the premaxilla and maxillae join, which is situated palatal to the maxillary central incisors; contains nasopalatine vessels and nerve.

foramen magnum, *n* a passage in the occipital bone through which the spinal cord enters the spinal column.

foramen, mandibular, *n* the opening on the medial aspect of the vertical ramus of the mandible approximately midway between the mandibular and gonial notches; may be located posterior to the middle of the ramus. It contains interior alveolar vessels and the inferior alveolar nerve.

foramen, mental, *n* a circular opening on the lateral aspect of the body of the mandible either below the apex of the first premolar or below the apex of the second premolar, but usually between the first and second premolars inferior to their apices. The mental vessels and nerve pass through this foramen to supply the

lip. In edentulous mandibles, the bone may have been resorbed, so that it is in such a position that the denture base will cover it.

foramen, nasopalatine, *n* See foramen, incisive.

force, *n* any application of energy, either internal or external to a structure; that which initiates, changes, or arrests motion.

force and stress, *n* pressure forcibly exerted on the teeth and on their investing and supporting tissues that is detrimental to tissue integrity. In occlusal trauma, the production of lesions of the attachment apparatus depends on an interrelationship of the strength, duration, and frequency of the application of the force.

force, centrifugal, *n* a force that tends to recede from the center.

force, chewing, *n* the degree of force applied by the muscles of mastication during the mastication of food.

force, component of, *n* **1.** one of the factors from which a resultant force may be compounded or into which it may be resolved. **2.** one of the parts of a force into which it may be resolved.

force, condensing, *n* **1.** the force required to compress gold-foil pellets, facilitating their cohesion, to fabricate or build up a gold-foil restoration. **2.** the force required to compact or condense a plastic material (for example, amalgam, wax).

force, constant, *n* a continuous force or pressure applied to the teeth.

force, counter-dislodgement, *n* any pressure which comes into play when food is evenly distributed in the mouth so that contact between the upper and lower teeth is equalized on both sides during mastication.

force, denture-dislodging, *n* an influence that tends to displace a denture from its intended position on supporting structures.

force, denture-retaining, *n* an influence that tends to maintain a denture in its intended position on its supporting structures.

force, electromotive, *n* the difference in potential in a roentgen-ray tube between the cathode and anode; usually expressed in kilovolts.

force, intermittent, *n* a force or pressure (applied to the teeth) that is alternated with a period of passiveness or rest.

force, line of, n the direction of the power exerted on a body.

force, masticatory, n the force applied by the muscles attached to the mandible during mastication.

force, occlusal (occlusal load), n 1. the result of muscular forces applied on opposing teeth. 2. the force transmitted to the teeth and their supporting structures by tooth-to-tooth contact or through a bolus of food or other interposed substance.

forced expiratory volume (FEV), n the volume of air that can be forcibly expelled in a fixed time period after full inspiration.

forceps, n 1. an instrument used for grasping or applying force to teeth, tissues, or other objects. 2. an instrument used for grasping and holding tissues or specific structures. (Objectionable term in restorative dentistry because of its association with the extraction of teeth.)

forceps, bone, n the force used for grasping or cutting bone.

forceps, chalazion, n a thumb forceps with a flattened plate at the end of one arm and a matching ring on the other. Originally used for isolation of eyelid tumors. It is useful for isolation of lip and cheek lesions, such as a mucocele, to facilitate removal.

forceps, dental extracting, n forceps used for grasping teeth.

forceps, hemostatic, n an instrument for grasping blood vessels to control hemorrhage.

forceps, insertion, n See forceps, point.

forceps, lock, n See forceps, point.

forceps, Magill, n.pr a tongs-shaped tool used to remove objects from the mouth.

forceps, mosquito, n a small hemostatic forceps.

forceps, point (lock forceps, insertion forceps), n a device used in filling root canals that securely holds the filling cones during their placement.

forceps, rubber dam clamp, n forceps whose beaks are designed to engage holes in the rubber dam retainer to facilitate its placement, adjustment, or removal.

forceps, suture, n See needle holder.

forceps, thumb, n forceps used for grasping soft tissue; used especially during suturing.

forceps, tissue, n a thumb forceps; an instrument with one or more fine teeth at the tip of each blade for controlling tissues during surgery, especially during suturing.

Fordyce's spots, n.pr See spots, Fordyce's.

forecasting, n the attempt to predict the future on the basis of expert opinion, market research, trend projection, leading indicators, and other modalities.

forehead, n that portion of the face directly above the orbits and extending posteriorly/superiorly to the hair line or crown of the head.

foreign body, n any object or substance found in the body in an organ or tissue in which it does not belong under normal circumstances, such as a bolus of food in the trachea or a particle of dust in the eye. See also body, foreign.

forensic, adj pertaining to the law or to legal proceedings.

forensic anthropology, n the use of anatomic structures and physical characteristics to identify a subject for legal purposes.

forensic dentistry, n the use of den tal characteristics for the purpose of identifying a subject for legal purposes. See also jurisprudence, dental.

foreshortening, n See distortion, vertical.

forging, n working or shaping heated metal; hot-working a metal.

fork, face-bow, n the part of the face-bow assembly used to attach an occlusion rim or transfer record of maxillary teeth to the face-bow proper.

form, n the configuration, shape, or particular appearance of anything.

form, acquaintance, n a registration sheet for new patients on which data (for example, the patient's name and address) are recorded and that contains a statement of the policies of the specific dentist's office and the responsibilities of the dentist to the patient.

form, anatomic, n the natural shape of a part.

Anatomic charting form. (Bird/Robinson, 2002)

form, anatomic charting, *n* one of three types of manually recorded dental documentation, features a graphic template displaying a representation of each tooth, as well as the roots and gums. Design provides for note taking associated with each tooth. The form becomes part of the patient's legal health records and is useful for planning patient care, ascertaining legal questions regarding treatment, and is relied upon for patient identification in the event of an emergency. See also form, examination.

form, arch, *n* the shape of the dental arch. See also arch, dental.

form, convenience, *n* the modifications necessary, beyond basic outline form, to facilitate proper instrumentation for the preparation of the cavity or insertion of the restorative material; also the placing of starting points or slight undercuts to retain the first portions of restorative material while succeeding portions are placed.

form, examination, *n* written documentation recording the thorough assessment of the oral cavity and surrounding structures. The form should include patient history and descriptions of observed abnormalities of visible characteristics. Also called *record form.*

form, face, *n* the outline form of the face from an anterior frontal view.

form, functional, *n* the shape that permits optimal performance.

form, geographic charting, *n* one of three types of manually recorded dental documentation, describes each tooth by either a number or a letter within a quadrant. The gums and roots of the teeth are not included, making this chart unsuitable for periodontal assessment.

Geographic charting form. (Bird/Robinson, 2002)

form, message, *n* a checklist form, by means of which auxiliary personnel can quickly make a record of telephone communications for the dentist to peruse later.

form, occlusal, *n* the form of the occlusal surface of a tooth, a row of teeth, or dentition.

form, outline, *n* the shape of the area of the tooth surface included within the cavosurface margins of a prepared cavity.

form, posterior tooth, *n* the distinguishing contours of the occlusal surface of the various posterior teeth.

form, registration, *n* a form used to gather personal (nonprofessional) data about a patient.

form, resistance, *n* the shape given to a prepared cavity to enable the restoration and remaining tooth structure to withstand masticatory stress.

form, retention, *n* the provision made in a cavity preparation to prevent displacement of the restoration.

form, root, *n* the shape of the root of the tooth. It is capable of being modified by such factors as resorption and cemental apposition.

form, tooth, *n* the characteristics of the curves, lines, angles, and contours of various teeth that permit their identification and differentiation.

formaldehyde, *n* a toxic, pungent water-soluble gas used in the aqueous form as a disinfectant, fixative, or tissue preservative.

formalin, *n* a clear aqueous solution of formaldehyde. A 37% solution is used to fix and preserve tissues for histologic and pathologic study.

format, *n* a predetermined computer arrangement of characters, fields, lines, page numbers, punctuation marks, and the like.

former, angle, *n* See angle former.

former, crucible, *n* See sprue former.

former, sprue, *n* See sprue former.

formocresol, *n* a compound consisting of formaldehyde, cresol, glycerin, and water used in vital pulpotomy of primary teeth and as a temporary intracanal medicament during root canal therapy. *Trade name:* Buckley's Formo Cresol.

fortified (fôrtə'fīd), *adj* containing additives more potent than the principal ingredient.

forward protrusion, *n* See protrusion, forward.

foscarnet sodium/phosphonoformic acid, *n trade name:* Foscavir; *drug class:* antiviral; *action:* antiviral activity is produced by selective inhibition at the pyrophosphate binding site on virus-specific DNA polymerases, inhibits replication of all known herpesviruses; *uses:* CMV retinitis in AIDS, acyclovir-resistant herpes zoster in HIV-infected patients.

Foshay's test, *n.pr* See test, Foshay's.

fosinopril, *n trade name:* Monopril; *drug class:* angiotensin-converting enzyme (ACE) inhibitor; *action:* selectively suppresses renin-angiotensin-aldosterone system; *uses:* hypertension alone or in combination with thiazide diuretics.

fossa (fos'ə), *n* a pit, hollow, or depression.

Fossa. (Bath-Balogh/Fehrenbach, 1997)

fossa, canine, *n* the concavity, or depression, in the maxilla superior to the apex of the canine tooth.

fossa, depth of, *n* the distance from the top of the shorter cusp downward into the bottom of the fossa.

fossa, nasal, *n* See cavity, nasal.

foundation, *n* **1.** a charitable organization usually established to allocate private funds to worthy projects or to provide other services. **2.** in dentistry, any device or material added to a remaining tooth structure to enhance the stability and retention of an overlying cast restoration. May be a pin retainer of amalgam, plastic cement, or a casting.

four-handed dentistry, *n* See dentistry, four-handed.

fovea, palatine (fō′vē-ə), *n* small depression at the junction between the hard and soft palates; plays a role in the gag reflex.

Fox scissors, *n.pr* See scissors, Fox.

Fox's knife, *n.pr* See knife, Goldman-Fox.

fractionation, *n* **1.** the separation of a substance into its basic constituents. **2.** the process of isolating a pure culture by sucessive culturing of a small portion of a colony of bacteria. **3.** the process of isolating different components of living cells by centrifugation. **4.** the process of administering a dose of radiation in smaller units over a period of time to minimize tissue damage.

fracture, *n* a break or rupture of a part. In the oral region, fracture is most frequently seen in teeth and bones.

fracture, avulsion, *n* the loss of a section of bone.

fracture, blow-out, *n* a fracture involving the orbital floor, its contents, and the superior wall of the maxillary antrum, in which orbital contents are incarcerated in the fracture area, producing diplopia.

fracture, cementum, *n* the tearing of fragments of the cementum from the tooth root.

fracture, clasp, *n* failure of a clasp arm because of stresses that have exceeded the elastic limit of the metal from which the arm was made.

fracture, closed reduction of, *n* a reduction and fixation of fractured bones without making a surgical opening to the fracture site.

fracture, comminuted, *n* a fracture in which the bone has several lines of fracture in the same region; a fracture in which the bone is crushed and splintered.

fracture, compound, *n* a fracture in which the bony structures are exposed to an external environment.

fracture, craniofacial dysjunction (transverse facial fracture), *n* a complex fracture in which the facial bones are separated from the cranial bones; a LeFort III fracture.

fracture, dislocation, *n* a fracture of a bone near an articulation, with dislocation of the condyloid process.

fracture, fissured, *n* a fracture that extends partially through a bone, with no displacement of the bony fragments.

fracture fixation, *n* the fractured fragments of bone are stabilized in close proximation to promote healing.

fracture, greenstick, *n* a fracture in which the bone appears to be bent; usually only one cortex of the bone is broken.

fracture, Guérin's, *n.pr* a LeFort I fracture of the facial bones in which there is a bilateral horizontal fracture of the maxillae.

fracture, impacted, *n* a fracture in which one fragment is driven into another portion of the same or an adjacent bone.

fracture, indirect, *n* a fracture at a point distant from the primary area of injury caused by secondary forces.

fracture, intraarticular, *n* a fracture of the articular surface of the condyloid process of a bone.

fracture, intracapsular, *n* a fracture of the condyle of the mandible occurring within the confines of the capsule of the temporomandibular joint.

fracture, LeFort, *n.pr* a transverse fracture involving the orbital, malar, and nasal bones.

LeFort III

LeFort II

LeFort I

LeFort classifications. (Liebgott, 2001)

fracture, midfacial, n fractures of the zygomatic, maxillary, nasal, and associated bones.

fracture, pyramidal, n a fracture of the midfacial bones, with the principal fracture lines meeting at an apex in the area of the nasion; a LeFort II fracture.

fracture, root, n a microscopic or macroscopic cleavage of the root in any direction.

fracture, simple, n a linear fracture that is not in communication with the exterior.

fracture, stress, n **I.** usually occuring from sudden, strong, violent, endogenous force, such as a simple fracture of the fibula in a runner. **2.** the fracture of metallic parts as a result of fatigue of prolonged or frequent stress.

fracture, tooth, n traumatic injury to a tooth that manifests itself as a chip, crack, or break. Manifestations may also include dislocation or complete displacement of a tooth.

Tooth fracture. (Daniel/Harfst, 2002)

fracture toughness, n the quality of the material used for brackets that indicates its ability to withstand applied force without cracking.

fracture, transverse facial, n See fracture, craniofacial dysjunction.

fragilitas ossium (frajil´ētəs os´ē-əm), *n* See osteogenesis imperfecta.

frail elderly, *n.pl* older persons (usually over the age of 75 years) who are afflicted with physical or mental disabilities that may interfere with the ability to independently perform activities of daily living.

frame, *n* a structure, usually rigid, designed to give support or attachment to a part, or to immobilize a part.

frame, implant, n See substructure, implant.

frame, occluding, n a device for relating casts to each other for the purpose of arranging teeth or for use in making an index of the occlusion of dentures; an articulator. See also articulator.

frame, rubber dam, n See holder, rubber dam.

framework, *n* the skeletal metal portion of a removable partial denture around which and to which the remaining units are attached.

franchise dentistry, *n* **I.** the practice of dentistry under a trade name, the rights of which have been purchased from another dentist or dental practice. Under a franchise license agreement, the franchiser may use the trade name, marketing products, and treatment techniques for a sum of money, as long as certain rules and regulations of the franchise are adhered to. **2.** reform to a system for marketing a dental practice, usually under a trade name, where permitted by state laws. In return for a financial investment or other consideration, participating dentists may also receive the benefits of media advertising, a national referral system, and financial and management consultation.

Francisella **(fran-sĭ-sel´ə),** *n* a type of gram-negative eubacteria with cell walls. It requires oxygen to survive.

Francisella tularensis **(too˝lə-ren´ sis),** *n.pl* the bacteria that causes the circulatory disease tularemia, which can be contracted via contaminated food or drink, physical contact, spray, or bug bite. Symptoms include fever, headache, swelling of the lymph nodes, and other pain or discomfort.

Frankel appliance, *n.pr* See appliance, Frankel removable orthodontic.

Frankfort horizontal plane, *n.pr* See plane, Frankfort horizontal.

Frankfort-mandibular incisor angle, *n.pr* See angle, Frankfort-mandibular incisor.

F-ratio (F-test), *n* a value used in determining whether the difference between two variables is statistically significant or stable. A larger variance is divided by a smaller variance, both of which are the results of analysis of variance procedures. The value for F is looked up in a table that shows the probability of occurrence of a ratio of this size.

fraud, *n* an intentional perversion of

truth for the purpose of inducing another, in reliance on it, to part with something valuable or to surrender a legal right; deliberate deception; deceit; trickery.

fraudulent concealment, *n* the deliberate attempt to withhold information or to conceal an act to avoid contractual responsibility. Fraudulent concealment as applied to health care providers arises when a treating doctor conceals from an aggrieved patient that a previous treating doctor may have committed malpractice.

freckle, *n* See ephelis.

free gingiva, *n* See gingiva, free.

free gingival groove, *n* See groove, gingiva, free.

free gingival margin, *n* See margin, free gingival.

free mandibular movement, *n* See movement, mandibular, free.

free radical, *n* a compound with an unpaired electron or proton. It is unstable and reacts readily with other molecules.

free-end, *n* See base, extension.

free-way space, *n* See distance, interocclusal.

freedom of choice, *n* a provision in a dental benefits program that permits the insured to choose any licensed dentist to provide his or her dental care and receive full benefits under the program.

freeze drying, *n* the freezing of heat-sensitive liquid materials in a vacuum to preserve the characteristics of the substrate and remove the volume of water or liquid by sublimation.

fremitus (frem′itus), *n* palpable vibrations of nonvascular origin that can be noted by placing the hand on the chest. See also thrill.

frenal pull, charting (frē′nəl), *n* notations made to a patient's chart concerning evidence of the forces exerted on the upper and lower teeth by the mucous membranes which attach the lips and cheeks to the jaw.

frenectomy (frənek′tōmē), *n* **1.** the excision of a frenum. **2.** the surgical detachment and/or excision of a frenum from its attachment into the mucoperiosteal covering of the alveolar processes.

frenoplasty (frē′nōplas′tē), *n* a correction of an abnormal frenum by repositioning it.

frenotomy (frənot′əmē), *n* the cutting of a frenum; especially the release of tongue-tie, or ankyloglossia.

frenulum (fren′yōōlum). *n* See frenum.

frenum (frē′num) (frenulum), *n* a fold of mucous membrane attaching the cheeks and lips to the mandibular and maxillary mucosa and limiting the motions of the lips and cheeks.

Frenum. (Newman/Takei/Carranza, 2002)

frenum, abnormal (enlarged labial frenum), *n* a labial frenum appearing to be unusually heavy, broad, or attached too near the crest of the ridge that may be an etiologic factor in the production, perpetuation, and/or modification of lesions of the marginal gingivae.

frenum, buccal, *n* a fold or folds of mucous membrane connecting the residual alveolar ridge to the cheek in the premolar region. They exist in both the upper and lower jaws and separate the labial vestibule from the buccal vestibule.

frenum, enlarged labial, *n* See frenum, abnormal.

frenum, labial, *n* the fold of mucous membrane connecting the lip of the residual alveolar ridge near the midline of both the upper and lower ridges.

frenum, lingual, *n* the vertical band of mucous membrane connecting the tongue with the floor of the mouth and the alveolar or residual alveolar ridge.

frequency, *n* the number of cycles per second of a wave or other periodic phenomenon.

frequency polygon, *n* a graphic representation of a frequency distribution constructed by plotting each frequency above the score or midpoint of a class interval laid out on a base line and connecting the points so plotted by a straight line.

Frey's syndrome (frīz), *n.pr* See syndrome, auriculotemporal.

friable (frī'-əbəl), *adj* brittle or fragile; easily damaged.

fricative (frik'ətiv), *n* any speech sound made by forcing the airstream through such a narrow orifice or opening that audible high-frequency air currents or vibrations are set up.

friction, *n* the resistance to movement as one object is moved across the other, usually creating heat.

Friedman's test (fred'mənz), *n.pr* See test, pregnancy.

fringe benefits, *n.pl* benefits, other than wages or salary, provided by an employer for employees (for example, health insurance, vacation time, disability income).

frit (frit), *n* a partly or wholly fused porcelain that has been plunged into water while hot. The mass cracks and fractures, and from this "frit," dental porcelain powders are made.

frontal (PA) cephalometric radiograph, *n* a cephalometric radiograph made with the subject facing the film (posteroanterior [PA] view); the axis between the ears is parallel to the film and perpendicular to the x-ray beam.

frontal bone, *n* a single cranial bone that forms the front of the skull from above the orbits posteriorly to a junction with the parietal bones at the coronal suture.

frontal lobe, *n* the largest of five lobes constituting each of the two cerebral hemispheres. The frontal lobe lies beneath the frontal bone. The frontal lobe significantly influences personality and is associated with the higher mental activities, such as planning, judgment, and conceptualizing.

frontal sinus, *n* one of a pair of small cavities in the frontal bone of the skull that communicates with the nasal cavity.

frozen sections, *n* a histologic section of tissue that has been frozen by exposure to dry ice.

fructose, *n* a yellowish-to-white, crystalline water-soluble levorotatory ketose monosaccharide that is sweeter than sucrose and is found in

honey, several fruits, and combined in many disaccharides and polysaccharides. Also called *fruit sugar* and *levulose.*

fructose intolerance, *n* an inherited disorder marked by an absence of enzymes needed to metabolize fructose. Symptoms include sweating, tremors, confusion, and digestive distress with vomiting, and failure of infants to grow.

fulcrum, extraoral, *n* a stabilizing support point outside of the mouth against which the hand or finger is placed for leverage during a dental procedure in order to ensure precise control of the instrument; usually the chin or cheek.

fulcrum, intraoral, *n* a stabilizing support point within the mouth against which a finger is placed for leverage during treatment in order to ensure precise control of the instrument; usually a tooth that is in close proximity to the one being treated.

fulcrum line, *n* See line, fulcrum.

fulguration (ful'gyərā'shən), *n* the destruction of soft tissue by an electric spark that jumps the gap from an electrode to the tissue without the electrode touching the tissue. See also electrocoagulation.

function, *n/v* the normal or special action of a part. As a noun, *function* has the following synonyms: *role, capacity, task, use, purpose, service, activity,* and *direction.* As a verb, it has the following synonyms: *act, operate, work, perform, go, take effect,* and *serve.* Use of the term to express intended purpose may be misleading.

function, auxiliary, *n* a function that is supplementary or additional to the function for which the part or organ is primarily intended.

function, dental, normal, *n* the correct action of opposing teeth in the process of mastication; sometimes referred to as *normal occlusion.*

function, group, *n* the simultaneous contact of opposing teeth in a segment or group.

function, heavy (occlusal function), *n* an increase in functional activities of the tooth, which may result in compensatory changes in the attachment apparatus (for example, a stronger periodontal ligament) with an

F

increase in the number of fibers, a reinforcement of the supporting bone by formation of new bone, and the formation of cemental spikes, which are calcifications of the cemental fibers. Such changes take place so that the increased stress may be withstood without damage.

function, impaired, *n* diminished, weakened, or less-than-optimal work or action.

function, insufficiency of, *n* hypofunction of the tooth, which may lead to regressive changes in the attachment apparatus and supporting bone. The severity of lesions varies with the degree of hypofunction. See also atrophy of disuse.

function, muscle, *n* the action of muscle, which is principally contraction.

function, occlusal, *n* See function, heavy.

function, physiologic, *n* the degree of activity that stimulates the physical structures but that is so limited as not to irritate those tissues.

function, skeletal, *n* the role of the skeleton in relation to the maintenance of body functions. The bony skeleton welds together and protects the softer vital visceral organs, supports and maintains the body form, and accomplishes body movement for locomotion, respiration, manual skills, and the functions associated with mandibular motion.

function, subcortical, *n* function controlled by all the structures of the brain except the outer cortical rim of the cerebrum; most of the nonconscious activities of a sensory and motor nature.

functional, *adj* **1.** pertaining to the movements and actions of a part. **2.** of or pertaining to the functions of an organ, part, or prosthesis.

functional jaw orthopedics, *n* the objectives of activator-type appliances.

functionally dependent elderly, *n.pl* persons who have experienced a deterioration of physical capacities due to advanced age and must rely on mechanical assistance or the assistance of others.

functionally independent elderly, *n.pl* persons who are physically well despite advanced age. Also called *well elderly.*

fundoplication, *n* a surgical procedure involving making tucks in the fundus of the stomach around the lower end of the esophagus. The operation is used in the treatment of gastric acid reflux into the esophagus.

fungal infection, *n* an infection caused by a fungus or yeast organism.

fungate (fung′gāt), *v* to produce fungus-like growths; to grow rapidly like a fungus.

fungus (fung′gəs), *n* a class of vegetable organisms of a low order of development, including mushrooms, toadstools, and molds. Many are saprophytic and/or pathogenic for humans (for example, *Candida albicans* and *Histoplasma, Trichophyton, Actinomyces,* and *Blastomyces* organisms). Oral and systemic moniliasis (thrush) is produced by overgrowth of *C. albicans,* which is a saprophytic resident in the oral cavity. When physiologic processes are sufficiently impaired, the organism may gain a foothold and assume a pathogenic role. Of the more than 100,000 identified species, 100 are common in humans and 10 are known pathogens.

furcal concavity (fur′kəl konkav′itē), *n* depression present in the furcation area of the root of a tooth.

furcation (furkā′shən), *n* the region of division of the root portion of a tooth.

furcation defects, *n.pl* structural de-

Furcation. (Daniel/Harfst, 2002)

fects that occur in the region of the division of the root of a tooth into two, three, or four divisions. Generally, these defects constitute a communication channel between the pulp and the periodontal space.

furcation invasion, n the loss of bone at the point where the roots of a multirooted tooth divide.

furcation probe (furkā′shən), n See probe, furcation.

furcation, root, n the interradicular bone resorption in multirooted teeth caused by periodontal disease.

furnace, n an apparatus in which to generate heat.

furnace, inlay, n a furnace used for eliminating the wax from an inlay mold and establishing the proper condition and temperature of the investment to receive the molten casting gold.

furnace, porcelain, n a furnace used for fusing, firing, or fusion.

furosemide, n *trade names:* Lasix, Lasix Special; *drug class:* loop diuretic; *action:* acts on loop of Henle to decrease reabsorption of chloride and sodium and resultant diuresis; *uses:* pulmonary edema, edema in CHF, liver disease, ascites, hypertension.

fused teeth, n.pl teeth that are joined together during tooth development by one or more of the hard tissues: enamel, dentin, or cementum.

fusiform bacilli, morphologic form of (fyōō′zifôrm), n.pl the fused strands of the narrow filaments of bacteria, tapered at both ends. See also *Fusobacterium, fusiforme.*

fusion, n **1.** the uniting or joining together of two or more entities. The fusion temperature of an alloy lies just below the lower limit of its melting range, which is particularly important in soldering operations because temperatures near or above fusion temperature will decrease ductility. **2.** the process of producing fused teeth. See also crescence and range, melting.

Fused teeth. (Neville/Damm/Allen/Bouquot, 2002)

fusion, nuclear, n the union of atomic nuclei to form heavier nuclei, resulting in the release of enormous quantities of energy when certain light elements unite.

fusion of metal, n See metal, fusion of.

Fusobacterium, n a genus of bacteria containing gram-negative, non-sporeforming, obligately anaerobic rods that produce butyric acid as a major metabolic product. These organisms are found in cavities of man and other animals; some species are pathogenic.

Fusobacterium fusiforme (fyōō′zōbaktir′ē-əm fyōozifôr′mā) **(Vincent's bacillus),** n a microorganism that, along with *Borrelia vincentii,* is implicated in the causation of necrotizing ulcerative gingivitis. Although *F. fusiforme* and *B. vincentii* are inhabitants of the oral cavity, they may become pathogenic when tissue resistance is impaired.

Fusobacterium nucleatum, n a genus of schizomycetes, an anaerobic gram-negative bacterium often seen in necrotic tissue and implicated, but not conclusively, with other organisms in the causation and perpetuation of periodontal disease.

g, n See gram.

gabapentin, n *trade name:* Neurontin; *drug class:* anticonvulsant; *action:* anticonvulsant action is unclear; *use:* adjunctive therapy in adults with partial seizures.

gadolinium (Gd), n a rare earth metallic element with an atomic number of 64 and an atomic weight of 157.25. Gadolinium is used as a phosphor to intensify x-ray screens.

gag, n a surgical device for holding the mouth open.

gag reflex, n a normal neural reflex elicited by touching the soft palate or posterior pharynx; the response is a symmetric elevation of the palate, a retraction of the tongue, and a con-

G

traction of the pharyngeal muscles. The reflex is used as a test of the integrity of the vagus and glossopharyngeal nerves.

gagging, *n* an involuntary retching reflex that may be stimulated by something touching the posterior palate or throat region.

gait (gāt), *n* a manner of walking; a cyclic loss and regaining of balance by a shift of the line of gravity in relationship to the center of gravity. A person's gait is as characteristic and as individual as a fingerprint.

gait, cerebellar, n an unsteady, irregular gait characterized by short steps and a lurching from one side to the other; most commonly seen in multiple sclerosis or other cerebellar diseases.

gait, festinating, n a gait characterized by rigidity, shuffling, and involuntary hastening. The upper part of the body advances ahead of the lower part. It is associated with paralysis agitans and postencephalitic Parkinson's syndrome.

gait, sensor ataxic, n an irregular, uncertain, stamping gait. The legs are kept far apart, and either the ground or the feet are watched, since there has been a loss of knowledge of the position of the lower limbs. This gait is caused by an interruption of the afferent nerve fibers and may be associated with tabes dorsalis and sometimes with multiple sclerosis and other lesions of the nervous system.

gait, spastic, n (creeping palsy) a slow, shuffling gait in which the patient appears to be wading in water. Knee and hip movements are restricted. This gait may be associated with multiple sclerosis, syphilis, combined systemic disease, or other diseases affecting the spinal pyramidal tracts.

gait, staggering, n a reeling, tottering, and tipping gait in which the individual appears as if he may fall backward or lose his balance. A staggering gait is associated with alcohol and barbiturate intoxication.

gait, waddling, n an exaggerated alteration of lateral trunk movements, with an exaggerated elevation of the hip, suggesting the gait of a duck; characteristic of progressive muscular dystrophy.

galactin (gəlak′tin), *n* See hormone, lactogenic.

galactosamine, *n* a chondrosamine; a derivative of galactose, occurs in various mucopolysaccharides, notably of chondroitin sulfuric acid and B blood group substance.

galactose, *n* a simple sugar found in the dextrorotatory form in lactose (milk sugar), nerve cell membranes, sugar beets, gums, seaweed, and, in the levorotatory form, in flaxseed mucilage. Galactose, a white crystalline substance, is less sweet and less soluble in water than glucose but is similar in other properties.

galactosemia (gə-lak″to-se′me-ə), *n* an inherited condition that prevents normal metabolism of galactose due to a lack of the galactose-*l*-phosphate uridyl transferase enzyme.

gallic acid, *n* an astringent used topically, made from tannic acid or nutgalls, and chemically known as 3,4,5-trihydroxybenzoic acid.

gallium, *n* a metallic element with an atomic number of 31 and an atomic weight of 69.72. Gallium is used in high temperature thermometers, and its radioisotopes are used in total-body scanning procedures.

galvanic current, *n* See current, galvanic.

galvanic skin response (GSR), *n* a reaction to certain stimuli as indicated by a change in the electric resistance of the skin. The GSR is used in some polygraph examinations.

galvanism, *n* See current, galvanic.

galvanotherapy, *n* See ionization.

gamma globulins, *n.pl* plasma proteins which are essential antibodies which circulate in the immune system.

gamma rays, *n* an electromagnetic radiation of short wavelength emitted by the nucleus of an atom during a nuclear reaction. Composed of high-energy photons, gamma rays lack mass and an electric charge and travel at the speed of light.

ganciclovir, *n trade names:* Cytovene, DHPG; *drug class:* antiviral; *action:* inhibits replication of most herpes viruses *in vitro;* in vivo by selective inhibition of human CMV DNA polymerase and by direct incorporation into viral DNA; *uses:* cytomegalovirus (CMV) retinitis in patients with AIDS.

ganglion(ia) (**gang'glē-on**), *n/n.pl* any collection or mass of nerve cells that serves as a center of nervous influence.

ganglion, basal, n a group of forebrain nuclei that, with the related structures of the brain, play an important role in the regulation of muscle tone and motor control. The cell groups of these ganglia and their respective nerve tracts are classified as the *extrapyramidal motor system* to differentiate them from the *pyramidal motor system,* which goes directly from the cerebral cortex to the lower motor neuron. Disease associated with the basal ganglia is manifested by three principal motor abnormalities: disturbance of muscle tone, derangement of movement, and loss of associated or automatic movement.

ganglion, ciliary, n a parasympathetic nerve ganglion in the posterior part of the orbit. The ciliary ganglion receives preganglionic fibers from the region of the oculomotor nucleus and sends postganglionic fibers via short ciliary nerves to (1) the constrictor muscle of the iris (constriction of pupil) and (2) circular fibers of the ciliary muscle (accommodation for vision).

ganglion, otic, n a ganglion located medial to the mandibular nerve just below the foramen ovale in the infratemporal fossa. It supplies the sensory and secretory fibers for the parotid gland. Its sensory fibers arise from the facial and glossopharyngeal nerves.

ganglion, sphenopalatine, n one of the four ganglia of the autonomic nervous system associated with the head and neck region. It is located deep in the pterygopalatine fossa and is intimately associated with the maxillary nerve. It lies distal and medial to the maxillary tuberosity. Its fibers supply the mucous membrane of the roof of the pharynx, tonsils, soft and hard palates, and nasal cavity. The mucous and serous secretions of all the mucous membranes in the oropharynx are also mediated by this ganglion.

ganglion, submandibular, n a ganglion located on the medial side of

the mandible between the lingual nerve and the submandibular duct. The submandibular ganglion is distributed to the sublingual and submandibular glands. The sensory fibers arise from the lingual branch of the trigeminal nerve; that is, the chorda tympani of the facial nerve.

ganglionectomy, n the excision of a ganglion.

ganglionitis, acute posterior (**gang'glē-ənītis**), n See herpes zoster.

gangrene, n the death of tissue *en masse,* usually the result of loss of blood supply, bacterial invasion, and subsequent putrefaction. For example, gangrene of the pulp is total death and necrosis of the pulp.

gangrene, dry, n a late complication of diabetes mellitus that is already complicated by arteriosclerosis in which the affected extremity becomes cold, dry, and shriveled and eventually turns black.

gangrene, gas, n necrosis accompanied by gas bubbles in soft tissue after trauma or surgery. It is caused by anaerobic microorganisms such as various species of *Clostridium,* particularly *C. perfringens.* If untreated, gas gangrene is rapidly fatal.

gangrene, moist, n a condition that may follow a crushing injury or an obstruction of blood flow by an embolism, tight bandages, or a tourniquet. This form of gangrene has an offensive odor, spreads rapidly, and may result in death in a few days. All types of gangrene require the removal of the necrotic tissue before healing can progress.

Gantrisin, *n.pr* the brand name for sulfisoxazole, an antibacterial sulfonamide, which is effective in the treatment of acute, recurrent, or chronic urinary tract infections, meningococcal meningitis, and acute otitis media.

gap arthroplasty, n the surgical correction of ankylosis by creation of a space between the ankylosed part and the portion in which movement is desired.

gap, interocclusal, n See distance, interocclusal.

Gardner-Diamond syndrome, *n.pr* a condition resulting from autoerythrocyte sensitization, marked by large, painful, transient ecchymoses that appear without apparent cause but often accompany emotional upsets, various collagen disorders, and abnormalities of protein metabolism. Treatment includes topical and systemic corticosteroids. Also called *autoerythrocyte sensitization syndrome.*

gargoylism, *n* See syndrome, Hurler's.

GAS, *n* See syndrome, general adaptation.

gas, *n* a fluid with no definite volume or shape whose molecules are practically unrestricted by cohesive forces.

gas, laughing, n See nitrous oxide.

gas, noble, n a gas that will not oxidize; the inert gases (for example, helium and neon).

gas, olefiant, n a machine that uses ethylene oxide gas to sterilize objects that cannot withstand high temperatures, such as soft plastic and cloth.

gasometer (gasäm′ətur), *n* a calibrated instrument or vessel for measuring the volume of gases. Used in clinical and physiologic investigation for measuring respiratory volume.

gastric acid, *n* hydrochloric acid secreted by the gastric glands in the stomach; aids in the preparation of food for digestion.

gastric intrinsic factor (GIF), *n* a substance secreted by the gastric mucosa that is essential for the intestinal absorption of vitamin B_{12}; also known as *intrinsic factor.*

gastric juice, *n* the digestive secretions of the gastric glands in the stomach, consisting chiefly of pepsin, hydrochloric acid, rennin, and mucin.

gastric mucosa, *n* the lining of the stomach.

gastrinoma, *n* a gastrin-secreting tumor associated with the Zollinger-Ellison syndrome.

gastritis, *n* an inflammation of the lining of the stomach that occurs in both acute and chronic forms. Acute gastritis may be caused by aspirin or other antiinflammatory agents, corticosteroids, drugs, foods, condiments, and alcohol and chemical toxins. The symptoms are anorexia, nausea, vomiting, and discomfort after eating. Chronic gastritis is usually a sign of underlying disease, such as peptic ulcer or pernicious anemia.

gastritis, atrophic, n a chronic form of gastritis with atrophy of the mucous membrane and destruction of the peptic glands, sometimes associated with pernicious anemia or gastric carcinoma.

gastroenteritis, *n* an inflammation of the stomach and intestines accompanying numerous gastrointestinal (GI) disorders. Symptoms are anorexia, nausea, vomiting, abdominal discomfort, and diarrhea.

gastroenterology, *n* the study of diseases affecting the GI tract, including the esophagus, stomach, intestines, rectum, gallbladder, and bile duct.

gastroesophageal reflux, *n* a backflow of the contents of the stomach into the esophagus that is often the result of incompetence of the lower esophageal sphincter. Gastric juices are acid and therefore produce burning pain in the esophagus.

gastrointestinal disease, *n* any abnormal state or function of the GI system.

gastrointestinal system, *n* the chain of organs of the GI tract, from the mouth to the anus.

gastroscopy, *n* the visual inspection of the interior of the stomach by means of a flexible fiberoptic tube inserted through the mouth and passing the length of the esophagus into the stomach.

gastrostomy, *n* the surgical creation of an artificial opening into the stomach through the abdominal wall, used to feed a patient who has cancer of the esophagus or other kind of barrier to oral feeding.

gate-keeper system, *n* a managed-care concept used by some alternative benefit plans, in which enrollees elect a primary care dentist, usually a general practitioner or pediatric dentist, who is responsible for providing nonspecialty care and managing referrals, as appropriate, for specialty and ancillary services.

gauge, *n* an instrument used to determine the dimensions or caliber of an object.

gauge, Boley, n.pr a vernier type of instrument used for measuring in the metric system. A Boley gauge is accurate to tenths of millimeters.

gauge, leaf, n a device for measuring the distance between two objects. A leaf gauge consists of a series of thin strips of plastic or metal, each calibrated and arranged in a sequential fashion in ascending or descending thicknesses, usually expressed in millimeters or fractions of millimeters. In dentistry, the leaf gauge is used to measure interocclusal space or the magnitude of an interocclusal interference.

gauge, undercut, *n* an attachment used in conjunction with a dental cast surveyor to measure the amount of infrabulge of a tooth in a horizontal plane.

gauze strip, for flossing, *n* folded 6- to 8-inch pieces of sterile gauze used to clean abutment teeth, teeth located at the end of a row, the space underneath dental appliances that cannot be completely removed, and between teeth that are exceptionally far apart.

gel (jel), *n* a colloid in solid form, jellylike in character. Hydrocolloid impression materials are examples of gels.

gel, brush-on, *n* gelatinous preparation used to promote remineralization of teeth and discourage further demineralization, intended to augment daily brushing and flossing. Formulas contain either 1.1% sodium fluoride or 0.4% stannous fluoride in a glycerin base.

gel strength, *n* See strength, gel.

gel time, *n* See time, gel.

gelatin, *n* a protein formed from collagen by boiling in water. Medically, gelatin is used as a hemostat, a plasma substitute, and a protein food adjunct in severe cases of malnutrition. Gelatin is used in the manufacture of capsules and suppositories. It is also used in the production of x-ray films as the medium for suspending the crystal salts on the surface of the acetate film.

gelation time (jelā′shən), *n* See time, gel.

gemfibrozil, *n trade name:* Lopid; *drug class:* antihyperlipidemic; *action:* reduces plasma triglycerides and very low density lipoproteins; *uses:* type IIb, IV, and V hyperlipidemia.

gene, *n* See family practice.

gene, homeobox (ho′me-o-boks″), *n* a gene containing a DNA sequence called the homeobox, which is very similar between species and encodes a DNA-binding domain in the resulting protein molecule. Homeobox genes usually play a role in controlling development of the organism.

gene locus, *n* See locus, gene.

gene, sex-linked, *n* a gene located in a sex chromosome.

gene therapy, *n* a procedure that involves injection of "health genes" into the bloodstream of a patient to cure or treat a hereditary disease or similar illness.

general supervision, *n* a circumstance of treatment in which the dentist must diagnose and authorize the work to be performed on the patient by the dental hygienist but is not required to be on the premises while the treatment is carried out.

generated path (chew-in), *n* See path, generated occlusal.

generator, *n* one who, or that which, begets, causes, or produces.

generator, electric, *n* a device that converts mechanical energy into electrical energy.

generator, x-ray, *n* a device that converts electrical energy into electromagnetic energy (photons).

genetic counseling, *n* the process of advising a patient with a genetic disease, or child-bearing parents of a patient with a genetic disease, about the probabilities and risks of future genetic accidents in conception, and counseling such persons about future family planning.

genetic disease, *n* a disease that is caused by a defect or anomaly in the genetic inheritance of the patient.

genetic effects of radiation (jənet′ik), *n.pl* those changes produced in the individual's genes and chromosomes of all nucleated body cells, both somatic and gonadal. The more common meaning relates to the effect produced in the reproductive cells. Radiation received by the gonads before the end of the reproductive period has the potential to add to the number of undesirable genes present in the population.

genetic marker, *n* any specific gene that produces a readily recognizable genetic trait that can be used in family and population studies or in linkage analysis.

genetics, *n* the science that deals with the origin of the characteristics of an individual.

genial tubercle, *n* See tubercle, genial.

genioplasty (jē′nē-ōplastē), *n* a surgical procedure, performed either intraorally or extraorally, to correct deformities of the mandibular symphysis.

genital wart (condyloma acuminatum), *n* a soft, wartlike growth found on the warm, moist skin and mucous membranes of the genitalia, caused by a virus and transmitted by sexual contact. Also called *acuminate wart.*

genome, *n* the total gene complement of a set of chromosomes found in higher life forms.

genome, human, n the complete set of genes in the chromosomes of each cell of a human being.

genotype (jē′nōtīp), *n* the aggregate of ordered genes received by offspring from both parents; for example, a person with blood group AB is of genotype AB.

gentamicin sulfate, *n* (ophthalmic), *trade names:* Garamycin Ophthalmic, Gentak; *drug class:* aminoglycoside antiinfective ophthalmic; *action:* inhibits bacterial protein synthesis; *use:* infection of external eye.

gentian violet (jen′shən), *n* See violet, gentian.

geographic tongue, *n* See tongue, geographic.

geometric unsharpness, *n* an impairment of image definition resulting from the geometric penumbra. See also penumbra, geometric and x-ray beam.

geometry of x-ray beam, *n* the effect of various factors on the spatial distribution of radiation emerging from an x-ray generator or source. See also law, inverse square; penumbra, geometric; and x-ray beam.

gerbil, *n* a small rodent used as a laboratory animal and/or household pet, native to Africa and Asia. The name applies to any of 13 genera of the subfamily Gerbillinae. They resemble kangaroo rats and can survive without drinking water.

geriatric assessment, *n* the evaluation of the physical, mental, and emotional health of elderly patients.

geriatric dentistry, *n* a branch of dentistry that deals with the special and unique dental problems of senior citizens.

geriatrics (jer′ē-at′riks), *n* the department of medicine or dentistry that treats health problems peculiar to advanced age and the aging, including the clinical problems of senescence and senility.

germ cell, *n* a sexual reproductive cell in any stage of development; that is, an ovum or spermatozoon or any of their preceding forms.

germanium, *n* a metallic element with some nonmetallic properties. Its atomic number is 32 and its atomic weight is 72.59.

germicide (jur′misīd), *n* a substance capable of killing a wide variety of microorganisms, more specifically, one capable of killing all microorganisms, except for spores, with which it is in contact for a standard period of time.

germination (jur′minā′shən), *n* the division of a tooth bud that results in the formation of double, or twin, crowns on a single root with a single pulp canal.

gerodontics (jer′ōdon′tiks), *n* (gerodontology) the branch of dentistry that deals with the diagnosis and treatment of the dental conditions of aging and aged persons.

gerodontology (jer′ōdontol′ōjē), *n* See gerodontics.

gerontology (jer″on-tol′ə-je), *n* the comprehensive (physical, psychological, and social) study of aging.

gestation, *n* the period of development between fertilization and birth.

gestational age, *n* the age of a fetus or newborn, usually expressed in weeks dating from the first day of the mother's last menstrual period.

giant cell, *n* an abnormally large tissue cell. It often contains more than one nucleus and may appear as a merger of several normal cells.

giantism, *n* (macrosomia), excessive growth resulting in a stature larger than the range that is normal for age and race.

giantism, infantile, n excessive growth occurring before adolescence.

giantism, primary, n excessive growth not attributable to a definite cause.

giantism, secondary, n excessive growth secondary to a disorder of the adrenal, pineal, gonadal, or pituitary gland.

Giardia, *n* a common genus of the flagellate protozoans. Many species of *Giardia* normally inhabit the digestive tract and cause inflammation in association with other factors that produce rapid proliferation of the organism.

giardiasis, *n* an inflammatory intestinal condition caused by overgrowth of the protozoan *Giardia lamblia.* The source of infection is usually contaminated water. Also called *traveler's diarrhea.*

GIF, *n* See gastric intrinsic factor.

gift, *n* **1.** a voluntary transfer of personal property without condition. *n* **2.** the abbreviation for gamete intrafallopian transfer.

Gillies' operation, *n.pr* See operation, Gillies'.

Gillmore needle, *n.pr* See needle, Gillmore.

Gilson fixable-removable bar, *n.pr* See connector, cross arch bar splint.

gingiva(e) (jin′jivə), *n/n.pl* the fibrous tissue covered by mucous membrane that immediately surrounds the teeth.

Vestibule and vestibular gingivae of oral cavity. A, Maxilla. B, Mandible. (Liebgott, 2001)

gingivae, attached, *n* the portion of the gingivae extending from the free gingival groove, which demarcates it from the free or marginal gingivae, to the mucogingival junction, which separates it from the alveolar mucosa. This tissue is firm, dense, stippled, and tightly bound down to the underlying periosteum, tooth, and bone.

 gingivae, attached, extension, *n* See extension, gingiva, attached.

gingiva, detached by calculus, *n* the recession and ultimate disconnection of gingival tissue from tooth surfaces which occurs as the result of calculus build-up.

gingivae, erythemic, *n.pl* unusually red gums which may be caused by either inflammation or excessive blood in the tissue. The condition may occur as a result of excess vitamin A.

gingivae, free, *n.pl* the unattached coronal portion of the gingiva that encircles the tooth to form the gingival sulcus.

gingivae hyperplasia, *n.pl* See hyperplasia, gingival, Dilantin.

gingiva, interdental, *n* (interproximal gingiva[e]), the soft supporting tissue, consisting of prominent horizontal collagen fibers, that normally fills the space between two contacting teeth.

Gingiva, interdental. (Bird/Robinson, 2002)

gingiva, interproximal, *n* See gingiva, interdental.

gingiva, lymphatic drainage of, *n* lymphatic drainage that follows the course of the gingival blood supply; that is, from the lymphatic vessels on the gingival side of the periosteum of the alveolar process to the lymphatic vessels in the periodontal membrane to vessels leaking into the alveolar bone.

gingiva, marginal, n the free gingiva at the labial, buccal, lingual, and palatal aspects of the teeth.

gingivae, microscopic appearance of, n.pl stratified squamous epithelium that varies in degree of keratinization and overlies a corium of connective tissue with interspersed blood vessels and nerves. Rete pegs of epithelium project downward into the connective tissue corium, except from the base of sulcular epithelium. The gingival fiber apparatus is readily discerned.

gingival, *adj* pertaining to or in relation to the gingiva.

gingival abrasion, n the attrition (scraping or wearing away) of the gingival tissue by harsh irritants such as coarse foods or faulty toothbrushing.

gingival anatomy, n the gingiva, which is a dense connective tissue covered by keratinized mucosa except in the sulcus, where it is nonkeratinized. The margin is arcuate buccolingually with the peaks (papillae) interdentally. The sulcus depth normally is the apical limit to the free (unattached) gingiva, the attached gingiva extending from the free gingiva to the oral mucosa.

gingival architecture, n gingival form.

gingival blanching, n the lightening of gingival color resulting from stretching with diminution of blood supply; usually of a temporary nature.

gingival bleeding, n a prominent symptom of periodontal disease produced by ulceration of the sulcular epithelium and an inflammatory process.

gingival blood supply, n the vascular supply to the gingivae arises from the vessels that pass on the gingival side of the outer periosteum of bone and anastomoses with blood vessels of the periodontal membrane and intraalveolar blood vessels.

gingival color, n the color of the gingival tissues in health and in disease. It varies with the thickness and degree of keratinization of the epithelium, blood supply, pigmenta-

tion, and alterations produced by diseased processes affecting the gingival tissues. In health often described as coral pink.

gingival consistency, n the visual and tactile characteristics of healthy gingival tissue. Visual consistency varies from a smooth velvet to that of an orange peel, either finely or coarsely grained. The tactile consistency of the gingival tissue should be firm and resilient.

gingival crater, n a concave depression in the gingival tissue. Especially seen in the area of the former apex of the interdental papilla as a result of gingival destruction associated with necrotizing ulcerative gingivitis or when food impaction occurs against the tissue subjacent to the contact points of adjacent teeth.

gingival crevicular fluid, n an altered serum transudate found in the gingival sulcus. Irritation and inflammation of the gingival tissue increase the flow and alter the constituents of crevicular fluid.

gingival cyanotic tissue, n gum tissue that appears slightly blue due to a reduction in oxygenated hemoglobin; may occur in conjunction with vitamin C deficiency. See also cyanosis.

gingival discoloration, n a change from the normal coloration of the gingivae; associated with inflammation, diminution of blood supply, and abnormal pigmentation.

gingival enlargement, drug influenced, n a swelling of the gingival tissues and papillae resulting from the use of drugs that block calcium channels; can be treated by prescribing an alternative drug.

gingival erythema, linear, n a characteristic of a necrotizing periodontal condition in an HIV-positive patient. A band of acute erythema located at the gingival margin.

gingival erythema, lingual, n a band of acute erythema located at the inside gingival margin (next to the tongue).

gingival fibroblast, n a formative cell that moderates wound healing and healing after treatment.

gingival hemorrhage, n bleeding of the gum tissues; usually at the interpapillary crest, the gingival margin, or in the crevicular sulcus.

gingival hormonal enlargement, n an enlargement of the gingivae associated with hormonal imbalance during pregnancy or puberty.

gingival mat, n the gingival connective tissue composed of coarse, broad collagen fibers that serve to attach the gingivae to the teeth and to hold the free gingivae in close approximation to the teeth.

gingival physiology, n the gingivae encircle the teeth and serve as a protective mucosal covering for the underlying tissues; the gingival fiber apparatus serves as a barrier to apical migration of the epithelial attachment and binds the gingival tissues to the teeth. The normal topography permits the free flow of food away from the occlusal surfaces and from the cervical and interproximal areas of the teeth.

gingival pigmentation, n variations in gingival color may be correlated with the complexion of an individual or may be a reflection of pathologic influences, such as the melanin pigmentation associated with hypoadrenocorticism (Addison's disease), nevi, and depositions of heavy metals.

gingival pocket, n a localized deepening of the gingival crevice of 2 mm or more.

gingival position, n the level of the gingival margin in relation to the tooth.

gingival recession, n the apical migration of the gingival crest.

gingival shrinkage, n the reduction in size of gingival tissue, principally by diminution of edema, usually as a result of therapeutic elimination of subgingival deposits and curettement of the soft tissue wall of the pocket.

gingival stippling, n a series of small depressions characterizing the surface of healthy gingivae, varying from a smooth velvet to that of an orange peel.

gingival sulcus, n the space between the free gingiva and the tooth.

gingival surface texture, n the texture of the attached gingivae, which normally is stippled; in inflammatory conditions, the edema, cellular infiltration, and concomitant swelling cause loss of the surface stippling,

and the gingivae take on a smooth, shiny, edematous appearance.

gingival third, n relating to the most apical one third of a given clinical crown or of an axial surface cavity or preparation.

gingival topography, n the form of the healthy gingival tissues. The marginal gingivae and the interdental papillae have a characteristic shape.

gingivectomy (jin′jivek′təmē), *n* the surgical excision of unsupported gingival tissue to the level where it is attached, creating a new gingival margin apical in position to the old. *gingivectomy in edentulous area, n* the elimination of periodontal pockets surrounding abutment teeth; requires the removal of gingival tissue on the adjacent edentulous area.

gingivitis (jin′jivī′tis), *n* any inflammation of the gingival tissue.

gingivitis and malposed teeth, n malposition may predispose the gingivae to inflammation by permitting food impaction or impingement, by providing irregular spaces in which calculus may be deposited, and by making cleaning difficult.

gingivitis, bacteria in, n the causative organisms in gingival inflammation. The common chronic forms of gingivitis, from a bacterial standpoint, are nonspecific, with the exception of acute necrotizing ulcerative gingivitis, in which there is an apparent specificity of the bacterial flora: the fusospirochetal organisms.

gingivitis, bismuth, n metallic poisoning caused by bismuth given for treatment of systemic disease; characterized by a dark, bluish line along the gingival margin.

gingivitis, chronic atrophic senile, n gingival inflammation characterized by atrophy and areas of hyperkeratosis; found primarily in elderly women.

gingivitis, desquamative, n an inflammation of the gingivae characterized by a tendency of the surface epithelium to desquamate. The disease is a clinical entity, not a pathologic entity. Desquamative gingivitis is most frequently associated with menopause but may be associated with any biologic stress.

gingivitis, eruptive (ērup′tiv), *n* gingival inflammation occurring at the time of eruption of the permanent teeth.

gingivitis, fusospirochetal, *n* See gingivitis, necrotizing ulcerative.

gingivitis gravidarum, *n* See gingivitis, pregnancy.

gingivitis, hemorrhagic, *n* gingivitis characterized by profuse bleeding, especially that associated with ascorbic acid deficiency.

gingivitis, herpetic, *n* an inflammation of the gingivae caused by herpesvirus. See also gingivostomatitis, herpetic.

gingivitis, hormonal, *n* gingivitis associated with endocrine imbalance, the endocrinopathy being modified, in most instances, by the influence of local environmental factors.

gingivitis, hyperplastic, *n* gingivitis characterized by proliferation of the various tissue elements. May be accompanied by dense infiltration of inflammatory cells.

gingivitis, idiopathic, *n* a gingival inflammation of unknown causation.

gingivitis, infectious, *n* gingivitis not caused by plaque, but instead originating from bacteria, fungi, or viruses.

gingivitis, inflammatory cells in, *n* since the gingival inflammatory process is usually chronic and progressive in nature, the inflammatory cells are, for the most part, lymphocytes, plasma cells, and some histiocytes. With acute exacerbations, polymorphonuclear leukocytes are also present.

gingivitis, marginal, *n* an inflammation of the gingivae localized to the marginal gingivae and interdental papillae.

gingivitis, necrotizing ulcerative, *n* (fusospirochetal gingivitis, NUG, trench mouth, ulcerative gingivitis, ulceromembranous gingivitis, Vincent's gingivitis, Vincent's infection) an inflammation of the gingivae characterized by necrosis of the interdental papillae, ulceration of the gingival margins, the appearance of a pseudomembrane, pain, and a fetid odor.

gingivitis, necrotizing ulcerative, inflammatory cells, *n* prevalent cellular infiltrate in necrotizing ulcerative gingivitis, including polymorphonuclear leukocytes, plasma cells, and lymphocytes. In the acute phase, polymorphonuclear leukocytes predominate.

gingivitis, nephritic, *n* (uremic gingivitis, uremic stomatitis), a membrane form of stomatitis and gingivitis associated with a failure of kidney function. Nephritic gingivitis is accompanied by pain, ammoniacal odor, and increased salivation.

gingivitis, non-plaque-induced, *n* gingivitis caused by factors other than plaque, such as allergic reaction, dermatologic disease, a genetic condition, infectious agents, response to a foreign body, or physical trauma.

gingivitis, plaque-induced, *n* gingivitis caused by the accumulation of plaque.

gingivitis, pregnancy, *n* (gingivitis gravidarum, hormonal gingivitis), an enlargement of hyperplasia of the gingivae resulting from a hormonal imbalance during pregnancy.

gingivitis, puberty, *n* an enlargement of the gingival tissues as a result of an exaggerated response to irritation resulting from hormonal changes.

gingivitis, scorbutic, *n* gingivitis associated with vitamin C (ascorbic acid) deficiency.

gingivitis, systemic disease-induced, *n* gingivitis occurring as a complication of a systemic disease, such as Type 1 diabetes mellitus or acute leukemia.

gingivitis, ulcerative, *n* See gingivitis, necrotizing ulcerative.

gingivitis, ulceromembranous, *n* See gingivitis, necrotizing ulcerative.

gingivitis, uremic, *n* See gingivitis, nephritic.

gingivitis, Vincent's, *n.pr* See gingivitis, necrotizing ulcerative.

gingivoplasty (jin′jivōplastē), *n* the surgical contouring of the gingival tissues to secure the physiologic architectural form necessary for the maintenance of tissue health and integrity.

gingivosis (jin′jivō′sis), *n* a noninflammatory degenerative condition of the gingivae. The term is applied to desquamative gingivitis.

gingivostomatitis (jin′jivōstō′mətī′tis), *n* an inflammation that involves the gingivae and the oral mucosa.

gingivostomatitis, acute herpetic, *n* See stomatitis, herpetic, acute.

gingivostomatitis, herpetic, n an inflammation of the gingivae and oral mucosa caused by primary invasion of herpesvirus. Herpetic gingivostomatitis occurs chiefly in childhood, one attack giving immunity to generalized stomatitis but not to isolated lesions (herpetic lesions). The symptoms are red and swollen gingivae; red mucosa, which soon shows vesicles and ulcers; painful mouth; and elevated temperature. The course is about 14 days.

gingivostomatitis, membranous, n a disease, or group of diseases, in which false membranes form on the gingivae and oral mucosa; the membranes are a grayish white color and are surrounded by a narrow red margin. Detachment of the membrane leaves a raw, bleeding surface. One cause is mixed pyogenic infection, in which *Streptococcus viridans* and *Staphylococcus* organisms predominate.

gingivostomatitis, white folded, n See nevus spongiosus albus mucosa.

ginglymus (hinge joint)
(jing′glimǝs), n a joint that allows motion around an axis.

glabella (glǝbel′ǝ), n the most anterior point on the frontal bone.

gland(s), n/n.pl an organ producing a specific product or secretion.

gland, parotid salivary, n the largest of the major salivary glands; its anterior position is situated between the ramus of the mandible, its posterior portion between the mastoid process and sternocleidomastoid muscle, and inferior to the zygomatic arch; irregularly wedge shaped, with the lateral surface flattened and the medial aspect more or less pointed toward the pharyngeal wall. Its secretion, which is serous, traverses Stensen's duct to empty into the mouth at the ductal orifice on the buccal mucosa opposite the maxillary molar teeth.

gland, pituitary, n (hypophysis), an endocrine gland located at the base of the brain in the sella turcica. The pituitary gland is composed of two parts: the pars nervosa, which is an extension of the anterior part of the hypothalamus, and the pars intermedia, which is an epithelial evagination of secretory tissue from the

stomodeum of the embryo. By its structural and functional relationships with the nervous system and the endocrine glands, it acts as a mediator of both the nervous system and the endocrine system.

gland, sublingual salivary, n the smallest of the major salivary glands. It lies inferior to the mucous membranes of the floor of the mouth bilateral to the lingual frenum and is in contact with the sublingual depression on the inner side of the mandible. Its numerous ducts open directly into the mouth bilateral to the lingual frenum and join to form the duct of Bartholin (sublingual duct), which enters into the Wharton's duct (submandibular duct). Its secretion is mucous in nature.

gland, submandibular salivary, n a major gland that has an irregular form and is situated in the submandibular triangle, bordered anteriorly by the anterior belly of the digastric muscle and posteriorly by the stylomandibular ligament. Its mucoserous section is carried by Wharton's duct, whose orifice lies at the summit of a small papilla (submandibular caruncle) bilateral to the lingual frenum.

gland, thymus, n See thymus.

glands, Blandin and Nuhn's, n.pr See spots, Fordyce's.

glands, endocrine, n.pl any one of the glands of internal secretion; a hormone-secreting gland (for example, the pituitary gland, thyroid gland, parathyroid glands, adrenal glands, ovaries, and testes).

glands, lacrimal, n.pl the ducted (exocrine) glands that produce lacrimal fluid, commonly called *tears.* See also lacrimal apparatus.

glands, minor salivary, n.pl glands located at the posterior aspect of the dorsum of the tongue behind the circumvallate papillae and along the lateral surface of the tongue; also located in the palate, labial mucosa, and buccal mucosa. The secretion is mucous. Also called *accessory salivary glands.*

glands, salivary, n.pl glands in the oral cavity that secrete saliva. Three major groups of salivary glands contribute their secretions to form the whole saliva; minor mucous glands found within oral mucosa contribute also in small part. The primary salivary glands are the parotid, submandibular, and sublingual.

glass ionomer cement, *n* a dental cement of low strength and toughness produced by mixing a powder prepared from a calcium aluminosilicate glass and a liquid prepared from an aqueous solution of prepared polyacrylic acid; used chiefly for small restorations on the proximal surfaces of anterior teeth and for restoration of eroded areas at the gingival margin.

glass, lead, *n* lead-impregnated glass used in windows of control booths and in protective shields to protect radiologists and their assistants from primary and scattered radiation.

glatiramer acetate (glah-tear′a-meer as′ə-tāt), *n* a medication used to decrease or stop a relapse of multiple sclerosis. It is typically used to treat individuals resistant to the effects of interferon-beta.

glaucoma, *n* an abnormal condition of elevated pressure within the eye because of obstruction of the outflow of aqueous humor.

glaucoma, acute, n (closed-angle) a condition that occurs if the pupil in an eye with a narrow angle between the iris and cornea dilates markedly, causing the folded iris to block the exit of aqueous humor from the anterior chamber.

glaucoma, chronic, n (open-angle) a condition that is much more common than closed-angle glaucoma and is often bilateral. Open-angle glaucoma develops slowly and is genetically determined and progressive with age. The obstruction is believed to occur within the canal of Schlemm.

glaze, *n* a critical stage in the final firing of dental porcelain when complete fusion takes place, with the formation of a thin, vitreous, glossy surface, or glaze.

glenoid, *n* the fossae in the temporal bone in which condyles of the mandible articulate with the skull.

gliadin, *n* a protein substance that is obtained from wheat and rye. Its solubility in diluted alcohol distinguishes gliadin from glutenin.

glide(s), *n* **I.** the passage of one object over another as guided by their contacting surfaces. *n.pl* **2.** the sounds *w, wh,* and *y,* which are

voiced as bilabial and palatal glides, respectively. The rapid movement of the lips or tongue from a set position toward a neutral vowel (*u,* as in up).

glide, mandibular, n side-to-side, protrusive, intermediate movement of the mandible that occurs when the teeth or other occluding surfaces are in contact.

gliding occlusion, *n* See occlusion, gliding.

glimepiride, *n trade name:* Amaryl; *drug class:* oral antidiabetic; *action:* a sulfonylurea type action; *use:* non-insulin-dependent diabetes, sometimes in combination with insulin support.

glioma, *n* any of the largest group of primary tumors of the brain, composed of malignant glial cells.

glipizide, *n trade name:* Glucotrol; *drug class:* oral antidiabetic (second generation); *action:* causes functioning β cells in pancrease to release insulin, leading to a drop in blood glucose levels; *use:* stable adult-onset diabetes mellitus (type 2).

globin, *n* a group of four globulin protein molecules that become bound by the iron in heme molecules to form hemoglobin or myoglobin.

globulin, *n* a class of proteins.

globulin, antihemophilic, n See factor VIII.

globulin, antihemophilic A, n See factor VIII.

globulin, antihemophilic B, n See factor IX.

glomerular disease, *n* any of a group of diseases in which the glomerulus of the kidney is affected.

glomerular filtration rate, *n* a kidney function test in which the results are determined from the amount of ultrafiltrate formed by plasma flowing through the glomeruli of the kidney. It may be calculated from insulin and creatinine clearance, serum creatinine, and blood urea nitrogen (BUN).

glomerulus, *n* a tuft or cluster of blood vessels or nerve fibers, such as the cluster of blood vessels in the kidney that function as filters of the plasma portion of the blood.

glossalgia (glôsal′jē-ə), *n* painful sensations in the tongue.

glossectomy (glôsek′təmē), *n* the surgical removal of the tongue, a portion of the tongue, or a lesion of the tongue.

glossitis (glôsī'tis), *n* an inflammation of the tongue.

Glossitis. (Regezi/Sciubba/Pogrel, 2000)

glossitis areata exfoliativa, n See tongue, geographic.

glossitis, atrophic, n (bald tongue, smooth tongue) atrophy of the glossal papillae, resulting in a smooth tongue. The tongue may be pallid or erythematous and may appear small or enlarged. Atrophic glossitis may be associated with anemias, pellagra, vitamin B complex deficiencies, sprue, or other systemic diseases or may be local in origin. Because atrophy may be one phase, and circumscribed, painful, glossal excoriations may be another phase of one or more of the same systemic disease(s), much confusion in terminology has arisen (for example, Moeller's glossitis; Hunter's glossitis; slick, glazed, varnished, glossy, or bald tongue; chronic superficial erythematous glossitis; glossodynia exfoliativa; beefy tongue; and pellagrous glossitis).

glossitis, benign migratory, n See tongue, geographic.

glossitis exfoliativa, n See glossitis, Moeller's.

glossitis, interstitial sclerous, n (Clarke-Fournier glossitis), nodular, lobulated, indurated tongue associated with terminal syphilis.

glossitis, median rhomboid, n a developmental defect appearing as a red, slightly elevated area of the tongue just anterior to the foramen cecum. It is of no clinical significance and results from trapping of the median lobe of the tongue (tuberculum impar) at the surface during development.

glossitis migrans, n See tongue, geographic.

glossodynia (glôs'ōdī'nē-ə), *n* painful sensations in the tongue; a sensation of burning in the tongue; a sore tongue.

glossopharyngeal nerve, *n* either of a pair of the ninth cranial nerves essential to the sense of taste. The nerve has both sensory and motor fibers that pass from the tongue, parotid gland, and pharynx; it communicates with the vagus nerve, and connects with a motor and sensory area of the brain. See also nerve(s).

glossoplasty (glôs'ōplastē), *n* a surgical procedure performed on the tongue.

glossoplegia (glôs'ōplē'jē-ə), *n* a paralysis of the tongue; may be unilateral or bilateral.

glossoptosis, *n* a downward displacement of the tongue; a severe displacement may occlude the airway.

glossopyrosis (glôs'ōpīrō'sis), *n* a burning sensation of the tongue.

glossorrhaphy (glôsôr'əfē), *n* the suture of a wound of the tongue.

glossotomy (glôsot'əmē), *n* an excision or incision of the tongue.

glottal (glot'əl), *adj* pertaining to, or produced in or by, the glottis. The sound of *h* is a voiceless glottal fricative. The airstream on the exhalation phase moves unimpeded through the larynx, pharynx, and oral cavities.

glottis (glot'is), *n* the vocal apparatus of the larynx, consisting of the true vocal cords (vocal folds and the opening between them [rima glottidis]).

gloves or surgical gloves, *n.pl* latex gloves used as an essential part of barrier protection in health care delivery.

glucagon (glōō'kəgon), *n* (hyperglycemic factor, hyperglycemic-glycogenolytic factor [HGF]) a hormone from the α cells of the pancreas that raises the blood sugar by increasing hepatic glycogenolysis.

glucans, *n.pl* polyglucose compounds such as cellulose, starch, amylose, glycogen amylose, and callose.

glucocorticoids (glōō'kōkôr'təkoidz), *n.pl* (antiinflammatory hormone, 11-oxycorticoids) adrenocortical steroid hormones that affect glycogenesis in the liver. They are antiinflammatory, are active in protection against stress, and affect carbohydrate and protein metabolism. Typical of the group are cortisol and cortisone.

glucokinase, *n* a hexokinase or phosphotransferase that catalyzes the conversion of glucose to glucose-6-phosphate by ATP.

gluconeogenesis (glŏŏ′kōnē′ōjen′əsis), *n* the formation of glycogen or glucose from noncarbohydrate sources (for example, the glycogenic amino acids, glycerol, lactate, and pyruvate) by pathways mainly involving the citric acid cycle and glycolysis.

glucose (glŏŏ′kōs), *n* a six-carbon (hexose) sugar that is the principal sugar in blood and serves as a major metabolic source of energy.

glucose, casual plasma, n the amount of glucose in the blood at any time, unrelated to eating.

glucose, fasting plasma (FPG), n a self-administered test of blood glucose levels for diabetes patients. The blood is tested after at least eight hours of fasting. If results of the test are consistently at or above 126 mg/dl, the patient is commonly diagnosed with diabetes.

glucose meter, n an electronic device used to measure blood glucose levels which can be used by a patient at home. The device provides an accurate reading of blood glucose level with only a drop of blood from a pricked finger.

glucose oxidase, n an antibacterial flavoprotein enzyme obtained from *Penicillium notatum* and other fungi. It is antibacterial in the presence of glucose and oxygen.

glucose, postprandial plasma, n the level of glucose in the blood plasma based on a sample of blood taken after ingesting a meal; used to diagnose diabetes.

glucose tolerance, impaired, n one category of oral glucose tolerance test results. The diagnosis is not necessarily indicative of diabetes, but the patient may be at risk of diabetes and heart disease.

glucose tolerance test, n a metabolic test that measures the ability of the body to metabolize carbohydrates. A patient is administered a standard dose of glucose, and blood and urine samples are measured for glucose levels at periodic intervals following administration. The test is most often used to assist in the diagnosis of diabetes.

glucoside (glŏŏ′kōsīd), *n* a glycoside in which the sugar component is glucose.

glucosuria (gloo″ko-su′re-ə), *n* See glycosuria.

glucuronidase, *n* an enzyme that acts as a catalyst in the hydrolysis of various glucuronides with the liberation of glucuronic acid.

glutamic acid, *n* a nonessential amino acid occurring widely in a number of proteins. Preparations of glutamic acid are used as aids for digestion.

glutaraldehyde, *n* a germicidal agent used for the disinfection and sterilization of instruments or equipment that cannot be heat sterilized. An effective agent used in solution for "cold" sterilization.

glutathione, *n* an enzyme whose deficiency is commonly associated with hemolytic anemia.

gluten, *n* an insoluble protein constituent of wheat and other grains consisting of a mixture of gliadin, glutenin, and other proteins. Gluten provides the elastic qualities of bread dough.

glyburide, *n* *trade names:* Apo-Glyburide, DiaBeta, Micronase; *drug class:* oral antidiabetic (second generation); *action:* causes functioning cells in pancreas to release insulin, leading to a drop in blood glucose levels; *use:* stable adult-onset diabetes mellitus (type 2).

glycemia (gli-se′me-ə), *n* existence of glucose in the bloodstream. See also hypoglycemia, hyperglycemia.

glyceride (glis′ərīd), *n* an ester of glycerin with one or more aliphatic acids.

glycerin, *n* a sweet, colorless, oily fluid that is a pharmaceutical grade of glycerol. Glycerin is used as a moistening agent for chapped skin, as an ingredient of suppositories for constipation, and as a sweetening agent and vehicle for drug preparation. It is also spelled glycerine.

glycerite (glis′ərīt), *n* a solution or suspension of a drug in glycerin.

Glycerol, *n.pr* an alcohol that is a component of fats. See also glycerin.

glycine, *n* a nonessential amino acid occurring widely as a component of animal and plant proteins. Synthetically produced glycine is used in solutions for irrigation, in the treatment of various muscle diseases, and as an antacid and dietary supplement.

glycogen (glī′kōjen), *n* a branched, homopolysaccharide of glucose held by α 1-4 and α 1-6 glucosidic bonds. Liver glycogen provides a ready source of blood glucose through glycogenolysis.

glycogen storage disease, *n* any of a group of inherited disorders of glycogen metabolism. An enzyme deficiency causes glycogen to accumulate in abnormally large amounts in various parts of the body. The full taxonomy of glycogen storage diseases runs from Type I to Type VII.

glycogenesis (gli′kōjen′əsis), *n* the synthesis of glycogen from glucose.

glycogenolysis (gli′kōjēnol′isis), *n* the formation of blood glucose by hydrolysis of stored liver glycogen.

glycolipids (gli″ko-lip′ids), *n.pl* fats found in the brain and nervous system which contain a carbohydrate constituent.

glycolysis (glīkol′isis), *n* **1.** oxidation of glucose or glycogen by cytoplasmic enzymes of the Embden-Meyerhof pathway to pyruvate and lactate. **2.** a series of enzymatically catalyzed reactions occurring within cells, by which glucose and other sugars are broken down to yield lactic acid or pyruvic acid, releasing energy in the form of adenosine triphosphate.

glyconeogenesis (gli″ko-ne″o-jen′ə-sis), *n* the synthetic creation of blood sugar from mediating metabolites. See also gluconeogenesis and glycogenolysis.

glycoprotein, *n* any of the large group of conjugated proteins in which the nonprotein substance is a carbohydrate. These include the mucins, the mucoids, and the chondroproteins.

glycopyrrolate, *n trade names:* Robinul, Robinul Forte; *drug class:* anticholinergic; *action:* inhibits acetylcholine at receptor sites in autonomic nervous system, which controls secretions, free acids in stomach; *uses:* decreased secretions before surgery, reversal of neuromuscular blockade, peptic ulcer disease, irritable bowel syndrome.

glycosaminoglycan, *n* See mucopolysaccharide.

glycoside (gli′kōsīd), *n* a compound that contains a sugar as part of the molecule.

glycosuria (gli′kōsŏŏr′ē-ə), *n* the presence of sugar in the urine. Glycosuria most commonly results from diabetes mellitus but may occur from a lowered renal threshold (renal glycosuria) in pregnancy, inorganic renal disease, and in patients taking adrenocortico-steroids.

glycosylated hemoglobin assay, *n* a laboratory test to determine the amount of glucose in the blood that is permanently bound to a molecule of hemoglobin; helps prevent development of long-term complications by monitoring glycemic control over a longer period.

Gm, *n* See gram.

gnathion (nā′thē-on), *n* the lowest point in the lower border of the mandible at the median plane. It is a point on the bony border palpated from below and naturally lies posterior to the tegumental border of the chin.

gnathodynamometer (nath′ōdī′nəmom′ətur), *n* an instrument used for measuring biting pressure.

gnathodynamometer, bimeter, *n* a gnathodynamometer equipped with a central bearing point of adjustable height.

Gnathograph (nath′ōgraf), *n.pr* an articulator designed by McCollum. It resembles the Hanau instrument but differs chiefly by having a provision for increasing the intercondylar distance, an important determinant of groove directions in the occlusal surfaces of teeth.

Gnatholator, *n.pr* an articulator designed by Granger that has since been succeeded by an improved instrument called the Simulator (or Gnathosimulator).

gnathologic instrument, *n* a term often used as a synonym for an articulator. Any dental instrument used for diagnosis and treatment, such as a probe for determining the depth of a periodontal pocket, is a gnathologic tool.

gnathology, *n* the study of the functional and occlusal relationships of the teeth; sometimes also used to identify a specific philosophy of occlusal function.

gnathoschisis (nathos′kisis), *n* See jaw, cleft.

gnathostatics (nath´ōstat´iks), *n* a technique of orthodontic diagnosis based on relationships between the teeth and certain landmarks on the skull. See also cast, gnathostatic.

goal, *n* the purpose toward which an endeavor is directed, such as the outcome of diagnostic, therapeutic, and educational management of a patient's health problem.

goggles, *n* protective eyewear worn by dental healthcare providers.

goiter (goi´tur), *n* an enlargement of the thyroid gland.

goiter, colloid, *n* (endemic goiter, iodine deficiency goiter, simple goiter) a visible enlargement of the thyroid gland without obvious signs of hypofunction or hyperfunction of the gland resulting from inadequate intake or from an increased demand for iodine.

goiter, endemic, *n* See goiter, colloid.

goiter, exophthalmic, *n* a disease of the thyroid gland consisting of hyperthyroidism, exophthalmos, and goiterous enlargement of the thyroid gland. A diffuse primary hyperplasia of the thyroid gland of obscure origin; may occur at any age. It produces nervousness, muscular weakness, heat intolerance, tremor, loss of weight, lid lag, and absence of winking and may lead to thyrotoxic heart disease and thyroid crisis.

Goiter, exophthalmic. (Zitelli/Davis, 2002)

goiter, iodine deficiency, *n* See goiter, colloid.

goiter, nodular, nontoxic, *n* recurrent episodes of hyperplasia and involution of colloid goiter, resulting in a multinodular goiter. Symptoms are related to pressure.

goiter, simple, *n* See goiter, colloid.

goitrogens (goi´trōjenz), *n.pl* agents such as thiouracil and related antithyroid compounds that are capable of producing goiter.

gold, *n* a precious or noble metal; yellow, malleable, ductile, nonrusting; much used in dentistry in pure and alloyed forms.

gold alloys, *n.pl* any alloy that contains gold; usually alloyed with copper, silver, platinum, palladium, and zinc. The alloying of gold enhances certain properties such as hardness, or creates a lower melting point for gold solder.

gold compound, *n* a drug containing gold salts, usually administered with other drugs in the treatment of rheumatoid arthritis. Various radioisotopes of gold have been used in diagnostic radiology and in the radiologic treatment of certain malignant neoplastic diseases.

gold, crystal, *n* See gold, mat.

gold, fibrous, *n* See foil, gold.

gold file, *n* See file, gold.

gold foil, *n* See foil, gold.

gold foil cylinder, *n* See foil cylinder.

gold foil pellet, *n* See pellet, foil.

gold, inlay, *n* **1.** an alloy, principally gold, used for cast restorations. Desired physical properties may be obtained by selecting those with varying ingredients and/or proportions. Acceptable alloys are classified by the American Dental Association (ADA) specifications according to Brinell hardness: Type A–soft, Brinell 40 to 75; Type B–medium, Brinell 70 to 100; Type C–hard, Brinell 90 to 140. *n* **2.** an intracoronal cast restoration of gold alloy fabricated outside the mouth and cemented into the prepared cavity.

gold knife, *n* See knife, gold.

gold, mat, *n* (crystal gold, sponge gold) a noncohesive form of pure gold prepared by electrodeposition. Sometimes used in the base of restorations and then veneered or overlaid with cohesive foil.

gold, powdered, n fine granules of pure gold, formed by atomizing the molten metal or by chemical precipitation. For clinical use, powdered gold is available either as clusters of the granules or as pellets of the powder contained in an envelope of gold foil.

gold saw, n See saw, gold.

gold sodium thiosulfate, n an antirheumatic used in the treatment of rheumatoid arthritis.

gold, sponge, n See gold, mat.

gold, white, n a gold alloy with a high palladium content. It has a higher fusion range, lower ductility, and greater hardness than a yellow gold alloy.

Goldent, n.pr the trade name for a direct gold restorative material. It consists basically of varying amounts of powdered gold contained in a wrapping or envelope of gold foil.

Goldman-Fox knife, n.pr See knife, Goldman-Fox.

Golgi apparatus, n.pr one of many small membranous structures found in most cells, composed of various elements associated with the formation of carbohydrate side chains of glycoproteins, mucopolysaccharides, and other substances. Also called *Golgi body* or *Golgi complex.*

Golgi's corpuscles (gol'jēz), n.pr See corpuscle, Golgi's.

gomphosis (gämfō'sis), n a form of joint in which a conical body is fastened into a socket, as a tooth is fastened into the jaw.

gonad (gō'nad), n an ovary or testis, the site of origin of eggs or spermatozoa.

gonadotrophin (gōnad'ōtrōf'in), n See gonadotropin.

gonadotropin (gōnad'ōtrōp'in), n (gonadotropic hormone) a gonadstimulating hormone derived either from the pituitary gland (for example, follicle-stimulating hormone [FSH] and luteinizing hormone [LH], which is also an interstitial cell-stimulating hormone [ICSH]) or from the chorion (for example, chorionic gonadotropin, which is found in the urine of pregnant women).

gonadotropin, chorionic, n See hormone, pregnancy.

gonion (Go), n the most posteroinferior point of the angle of the mandible near the lower border of the ramus.

gonorrhea, n a sexually transmitted disease of the genitourinary tract which is spread by direct contact with an infected person or fluids containing the infectious microorganism. The disease may also affect the conjunctiva, oral tissue, and other tissues and organ systems.

good faith, n honesty of intention. Generally, not a sufficient defense in a dental malpractice lawsuit.

good samaritan legislation, n statutes enacted in some states protecting physicians, dentists, and some other health professionals from liability for aid rendered in emergency situations, unless there is a showing of willful wrong or gross negligence.

goodwill, n the intangible assets of a firm established by the excess of the price paid for the ongoing concern over its book value.

gothic arch tracer, n See tracer, needle point.

gothic arch tracing, n See tracing, needle point.

gout, n a disease associated with an inborn error of uric acid metabolism that increases production or interferes with the excretion of uric acid. Excess uric acid is converted to sodium urate crystals that precipitate from the blood and become deposited in joints and other tissues. The great toe is a common site for the accumulation of urate crystals. This condition can be exceedingly painful with swelling of a joint and may be accompanied by chills and fever.

gown, n protective garment worn by healthcare provider designed to prevent the spread of infection between the healthcare provider and the patient.

gr, n See grain.

grace period, n a specified time, after a plan's premium payment is due, in which the protection of the plan continues subject to actual receipt of the premium within that time.

graft, n a slip or portion of tissue used for implantation. See also donor site; recipient site.

graft, allo-, n a graft between genet-

G

G

ically dissimilar members of the same species.

graft, alloplast, n a graft of an inert metal or plastic material.

graft, auto-, n See graft, autogenous.

graft, autogenous, n a graft taken from one portion of an individual's body and implanted into another portion of the individual's body.

graft, bone, n the transplantation of healthy bone tissue to a defective bone cavity so that the new bone tissue meets the surrounding, unaffected surface and promotes healing and new growth.

graft, bone, allograft, n a bone graft using tissue obtained from an individual other than, but of the same species as, the host of the bone graft; sources include human cadavers, living relatives, and nonrelatives. Also called *allogeneic graft* and *homograft.*

graft, bone, autogenous, n See graft, autogenous.

graft donor site, n the site from which graft material is taken.

graft, filler, n the filling of defects, such as bone chips used to fill a cyst.

graft, free, n a graft of tissue completely detached from its original site and blood supply.

graft, full-thickness, n a skin graft consisting of the full thickness of the skin with none of the subcutaneous tissues.

graft, hetero-, n See graft, heterogenous.

graft, heterogenous, n a graft implanted from one species to another.

graft, homo-, n See graft, homogenous.

graft, homogenous, n a graft taken from a member of a species and implanted into the body of a member of the same species.

graft, iliac, n a bone graft whose donor site is the crest of the ilium. Various locations of the iliac crest duplicate areas of the mandible and curvatures of the midfacial skeleton.

graft, iso-, n a graft between individuals with identical or histocompatible antigens.

graft, kiel, n a denatured calf bone used to fill defects or restore facial contour.

graft, mucosal, n a split-thickness graft involving the mucosa.

graft, onlay bone, n a graft in which the grafted bone is applied laterally to the cortical bone of the recipient site, frequently to improve the contours of the chin or the malar eminence of the zygomatic bone.

graft, pedicle, n a stem or tube of tissue that remains attached near the donor site to nourish the graft during advancement of a skin graft.

graft, split-thickness, n a graft with varying thickness containing only mucosal elements and no subcutaneous tissue.

graft, swaging, n a procedure analogous to bone grafting. Also referred to as a *contiguous transplant,* which involves a greenstick fracture of bone bordering on an infrabony defect and the displacement of bone to eliminate the osseous defect.

graft, Thiersch's skin, n.pr a split-thickness skin graft containing cutaneous and some subcutaneous tissues, the line of cleavage through the rete peg layer.

grain (gr), n **1.** a unit of weight equal to 0.0648 g. n **2.** a crystal of an alloy.

grain boundary, n the junction of two grains growing from different nuclei, impinging and causing discontinuity of the lattice structure. Important in corrosion and brittleness of metals.

grain growth, n See growth, grain.

gram (Gm, g), n the basic unit of mass of the metric system. Equivalent to 15.432 gr.

gram-negative, n having the pink color of the counterstain used in Gram's method of staining microorganisms. Staining property is a common method of classifying bacteria. See also Gram's stain.

gram-positive, n retaining the violet color of the stain used in Gram's method of staining microorganisms. Staining property is a common method of classifying bacteria. See also Gram's stain.

gramicidin, n an antibacterial agent generally used in conjunction with nystatin, a specific anticandidal agent, and neomycin, a complementary antibacterial agent, in the treatment of angular cheilosis.

Gram's stain, n.pr also called *Gram's method.* A sequential process for staining microorganisms in which a violet stain is followed by a wash and then a counterstain of safranin. Gram-positive organisms appear violet or blue; gram-negative organisms appear rose pink.

granulation tissue, *n* any soft, pink, fleshy projections that form during the healing process in a wound not healing by first intent. Granulation tissue consists of many capillaries surrounded by fibrous collagen. Overgrowth is termed *proud flesh.* Such tissue is evident at the opening to a fistulous tract or at the site of a recent tooth extraction.

granules, sulfur, *n.pl* See actinomycosis.

granulocyte, *n* a type of leukocyte (white blood cell) characterized by the presence of cytoplasmic granules.

granulocytopenia (gran′yōōlōsī′tōpē′nē-ə), *n* a deficiency in the number of granulocytic cells in the bloodstream. See also agranulocytosis.

granuloma (gran′yōōlō′mə), *n* a localized mass of granulation tissue characterized by an accumulation of macrophages, epithelioid macrophages, with or without lymphocytes, and giant cells into a discrete mass.

Midline granuloma. (Regezi/Sciubba/Jordan, 2003)

granuloma, chronic, n (chronic apical periodontitis) chronic inflammatory tissue surrounding the apical foramina as a result of irritation from within the root canal system.

granuloma, dental, n a mass of granulation tissue surrounded by a fibrous capsule attached at the apex of a pulp-involved tooth. It produces a radiolucency that is fairly well demarcated.

granuloma, eosinophilic (ē′-əsin′ōfil′ik), n a granulomatous inflammatory disease of unknown etiology, usually monofocal in bone but sometimes affecting soft tissues. Sheets of histiocytes and masses of eosinophils characterize the lesion histologically.

granuloma, giant cell reparative, n an inflammatory lesion located near the gingival margin. It takes the shape of a mushroom, has a smooth, glossy surface, bleeds easily, and tends to reoccur after removal. It generally occurs in the third trimester of pregnancy. See also granuloma, pyogenic.

granuloma inguinale, n a sexually transmitted disease characterized by ulcers of the skin and subcutaneous tissues of the groin and genitalia. It is caused by infection with *Calymmatobacterium granulomatis,* a small, gram-negative, rod-shaped bacillus.

granuloma, pyogenic, n a tumorlike mass of granulation tissue produced in response to minor trauma in some individuals. It is not pus-producing, as the name suggests, but is highly vascular and bleeds readily. Pyogenic granulomas are histologically identical to pregnancy granulomas, but they may be found in either gender in any location, and may occur at any age.

granuloma, reticuloendothelial, n See disease, lipoid storage.

graph, *n* a diagram used to compare numerical relationships.

graphite, *n* a soft carbon substance with a metallic black or gray sheen and a greasy feel. It is used in pencils, as a constituent of lubricants, and for making refractories such as crucibles in which to melt gold and other metals.

grasp, *n* the manner in which an instrument is held.

grasp, finger, n a modification of the palm and thumb grasp; it is more useful with modern, smaller handled instruments. The handle is held by the four flexed fingers rather than allowed to rest in the palm, and the thumb is used to secure a rest. Used when working indirectly on the upper arch.

grasp, instrument, n a method of holding the instrument with the fingers in such a manner that freedom of action, control, tactile sensitivity, and maneuverability are secured. The most common grasp is the pen grasp.

grasp, modified pen, *n* a method for holding instruments that is designed to enhance control and sensitivity. The grasp consists of the tips of the thumb, index finger, and middle finger holding the instrument while the ring finger provides support. See also grasp, pen.

grasp, palm-and-thumb, *n* a grasp that is similar to the hold on a knife when one is whittling wood; the handle rests in the palm and is grasped by the four fingers, while the thumb rests on an adjoining object.

grasp, pen, *n* a grasp in which the instrument is held somewhat as a pen is held, with the handle in contact with the bulbous portion of the thumb and index finger and the shank in contact with the radial side of the bulbous portion of the middle finger (not crossing the nail), while the handle rests against the phalanx of the index finger.

gratis, *adj* free, without reward or consideration.

Graves' disease, *n.pr* See goiter, exophthalmic.

gravity, specific, *n* a number indicating the ratio of the weight of a substance to that of an equal volume of water.

Gray (Gy), *n* unit of measurement for an absorbed dose of radiation, from the French *Systéme International d'Unités;* converts to the traditional rad by the formula 100 rad = 1 Gy.

grid, *n* a device used to prevent as much scattered radiation as possible from reaching an x-ray film during the making of a radiograph. It consists essentially of a series of narrow lead strips closely spaced on their edges and separated by spacers of low-density material.

grid, crossed, *n* an arrangement of two parallel grids rotated in position at right angles to each other. See also grid, parallel.

grid, focused, *n* a grid in which the lead foils are placed at an angle so that they all point toward a focus at a specified distance.

grid, moving, *n* a grid that is moved continuously or oscillated throughout the making of a radiograph.

grid, parallel, *n* a grid in which the lead strips are oriented parallel to each other.

grid, Potter-Bucky, *n.pr* a grid using the principle of the moving grid, with an oscillating movement.

grid, stationary, *n* a nonoscillating or nonmoving grid; the image of its strips will be visible on the radiograph for which it is used.

grinding, selective, *n* a modification of the occlusal forms of teeth by grinding at selected places to improve function.

grinding-in, *n* the process of correcting errors in the centric and eccentric occlusions of natural or artificial teeth.

griseofulvin microsize/griseofulvin ultramicrosize, *n trade names:* Fulvicin U/F, Grifulvin V, Gris-PEG; *drug class:* antifungal; *action:* arrests fungal cell division at metaphase; binds to human keratin, making it resistant to disease; *uses:* mycotic infections: tinea corporis, tinea pedis, tinea cruris, tinea barbae, tinea capitis, tinea unguium if caused by *Epidermophyton, Microsporum, Trichophyton.*

grit, *n* the measurement of the abrasive particle size.

groin, *n* each of two areas where the abdomen joins the thighs.

groove, *n* a linear channel or sulcus.

groove, abutment, *n* a transverse groove that may be cut in the bone across the alveolar ridge to furnish positive seating for the implant framework and to prevent tension of the tissue.

groove, developmental, *n* a fine depressed line in the enamel of a tooth that marks the union of the lobes of the crown in its development.

groove, gingiva, free, *n* the shallow line or depression on the surface of the gingiva at the junction of the free and attached gingivae.

groove, interdental, *n* a linear, vertical depression on the surface of the interdental papillae; functions as a sluiceway for the egress of food from the interproximal areas.

groove, labiomental, *n* a natural indentation in the chin, just below the lips, that takes its form from the muscles and bones lying beneath the skin.

groove, linguogingival, n vertical groove on the lingual surface of certain anterior teeth that originates in the lingual pit and extends cervically and slightly distal onto the cingulum.

groove, marginal, n developmental furrow that forms across the marginal ridges of posterior teeth.

groove, retention, n a groove formed by opposing vertical constrictions in the preparation of a tooth that provides improved retention of the restoration.

ground, electrical, *n* an electrical connection with the earth (or other ground).

ground state, *n* the state of a nucleus, an atom, or a molecule when it has its lowest energy. All other states are termed *excited.*

ground substance, *n* See matrix.

ground substance, of bone, n major component of bone consisting of proteoglycans that contain chondroitin sulfate and hydroxyapatite.

grounded, *adj* pertaining to an arrangement whereby an electrical circuit or equipment such as an x-ray generator is connected by an electrical conductor with the earth or some similarly conducting body.

group, blood, *n* See blood groups.

group function, *n* See function, group.

group practice, *n* the association of several health care providers to complement, facilitate, and extend their scope of health care delivery, not possible in a sole or single practice. See also practice, group.

group purchase, *n* the purchase of dental services, either by postpayment or prepayment, by a large group of people.

growth, *n* an increase in size.

growth and development, n growth is defined as an increase in size; *development* is defined as a progression toward maturity. Thus the terms are used together to describe the complex physical, mental, and emotional processes associated with the "growing up" of children.

growth factor, n one of about a hundred chemical messengers that induces cell growth by tissue type (for example, osteoinductive factor, epidermal growth factors).

growth failure, n a lack of normal physical and psychologic development as a result of genetic, nutritional, pathologic, or psychosocial factors. See also failure to thrive.

growth, grain, n a phenomenon resulting from heat treatment of alloys. In excessive amounts, this growth produces undesirable physical properties.

growth hormone, n (GH) a single-chain peptide secreted by the anterior pituitary gland in response to growth hormone releasing factor (GHRF) from the hypothalamus. Growth hormone promotes protein synthesis in all cells, increased fat mobilization and use of fatty acids for energy, and decreased use of carbohydrates.

GTT, *n* See test, glucose tolerance.

guaiacol, *n* catecholomonomethyl ether, which is used as an expectorant and intestinal disinfectant

guaifenesin, *n trade names:* Anti-Tuss, Robitussin; *drug class:* expectorant; *action:* acts as an expectorant by stimulating mucosal reflex to increase production of less viscous lung mucus; *use:* dry, nonproductive cough.

guanabenz acetate, *n trade names:* Wytensin; *drug class:* centrally acting antihypertensive; *action:* stimulates central α_2-adrenergic receptors, resulting in decreased sympathetic outflow from the brain; *use:* hypertension.

guanadrel sulfate, *n trade name:* Hylorel; *drug class:* antihypertensive; *action:* inhibits sympathetic vasoconstriction by inhibiting release of norephinephrine, depleting norepinephrine stores in adrenergic nerve endings; *use:* hypertension.

guanethidine sulfate, *n trade name:* Ismelin; *drug class:* antihypertensive; *action:* inhibits norepinephrine release, depleting norepinephrine stores in adrenergic nerve endings; *use:* moderate-to-severe hypertension.

guanfacine HCl, *n trade name:* Tenex; *drug class:* antihypertensive; *action:* stimulates central α-adrenergic receptors, resulting in decreased sympathetic outflow from the brain; *use:* hypertension in individuals using a thiazide diuretic.

guanosine, *n* a compound derived from a nucleic acid, composed of guanine and a sugar, D-ribose. Guanosine is a major molecular component of the nucleotides guanosine monophosphate and guanosine triphosphate and of DNA and RNA.

guanosine triphosphate, n (GTP) a high-energy nucleotide, similar to adenosine triphosphate, that functions in various metabolic reactions such as the activation of fatty acids and the formation of the peptide bond in protein synthesis.

guaranty, n a contract that some certain and designated thing shall be done exactly as it is agreed to be done.

guard, bite, n an acrylic resin appliance designed to cover the occlusal and incisal surfaces of the teeth of a dental arch to stabilize the teeth and/or provide a flat platform for the unobstructed excursive glides of the mandible. See also plane, bite.

guard, mouth, n a resilient intraoral device worn during participation in contact sports to reduce the potential for injury to the teeth and associated tissue.

guard, night, n See guard, bite.

guardian, n a person appointed to take care of the person or property of another; one who legally has the care and management of the person or the property or both of a child until the child attains adulthood.

Guérin's fracture (gāranz'), *n.pr* See fracture, Guérin's

guidance, n a mechanical or other means for controlling the direction of movement of an object.

guidance, angle, n See angle, incisal guidance.

guidance, condylar, n See guide, condylar.

guidance, condylar, inclination, n See guide, condylar, inclination.

guidance, developmental, n comprehensive dentofacial orthopedic control over the growth of the jaws and eruption of the teeth, with the objective of optimizing the achievement of the genetic potential of the individual. Requires a combination of carefully timed active appliance therapy and supervisory examinations, including radiography and other diagnostic records, at various stages of development. May be required throughout the entire period of

growth and maturation of the face, beginning at the earliest detection of a developing malformation.

guidance, incisal, n the influence on mandibular movements of the contacting surfaces of the mandibular and maxillary anterior teeth.

guide, n a device for directing the motion of something.

guide, adjustable anterior, n an anterior guide, the superior surface of which may be varied to provide desired separation of the casts in various eccentric relationships.

guide, anterior, n the part of an articulator contacted by the incisal guide pin to maintain the selected separation of the upper and lower members of the articulator. The guide influences the changing relationships of mounted casts in eccentric movements. See also guide, incisal.

guide, condylar, n (condylar guidance) the mechanical device on an articulator; intended to produce guidance in articulator movement similar to that produced by the paths of the condyles in the temporomandibular joints.

guide, condylar, inclination, n (condylar guidance inclination) the angle of inclination of the condylar guide mechanism of an articulator in relation to the horizontal plane of the instrument.

guide, incisal, n (anterior guide) the part of an articulator that maintains the incisal guide angle.

guide, incisal, adjustment, n occlusal adjustment that produces a minimum of overbite (vertical overlap) and a maximum of overjet (horizontal overlap), eliminates fremitus and racking effects on the anterior segment of teeth in the protrusive glide, and attains maximal incisive group function.

guide, incisal, angle, n See angle, incisal guide.

guide plane, n a fixed or removable orthodontic appliance designed to deflect the functional path of the mandible and alter the positions of specific teeth.

guide dog, n carefully trained dog used to assist an individual with limited vision with daily living skills.

guidelines, *n.pl* a set of standards, criteria, or specifications to be used or followed in the performance of certain tasks.

gum(s), *n* the fibrous and mucosal covering of the alveolar process or ridges. See also gingiva.

gum pads, n edentulous segments of the maxillae and mandible that correspond to the underlying primary teeth.

gumboil, *n* an abscess of the gingiva and periosteum resulting from injury, infection, impacted food particles, or periapical infection. The gum is characteristically red, swollen, and tender. The abscess may rupture spontaneously, or it may require incision, as well as treatment of the underlying cause.

gumma (gum´ə), *n* a granulomatous, gummy lesion of tertiary syphilis. The palate and tongue are sites of predilection in the oral region. A similar lesion occurring with tuberculosis is designated a tuberculous gumma.

Gunn's syndrome, *n.pr* See splint, Gunning's.

gutta-percha (gut´əpur´chə), *n* the coagulated juice of various tropical trees that has certain rubberlike properties. Used for temporary sealing of dressings in cavities; also used in the form of cones for filling root canals and in the form of sticks for sealing cavities over treatment.

gutta-percha, baseplate, n gutta-percha combined with fillers and coloring materials and rolled into sheets that are used as temporary bases for denture construction.

gutta-percha points, n.pl fine, tapered cylinders of gutta percha used, because of their radiopacity, for radiographic ascertainment of pocket depth and topography; used also as a root canal filling material.

gutta-percha, temporary stopping, n gutta-percha mixed with zinc oxide and white wax. Used for temporary sealing of dressings in cavities.

gynecologist, *n* a physician whose practice of medicine focuses on the care of women, including the treatment of conditions related to the female genitourinary tract, endocrine system, and reproductive organs.

gypsum (jip´sum), *n* the dihydrate of calcium sulfate ($CaSO_4 \cdot 2H_2O$). α Hemihydrate and β hemihydrate are derived from gypsum. See also plaster of paris.

h II., *n* See *hemophilia B.*

h.s., *n* the abbreviation for the Latin term *hora somni,* meaning "at bedtime."

habilitation, *n* See *rehabilitation.*

habit, *n* the tendency toward an act that has become a repeated performance, relatively fixed, consistent, easy to perform, and almost automatic. Once learned, habits may occur without the intent of the person or may appear to be out of control and are difficult to change. In dentistry, habits such as bruxism, clenching, tongue thrusting, and lip and cheek biting may produce injury to the teeth, their attachment apparatus, oral mucosa, mandibular and temporomandibular musculature, and articulation.

habituation, *n* a state in which an individual involuntarily tends to continue the use of a drug. Generally refers to the state in which an individual continues self-administration of a drug because of psychologic dependence without physical dependence.

Haemophilus, *n* a genus of gram-negative pathogenic bacteria, frequently found in the respiratory tract of humans and other animals. *Hae mophilus* species are generally sensitive to cephalosporins, tetracyclines, and sulfonamides.

Haemophilus influenzae, *n* a small, gram-negative, nonmotile, parasitic bacterium that occurs in two forms, encapsulated and nonencapsulted, and in six types: A, B, C, D, E, and F. Almost all infections are caused by the encapsulated type B organisms. *H. influenzae* is found in the throats of 30% of healthy, normal people. It may cause destructive inflammation of the larynx, trachea, and bronchi in children and debilitated older people.

Hageman trait (hä′gə-mən), *n* See *factor XII.* (not current)

hair covering, *n* part of an overall contamination limiting strategy; hair should be pulled back from the shoulders and face. Longer hair may be completely concealed beneath a cap made from an approved material.

halazepam, *n trade name:* Paxipam; *drug class:* benzodiazepine (Controlled Substance Schedule IV); *action:* produces central nervous system depression by interaction with benzodiazepine receptor to facilitate action of inhibitory neurotransmitter γ-aminobutyric acid; *use:* anxiety.

halcinonide, *n trade names:* Halog-E, Halog; *drug class:* corticosteroid, synthetic topical; *action:* interacts with steroid cytoplasmic receptors to induce antiinflammatory actions; *use:* inflammation of corticosteroid-responsive dermatoses.

half-life, *n* the time in which a radioactive substance will lose half of its activity through disintegration.

half-life, biologic, n the time in which a living tissue, organ, or individual eliminates, through biologic processes, half of a given amount of a substance that has been introduced into it.

half-life, effective, n the half-life of a radioactive isotope in a biologic organism, resulting from the combination of radioactive decay and biologic elimination.

half-life, physical, n the average time required for the decay of half the atoms in a given amount of a radioactive substance.

half-value layer (HVL), *n* the thickness of a specified material (usually aluminum, copper, or lead) required to decrease the dosage rate of a beam of x-rays at a point of interest to half its initial value. A determination of the half-value layer of a given x-ray beam is used to denote the quality of the x-ray beam. The half-value layer will vary depending on kilovolt peak and the amount of filtration at the source.

halisteresis (həl-is′tər-ē′sis), *n* a theory of the method of bone resorption according to which bone salts can be removed by a humoral mechanism and returned to the tissue fluids, leaving behind a decalcified bone matrix; osteolysis. This is not considered to be the mechanism under which resorption occurs in periodontal disease.

halitophobia (hal′it-ō-fō′bē-ə), *n* an abiding fear of having fetid breath, whether a valid concern or not. In some cases it may be symptomatic of mental illness.

halitosis (bad breath, bromopnea, fetor ex ore, offensive breath) (hal′i-tō′sis), *n* an offensive odor of the breath resulting from local and metabolic conditions (for example, poor oral hygiene, periodontal disease, sinusitis, tonsilitis, suppurative bronchopulmonary disease, acidosis, uremia).

Haller's plexus, *n.pr* See *plexus, Haller's.*

hallucination (həl-ōō′sin-ā′shən), *n* an artificial sensory experience without the presence of an external cause.

hallucinogens, abuse of (həl-ōō′sin-ə-jenz), *n* a regular use of mescaline or *d*-lysergic acid diethylamide (LSD) for reasons other than recognized medical applications. Street names include *cubes, acid, blue dragon, cupcake, big chief, sunshine, mesc,* and *buttons.*

halobetasol propionate, *n trade name:* Ultravate; *drug class:* topical corticosteroid, group VI potency; *action:* interacts with steroid cytoplasmic receptors to induce antiinflammatory effects, possesses antipruritic/antiinflammatory actions; *uses:* psoriasis, eczema, contact dermatitis, pruritus.

halogen (hal′ō-jen), *n* an element of a closely related group of elements consisting of fluorine, chlorine, bromine, and iodine.

halogenated hydrocarbons (hal′jən-āt-əd hī′drō-kär-bənz), *n.pl* general anesthetic agents such as halothane and isoflurane, which work with a minimum of nausea and mucous membrane irritation. They produce drowsiness for several hours after the primary effects wear off.

haloperidol/haloperidol decanoate, *n trade name:* Haldol; *drug class:* antipsychotic/butyrophenone; *action:* blocks neurotransmission at dopaminergic synapses at the cerebral cortex, hypothalamus, and limbic system; *uses:* psychotic disorders, control of tics and vocal utterances in Gilles de la Tourette syndrome, short-term treatment of hyperactive children showing excessive motor activity.

halothane (hal'ə-thān), n a potent nonflammable and nonexplosive liquid anesthetic agent administered by inhalation. Common complications associated with other inhalation anesthetic agents are generally absent. Chemical name is 2-bromo-2-chloro-1, 1, 1-trifluoroethane.

hamartoma (ham'är-tō'mə), n a localized error in the composition of the tissue elements of an organ. May be automatically manifested in three ways, either singly or in combination: abnormal quantity, abnormal structure, or degree of maturation of the tissue components.

hamster, n any of four genera of small rodents widely used in research and commonly kept as pets. All hamsters are seed and plant feeders, store away their food, hibernate in winter, and breed throughout the year under laboratory conditions.

hamular notch, n See *notch, pterygomaxillary.*

hamular process, n See *process, hamular.*

hand condenser, n See *condenser, hand.*

hand pressure, n See *pressure, hand.*

Hand-Schüller-Christian disease (hand-shül'er-kris'chən), n.pr See *disease, Hand-Schuller-Christian.*

handicap, n a disability that hinders effective function; may involve any combination of physical, emotional, or social factors.

handpiece, n an instrument that is used to hold rotary instruments in the dental engine or condensing points in mechanical condensing units. It is connected by an arm, cable, belt, or tube to the source of power (e.g., motor, air, water).

handpiece, air-turbine, n a handpiece with a turbine powered by compressed air.

handpiece, contra-angle, n a binangled instrument for use with the dental engine; permits access to areas difficult or impossible to reach with a straight handpiece.

handpiece, high-speed, n a type of rotary or vibratory cutting tool that operates at speeds above 12,000 rpm. It is propelled by gears, a belt, or a turbine. Generally classified as an air turbine, a hydraulic turbine, or a high-speed handpiece on a conventional dental engine.

handpiece, high-speed, ultra, n a handpiece designed to permit rotational speeds of 100,000 to 300,000 rpm.

handpiece, right-angle, n a monangled instrument used with mechanical condensers to reach some operating areas.

handpiece, straight, n a handpiece whose axis is in line with the rotary instrument.

handpiece, water-turbine, n a handpiece with a turbine powered by water under pressure.

handwashing, n a fundamental part of sterilization procedures and disease control for dental workers; helps reduce or prevent infection and transmittal of microbes among people and objects; for regular dental procedures, liquid soap and water is sufficient but for surgical procedures, antimicrobial cleansers should be used.

Hansen's disease, n.pr See *leprosy.*

hapten, n a nonproteinaceous substance that acts as an antigen by combining with particular bonding sites on an antibody. Unlike a true antigen, it does not induce the formation of antibodies. A hapten bonded to a carrier protein may induce an immune response. Also called *haptene.*

hard copy, n readable output from a computer generated in a storable form such as printed on paper or on microfiche; contrasts with soft copy in which the data are displayed on a video terminal or presented in some other transitory form.

hard of hearing, adj a term applied to persons whose hearing is impaired but who have enough hearing left for practical use.

hard palate, See *palate, hard.*

hardener, n an ingredient (potassium alum) of the photographic and radiographic fixing solution that serves to harden the gelatin of the film to prevent softening and swelling of the gelatin.

hardening, *n* the process of setting or becoming firm.

hardening, age, n the precipitation of intermetallic compounds that alters certain physical properties in alloys; usually brought about through heat treatment.

hardening, precipitation, See *tempering.*

hardening solution, See *solution, hardening.*

hardening, strain, an increase in proportional limit resulting from distortion of the space lattice and fracture of grain boundaries through cold working. Ductility is markedly reduced.

hardening, work, n the hardening of a metal by cold work, such as repeated flexing.

hardness (of a substance), *n* the ability of a material to resist an indenting type of load.

hardness (of x-rays), n term used to indicate in a general way the quality of x radiation, with hardness being a function of the wavelength; the shorter the wavelength, the harder the x radiation.

hardness, Mohs, n relative scratch resistance of minerals based on an arbitrary scale: 10, diamond; 9, corundum; 8, topaz; 7, quartz; 6, orthoclase; 5, apatite; 4, fluorite; 3, calcite; 2, gypsum; and 1, talc.

hardness tests, See *tests, hardness.*

hardware, *n* the mechanical, magnetic, electronic, and electric devices or components of a computer.

harelip (cheiloschisis, cleft lip, congenital cleft lip) (her'lip), *n* a congenital nonunion or inadequacy of soft and hard tissues related to the lip. The deformity may be extensive enough to involve the nose, alveolar process, hard palate, and velum. The extent of the deformity varies among individuals. Various classifications have been established to identify the extent of a cleft. A rare midline cleft may occur in the lower lip at the embryonal junction of the two mandibular processes. Outdated term. See also *lip, cleft* and *lip, congenital cleft.*

harmony, functional occlusal, *n* an occlusal relationship of opposing teeth in all functional ranges and movements that will provide the greatest masticatory efficiency without causing undue strain or trauma on the supporting tissues.

harmony, occlusal, *n* the nondisruptive relationship of an occlusion to all its factors (for example, the neuromuscular mechanism, temporomandibular joints, teeth and their supporting structures).

hashish, abuse of (hash'ish, həsh-ēsh), *n* a regular use of the cannabis derivative hashish for reasons other than recognized medical applications. Street names are *hash* and *soles.*

Hatch clamp, See *clamp, gingival, Hatch.* (not current)

hatchet, *n* an angled cutting hand instrument in which the broad side of the blade is parallel with the angle(s) of the shank. Used to develop internal cavity form. May be bibeveled or single beveled like a chisel, in which case the instrument is paired with another.

haversian system, See *osteon.*

Hawley appliance, chart, retainer, (See under appropriate noun.)

Hawley retainer, See *retainer, Hawley.*

hay fever, *n* an acute seasonal allergic rhinitis, stimulated by tree, grass, or weed pollens. Also called *allergic rhinitis.*

hay rake, See *appliance, hay rake.*

hazard communication plan, *n* a set of written standards designed to reduce workplace illness and injury by ensuring that all employees are familiar with the names and potential hazards of the chemicals they handle and understand the precautions necessary for protecting themselves and others against any possible risks.

hazard, radiation, *n* the hazard that exists in any area in which a person is subject to radiation.

hazardous waste, *n* any material, gas, liquid, or solid substance that has the potential to cause injury or illness; that in an unprotected state poses a risk to the environment, including plant or animal life.

HDL, *n* the abbreviation or acronym for high-density lipoproteins. HDL molecules are considered a protective factor in coronary heart disease.

head and neck, anatomical nomenclature, *n* naming system based on the anatomic position of a structure in the body.

head covering, n part of an overall contamination limiting strategy, a protective accessory that conceals most of the hair and head

head, steeple, See *oxycephalia.*

headache, n pain in the cranial vault resulting from intracranial, extracranial, or psychogenic causes: intracranial vascular dilation; space-occupying lesions; diseases of the eyes, ears, and sinuses; extracranial vascular dilation; sustained muscular contraction; hysteria; certain habit patterns (clenching); and reaction to stress.

headache, cluster, See *neuralgia, facial, atypical.*

headache, lower-half, See *neuralgia, facial, atypical.*

headache, migraine, n a vascular type of headache, typically unilateral in the temporal, frontal, and retroorbital area, but may occur midface. It is described as throbbing, burning, pulsating, exploding, or pressure and may become generalized and persist for hours or days. Onset of pain is usually preceded by prodromal symptoms that may include visual disturbances, scotomas, vomiting, and nausea. A migraine headache is usually considered to be a psycho-physiologic (psychosomatic) disorder.

headcap, n the part of an extraoral orthodontic appliance that engages the back of the head, incorporating the skull as a source of resistance for tooth movement, and gives attachment to the intraoral element of the appliance.

headcap, plaster, n a cap that is constructed of plaster-of-paris gauze and embodies points for applying fixation and traction appliances in the treatment of mandibular and maxillofacial injuries.

headgear, n the apparatus encircling the head or neck and providing attachment for an intraoral appliance in use of extraoral anchorage.

headgear, radiologic, n a device that is used to protect the head from injury by radiation.

health, n a bodily state in which all parts are functioning properly. Also refers to the normal functioning of a part of the body. A state of normal functional equilibrium; homeostasis.

health ASA classification, n a system for ranking the level of a patient's health, established in 1962 by the American Society of Anesthesiologists. Patients are classified as ASA I, indicating a patient in a normal state of health, with no apparent disease. ASA II indicates a patient with a mild disease. ASA III indicates a patient with a serious disease, which may limit normal activity, but does not cause incapacitation. ASA IV indicates a patient with a life-threatening and incapacitating disease. ASA V indicates a declining patient who is not expected to live beyond a day, regardless of medical attention. ASA E indicates emergency status when added to any of the normal status designations.

health assessment, n an evaluation of the health status of an individual by performing a physical examination after obtaining a health history. Various laboratory and functional tests may also be ordered to confirm a clinical impression or to screen for dysfunction.

health behavior, n an action taken by a person to maintain, attain, or regain good health and to prevent illness. Health behavior reflects a person's health beliefs.

health care clearing house, n an entity used to process or aid in the processing of information; may also be called a repricing company, billing service, community health information system, community health management information system, or "value-added" switch or network.

health care operations, n.pl functions performed by a health care provider, health plan, or health care clearing house to conduct administrative and business management activities.

health care provider, n any individual who provides health services to health care consumers (patients).

health education, n an educational program directed to the general public that attempts to improve, maintain, and safeguard the health of the community.

health hazard, n a danger to health resulting from exposure to environmental pollutants such as asbestos or ionizing radiation, or to a lifestyle influence such as cigarette smoking or chemical abuse.

health history, *n* previously diagnosed physical or mental condition of an individual. See also *health assessment* and *chart, history.*

health information, *n* recorded information in any format (e.g., oral, written, or electronic) regarding the physical or mental condition of an individual, health care provision, or health care payment. See also *health assessment* and *health, patient.*

health information, individually identifiable, *n* recorded information in any format (e.g., oral, written, or electronic) regarding the physical or mental condition of an individual, health care provision, or health care payment. It contains demographic information able to specifically distinguish an individual. In some cases, this information may not be considered "protected." See also *health information, protected.*

health information, protected (PHI), *n* recorded information in any format (e.g., oral, written, or electronic) regarding the physical or mental condition of an individual, health care provision, or health care payment. It contains demographic information able to specifically distinguish an individual. See also *health information, individually identifiable.*

health maintenance organization (HMO), *n* a legal entity that accepts responsibility and financial risk for providing specified services to a defined population during a defined period at a fixed price. An organized system of healthcare delivery that provides comprehensive care to enrollees through designated providers. Enrollees are generally assessed a monthly payment for health care services and may be required to remain in the program for a specified amount of time.

health, patient, *n* the state of bodily soundness of the patient; the patient's absolute or relative freedom from physical and mental disease.

health physics, *n* the study of the effects of ionizing radiation on the body and the methods for protecting people from the undesirable effects of radiation.

health policy, *n* **1.** a statement of a decision regarding a goal in health care and a plan for achieving that goal; for example, to prevent an epidemic, a program for inoculating a population is developed and implemented. *n* **2.** a field of study and practice in which the priorities and values underlying health resource allocation are determined.

health professional, *n* a person who by education, training, certification, or licensure is qualified to and is engaged in providing health care.

health promotion, *n* an educational program or effort directed at a targeted population to improve, maintain, and safeguard the health of that segment of society. See also *health education.*

health resources, *n* all materials, personnel, facilities, funds, and anything else that can be used for providing health care and services.

health risk, *n* a disease precursor associated with a higher than average morbidity or mortality. The disease precursors may include demographic variables, certain individual behaviors, familial and individual histories, and certain physiologic changes.

health risk appraisal, *n* a process of gathering, analyzing, and comparing an individual's prognostic characteristics of health with a standard age group, thereby predicting the likelihood that a person may develop prematurely a health problem associated with a high morbidity and mortality rate.

hearing, *n* the sense by which sound perception occurs; happens after sound waves are converted into impulses of the nerves and translated by the brain.

hearing aid, *n* electronic device used to amplify and shape waves of sound entering the external auditory canal.

hearing aid, behind-the-ear, *n* an electronic device, situated over the ear, for amplifying and shaping sound waves entering the external auditory canal.

hearing aid, eyeglass model, *n* an electronic device, attached to the eyeglasses' thickened temple bar, for amplifying and shaping sound waves entering the external auditory canal.

hearing disorders, *n.pl* any structural or functional impairment of the ability to detect and recognize sound.

hearing disorders, indications of, *n.pl* symptoms such as an inability to pay attention or respond appropriately to spoken dialogue, heightened focus, increased use of a specific ear, frequent requests for repetition of spoken statements, and abnormal quality of speech.

hearing disorders, types of, n.pl classifications include a loss of central, mixed, sensorineural, or conductive hearing.

hearing loss, *n* a reduction in the acuity to detect and recognize sound.

hearing loss, conductive, n a hearing impairment of the outer or middle ear, which is due to abnormalities or damage within the conductive pathways leading to the inner ear.

hearing loss, mixed, n a hearing impairment that is the result of damage to both conductive pathways or the middle ear and to the nerves or sensory hair cells of the inner ear.

hearing loss, sensorineural, n a hearing impairment of the inner ear resulting from damage to the sensory hair cells or to the nerves that supply the inner ear.

hearsay, *n* **1.** the testimony given by a witness who relates not what is known personally but what others have stated *n* **2.** evidence that does not derive its value solely from the credit of the witness, but rests mainly on the veracity and competency of other persons and is admitted in court only in specified cases, from necessity.

heart, *n* the muscular pump that maintains and regulates the flow of blood through the body.

heart, artificial, n a mechanical device that acts to pump blood to and from the body tissues during repair of the heart.

heart attack, n See *myocardial infarction; thrombosis, coronary;* or *occlusion, coronary.*

heart block, n the condition in which the muscular interconnection between the auricle and ventricle is interrupted so that the auricle and ventricle beat independently of each other.

heart, compression of, n See *massage, cardiac.*

heart defect, n a fault in the structural integrity of the heart.

heart defect, congenital, n structural errors in the heart formed during embryonic and fetal life.

heart disease, n a disorder in the normal functioning of the heart.

heart disease, dental hygiene concerns, n.pl special considerations taken to eliminate oral disease by maintaining an elevated level of oral health and prevent infective endocarditis, an infection of the heart valves that may be caused by bacteremia created during dental treatments.

heart disease risk factors, n.pl hereditary, lifestyle, and environmental influences that increase one's chances of developing heart disease.

heart massage, n See *massage, cardiac.*

heart murmur, n the sound of blood flowing back through a defective heart valve.

heart, normal, n a heart without anatomic defects that could cause an impairment in the function of the organ.

heart rate, n the rate or tempo of heart contractions recorded in beats per minute.

heart sounds, n.pl normal noises produced within the heart during the cardiac cycle that can be heard over the precordium and may reveal abnormalities in cardiac structure or function. The use of the stethoscope over the left side of the chest is a common clinical technique to assess heart function. The typical sounds are a rythmic lub dup; abnormal sounds include clicks, murmurs, rubs, snaps, and gallops.

heart surgery, n any surgical procedure involving the heart, performed to correct acquired or congenital defects, to replace diseased valves, to open or bypass blocked vessels, or to graft a prosthesis or a transplant in place.

heart valves, n.pl one of the four structures within the heart that prevent backflow of blood by opening and closing with each heartbeat. The valves include two semilunar valves, the aortic and pulmonary; the mitral, or bicuspid, valve; and the tricuspid valve. The valves permit the flow of blood in only one direction, and any one of the valves may become defective, permitting the backflow associated with heart murmurs.

heart failure (härt' fāl-yur), *n* a sudden, sometimes fatal, cessation of the heart's action.

heart failure, acute, n a rapid and marked impairment of the cardiac output.

heart failure, backward, n congestive heart failure in which the initiating factor is increased venous pressure resulting from ventricular failure to empty the atria.

heart failure, congestive, n a clinical syndrome resulting from chronic cardiac decompensation associated with left-sided or right-sided heart failure. Left-sided failure may result from rheumatic mitral valvular disease, aortic valvular disease, systemic hypertension, or arteriosclerotic disease. Manifestations include orthopnea, paroxysmal dyspnea, pulmonary edema, cough, and cardiac asthma. Right-sided failure results most commonly from pulmonary congestion and hypertension associated with left-sided failure but may result from anemia, myocarditis, beriberi, or dysrhythmia. Manifestations include peripheral pitting edema, ascites, cyanosis, oliguria, and hydrothorax.

heart failure, forward, n heart failure initiated by decreased cardiac output that leads to decreased blood supply to tissues, decreased excretion of salt (Na1) and salt retention, elevated venous pressure, and edema.

heartburn, *n* a painful burning sensation in the esophagus just below the sternum. Heartburn is usually caused by the reflux of gastric contents into the esophagus, but it may be caused by gastric hyperacidity or peptic ulcer.

heat, *n* the state of a body or of matter that is perceived as being opposite of cold and is characterized by elevation of temperature.

heat, applied, n the therapeutic application of wet or dry heat to increase circulation and produce hyperemia, accelerate the dissolution of infection and inflammation, increase absorption from tissue spaces, relieve pain, relieve muscle spasm and associated pain, and increase metabolism.

heat, applied, and cold, n the most commonly employed physical agents in dental practice; they modify the physiologic processes and have both a systemic and a local effect. The principal effect on the tissues is mediated by the alteration in the circulatory mechanisms. Properly used, heat and cold have a salutary therapeutic result; improperly used, they may produce serious pathologic consequences.

heat, applied, contraindications, n.pl conditions that preclude the use of heat application: peripheral neuropathy, conditions in which maximum vasodilation and inflammation are already present, acute inflammatory conditions in which more swelling will cause acute pain and pulpitis, septicemia, and malignancies.

heat, applied, general physiologic effects, n.pl the physiologic effects of generally applied wet or dry heat; increase in body temperature, generalized vasodilation, rise in metabolism, decrease in blood pressure, increase in pulse rate and circulation, and increase in depth and rate of respiration.

heat, applied, local physiologic effects, n.pl the physiologic effects of locally applied wet or dry heat to the intraoral or extraoral tissues: increase in caliber and number of capillaries, increased absorption resulting from capillary dilation, increased lymph formation and flow, relief of pain, relief of spasm, increase of phagocytes, and a rise in local metabolism.

heat loss, metabolic causes, n.pl biologic factors that influence heat loss: redistribution of blood vasodilation and vasoconstriction, variations in blood volume, tendency of fat to insulate the body, and evaporation.

heat loss, physical causes, n.pl physical factors that influence heat loss: radiation, convection, and conduction; evaporation from the lungs, skin, and mucous membranes; the raising of inspired air to body temperatures; and the production of urine and feces.

heat production, metabolic causes, n.pl chemical factors of the body that cause heat production: specific dynamic action of food, especially protein, that results in a rise of metabolism; a high environmental temperature that, by raising temperatures of the tissues, increases the velocity of reactions and thus increases heat production; and stimulation of the adrenal cortex and thyroid glands by the hormones of the pituitary glands.

heat treatment, See *treatment, heat.*

heat stabile, *adj* heat resistant. Also called *thermostabile.*

heavy function, *n* See *function, heavy.*

hebephrenia (hē′bə-frē′nē-ə), *n* a form of schizophrenia in which the individual behaves like a child (for example, inappropriate laughter and silliness).

heel effect, *n* See *effect, heel.*

Heerfordt's syndrome, *n pr* See *fever, uveoparotid.*

height of contour, *n* See *contour, height of.*

Heimlich maneuver, *n.pr* an emergency procedure for dislodging a bolus of food or other obstruction from the trachea to prevent asphyxiation. The choking person is grasped from behind by the rescuer, whose fist, thumb side in, is placed just below the victim's sternum and whose other hand is placed firmly over the fist. The rescuer then pulls the fist firmly and abruptly into the epigastrium, forcing the obstruction up the trachea.

Heimlich sign, *n.pr* a universal distress signal that a person is choking and unable to speak, made by grasping the throat with a thumb and index finger, thereby attracting the attention of others nearby.

Helicobacter, n a genus of gram-negative, spiral-shaped bacteria that is pathogenic and has been isolated from the intestinal tract of mammals, including humans.

Helicobacter pylori, n a newly classified spiral bacterium active as a human gastric pathogen. It is a gram-negative, urease-positive, curved or slightly spiral organism initially isolated in 1982 from patients with lesions of gastritis or peptic ulcers in Western Australia.

helium (hē′lē-um), *n* a colorless, odorless, tasteless gas; one of the inert gaseous elements. Symbol, He; atomic number, 2; atomic weight, 4.003. Used in medicine as a diluent for other gases.

hellac base, See *base, shellac.* (not current).

helminths (hel′minths), *n.pl* parasitic worms that cause disease and illness in humans such as tapeworm, pinworm, and trichinosis. They are usually transmitted via contaminated food, water, soil, or other objects. Adult worms live in the intestines and other organs. Minor infections may be asymptomatic, whereas stronger cases may cause dietary deficiencies or digestive, muscular, and nervous disorders.

Helsinki declaration (accords), *n.pr* a declaration signed by the representatives of 35 member nations of the Conference on Security and Cooperation in Europe in Helsinki, Finland, on August 1, 1975. The declared goals of the nonbinding document comprise four principal aspects of European security: economic cooperation, humanitarian issues, contact between East and West, and provision for a later follow-up conference. The principle and practice of informed consent in health care grew from the Helsinki accords.

hemangioameloblastoma (hē-man′jē-ō-ə-mel′ō-blast-ō′mə), *n* a neoplasm in the jaw that has characteristics of ameloblastoma and hemangioma.

hemangioendothelioma (hē-man′jē-ō-en′dō-thē′lē-ō′mə), *n* a malignant tumor formed by proliferation of endothelium of the capillary vessels.

hemangiofibroma (hē-man′jē-ō-fī-brō′mə), *n* a benign neoplasm characterized by proliferation of blood channels in a dense mass of fibroblasts.

hemangioma (hē-man′jē-ō′mə), *n* **1.** a benign neoplasm characterized by blood vascular channels. A cavernous hemangioma consists of large vascular spaces. A capillary hemangioma consists of many small blood vessels. *n* **2.** a benign tumor composed of newly formed blood vessels.

H

Hemangioma. (Neville/Damm/Allen/Bouquot, 2002)

hemangiopericytoma (hē-man′jē-ō-per′i-sī-tō′mə), *n* a vascular tumor composed of pericytes.

hemarthrosis (he″mahr-thro′sis), *n* the blood found in the cavity of a joint.

hemataerometer, *n* a device for determining the pressure of the gases in the blood (not current).

hematemesis (hē′mə-tem′e-sis), *n* vomiting of blood.

hematocrit (hē-mat′ō-crit), *n* (packed-cell volume), **1.** the percentage of the total blood volume composed of red blood cells (erythrocytes). Normal values are 42% to 45%. *n* **2.** the percentage of the total volume of a blood sample that is taken up by the red blood cells. Normal values: children, 32% to 65%; adult men, 42% to 53%; adult women, 38% to 46%.

hematogenous (hē′mət-o-jəə-nus), *adj* part of or originating in the blood, or distributed through the bloodstream.

hematologic disorders, *n.pl* diseases of the blood and blood-forming tissues.

hematology, *n* the scientific study of blood and blood-forming tissues.

hematology tests, *n.pl* diagnostic tests of the blood and its constituent parts.

hematoma (hē′mə-tō′mə), *n* a mass of blood in the tissue as a result of trauma or other factors that cause the rupture of blood vessels.

hematoma, subdural, *n* a collection of extravasated blood trapped below the dural membranes of the brain causing pressure on the brain, resulting in pain and neural dysfunction. Subdural hematomas may be life threatening.

hematopoiesis, *n* the normal formation and development of blood cells in the bone marrow.

hematosis (hē′mə-tō′sis), *n* oxygenation or aeration of the venous blood in the lungs.

hematoxylin, *n* a dye or stain commonly used to treat tissue sections for microscopic examination, usually used in combination with eosin.

hematuria (hē′mə-tōō′rē-ə), *n* blood in the urine.

hematuria, gross, *n* visible evidence of blood in the urine. It may occur from neoplasms of the kidney and bladder, hemorrhagic diathesis, hypertension with renal epistaxis, or acute glomerular nephritis.

hematuria, microscopic, *n* the demonstration of hematuria during the microscopic examination of centrifuged urine. It may result from the same causes as gross hematuria or from toxicity of drugs, embolic glomerulitis, vascular diseases, or chronic glomerular nephritis.

heme, *n* the pigmented, iron containing, nonprotein portion of the hemoglobin molecule.

hemiachromatosia, *n* a state of being color blind in only one half of the visual field.

hemianesthesia (hem′ē-an′es-thē′zh-ə), *n* anesthesia or loss of tactile sensibility on one side of the body.

hemiatrophy (hem′ē-at′rō-fē), *n* atrophy of one half of the body, an organ, or a part (for example, facial hemiatrophy).

hemidesmosome (hem′ē-dez′mō-sōm), *n* one-half of a cell junction (desmosome), the connection site between the surface of the tooth and the epithelium.

hemiglossectomy (hem′ē-glôs-ek′tə-mē), *n* the surgical removal of half of the tongue.

hemihypertrophy (hem′ē-hī-pur′ trə-fē), *n* an excessive growth of half of the body, an organ, or a part (for example, hemihyperplasia of the tongue).

Hemihypertrophy. (Neville/Damm/Allen/ Bouquot, 2002. Courtesy Dr. George Blozis)

hemiplegia (hem′ē-plē′jē-ə), *n* in medical jurisprudence, paralysis of one side of the body.

hemisection, *n* the complete sectioning through the crown of a tooth into the furcation region.

hemochromatosis (hē′mō-krō′mə-tō′sis), *n* an uncommon disorder, usually a complication of hemolytic anemia, that results in a surplus of iron deposits throughout the body. See also *hemosiderosis; iron metabolism; siderosis;* and *thalassemia.*

hemocyte, *n* a generic term referring to any cellular or formed element of the blood. Synonym: hematocyte.

hemodialysis, *n* a procedure in which impurities or wastes are removed from the blood. This procedure is used in treating renal failure and various toxic conditions. The patient's blood is shunted from the body through a machine for diffusion and ultrafiltration and returned to the patient's circulation.

hemodynamics, *n* the study of the physical aspects of blood circulation, including cardiac function and peripheral vascular physiology.

hemoglobin (hē′mō-glōb-in), *n* the oxygen-carrying red pigment of the red blood corpuscles. Hemoglobin is a reddish, crystallizable conjugated protein consisting of the protein globulin combined with the prosthetic group, heme.

hemoglobin A (HBA), n a normal hemoglobin. Also called *adult hemoglobin.*

hemoglobin estimation, n a determination of the hemoglobin content of the blood. By the Sahli method, 14 to 17 g/100 mL of blood is normal, and 15.1 Sahli units are taken as 100% for estimation of hemoglobin percentages.

hemoglobinopathy (hē′mō-glō′bin-op′ə-thē), *n* any one of a group of genetically determined diseases involving abnormal hemoglobin (for example, sickle cell disease, in which hemoglobin S occurs, and hemoglobin C disease).

hemoglobinopathy, paroxysmal nocturnal, n an acquired hemolytic anemia of unknown cause characterized by increased hemolysis during sleep, resulting in the presence of hemoglobin in the urine on awakening.

hemohydremia, anhydremia, a decrease in blood volume resulting from a decrease in the serum component of blood; occurs in shock or any condition in which blood fluid is passed into the tissue and results in hemoconcentration. (not current).

hemolysin (hēm-ol′i-sin), *n* an antibody that causes hemolysis of red blood cells in vitro.

hemolysis, *n* the breakdown of red blood cells and the release of hemoglobin that occurs normally at the end of the life span of a red blood cell.

hemophilia (bleeder's disease) (hē′mō-fil′ē-ə), *n* a sex-linked genetic disease manifested in males and characterized by severe hemorrhage.

hemophilia A (classic hemophilia), n a hemorrhagic diathesis resulting from a deficiency of antihemophilic globulin (AHG); inherited as a recessive sex-linked characteristic and characterized by recurrent bouts of bleeding from even trivial injury. The coagulation time is prolonged, but the bleeding time is normal.

hemophilia B (Christmas disease, hemophilia II, hemophilioid state C), n a hemorrhagic diathesis resulting from a deficiency of plasma thromboplastin component (PTC); transmitted as a sex-linked recessive characteristic and characterized clinically by the same manifestations as classic hemophilia. There is a delay in the generation of thromboplastin. The platelet count, bleeding time, tourniquet test, and thrombin and prothrombin times are normal.

hemophilia C (plasma thromboplastin antecedent [PTA] deficiency, Rosenthal's syndrome), n a hemophilia-like condition believed to result from a deficiency of plasma thromboplastin antecedent (PTA), transmitted as a simple autosomal dominant trait and characterized by a moderate bleeding tendency after extraction of teeth or after tonsillectomy. Prothrombin consumption and thromboplastin generation are abnormal. See also *factor XI.*

hemophilia, classic, n See *hemophilia A.*

hemophilia, vascular, n a hereditary hemorrhagic disorder affecting both sexes and associated with a deficiency of antihemophilic globulin and vascular abnormalities characteristic of pseudohemophilia (von Willebrand's disease). The bleeding time is prolonged, and severity of bleeding varies considerably among persons with this condition.

hemophilioid state C (hē′mō-fil′ē-oid), *n* See *hemophilia B.*

hemopoiesis (hē′mō-pō-ē′sis), *n* See *hematopoiesis.*

hemoptysis (hēm-op′ti-sis), *n* the expectoration of blood, by coughing, from the larynx or lower respiratory tract.

hemorrhage (hem′ər-əj), *n* the escape of a large amount of blood from the blood vessels in a short period; excessive bleeding.

hemorrhagic bone cyst, *n* See *cyst, hemorrhagic.*

hemorrhagic diathesis, *n* an inherited predisposition to any one of a number of abnormalities characterized by excessive bleeding.

hemosiderin (hē′mō-sid′ər-in), *n* an intracellular storage form of iron; the granules consist of an ill-defined complex of ferric hydroxides, polysaccharides, and proteins having an iron content of approximately 33% by weight. It appears as a dark yellow-brown pigment.

hemosiderosis, *n* a focal or general increase in tissue iron stores without associated tissue damage.

hemostasis (hē′mō-stā′sis), *n* the arrest of an escape of blood.

hemostat (hē′mō-stat), *n* a procedure or device that stops the flow of blood.

hemostatic (hē′mō-stat′ik), *n* an agent used to reduce bleeding from minute vessels by hastening the clotting of blood or by the formation of an artificial clot.

Hepadnaviridae **(hep-ad″nə-vir′ĭ-de),** *n* one of the major virus families, to which the hepatitis B virus belongs. Viruses in this family have a double-stranded incomplete circular molecular structure with icosahedral symmetry.

heparin/heparin calcium/heparin sodium, *n trade names:* Hep Lock, Liquaemin Sodium; *drug class:* anticoagulant; *action:* acts in combination with antithrombin III (heparin cofactor) to inhibit thrombosis; inactivates factor Xa and inhibits conver-

sion of prothrombin to thrombin; affects both intrinsic and extrinsic clotting pathways; *uses:* anticoagulant in thrombosis, embolism, coagulopathies, deep vein thrombosis, dialysis, maintenance of patency of indwelling intravenous lines.

heparinized lock system, *n* an indwelling intravenous system by which multiple daily intravenous accesses can be accomplished and multiple penetrations of the veins can be avoided. The heparin chamber prevents the formation of a clot or thrombus at the needle site.

hepatitis (hep′ə-tī′tis), *n* an inflammation of the liver.

hepatitis C (HCV non-A, non-B hepatitis), *n* a type of hepatitis transmitted largely by blood transfusion or percutaneous inoculation, such as with intravenous drug users sharing needles. The disease progresses to chronic hepatitis in up to 50% of the patients acutely infected.

hepatitis, chronic active, *n* a subacute hepatitis with chronic portal inflammation with regional necrosis and fibrosis, which may progress to nodular postnecrotic cirrhosis.

hepatitis, delta, *n* a particularly virulent form of hepatitis caused by the delta hepatitis virus in conjunction with the hepatitis B virus, which is spread by contaminated needles or by direct exposure to blood or other body fluids from infected individuals. It occurs primarily in persons who have been repeatedly exposed to the hepatitis B virus either through frequent blood transfusions or intravenous drug use. It may also be spread during the birthing process.

   hepatitis delta virus (HDV), *n* the infectious agent that causes delta hepatitis, but only in the presence of the hepatitis B virus. The virus is usually superimposed on carriers of the hepatitis B surface antigen (HBsAg). It is also called the *delta agent.*

hepatitis E (HEV, epidemic non-A, non-B hepatitis), *n* a self-limited type of hepatitis that may occur after natural disasters because of fecal-contaminated water or food. There is currently no serologic test available.

hepatitis G, *n* a viral infection of the stomach and intestines, transmitted via blood and coinfection with the hepatitis C virus. The duration of the incubation period and range of symptoms are unknown, and no vaccine is available.

hepatitis, homologous serum (homologous serum jaundice, serum hepatitis, syringe jaundice, type B hepatitis), n a viral hepatitis clinically difficult to distinguish from epidemic infectious hepatitis. It is transmitted by human serum (that is, through parenteral injection, transfusions, lacerations). The incubation period is 40 to 90 days or longer. Principal manifestations are jaundice, gastrointestinal symptoms, anorexia, and malaise.

hepatitis, infectious (IH, type A hepatitis), n a viral hepatitis that is frequently epidemic in nature and has an incubation period of 1 to 4 or even 7 weeks. It is usually transmitted by the virus in fecal matter but may be transmitted by human serum (transfusions, lacerations, needle punctures).

hepatitis, non-ABCDE, n a viral infection of the stomach and intestines that is diagnosed by ruling out other forms of hepatitis. It may be transmitted orally, via injection, sexual contact, or fecal matter.

hepatitis, serum, n See *hepatitis, homologous serum.*

hepatitis, viral, n **1.** hepatitis caused by any one of three immunologically unrelated viruses: hepatitis A virus; hepatitis B virus; and non-A, non-B virus. n **2.** hepatitis caused by a viral infection, including that by Epstein-Barr virus and cytomegalovirus.

hepatomegaly, abnormal, n an enlargement of the liver that is usually a sign of liver disease. It is usually discovered by percussion and palpation as part of a physical examination. It may be caused by hepatitis, fatty infiltration, alcoholism, biliary obstruction, or malignancy.

Herbst appliance, n.pr the only fixed, tooth-borne, functional orthodontic appliance in which jaw position is influenced by a pin-and-tube spring-loaded appliance that is cemented or bonded to the teeth.

hereditary benign intraepithelial dyskeratosis, n a hereditary disease seen in triracial isolates (whites, Native Americans, blacks). It involves the oral mucosa and may

cause periodic seasonal keratoconjunctivitis.

hereditary opalescent dentin, n a developmental disturbance in the formation of dentin, better known as dentiogenesis imperfecta. The teeth range from gray to brownish violet and are translucent or opalescent. The crowns fracture easily because of an abnormal dentinoenamel junction.

heredity (her-ed'i-tē), n the inheritance of resemblance, physical qualities, or disease from a familial predecessor; the passage of characteristics from one generation to its progeny by genetic linkage.

Hering-Breuer reflex (her'ing broi'ur), n.pr See *reflex, Hering-Breuer.*

hermetic seal, n See *seal, hermetic.*

hernia, n the protrusion of an organ through an abnormal opening in the muscle wall of the cavity that surrounds it. A hernia may be congenital, may result from the failure of certain structures to close after birth, or may be acquired later in life because of obesity, muscular weakness, surgery, or illness.

hernia, hiatal, n a protrusion of a portion of the stomach upward through the diaphragm. The condition occurs in approximately 40% of individuals and most people display few, if any, symptoms. The major difficulty is gastroesophageal reflux, which is the backflow of the acid contents of the stomach into the esophagus.

hernia, inguinal (direct), n a protrusion of the intestines into an opening between the deep epigastric artery and the edge of the rectus muscle; (indirect) involves the internal inguinal ring and passes into the inguinal canal.

heroin (her'ō-in), n a highly addictive alkaloid prepared from morphine, previously used for cough relief. Use of heroin is prohibited by federal law because of its highly addictive properties and potential for abuse.

herpangina (hur'pan-jī'nə), n (Coxsackie A disease), a viral disease of children, usually occurring in summer, and characterized by sudden onset, fever (100° to 105° F; 38° to 40.5° C), sore throat, and oropharyngeal vesicles. Herpangina results from Coxsackie A viruses and is self-limiting.

Herpangina. (Sams/Lynch, 1990)

herpangina aphthous ulcer, *n* See *aphthous pharyngitis.*

herpes labialis (hur'pēz lā'bē-al'is), (cold sore), a disease of the lips caused by herpes virus and characterized by vesicles that rupture, leaving ulcers. The local lesions are often called *fever blisters* or *cold sores.* Herpes simplex of the lips.

Herpes labialis. (Neville/Damm/Allen/Bouquot, 2002)

herpes simplex (hur'pēz sim'plex), *n* an infection caused by the herpes simplex virus. Primary infection, occurring most often in children between 2 and 5 years of age, may result in apparent clinical disease or such manifestations as acute herpetic gingivostomatitis, keratoconjunctivitis, vulvovaginitis, or encephalitis. Recurrent manifestations may include herpes labialis (fever blisters or cold sores), dendritic corneal ulcers, or genital herpes simplex.

Herpes simplex. (Neville/Damm/Allen/Bouquot, 2002)

herpes zoster (hur'pēz zos'tur), *n* (acute posterior ganglionitis, shingles), an acute viral disease involving the dorsal spinal root or cranial nerve and producing vesicular eruption in areas of the skin corresponding to the involved sensory nerve. Pain is a prominent feature and may persist, although skin lesions subside in 1 to 2 weeks.

Herpes zoster. (Ibsen/Phelan, 2000)

Herpesviridae (hər"pēz-vi'ri-de), *n* one of the major virus families, to which the herpes simplex, varicella zoster, and Epstein-Barr viruses belong. Viruses in this family have a double-stranded linear molecular structure with icosahedral symmetry.

herpetic lesion, *n* See *lesion, herpetic.*

Hertwig's root sheath, *n* an elongation of the cervical loop, which helps determine the shape, size, and number of roots and which influences the formation of dentin during the developmental stages of a tooth.

heteresthesia (het'ər-es-thē'zē-ə, -zhə), *n* a variation in the degree of cutaneous sensibility on adjoining areas of the body surface.

heterograft, *n* See *graft, heterogenous.*

heteropolysaccharides (het'ər-ō-pol'ē-sak'ə-rīdz), *n.pl* complex carbohydrates formed by combining carbohydrates with noncarbohydrates or carbohydrate derivatives; examples include pectin, lignin, glycoproteins, glycolipids, and mucopolysaccharides.

heterosexual, *n* a person with a sexual attraction to or preference for persons of the opposite gender; *adj* having erotic attraction to, predisposition to, or sexual activity with a person of the opposite gender.

heterotrophic (het'ər-ō-trof'ik), *adj* pertaining to a organism that must depend on others to provide sustenance. Parasitic.

heterozygote, *n* an organism whose somatic cells have two different allelomorphic genes on the same locus of each pair of chromosomes. It can produce two different types of gametes.

heterozygous (het'ər-ō-zī'gus), *adj* a term indicating that genes lying at equivalent loci on chromosome pairs are different.

hexamethonium, *n* a cholinergic blocking agent used to control bleeding and used in the treatment of peptic ulcers and hypertension. It produces ganglion blocking by occupying receptor sites.

hexosamine, *n* the amine derivative (NH2 replacing OH) of a hexose such as glucosamine.

HGF, *n* See *glucagon.*

HIAA, *n.pr* the abbreviation for Health Insurance Association of America.

hiccup, *n* an involuntary spasmodic contraction of the diaphragm that causes a beginning inspiration that is suddenly checked by closure of the glottis, thus producing a characteristic sound.

hidradenoma, *n* a benign neoplasm derived from epithelial cells of sweat glands.

hidrocystoma, *n* a cystic form of sweat gland adenoma. A hidrocystoma is produced by the cystic proliferation of apocrine secretory glands. It is not uncommon, occurring in adult life in no particular age group, with males and females equally affected. The most common site is around the eye. Hidrocystomas are cured by surgical removal.

hierarchy, *n* **I.** any system of persons or things ranked one above the other. *n* **2.** in psychology and psychiatry, an organization of habits or concepts in which simpler components are combined to form increasingly complex integrations.

hierarchy, Maslow's, See *Maslow's hierarchy.*

high labial arch, *n* See *arch, high labial.*

high lip line, *n* See *lip line, high.*

high speed, *n* See *speed, high.*

high-pull headgear, *n* apparatus de-

signed to give an upward pull on the face-bow.

high-speed handpiece, *n* See *handpiece, high-speed.*

hilus (hī'lus), *n* an indentation appearing on an organ or other internal structure, such as a lymph node, at the point where nerves and vessels enter. Also called *hilum.*

hinchazon (hinch'əzon), *n* See *beriberi.*

hinge axis, *n* See *axis, hinge.*

hinge axis, determination, *n* See *axis, condylar, determination.*

hinge axis, orbital plane, *n* See *axis, hinge, orbital plane.*

hinge axis point, *n* See *point, hinge axis.*

hinge movement, *n* See *movement, hinge.*

hinge position, *n* See *position, hinge.*

hinge-bow, *n* the kinematic face-bow used to determine the location of the hinge axis. The hinge-bow is a three-piece instrument with independently adjustable arms controlled by micrometer screws that lengthen or shorten them. Other micrometer screws raise or lower the caliper points to find the spots in or on the skin near the tragi where only rotary movements occur when the jaw is opened and closed at the rearmost point. See also *face-bow, kinematic.*

hippocampus, *n* a curved convoluted elevation of the floor of the inferior horn of the lateral ventricle of the brain. The hippocampus is composed of gray substance covered by a layer of white fibers, or the alveus, and functions as an important component of the limbic system.

hippus, respiratory (hip'əs), *n* a dilation of the pupils occurring during inspiration and a contraction of the pupils occurring during expiration; often associated with pulsus paradoxus.

Hirschfeld-Dunlop file, *n.pr* See *file, Hirschfeld-Dunlop.*

Hirschfeld's method, *n.pr* See *point, Hirschfeld's silver.*

hirsutism (hir'sōō-tiz-əm), *n* increased body or facial hair, which is especially noted in the female.

histamine, *n* a compound found in all cells that is produced by the breakdown of histidine. Histamine is released in allergic, inflammatory reactions and causes dilation of capillaries, decreased blood pressure, increased secretion of gastric juice, and constriction of smooth muscles of the bronchi and uterus.

histamine blocker, *n* a drug used in the treatment of gastroesophageal reflux disease, including cimetidine, nizatidine, and ranitidine. The drug inhibits the release of stomach acid and reduces pain caused by introduction of stomach acids to esophagus.

histidine, *n* one of the essential amino acids for infants and children. See also *amino acid.*

histiocyte (his′tē-ō-sīt), *n* a large phagocytic cell found in the interstices of the tissues; of reticuloendothelial origin.

histiocytosis, acute disseminated, X, *n* See *disease, Letterer-Siwe.*

histiocytosis, chronic disseminated X, *n* See *disease, Hand-Schuller-Christian.*

histiocytosis, nonlipid (his′tē-ō-sī-tō′sis), *n* See *disease, Letterer-Siwe.*

histiocytosis X, *n* a group of diseases characterized by abnormal histiocyte activity. Includes a chronic disseminated type (Hand-Schuller-Christian disease) and a chronic localized type (eosinophilic granuloma).

histoclasia, implant (his′tō-klā′zē-ə), *n* a condition of the tissues existing in the presence of an implant, in which the implant is not directly involved. It is a condition of the oral mucosal tissues, in which the pathologic condition results from some external cause (for example, salivary calculus, attached prosthetic appliances).

histocompatibility, *n* the compatibility of the antigens of donor and recipient of transplanted tissue.

histocompatibility testing, *n* the determination of the compatibility of the antigens of donor and recipient before tissue transplantation. Usually follows a blood typing protocol.

histocytoma, *n* a tumor composed of histiocytes.

histodifferentiation (his′tō-dif′ər-en′shē-ā′shən), *n* the process in which cells develop the distinctive characteristics of the tissues to which they are to belong.

histogram, *n* a bar graph; a graphic representation of a frequency distribution.

histology, *n* microanatomy, which is the microscopic study of normal tissue and organs at the cellular level. *histology, oral, of soft tissues,* *n* See *epithelium, oral; lamina, propria; submucosa;* and *membrane, basement.*

histopathology, *n* the microscopic study of abnormal tissue and organs at the cellular level.

histoplasmosis (his′tō-plaz-mō′sis), *n* a disease caused by the fungus *Histoplasma capsulatum* and affecting the reticuloendothelial system. Ulceration of the oral mucosa may occur.

Histoplasmosis. (Regezi/Sciubba/Pogrel, 2000)

history, case, *n* a detailed and concise compilation of all physical, dental, social, and mental factors relative and necessary to diagnosis, prognosis, and treatment.

history, case, forms, *n.pl* questionnaires to aid the practitioner in taking medical history; should cover all aspects of patient's prior medical history; the American Dental Association distributes a basic health form that may provide a baseline.

history, case, hepatic disease, *n* as part of the process of taking a medical history, practitioner should ask patient for details and occurrences of liver disease or drug metabolism problems.

history case, self-medication, *n* as part of the medical history process, practitioner should ask patient for descriptions of the type and frequency of self-administered medication as well as any history of substance abuse; this information can help eliminate complications in patient treatment schedules.

histotoxic (his'tō-täk'sik), *adj* relating to poisoning of the respiratory enzyme system of the tissues.

HIV gingivitis (HIV-G), *n* a distinct type of gingivitis found in HIV-infected patients, characterized by an intensely red linear erythemic band around the free gingiva that extends 2 to 3 mm apically into the attached gingiva. The involved gingiva tends to bleed spontaneously and may be present even in AIDS patients with good plaque control.

HIV periodontitis (HIV-P), *n* an aggressive form of periodontal disease with all of the characteristics of HIV-G combined with soft tissue ulceration and necrosis and rapid destruction of the periodontium and bone. The condition is very painful. HIV-P may resemble acute necrotizing ulcerative gingivitis (ANUG). However, ANUG is limited to the soft tissue, whereas HIV-P disease extends into the crestal bone.

HIV-1, *n* the abbreviation for *human immunodeficiency virus type 1,* which is widely recognized as the causal agent of acquired immunodeficiency syndrome (AIDS). HIV-1 is characterized by its cytopathic effect and affinity for the T4-lymphocyte.

HIV-2, *n* the abbreviation *for human immunodeficiency virus type 2,* which is related to HIV-1 but carries different antigenic components with differing nucleic acid composition. It shares serologic reactivity and sequence homology with the simian lentivirus Simian immunodeficiency virus (SIV) and infects only T4-lymphocytes expressing the CD4 phenotypic marker.

HIV-G, *n* See *HIV gingivitis.*

HIV-P, *n* See *HIV periodontitis.*

HIV-wasting syndrome, *n* a constitutional disease associated with AIDS, also known as the *slim disease.* Patients in this subgroup have a history of fever of more than 1 month, involuntary weight loss of more than 10%, or diarrhea persisting for more than 1 month.

hives, *n* See *urticaria.*

hockey, *n* a team contact sport played on ice skates or with roller blades. Because limited facial protection for the players exists (except for the goalie), there is opportunity for traumatic injury to the face and teeth.

Hodgkin's disease, *n.pr* See *disease, Hodgkin's.*

hoe, *n* an angled instrument with the broad dimension of its blade perpendicular to the axis of the shank of the shaft.

hold, *v* to possess by reason of a lawful title.

hold harmless clause, *n* a contract provision in which one party to the contract promises to be responsible for liability incurred by the other party. Hold harmless clauses frequently appear in the following contexts: (1) Contracts between dental benefits organizations and an individual dentist often contain a promise by the dentist to reimburse the dental benefits organization for any liability the organization incurs because of dental treatment provided to beneficiaries of the organization's dental benefits plan. This may include a promise to pay the dental benefits organization's attorney fees and related costs. (2) Contracts between dental benefits organizations and a group plan sponsor may include a promise by the dental benefits organization to assume responsibility for disputes between a beneficiary of the group plan and an individual dentist when the dentist's charge exceeds the amount the organization pays for the service on behalf of the beneficiary. If the dentist takes action against the patient to recover the difference between the amount billed by the dentist and the amount paid by the organization, the dental benefits organization will take over the defense of the claim and will pay any judgments and court costs.

holder, *n* an apparatus or instrument that is used to hold something.

film holder, precision, *n* a stainless steel device used to hold the film firmly in place during a dental x-ray procedure, which provides the rectangular collimation necessary for the paralleling technique.

film holder, Rinn X-C-P, *n* a film-positioning device with aiming capability made from a combination of plastic and stainless steel that is especially suited to the paralleling technique.

film holder, Stabe, *n.pr* a disposable film-positioning device made from styrofoam that is especially suited to the paralleling or bisecting angle techniques.

holder, broach, n See *broach holder.*

holder, clamp, n See *holder, rubber dam clamp.*

holder, matrix, n See *retainer, matrix.*

holder, rubber dam, n an apparatus used to hold a rubber dam in place on the face and to secure the edges of the dam clear of the field of operation.

holder, rubber dam clamp (clamp holder), n See *forceps, rubber dam clamp.*

holistic health, n a concept in which concern for health requires a perspective of the individual as an integrated system rather than as a collection of parts and functions.

Hollenback condenser, n.pr See *condenser, pneumatic.*

hollow bulb, n that portion of a prosthesis made hollow to minimize weight.

holograph, n a writing completely in a person's handwriting, such as a deed, will, or letter. A holograph may have legal standing without witnesses.

holoprosencephaly, n a congenital defect caused by the failure of the prosencephalon to divide into hemispheres during embryonic development. It is characterized by multiple midline facial defects, including cyclopia in severe cases.

homatropine hydrobromide (optic), n   *trade names:* AK-Homatropine, Isopto Homatropine; *drug class:* mydriatic (topical); *action:* blocks response of iris sphincter muscle and muscle of accommodation of ciliary body to cholinergic stimulation, resulting in dilation and paralysis of accommodation; *uses:* cycloplegic refraction, uveitis, mydriatic lens opacities.

home care, n the physiotherapeutic measures employed by the patient for the maintenance of dental and periodontal health. Includes proper cleaning with a toothbrush, floss, or other device.

home health agency, n an organization that provides health care in the home. Medicare certification for a home health agency depends on the providing of skilled nursing services and of at least one additional therapeutic service, usually physical or occupational therapy.

homeless person, n a person without a home, legal residence, or shelter either by choice or circumstances.

homeostasis (hō′mē-ō-stā′sis), n the term used to describe the tendency toward physiologic equilibration (for example, acid-base balance, pH level of blood, blood sugar level).

homeostasis, cell, n the tendency of biologic tissues and processes to maintain a constancy of environment consistent with their vitality and well being. For cells to maintain their stability or equilibrium, the cell membranes must be in continuous interaction with both the internal (intracellular) environment and the external (extracellular) environment. When the equilibrium of any component is disturbed, the interaction permits automatic readjustment by giving rise to stimuli that result in restoration of the equilibrium.

homicide, n the killing of one human being by another. Legally there are differing degrees of homicide based on motive, opportunity, and circumstances.

Hominidae, n the primate family, which includes humans.

homocystinuria (hō′mō-sis′tin-yōō′rē-ə), n a genetic disorder of amino acid metabolism in which the amino acid homocystine appears in the blood and urine; may respond to a low-protein diet and the administration of synthetic amino acids.

homograft, n See *graft, homogenous.*

homopolysaccharides (hō′mō-pol′ē-sak′ər-ēdz), n.pl complex carbohydrates formed from at least six identical monosaccharides; examples include starch, glycogen, cellulose, and insulin.

homosexual, n a person with a sexual attraction to or preference for persons of the same gender; *adj* having erotic attraction to, predisposition to, or sexual activity with a person of the same gender.

homovanillic acid, n an acid that is produced by normal metabolism of dopamine and may be elevated in the urine in association with tumors of the adrenal gland.

homozygous (hō′mō-zī′gus), adj a

term indicating that genes lying at equivalent loci on chromosome pairs are the same.

hone, *v* to sharpen.

hook, skin, *n* a metallic instrument ending in a fine, sharp hook for handling soft tissues during surgery.

Hoover's sign, *n.pr* See *sign, Hoover's.*

HOP, *n* the abbreviation for high oxygen pressure.

horizontal overlap, *n* See *overlap, horizontal.*

horizontal plane, *n* See *plane, horizontal.*

horizontal position, *n* a posture in which the body lies flat and the feet and head remain on the same level. Also called *supine.*

hormone(s) (hôr'mōn[z]), *n.pl* the biochemical secretions of the endocrine glands that, in relatively small quantities, partially regulate the physiologic activity of the tissues, organs, organ systems, and other endocrine glands, and of the nervous system itself. The hormonal secretions are conducted and distributed throughout the body by the circulation of the bloodstream and tissue fluids.

hormones, adenohypophyseal, *n.pl* hormones secreted by the adenohypophysis. Includes seven distinct hormones: somatotropin (STH), thyrotropin (TSH), prolactin, follicle-stimulating hormone (FSH), luteinizing hormone (LH), melanocyte-stimulating hormone (MSH), and adrenocorticotropic hormone (ACTH).

hormones, adrenal medullary, *n.pl* hormones secreted by adrenal medulla, including two catecholamines: epinephrine and norepinephrine.

hormones, adrenocortical, *n* steroid hormones secreted by the adrenal cortex that are biologically active in one or more of the following states: stress, inflammation, metabolism of carbohydrates, proteins, electrolytes, and water.

hormones, adrenocorticotropic, *n* See *ACTH.*

hormones, adrenotropic, *n* See *ACTH.*

hormones, anabolic, *n.pl* hormones that decrease blood glucose; an example is insulin. See also *anabolic steroids.*

hormones, androgenic, *n.pl* See *hormones, sex, male.*

hormones, anterior pituitary-like, *n* See *hormone, pregnancy.*

hormones, antidiabetic, *n* See *insulin.*

hormones, antidiuretic (ADH, vasopressin), *n* a hormone of the posterior pituitary gland that encourages resorption of water by acting on the epithelial cells of the distal portion of the renal tubule. It raises blood pressure by its effect on the peripheral blood vessels and exerts an antidiuretic effect (antifacultative resorption of water in the renal tubules). An absence of antidiuretic hormone causes diabetes insipidus.

hormones, antiinflammatory, *n.pl* See *glucocorticoids.*

hormones, catabolic, *n.pl* hormones that increase blood glucose; examples include glucagon, epinephrine, steroid and growth hormones, and thyroxine.

hormones, chorionic gonadotropic, *n* a glycoprotein secreted by placental tissue early in normal pregnancy. This protein is also found in the urine or blood in association with chorioepitheliomas and some neoplastic diseases of the testes.

hormones, corticosteroid, *n* See *steroid, adrenocortical.*

hormones, corticotropic, *n* any one of the ovarian or adrenal hormones (for example, estradiol, estrone, estriol) that is capable of stimulating changes of a cyclic nature in the genital system. One of the ovarian or adrenal hormones capable of affecting the cyclic changes of the female genital system. See also *ACTH.*

hormones, female sex, *n.pl* hormones secreted by the ovary. They include two main types: the follicular, or estrogenic, hormones produced by the graafian follicle, and the progestational hormones from the corpus luteum.

hormones, follicle-stimulating, a pituitary tropic hormone that promotes the growth and maturation of the ovarian follicle and, with other gonadotropins, induces secretion of estrogens and possibly spermatogenesis.

hormones, gastrointestinal, *n* hormones that regulate motor and secretory activity of the digestive organs; that is, gastrin, secretin, and cholecystokinin.

hormones, gonadotropic, *n* See *gonadotropin.*

hormones, growth (somatotropic hormone, somatotropin), *n* a growth, or somatotropic, hormone that is secreted by the anterior lobe of the pituitary gland and that exerts an influence on skeletal growth. As long as the growth apparatus is functional, it is responsive to the effects of the hormone.

hormones, ketogenic, *n* the term used to describe a factor of the anterior pituitary hormone responsible for ketogenic effect. It is probably not an entity differing from known pituitary hormones.

hormones, lactogenic (galactin, mammotropin, prolactin), *n* a pituitary hormone that stimulates lactation.

hormones, luteal, *n* See *hormones, progestational.*

hormones, luteinizing, *n* a pituitary hormone that causes ovulation and development of the corpus luteum from the mature graafian follicle. It is called an *interstitial cell and stimulating hormone* because of its action on the testis in maintaining spermatogenesis and because of its role in the development of accessory sex organs.

hormones, male sex (androgenic hormone, C-19 steroids), *n.pl* hormones found in the testes, urine, and blood. Included are testosterone found in the testes, andosterone excreted into the urine, and dehydro-3-epiandrosterone found in the blood.

hormones, melanocyte-stimulating (MSH, intermedin), *n* a hormone of the middle lobe of the pituitary gland that increases melanin deposition by the melanocytes of the skin.

hormones, N, *n* See *hormone, nitrogen and steroid, C-19 cortico.*

hormones, neurohypophyseal, *n.pl* octapeptides of the neural lobe: oxytocin and vasopressin.

hormones, nitrogen (N hormone), *n.pl* C-19 corticosteroids that have androgenic and protein anabolic effects.

hormones, parathyroid, *n* the secretory product of the parathyroid glands that promotes bone resorption and increases renal resorption of calcium and magnesium and diminishes that of phosphate. Excessive secretion of the parathyroid hormone produces generalized bone resorption, formation of fibrous marrow in the spongiosa, and, in young individuals, hypocalcification of the teeth.

hormones, pituitary, *n.pl* hormones of the anterior lobe of the pituitary gland, including the growth hormones (somatotropin 1, lactogenic hormone, prolactin, galactin, mammotropin) and pituitary tropins (gonadotropins, thyrotropic hormone, and ACTH). Whether or not a true diabetogenic pituitary hormone exists is a question. The melanocyte-stimulating hormone is secreted by the middle lobe of the pituitary gland, and vasopressin and oxytocin are secreted by the posterior lobe of the pituitary gland.

hormones, pregnancy (anterior pituitary-like hormone, antuitrin S, chorionic gonadotropin), *n* a gonadotropic hormone found in the urine during pregnancy; it is a product of the very early placenta.

hormones, progestational (luteal hormone), *n.pl* hormones produced during the phase of the menstrual cycle just preceding menstruation. Includes progesterone, pregnanediol, and pregneninolone.

hormones, proinflammatory, *n* See *mineralocorticoids.*

hormones, "S" (glucocorticoid factor, sugar hormone), *n* a factor in the secretions of the adrenal cortex related to the regulation of carbohydrate metabolism.

hormones, sex, *n.pl* steroid hormones that are produced by the testes and ovaries and that control secondary sex characteristics, the reproductive cycle, development of the accessory reproductive cycle, and development of the accessory reproductive organs. Also included are the gonadotropins produced by the pituitary gland.

hormones, somatotropic, *n* See *hormone, growth.*

hormones, steroid, *n.pl* a group of biologically active organic compounds that are secreted by the adrenal cortex, testes, ovary, and placenta, and that have in common a cyclopentanoperhydrophenanthrene nucleus.

hormones, sugar, n See *hormone, "S" and steroid, C-21 cortico-.*

hormones, testicular, n.pl hormones elaborated by the testes (chiefly testosterone) that promote the growth and function of the male genitalia and secondary sex characteristics and that have potent protein anabolic effects.

hormones, thyroid, n.pl hormonal variants, including thyroxin and triiodothyronine, derived from the thyroid gland. Thyroid hormone acts as a catalyst for oxidative processes of the body cell and thus regulates the rates of body metabolism and stimulates body growth and maturation.

hormones, thyroid, thyroid-stimulating, n See *hormone, thyrotropic.*

hormones, thyrotropic (thyroid-stimulating hormone [TSH]), n a pituitary hormone that regulates the growth and activity of the thyroid gland.

horn, pulp, n a small projection of vital pulp tissue directly under a cusp or developmental lobe.

hospice, n a program under medical direction and nurse coordination that provides a variety of inpatient and home care for individuals who are terminally ill and their family members; provides calming and accommodating care that meets the special needs arising from the variety of stresses experienced during the final phases of illness, death, and grieving (e.g., emotional, physical, social, economic, and spiritual).

hospital, n an institution for the care of sick, wounded, infirm, or aged persons; generally incorporated as a nonprofit organization.

host site, n an anatomic area surgically prepared to receive an implant or graft.

hostility, n the tendency of an organism to threaten harm to another or to itself.

Howard's method, n.pr See *method, Howard's.*

Howe's silver nitrate, n.pr See *silver nitrate, ammoniacal.*

Howe's silver precipitation method, n.pr See *method, Howe's silver precipitation.*

Howship's lacuna, n.pr See *lacuna, absorption.*

human genome project, n a federally sponsored research project to identify and map the entire human gene pool.

human herpes virus-6 (HHV-6), n the herpes virus responsible for causing a skin rash similar to the type seen in persons infected with mononucleosis.

human immunodeficiency virus (HIV), n a type of retrovirus that causes AIDS. Retroviruses produce the enzyme reverse transcriptase, which allows transcription of the viral genome onto the DNA of the host cell. It is transmitted through contact with an infected individual's blood, semen, cervical secretions, cerebrospinal fluid, or synovial fluid. HIV infects T-helper cells of the immune system and results in infection with a long incubation period, averaging 10 years.

human needs diagnostic model, n one of four approaches to patient care, employs an eight-point analysis of human needs to gauge the status of the patient's mouth, teeth, and gums.

human parvovirus B19, n also called *Erythema infectiosum* or *fifth disease;* spread via the upper respiratory tract, this virus impacts on children more strongly than adults.

human rights, n.pl the legal and moral rights of humans recognized by national and international laws.

humectant (hyōōmek'tənt), n 1. a substance that prevents loss of moisture. n.pl 2. substance contained in toothpastes, gels, and powders that prevents their chemical or physical decomposition by maintaining moisture.

humidifier, n a device for adding moisture to dry air inside the home to help counteract the reduction in saliva that often occurs as a result of hyposalivation, radiation therapy, or other treatments that cause xerostomia.

humidity, n pertaining to the level of moisture in the atmosphere, the amount varying with the temperature. The percentage is usually represented in terms of relative humidity, with 100% being the point of air saturation or the level at which the air can absorb no additional water without an increase in temperature.

Hunt's syndrome, *n.pr* See *syndrome, Hunt's.*

Hunter's glossitis, *n.pr* See *glossitis, Moeller's.*

Huntington's chorea, *n.pr* a rare, abnormal hereditary condition characterized by chronic, progressive chorea and mental deterioration that terminates in dementia. The individual afflicted usually shows the first signs in the fourth decade of life and dies usually within 15 years. There is no known effective treatment but symptoms can be relieved with medications.

hurt, *v* to molest or restrain; not restricted to physical injuries; also includes mental pain, discomfort, or annoyance.

husband, *n* a man who has a spouse.

Hutchinson triad, *n.pr* See *triad, Hutchinson.*

Hutchinson's incisors, *n.pr* See *incisors, Hutchinson's.*

Hutchinson-Gilford syndrome, *n.pr* See *syndrome, Hutchinson-Gilford.*

HVL, *n* See *half-value layer.*

hyalinization (hī′-əl-in′i-zā′shən), *n* the appearance of an acellular, avascular, homogeneous area in the periodontal ligament, in which compression of the ligament between bone and tooth occurs as a result of orthodontic forces.

hyalinization of periodontal ligament, *n* a degenerative process resulting from long-continued occlusal trauma, in which the fibers become hyalinized into a homogeneous mass.

hyaluronic acid, *n* a mucopolysaccharide that forms the gelatinous substance in the tissue spaces. Hyaluronic acid is the intercellular cementing substance found throughout the tissues of the body.

hyaluronidase (hī′-əl-yōōr-on′ə-dās), *n* an enzyme that produces hydrolysis of hyaluronic acid, the cementing substance of the tissues. Produced by certain pathogenic bacteria and also formed by sperm.

hybridization, *n* crossbreeding; the process of breeding a hybrid, such as crossbreeding a horse with a donkey to produce a mule.

hydralazine HCl, *n trade name:*

Apreso-line; *drug class:* antihypertensive, direct-acting peripheral vasodilator; *action:* vasodilates arteriolar smooth muscle by direct relaxation; *uses:* essential hypertension.

hydraulic pressure, *n* See *pressure, hydraulic.*

hydremia (hī′drē′mē-ə), *n* an increase in blood volume caused by an increase in serum volume. This may result from cardiac failure, renal insufficiency, pregnancy, or the intravenous administration of fluids.

hydroalcoholic (hī′drō-al′kō-hol′ik), *adj* containing both water and alcohol. See also *solution.*

Hydrocal (hī′drō-kal), *n* the trade name for a gypsum product, a-hemihydrate, known as artificial stone. It is used for making casts.

hydrocele, *n* an accumulation of fluid in any saclike cavity or duct, specifically in the tunica vaginalis testis or along the spermatic cord.

hydrocephalus (hī′drō-sef′əl-us), *n* an abnormal accumulation of cerebrospinal fluid in the cranial vault, resulting in a disproportionately large cranium.

hydrochloric acid, *n* a compound consisting of hydrogen and chlorine. Hydrochloric acid is secreted in the stomach and is a major component of gastric juice.

hydrochlorothiazide, *n trade names:* Esidrix, HydroDIURIL; *drug class:* thiazide diuretic; *action:* acts on distal tubule by increasing excretion of water, sodium, chloride, potassium; *uses:* edema, hypertension, diuresis, congestive heart failure.

hydrocodone, *n* a semisynthetic narcotic analgesic and antitussive with multiple actions similar to those of codeine. Hydrocodone is an ingredient in prescription analgesics and cough medicines.

hydrocodone bitartrate, *n trade name:* Hycodan; *drug class:* narcotic analgesic, controlled substance schedule III; *action:* interacts with opioid receptor in the central nervous system to alter pain perception; acts directly on cough center in medulla to suppress cough; *uses:* hyperactive and nonproductive cough; mild to moderate pain.

hydrocolloid (hī′drō-kol′oids), *n.pl*
l. the materials listed as colloid

solids with water; used in dentistry as elastic impression materials. Hydrocolloids can be reversible or irreversible. *n.pl* **2.** an agar-base impression material.

hydrocolloid, irreversible (alginate), *n* a hydrocolloid whose physical condition is changed by a chemical action that is not reversible. It is an impression material that is elastic when set. See *also alginate.*

hydrocolloid, reversible (agar-agar type), *n* a hydrocolloid whose physical condition is changed by temperature. The material is made fluid by heat and becomes an elastic solid on cooling.

hydrocortisone (hīʹdrō-kôrʹti-sōn), *n* (cortisol), a glucocorticosteroid secreted by the adrenal cortex in response to stimulation by ACTH. Hydrocortisone is antianabolic, stimulates gluconeogenesis, and probably acts on some cellular system in response to a need for adaptation to change (stress).

hydrocortisone acetate/hydrocortisone sodium phosphate/hydrocortisone sodium succinat, *n trade names:* Cortef, Cortifoam, Cortenema; *drug class:* corticosteroid; *action:* decreases inflammation by suppression of macrophage and leukocyte migration; reduces capillary permeability and inhibits lysosomal enzymes; *uses:* severe inflammation, shock, adrenal insufficiency, ulcerative colitis, collagen disorders.

hydrocortisone acetate/hydrocortisone valerate, *n trade names:* Acticort, Cortaid, Cort-Dome, Dermicort; *drug class:* topical corticosteroid; *action:* interacts with steroid cytoplasmic receptors to induce antiinflammatory effects; possesses antipruritic, antiinflammatory actions; *uses:* psoriasis, eczema, contact dermatitis, pruritus.

hydrofluoric acid, *n* a compound consisting of hydrogen and flourine. It is a very active, corrosive compound, used to etch glass and precious metals.

hydrogen (H), *n* a gaseous, univalent element. Its atomic number is 1 and its atomic weight is 1.008. It is the simplest and lightest of the elements and is normally a colorless, odorless, highly flammable diatonic gas.

hydrogen peroxide, *n* an unstable compound of hydrogen and oxygen that is easily broken down into water and oxygen. A 3% solution is used as a mild antiseptic for the skin and mucous membranes; more concentrated solutions may be used as a bleach. May be used to reduce gingival inflammation, but may not eliminate the responsible bacteria.

hydrogenation (hī-drojʹə-nāʹshən), *n* the infusion of hydrogen into a compound. Also called *reduction.*

hydrokinetic activity (hīʹdrō-ki-netʹik), *n* refers to the movement or source of movement that causes fluid to be in motion.

hydrolysis (hī-drolʹis-is), *n* **1.** a reaction between the ions of salt and those of water to form an acid and a base, one or both of which is only slightly dissociated. A process whereby a large molecule is split by the addition of water. The end products divide the water, the hydroxyl group being attached to one and the hydrogen ion to the other. *n* **2.** the splitting of a compound into two parts with the addition of the elements of water.

hydromorphone HCl, *n trade names:* Dilaudid; *drug class:* synthetic narcotic analgesic (controlled substance schedule II); *action:* inhibits ascending pain pathways in the central nervous system, increases pain threshold, alters pain perception; *uses:* moderate to severe pain.

hydrophilic (hīʹdrō-filʹik), *adj* having an affinity for water. Opposite of lipophilic. See also *ointment, hydrophilic.*

hydroquinone (hī-drō-kwinʹōn), *n* **1.** a reducing agent used as an inhibitor in resin monomers to prevent polymerization during storage. *n* **2.** one of the two chemicals used as reducing agents in film-developing solutions. Hydroquinone is made from benzene (paradihydroxybenzene) and is sensitive to thermal changes. Above 70° F (21° C), the action of hydroquinone is rapid; below 60° F (15.5° C), hydroquinone becomes inactive. Its action is to control the contrast of the film.

hydrostatic pressure (hīʹdrō-statʹik), *n* See *pressure, hydrostatic.*

hydrotherapy (hīʹdrō-therʹə-pē), *n*

H

an empirical adjunct to oral physiotherapy where forced water irrigation is used to cleanse subgingival spaces, remove debris from interproximal spaces, and cleanse pockets.

hydroxide, *n* an ionic compound that contains the OH_2 ion, usually consisting of metals or the metal equivalent of the ammonium cation (NH42) that inactivates an acid.

hydroxyapatite (hī-drok´sē-ap´ət-īt), *n* a mineral compound of the general formula 3Ca3(PO4)2-Ca(OH)2, which is the principal inorganic component of bone, teeth, and dental calculus.

hydroxyapatite ceramic, n a synthetic substance composed of calcium and phosphate that is similar to a naturally occurring compound found in bones and teeth; used as the primary fabricating material or coating for dental implants.

hydroxychloroquine sulfate, *n trade name:* Plaquenil Sulfate; *drug class:* antimalarial; *action:* inhibits parasite replications, transcription of DNA to RNA by forming complexes with DNA of the parasite; *uses:* malaria, lupus erythematosus, rheumatoid arthritis.

hydroxyurea, *n trade name:* Hydrea; *drug class:* antineoplastic; *action:* acts by inhibiting DNA synthesis without interfering with synthesis of RNA or protein; *uses:* melanoma, chronic myelocytic leukemia, recurrent or metastatic ovarian cancer.

hydroxyzine HCl/hydroxyzine pamoate, *n trade names:* Atarax, Quiess, Visaject, Hyzine; *drug class:* antianxiety antihistamine; *action:* depresses subcortical levels of the central nervous system, antagonist for histamine H1-receptors; *uses:* anxiety; preoperatively, postoperatively to prevent nausea, vomiting; to potentiate narcotic analgesics; sedation; pruritus.

hygiene (hī´jēn), *n* the science of health and its preservation.

hygiene, dental, continuing care, n a regular and continuing program of monitoring, evaluation, and therapy that strives to maintain a patient's optimal dental health by combining diligent self-care with periodic professional treatment.

hygiene, oral (mouth hygiene), n the practice of personal maintenance of oral cleanliness.

hygiene, oral, special needs persons, n procedures using special skills and devices (e.g., suction or power-assisted toothbrushes) that are designed to promote the personal oral care of an individual who cannot participate in the cleaning process.

hygiene, radiation, n the art and science of protecting human beings from injury by radiation. Because any amount of radiation is potentially harmful, the ideal objective is to prevent the exposure of any person without a definite medical purpose.

hygienist, dental, *n* a licensed professional trained in an accredited postsecondary education program to provide oral health services, including scaling and polishing teeth, health education and training, and taking x-ray films, all under the direction of a licensed dentist.

hygroma (hī-grō´mə), *n* a sac or cyst swollen with fluid.

hygroma colli cysticum (cystic hygroma, cystic lymphangioma), n a cavernous lymphangioma involving the neck. It may be large, thereby impairing breathing and swallowing.

hygroscopic (hī´grō-skop´ik), *adj* having the property of absorbing moisture. When applied to gypsum products in contact with free water during their set, the resultant expansion is implied. See also *expansion, hygroscopic.*

hygroscopic investment, n See *investment, hygroscopic.*

hyoid bone, *n* a single U-shaped bone suspended from the styloid processes of the temporal bone behind and lower border of the mandible in front by a system of muscle and ligament attachments.

hyoscyamine sulfate, *n trade names:* Anaspaz, Levsin, Levsinex, Gastrosed; *drug class:* anticholinergic; *action:* inhibits muscarinic actions of acetylcholine at postganglionic parasympathetic neuroeffector sites; *uses:* treatment of peptic ulcer disease in combination with other drugs; other gastrointestinal disorders; other spastic disorders such as parkinsonism; also preoperatively to reduce secretions.

hypalgesia (hī'pal-jē'zē-ə), *n* diminished sensitivity to pain that results from a raised pain threshold.

hyper- (hī'pur), *pref* a prefix signifying above, beyond, or excessive.

hyperactivity, *n* abnormally heightened behaviors.

hyperadrenocorticism (hī'pər-əd-rē'nō-kôr'ti-siz-əm), *n* adrenocortical hyperfunction resulting from neoplasia of the cortex or hyperplasia of the cortex secondary to an increase in ACTH. Manifestations include hyperglycemia, edema, hypertension, glycosuria, negative nitrogen balance, acne, and hirsutism. See also *syndrome, adrenogenital and syndrome.*

hyperalgesia (hī'pər-al-jē'zē-ə), *n* a greater-than-normal sensitivity to pain that may result from a painful stimulus or a lowered pain threshold.

hyperalgia (hī-pər-al'jē-ə), *n* an abnormal sensitivity to pain.

hyperandrogenism, *n* a state characterized or caused by an excessive secretion of androgens by the adrenal cortex, ovaries, or testes. The clinical significance in males is negligible, so the term is used most commonly with reference to the female. The common manifestations in women are hirsutism and virilism. Hyperandrogenism is often caused by either ovarian or adrenal diseases.

hyperbaric oxygen (hī'pur-ber'ik), *n* oxygen delivered to a patient in an airtight chamber at an atmospheric pressure that is greater than normal to equalize internal and external pressure on the body for the purpose of treating decompression sickness (the bends) and certain types of infections or tumors.

hyperbilirubinemia, *n* greater than normal amounts of the bile pigment bilirubin in the blood, often characterized by jaundice, anorexia, and malaise. Hyperbilirubinemia is associated with liver disease and biliary obstruction, but it also occurs when there is excessive destruction of red blood cells, as in hemolytic anemia.

hypercalcemia (hī'pər-kal-sē'mē-ə), *n* (hypercalcinemia), **1.** an elevated blood calcium level. *n* **2.** an abnormal elevation of calcium in the blood. Causes include primary hyperparathyroidism, sarcoidosis, multiple my-eloma, malignant neoplasms, prolonged androgen therapy, and massive doses of vitamin D. Symptoms suggestive of hypercalcemia are nausea, vomiting, constipation, polyuria, weight loss, muscular weakness, and polydipsia. The normal level of total serum calcium is 8.5 to 10.5 mg/100 mL.

hypercalcinuria, *n* See *hypercalciuria.*

hypercalciuria (hī'pər-kal'sē-ōō'rē-ə), (hypercalcinuria), a condition in which there is an excessive increase in urinary calcium excretion. Major causes include primary hyperparathyroidism, hypervitaminosis D, excessive milk intake, metastatic malignancy, immobilization, and renal tubular acidosis. See also *hypercalcemia.*

hypercapnia (hī'pər-kap'nē-ə), *n* the presence of more than the normal amount of carbon dioxide in the blood tissues resulting from an increase of carbon dioxide in the inspired air or a decrease in elimination.

hypercementosis (hī'pur-se'men-tō'sis), *n* an excessive formation of cementum on the roots of one or more teeth.

hypercenesthesia (hī'pur-sen'es-thē'zh-ə), *n* a feeling of exaggerated well being such as is seen in general paralysis and sometimes in mania.

hyperchloremia (hī'pur-klôr-ē'mē-ə), *n* an excessive concentration of chloride in the plasma. Normal range is 98 to 100 mEq/L. It may occur in water depletion, dehydration, decreased bicarbonate concentration, or metabolic acidosis.

hypercholesterolemia, *n* the presence of an abnormally large amount of cholesterol in the cells and plasma of the circulating blood.

hyperemia (hī'pər-ē'mē-ə), *n* an increased and excessive amount of blood in a tissue. The hyperemia may be active or passive.

hyperemia, active, n hyperemia caused by an increased flow of blood to an area by active dilation of both the arterioles and capillaries. It is associated with neurogenic, hormonal, and metabolic function.

hyperemia, passive, n hyperemia caused by a decreased outflow of blood from an area. It may be generalized, resulting from cardiac, renal, or pulmonary disorders, or it may be localized, as in the oral cavity, and caused by pressure from mechanical or physical obstruction or by pressure from a tumor, denture, filling, or salivary calculus.

hyperesthesia (hī′pər-es-thē′zhə), *n* an excessive sensitivity of the skin or of a special sense.

hyperesthetic (hī′pər-es-thet′ik), *adj* pertaining to or affected with hyperesthesia.

hyperfunction, *n* an increase in activity of a part or in the stresses applied to a part.

hypergammaglobulinemia (hī′pur-gam′ə-glob′yōōlin-ē′mē-ə), *n* an excess of gammaglobulin in the blood. It occurs in chronic granulomatous inflammations, chronic bacterial infections, liver disease, multiple myeloma, lymphomas, and dysproteinemias.

hyperglobulinemia (hī′pur-glob′yōō-lin-ē′mē-ə), *n* an abnormally high concentration of globulins in the blood.

hyperglycemia (hī′pur-glī-sē′mē-ə), *n* an increase in the concentration of sugar in the blood. It is a feature of diabetes mellitus.

hypergonadism (hī′pər-gō′nad-iz-əm), *n* an excessive secretion of hormonal agents by the testes or ovaries. Gingival changes induced by the administration of estrogens and androgens include an increase in keratinization and hyperplasia of epithelial and connective tissue (not current).

hyperhidrosis (hī′pur-hī-drō′sis), *n* excessive sweating, which may be generalized or localized.

hyperhidrosis, gustatory, n increased sweating in the preauricular region, forehead, or face associated with eating. See also *syndrome, auriculotemporal.*

hyperhidrosis, masticatory, n excessive sweating associated with chewing. The cause is traumatic injury producing anastomosis of the facial nerve with a sympathetic branch.

hyperkalemia (hī′pur-kəl-ē′mē-ə), *n* an abnormally elevated concentration of serum potassium. It may occur in renal failure, shock, and advanced dehydration, and in association with high intracellular potassium in Addison's disease. The nor-

mal adult range of serum potassium is 4.0 to 5.5 mEq/L.

hyperkeratosis (hī′pur-ker′ə-tō′sis), *n* an excessive formation of keratin (for example, as seen in leukoplakia).

Hyperkeratosis. (Regezi/Sciubba/Pogrel, 2000)

hyperkeratosis, benign, n a nonmalignant form of a thickening condition that affects the keratin layer of the oral mucous membrane; generally appears as a white lesion.

hyperkinesis (hī′pur-kin-ē′sis), *n* excessive or frequent movement; fidgetiness.

hyperlipidemia, *n* an excess of lipids in the plasma, including the glycolipids, lipoproteins, and phospholipids.

hyperlipoproteinemia (hī′pur-lip′ō-prō′tēn-ē′mē-ə), *n* a metabolic disorder in which large amounts of certain fatty substances accumulate in the blood along with small amounts of high-density lipoproteins (HDLs).

hypermagnesemia (hī′pur-mag′nəs-ē′mē-ə), *n* an excess of magnesium in the blood serum. Normal range is 1.5 to 2.5 mEq/L. It may result in respiratory failure and coma and may occur in untreated diabetic acidosis, renal failure, and severe dehydration.

hypernasality (hī′pur-nāz-al′itē), *n* an excessive nasal resonance usually accompanied by emission of air through the nasal passageways.

hypernatremia (hī′pur-nə-trē′mē-ə), *n* an abnormally elevated concentration of serum sodium. It may occur rarely in nephrosis, congestive heart failure, and Cushing's disease and after administration of adrenocorticotropic hormone (ACTH), cortisone, or deoxycorticosterone. Normal adult range of serum sodium is 135 to 145 mEq/L.

hyperocclusion (traumatic), *n* premature tooth contact during mouth closure.

hyperopia (hī′pər-ō′pē-ə), *n* a condition in which vision improves for far objects rather than near.

hyperostosis (hī′pər-os-tō′sis), *n* **1.** an excessive growth of bone, as in infantile cortical hyperostosis. *n* **2.** hypertrophy of bone.. See also *exostosis.*

hyperostosis, infantile cortical (Caffey's disease, Smyth's syndrome), *n* a disease of infants; of unknown cause and characterized by tender, soft tissue swelling that is followed by hyperostosis of the cortex of the underlying bone. The mandible, clavicle, and ulna are most frequently affected.

hyperoxaluria, *n* an excessive level of oxalic acid or oxalates, primarily calcium oxalate, in the urine. The cause is usually an inherited deficiency of an enzyme needed to metabolize oxalic acid, which is present in many fruits and vegetables, or a disorder of fat absorption in the small intestine. An excess of oxalates may lead to the formation of renal calculi. Treatment may include pyridoxine, forced fluid, and a low-oxalate diet.

hyperoxaluria, primary, *n* an inherited deficiency of the enzyme that metabolizes oxalic acid, resulting in an excessive level of oxalic acid or oxalates in the urine.

hyperoxia (hī′pər-ok′sē-ə), *n* an excess of oxygen in the system.

hyperparathyroidism (hī′pur-per′e-thī′roid-iz-əm), *n* (generalized osteitis fibrosa cystica, von Recklinghausen's disease of bone), **1.** increased parathyroid function resulting from primary hyperplasia, a functioning neoplasm of the parathyroid glands, or secondary hyperplasia related most often to chronic renal insufficiency. Manifestations are related to abnormalities of the bones, kidneys, and blood vessels. Skeletal changes are referred to as *generalized osteitis fibrosa cystica or von Recklinghausen's disease.* Brown tumors, which are essentially giant cell tumors, may develop generally, as well as in the jaws. Kidney changes include renal stones and nephrocalcinosis. Calcification of muscles in arteries occurs. Renal rickets is associated with secondary hyperparathyroidism in children with chronic renal disease. Laboratory findings include a high serum calcium level, low phosphorus level, and a normal or high alkaline phosphatase level. Renal impairment, such as occurs in secondary hyperparathyroidism, tends to nullify hypercalcemia because of an increased loss of calcium in the urine. *n* **2.** an abnormal increase in activity of the parathyroid glands, causing loss of calcium from the bones and resulting in tenderness in bones, spontaneous fractures, muscular weakness, and osteitis fibrosa. **3.** excessive production of parathormone by the parathyroid gland (as in parathyroid hyperplasia and/or adenoma), resulting in increased renal excretion of phosphorus by lowering of the renal threshold for this substance. The pathologic changes produced are osteoporotic or osteodystrophic in nature as a consequence of withdrawal of calcium and phosphorus from osseous tissues.

hyperparathyroidism, brown node of, *n* See *node, brown, of hyperparathyroidism.*

hyperphosphatemia (hī′pur-fos′fə-tē′mē-ə), *n* an increased concentration of inorganic phosphates in the blood serum. Hyperphosphatemia may occur in childhood and also in acromegaly, renal failure, and vitamin D intoxication. Normal adult range of serum inorganic phosphorus is 2.5 to 4.2 mg/100 mL.

hyperphosphaturia (hī′pur-fos′fə-tōō′rē-ə), *n* an excessive excretion of phosphate in the urine.

hyperpigmentation, *n* an unusual darkening of the skin. Causes include heredity, drugs, exposure to the sun, and adrenal insufficiency.

hyperpituitarism (hī′pur-pit-ōō′it-er-iz-əm), *n* a condition caused by excessive production of the hormones secreted by the pituitary gland. An excess of the growth hormone results in giantism or acromegaly; an excess of ACTH produces Cushing's syndrome.

hyperplasia (hī′pur-plā′zē-ə, -zhə), *n* the abnormal multiplication or increase in the number of normal cells in normal arrangement in a tissue or organ, resulting in a thickening or enlargement of the tissue or organ.

hyperplasia, denture (denture hypertrophy), *n* an enlargement of tissue beneath a denture that is traumatizing the soft tissue.

hyperplasia, Dilantin gingival (dilantin) (Dilantin enlargement), *n* an enlargement of the gingivae caused by the use of diphenylhydantoin sodium (Dilantin sodium) in the treatment of epilepsy.

hyperplasia, focal fibrous, *n* a small, firm nodule originating in the fibrous connective tissue, which forms on the tongue, lower lip, or mucous membrane lining of the mouth as the result of injury or chronic irritation.

hyperplasia, gingival, *n* **1.** an enlargement of the gingival tissue resulting from proliferation of its cellular elements. Hereditary or inflammatory causes may be involved. *n* **2.** the proliferation of gingival epithelium to form elongated rete pegs and proliferation of fibroblasts with increased collagen formation in the underlying connective tissue; leads to nodular enlargement of the gingiva in diphenylhydantoin sodium therapy. *n* **3.** gingival enlargement, primarily produced by proliferation of connective tissue elements; often accompanied by gingival inflammation as a result of trauma to the hyperplastic tissues and coincidental with or following the ingestion of diphenylhydantoin sodium and other medications.

hyperplasia, idiopathic gingival, *n* See *fibromatosis gingivae.*

hyperplasia, inflammatory fibrous, *n* See *epulis fissurata.*

hyperplasia, inflammatory papillary (inflammatory papillomatosis, multiple papillomatosis, papillary hyperplasia), *n* a condition of unknown cause but associated with the presence of maxillary dentures. Characterized by numerous red papillary projections on the hard palate.

hyperplasia, papillary, *n* a growth in the midline of the hard palate, usually in the relief area of a denture; characterized by a papillary, or raspberry, appearance.

hyperplastic tissue, *n* See *tissue, hyperplastic.*

hyperpnea (hī′purp-nē′-ə), *n* an abnormal increase in respiratory volume; an abnormal increase in the rate and depth of breathing.

hyperpotassemia (hī′pur-po-t′əsē′mē-ə), *n* See *hyperkalemia.*

hyperproteinemia (hī′pur-prō′tēn-ē′mē-ə), *n* an abnormal increase in serum and plasma proteins.

hyperproteinuria (hī′pur-prō′tēn-yōō′rē-ə), *n* See *albuminuria.*

hypersalivation, *n* See *sialorrhea.*

hypersensitive, *n* abnormally sensitive.

hypersensitiveness (hī′pur-sen′sitiv-nes), *n* a state of altered reactivity in which the body reacts more strongly than normal to a foreign agent.

hypersensitivity, *n* **1.** an adverse reaction to contact with specific substances in quantities that usually produce no reaction in normal individuals. *n* **2.** usually, an allergic tendency. In general, a tendency to react with unusual violence to stimuli. *n* **3.** a common complaint after periodontal therapy in which dentin may be exposed, resulting in pain in the teeth or sensitivity to heat, cold, and sweet substances.

Contact hypersensitivity. (Regezi/Sciubba/ Pogrel, 2000)

hypersensitivity, atopic, *n* See *atopy.*

hypersensitivity, bacterial, *n* delayed inflammatory reaction resulting from previous sensitization of the host by an antigen.

hypersensitivity, delayed, *n* hypersensitivity involving a latent period between the antigen introduction and the reaction; cellular reactions mediated by the T lymphocytes

hypersensitivity, immediate, *n* a humoral reaction, mediated by the circulating B lymphocytes, which causes any of three immediate responses: anaphylactic hypersensitivity, cytotoxic hypersensitivity, and immune system hypersensitivity.

hypersensitivity reaction, cytotoxic, *n* surface antigens of a cell join with an antibody, causing complement-mediated cell destruction, or other types of cell-membrane damage.

hypersensitivity reactions, immune complex, n.pl one of four types of hypersensitivity reactions to antigens in the body, that acts as a barrier to disease. The reactions can cause tissue damage.

hypersensitization, n the process of rendering abnormally sensitive or the condition of being abnormally sensitive.

hypersplenism, n a syndrome consisting of splenomegaly and a deficiency of one or more types of blood cells.

hypersthenuria (hī′purs-then-yŏŏ′rē-ə), n urine with an abnormally high specific gravity. It is seen in uncontrolled diabetes mellitus and in severe dehydration.

hypersusceptibility (hī′pur-sə-sep′ti-bil′it-ē), n a condition of abnormal susceptibility to poisons, infective agents, or agents that are entirely innocuous in the normal individual.

hypersympathicotonus (hī′pur-sim-path′ik-ō-tō′nus), n an increased tonicity of the sympathetic nervous system. See also *sympathetic otonia.*

hypertarachia (hī′pur-tər-ak′ē-ə), n extreme irritability of the nervous system.

hypertelorism (hī′pur-tel′ər-iz-əm), n an excessive distance between paired organs. See also *syndrome, Greig's.*

hypertension (hī′pur-ten′shən), n an abnormal elevation of systolic or diastolic arterial pressure. Systolic hypertension is generally related to emotional stress, sclerosis of the aorta and large arteries, or aortic insufficiency. Diastolic hypertension may result from obscure causes (essential), renal disease, or endocrine disorders.

hypertension, essential, n an elevated blood pressure of unknown cause.

hypertension, malignant, n an elevated blood pressure characterized by a progressive course uncontrollable by medication.

hypertension, orthostatic, n plummeting blood pressure that occurs upon standing up which may be accompanied by dizziness or fainting.

hypertension, portal, n hypertension originating in the portal system as occurring in cirrhosis of the liver and other conditions caused by an obstruction of the portal vein.

hypertension pulmonary, n hypertension resulting from pulmonary or cardiac disease such as fibrosis of the lung or mitral stenosis.

hypertensive agents, n.pl agents that reduce or control blood pressure.

hyperthermia (hī′pur-thur′mē-ə), n an extremely high fever brought on by treatment.

hyperthermia, malignant (mə-lig′nənt), n an extremely high fever accompanied by muscle rigidity that occurs rapidly in susceptible individuals when they are exposed to certain types of anesthesia; may be fatal.

hyperthyroidism, n (Parry's disease), abnormalities of calorigenic mechanisms, body tissues, blood, and body fluids and of the circulatory, muscular, and nervous systems resulting from an excessive elaboration of thyroid hormone. Manifestations include increased sweating, increased appetite, intolerance to heat, weight loss, increased protein-bound iodine (PBI), early shedding of primary teeth and early eruption of permanent teeth, tachycardia, palpitation, tremors, nervousness, muscular weakness, diarrhea, increased excretion of calcium and phosphorus, hypocholesterolemia, creatinuria, and osteoporosis. May occur as the result of primary hyperplasia, hyperfunctioning nodular goiters, functional benign tumor, or adenoma of the thyroid gland. See also *goiter, exophthalmic.*

hypertonic (hī′pur-ton′ik), adj having an osmotic pressure greater than that of the solution with which it is compared.

hypertrichosis (hī′pur-trik-ō′sis), n an excessive growth of hair on the body, possibly as a result of endocrine dysfunction, as in the hirsutism accompanying excessive adrenocortical function.

hypertrophy (hī-pur′trō-fē), n a morbid enlargement or overgrowth of an organ or part resulting from an increase in size of its constituent cells.

hypertrophy, denture, n See *hyperplasia, denture.*

hypertrophy, muscle, n hypertrophy denotes an increase in the size or number of constituent fibers of a muscle. Any other condition such as inflammation, tumor, and fatty infiltration that increases the size of a muscle is called *pseudohypertrophy.*

H

True or physiologic hypertrophy results from excessive activity of muscle. Genetic and hormonal factors play a role in determining the size of muscles; for example, muscles in a man tend to be larger than in a woman in the temporal and facial regions. The histologic characteristics of hypertrophied muscle are normal. The fibrils are slightly wider in diameter than is normal, and the only change might be a slight increase in vascularity.

hyperventilation, *n* **1.** an abnormally prolonged, rapid, and deep breathing; also the condition produced by overbreathing of oxygen at high pressures. It is marked by confusion, dizziness, numbness, and muscular cramps brought on by such breathing. *n* **2.** Rapid, deep, forced breathing frequently resulting from anxiety. It results in a transient loss of carbon dioxide and respiratory alkalosis. Symptoms include anxiety, circumoral numbness, tingling sensation, faintness, and occasionally, carpopedal spasms, tetany, and syncope.

hyperventilation, managing, *n* steps that may be taken to assist a patient who experiences sudden, increased respiration that may be the result of anxiety or pain; may include verbal reassurances, repositioning, or deep breathing exercises.

hypervitaminosis A (hī-pur-vī´təm-i-nō´sis), *n* the effects of toxic doses of vitamin A. Manifestations include bone fragility, xeroderma, nausea, headache, and loss of hair.

hypervitaminosis D, *n* the toxic effects of ingesting large amounts of vitamin D. Manifestations include symptoms resulting from hypercalcemia, impairment of renal function, and metastatic calcification.

hypervolemia, *n* increased blood volume.

hypesthesia (hī´pes-thē´zhə), *n* a condition characterized by atypically decreased sensation.

hypnic (hip´nik), *adj* inducing or pertaining to sleep.

hypno- (hip´nō), *comb.* a combining form denoting a relationship to sleep.

hypnosis (hip-nō´sis), *n* a condition of artificially induced sleep or of a trance resembling sleep induced by drugs, psychologic means, or both. Generally creating a condition of heightened suggestibility in the subject.

hypnotic (hip-not´ik), *n* **1.** a drug that induces sleep or depresses the central nervous system at a cortical level. *adj* **2.** causing sleep or a trance. See also *sedative*.

hypnotism (hip´nō-tiz-əm), *n* **1.** the method or practice of inducing sleep. *n* **2.** in medical jurisprudence, a mental state rendering the patient susceptible to suggestion at the will and inducement of another.

hypnotize (hip´nō-tīz), *v* to put into a state of hypnosis in which there is a condition of heightened suggestibility.

hypo (hī´pō), *n* an abbreviated form of the term hyposulfite, which is a synonym of sodium thiosulfate (Na2S2O3), a solution used in photography and radiography to fix and harden the manifest image. See also *fixation*.

hypo- (hī´pō), *pref* a prefix signifying beneath, under, or deficient.

hypoadrenocorticalism (hī´pō-ə-drē´nō-kôr´tik-əl-iz-əm), *n* acute or chronic adrenocortical hypofunction, as in Waterhouse-Friderichsen syndrome or Addison's disease.

hypoadrenocorticism (hī´pō-ə-drēn-ō-kôr´tis-iz-əm), *n* See *hypoadrenocorticalism*.

hypoalgesia (hī´pō-al-jē´zē-ə), *n* a diminished sensation of pain resulting from a raised pain threshold.

hypoallergenic (hī´pō-al´ur-jen´ik), *adj* descriptor of a substance ensuring a generally nonactivating property with regard to allergy-producing symptoms in individuals with certain chemical sensitivities.

hypobranchial eminence (hī´pō-brang´kə-əl), *n* a small tissue structure formed from the second, third, and fourth pharyngeal arches during early embryonic development of the head and neck from which the tongue eventually takes shape.

hypocalcemia (hī´pō-kal-sē´mē-ə), *n* an abnormally low concentration of calcium in the blood; may be associated with hypoparathyroidism, rickets, osteomalacia, renal rickets, pancreatic disease, sprue, obstructive jaundice, or tetany.

hypocalcification (hī´pō-kal´si-fi-kā´shən), *n* reduced calcification, especially of enamel. It produces opaque white spots that may be discolored later. See also *fluorosis*.

Hypocalcification. (Zitelli/Davis, 2002)

hypocalcification, hereditary enamel, *n* a hereditary anomaly of enamel formation affecting the primary and permanent dentition in which the enamel peels off after tooth eruption and exposes dentin, giving the teeth a yellow appearance.

hypocalciuria (hī′pō-kal′sē-ŏŏ′rē-ə), *n* a decrease in urinary calcium. Normal values vary considerably but are roughly related to calcium intake. Various values are given (for example, 100 to 200 mg/day on a normal diet, or 350 to 400 mg/day for calcium intake of 10 mg/kg of body weight in children). Hypocalciuria may occur in hypoparathyroidism, rickets, osteomalacia, metastatic carcinoma of the prostate, and renal failure. See also *test, Sulkowitch's*.

hypocapnia (hī′pō-kap′nē-ə), *n* a deficiency of carbon dioxide in the blood.

hypocarbia, *n* See *hypocapnia*.

hypochloremia (hī′pō-klôr-ē′mē-ə), *n* a decrease below normal of chloride concentration in the plasma. The normal range is 98 to 100 mEq/L. It may occur in adrenal insufficiency, persistent vomiting, renal failure, acute infections, and dehydration with sodium depletion.

hypochlorous acid, *n* a greenish-yellow liquid derived from an aqueous solution of lime. An unstable compound that decomposes to hydrochloric acid and water; hypochlorous acid is used as a bleaching agent and disinfectant.

hypochondria (hī′pō-kon′drē-ə), *n* anxiety about disease; a type of neurosis characterized by fear of disease or by simulated disease.

hypochondriasis (hī′pō-kon-drī′-ə-sis), *n* See *hypochondria*.

hypochromia (hī-pō-krō′mē-ə), *n* a reduced staining quality of cells, particularly pale staining red blood cells associated with hemoglobin deficiency.

hypodermoclysis (hī′pō-dur-mok′lis-is), *n* a subcutaneous injection of fluid in large volume.

hypodontia (hī′pō-don′shē-ə), *n* fewer teeth than normal.

hypoesthesia (hī′pō-es-thē′zē-ə, -zhə), *n* a decreased sensitivity to touch or pressure.

hypoestrogenism (hī′pō-es′trō-jen-iz-əm), *n* diminished production of estrogenic substances by the ovaries, such as that which occurs during menopause. May produce desquamative lesions on the oral mucous membranes. See also *gingivitis, desquamative*.

hypofibrinogenemia (hī′pō-fĭb-rin′ō-jən-ē′mē-ə), *n* a reduction of fibrinogen in the blood. Excessive bleeding may occur following trauma. The deficiency of fibrinogen may be congenital or may result from faulty synthesis associated with liver disease and defibrinogenation resulting from disorders of pregnancy involving the placenta and amniotic fluid. The normal range is 200 to 600 mg/100 mL of plasma. Clotting deficiencies do not occur until the concentration falls below 75 mg/100 mL.

hypogammaglobulinemia (hī′pō-gam′ə-glob′yōō-linē′mē-ə), *n* a deficiency of gammaglobulin, usually manifested by recurrent bacterial infections.

hypogeusia (hī′pō-gōō′zē-ə), *n* a decreased sense of taste.

hypoglossal nerve (XII), *n* paired twelfth cranial nerve, essential for swallowing and moving the tongue. Each nerve has four major branches, communicates with the vagus nerve, and connects to the nucleus XII in the brain. See *nerve*.

hypoglycemia (hī′pō-glī-sē′mē-ə), *n* a condition existing when the concentration of blood sugar (true blood sugar) is 40 mg/100 mL or less. Symptoms may not occur even when the concentration is considerably less.

Symptoms include nervousness, hunger, weakness, vertigo, and faintness. Hypoglycemia may occur in the fasting state or following the injection of insulin.

hypoglycemia, fasting, n hypoglycemia occurring in the postabsorptive state; occurs in renal glycosuria, lactation, hepatic disease, and in central nervous system lesions.

hypoglycemia, insulin, n hypoglycemia resulting from improper administration of insulin. If hypoglycemia is severe, convulsions, coma, and death may occur. See also *shock, insulin.*

hypoglycemia, mixed, n hypoglycemia occurring during the fasting state and after the ingestion of carbohydrates; occurs in idiopathic spontaneous hypoglycemia of infancy, in anterior pituitary and adrenocortical insufficiency, and with tumors of the islet cells of the pancreas.

hypoglycemia, reactive, n hypoglycemia occurring after the ingestion of carbohydrates with an excessive release of insulin, as in functional hyperinsulinism.

hypoglycemia, spontaneous, n hypoglycemia that is functional (such as in renal glycosuria, lactation, and severe muscular exertion) or is caused by organic disease such as in hepatic disease and adrenocortical insufficiency.

hypoglycemic agents, *n.pl* a large heterogeneous group of drugs prescribed to decrease or control the amount of glucose circulating in the blood; used in the prevention and treatment of diabetes.

hypogonadism (hī′pō-gō′nad-iz-əm), n a gonadal deficiency resulting from abnormalities of the testes and ovaries or to pituitary insufficiency. Manifestations include eunuchism, eunuchoidism, Frohlich's syndrome, amenorrhea, and incomplete development or maintenance of secondary sex characteristics.

hypohidrotic ectodermal dysplasia (hī′pō-hī-drot′ik ek-tō-dur′məl dis-plā′zhə), n a syndrome consisting of hypodontia, hypotrichosis, hypohidrosis, and other defects related to the development of ectodermal structures.

hypokalemia (hī′pō-kəl-ē′mē-ə), n an abnormally low serum potassium level. Hypokalemia may occur in metabolic alkalosis, chronic diarrhea,

Cushing's syndrome, primary aldosteronism, and excessive use of deoxycorticosterone, cortisone, or ACTH.

hypolarynx (hī′pō-ler′inks), n the infraglottic compartment of the larynx that extends from the true vocal cords to the first tracheal ring.

hypolethal (hī′pō-lē′thəl), adj not quite lethal; said of dosage.

hypomagnesemia (hī′pō-mag′nəs-ē′mē-ə), n a deficiency of magnesium in the blood serum (normal values range from 1.5 to 2.5 mEq/L). It may be associated with chronic alcoholism, starvation, and prolonged diuresis in congestive heart failure. Manifestations include muscular twitching, convulsions, and coma.

hyponasality (hī′pō-nāz-al′itē), n a lack of nasal resonance necessary to produce acceptable voice quality. The type of voice quality heard when the speaker's nose is occluded or when the speaker is suffering from a severe cold.

hyponatremia (hī′pō-nə-trē′mē-ə), n an abnormally low concentration of sodium in the blood serum. It may develop in adrenocortical insufficiency and chronic renal disease or with extreme sweating.

hypoparathyroidism (hī′pō-per′ə-thī′roid-iz-əm), n a decrease in parathyroid function, usually the result of surgical removal. Symptoms include tetany, irritability, and muscle weakness. The serum calcium is low, the blood phosphorus elevated, the blood magnesium reduced, and the alkaline phosphatase normal.

hypopharyngoscope (hī′pō-fər-ing′gō-skōp), n an apparatus devised for bringing the lower part of the pharynx or hypopharynx into view.

hypopharynx (hī′pō-fer′inks), n the division of the pharynx that lies below the upper edge of the epiglottis and opens into the larynx and esophagus.

hypophosphatasia (hī′pō-fos′fə-tā′zhə), n a familial disease in which the children may have very low serum alkaline phosphatase levels, total or partial aplasia of the cementum, and an abnormal periodontal ligament in the primary teeth; a decreased phosphatase level that has been linked to a premature loss of primary teeth in children. Examination reveals absence, hypoplasia, or dysplasia of cementum.

hypophosphatemia (hī′pō-fos′fə-tē′mē-ə), *n* an abnormally low concentration of serum phosphates. Blood phosphorus levels are low in sprue, celiac disease, and hyperparathyroidism and in association with an elevated alkaline phosphatase in vitamin D-resistant rickets and other diseases involving a renal tubular defect in resorption of phosphate.

hypophysis, *n* See *gland, pituitary.*

hypopituitarism (hī′pō-pit-ōō′it-er-iz-əm), *n* a decrease in the hormonal secretions of the pituitary gland.

hypoplasia (hī′pō-plā′zhə), *n* the defective or incomplete development of any tissue or structure.

Hypoplasia. (Regezi/Sciubba/Pogrel, 2000)

hypoplasia, enamel, chronologic, n a prenatal or postnatal systemic hypoplasia affecting amelogenesis occurring at the time of the systemic disorder.

hypoplasia, enamel, hereditary (hereditary brown tooth), n a hereditary anomaly of the enamel affecting the primary and permanent dentition in which a thin layer of hard enamel covering the yellow dentin gives the tooth a brown appearance.

hypoplasia, mandibular, n an abnormally small mandibular development (for example, in micrognathia or brachygnathia).

hypopnea (hī-pop′nē-ə), *n* abnormally shallow and rapid respirations.

hypopotassemia (hī′pō-pot′ə-sē′mē-ə), *n* See *hypokalemia.*

hypoproteinemia (hī′pō-prō′tēn-ē′mē-ə), *n* a decrease in serum and plasma proteins.

hypoprothrombinemia (hī′pō-prō-throm′binē′mē-ə), *n* a deficiency of prothrombin in the blood. It may be congenital or associated with vitamin K deficiency, large doses of salicylates, liver disease, or excessive anticoagulant. The normal level ranges from 70% to 120% plasma prothrombin concentration. There is little danger of hemorrhage if the prothrombin concentration is greater than 20% of normal.

hyposalivation (hī′pō-sal′i-vā′shən), *n* a decreased flow of saliva. It may be associated with dehydration, radiation therapy of the salivary gland regions, anxiety, the use of drugs such as atropine and antihistamines, vitamin deficiency, various forms of parotitis, and various syndromes (Sjögren's, Riley-Day, Plummer-Vinson, and Heerfordt's disease). See also *asialorrhea.*

hyposensitive (hī′pō-sen′si-tiv), *adj* less *sensitive.*

hyposthenuria (hī′pōs-then-yōō′rē-ə), *n* a condition in which the urine has an abnormally low specific gravity. Hyposthenuria may occur in cases in which renal damage impairs concentrating power or when the kidneys are normal but lack hormonal stimulus for concentrations, as in diabetes insipidus.

hypotension (hī′pō-ten′shən), *n* abnormally low tension, especially low blood pressure.

hypotension, orthostatic (postural) (ôr′thō-stat′ik), n plummeting blood pressure that occurs when standing; dizziness and fainting may result.

hypothalamus (hī′pō-thal′ə-mus), *n* a small extension of the brain that lies in the sella turcica in the cranium. The hypothalamus lies just at the superior level of the body of the sphenoid bone. It is intimately related structurally and functionally with the pituitary gland and is important in the central regulation of the endocrine glands, including the thyroid gland, pancreas, adrenal glands, and gonads. The most important visceral functions are under control of the hypothalamus because it functions in such close coordination with the endocrine glands. The control is mediated through its structural communication with the pituitary gland.

hypothermia, *n* body temperature significantly below normal; that is, 98.6° F, 37° C.

hypothetical question, *n* assumed or proved facts and circumstances, stated to constitute a specific situation or state of facts, on which the opinion of an expert is asked, in producing evidence at a trial.

hypothyroidism (hī′pō-thī′roid-iz-əm), *n* diminished activity of the thyroid gland with decreased secretion of thyroxin, resulting in lowered basal metabolic rate, lethargy, sleepiness, dysmenorrhea in females, and a tendency toward obesity. Occasionally there is accompanying gingival hyperplasia. The condition is called cretinism in children and myxedema in adults.

hypotonic (hī′pō-ton′ik), *adj* exhibiting less tension or firmness.

hypotrichosis, *n* a less-than-normal amount of hair on the head or body.

hypoventilation, *n* an abnormal condition of the respiratory system, characterized by cyanosis, polycythemia, increased carbon dioxide arterial tension, and generalized decreased respiratory function. Hypoventilation occurs when the volume of air that enters the alveoli and takes part in gas exchanges is not adequate for the metabolic needs of the body.

hypoxanthine, *n* a purine present in the muscles and other tissues, formed during purine catabolism by deamination of adenine.

hypoxanthine phosphoribosyl-trans-ferase, *n* an enzyme present in human tissue that converts hypoxanthine and guanine to their respective 5 nucleotides, with 5-phosphoribose 1-diphosphate as the ribose-phosphate donor.

hypoxemia (hī′pok-sē′mē-ə), *n* deficient oxygenation of the blood.

hypoxia (hī-pok′sē-ə), *n* low oxygen content or tension.

hypoxia, anemic, n hypoxia brought about by a reduction of the oxygen-carrying capacity of the blood because of a decrease in the complete blood counts or an alteration of the hemoglobin constituents.

hypoxia, anoxic, n hypoxia resulting from inadequate oxygen in inspired air or interference with gaseous exchange in the lungs.

hypoxia, histotoxic, n hypoxia resulting from the inability of the tissue cells to use the oxygen that may be present in normal amount and tension.

hypoxia, metabolic, n hypoxia resulting from an increased tissue demand for oxygen.

hypoxia, stagnant, n hypoxia resulting from decreased circulation in an area.

hyrax appliance, *n* a fixed orthodontic appliance used for the bilateral expansion of the maxillary posterior teeth or the bilateral expansion of the palate.

hysteresis (his-ter-ē′sis), *n* a physical phenomenon whereby a material such as a reversible hydrocolloid passes from a solid to a gel state at one temperature and a gel to a solid state at another.

hysteria (his-ter′ē-ə), *n* **1.** a disease or disorder of the nervous system, more common in females than males, not originating in lesions and resulting from psychic rather than physical causes. *n* **2.** a psychoneurosis characterized by lack of control over emotions or acts, exaggeration of sensory impression, and simulation of disease or pain associated with disease. In some patients, trismus, neuralgia, and temporomandibular joint disturbance may be hysterical in origin.

I and D (surgical fistulation), *n* the abbreviation for **incision and drainage,** which is the procedure of incising a fluctuant mucosal lesion to allow for the release of pressure and drainage of fluid exudate.

I cell disease, *n* a congenital disease, also known as *mucolipidosis II*. It is characterized by shortness of stature, psychomotor retardation, coarse facial features, and gingival enlargement. The progressive gingival enlargement may delay tooth eruption and may impair closure of the mouth.

iatrogenic (ī´-atrōjen´ik), *adj* originating as a result of professional care; for example, an iatrogenic dermatitis.

iatrosedation (ī-ətrōsēdā´shən), *n* a relaxed state induced by actions rather than drugs; a method of anxiety reduction that is psychologically based.

ibuprofen, *n trade names:* Advil, Excedrin-IB, Midol-IB, Motrin IB; *drug class:* nonsteroidal antiinflammatory; *action:* inhibits prostaglandin synthesis by interfering with cyclooxgenase needed for biosynthesis, possesses analgesic, antiinflammatory, antipyretic properties; *uses:* rheumatoid arthritis, osteoarthritis, mild-to-moderate pain. Ibuprofen is useful for the temporary relief of minor aches and pains associated with the common cold, toothache, muscular aches, minor arthritic pain, and menstrual cramps, and for the reduction of fever.

Ichthyosis, *n* any of several inherited dermatologic conditions in which the skin is dry, hyperkeratotic, and fissured, resembling fish scales. It usually appears at or shortly after birth and may be part of one of several rare syndromes. Some types respond temporarily to bath oils, topical retinoic acid, or propylene glycol. Also called *xeroderma.*

icterus (ik´terəs), *n* See jaundice.

icterus, acholuric, *n* See jaundice, hemolytic, congenital.

id, *n* the part of the psyche functioning in the unconscious that is the source of instinctive energy, impulses, and drives. It is based on the pleasure principle and has strong tendencies toward self-preservation. The full taxonomy includes the id, the ego, and the superego.

identity, *n* sameness; the fact that a subject, person, or thing before a court is the same as it is claimed to be.

idiopathic (id˝e-o-path´ik), *adj* without apparent cause; of unknown origin.

idiopathic disease, *n* See disease, idiopathic.

idiopathic enlargement (id´ē-ōpath´ik), *n* See enlargement, idiopathic.

idiosyncrasy (id´ē-ōsing´krəsē), *n* **1.** the tendency to react atypically or with unusual violence to a food, drug, or cosmetic. **2.** any characteristic that is peculiar to an individual.

idoxuridine-IDU (ophthalmic), *n trade name:* Herplex; *drug class:* antiviral; *action:* inhibits viral replication by interfering with viral DNA synthesis; *uses:* herpes simplex keratitis, vaccinia virus keratitis, herpes simplex keratoconjunctivitis.

IgA, *n* the abbreviation for **immunoglobulin A.**

IgA deficiency, *n* a selective lack of immunoglobulin A, which constitutes the most common type of immunoglobulin deficiency, appearing in about 1 in 400 individuals. Immunoglobulin A is a major protein antibody in the saliva and the mucous membranes of the intestines and bronchi. It protects against bacterial and viral infections. IgA deficiency is common in patients with rheumatoid arthritis and in patients with systemic lupus erythematosus.

IgE, *n* the abbreviation for **immunoglobulin E.**

IgG, *n* the abbreviation for **immunoglobulin G.**

IgM, *n* the abbreviation for **immunoglobulin M.**

ignorance of law, *n* See law, ignorance of.

ilium, *n* the uppermost of the three bones that make up the innominate bone. The ilium forms part of the acetabulum. The iliac crest is a source of bone for mandibular and chin reconstruction and enhancement.

illegal, *adj* not authorized by law; illicit.

illuminator (light box), *n* a source of light with uniform intensity for viewing radiographs.

illusion, *n* a mistaken or erroneous perception of an object external to the individual. In some cases, the laws of physics explain the errors. In others, the explanation lies with the perceiver. Illusions should be distinguished from *hallucinations,* which are perceptions that lack external stimuli, and *delusions,* which are false beliefs. Illusions are seen in certain reactions to general anesthesia or intoxication.

illustration, *n* a drawing or photograph used to help clarify the patient's concept of proposed treatment and conditions present.

image enhancement, *n* the use of computer digital technology to improve the resolution of cathode ray images.

image, latent, *n* the invisible image produced on photographic or radiographic film by the action of light or radiation before development.

imaging, *n* the creation of digital, print, or film representations of anatomical structures for the purpose of diagnosis.

imbedded, *adj* See embedded.

imbibition (im'bibish'ən), *n* the absorption of liquid. Gel structures are particularly susceptible to imbibition.

imbrication lines (im″brĭ-ka′shən līnz), *n.pl* **1.** the seams which are formed by overlapping layers of tissue in order to close a surgical wound. **2.** slight mesiodistal ridges in the cervical third of a tooth. They are associated with the lines of Retzius in the enamel.

imipramine HCl, *n trade names:* Norfranil, Tipramine; *drug class:* tricyclic antidepressant; *action:* inhibits both norepinephrine and serotonin (5-HT) uptake in the brain; *uses:* depression, enuresis in children.

immediate denture, *n* See denture, immediate.

immersion, *n* the placing of a body or an object into water or other liquid so that it is completely covered by the liquid.

immobilization, *n* the act of securing in a fixed relationship to prevent damage and to promote healing, such as the use of a splint or cast to maintain the fractured pieces of bone in proper relationship to each other for healing to occur.

immune reaction, *n* See reaction, immune.

immune system, *n* a biochemical complex that protects the body against pathogenic organisms and other foreign bodies. The system incorporates the humoral immune response, which produces antibodies to react with specific antigents, and the cell-mediated response, which uses T cells to mobilize tissue macrophages in the presence of a foreign body. The immune system also protects the body from invasion by creating local barriers and inflammation. The principal organs of the immune response system include the bone marrow, the thymus, and the lymphoid tissues.

immune system, duality of, *n* the division of lymphocyte white blood cells into two classes of cells, types B and T. Type B cells help develop humoral immunities, while type T cells are active in cellular immunity.

immunity (imyōō′nitē), *n* **1.** exemption from service or from duties that the law ordinarily requires most citizens to perform (for example, jury duty). **2.** the condition of an organism whereby it successfully resists or is not susceptible to injury or infection.

immunity, acquired, *n* **1.** resistance to a particular disease (e.g., chicken pox) after recovering from that disease. **2.** resistance to poisons or medications developed over a usually long period of gradually increasing exposure.

immunity, active, *n* resistance to a disease or other biological or chemical agents acquired naturally as a result of exposure to the disease or agent; can also be acquired artificially by use of a vaccine containing a weakened or deadened form of the agent, stimulating the immune system to produce antibodies long after the initial exposure. See also passive immunity.

immunity, natural, *n* the inherited ability to remain resistant to or unaffected by a specific disease.

immunity, passive, *n* short-term resistance to a specific disease that has been acquired either through the placenta from mother to fetus or as the result of receiving an injection of serum antibodies taken from an immune person or animal (innoculation).

immunization, *n.pl* **1.** a fundamental element of preventative healthcare for dental workers, who should be fully immunized against influenza, hepatitis B, and all regular childhood diseases. HIV and hepatitis C vaccines are not available. **2.** a process by which resistance to an infectious disease is induced or augmented.

immunoassay, *n* a competitive-binding assay in which the binding protein is an antibody.

immunoblotting, *n* immunologic methods for isolating and quantitatively measuring immunoreactive substances. When used with immune reagents such as monoclonal antibodies, the process is known generically as *western blot analysis.*

immunocompromised, *adj* having the quality of an immune response that has been weakened by a disease or immunosuppressive agent.

immunodeficiency, *n* a condition resulting from a defective immunologic mechanism. Primary immunodeficiency is caused by a defect in the immune system; secondary immunodeficiency is a result of another disease process such as HIV infection.

immunodiffusion, *n* a technique for the identification and quantification of any of the immunoglobulins.

immunoelectrophoresis, *n* a technique that combines eletrophoresis and immunodiffusion to separate and allow identification of complex proteins.

immunogens (im'u-no-jəns), *n.pl* agents that may be used to trigger the body's immune response, such as vaccines; antigens.

immunoglobulins (Ig) (im'yōōnō-glob'yōōlinz), *n.pl* serum proteins (g globulins) synthesized by plasma cells that act as antibodies and are important in the body's defense mechanisms against infection. Main classes are designated as IgG, IgA, and IgM.

immunohistochemistry, *n* the demonstration of specific antigens in tissues by the use of markers that are either fluorescent dyes or enzymes, especially horseradish peroxidase. See also peroxidase, horseradish.

immunology, *n* the study of the reaction of tissues of the immune system of the body to antigenic stimulation.

immunosuppressants, *n.pl* agents that lower or reduce immune response; useful in organ transplant surgery to prevent organ rejection. Corticosteroid hormones given in large amounts; cytotoxic drugs, including antimetabolites and alkylating agents; antilymphocytic serum; and irradiation may result in immunosuppression.

immunosuppression, *n* **1.** the administration of agents that significantly interfere with the ability of the immune system to respond to antigenic stimulation by inhibiting cellular and humoral immunity. Immunosuppression may be deliberate, such as in preparation for bone marrow or other transplantation to prevent rejection by the host of the donor tissue. **2.** an abnormal condition of the immune system characterized by markedly inhibited ability to respond to antigenic stimuli.

immunotherapy, *n* a special treatment of allergic responses that administers increasingly large doses of the offending allergens to gradually develop immunity.

impact strength, *n* See strength, impact.

impacted tooth, *n* See tooth, impacted.

impaction, *n* pressed closely together to be immovable.

impaction, food, n the impaction of food generally interproximally because of open contact areas, uneven marginal ridge height, or "plunger" cusps.

impaction, tooth, n a situation in which an uncrupted tooth is wedged against another tooth or teeth or otherwise located so that it cannot erupt normally.

impaired function, *n* See function, impaired.

impairment, *n* See function, impaired.

impeachment of witness, *n* the questioning of the veracity of a witness by means of evidence obtained for that purpose.

impetigo (im'pəti'gō), *n* an inflammatory disease of the skin; characterized by pustules.

Impetigo. (Zitelli/Davis, 2002. Courtesy of Michael Sherlock, MD, Lutherville, MD)

impingement, *n* the striking or application of excessive pressure to a tissue by food or a prosthesis.

implant, *n* a device, usually alloplastic, that is surgically inserted into or onto the jawbone. To be used as a prosthodontic abutment, it should remain quiescent and purely incidental to local tissue physiology.

implant, abutment of, *n* the portion of an implant that protrudes through the gingival tissues and is designed to support a prosthodontic appliance.

implant, anchor endosteal, *n* an implant with a narrow buccolingual wedge-shaped infrastructure that is designed to be placed deep into the bone. The outline of the implant appears similar to a nautical anchor, and there is a variety of sizes and shapes to satisfy many anatomic and prosthodontic needs. Endosteal anchor implants are cast of chromium-cobalt surgical alloy and annealed.

implant, anterior subperiosteal, *n* an implant placed in the anterior part of an edentulous mandible and designed to supply abutments in the two canine regions.

implant, arms of anchor endosteal, *n* the major portion of the implant infrastructure.

implant, arthroplastic, *n* a cast chrome-alloy glenoid fossa prosthesis available in right and left models.

implant, blade endosteal, *n* an implant with a narrow (buccolingually) wedge-shaped infrastructure bearing openings or vents through which tissue grows to obtain retention.

implant, bone, *n* See graft, autogenous, bone; graft, iliac; graft,

implant, ceramic endosteal, *n* an endosteal implant of a variety of designs constructed of silicate or porcelain.

implant, cervix of, *n* that portion of an implant that connects the infrastructure with the abutment as it passes through the mucoperiosteum.

implant, CM (crête manche) spiral end-osteal, *n* a narrow-diameter screw implant designed for thin ridges.

implant, complete subperiosteal, *n* an implant used for an entire edentulous jaw.

implant, complete-arch blade endosteal, *n* a blade type of implant designed to be inserted into a completely edentulous ridge as a single appliance bearing multiple abutments.

implant, crown of anchor endosteal, *n* the abutment part of an anchor implant.

implant, endodontic endosteal, *n* an implant with a threaded or non-threaded pin that fits into a root canal and extends beyond the dental apex into the adjacent bone, thereby lengthening the clinical root.

implant, endosseous, *n* See implant, endosteal.

implant, endosteal, *n* an implant that is placed into the alveolar and/or basal bone and that protrudes through the mucoperiosteum.

implant, fabricated, *n* a custom-designed implant constructed for a specific operative site.

implant, fixation screw of subperiosteal, *n* screws, 5 to 7 mm long, that are made of the same surgical alloy as the implant and are used to affix the implant to the underlying bone.

implant, flukes of anchor endosteal, *n* the end portions of the arms that rise to the most superficial portion within the bone.

implant, frame type of ramus endosteal, *n* a prefabricated mandibular full-arch implant consisting of two posterior ramus implants: an anterior (symphyseal) endosteal component and a conjunction bar.

implant, helicoid endosteal, *n* a two-piece end-osteal implant consisting of a helical steel spring that is inserted into bone as a female and a male that may be placed postoperatively and serves as the abutment.

implant, infrastructure of, *n* the part of an implant that is designed to give it retention.

implant, intraperiosteal, *n* an artificial appliance made to conform to the shape of a bone and placed beneath the outer, or fibrous, layer of the periosteum.

implant, mandrel of needle endosteal, *n* a hollow device available in full, half, and shallow depths into which needle implants fit. The mandrel, in turn, is used in the contraangle to drive the needle implant into place.

implant, mesostructure, n an intermediate superstructure. A series of splinted copings, each of which fits over an implant abutment or natural tooth and over which fits the completed prosthodontic appliance.

implant, needle endosteal, n (pin endosteal) a smooth, thin shaft (self-perforating) that serves as an implant usually in conjunction with two others, the three being placed in bone in tripodal conformity.

implant, oral, n See implant.

implant, polymer tooth replica, n an acrylic resin implant, shaped like the tooth recently extracted, that is placed into the tooth's alveolus.

implant, ramus endosteal, n a blade type of implant designed for the anterior part of the ramus. See also implant, endosteal, blade.

implant, seating instrument of anchor endosteal, arm type, n a bayonet-shaped device designed to assist in seating an anchor implant by straddling its arms over a specially designed *seating notch.*

implant, seating instrument of anchor endosteal, crown type, n a bayonet-shaped, double-ended device designed to assist in seating an anchor implant by cupping its crown or abutment.

implant, seating instrument of endosteal, n a device designed to be placed on a portion of an implant so that malleting on it will seat the implant into the bone. It usually has an angled or bayoneted shaft to enable it to protrude from the mouth in a more-or-less vertical direction.

implant, shaft of anchor endosteal, n the cervix of an anchor implant.

implant, shoulder of blade endosteal, n that unbroken surface of the wedge-shaped infrastructure that is widest and most superficial. This part is tapped during the seating of the implant.

implant, single-tooth subperiosteal, n an implant designed to replace a single missing tooth; usually unsupported by adjacent natural teeth.

implant, spiral endosteal, n a screw type of implant, either hollow or solid, usually consisting of abutment, cervix, and infrastructure.

implant, stock, n an implant, usually endosteal, that is available in manu-

factured form in uniform sizes and shapes.

implant, strut of subperiosteal, n a thin, striplike component of an infrastructure.

implant, subperiosteal, n an appliance consisting of an open-mesh frame designed to fit over the surface of the bone beneath the periosteum.

implant, superstructure of, n a completed prosthesis that is supported entirely or in part by an implant. It may be a removable or fixed prosthesis but may be a single crown or a complete arch splint.

implant, two-piece, n an implant, either end-osteal or subperiosteal, having its infrastructure and abutment in separate parts. Generally, the abutment, which is threaded, is screwed to the infrastructure some weeks after its incision, so that healing has taken place.

implantology, oral (im'plantol'əjē), n the art and science of dentistry concerned with the surgical insertion of materials and devices into, onto, and about the jaws and oral cavity for purposes of oral maxillofacial or oral occlusal rehabilitation or cosmetic correction.

implied, *adj* inferred; conceded.

Impression, n an imprint or negative likeness of an object from which a positive reproduction may be made.

impression, anatomic, n an impression that records tissue shape without distortion.

impression, area, n See area, impression.

impression, boxing of an, n See boxing.

impression, bridge, n an impression made for the purpose of constructing or assembling a fixed restoration, fixed partial denture, or bridge.

impression, cleft palate, n an impression of the upper jaw of a patient with a cleft (incomplete closure, or union) in the palate.

impression, closed mouth, n an impression made while the mouth is closed and with the patient's muscular activity molding the borders.

impression, complete denture, n an impression (negative record) of an edentulous arch made for the purpose of constructing a complete denture.

impression, composite, n an impression consisting of two or more parts.

impression, correctable, n an impression with a surface that is capable of alteration by the removal from or addition to some area of its surface or border.

impression, dual, n See technique, impression, dual.

impression, duplicating, n See duplication.

impression, elastic, n an impression made in a material that will permit registration of undercut areas by springing over projecting areas and then returning to its original position.

impression, final (secondary impression), n an impression used for making the master cast.

impression, fluid wax, n an impression of the functional form of subjacent structures made with selected waxes that are applied (brushed on) to the impression surface in fluid form.

impression, functional, n an impression of the supporting structures in their functional form. See also structure, supporting, functional form of.

impression, hydrocolloid, n an impression made of a hydrocolloid material.

impression, lower, n See impression, mandibular.

impression, mandibular (lower impression), n an impression of the mandibular jaw and related tissues and dental structures.

impression, material, n See material, impression.

impression, maxillary (upper impression), n an impression of the maxillary jaw and related tissues and dental structures.

impression, mercaptan, n an impression made of mercaptan (polysulfide), a rubber-base elastic material.

impression, partial denture, n an impression of part or all of a partially edentulous arch made for the purpose of designing or constructing a partial denture.

impression, pickup, n an impression made with the superstructure frame in place on the abutments in the mouth after the implant has been surgically inserted and the mouth has healed. The superstructure frame is included in the impression material, and an accurate impression of the oral mucosal tissue over the implant is obtained.

impression, preliminary, n (primary impression) an impression made for the purpose of diagnosis or the construction of a tray for making a final impression.

impression, primary, n See impression, preliminary.

impression, secondary, n See impression, final.

impression, sectional, n an impression that is made in sections.

impression, silicone, n a rubber-base elastic impression using a material that contains a silicone. See also silicone.

impression, snap, n See impression, preliminary.

impression, surface, n See denture foundation area and surface, basal.

impression, surgical bone, n a negative likeness of the exposed bony surfaces necessary to support the implant substructure.

impression technique, n See technique, impression.

impression tray, n See tray, impression.

impression, upper, n See impression, maxillary.

impulse, *n* a surge of electric current for a short time span; for example, in a 60-cycle AC current, there are 120 impulses per second. See also impression, maxillary.

impulse, muscle, n a wave of excitation along a muscle fiber initiated at the neuromuscular endplate; accompanied by chemical and electrical changes at the surface of the muscle fiber and by activation of the contractile elements of the muscle fiber; detectable electronically (electromyographically); and followed by a transient refractory period.

impulse, nerve, n a wave of excitation along a nerve fiber initiated by a stimulus; accompanied by chemical and electrical changes at the surface of the nerve fiber and followed by a transient refractory period during which further stimulation has no effect.

impulsive behavior, *n* action initiated without due consideration or thought as to the costs, results, or consequences.

IMZ implant system, *n* an endosseous implant system provisionally accepted by the ADA.

in chief principal; directly obtained, *n* evidence obtained from a witness on examination in court by the party producing the witness.

in pais (in pā′), *adj* a legal transaction that has been accomplished without legal proceedings.

in potestate parentis (in pōtestä′tā pərən′tis), *adj* under the authority of the parent.

in utero **(in yōōtərō),** *adj/adv* pertaining to or occurring before birth, i.e., during the gestation period.

in vitro **(in ve′tro),** *adj/adv* occurring in a laboratory.

in vivo **(in ve′vo),** *adj/adv* occurring withing a living organism; alive.

in-house, *adj* describes personal, mechanical, or electronic services that are located in the building where they are used instead of being located remotely.

inactivate, *v* to render inactive; to destroy the activity of.

inactivator, *n* a substance added to a culture medium to prevent the activity of an inoculant. Penicillinase is added to the culture medium to prevent the activity of penicillin that might be carried over from a root canal treatment.

inadequacy, velopharyngeal (vel′ōfərin′jē-əl), *n* a lack of functional closure of the velum to the postpharyngeal wall.

inadmissible, *adj* that which cannot be admitted into evidence in a legal proceeding under the established rules of law.

inbreeding, *n* the production of offspring by the mating of closely related individuals, organisms, or plants; self-fertilization is the most extreme form, which normally occurs in certain plants and lower animals. The practice provides a greater chance for recessive genes for both desirable and undesirable traits to become homozygous and to be expressed phenotypically.

incentive plan, *n* a plan whereby the insurer pays an increasing share of the claim cost provided the covered individual visits the dentist as stipulated during each incentive period (usually a year) and receives the prescribed treatment.

incentive program, *n* a dental benefits program that pays an increasing share of the treatment cost provided that the covered individual uses the benefits of the program during each incentive period (usually a year) and receives the treatment prescribed. For example, a 70% to 30% copayment program in the first year of coverage may become an 80% to 20% program in the second year if the subscriber visits the dentist in the first year as stipulated in the program. Most frequently, there is a corresponding percentage reduction in the program's copayment level if the covered individual fails to visit the dentist in a given year (but never below the initial copayment level).

incidence, *n* **1.** the number of times an event occurs. **2.** the number of new cases in a particular period of time. Incidence is often expressed as a ratio, in which the number of cases is the numerator and the population at risk is the denominator.

incipient (insip′ē-ent), *adj* beginning, initial, commencing.

incisal (insī′zəl), *adj* relating to the cutting edge of the anterior teeth, incisors, or canines.

incisal angle, *n* See angle, incisal.

incisal guidance angle, *n* See angle, incisal guidance.

incisal guide, *n* See guide, incisal.

incisal guide pin, *n* See pin, incisal guide.

incisal rest, *n* See rest, incisal.

incisal guidance, *n* See guidance, incisal.

incision (insizh′ən), *n* the act of cutting or biting.

incision and drainage, *n* See I and D.

incision of food, *n* the phase of the masticatory cycle, using the incisor teeth, that cuts or separates the bolus of food.

incision, preauricular, *n* the incision of the soft tissue anterior to the external ear that permits access to the temporomandibular joint.

incision, relieving, *n* a cut into the soft tissues adjacent to a wound to permit a tension-free closure.

incision, Risdon's, *n* the incision of the soft tissues in the area of the mandibular angle that permits access to the lateral surface of the mandibular ramus, subcondylar neck, and condylar area.

incisive foramen, *n* See foramen, incisive.

incisive papilla, *n* See papilla, incisive.

incisor(s) (insī´zur), *n* a cutting tooth, one of the four anterior teeth of either jaw.

incisor, central, *n* the first incisor.

incisor, Hutchinson's, *n* malformed teeth caused by the presence of congenital syphilis during tooth development. The incisors usually are shorter than normal, show a single permanent notch on each incisal edge, and are screwdriver-shaped.

incisor, lateral, *n* the second incisor.

incisor point, *n* See point, incisor.

inclination (in´klinā´shən), *n* the angle of slope from a particular item of reference.

inclination, axial, *n* the alignment of a tooth in a vertical plane in relationship to its basal bone structure.

inclination, lateral condylar, *n* the direction of the lateral condyle path.

inclination of tooth, *n* See tooth, inclination of.

inclusion cyst, *n* an epidermal cyst formed of a mass of squamous epithelium cells with concentric layers of keratin.

income, *n* the return in money from one's business, practice, or capital invested; gains, profit.

income tax, *n* a tax upon an adjusted gross income (individual or corporate) imposed as a major source of governmental revenue at the state and federal levels.

incompatibility (in´kəmpat´ibil´itē), *n* a disharmonious relationship among the ingredients of prescriptions or other drug mixtures.

incompatibility, chemical, *n* a situation in which two or more of the ingredients of a drug interact chemically, with resulting deterioration of the mixture.

incontinentia pigmenti, *n* See syndrome, Bloch-Sulzberger.

incubation (in´´ku-ba´shən), *n* the maintenance of an ideal environment with regard to temperature, light, air, and humidity in order to foster development of an organism or culture.

incubation period, *n* the lapsed time between exposure to an infectious agent and the onset of symptoms of a disease.

incubator (in´kyōōbātur), *n* a laboratory container with controlled temperature for the cultivation of bacteria.

incurred claims, *n.pl* outstanding obligations of the insurer for dental services rendered to the insured.

indapamide, *n* *trade name:* Lozol; *drug class:* diuretic, thiazide-like; *action:* acts on distal tubule by increasing excretion of water, sodium, chloride, potassium; *uses:* edema, hypertension.

indemnification schedule, *n* See table of allowances.

indemnity benefit, *n* a contract benefit that is paid to the insured to meet the cost of dental services received.

indemnity plan, *n* **1.** a plan that provides payment to the insured for the cost of dental care but makes no arrangement for providing care itself. **2.** a dental plan in which a third-party-payer provides payment of an amount for specific services regardless of the actual charges made by the provider. Payment may be made to enrollees or by assignment directly to dentists. Schedule of allowances, table of allowances, and reasonable and customary plans are examples of indemnity plans.

index, *n* **1.** the ratio of a measurable value to another. **2.** a core or mold used to record or maintain the relative position of a tooth or teeth to one another or to a cast. See also splint.

index, Broders's (Broders's classification), *n.pr* **1.** a system of grading of epidermoid carcinoma suggested by Broders. Tumors are graded from I to IV on the basis of cell differentiation. Grade I tumors are highly differentiated, with much keratin production; Grade IV tumors are poorly differentiated; the cells are highly anaplastic, with almost no keratin formation. *n* **2.** the classification and grading of malignant neoplasms according to the proportion of malignant cells to normal cells in the lesion.

index, cardiac, *n* the minute volume of blood per square meter of body surface.

index, carpal, *n* the degree of ossification of the carpal bones noted in radiographs of the wrist; a method of determining the state of skeletal maturation.

index, cephalic, n head shape and size.

index, DEF (decayed, extracted, filled), n.pr a dental caries index applied to the primary dentition in somewhat the same manner as the DMF index is used for classifying permanent teeth. Missing primary teeth are ignored in this index because of the uncertainty in determining whether they were extracted because of advanced caries or exfoliated normally.

index, DMF (decayed, missing, filled), n.pr a technique for managing statistically the number of decayed, missing, or filled teeth in the mouth. Analysis may be based on the average number of DMF teeth (sometimes called DMFT) per person or the average number of DMF tooth surfaces (DMFS).

index, gingiva and bone count (Dunning-Leach index), n an index that permits differential recording of both gingival and bone conditions to determine gingivitis and bone loss.

index, gingival (GI), n an assessment tool used to evaluate a case of gingivitis based on visual inspection of the gingivae that takes into consideration the color and firmness of gingival tissue along with the presence of blood during probing.

index, gingival bleeding (GBI), n an assessment tool used to verify the presence of gingival inflammation based on any bleeding that occurs at the gingival margin during or immediately after flossing.

index, gnathic, n the relationship of jaw size to head size.

index, icterus, n See test, Meulengracht's.

index, malocclusion, n a measure of the severity of a malocclusion, obtained by assigning values to a series of defined observations.

index, measuring, n an expression of relationship of one measurable value to another, or a formula based on measurable values.

index, missing teeth, n See index, DMF.

index, oral hygiene, simplified (Greene-Vermillion index), n an index made up of two components, the debris index and the calculus index, which are based on numerical determination representing the amount of debris or calculus found on six preselected tooth surfaces.

index, periodontal (Ramfjord index), n a thorough clinical examination of the periodontal status of six teeth, with an evaluation of the gingival condition, pocket depth, calculus and plaque deposits, attrition, mobility, and lack of contact.

index, periodontal disease (Russell index), n an index that measures the condition of both the gingiva and the bone individually for each tooth and arrives at the average status for periodontal disease in a given mouth.

index, plaque, n an assessment tool used to evaluate the thickness of plaque at the gingival margin that may be applied to selected teeth or to the entire mouth.

index, PMA (Schour-Massler index), n an index used for recording the prevalence and severity of gingivitis in schoolchildren by noting and scoring three areas: the gingival papillae (P), the buccal or labial gingival margin (M), and the attached gingiva (A).

index, Pont's, n the relation of the width of the four incisors to the width between the first premolars and the width between the first molars.

index, Russell, n.pr See index, periodontal disease.

index, salivary **Lactobacillus,** *n* a count of the lactobacilli per milliliter of saliva; used as an indicator of present dental caries activity. The test is of questionable value in individual patients, although its use in large groups has led to valuable information on caries activity.

index, saturation, n a number indicating the hemoglobin content of a person's red blood cells as compared with the normal content.

index, sulcus bleeding, n.pr an assessment tool used to evaluate the existence of gingival bleeding in individual teeth and/or regions of the mouth upon gentle probing by assigning a score of 0–5, with 0 indicating a healthy appearance and no bleeding.

index, therapeutic, n the ratio of toxic dose to effective dose.

index, ventilation, *n* the index obtained by dividing the ventilation test by the vital capacity.

indication, *n* that which serves as a guide or warning.

indicator, *n* a mark or symptom specific to a condition or disease.

indicator, biologic, *n* a small quantity of harmless bacteria placed into an object prior to sterilization, the subsequent death of which indicates that sterilization has taken place.

indicator chemical, *n* a temperature-sensitive mark that changes color when a specific temperature has been reached. Used in the heat sterilization process but is by itself not proof that an object has been sterilized.

indicator diseases, *n* opportunistic infectious diseases or neoplastic diseases that are associated with primary immunodeficiency disease, such as caused by the retrovirus HIV-1.

indirect method, *n* See method, indirect restorative.

indirect pulp capping, *n* See capping, pulp, indirect.

indirect retention, *n* See retention, indirect.

indirect vision, *n* See vision, indirect.

indium, *n* a silvery metallic element with some nonmetallic chemical properties. Its atomic number is 49, and its atomic weight is 114.82. It is used in electronic semiconductors.

individual practice association (IPA), *n* **1.** organization for the maintenance of the solo private practitioner as a lobbying force and springboard. **2.** legal entity organized and operated on behalf of individual participating dentists for the primary purpose of collectively entering into contracts to provide dental services to enrolled populations. Dentists may practice in their own offices and may provide care to patients not covered by the contract as well as to IPA patients.

individual retirement account (IRA), *n* a savings certificate exempt from income tax until the time of withdrawal. There are limits to the amount that can be saved annually under this plan, and there are conditions of withdrawal for maximal interest and tax advantage.

individuality, *n* the aggregate of char-

acteristics or traits that distinguish one person or thing from all others.

indomethacin/indomethacin sodium trihydrate, *n trade names:* Indocin, Indocin SR, Indameth; *drug class:* nonsteroidal antiinflammatory; *action:* inhibits prostaglandin synthesis by interfering with cyclooxygenase needed for biosynthesis; possesses analgesic, antiinflamatory, antipyretic properties; *uses:* rheumatoid arthritis, osteoarthritis, ankylosing rheumatoid spondylitis, acute gouty arthritis.

induced, *adj* artificially caused to occur.

induction, *n* the act or process of inducing or causing to occur.

inductive reasoning, *n* analyzing a problem by working from specific facts and discovering general principles. See also deductive reasoning.

indurated, *adj* hardened.

indurated tissue, *n* soft tissue that is abnormally firm because of an influx of exudate or fibrous tissue elements.

industrial dentistry, *n* **1.** dentistry that is concerned with the dental health of the worker as it affects the working environment. **2.** dental service provided in the plant, usually restricted to emergency care.

inert, *adj* inactive; without the ability to act, move, change, or resist.

inertia (inur′shə), *n* according to Newton's law of inertia, the tendency of a body that is at rest to remain at rest and a body that is in motion to continue in motion with constant speed in the same straight line unless acted on by an outside force.

infant, *n/adj* a child who is in the earliest stage of extrauterine life, a time extending from the first month after birth to approximately 12 months of age, when the baby is able to assume an erect posture; some extend the period to 24 months of age.

infant mortality, *n* the statistical rate of infant death during the first year after live birth, expressed as the number of such births per 1,000 live births in a specific geographic area. Neonatal mortality accounts for 70% of infant mortality.

infantilism (infan′tilizəm), *n* a disturbance marked by mental retardation and retention of childhood characteristics into adult life. Teeth may be delayed in eruption or absent.

infarct (in'färkt), *n* the death of a tissue caused by partial occlusion of a vessel or vessels supplying the area.

infection (infek'shen), *n* an invasion of the tissues of the body by disease-producing microorganisms and the reaction of these tissues to the microorganisms and/or their toxins. The mere presence of microorganisms without reaction is not evidence of infection.

infection, adenovirus, n a proliferation of the adenovirus that may cause any number of illnesses, including "swimming pool conjunctivitis," gastrointestinal or respiratory diseases, among others; it is possible to be infected without manifesting any symptoms.

infection, airborne, n infection contracted by inhalation of microorganisms contained in air or water particles.

infection control, n procedures and protocols designed to prevent or limit cross-contamination in the health care delivery environment.

   infection control, blood bank and blood transfusion, n.pl the precautions taken to ensure that bloodborne pathogens are not transmitted via donated blood; includes rejection of potential donors whose medical history shows evidence of viral hepatitis, drug addiction or recent blood transfusions or tattoos, as well as laboratory testing of all donated blood for the presence of hepatitis B and C, syphilis, and the HIV-1 antibody.

   infection control, surveillance, n the monitoring of the transmission of a disease in order to limit its occurrence.

infection, focal, n the process in which microorganisms located at a certain site, or focus, in the body are disseminated throughout the body to set up secondary sites, or foci, of infection in other tissues.

infection, hemolytic streptococcal, n **1.** an infection usually caused by Group A hemolytic streptococci. Such infections include scarlet fever, streptococcal sore throat, cellulitis, and osteomyelitis. **2.** an infection caused by streptococci that produce a toxic substance (hemolysin) that will lyse the erythrocytes and liberate hemoglobin from red blood cells.

infection, inflammatory, n an influx or accumulation of inflammatory elements (cellular and exudative) in the interstices of the tissues as a result of tissue injury by physical, chemical, microbiologic, and other irritants. Cellular elements include lymphocytes, plasma cells, polymorphonuclear leukocytes, and the macrophages of reticuloendothelial origin.

infection, latent, n a lingering infection that may lie dormant in the body for a period of time but may become active under certain conditions.

infection, local, n the prevention of excitation of the free nerve endings by literally flooding the immediate area with a local anesthetic solution.

infection, marginal, n an inflammation of the free and attached edges of tissue along the gum line of a single tooth or several teeth.

infection, nosocomial, n any infection that first occurs during a patient's stay at a health-care facility, regardless of whether it is detected during the stay or after.

infection, opportunistic, n an illness or condition that occurs when pathogens are able to exploit a vulnerable host. An infection that is able to take hold because resistance is low.

infection, papillary, n an inflammation of the gum tissue between two teeth, but not the surrounding area. It may be confined to a single interdental area or encompass the entire mouth.

infection, primary, n the original outbreak of an illness against which the body has had no opportunity to build antibodies; the originating infection.

infection, recurrent, n a reoccurrence of the same illness from which an individual has previously recovered.

infection, Vincent's, n.pr See gingivitis, necrotizing ulcerative.

infection, waterborne, n illness that occurs as the result of drinking contaminated water or of eating fish that has been taken from contaminated waters.

infection resistance, *n* the ability of an individual to fight off the detrimental effects of microorganisms and their toxic products. A complexity involving individual and interacting factors—for example, antibody formation, adequate nutrition, tissue tone, circulation, and emotional stability.

infection susceptibility, *n* the degree of capability of being influenced by or involved in the pathologic processes produced by microorganisms and/or their toxins.

infectious, *adj* contagious; communicable; capable of causing infection.

infectious mononucleosis, *n* a benign lymphadenosis caused by the Epstein-Barr virus and characterized by fever, sore throat, enlargement of lymph nodes and spleen, and prolonged weakness with a characteristic shift in the white blood cells during the course of the disease.

inferior alveolar nerve, *n* See nerve, inferior alveolar.

infertile, *adj* unable to produce offspring.

infiltrate (infil´trāt), *n* **1.** material deposited by infiltration. *v* **2.** to deposit material in a location.

infiltration (in´filtrā´shən), *n* an accumulation in a tissue of a substance not normal to it.

inflammation (in´fləmā´shən), *n* the cellular and vascular response or reaction to injury. Inflammation is characterized by pain, redness, swelling, heat, and disturbance of function. It may be acute or chronic. The term is not synonymous with *infection,* which implies an inflammatory reaction initiated by invasion of living organisms.

inflammation, gingival, n See gingivitis.

inflammation, granulomatous, n a chronic inflammation in which there is formation of granulation tissue.

inflammation, periodontal, n See periodontitis.

inflation (inflā´shən), *n* the act of distending with air or a gas.

influences, local environmental, *n.pl* factors or agents within the oral cavity that are responsible for the initiation, perpetuation, or modification of a pathologic state within the stomatognathic system.

influences, systemic environmental, *n.pl* systemic factors that may initiate, perpetuate, or modify disease processes within the stomatognathic system. Generally, the oral manifestations of systemic disease are modified by the influence of local environmental factors.

influenza, *n* a highly contagious infection of the respiratory tract caused by a myxovirus and transmitted by airborne droplet infection. Symptoms include sore throat, cough, fever, muscular pains, and weakness. Fever and constitutional symptoms distinguish influenza from the common cold. Three main strains of influenza virus have been recognized: Type A, Type B, and Type C. New strains of the virus emerge at regular intervals and are named according to geographic origin. Asian flu is a Type A influenza.

influenza-virus vaccine, n an active immunizing agent prescribed for immunization against influenza, generally recommended for at-risk populations, such as the elderly.

information, *n* a meaningful collection of data as perceived by its user.

information retrieval, n the methods and procedures for recovering specific information from stored data.

information system, n a computerized system with the capability of manipulating and processing data in different ways to facilitate their interpretation and use.

informed consent, *n* an agreement by a patient, verbal or written, after being told in sufficient detail of possible risks, to have a procedure performed.

infrabony pocket (in´frəbōnē) See pocket, infrabony.

infrabulge (in´frəbulj), *n* the surface of the crown of a tooth cervical to the clasp guide line, survey line, or surveyed height of contour.

infraclusion (in´frəklōō´zhən), *n* (infraversion) the position occupied by a tooth when it has failed to erupt sufficiently to reach the occlusal plane.

infradentale (in´frədental´ē), *n* the most anterior point of the alveolar process of the mandible.

infrahyoid muscles (in´frəhī´-oid), *n.pl* See muscle, suprahyoid and infrahyoid.

infraversion (in´frəvur´zhən), *n* See infraclusion.

infusion, *n* **1.** the therapeutic introduction of a fluid, such as saline solution, into a vein. In contrast to injection, infusion suggests the introduction of a larger volume of a less concentrated solution over a more protracted period. **2.** a term used in pharmacy for a liquid extract prepared by steeping a plant substance in water.

ingate, *n* See sprue.

inhalant (inhā′lənt), *n* a medicine to be inhaled.

inhalation (inhəlā′shən), *n* the drawing of air or other gases into the lungs.

inhalation, endotracheal, *n* the inhalation of an anesthetic mixture into the lungs through an endotracheal catheter at low or atmospheric pressure.

inhaler, nasal, *n* a device that is placed over the nose to permit inhalation of anesthetic agents.

inhibition (in′hibish′ən), *n* a neurologic phenomenon associated with the transmission of an impulse across a synapse. An impulse can be blocked from passing a synapse in a reflex situation by the firing of another, more dominant nerve. Inhibition can be achieved directly by preventing the passage of an impulse along an axon, or it can be achieved by liberation of a chemical substance at the nerve ending. This chemical inhibition is demonstrated by the sympathetic-parasympathetic control over smooth muscle activity in a blood vessel. Inhibition is the restraining of a function of a tissue or organ by some nervous or hormone control. It is the opposite of *excitation.*

inhibitor, *n* a substance that slows or stops a chemical reaction.

inhibitor of cholinesterase (inhib′itur əv kō′lines′terās), *n* a chemical that interferes with the activity of the enzyme cholinesterase.

inhibitor, proton pump, *n* pharmacologic agent used to control heartburn by suppressing the production of stomach acid by blocking the action of the proton pump.

inion (in′ē-on), *n* the most elevated point on the external occipital protuberance in the midsagittal plane.

initialize, *v* to set counters, switches, and addresses to 0 or other starting values at the beginning of, or at prescribed points in, a computer routine.

initiation stage, *n* the primary stage in the development of a tooth.

initiator (inish′ē-ātur) *n* a chemical agent added to a resin to initiate polymerization.

injection (Injek′shən), *n* the act of introducing a liquid into the body by means of a needle and syringe. Injections are designated according to the anatomic site involved. The most common injections are intraarterial, intradermal, intramuscular, intravenous, and subcutaneous.

Injection into skin. (Chester, 1998)

injection, anterior middle superior alveolar (AMSA), n See nerve block, anterior middle superior alveolar.

injection, anterior superior alveolar (ASA), n See nerve block, anterior superior alveolar.

injection, Gow-Gates (GG), n See technique, Gow-Gates (GG) anesthetic.

injection, greater palatine (GP) anesthetic, n See nerve block, greater palatine.

injection molding, n See molding, injection.

injury, *n* the insult, harm, or hurt applied to tissues; may evoke dystrophic or inflammatory response from the affected part.

injury, root, n damage to the root, especially to the cementum, when an excessive force is placed on the tooth.

injury, toothbrush, n an insult or damage to the teeth and their investing structures produced by faulty toothbrushing.

inlay, *n* **1.** a restoration of metal, fired porcelain, or plastic made to fit a tapered cavity preparation and fastened to or luted into it with a cementing medium. *v* **2.** to perform such a procedure.

inlay furnace, n See furnace, inlay.

inlay, setting, n the procedure of fitting a casting to a preparation; adjusting the occlusal function and contact areas; securing the proper, clean dry field; cementing the cleaned, polished casting in an aseptic, dry prepared cavity; and completing the final finishing and polishing of the restoration.

inlay wax, n See wax, inlay.

innervation (in′urvā′shən), *n* the distribution or supply of nerves to a part.

innervation, reciprocal, n the simultaneous excitation of one muscle with the inhibition of its antagonist. Rhythmic chewing is achieved efficiently when the masticatory muscles are reciprocally innervated, permitting alternate elevation and depression of the mandible in a smooth, coordinated sequence of actions.

inoculation (ĭ-nok″u-la′shən), *n* a procedure in which a disease-causing substance is introduced into other-

wise healthy tissue for the sole purpose of inducing immunity.

inorganic, *adj* having no derivation from living organisms; chemical compounds that generally do not contain carbon.

inositol, *n* an essential growth factor in tissue culture with no known human requirement. It has been used therapeutically in the management of diseases associated with the metabolism of fat.

input, computer, *n* the data to be processed.

input/output control (I/O control), *n* the portion of the central processor of some computer systems that contains software/firmware for supervising data flow between memory and the input/output devices connected to the CPU.

inquiry, *n* a request for information from storage in a computer.

insert, intramucosal (in′trəmyōōkō′səl), *n* (mucosal insert, implant button), a nonreactive metal appliance that is affixed to the tissue-bone surface of a denture and offers added retentive qualities to the denture. An intramucosal insert consists of a base, cervix, and head.

insert, mucosal, *n* See insert, intramucosal.

insertion (insur′shən), *n* the act of implanting, placing, or introducing the needle into the tissues.

insertion, path of, n the direction in which a prosthesis is inserted and removed.

insidious (insid′ē-us), *adj* coming on in a stealthy manner, in reference to the onset of a disease state.

insoluble, *adj* not susceptible to being dissolved.

insomnia, *n* the chronic inability to sleep or remain asleep throughout the night.

inspection, *n* the visual examination of the body or portions thereof, which is an integral phase of the physical or dental examination procedure.

inspiration (in″spĭ-ra′shən), *n* the act of drawing air into the lungs.

inspirometer (in′spirom′ətur), *n* an instrument for measuring the force, frequency, or volume of inspirations.

institutionalize, *v* to place a person in a health care or custodial facility for psychologic or physical treatment or for the protection of the person or society.

instruction, *n* a set of characters, together with one or more addresses, that defines a computer operation and, as a unit, causes the computer to operate accordingly on the indicated quantities; a term associated with software operation.

instruction of partial denture patient, *n* See denture, partial, instruction of patient.

instrument(s), *n* a tool or implement, especially one used for delicate or scientific work. See under the specific type of instrument (e.g., knife). See also instrumenting, instrumentarium.

instrument, air application, *n* any tool used to apply air in order to dry teeth, remove debris, and control saliva during treatment or in preparation for a specific procedure.

instrument, bibeveled cutting **(bī'bevəld),** *n* an instrument in which both sides of the end of the blade are beveled to form the cutting edge, as in a hatchet.

instrument blade, *n* the part bearing a cutting edge; it begins at the terminal angle of the shank and ends at the cutting edge.

instrument, blade face, *n* the innermost surface of a scaler or curet blade.

The face blade of a curet. (Daniel/Harfst, 2002)

instrument, carving, *n* See carver.

instrument, classification of, names, *n* the classification of instruments by name to denote purpose (for example, excavator), to denote position or manner of use (for example, hand condenser), to describe the form of the point (for example, hatchet), or to describe the angle of the blade in relation to the handle.

instrument, cutting, *n* an instrument used to cut, cleave, or plane the walls of a cavity preparation; the blade ends in a sharp, beveled edge. Unless otherwise specified, it refers to a hand instrument rather than to a rotary type.

instrument, diamond, *n* a rotary abrasive instrument, wheel, or mounted point. Made of fine diamond chips bonded into a desired form; used to reduce tooth structure.

instrument, double-ended, *n* a hand-held tool with two functional ends that are identical or complementary

instrument, double-plane, *n* an instrument with the curve of the blade in a plane perpendicular to that of the angles of the shank.

instrument, formula name of, *n* a method of naming and describing dental hand instruments. Measurements are in the metric system. The working point is described first; then the formula is given, in three (or sometimes four) units. The first figure denotes the width of the blade, in tenths of millimeters; the second shows the length of the blade, in millimeters; and the third indicates the angle of the blade in relation to the shaft, in centigrades or hundredths of a circle. Whenever it is necessary to describe the angle of the cutting edge of a blade with its shaft, the number is entered in brackets as the second number of the formula. Paired instruments are also designated as right or left. In lateral cutting instruments the one used to cut from right to left is termed *right;* in direct cutting instruments with right and left bevels, the one having the bevel on the right side of the blade as it is held with the cutting edge down and pointing away from the observer is termed *right.*

instrument grasp, *n* See grasp, instrument.

instrument, hand, *n* an instrument used principally with hand force.

instrument, holding, *n* an instrument used to support gold foil while a foil restoration is inserted.

instrument, McCall's, *n.pr* periodontal instruments designed by John Oppie McCall; used for gingival curettage and for removing accretions from the tooth surfaces.

instrument nib, *n* the counterpart of the blade in the condensing instrument; the end of the nib is the face.

Parts of an instrument. (Bird/Robinson, 2002)

instrument, parts, *n.pl* handle or shaft, blade or nib, and shank.

instrument, plastic, *n* an instrument used to manipulate a plastic restorative material.

instrument, rotary cutting, *n* a power-activated instrument used in a dental handpiece, such as a bur, mounted diamond point, mounted carborundum point, wheel stone, or disk.

instrument, screwdriver, *n* an instrument made of surgical alloy; it may have at its tip a screw holder that is designed to drive screws into the bone.

instrument shaft/handle, *n* the part that is grasped by the operator's hand while using the instrument.

instrument shank, *n* the part that connects the shaft and the blade or nib.

instrument sharpening, *n* See sharpening, instrument.

instrument, single-beveled cutting, *n* an instrument in which one side of the end of the blade is beveled to form the cutting edge, as in a wood chisel.

instrument, single-plane, *n* an instrument with all its angles and curves in one plane; when the instrument lies on a flat surface, the cutting edge and the blade will parallel the surface.

instrument stop, *n* a device, usually metal, that can be placed on a reamer or file to mark the measurement of the root.

instrument, toe, *n* the tip or terminating end of the blade, may be rounded (blunt) or pointed (sharp).

instrumentarium, *n* the exact instruments required to perform a specific procedure.

instrumentation (in´strōōmentā´shən), *n* the use of, or work done by, instruments in the treatment of a patient.

instrumentation, endpoint of, *n* the ultimate goal of instrument use in the periodontal process, which is to prepare the teeth and surrounding structures for healing and to maintain optimal oral health.

instrumentation zone, *n* the section of a tooth requiring the use of an instrument to remove deposits and debris.

instrumenting, *n* clinical jargon for the use of hand-activated tools to remove debris, plaque, and overhangs from the teeth.

insufficiency, adrenocortical (ədrē´nōkôr´tikəl), *n* See hypoadrenocorticalism.

insufficiency, functional, *n* the inadequacy of usage of stimulation to a part of the body, often resulting in atrophic tissue changes.

insufflation (in´səflā´shən), *n* the act of blowing a powder, vapor, gas, or air into a cavity such as the lungs.

insufflation, endotracheal, *n* the forcing of an anesthetic mixture into the lungs through an endotracheal catheter under pressure.

insufflation, mouth-to-mouth, *n* the oldest recorded procedure for artificially ventilating the lungs. The lungs are inflated by blowing into the mouth, and expiration either is passive or is assisted by compressing the thorax. Adequate ventilation is produced, and the procedure should be used when other techniques are not applicable; for example, in thoracic injury. Auxiliary airway tubes are available for use when mouth-to-mouth insufflation is required. Such tubes maintain the airway and prevent the tongue from obstructing the glottis.

insufflator (in´sə-fla˝tər), *n* an instrument used in insufflation.

insulator, thermal (in´səflātur), *n* a material having a low thermal conductivity.

insulin (antidiabetic hormone), *n* a hormone produced by the β cells of the islets of Langerhans in the pancreas. It promotes a decrease in blood sugar. Its action may be influenced by the pituitary growth hormone, adrenocorticotropic hormone; hormones of the adrenal cortex; epinephrine; glucagon; and thyroid hormone.

insulin (obtained from beef or pork, or human recombinant technology), *n trade names:* Velosulin, Humulin R, Novolin R, Lente Insulin; *drug class:* exogenous insulin, antidiabetic; *action:* decreases blood glucose; important in regulation of fat and protein metabolism; *uses:* ketoacidosis; type 1, type 2 diabetes mellitus; hyperkalemia; hyperalimentation.

insulin, exogenous, n insulin that comes from a source external to a diabetic patient's body, taken to offset the patient's natural deficiency of insulin.

insulin, intermediate acting, n a type of insulin that is a medium between rapid-acting and long-acting insulins; the onset is not as fast as rapid acting insulin, but it reaches its peak action over a four-to-twelve-hour period.

insulin, Lente, n.pr one type of intermediate-acting insulin, reaches its peak action over a four-to-twelve-hour period.

insulin, Lispro, n.pr a rapid-acting insulin that reaches its peak action in thirty to ninety minutes.

insulin, long acting, n an insulin that has a slow onset but reaches its peak action from twelve to sixteen hours after administration.

insulin, NPH, n a synthetic type of insulin used to treat diabetes. Classified as intermediate acting; peak action occurs 4–10 hours after administering.

insulin, rapid acting, n a synthetic type of insulin used to treat diabetes. Reaches peak action 30–90 minutes after administering.

insulin, regular, n a synthetic type of insulin used to treat diabetes. Classified as short acting; peak action occurs 2–3 hours after administering.

insulin resistance, n a complication of diabetes mellitus characterized by a need for more than 200 units of insulin per day to control hyperglycemia and ketosis. The cause is associated with insulin binding by high levels of antibody.

insulin shock, n See shock, insulin.

insulin, short acting, n a synthetic type of insulin used to treat diabetes. Reaches peak action 2–3 hours after administering. Also called *regular insulin.*

insulin, ultralente, n a synthetic type of insulin used to treat diabetes. Classified as long acting, with peak action occurring 12–16 hours after administering.

insurance, *n* a contract, or policy, whereby, for a stipulated consideration, or premium, one party (the insurer or underwriter) promises to compensate the other (the insured or assured) for loss on a specified subject (insurable interest) by specified perils or risks.

insurance benefits, n the contractual pay-out agreed to by the carrier for the policy holder.

insurance carriers, n.pl organizations that for a contractual fee underwrite the payment of losses or costs incurred by the policy holder within the conditions of the policy.

insurance, group, n insurance covering a group of persons, usually employees of a single employer or members of a union local, under one contract for the benefit of the members of the group.

insurance, guaranteed renewable, n a policy that is renewable at the option of the insured until a stated time, such as the 70th birthday of the insured. See also noncancellable insurance.

insurance, health, n insurance that provides financial return when the dentist is unable to practice because of prolonged illness.

insurance, liability, n insurance protecting the dentist from financial loss resulting from liability suits.

insurance, life, n a protective contract providing for compensation to the beneficiaries of the insured.

insurance, malpractice, n in dentistry, insurance covering accidents or catastrophes that may occur during the performance of professional duties.

insurance, retirement, n life insurance that carries, as an additional benefit, payments to the insured when he or she reaches a specific age.

insured, *n* a person covered by an

insurance program. See also beneficiary.

insurer, *n* an organization that bears the financial risk for the cost of defined categories or services for a defined group of beneficiaries. See also third party.

intake, *n* the substance or quantities thereof taken in and used by the body.

integral endosseous implant system, *n* an endosseous implant system provisionally accepted by the ADA. See IMZ implant system.

intelligence, *n* mental potential or capacity; an individual's total repertoire of problem-solving and cognitive discrimination responses that are usual and expected at a given age level and in the large population unit; that which is measured by an intelligence test.

intelligence dental, quotient, *n* an estimated appraisal of a patient's knowledge and appreciation of dental services.

intelligence quotient (IQ), *n* an estimate of intelligence level; an index determined by dividing the mental age in months by the chronologic age in months and multiplying the result by 100. Thus, the IQ of a child of 100 months with a mental age of 110 months would be 110.

intensifying screen, *n* See screen, intensifying.

intensity of an x-ray beam, *n* the amount of energy in an x-ray beam per unit volume or area.

intensity, radiation, *n* the energy flowing through a unit area perpendicular to the beam per unit of time. It is expressed in ergs per square centimeter or in watts per square centimeter.

intensive care, *n* the constant, complex, detailed health care as provided in various acute life-threatening conditions, such as multiple trauma, severe burns, and myocardial infarction, and after certain kinds of surgery.

interaction, *n* according to Newton's law of interaction, the phenomenon in which every force is accompanied by an equal and opposite force. For every force there are two bodies—one to exert the force and one to receive it. Furthermore, whenever there is one force, another force must also be involved. If there is force to the right on one body, there is force to the left on another. Since the one force acts as long as the other, the impulses are equal. The total momentum of the two interacting bodies cannot change. Continuous interaction is demonstrated between the food that is masticated and the force applied to the food.

interalveolar space (in′təralvē′-ōlur), *n* See distance, interarch.

interarch distance, *n* See distance, interarch.

intercellular (in′tursel′yōōlur), *adj* taking place between or among cells.

interceptive orthodontics, *n* an extension of preventive orthodontics that may include minor local tooth movement in an otherwise normally developing dentition.

intercondylar distance (in′turkon′ dilur), *n* the distance between the vertical axes of a pair of condyles.

intercuspation (in′turkuspā′shən), *n* the cusp-to-fossa relationship of the upper and lower posterior teeth to each other.

Intercuspation. (Roberson/Heymann/Swift, 2002)

interdental (in′turden′təl), *adj* situated between the proximal surfaces of adjacent teeth.

interdental canal, *n* See canal, interdental.

interdental embrasure, *n* See embrasure, interdental.

interdental gingiva, *n* See gingiva, interdental.

interdental septum, *n* See septum, interdental.

interdental splint, *n* See splint, interdental.

interdental tip, *n* an oral hygiene tool that features a rubber tip shaped like a small cone or pyramid; used to remove plaque and other matter from between teeth. Also effective in and around the gingival area.

interdigitation (in'turdij'itā'shən), *n* See intercuspation.

interdisciplinary team, *n* a group that consists of specialists from several fields combining skills and resources to present guidance and information.

interface (in'turfās), *n* the surface, such as a plane surface, formed between the walls of a prepared cavity or extracoronal preparation and a restoration. It forms a common boundary between the tooth structure and the restorative material.

interface, computer, n a common boundary (connection) between automatic data processing systems or parts of a system.

interfacial surface tension, *n* See tension, interfacial surface.

interference, cuspal, *n* See contact, deflective occlusal.

interference, occlusal, *n* any tooth-to-tooth contact that interferes with jaw movement.

interferon, *n* a small class of glycoproteins capable of exerting antiviral activity in homologous cells through metabolic processes involving synthesis of RNA.

interferon alpha, n formed by leukocytes in response to viral infection or by stimulation with double-stranded RNA. These protein products are used as antineoplastic agents. Specifically used as an antineoplastic agent for the treatment of Kaposi's sarcoma in AIDS patients. See also interferon alfa-2a.

interferon alfa-2a/interferon alfa-2b/interferon alfa-n1/interferon alfa-n3, n trade names: Roferon-A, Intron-A, Alferon N; *drug class:* biologic response modifier; *action:* antiviral action inhibits viral replication by reprogramming virus; antitumor action suppresses cell proliferation; immunomodulating action phagacytizes target cells; *uses:* hairy-cell leukemia in persons older than 18 years, metastatic melanoma, AIDS, Kaposi's sarcoma, bladder carcinoma, lymphomas, malignant myeloma, mycosis fungoides.

interferon beta, n formed by fibroblasts by stimulation similar to the alpha form.

interferon gamma, n formed by lymphocytes in response to mitogenic stimulation. See also interferon gamma-1b.

interferon gamma-1b, n trade name: Actimmune; *drug class:* biologic response modifier; *action:* species-specific protein synthesized in response to viruses, enhances antibody-dependent cellular cytotoxicity, enhances natural killer cell activity; *uses:* serious infections associated with chronic granulomatous disease.

interim denture, *n* See denture, interim.

interim prosthesis, *n* See prosthesis, temporary.

interincisal angle, *n* the A-P angle made by the intersection of the long axis of the maxillary central incisor with the mandibular central incisor. Statistically, a normal angle is about 130 degrees. A more acute angle may indicate a proclined incisor, and a more obtuse angle may indicate a retracted incisor.

interleukin-1 (IL-1), *n* a protein with numerous immune system functions, including activation of resting T cells, and endothelial and macrophage cells, mediation of inflammation, and stimulation of synthesis of lymphokines, collagen, and collagenases. It can also induce fever, sleep, and nonspecific resistance to infection. A number of interleukin proteins with varying immune-response properties exist. They are identified by numbers of 1 through 8.

interleukin-2, *n* a hormone produced by T helper and suppressor lymphocytes that functions to control the expansion and reactivity of T lymphocytes. Used to boost the immune system in HIV-positive patients.

intermaxillary, *adj* between the maxillae and mandible.

intermaxillary anchorage, n See anchorage, intermaxillary.

intermaxillary elastic, n See elastic, maxillomandibular.

intermaxillary fixation, n See fixation, maxillomandibular.

intermaxillary relation, n See relation, maxillomandibular.

intermaxillary traction, n See traction, maxillomandibular.

intermedin (inturmē′d), n See hormone, melanocyte stimulating.

intern, n a dental or medical college graduate serving and residing for 12 months in a hospital, usually during the first year after receiving a D.D.S., D.M.D., or M.D. degree.

internal medicine, n the branch of medicine concerned with the study of the physiology and pathology of the internal organs and with the medical diagnosis and treatment of diseases and disorders of these organs.

International Classification of Diseases (ICD), n.pr diagnostic codes designed for the classification of morbidity and mortality information for statistical purposes, for the indexing of hospital records by disease and operations, and for data storage and retrieval.

interneurons, n.pl combinations or groups of neurons between sensory and motor neurons, which govern coordinated activity.

interocclusal (in′tərəklōō′səl), adj between the occlusal surfaces of the maxillary and mandibular teeth.

interocclusal clearance, n See clearance, interocclusal.

interocclusal contacts, n tooth contact between maxillary and mandibular teeth in closure.

interocclusal distance, n the distance between the maxillary and mandibular teeth when the mandible is in the rest position or other defined position of the mandible to maxillary. See also distance, interocclusal.

interocclusal gap, n See distance, interocclusal.

interocclusal record, n See record, interocclusal.

interocclusal rest space, n See distance, interocclusal.

interoceptors (inter′ōsepturz), n.pl those sensory nerve end receptors lining the mucous membrane of the respiratory and digestive tracts. They are similar to exteroceptors but differ from them essentially in their location in the viscera.

interphase, n the metabolic stage in the cell cycle during which the cell is not dividing.

interpolate (intur′pōlāt), v to insert intermediate terms in a series according to the trend of the series; to calculate intermediate values according to observed values.

interposition arthroplasty (är-th′rōplastē), n the surgical correction of ankylosis by the separating of the immobile fragment from the mobilized fragment and the interpositioning of a substance, such as fascia, cartilage, metal, or plastic, between them. See also ankylosis.

interpretation, n the translation of radiographic changes seen by the dentist into real variations in the object radiographed for diagnostic purposes.

interpretation, radiographic (radiologic interpretation, roentgenographic interpretation), n an opinion formed from the study of a radiograph.

interpretation, radiographic, external oblique ridge, n radiopaque line formed by an elevated bony surface on the mandible.

interpretation, radiographic, genial tubercles, n submandibular radiopaque structures that represent the attachment site for genohyoid and genioglossus muscles.

interpretation, radiographic, inferior border on mandible, n radiopaque area that represents the cortical bone.

interpretation, radiographic, internal oblique ridge, n radiopaque line that represents a bony ridge on the mandibular surface, the attachment site of the mylohyoid muscles.

interpretation, radiographic, lingual foramen, n small area of radiolucency located centrally in the genial tubercles.

interpretation, radiologic, n See interpretation, radiographic.

interproximal, adj between the proximal surfaces of adjoining teeth.

interradicular alveoloplasty (in′tur-rədik′yōōlur alvē′-ōlōplastē), n (intraseptal alveoloplasty), the removal of the interradicular bone and the collapsing of the cortical plates to a more normal alveolar contour. See also alveolectomy.

interradicular osseous defect, n radiographic evidence of a discontinuity in the bony image in the area between the roots of a multirooted tooth.

interradicular septum, *n* a thin, bony divider within the tooth socket that separates the roots of a multirooted tooth.

interridge distance, *n* See distance, interarch.

interstitial (in'turstish'əl), *adj* pertaining to the tiny spaces between tissues.

intervention studies, *n.pl* epidemiologic investigations designed to test a hypothesized cause and effect relation by modifying the supposed causal factor(s) in the study population.

interview, *n* **1.** a question-and-answer conference at which the parties concerned state the principles and facts regarding their relationship. In dental practice, this usually refers to the relationship between dentist and employee, and between dentist and patient. *v* **2.** to query a potential employee.

intolerance, *n* inability to endure or withstand.

intraarterial, *adj* situated within an artery or arteries.

intracellular (in'trəsel'yōōlur), *adj* situated or occurring within a cell or cells.

intracoronal (in'trəkôrō'nəl), *adj* pertaining to the inside of the coronal portion of a natural tooth.

intracoronal attachment, *n* See attachment, intracoronal.

intracoronal retainer, *n* See retainer, intracoronal.

intracranial pressure, *n* pressure that occurs within the cranium. Trauma to the head, inflammation, or infection of the linings of the brain may cause an increase in pressure within the cranium, which is painful, dysfunctional, and may become life-threatening.

intramaxillary anchorage, *n* See anchorage, intramaxillary.

intramaxillary elastic, *n* See elastic, intramaxillary.

intramucosal insert, *n* See insert, intramucosal.

intramuscular (in'trəmus'kyōōlur), *adj* situated in the substance of a muscle.

intraocular pressure, *n* the internal pressure of the eye, regulated by resistance to the flow of aqueous humor through the fine sieve of the trabecular meshwork. Obstruction within the trabecular meshwork will cause an increase in the intraocular pressure. High persistent intraocular pressure may lead to blindness.

intraoral (in'trə-ôr'əl), *adj* within the mouth.

intraoral tracing, *n* See tracing, intraoral.

intraosseous fixation (in'trə-os'ē-us), *n* See fixation, intraosseous.

intrapartum, *adj/adv* pertaining to or occurring during the delivery of offspring.

intrapulmonary (in'trəpul'mənerē), *adj* situated in the substance of a lung.

intrathecal (in'trəthē'kəl), *adj* pertaining to a structure or substance contained within a sheath; in drug delivery, the injection of a therapeutic agent into the sheath surrounding the spinal cord.

intravascular (in'trəvas'kyōōlur), *adj* within a blood vessel.

intravenous (in'trəvē'nus), *adj* in, into, or from within a vein or veins.

intraversion, *n* indicating teeth or other maxillary structures that are too near the medial plane.

intrinsic, *adj* naturally occurring within; inherent; essential.

intrinsic coloring, *n* coloring from within; the incorporation of pigment within the material of a prosthesis.

intrude, *v* to move a tooth apically.

intrusion, *n* a depression; an inward projection.

intrusion upon seclusion, *n* an offensive invasion of someone's personal affairs or property.

intubate (in'tōōbāt), *v* to treat by intubation.

intubation (in'tōōbā'shən), *n* the insertion of a tube; especially the introduction of a tube into the larynx through the glottis for the introduction of an anesthetic gas or oxygen.

intubator (in'tōōbātur), *n* an instrument used in intubation.

inulin, *n* a fructose-derived substance used as a diagnostic aid in tests of kidney function, specifically glomerular filtration. Inulin is not metabolized or absorbed by the body but is readily filtered through the kidney.

inunction (inungk′shən), *n* the local application of a drug in an oily or semisolid vehicle, such as an ointment, or the preparation that is thus applied.

invagination, epithelial, *n* the downgrowth of epithelium along the cervical tract of an implant.

invasion of privacy, *n* legal term defining any mistreatment of another's private life. See also false light, intrusion upon seclusion, and appropriation.

inventory, *n* an itemized compilation of materials on hand.

inventory, equipment, *n* a detailed listing of all the nonexpendable items owned by the dentist and used in the practice of the profession.

inventory, materials, *n* a detailed listing of expendable supplies that are on hand in the practice. This is a constantly fluctuating list, depending on the quantity of the various materials presently on hand.

inverse-square law, *n* See law, inverse-square.

inversion, *n* the state of being upside down.

invest (invest′), *v* to surround, envelop, or embed in an investment material; for example, a gypsum product.

investing (inves′ting), *n* the process of covering or enveloping an object wholly or in part.

investing, vacuum, *n* the investing of a pattern within a vacuum to form a mold.

investment (invest′ment), *n* the material used to enclose or surround a pattern of a dental restoration for casting or molding or to maintain the relations of metal parts during soldering.

investment, casting, *n* the material from which the casting mold is made in fabrication of gold or cobalt-chromium castings.

investment, gypsum-bonded casting, *n* a casting investment that can be bonded by a-hemihydrate, a derivative of gypsum, because the fusion temperatures of the metal alloys to be cast in it are relatively low. All gold alloy investments and some low-fusing cobalt-chromium alloy investments are gypsum bonded.

investment, hygroscopic, *n* an investment specially designed for use with the hygroscopic investing techniques.

investment, phosphate-bonded casting, *n* a casting investment that is bonded by a phosphate and a metallic oxide that react to form a hard mass; generally used for high-fusing alloys.

investment, refractory, *n* an investment material that can withstand the high temperatures used in soldering or casting.

investment, sectional, *n* a mold made in sections.

investment, silica-bonded casting, *n* a casting investment that is bonded by a silica gel that reverts to cristobalite in heating and is generally used for high-fusing alloys.

investment, soldering, *n* a quartz investment, preferably one with a very low thermal expansion, used for the investment of appliances during the soldering procedure.

involucrum (in′vəlōōkrum), *n* a covering; usually a covering of new bone around a sequestrum.

involuntary, *adj* performed independently of the will.

involute (in′vəlōōt), *v* to decrease normally, in size and functional activity, an organ whose role in the body economy is temporary or confined to certain periods of life. Involute should be distinguished from *atrophy,* which means to waste away from abnormal causes.

involvement, *n* the state of becoming involved.

involvement, bifurcation (bīfurkā′shən), *n* the extension of pocket formation into the interradicular area of multirooted teeth in periodontitis.

involvement, pulp, *n* a condition wherein consideration of the vitality or health of the dental pulp is a factor.

involvement, trifurcation, *n* See involvement, bifurcation.

iodine, *n* a halogen element that is nonmetallic in nature; atomic weight is 126.91. As a nutritional element, iodine is vital to the production of thyroxin by the thyroid gland. In radioactive form, iodine is used as a diagnostic substance to determine the ability of the thyroid gland to take up iodine. In tincture form, iodine is used as a locally applied antiseptic, germicide, and disclosing solution.

iodine number, *n* measured in grams, the amount of iodine absorbable by 100 grams of a fat or an oil; the lower the level of unsaturated fatty acids in the fat or oil, the higher the iodine number.

iodine, protein-bound (PBI), *n* iodine bound to protein, mainly thyroxin in the plasma. The thyroid hormone is precipitated by protein-denaturing agents, and, in general, the amount of iodine in a protein precipitate indicates the amount of thyroid hormone present and is thus an index of thyroid activity. Various values are given for thyroid function: hypothyroidism, 0 to 3.5 µg/ml of protein-bound iodine; euthyroidism 3.5 to 8 µg/ml; hyperthyroidism, values higher than 8 µg/ml.

iodism (iodine poisoning), *n* acute or chronic intoxication caused by the ingestion or absorption of iodides. Manifestations of acute poisoning include abdominal pain, nausea, vomiting, hypersalivation, conjunctivitis, and collapse. Chronic manifestations include hypersalivation, fever, acute rhinitis, swelling and tenderness of the salivary glands, and dermatitis and stomatitis in hypersensitive individuals. Iodism is a toxic condition that sometimes follows the use of preparations containing iodine.

iodophor (ī-ō′dəfôr), *n* a loose chemical compound of iodine with certain organic compounds; for example, polyvinylpyrrolidone.

iodoquinol (ī′-ōdō′kwinôl), *n* an antimicrobial agent that acts against the parasite *Entamoeba histolytica.* It is used in the treatment of intestinal disease.

ion (ī′-on), *n* an atomic particle, atom, or chemical radical bearing an electrical charge, either negative or positive.

ion exchange chromatography, *n* the process of separating and analyzing different substances according to their affinities for chemically stable but very reactive synthetic exchangers, which are composed largely of polystyrene and cellulose. The process uses an absorbent containing ionizing groups and accommodates the exchange of ions between a solution of substances to be analyzed and the absorbent. Ion exchange chromatography is often used to separate components of nucleic acids and proteins.

ion pair, *n* two particles of opposite charge, usually the electron and the positive atomic residue resulting after the interaction of ionizing radiation with the orbital electrons of atoms. The average energy required to produce an ion pair is approximately 33 (or 34) electron volts.

ion-selective electrode, *n* a potentiometric electrode that develops a potential in the presence of one ion (or class of ions), but not in the presence of a similar concentration of other ions.

ionization (ī′-ănīzā′shən), *n* the process or the result of a process by which a neutral atom or molecule acquires either a positive or negative charge.

ionization chamber, *n* See chamber, ionization.

ionization, chamber, air-equivalent, *n* See chamber, ionization, air-equivalent.

ionization density, *n* the number of ion pairs per unit volume.

ionization path (ionization track), *n* the trail of ion pairs produced by ionizing radiation in its passage through matter.

ionization potential, *n* the potential necessary to separate one electron from an atom, resulting in the formation of an ion pair.

ionizer, *n* See electrolyzer.

iontophoresis (ī-on′tōfôrē′sis), *n* application, by means of an appropriate electrode, of a galvanic current to an ionizable agent in contact with a surface to hasten the movement into the tissue of the ion of opposite charge to that of the electrode. See also ionization.

ipratropium bromide, *n* *trade name:* Atrovent; *drug class:* anticholinergic bronchodilator; *action:* inhibits interaction of acetylcholine at receptor sites on the bronchial smooth muscle, resulting in bronchodilation; *uses:* bronchodilation during bronchospasm in those with chronic obstructive pulmonary disease, bronchitis, emphysema, asthma; not for rapid bronchodilation; maintenance treatment only.

ipsilateral (ip″sĭ-lat′ər-əl), *adj* originating or occurring on the same side of the body.

IQ, *n* See intelligence quotient.

iridium, *n* a silvery-bluish metallic element. Its atomic number is 77 and its atomic weight is 192.2.

iris, *n* a circular, contractile disc suspended in aqueous humor between the cornea and the crystalline lens of the eye and perforated by a circular pupil. The iris regulates the amount of light passing into the chambers of the eye.

iron, (Fe), *n* a common metallic element essential for the synthesis of hemoglobin. Its atomic number is 26 and its atomic weight is 55.85. Normal blood levels of iron range between 60 and 190 micrograms.

iron oxide, *n* a compound of iron and oxygen which is often used for laboratory polishing of precious metals. See also jeweler's rouge.

irradiation (irā′dē-ā′shən), *n* **1.** the exposure of material to roentgen or other radiation. (One speaks of *radiation therapy* but of *irradiation of the patient.*) **2.** the exposure to radiation.

irreversibility (ir′ēvur′sibil′itē), *n* incapable of being returned to the original state.

irreversible (ir′ēvur′sebəl), *adj* incapable of being reversed or returned to the original state.

irreversible hydrocolloid, adj See hydrocolloid, irreversible.

irrigation (ir′igā′shən), *n* the technique of using a solution to wash or flush debris from the root canal or from a wound.

irrigation, supragingival, n the flushing of liquid using a handheld device to remove bacterial plaque from dental surfaces above or even with the gum line.

irrigator, *n* dental tool used to force liquid through a given area; features a soft tube that draws liquid from a contained source.

irritability, *n* the quality of being irritable or of responding to a stimulus.

irritant, *n* **1.** an agent that causes an irritation or stimulation. **2.** an agent that is toxic, bacterial, physical, or chemical and is capable of inducing functional derangements or organic lesions of the tissues.

irritant, chemical, n a chemical agent that causes irritation. The primary agents that have an etiologic relationship to periodontal disease are plaque and calculus. Other agents that serve as a medium for the growth of microorganisms include food debris, sloughed cells, and necrotic material.

irritation, *n* the act of stimulating. Any condition of functional derangement and nervous irritability.

irritation from overstimulation, n See impingement.

irritation, mechanical, n tissue damage, injury, or insult by physical forces directed against the tissue—for example, tissue irritation produced by faulty toothbrushing.

irritation of gingival tissues, n See impingement.

ischemia (iskē′mē-ə), *n* a focal deficiency of blood to a part of the body or simply a local anemia. It results from encroachment of the lumen of an artery or the capillaries supplying the affected area. The reduction in the lumen may be caused by allergic hypersensitivity, degeneration of the tunica intima (atherosclerosis), inflammation, physical pressure, pharmacologic and toxic agents, or neurogenic disorders.

isobar (ī′sōbär), *n* in radiochemistry, one of two or more different nuclides having the same mass number.

isoelectric focusing, *n* the ordering and concentration of substances according to their isoelectric points.

isoelectric point, *n* the pH at which a molecule containing two or more ionizable groups is electrically neutral.

isoetharine HCl/isoetharine mesylate, *n trade names:* Bronkosol, Bron-kometer, Dispos-a-Med; *drug class:* adrenergic beta$_2$-agonist; *action:* causes bronchodilation by beta$_2$ stimulation, resulting in increased levels of cAMP and causing relaxation of bronchial smooth muscle with very little effect on heart rate; *uses:* bronchospasm or asthma.

isogenic (ī′sōjen′ik), *adj* originating from a common source; possessing the same genetic composition.

isolation of a tooth, *n* a technique to

protect a tooth against contamination from oral fluids during a surgical or restorative procedure, usually through the application of a rubber dam or the use of cotton rolls.

isoleucine, *n* one of the essential amino acids occurring in most dietary proteins. Isoleucine is essential for proper growth in infants and for nitrogen balance in adults. See also amino acid.

isomers (ī'sōmurz), *n.pl* **1.** organic compounds having the same empirical formula—that is, the same number of the same atoms but different structural formulas and therefore different physical and chemical properties. *n* **2.** one of several nuclides having the same number of neutrons and protons but capable of existing, for a measurable time, in different quantum states with different energies and radioactive properties. The isomer of higher energy commonly decays to one with lower energy by a process known as isomeric transition.

isomers, optical, n.pl two isomers whose structures, dextro- and levo-, differ only in a spatial arrangement that makes them mirror images. This occurs only when there is an asymmetric carbon atom—that is, one attached to four different substituents. The pharmacologic activity often resides very largely in one of the two forms.

isomers, stereo-, n.pl molecules that differ only in the spatial arrangement of the atoms. This term includes optical isomers.

isometric muscle contraction (ī'sōmet'rik), *n* See contraction, muscle, isometric.

isoniazid (INH), *n trade names:* Laniazid, Nydrazid; *drug class:* antitubercular; *action:* bactericidal interference with lipid, nucleic acid biosynthesis; *uses:* treatment and prevention of tuberculosis.

isoproterenol HCl/isoproterenol sulfate, *n trade names:* Isuprel, Vapo-Iso, Aerolone; *drug class:* adrenergic beta$_1$- and beta$_2$-agonist; *action:* relaxes bronchial smooth muscle and dilates trachea and main bronchi by increasing levels of cAMP, which relaxes smooth muscles; causes increased contractility and heart rate; *uses:* broncho-

spasm, asthma, heart block, bradycardia, or shock.

isosorbide dinitrate, *n trade names:* Iso-Bid, Isotrate, Dilatrate-SR, Isordil; *drug class:* nitrate antianginal; *action:* decreases preload/afterload, which is responsible for decreasing left ventricular end-diastolic pressure, systemic vascular resistance; *uses:* chronic stable angina pectoris, prophylaxis of angina pain.

isosorbide mononitrate, *n trade name:* ISMO; *drug class:* antianginal, organic nitrate; *action:* decreases preload/afterload, which is responsible for decreasing left ventricular end-diastolic pressure, systemic vascular resistance; arterial and venous dilation; *use:* prevention of angina pectoris caused by coronary artery disease.

isosthenuria (ī'sōsthənyōō'rē-ə), *n* the excretion of urine with fixed specific gravity. It may occur in terminal renal disease when the specific gravity reaches that of the glomerular filtrate, 1.010.

isotone (ī'sōtōn), *n* one of several different nuclides having the same number of neutrons in their nuclei, but different mass numbers.

isotonic (ī'sōton'ik), *adj* equivalence in osmotic pressure. Specifically used in reference to a solution whose osmotic pressure is equal to that of a body fluid, such as blood plasma or tears, to which the solution is compared.

isotonic muscle contraction, n See contraction, muscle, isotonic.

isotope (ī'sōtōp), *n* one of several nuclides having the same number of protons in their nuclei, and hence having the same atomic number but differing in the number of neutrons, and therefore in the mass number. The isotopes of a particular element have virtually identical chemical properties.

isotope, stable, n a nonradioactive isotope of an element.

isotretinoin, *n trade name:* Accutane; *drug class:* retinoic acid isomer, vitamin A derivative; *action:* decreases sebum secretion, improves cystic acne; *uses:* severe recalcitrant cystic acne.

isoxsuprine HCl, *n trade name:* Vasodilan; *drug class:* peripheral vasodilator; *action:* beta-adrenoreceptor antagonist with beta-adrenoreceptor-stimulating properties; may also act directly on vascular smooth muscle; causes cardiac stimulation, uterine relaxation; *uses:* symptoms of cerebrovascular insufficiency, peripheral vascular disease including arteriosclerosis obliterans, or Raynoud's disease.

Isradipine, *n.pr trade name:* Dyna-Circ; *drug class:* calcium channel blocker; *action:* inhibits calcium ion influx across cell membrane during cardiac depolarization; produces relaxation of coronary vascular smooth muscle, peripheral vascular smooth muscle; increases myocardial oxygen delivery in patients with vasospastic angina; *use:* essential hypertension.

itraconazole, *n trade name:* Sporanox; *drug class:* antifungal, systemic; *action:* inhibits cytochrome P-450 enzyme's blocking synthesis of essential membrane sterols in fungal organism; *uses:* blastomycosis, histoplasmosis.

Ivalon sponge, *n.pr* a polyvinyl alcohol sponge.

Ivy loop wiring, *n.pr* See wiring, Ivy loop.

Ivy's test, *n.pr* See test, Ivy's.

jacket, *n* See crown, complete, veneer, acrylic resin and crown, complete, veneer, porcelain.

jackscrew, *n* a threaded device used in appliances for separation or approximation of teeth or jaw segments.

Jackson's sign, *n.pr* See sign, Jackson's.

Janet's test, *n.pr* See test, Janet's.

jaundice (jändis), *n* a condition characterized by an abnormal accumulation of bilirubin (red bile pigment) in the blood and manifested by a yellowish discoloration of the skin, mucous membranes, and cornea. Seen in hemolytic anemias, biliary obstruction, hepatitis, cholangiolitis, and cirrhosis of the liver. Oral mucous membranes may be pigmented.

Jaundice. (Neville/Damm/Allen/Bouquot, 2002)

jaundice, acholuric, n jaundice without bile in the urine.

jaundice, congenital hemolytic (acholuric icterus, spherocytic anemia, hereditary spherocytosis), n a familial hemolytic anemia transmitted as a Mendelian dominant trait. The intrinsic defects of the red blood cells include a spheroidal shape, which allows them to be trapped by the spleen, and increased mechanical fragility.

jaundice, epidemic, n See disease, Weil's.

jaundice, hemolytic (prehepatic jaundice), n excess bile pigments in the blood resulting from increased destruction of erythrocytes.

jaundice, hepatic, n See jaundice, hepatocellular.

jaundice, hepatocellular (hepatic jaundice, infective jaundice, medical jaundice, toxic jaundice), n jaundice resulting from disease of liver cells by infectious agents or toxins, decreasing the ability of the liver to handle the bile pigments that are continually produced by the destruction of red blood cells.

jaundice, homologous serum, n See hepatitis, homologous serum.

jaundice, infective, n See jaundice, hepatocellular.

jaundice, latent, n increased bilirubin in the blood without clinical signs of jaundice.

jaundice, medical, n See jaundice, hepatocellular.

jaundice, obstructive (posthepatic jaundice), n extrahepatic and intrahepatic obstruction of the biliary tract, resulting in retrograde retention of bile pigments and jaundice.

jaundice, posthepatic, n See jaundice, obstructive.

jaundice, prehepatic, n See jaundice, hemolytic.

jaundice, regurgitating, n jaundice resulting from reentry of conjugated bilirubin into the blood as a result of obstruction of the biliary tract or hepatocellular damage and failure to excrete conjugated bilirubin from liver cells.

jaundice, retention, n an increase in bilirubin in the blood from hemolysis; failure of the liver cells to conjugate bilirubin or remove free bilirubin.

jaundice, surgical, n extrahepatic obstruction of the biliary tract.

jaundice, syringe, n See hepatitis, homologous serum.

jaundice, toxic, n See jaundice, hepatocellular.

jaw, *n* a common name for either the maxillae or the mandible; the meaning is usually extended to include their soft tissue covering.

jaw, cleft (gnathouschisis), n See palate, cleft.

jaw cyst, n an abnormal bladder-like sac within the jaw. May occur in either the maxilla or mandible associated with or not associated with the dentition and its formation. See also cyst.

jaw fracture, n a break in the continuity of the bone of the maxilla or mandible. See also fracture.

jaw, lumpy, n See actinomycosis.

jaw movement, n See movement, jaw.

jaw, phossy, n See poisoning, phosphorus.

jaw reflex, n See reflex, jaw.

jaw relation, n See relation, jaw.

jaw-to-jaw relationship, n See relation, jaw.

JCAHO, *n.pr* an acronym for the **Joint Commission on Accreditation of Healthcare Organizations.**

jealousy, *n* resentment against a rival or competitor. Jealousy may be a significant barrier to functional interpersonal relationships within any group.

jejunum, *n* the middle or intermediate of the three portions of the small intestine, connecting proximally with the duodenum and distally with the ileum. The jejunum has a slightly larger diameter, a deeper color, and a thicker wall than the ileum, and it contains heavy, circular folds that are absent in the lower part of the ileum.

jelly, petroleum, *n* See petrolatum.

jet tips, *n* the end of an oral irrigating device; engineered to deliver a directed flow of water into the subgingival area. Designs include monojet (single flow) and fractionated microjet (similar to a showerhead), and flow may be pulsating or nonpulsating.

jeweler's rouge, *n* iron oxide which has been pressed into a fine red powder, used to polish gold and metal alloys.

job satisfaction, *n* the state of finding fulfillment in one's work.

Johnston's method, *n.pr* See method, chloropercha.

Joint Commission on Accreditation of Healthcare Organizations (JCAHO), *n.pr* formerly the Joint Commission on Accreditation of Hospitals. The JCAHO conducts accreditation programs for most of the health care facilities in the United States. The American Dental Association is a corporate member of the JCAHO. Hospitals and clinics are surveyed on a regular basis for compliance with the standards and criteria for accreditation.

Joint Commission on Accreditation of Hospitals, *n.pr* See Joint Commission on Accreditation of Healthcare Organizations.

joint(s), *n* the junction of union between two or more bones or cartilages of the skeleton.

joint(s), Charcot's (shärkōz′), n a manifestation of late syphilis in which there is degeneration, hypertrophy, hypermobility, and loss of contour of a joint, usually a weight-bearing joint. It is most common in tabes dorsalis.

joint(s) diarthrosis (dī-ärthrō′sis), n a joint that moves freely in contact. The adjacent bone surfaces are typically covered by a film of cartilage and are bound by stout connective tissues, frequently enclosing a liquid-filled joint cavity.

joint(s) disease, n any inflammatory, infectious, or functional disorder within a joint

joint(s), hinge, n See ginglymus.

joint(s) mice, n cartilaginous material present in the synovial spaces of a joint.

joint(s) prosthesis, n the addition to or replacement of a member(s) or of structural elements within a joint to improve and enhance the function of the joint. Principal joint prostheses include hip replacement and knee replacement. Less common is a joint prosthesis for the TMJ.

joint(s) synarthrosis **(sin´ärthrō´sis)** n (junctura fibrosa, fibrous joint) a joint in which the bony elements are connected by thin intervening layers of cartilage, connective tissue, or direct contact of bone to bone such as the rigid unions in the adult skull.

joint(s), temporomandibular, n See articulation, temporomandibular.

Jones protein, *n.pr* See protein, Bence Jones.

Jorgensen's drug administration principles, *n.pr* principles employed in the selection and administration of intravenous sedative agents that have a wide margin of safety and predictable effects and that, in combination, can elevate the pain threshold, produce euphoria, have an antisialogogue effect, and promote an amnesic response. The principles include the sequence and rate of administration while monitoring patient response signs.

judgment, n **1.** a legal finding. n **2.** the ability to discriminate between or among two or more states or conditions.

judicial process, n the rules which determine the role of judge and jury in the courtroom as well as the jurisdiction of the individual courts over specific areas of law.

junction (jungk´shən), n a place of coming together, or union.

junction, cementoenamel (cervical line), n the junction of the enamel of the crown and the cementum of the root of a tooth. The area above the junction corresponds to the anatomic crown of the tooth; the area apical to the junction constitutes the anatomic root of the tooth.

junction, dentinocemental, n the line of union or apposition of the cementum and dentin of a tooth.

junction, dentinoenamel (dentoenamel junction), n the interface of enamel and dentin of the tooth crown, conforming in a general way to the shape of the crown.

junction, dentoenamel, n See junction, dentinoenamel.

junction, dentogingival, n the junction between the gingival attachment, a nonkeratinized epithelium, and the tooth surface.

junction, mucogingival, n the scalloped linear area denoting the approximation or separation of the gingivae and alveolar mucosa.

junctional epithelium, n a band of epithelial cells that surrounds the tooth and creates a seal at the gingival sulcus to hold it firmly in place.

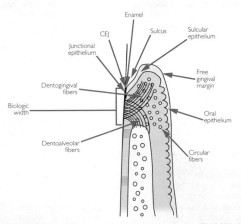

Tissues and fibers of the gingiva and attachment apparatus. (Daniel/Harfst, 2002)

jurisprudence, *n* the philosophy of law.

jurisprudence, dental (forensic dentistry), *n* **1.** the science that teaches the application of every branch of dental knowledge to the purposes of the law; this also includes the elucidation of doubtful legal questions. *n* **2.** the state laws and codes covering the legal limitations of the practice of the profession of dentistry.

jurisprudence, medical *n* the science that applies the principles and practice of the different branches of medicine in the elucidation of doubtful questions in a court of justice. Also called *forensic medicine.*

jury, *n* a certain number of citizens selected according to law and sworn to inquire of certain matters of fact and to declare the truth on evidence submitted to them.

just, *adj* right; according to law and justice.

justice, *n* the constant and perpetual disposition to render every person his or her due. Also, the conformity of one's actions and will to the law.

juvenile periodontitis, *n* a distinct form of periodontal disease that may present with symptoms such as localized or generalized inflammatory changes in the periodontium of prepubertal children. The disease is characterized by severe pocketing and rapid destruction of alveolar bone. Several subtypes of the disease are recognized (formerly called *periodontosis*).

juxtaposition, *n* adjacent situation; apposition or contact.

kakke (käk′kā), *n* See *beriberi.*

kallikrein, *n* a group of enzymes (plasma, tissue, pancreatic, urinary, submandibular kallikrein) that can convert kininogen to bradykinin or kallidin; trypsin and plasmin can also affect the conversion.

kallikrein-kinin system, *n* a proposed hormonal system that functions within the kidney, with the enzyme kallikrein in the renal cortex mediating production of bradykinin, which acts as a vasodilator peptide.

kanamycin, *n* an aminoglycoside antibiotic that acts by inhibiting the synthesis of protein in susceptible organisms. Kanamycin requires close clinical supervision because of its potential toxicity and adverse side effects to the auditory and vestibular branches of the eighth cranial nerve and to the renal tubules.

kaolin (kā′ə-lin), *n* a fine, pure-white clay (hydrated aluminum silicate) used in porcelain teeth.

Kaposi's sarcoma, *n.pr* See *sarcoma, Kaposi's.*

karyotype (ker′ē-ō-tīp) *n* the chromosomal arrangement of a single cell. The schematic representation of an individual's chromosomes, arranged in pairs according to number, form, and size.

Kazanjian's operation (kəz-an′jē-ənz), *n.pr* See *operation, Kazanjian's.*

Kazanjian's procedure, *n.pr* See *operation, Kazanjian's.*

keloid (kē′loid), *n* a dense, proliferative growth on the skin (hypertrophy of scar tissue) that appears to be an abnormal reaction to trauma, especially burns. Keloids tend to recur after excision and occur more frequently in blacks than in whites.

Keloids. (Zitelli/Davis, 2002)

keloplasty (kē′lō-plast-ē), *n* the excision of scar tissue in the skin.

Kendall's compound B, *n.pr* See *corticosterone.*

Kendall's compound E, *n.pr* See *cortisone.*

Kennedy bar, *n.pr* See *connector, minor, secondary lingual bar.*

Kennedy classification, *n.pr* a method of classifying partially edentulous conditions and partial dentures; based on the location of the edentulous spaces in relation to the remaining teeth.

keratin (ker′ə-tin), *n.* an insoluble sulfur-containing protein with a high content of the amino acids tyrosine and leucine; the main component of epidermis, hair, nails, keratinized epithelium. It contains a relatively large amount of sulfur, is insoluble in the gastric juices, and is sometimes used for coating enteric pills that are intended to be dissolved only in the intestine.

keratinization (ker′ə-tin′i-zā′shən), *n* the process of becoming keratinized.

keratinocytes, *n.pl* a cell of the living epidermis and certain oral epithelia that produces keratin in the process of differentiating into the dead and fully keratinized cells of the stratum corneum.

keratitis, *n* any inflammation of the cornea.

keratoacanthoma (ker′ət-ō-ak′anth-ō′mə), *n* a rapidly growing papular lesion with a superficial crater filled with keratin.

Keratoacanthoma. (Regezi/Sciubba/Pogrel, 2000)

keratoconjunctivitis sicca (ker′ə-tō-kən-jungk′ti-vī′tis sik′ə), *n* See *syndrome, Sjögren's.*

keratocyst (ker′ə-tō-sist), *n* a hornified cyst.

keratohyalin granules (ker′ə-tō-hī′ə-lin), *n.pl* basophilic granules (0.2 to 4.5 micron) found in cells of the stratum granulosum that are presumed to play a role in keratinization.

keratolytic agents, *n.pl* agents that loosen or remove the horny outer layer of the skin.

keratoplasty, *n* corneal transplantation.

keratosis (ker′ə-tō′sis), *n* **1.** a horny or cornified growth (for example, wart, callosity). *n* **2.** a condition characterized by cornification, or hyperkeratinization, of the tissues.

keratosis, actinic, n an overgrowth of the horny layer of the epidermis caused by excessive exposure to the sun.

keratosis blennorrhagia, n a skin condition found in Reiter's syndrome characterized by pustules and crusting; once incorrectly associated with gonorrhea; more recently considered a genetic disorder occurring mostly in men between the ages of 20 and 25.

keratosis, chronic senile, n keratosis of the lips in elderly individuals. These lesions should be considered precancerous.

keratosis, focal, n localized areas of increased cornification (hyperkeratinization). Such lesions are seen particularly on the lips.

keratosis follicularis, n See *disease, Darier's.*

keratosis, seborrheic (basal cell papilloma, verruca senilis), n benign, pigmented, superficial epithelial tumors that clinically appear to be pasted on the skin of the trunk, arms, or face. Characterized histologically by marked hyperkeratosis, with keratin cyst formation, acanthosis of basal cells, and melanin pigmentation, all above the level of the adjacent epidermis.

keratosis, senile, n small, firm lesions occurring principally on the face and back of the hands in elderly people or those exposed to the sun. There is hyperkeratosis with irregular and atypical proliferation of the cells of the rete Malpighi. The condition is one of premalignancy with tendency toward epidermoid carcinoma. See also leukoplakia.

ketamine, *n* a parenterally administered anesthetic that produces catatonia, profound analgesia, increased sympathetic activity, and little relaxation of skeletal muscles.

ketoacidosis (kē′tō-as′i-dō′sis), *n* a form of acidosis characterized by an increased accumulation of ketone bodies (acetoacetic acid, β-hydroxy-butyric acid, acetone) in the blood (for example, the acidosis of uncontrolled diabetes mellitus).

ketoconazole, *n* a broad-spectrum synthetic antifungal agent applied to the skin to inhibit the growth of dermatophytes and yeasts, effective in *Candida* infections and in the treatment of seborrheic dermatitis; *trade name:* Nizoral; *drug class:* imidazole antifungal; *action:* alters cell membranes and inhibits several fungal enzymes; *uses:* systemic candidiasis, chronic mucocutaneous candidiasis, candiduria, coccidioidomycosis, histoplasmosis, chromomycosis, para-coccidioidomycosis, tinea pedis.

ketone, *n* an organic chemical compound characterized by having in its structure a carbonyl or keto group attached to two alkyl groups. It is produced by oxidation of secondary alcohols.

ketone body, n See *body, ketone.*

ketonuria (kē'tō-nyōō'rē-ə) *n* the indication of extra bodies of ketone within urine caused by decreased or unstable metabolism of carbohydrates; occurs more frequently in certain medical conditions (e.g., starvation acidosis and diabetes mellitus); may also be called *acetonuria.*

ketoprofen, *n trade names:* Orudis, Oruvail, Actron; *drug class:* nonsteroidal antiinflammatory; *action:* inhibits prostaglandin synthesis by interfering with cyclooxygenase needed for biosynthesis; possesses analgesic, antiinflammatory, antipyretic properties; *uses:* osteoarthritis, rheumatoid arthritis, dysmenorrhea.

ketorolac/ketorolac trometha-mine injection, *n trade name:* Toradol; *drug class:* nonsteroidal antiinflammatory; *action:* inhibits prostaglandin synthesis by interfering with cyclooxygenase needed for biosynthesis; possesses analgesic, antiinflammatory, antipyretic properties; *use:* acute mild-to-moderate pain; not for chronic pain use.

ketosis, *n* See *ketoacidosis.*

kev, *n* the abbreviation for 1000 electron volts.

keyway, *n* the slot into which the male portion of precision attachments fits.

kg, *n* See *kilogram.*

KHN, *n.pr* the abbreviation for Knoop hardness number. See also *test, Knoop hardness.*

kidney, *n* one of a pair of bean-shaped urinary organs in the dorsal part of the abdomen, one on each side of the vertebral column. The kidneys produce and eliminate urine through a complex filtration network and reabsorption system comprising more than 2 million nephrons. More than 2500 pints of blood pass through the kidneys every day.

killer cell, *n* a lymphocyte that develops in the bone marrow and lacks the characteristic surface markers of the B and T lymphocytes. Killer or null cells represent a small proportion of the lymphocyte population. Stimulated by the presence of an antibody, null cells can attach certain cellular targets directly and are known as *natural killer cells.*

kilo- (kil'ō), *pre* 1000.

kilocalorie, *n* 1000 calories, a unit of measure of the energy value in foodstuffs.

kilogram (kil'ə-gram), *n* 1000 g, or equivalent to approximately 2.2 pounds avoirdupois.

kilohertz (kil'ō-hurts) *n* a frequency unit of 1000 cycles per second.

kilovolt (kil'ə-vōlt), *n* the unit of electrical potential equal to 1000 volts.

kilovolt peak (kvp), n the crest value of the potential wave in kilovolts in an alternating current cycle. When only half of the wave is used, the value refers to that of the useful half of the wave.

kilovolt potential, n refers to the intensitiy of the x-ray beam and the resulting image on the film. A higher kilovoltage x-ray increases the film density, whereas a lower kilovoltage x-ray increases contrast.

kilovoltage (kil'ə-vōl'təj), *n* the electrical potential difference between the anode and cathode of an x-ray tube.

kilovoltage, constant potential, n the potential of a constant voltage generator, in constant potential kilovolts (kvcp).

kilovoltage, equivalent (effective kilovoltage), n the kilovoltage of monoenergetic radiation having the same half-value layer (HVL) as the heterogeneous beam produced by the peak kilovoltage in question.

kinematic face-bow (kin-ə-mat′ik), *n* See *face-bow, kinematic.*

kinesiology (kin-ē′sē-ol′ə-jē), *n* the study of human motion that attempts to explain the manner in which movements of the body occur. The principles of kinesiology may be used to describe the laws of articulation and the several theories of mandibular movement.

kinetics, *n* the study of the forces that produce, arrest, or modify the motions of the body. Kinetics is the application of Newton's first and third laws of inertia to body dynamics. The reaction forces of the muscles contribute to the equilibrium and motion of the body.

kinin, *n* one of a number of widely differing substances having pronounced and dramatic physiologic effects. Some are formed in blood by proteolysis secondary to some pathologic process. Kinins stimulate visceral smooth muscle but relax vascular smooth muscle, thus producing vasodilation.

kink, *n* a bend or twist.

Kirkland cement dressing, *n.pr* knife. See *knife, Kirkland.*

Kirschner wire, *n.pr* See *wire, Kirschner.*

Kirstein's method, *n.pr* See *method, Kirstein's.*

kissing disease, *n* a vernacular term for *infectious mononucleosis,* a viral infection frequently occurring in teenagers and young adults. See also *infectious mononucleosis.*

kleptomania (klep′tō-mā′nē-ə) *n* an impulse control disorder distinguished by an uncontrollable urge to steal typically unnecessary objects.

Kline's test, *n.pr* See *test, Kline's.*

Klinefelter syndrome, *n.pr* a syndrome of gonadal defects, appearing in males with an extra X chromosome in at least one cell line. Characteristics are small, firm testes, long legs, gynecomastia, poor social adaptation, subnormal intelligence, chronic pulmonary disease, and varicose veins.

Kloehn headgear, *n.pr* an extraoral orthodontic appliance consisting of a facebow and a cervical strap used to retract maxillary teeth or to reinforce the anchorage during tooth retraction.

knee, *n* a joint complex that connects the thigh with the lower leg. It consists of 3 condyloid joints, 12 ligaments, 13 bursae, and the patella.

knife, *n* an instrument used for cutting that consists of a sharp-edged blade with a handle.

knife, amalgam, n a bladed metal instrument used in the margination process to remove excess amalgam and overhangs.

knife, buck, n a periodontal knife possessing spear-shaped cutting points; used for interdental incision during gingivectomy.

knife, electronic, n an electrosurgical scalpel used to incise or shave tissue.

knife, gold, n an instrument sometimes contraangled, with a blade or cutting edge; used to trim excess metal and develop contour in foil restorations.

knife, Goldman-Fox, n.pr any of a group of surgical instruments designed for the incision and contouring of gingival tissue.

knife, Kirkland, n.pr a heart-shaped knife, sharp on all edges, used for the primary gingivectomy incision.

knife, Merrifield's, n.pr a knife that has a long, narrow, triangular blade in a shank; used for gingivectomy incisions.

knitting yarn, *n* an alternative to floss, used to clean surfaces of teeth that are exceptionally far apart; also effective for cleaning isolated teeth, including those at the end of a row. Sometimes used with a floss threader to reach the difficult areas under pontics and around fixed and cantilevered dentures.

Knoop hardness test, *n.pr* See *test, Knoop hardness.*

Kobayashi ties, *n.pr.pl* orthodontic ligature ties used to fix an orthodontic arch wire to the brackets attached to the teeth; also provides attachment for the use of inter- and intramaxillary elastic traction.

Koeber's saw, *n.pr* See *saw, Koeber's.*

koilocytosis, *n* a histologic feature of the mucosal changes associated with the intraoral use of smokeless tobacco. The spinous cells of the squamous epithelium present with pyknotic, irregularly shaped nuclei surrounded by a perinuclear clear zone.

Koplik spots, *n.pr.pl* See *spots, Koplik.*

Korotkoff sounds (kô-rot′kôf), *n.pr* the noises heard when taking a blood pressure reading, originated by blood passage causing vibrations in the walls of the blood vessel.

Kryptex, *n* See *cement, silicophosphate.*

krypton, *n* one of the inert gases, present in small amounts in the atmosphere with an atomic number of 36 and an atomic weight of 83.80.

KS, *n.pr* See *sarcoma, Kaposi's.*

Kurer anchor system, *n.pr* an endodontic post system with parallel sides, threaded and made of stainless material

kv, *n* See *kilovolt.*

kvcp, *n* See *kilovoltage, constant potential.*

kvp, *n* See *kilovolt peak.*

kVp (kilovoltage peak) selector, n the control on an x-ray machine that selects the kilovoltage for a given x-ray film. See also *radiograph, high kilovoltage radiograph, low kilovoltage.*

kwashiorkor (kwä′shē-ôr′kôr), *n* a wasting disease of malnutrition that occurs in children after weaning as a result of severe protein deficiency. The word is Ghanan, meaning "the displaced child's visible condition."

Kwashiorkor. (Zitelli/Davis, 2002)

kyphosis (kī-fō′sis), *n* (humpback), an abnormal curvature of the spine with the convexity backward.

label (lā′bəl), *n* **1.** the portion of the prescription in which the directions for use are stated. **2.** one or more characters used to identify an item of data. Also called *key.* See also signa.

labetatol, *n* *trade names:* Normodyne, Trandate; *drug class:* nonselective adrenergic β-blocker and α-blocker; *action:* produces falls in BP without reflex tachycardia or significant reduction in heart rate through mixture of α-blocking and β-blocking effects; elevated plasma renins are reduced; *use:* mild-to-severe hypertension.

labial (lā′bē-əl), *n* of or pertaining to a lip.

labial commissures, n.pl the lateral angles formed where the lips meet at the outer edges of the mouth; the corners of the mouth.

labial developmental depressions, n.pl indentations extending from the cervix to the occusal surface on the crown of an anterior tooth in order to separate the tooth into labial developmental lobes.

labial mucosa, n tissue lining located beneath the lip within the oral cavity comprising the basement membrane, epithelium, lamina muscularis mucosae, and lamina propria mucosae.

labial notch, n See notch, labial.

labile (lā′bīl), *adj* unstable, as labile fever.

labioversion (lā′bē-ō-vur′zhən), *n* any deviation of a tooth toward the lips from the line of occlusion.

labium superius oris (lā′bē-um sōōpir′ē-us ō′ris), *n* the point of the upper lip lying in the midsagittal plane and a line drawn across the boundary of the mucous surface tangent to the curves.

laboratory, dental, *n* a room in which the dentist or auxiliaries perform technical procedures related to dental treatment but not done directly in the patient's mouth.

laceration, *n* a wound produced by tearing; the process of tearing.

laches (lach′iz), *n* negligence; inexcusable delay; a failure to claim or enforce a claim or right at a proper time.

lacquer, *n* a resin dissolved in a volatile solvent used to create a protective coating on the surface of an object.

lacrimal apparatus, *n* a network of structures of the eye that secrete tears and drain them from the surface of the eyeball. The parts include the lacrimal glands, the lacrimal ducts, the lacrimal sacs, and the nasolacrimal ducts.

lacrimal glands, *n.pl* exocrine glands situated in the lacrimal fossa whose function is to secrete tears. See also lacrimal apparatus.

lacrimation, gustatory, *n* See syndrome, auriculotemporal.

lactalbumin, *n* a simple, highly nutritious protein found in milk. Lactalbumin is similar to serum albumin.

lactate dehydrogenase, *n* an enzyme found in the cytoplasm of almost all body tissues, where its main function is to catalyze the oxidation of L-lactate to pyruvate.

Lactobacilli, **cariogenic,** *n* a type of bacteria that may play an important role in tooth decay. It is usually found in small amounts in dental plaque. Its concentration increases with high sugar intake.

Lactobacillius acidophilus, *n* a species of the genus *Lactobacillius* of the family Lactobacillaceae characterized by gram-positive rods found in cultured buttermilk and in the gastrointestinal tract of persons on a high milk, lactose-, or dextrin-containing diet. *L. acidophilus* preparations may be effective in the treatment of some recurrent aphthous ulcers and for the prevention of candidiasis secondary to tetracycline and/or steroid therapy.

Lactobacillius casei, *n* a species of *Lactobacillius* found in milk and cheese.

lactoferrin, *n* an iron binding protein found in the specific granules of neutrophils where it apparently exerts an antimicrobial activity by withholding iron from ingested bacteria and fungi. It also occurs in many secretions and exudates such as milk, tears, mucus, saliva, and bile.

lactone, *n* an organic anhydride formed from a hyroxyacid by the loss of water between an 2OH and a 2COOH group.

lactoperoxidase, *n* a peroxidase enzyme obtained from milk.

lactose, *n* a disaccharide found in the milk of all mammals. Lactose is used as a component of formulas for infants; it is also used as a laxative and a diuretic.

lactose intolerance, *n* an inability to digest the lactose in milk and milk products.

lacuna (ləkōō′nə), *n* a term used in anatomic nomenclature to designate a small hollow cavity or pit.

lacuna, absorption (Howship's lacuna), *n* an area (pit) of bone resorption, usually irregular in outline, and often containing osteoclasts.

lacuna, osteocyte, *n* a hollow cavity within bone, containing osteocytes, from which canaliculi, containing protoplasmic processes of the osteocytes, radiate.

lambda (lam′də), *n* **1.** the eleventh letter of the Greek alphabet. **2.** the point in the skull at which the sagittal and lambdoid sutures meet. The strap of a rubber dam holder placed at this level will hold its position without slipping up or down.

lamella, cemental (ləmel′ə), *n* the arrangement and deposition of cementum in incremental layers more or less parallel to the root configuration.

lamina (lam′inə), *n* a flat, thin plate.

lamina dura, *n* a radiographic term denoting the plate of compact bone (alveolar bone) that lies adjacent to the periodontal membrane.

lamina propria, *n* the zone of connective tissue subjacent to the epithelium of a mucous membrane.

laminagraphy (lam′inäg′rəfē), *n* body-section radiography.

laminate veneer restoration, *n* a conservative esthetic restoration of anterior teeth to mask discoloration, restore malformed teeth, close diastemas, and correct minor tooth alignment. The materials of choice are acrylic veneers, processed composite resin veneers, and/or porcelain veneers that are bonded directly to a properly prepared tooth.

laminectomy, *n* the excision of a vertebral lamina, commonly used to denote the removal of the posterior arch.

laminin, *n* a large polypeptide glycoprotein component of the basement membrane.

lamivudine (3TC), *n* *trade name:* Epivir; *drug class:* antiviral, nucleoside analog; *action:* inhibition of

HIV reverse transcriptase; also inhibits RNA- and DNA-dependent DNA polymerase; *use:* in combination with zidovudine for the treatment of HIV infection.

lamotrigine, *n trade name:* Lamictal; *drug class:* antiepileptic; *action:* may be result of blockage of voltage-dependent sodium channels with inhibition of excitatory amino acids; *uses:* adjunctive treatment of refractive partial seizures in adults.

lamp, mouth, *n* a device to produce light or illumination directly in the oral cavity and transilluminate the dental tissues.

lance, *v* to cut open with a lancet; to incise.

lancinating, *adj* pertaining to a stabbing pain (for example, the pain occurring in tic douloureux).

landmark, *n* an anatomic structure used as a guide for anatomic relationships.

landmark, cephalometric **(sef′ əlōmet′rik),** *n* one of the points located on oriented-head radiographs from which lines, planes, and angles may be constructed to analyze the configuration and relationship of elements of the craniofacial skeleton.

Langerhans cells, *n.pl* the cells of the pancreas that produce insulin.

language, *n* a defined set of characters that is used to form symbols and words and the rules and connections for combining these into meaningful communications.

language, machine, *n* a language designed for interpretation and use by a computer system without translation. Also called *machine code.*

lansoprazole, *n trade name:* Prevacid; *drug class:* antisecretory, proton pump inhibitor; *action:* suppresses gastric secretion by inhibiting hydrogen/ potassium ATPase enzyme system in gastric parietal cell; *uses:* short-term treatment for healing and symptomatic relief of active duodenal ulcer and erosive esophagitis.

lanthanum, *n* a rare-earth metallic element. Its atomic number is 57, and its atomic weight is 138.91

laparotomy, *n* any surgical incision into the peritoneal cavity, usually performed under general or regional anesthesia, often on an exploratory basis.

large intestine, *n* the portion of the digestive tract comprising the cecum; the appendix; the ascending, transverse, and descending colons; and the rectum. The ileocecal valve separates the cecum from the ileum.

laryngectomy, *n* the surgical removal of the larynx, performed to treat cancer of the larynx.

laryngitis, *n* an inflammation of the mucous membrane lining the larynx, accompanied by edema of the vocal cords with hoarseness or loss of voice.

laryngopharyngeal (ləring′gōfərin′jē-əl), *adj* related jointly to the larynx and the pharynx.

laryngopharynx (ləring′gōfer′ingks), *n* the lower portion of the pharynx, which extends from the corner of the hyoid bone or the vestibule of the larynx to the lower border of the cricoid cartilage.

Pharyngeal tonsils
NASOPHARYNX
Uvula
Mouth of auditory tube
Soft palate
Salpingopharyngeal fold
OROPHARYNX
Laryngeal inlet
LARYNGOPHARYNX
LARYNX
Esophagus   Trachea

Laryngopharynx. (Liebgott, 2001)

laryngoscope (ləring′gōskōp), *n* a hollow tube equipped with electrical lighting, used to examine or operate upon the interior of the larynx through the mouth.

laryngoscopy, *n* the use of a laryngoscope to view the larynx.

laryngospasm (ləring′gōspazəm), *n* the spasmodic closure of the larynx, sometimes noted during the induction phase of general anesthesia or during the recovery period.

larynx, *n* the organ of voice that is part of the air passage connecting the pharynx with the trachea.

laser, *n* a high-energy coordinated light source used in surgery, including for the experimental removal of the hard tissues of the teeth.

last will and testament, *n* the legal document describing the desires of a person for the distribution of that person's worldly goods after death.

latent, *adj* hidden; beneath the surface; not obvious or active.

latent image, *n* See image, latent.

latent period, *n* See period, latent.

lateral (lat′ərəl), *adj* a position either to the right or the left of the midsagittal plane.

lateral abscess, *n* See abscess, periodontal.

lateral cervical cysts, *n.pl* slowly growing cyst commonly developing on the mouth floor in children and teenagers, near the sternocleidomastoid muscle; removable by surgery. Also called *lymphoepithelial cyst* or *branchial cleft cyst.* See also lymphoepithelioma.

lateral checkbite, *n* See record, interocclusal.

lateral condylar inclination, *n* See inclination, lateral condylar.

lateral condyle path, *n* See path, lateral condyle.

lateral deviation, *n* **1.** a frontal asymmetry of the face in which one portion, usually the lower face, is lateral to the midsagittal plane. **2.** a condition of the temporo-mandibular joint, muscles of mastication, and the teeth that causes the lower jaw to move to one side on opening or forward thrust.

lateral excursion, *n* See excursion, lateral.

lateral lingual swellings, *n.pl* puffy sections of tongue that appear along the midline during embryonic development of the tongue structure.

lateral movement, *n* See movement, lateral.

lateral nasal processes, *n.pl* protrusions of tissue that border the olfactory pits during early embryonic development of the face.

lateral pressure, *n* the minimum amount of pressure that must be exerted by an instrument against teeth or tissue to achieve the desired effect.

lateral protrusion, *n* See protrusion, lateral.

lateroretrusive (lat′ərōrētrōō′siv), *n* pertaining to a movement direction in cusp or condyle thrusts that has both lateral and backward components of movement.

laterotrusion (lat′ərōtrōō′zhən), *n* the outward thrust given by the muscles to the rotating condyle or the condyle on the bolus side.

laterotrusion, precurrent, *n* laterotrusion in which the working side condyle is rotated as it is thrust laterally.

latex (lā′teks), *n* natural rubber.

latex allergy, *n* a hypersensitivity to natural rubber latex in which symptoms may range from minor skin irritations, hives, itchy eyes, and runny nose to asthma and life-threatening anaphylaxis. Since many items used during dental procedures contain rubber latex, patients should be routinely screened for this allergy.

latitude (lat′itōōd), *n* the range between the minimum and maximum film exposures to radiation that yields images of structures of which photographic density differences are discernible under normal viewing conditions. Latitude chiefly varies directly with kilovoltage and inversely with contrast. See also contrast.

lattice, space (lat′is), *n* an arrangement of atoms in a definite relationship to each other, forming a lattice.

lavage (ləväzh′), *n* irrigation, or washing out, as in oral lavage.

lavage, fluid, *n* spray washing of the periodontal pocket that occurs as the result of fluid flowing through the tip of a mechanized instrument.

law(s), *n* **1.** that which is laid down or established. An enforceable rule of conduct. *n.pl* **2.** that which must be obeyed and followed by citizens, subject to sanctions or legal consequences. The term is also used in opposition to fact. For example, in a lawsuit, questions of law are to be decided by the court, whereas the jury decides questions in fact.

law, administrative, *n* a set of specific rules and regulations overseen by an administrative agency in order to enforce the law.

law, case, *n* the use of citations of previous court opinions in a court case, taken from the court decisions published by the state and federal government.

law, Charles's, n the principle that states that all gases expand equally upon heating and contract equally upon cooling.

law, constitutional, n the set of supreme laws set out in the U.S. Constitution. All other state and federal laws must be in accordance with the laws of the Constitution. The Constitution designates the roles of the three branches of government as well as setting forth which areas of law are in federal jurisdiction and which are left to the states.

law, Dalton's, n the principle that states that the pressure of a mixture of gases equals the sum of the partial pressures of the constituent gases.

law, ignorance of, n a want of knowledge or acquaintance with the laws of the land insofar as they apply to the act, relation, duty, or matter under consideration.

law, inverse-square, n principle stating that the strength of radiation from a point source varies inversely as the square of the distance.

law, judicial, n the interpretation of the written law by the courts. Decisions are often based on *stare decisis,* the doctrine that allows the court to follow the decision made in a previous case in the same jurisdiction. A departure from the legal precedents is known as a *landmark decision.*

law, moral, n the aggregate of rules and principles of ethics that relate to right and wrong conduct and prescribe the standards to which the actions of persons should conform in their dealings with each other.

law, neurologic, n See law of specific energy.

law of radiosensitivity, Bergonie-Tribondeau, n.pr law stating that the resistance or sensitivity to radiation depends on the metabolic state of a cell, tissue, or an organ.

law of specific energy (neurologic law), n principle that states, in essence, that sensory quality is perceived according to the nerve that is excited, not according to the object that excites. If pressure placed on the eyeballs stimulates the retina, light is perceived, not pressure; similarly, electrical stimulation will produce sensations of smell, taste, touch, or pain in accordance with the nerve stimulated but not a sensation of electricity as such. The special as well as the general senses maintain this principle.

law, tort, n area of law that deals with civil wrongs perpetrated against another person or private property. The primary concerns in dentistry are negligence and malpractice. Any lapse in professional standards may be subject to proceedings for negligence or malpractice.

law, Wolff's, n principle that states that all changes in the function of bone are attended by definite alterations in its internal structure.

law(s), written, n/n.pl law or laws created by express legislation or enactment, as distinguished from *unwritten* or *common law,* which includes all law or laws from any other legal source.

lay, adj nonprofessional.

layer, Beilby's (bil′bēz), n.pr an amorphous layer formed on the surface of metals by a disorientation of the crystalline structure during polishing.

LD50, n See dose, lethal, median.

LD$_{50}$ time, n See time, median lethal.

LDL, n.pl See lipoproteins, low-density.

lead, n a common soft, blue-gray, metallic element. Its atomic number is 82, and its atomic weight is 207. In its metallic form, lead is used as a protective shielding against x-rays. Lead is poisonous, a characteristic that has led to a reduction in the use of lead compound as pigments for paints and inks.

lead apron, n See apron, lead.

lead glass, n See glass, lead.

lead-lined cylindrical position-indicating device, n an cylinder open at both ends that is lined with lead and used to aim an x-ray beam.

lead poisoning, n See plumbism.

leadership, n the ability to influence others to achieve individual and group goals. Kinds of leadership include authoritarian, democratic, participative, and permissive.

leaf gauge, n See gauge, leaf.

learning, n the process of acquiring knowledge or some skill by means of study, practice, and/or experience.

learning disability, n inability to learn at a rate comparable to most members of a peer group. Some learning disorders have been traced to nutritional and behavioral causes, others stem from trauma or disease, and still others have genetic origins.

learning domains, n.pl the three spheres of learning—cognitive, affective, and psychomotor—that must be addressed by a teacher in order to influence behavioral change on the part of the learner. May be applied to the teaching of disease control.

learning-ladder continuum, *n* theory suggesting that learning takes place in sequential steps beginning with ignorance and culminating with habit. The process may be applied to the teaching of effective plaque control.

lease, *n* **1.** a conveyance of lands or tenements to a person for life, for a stated number of years, or at will, in consideration of rent or some other recompense. **2.** any agreement that gives rise to a landlord and tenant relationship.

least expensive alternative treatment (LEAT), *n* a limitation in a dental benefits plan that will only allow benefits for the least expensive treatment. Also referred to as *least expensive professionally acceptable alternative treatment (LEPAAT).*

lecithin (les´ithin), *n* a class of phosphatides containing glycerol, phosphate, choline, and fatty acids. Lecithins are widely distributed in cells and possess both metabolic and structural functions in membranes. Dipalmityl lecithin is an important surface-active agent in the lungs.

ledger sheet, *n* an accounting form for keeping track of debits, expenditures, credits, and charges.

leeway space, *n* the arch circumference difference between the primary canine, first primary and second primary molars, and the permanent canine and the first and second premolars. According to Black's means, the maxillary arch leeway space is 1.9 mm, and the mandibular arch leeway space is 3.4 mm.

LeFort fracture, *n.pr* See fracture, LeFort.

left justified, *n* data are left-justified when the left-most digit or character occupies the left-most position of the space allotted for those data.

legal, *adj* **1.** in compliance with the law. **2.** not forbidden by law.

Legionella *n* a genus of areobic, motile, non–acid fast, nonencapsulated, gram-negative bacilli that have a nonfermentative metabolism. They are water dwelling, airborne spread, and pathogenic for man.

Legionella pneumonia, *n* a form of pneumonia caused by a gram-negative bacillus identified as *Legionella pneumophila.* It was discovered after an outbreak of the disease among veterans attending a 1976 convention of the American Legion.

Legionella pneumophila, *n* a small, gram-negative, rod-shaped bacterium that is the causative agent of Legionnaires' disease.

Legionnaires' disease, *n.pr* an acute bacterial pneumonia caused by infection with *L. pneumophila* and characterized by an influenza-like illness followed within a week by high fever, chills, muscle aches, and headache. Contaminated air conditioning cooling towers and stagnant water supplies, including water vaporizers and water sonicators, may be a source of organisms.

legislation, *n* the act of making or forming law, or the laws and/or statutes formed by the legislative process.

legumes (ləgyōōmz´), *n* any plant belonging to the order Fabales and family Leguminosae. Examples of legumes are beans, peas, and lentils.

leiomyoma (lī´-ōmī-ō´mə), *n* a benign tumor derived from smooth muscle.

leiomyosarcoma, *n* a malignant neoplasm of muscle that contains spindle cells of unstriated muscle.

leishmaniasis, *n* an infection with any species of protozoan of the genus *Leishmania.*

length, *n* the longest measure of an object, or the measurement between the two ends.

length, muscle, n the variable end-to-end measurement of a muscle. The physical changes in muscle observed in the isotonic and isometric states of contraction are related to the alteration in the striated bands of muscle.

length of stay, n the expected length of time, usually a median, that institutionalized patients of similar age and diagnosis or condition in a hospital or other health care facility would be expected to remain.

length, tooth, n the distance along the long axis of the tooth from the apex of the root to the tip, or incisal edge, of the tooth.

lens, crystalline, n the lens of the eye.

lenses, curved, *n.pl* transparent pieces of plastic or glass that are shaped, molded, or ground to refract light in a specific way, as in eyeglasses, microscopes, or cameras.

lentulo (lentōō´lə), n a flexible spiral-wire instrument used in a handpiece to apply paste filling materials in root canals.

leontiasis ossea (lē´ontī´-əsis ŏs´ē-ə), n an enlargement of the bones of the face, leading to a lionlike appearance. Osseous encroachment may cause obliteration of sinuses, blindness, and malocclusion.

leproma, n a nodular lesion of leprosy seen on the skin, mucous membranes (including those of the eyes), upper respiratory tract, tongue, and palate.

leprosy (lep´rōsē), n a chronic granulomatous infection caused by *Mycobacterium leprae.* It may exist in lepromatous (contagious), tuberculoid (noncontagious), and intermediate forms.

Leprosy. (Neville/Damm/Allen/Bouquot, 2002)

leptocytosis, hereditary (lep´tōsī-tō´sis), n See thalassemia.

Leptothrix **(lep´tōthriks),** n a filamentous microorganism, apparently not directly capable of pathogenicity, that may act as a nidus for the formation of dental calculus and its attachment to the tooth structure. Some investigators have associated

this organism with the presence of periodontitis in human beings.

Lesch-Nyhan syndrome, *n.pr* a hereditary disorder of purine metabolism, characterized by mental retardation, self-mutilation of the fingers and lips by biting, impaired renal function, and abnormal physical development. It is transmitted as a recessive, sex-linked trait.

lesion (lē´zhən), n any pathologic disturbance of a tissue, with loss of continuity, enlargement, and/or function.

lesion, extravasation, n See cyst, traumatic.

lesion, flat oral, n a regularly or irregularly shaped laceration developing on the surface of the oral mucosa or normal skin.

Flat oral lesions. (Regezi/Sciubba/Jordan, 2003)

lesion, herpetic, n a vesicle and/or ulceration of the mucosa caused by the herpes virus.

lesion, herpetiform, n a painful ulceration of the oral mucosa with a red center and yellow border; occurs as a solitary lesion or in groups and appears similar to those lesions caused by herpes virus. The term *herpetiform* is used as a clinical designation unless the viral cause has actually been demonstrated.

lesion, indefinite bone, n See cyst, extravasation.

lesion, mucous extravasation, n.pl See cyst, mucous.

lesion, noncarious dental, n.pl abnormalities occurring on the surfaces of teeth that do not fall under the category of dental cavities. They may include enamel hypoplasia, attrition, erosion, abrasion, or tooth fractures.

lesion, precancerous, n a tissue abnormality or wound that although not yet malignant shows signs indicating the likely development of cancer in the future.

lesion, subsurface, *n* an area of softness below the tooth enamel that occurs as the result of acid retention. Can be corrected by fluoride administration.

lesion, traumatic bone, *n* See cyst, traumatic.

LET, *n* See transfer, linear energy.

lethargy (leth´ärjē), *n* sluggishness or fatigue; a feeling of listlessness.

Letterer-Siwe disease, *n.pr* See disease, Letterer-Siwe.

leucine, *n* one of the essential amino acids. See also amino acid.

leucovorin calcium (citrovorum factor/folinic acid), *n trade name:* Wellcovorin; *drug class:* folic acid antagonist antidote, antineoplastic adjunct; *action:* chemically reduced derivative of folic acid, converted to tetrahydrofolate; *counteracts* folic acid antagonists; *uses:* megaloblastic or macrocytic anemia caused by folic acid deficiency, overdose of folic acid antagonist, methotrexate toxicity caused by pyrimethamine or trimethoprim, or in colorectal cancer with fluorouracil.

leukemia (lōōkē´mē-ə), *n* a usually fatal disease of the blood-forming tissues characterized by the abnormal proliferation of leukocytes and their precursors and attended by fatigue, weakness, fever, lymphadenopathy, splenomegaly, and a tendency toward profuse tissue hemorrhage. Oral lesions include gingival enlargement, severe gingivitis, and necrosis. Lymphatic, monocytic, and myelogenous leukemias are the chief types.

Leukemia. (Regezi/Sciubba/Jordan, 2003)

leukemia, aleukemia, *n* a phase of the leukemic state marked by proliferation of leukocytes within the blood-forming tissues but without an increase in the white blood cell count: relatively few precursor cells are found in the blood smear until the phase passes and the blood becomes flooded with white cells. Oral lesions, when present, are ulceronecrotic and hypertrophic.

leukemia, lymphatic (lymphoid leukemia), *n* a hyperplasia, of undetermined origin, affecting lymphoid tissue. Predominating cells are lymphocytes and lymphoblasts. Generally assumes a more chronic course than other forms of leukemia but may be acute. Oral lesions include swollen and hyperplastic gingivae, ulceronecrotic lesions, and marked tendency to gingival hemorrhage.

leukemia, monocytic, *n* a form of leukemia characterized by an abnormal increase in the number of monocytes. Manifestations include progressive weakness, anorexia, lymphadenopathy, hepatomegaly, splenomegaly, and secondary anemia. Oral lesions may be ulceronecrotic or hemorrhagic.

leukemia, myelogenous, *n* leukemia in which the leukocytes are of bone marrow origin (for example, polymorphonuclear leukocytes, myelocytes, myeloblasts). Oral manifestations may include gingival enlargement and necrosis.

leukocyte (lōō´kōsīt), *n* **I.** a white blood cell. **2.** a white blood cell; a nucleated ameboid mass of protoplasm circulating in the blood. See also lymphocyte and monocyte.

leukocyte, basophilic, *n* a basophil; a leukocyte that has coarse granules stainable with basic dyes and a bent lobed nucleus.

leukocyte count, *n* the number of leukocytes in a cubic millimeter of blood. Normal values range from 5,000 to 10,000/mm^3.

leukocyte, eosinophilic, *n* an eosinophil; a leukocyte that has coarse granules stainable with eosin and a bilobed nucleus.

leukocyte, immature, *n* one of several forms of leukocyte usually found in disease (for example, myelocytes, myeloblasts, lymphoblasts).

leukocyte, polymorphonuclear, *n* **I.** a neutrophil; a white blood cell with finely granular cytoplasm, an irregularly lobulated nucleus, and the appearance of a microphage. It is found in the tissues during acute inflammatory processes and in the superficial surface aspects of a lesion during subacute or chronic inflammation. It is the predominating leukocyte of the blood. Blood levels may be increased during acute inflammatory states and myelogenous leukemia, and decreased in agranulocytosis (malignant neutropenia). **2.** a neutrophil; a polymorph; a leukocyte that has fine granules stainable with neutral dyes and an irregularly lobed nucleus.

leukocytosis (lōō′kōsītō′sis), *n* an increase in the normal number of white blood cells; may be a defensive reaction, as in inflammation, or may result from a disturbance in white blood cell formation, as in leukemia. Various limits are given; for example, leukocytosis in the adult is indicated when there are more than 10,000 white blood cells per cubic millimeter. See also eosinophilia; lymphocytosis; neutrophilia.

leukoedema (lōō′kō-ədē′mə), *n* an innocuous oral condition characterized by a filmy, opalescent, white covering of the buccal mucosa consisting of a thickened layer of parakeratotic cells. It is most commonly associated with mechanical and chemical irritation.

leukopenia (lōō′kōpē′nē-ə), *n* a decrease in the normal number of white blood cells in the circulating blood. Various lower limits are given; for example, leukopenia signifies less than 4,000 white blood cells per cubic millimeter. See also lymphocytopenia; neutropenia.

leukoplakia (lōō′kōplā′kē-ə), *n* **I.** a white plaque formed on the oral mucous membrane from surface epithelial cells. It is leathery, opaque, and somewhat thickened. Excluded from this are the white lesions of lichen planus, white sponge nevus, burns, thrush, and other clinically recognizable entities. Histologically, hyperkeratosis, acanthosis, and subepithelial and perivascular infiltrate of round cells may be seen. Dyskeratosis may be present. Leukoplakia lesions may progress to malignancy, with cellular atypicism, dyskeratosis, epithelial pearl formation, and infil-

tration of malignant cells into connective tissue corium. **2.** a premalignant surface lesion of the mucous membrane characterized by hyperkeratosis and dyskeratosis of the stratified squamous epithelium. See also dyskeratosis; hyperkeratosis.

Leukoplakia. (Regezi/Sciubba/Pogrel, 2000)

leukoplakia, hairy, *n* a white lesion appearing on the lateral surface of the tongue and occasionally on the buccal mucosa of patients with AIDS. The lesion appears raised, with a corrugated or "hairy" surface as a result of keratin projections.

leukotaxine (lōō′kōtak′sin), *n* a substance that appears when tissue is injured and can be removed from inflammatory exudates. Increases capillary permeability and the diapedesis of leukocytes.

lev-, *pref* See levo-.

levamisole HCl, *n* *trade name:* Ergamisol; *drug class:* immunomodulator; *action:* may increase the action of macrophages, monocytes, and T cells, which will restore immune function; *uses:* Dukes's stage C colon cancer, given with fluorouracil after surgical resection.

level (lev′əl), *v* to reduce the curve of Spee by intrusion and/or extrusion of the teeth in an arch.

leveling arch wire, *n* an arch wire used to align teeth in the same plane.

lever (lev′ur), *n* a bar or rigid body that is capable of turning about one joint or axis and in which are two or more other points where forces are applied. There are three classes of levers, and each has its own most effective use.

lever leverage (lev′ərəj), *n* the mechanical advantage gained by the use of a lever. A factor in the magnification of stresses generated by an extension-base partial denture.

lever, second-class, n a lever in which the force arm is longer than the work-producing arm; thus the work produced is always greater than the energy used, with a resultant high efficiency.

lever, third-class, n a lever in which the axis is at one end, the load at the other end, and the effort is exerted in between, as in a treadle.

levigated aluminum, n fine particles of aluminum oxide used to polish metals, but unsuitable for polishing teeth. See emery.

levo- (lev) (lē′vō), *pref* a prefix applied to the name of optical isomers that rotate the plane of polarized light to the left.

levobunolol hydrochloride, n *trade name:* Akbeta, Betagan C Cap BID, Betagan C Cap QD, Betagan Standard; *drug class:* b-adrenergic blocker; *action:* reduces production of aqueous humor by unknown mechanisms; *uses:* chronic open-angle glaucoma, ocular hypertension.

levocabastine HCl, n *trade name:* Livostin; *drug class:* antihistamine, H_1-receptor antagonist; *action:* selective antagonist for histamine at H_1 receptors; little or no systemic absorption; intended for topical effect; *uses:* temporary relief of seasonal allergic conjunctivitis.

levodopa, n *trade names:* Larodopa, Dopar; *class drug:* antiparkinson agent; *action:* levodopa is decarboxylated to dopamine, which can interact with dopamine receptors; *uses:* parkinsonism or parkinsonian symptoms.

levodopa-carbidopa, n *trade names:* Sinemet, Sinemet CR; *drug class:* antiparkinson agent; *action:* decarboxylation of levodopa to periphery is inhibited by carbidopa; more levodopa is made available for transport to brain and conversion to dopamine in the brain; *uses:* treatment of idiopathic, symptomatic, or postencephalitic parkinsonism.

levomethadyl acetate HCl, n *trade name:* ORLAAM; *drug class:* synthetic opioid; *action:* mimics the action of opioid analgesics by interacting with CNS opioid receptors;

use: management of opioid dependence.

levonordefrin (lē′vōnôrdef′rin), n an ingredient that may be added to a local anesthetic for the purpose of constricting blood vessels. It helps to contain the anesthetic in a specific area by reducing systemic absorption, decreasing blood flow, and prolonging effectiveness. *Brand name:* Neo-Cobefrin (no longer produced under this brand).

levonorgestrel implant, n *trade name:* Norplant System; *drug class:* contraceptive system; *action:* as a progestin, transforms proliferative endometrium into secretory endometrium; inhibits secretion of pituitary gonadotropins, which prevents follicular maturation and ovulation; *use:* prevention of pregnancy.

levothyroxine sodium, n *trade names:* Levo-T, Synthroid; *drug class:* thyroid hormone; *action:* increases metabolic rate, with increase in cardiac output, O_2 consumption, body temperature, blood volume, growth/development at cellular level; *uses:* hypothroidism, myxedema coma, thyroid hormone replacement, cretinism.

Leydig cells, *n.pr* cells of the interstitial tissue of the testes that secrete testosterone.

liabilities, *n.pl* all claims against a corporation. Liabilities include accounts and wages and salaries payable, dividends declared payable, accrued taxes payable, and fixed or long-term liabilities, such as mortgage bonds, debentures, and bank loans.

liabilities, current, *n.pl* short-term debts and obligations that must be paid within a period of 1 year.

liability (lī-əbil′itē), n the state of being bound by law or justice to do something or to make good something; legal responsibility.

libel (lī′bəl), n **1.** that which is written and published in order to injure the character of another by ridicule or contempt. **2.** defamation expressed by print, writing, pictures, or signs.

library, n a place established to contain books, manuscripts, and other material for reading, study, viewing, listening, or reference, usually consisting of organized stacks and files to contain reference materials as well as places to read, copy, view, or listen to the selected material.

license, *n* permission, accorded by a competent authority, granting the right to perform some act or acts that without such authorization would be contrary to law.

licensure, *n* the granting of permission by a competent authority (usually a government agency) to an organization or individual to engage in a practice or activity that would otherwise be illegal. Licensure is usually granted on the basis of education and examination rather than performance. It is usually permanent, but a periodic fee, demonstration of competence, or continuing education may be required. Licensure may be revoked by the granting agency for incompetence, criminal acts, or other reasons stipulated in the statutes or rules governing the specific area of licensure.

licensure, dental, n the permission to practice dentistry in a specific geopolitical area, granted by a government agency.

lichen planus (lī′kən plā′nəs), *n* **1.** a disease of unknown etiology affecting the skin and oral mucous membranes, either alone or concomitantly. The oral lesions are most common on the buccal mucous membrane, where they appear as a lacy pattern or bilateral network of raised white or bluish-white, porcelain-like fine lines or a series of small, similarly appearing dots. The lesions are painless. On the tongue the lesions may appear as flat white plaques resembling leukoplakia. **2.** a dermatologic disease affecting the skin and mucous membranes; of unknown etiology but often associated with nervousness, fatigue, emotional depression, and allergy and considered to be a manifestation of quinacrine (Atabrine) therapy. Oral lesions often appear as white or blue-white striae forming an interweaving lacelike network of lines of epithelial thickening. Associated with the striated network; bullous or erosive lesions may be found. Histologically, varying degrees of hyperkeratosis and epithelial acanthosis may be found, with formation of sawtooth-shaped rete pegs of epithelium projecting into connective tissue corium. Subjacent to the epithelium is a bandlike infiltrate of round cells with perivascular accumulation of leukocytes. Treatment is symptomatic.

Lichen planus. (Regezi/Sciubba/Jordan, 2003)

lichen planus, oral, n See lichen planus.

lidocaine HCl (cardiac), *n trade names:* Lidopen, Xylocaine, Xylocard; *drug class:* antidysrhythmic (Class IB); *action:* increases electrical stimulation threshold of ventricle and His-Purkinje system, which stabilizes cardiac membrane and decreases automaticity and excitability of ventricles; *uses:* ventricular tachycardia, ventricular dysrhythmias during cardiac surgery, cardiac catheterization.

lidocaine HCl (local), *n trade names:* Dalcaine, Dilocaine, Lidoject, Octocain, Xylocaine, Xylocaine-MPF; *drug class:* amide local anesthetic; *action:* inhibits ion fluxes across membranes, particularly sodium transport across cell membrane, decreases rise of depolarization phase of action potential, blocks nerve action potential; *uses:* local dental anesthesia, peripheral nerve block; caudal anesthesia; epidural, spinal, surgical anesthesia.

lidocaine HCl (topical), *n generic name:* Xylocaine Viscous; *drug class:* topically acting local anesthetic, amide; *action:* inhibits nerve impulses from sensory nerves, which produces anesthesia; *uses:* topical anesthesia of inflamed or irritated mucous membranes; to reduce gag reflex in dental radiologic examination or in dental impressions.

lien (lēn), *n* a qualified right of property that a creditor has in specific property of the debtor as security for the debt or for performance of some act.

life, effective half-, *n* See half-life, effective.

life expectancy, *n* the probable number of years a person will live after a given age, as determined by the mortality rate in a specific geographic area. This number may be individually qualified by the person's condition, race, sex, age, and other demographic factors.

life, radioactive, *n* See half-life.

ligament (lig´əment), *n* any tough, fibrous connective tissue band that connects bones or supports viscera. Some of the ligaments are distinct fibrous structures, others are folds of fascia or of indurated peritoneum; still others are the relics of unused fetal organs.

ligament, biologic width of periodontal, *n* the width of the periodontal ligament in normal, functioning teeth. It varies with the age of the individual and the functional demands made on the tooth. In normalcy, the periodontal ligament is about 0.25 and 0.1 mm in width, narrowest at the center of the alveolus and widest at the margin and apex.

ligament, periodontal (PDL), *n* the mode of attachment of the tooth to the alveolus. The ligament consists of numerous bundles of collagenous tissue (principal fibers) arranged in groups, between which is loose connective tissue, together with blood vessels, lymph vessels, and nerves. It functions as the investing and supportive mechanism for the tooth.

ligament, sphenomandibular, *n* the ligament extending from the spine of the sphenoid bone to the mandibular lingula.

ligament, stylohyoid, *n* a fibroelastic cord attached superior to the styloid process of the sphenoid bone.

ligament, stylomandibular, *n* a ligament extending from the styloid process of the temporal bone and attached to the mandibular gonial angle.

ligament, temporomandibular, *n* a triangular-shaped fibrous band extending from the lateral aspects of the root of the zygomatic process of

the temporal bone to the mandibular subcondylar neck.

ligand, *n* **I.** a molecule, ion, or group bound to the central atom of a chemical compound, such as the oxygen molecule in hemoglobin, which is bound to the central iron atom. **2.** an organic molecule attached to a specific site on a surface or to a tracer element.

ligate (lī´gāt), *v* to tie or bind with a ligature or suture.

ligation (līgā´shən), *n* the binding together of tissue or teeth with wire, string, or thread for stabilization and immobilization.

ligation, surgical, *n* the exposure of an unerupted tooth with placement of a metal ligature across its cervix. The free ends of the ligature are fixed to a fine, precious-metal chain, which in turn is fixed to an orthodontic appliance for the purpose of placing traction on the unerupted tooth to cause its eruption.

ligature (lig´əchur), *n* **I.** a cord, thread, or fine wire tied around teeth for the purpose of holding a rubber dam in place on retained teeth with fractured roots or split crowns or on teeth that have been replanted. **2.** a wire or threadlike substance used to tie a tooth to an orthodontic appliance or to another tooth.

ligature, grass-line, *n* a ligature composed of the fibers of a grass-cloth plant (ramie); used for minor tooth movement. It depends for its activation in movement on the property of shrinkage of the ligature when it is wet by the saliva of the patient.

ligature, steel, *n* a form of ligature, available as steel filaments in several useful diameters.

light, *n* **I.** electromagnetic radiation of the wavelength and frequency that stimulate visual receptor cells in the retina to produce nerve impulses that are perceived as vision. **2.** visible light ranges from 400 to 800 nm.

light box, *n* See illuminator.

light, chemiluminescent, *n* light produced by the conversion of chemical energy into light energy.

light fog, *n* See film fault, fogged.

light leaks, *n.pl* See film fault, dark.

light, operating, *n* a light with a strong beam that may be directed for concentrated illumination of a part being operated on.

light pen, *n* a pointerlike device available with some computer terminals. A light pen selects data displayed on the screen by being pointed at any desired item.

light touch, *n* See touch, light.

lighting, *n* the arrangement of a light source to create a certain effect. The lighting of a dental operatory is done to achieve a sufficient level of lighting to reduce eye strain in shifting from one field of vision to another and to achieve a light intensity across the spectrum to mimic natural light.

lignin (lig′nin), *n* one of several heteropolysaccharides contained in the cell walls of plants which provides dietary fiber for digestion.

limbic system, *n* a group of structures within the rhinencephalon of the brain that are associated with various emotions and feelings, such as anger, fear, sexual arousal, pleasure, and sadness. Unless the limbic system is modulated by other cortical areas, periodic attacks of uncontrollable rage may occur in some individuals. The function of the system is poorly understood.

limit, *n* restriction.

limit, elastic (proportional limit), *n* the greatest stress to which a material may be subjected and still be capable of returning to its original dimensions when the forces are released.

limit, proportional, *n* See limit, elastic.

limitations, *n* restrictive conditions stated in a dental benefits contract, such as age, length of time covered, and waiting periods, which affect an individual's or group's coverage. The contract may also exclude certain benefits or services, or it may limit the extent or condition under which certain services are provided. See also exclusions.

limited treatment, *n* treatment directed at a limited objective; not involving the entire dentition. It may be directed at the only existing problem, or at only one aspect of a larger problem in which a decision is made to defer more comprehensive therapy.

lincomycin, *n* *trade names:* Lincocin, Lincorex; *drug class:* antibacterial; *action:* binds to 50S subunit of bacterial ribosomes; suppresses protein synthesis; *uses:* infections caused by group A β-hemolytic streptococci, pneumococci, staphylococci (respiratory tract, skin, soft tissue, urinary tract infections; osteomyelitis; septicemia), and anaerobes. Lincomycin should be reserved for pencillin-allergic patients. Close clinical supervision is required because of severe colitis has been associated with lincomycin therapy. *Brand name:* Lincocin.

lindane, *n* γ-benzene hexachloride prescribed in the treatment of pediculosis and scabies.

line, *n* a boundary; demarcation.

line angle, *n* See angle, line.

line, basophilic, *n* a group of microscopic sections of bone that stains darkly with hematoxylin. Represents periods of bone inactivity.

line, Camper's, *n.pr* the line running from the inferior border of the ala of the nose to the superior border of the tragus of the ear.

line, cement, *n* the line of cement exposed at the margin of an inlay or crown.

line, cementing, *n* a basophilic line distinguishing adjacent lamellae of bone; represents periods of inactivity of bone formation and resorption.

line, cervical, *n* See junction, cementoenamel.

line, cross arch fulcrum, *n* See line, fulcrum, cross arch.

line, external oblique, *n* a ridge of osseous structure on the body of the mandible extending from the anterolateral border to the mandibular ramus, passing downward and forward, after covering the buccocervical portion of the third molar, and ending by blending into the molar teeth.

line, finish, *n* in cavity preparations, a minimal line of demarcation of the wall of the preparation at the cavosurface angle; usually results from a slice made by an abrasive disk.

line focus, *n* a principle employed in the design of x-ray tubes, by which the effective focal spot is sharply reduced relative to the actual (larger) focal spot desirable to deal with the heat generated. It involves focusing the cathode stream, in the pattern of a thin rectangle, onto an anode truncated at about 20 degrees to the transverse axis of the tube. See also spot, focal, effective.

line, fulcrum, n any imaginary line around which a removable partial denture tends to rotate.

line, fulcrum, anteroposterior, n an imaginary line of rotation extending through the rest and other support areas along the same side of a removable partial denture.

line, fulcrum, cross arch, n an imaginary line through the tooth-supported rest areas nearest to soft tissue-supported areas and around which the partial denture will tend to rotate when forces are applied to the soft tissue-supported areas.

line, lead, n a bluish-black patch on the gingival tissues, usually about 1 mm from the gingival crest. Caused by the deposition of fine granules of lead sulfide in the tissues. A sign of lead absorption in lead poisoning (plumbism).

line, median, n the intersection of the midsagittal plane with the maxillary and mandibular dental arches. The center line divides the central body surface into right and left.

line, mercurial, n a linear area of abnormal pigmentation of the gingival tissues associated with mercury poisoning. Seen along the gingival margin, it has been variously described as bluish, brownish, dirty reddish, or purplish in coloration.

line, neonatal, n line on a primary tooth marking the point at which prenatal growth stops and postnatal growth begins. See line, Owen contour.

line of credit, n an arrangement whereby a financial institution (bank or insurance company) commits itself to lend up to a specified maximum amount of funds during a specified period. The interest rate on the loan may be specified or not. Sometimes a commitment fee is imposed for obtaining the line of credit.

line of draw, n the direction or plane of withdrawal or seating of a removable or cemented restoration.

line of force, n See force, line of.

line of occlusion, n the alignment of the occluding surfaces of the teeth in the horizontal plane. See also plane, occlusal line.

line of Retzius, n.pr one of several

incremental lines appearing in the mature enamel, named for the Swedish anatomist and anthropologist who first described the line in 1873.

line, Owen contour, n.pr one of a series of adjoining imbrication lines in dentin that demonstates a disturbance in body metabolism. See line, neonatal.

line printer, n a fast printing device. A line printer prints on paper each line of characters in one operation, rather than character by character.

line, protrusive, n one of the three tracings made on each of the six projection planes of a jaw motion data recorder.

line, survey, n a line produced on the various portions of a dental cast by a surveyor, scriber, or marker. It designates the greatest height of contour in relation to the orientation of the cast to the vertical scriber.

line, vibrating, n the imaginary line across the posterior part of the palate marking the division between the movable and relatively immovable tissues of the palate.

linea alba buccalis, n a normal variation in the buccal mucosa that appears as a white line beginning at the corners of the mouth and extending posteriorly at the level of the occlusal plane.

Linea alba buccalis. (Daniel/Harfst, 2002. Courtesy Dr. Alice Curran, Jackson, Miss.)

linear energy transfer (LET), n the linear rate of loss of energy by an ionizing particle traversing a material medium.

linear models, n.pl statistical models in which the value of a parameter for a given value of a factor is assumed to be equal to $a + bx$, where a and b are constants. The models predict a linear regression.

linen strip, n See strip, abrasive.

liner, cavity, n See varnish, cavity.

lines, *n.pl* elongated marks traced by a stylus on a gnathic projection plane, indicating direction of movement related variously to condyle movements.

lingua alba, *n* See tongue, white hairy.

lingua nigra, *n* See tongue, black hairy.

lingual (ling′gwəl), *adj* pertaining to the tongue.

lingual appliances, *n.pl* orthodontic appliances that apply force from the lingual aspect of the anterior teeth. This mode of treatment is used to reduce the visibility of the appliance and thus improve the appearance of the smile during treatment.

lingual arch, *n* a space-holding arch or the basic arch for an active lingual orthodontic appliance. The arch usually spans around the inside of the dental arch from one first permanent molar to its antimere.

lingual bar, major connector, *n* See connector, major, lingual bar.

lingual button, *n* an attachment welded to the lingual side of the canine, premolar, or molar bands.

lingual fossa(e), *n* a depressed area that may appear on the lingual surface of selected anterior teeth.

lingual frenum, *n* a band of tissue that extends from the floor of the mouth to the inferior surface of the tongue.

lingual groove, *n* a furrow or channel that forms on the tongue side of selected front teeth.

lingual nerve, *n* See nerve(s).

lingual papillae, *n* the tiny, red protrusions covering the top surface of the tongue on which most of the taste buds can be found.

lingual peak, gingival, *n* a lingual peak that characterizes the normal interproximal tissue, which is composed of a lingual papilla and a buccal papilla connected interdentally in a triangular ridge depression termed a col.

lingual plate, *n* See connector, major, linguoplate.

lingual ridge, *n* a linear elevation that extends vertically from the chewing surface to the lingual developmental lobe on the tongue side of a canine tooth.

lingual tonsil, *n* a small nodule of lymphoid tissue that can be found just behind the circumvallate papillae at the base of the tongue.

lingula (ling′gyōōlə), *n* a small, tonguelike projection of bone forming the anterior border of the mandibular foramen.

linguocclusion (ling-gwəklōō′zhən), *n* an occlusion in which the dental arch or group of teeth is lingual to normal.

linguoplate, *n* See connector, major, linguoplate.

linguoversion, *n* the state of being displaced toward the tongue.

linkage (ling′kəj), *n* the connection between two or more objects. In computer programming, coding that connects two separately coded routines.

linkage, cross, *n* See polymerization, cross.

linkage, sex, *n* the inheritance of certain characteristics that are determined by genes located in the sex chromosomes.

linoleic acid, *n* an unsaturated fatty acid essential to nutrition. Linoleic acid occurs in many plant glycerides.

liothyronine sodium (T₃), *n trade names:* Cytomel, Triostat; *drug class:* thyroid hormone; *action:* increases metabolic rate with increase in cardiac output, O₂ consumption, body temperature, blood volume, growth/development at cellular level; *uses:* hypothyroidism, myxedema coma, thyroid hormone replacement, cretinism, nontoxic goiter.

liotrix, *n trade names:* Euthroid, Thyrolar; *drug class:* thyroid hormone; *action:* increases metabolic rates, cardiac output, O₂ consumption, body temperature, blood volume, growth/development at cellular level; *uses:* hypothyroidism, thyroid hormone replacement.

lip, *n* **1.** either the upper or lower fleshy structure surrounding the opening of the oral cavity. **2.** any rimlike structure bordering a cavity or groove.

lip biting, *n* an oral habit in which either lip is placed between the teeth with more or less forcible application of the teeth to the lips.

lip, cleft, *n* See harelip.

lip, congenital cleft, *n* See harelip.

lip, double, *n* a redundant fold of tissue on the mucosal side of the upper lip that gives the appearance of a second lip and that may become accentuated by habitually being sucked between the teeth.

lip line, high, *n* the greatest height to which the lip is raised in normal function or during the act of smiling broadly.

lip line, low, *n* the lowest position of the lower lip during the act of smiling or voluntary retraction. The lowest position of the upper lip at rest.

lip pits (congenital lip fistulas), *n.pl* congenital depressions, usually bilateral and symmetrically placed, on the vermilion portion of the lower lip. These pits may be circular or may be present as a transverse slit. The depression represents a blind fistula that penetrates downward into the lower lip to a depth of 0.5 to 2.5 cm. They often exude viscid saliva on pressure.

lip retractor, *n* an apparatus to retract the lips when taking intraoral photographs.

lip, structures of, *n.pl* See vermilion border; vestibule, labial; frenum, labial.

lipase, *n* any fat-splitting or lipolytic enzyme.

lipid (lip′id), *n* a heterogeneous group of substances related actually or potentially to the fatty acids that are soluble in nonpolar solvents such as benzene, chloroform, and ether and are relatively insoluble in water. Included are the fatty acids, acylglycerols, phospholipids, cerebrosides, and steroids.

lipid, plasma, *n* the various plasma lipid classes include triacylglycerols, phospholipids, cholesterol, cholesterol esters, and unesterified fatty acids. Because of their hydrophobic nature, plasma lipids are carried in association with specific plasma proteins, the lipoproteins.

lipidosis (lip′ido̅′sis), *n* See disease, lipid storage.

Lipiodol (lipe̅′o̅dəl), *n.pr* the trade name for an iodized oil used as an opaque contrast medium in radiography. When it is laced within periodontal pockets and radiographs are made, the depth and topography of periodontal pockets may be ascertained.

Lip structures. (Liebgott, 2001)

lipodystrophy, *n* any abnormality in the metabolism or deposition of fats.

lipogenesis (lip'ōjen'əsis), *n* the process that converts excess dietary carbohydrates into fat for storage as a source of long-term energy.

lipoids (lip'oidz), *n* a fatlike substance that may not actually be related to the fatty acids, although lipid and lipoid are occasionally used synonymously.

lipoma (lipō'mə), *n* a benign tumor characterized by fat cells.

Lipoma of the lip. (Regezi/Sciubba/Pogrel, 2000)

lipophilic (lipōfil'ik), *adj* **1.** showing a marked attraction to, or solubility in, lipids. **2.** having an affinity for oil or fat.

lipopolysaccharides, *n.pl* a compound or complex of lipid and carbohydrate.

lipoproteins, *n.pl* biochemical compounds that contain both lipid and protein. Most lipids in plasma are present in the form of lipoproteins.

lipoproteins, high-density (HDLs), *n.pl* lipoproteins containing approximately 50% protein that transport cholesterol to the liver for disposal. High HDL levels are associated with low body cholesterol and decreased risk of heart disease.

lipoproteins, low-density (LDLs), *n.pl* lipoproteins containing approximately 21% protein that deliver cholesterol from the liver to cells throughout the body. High amounts of LDLs may raise cholesterol levels in the body and increase the risk of developing atherosclerosis.

liposomes, *n.pl* multilayered spherical particles of a lipid in an aqueous medium within a cell.

lipoxygenase, *n* an enzyme that catalyzes the oxidation of unsaturated fatty acids with O_2 to form peroxides of the fatty acids.

lisinopril, *n trade name:* Zestril; *drug class:* angiotensin-converting enzyme (ACE) inhibitor; *action:* selectively suppresses renin-angiotensin-aldosterone system; inhibits ACE, which prevents conversion of angiotensin I to angiotensin II; *uses:* mild to moderate hypertension, post myocardial infarction if hemodynamically stable.

literature, *n* the entire body of writings on a given subject.

literature, dental, *n* the entire body of writing on dentistry. Most specifically, those writings published following a referee process to validate the scientific discipline in which the writings were produced.

lithium carbonate/lithium citrate, *n trade names:* Eskalith, Lithane, Lithobid, Lithotabs Cibalith-S; *drug class:* antimanic, inorganic salt; *action:* may alter sodium and potassium ion transport across cell membrane in nerve, muscle cells; may affect both norephinephrine and serotonin in CNS; *uses:* manic depressive illness (manic phase), prevention of bipolar manic depressive psychosis.

litigation, *n* the act or process of engaging in a lawsuit.

live birth, *n* the birth of an infant, irrespective of the duration of gestation, that exhibits any sign of life, such as respiration, heartbeat, umbilical pulsation, or movement of voluntary muscles. A live birth is not always a viable birth.

liver, *n* the largest gland of the body and one of the body's most complex organs. More than 500 functions of the liver have been identified. It is divided into four lobes, contains as many as 100,000 lobules, and is served by two distinct blood supplies. The hepatic artery conveys oxygenated blood to the liver, and the hepatic portal vein conveys nutrient-filled blood from the stomach and the intestines. At any given moment the liver holds about one pint of blood or approximately 13% of the total blood supply of the body.

liver cirrhosis, *n* a degenerative disease of the liver in which hepatic tissue is replaced with connective tissue, commonly a result of chronic alcoholism.

liver failure, *n* a condition in which the liver fails to fulfill its function or is unable to meet the demand made on it. Liver failure may occur as a result of trauma, neoplastic invasion, prolonged biliary obstruction, viral infections, or chronic alcoholism.

LJP, *n.pr* See localized juvenile periodontitis.

load, *n* an external force applied to an object.

load, occlusal, *n* the stresses generated by functional or habitual contacting of the occlusal surfaces of the upper and lower teeth. There are two components of such stress loads: the vertically directed components and those components that tend to move a tooth or denture laterally. See also force, occlusal.

loading, *n* the amount included in the premiums to meet liabilities beyond anticipated claims payments to provide administrative costs and contributions to reserve funds and to cover contingencies such as unexpected loss or adverse fluctuation.

lobbying, *n* the act of influencing, by argumentation, the course of action of a legislator.

lobectomy (lōbek′təmē), *n* the excision of a lobe of an organ, such as the submandibular gland or the lung.

Lobstein's disease (lōb′stīnz), *n.pr* See osteogenesis imperfecta.

local analgesia, *n* the loss of pain sensation over a specific area, caused by local administration of a drug that blocks nerve conduction.

localization, *n* a direct, exact site or restriction to a limited area, such as localization of abscess.

localization, radiographic, *n* determination, by means of radiographs, of the location of an object or structure in the body or head. Usually accomplished by obtaining radiographs made from different angulations to the part in question.

localization, tactile, *n* the property of localization associated with the sense of touch. Perception of the location of a stimulus is more precise in the regions of the lips and the fingertips than elsewhere. This more precise perception results from a greater density of special touch receptors in a given area.

localized juvenile periodontitis (LJP), *n* a localized periodontal tissue breakdown in young children in the primary or mixed dentition stage, apparently resulting from gingival pocket infection with *Haemophilus actinomycetemcomitans.* See also juvenile periodontitis.

location, practice, *n* place where equipment is set up to practice dentistry.

locking gate, *n* a portion of the peripheral frame of a maxillary subperiosteal implant; attached by a hinge. This device permits the implant to be placed into an area of undercut. After the implant is seated, the gate is closed and locked, and wire is wrapped around two locking buttons.

lockpin, *n* a soft metal pin used to attach an archwire to an orthodontic bracket.

locomotion, *n* the act or power to move from one place to another.

locomotor ataxia, *n* See tabes dorsalis.

locus, gene, *n* the position of a gene on the chromosome.

locus minoris resistentiae (lō′kus minôr′is rēsisten′chē-ā), *n* an area offering little resistance to invasion by microorganisms and/or their toxins. The junction between reduced enamel epithelium and oral epithelium within the epithelial wall of the gingival sulcus has been described as a weak link, providing a portal of entry for microorganisms and their toxins with initiation of pocket formation.

Lod score, *n* "Logarithm of the odds" score, which measures the likelihood of two genes being within measurable distance of each other.

lodoxamide tromethamine, *n* *trade name:* Alomide; *drug class:* mast cell stabilizer; *action:* prevents release of mediators of inflammation from mast cells involved with Type 1 immediate hypersensitivity reactions; *uses:* vernal keratoconjunctivitis, vernal conjunctivits, keratitis.

logic, *n* a disciplined method of reasoning or argumentation that employs the principles governing correct or reliable inference.

logistic models, *n.pl* statistical models that describe the relationship between a qualitative dependent variable (that is, one that can take only certain discrete values, such as the presence or absence of a disease) and an independent variable. A common application is in epidemiology for estimating an individual's risk (probability of contracting a disease) as a function of a given risk factor.

logopedics (lôg′ōpē′diks), *n* the study and treatment of speech defects in children, involving habilitation or rehabilitation of speech.

lomefloxacin HCl, *n trade name:* Maxaquin; *drug class:* fluoroquinolone antiinfective; *action:* a broad-spectrum bactericidal agent that inhibits the enzyme DNA gyrase needed for DNA synthesis; *uses:* lower respiratory tract infections (pneumonia, bronchitis); genitourinary infections (prostatitis); preoperatively to reduce UTIs in transurethral surgical procedures due to susceptible gram-negative organisms.

lomustine, *n trade name:* CeeNU; *drug class:* antineoplastic alkylating agent; *action:* interferes with RNA and DNA strands, which leads to cell death; *uses:* Hodgkin's disease; lymphomas; melanomas; multiple myeloma; brain, lung, bladder, kidney, colon cancer.

long face syndrome, *n* a malocclusion characterized by a long, narrow face; steep mandibular plane angle; and Class II Division 1 dental/skeletal relationship with anterior crowding and associated mouth breathing. A contemporary name for adenoid facies.

long-term care (LTC), *n* the provision of medical, social, and personal care services on a recurring or continuing basis to persons with chronic physical or mental disorders.

longevity, *n* length of life.

longitudinal studies, *n.pl* epidemiologic studies that record data from a respresentative sample at repeated intervals over an extended span of time rather than at a single or limited number over a short period.

loop, programming, *n* a programming technique whereby a group of instructions is repeated with modification of some of the instructions in the group and/or with modification of the data being operated on.

loop, vertical, *n* a U-shaped bend in the archwire that aids in the opening or closing of spaces in the arch.

loose premaxilla, *n* See premaxilla, loose.

loperamide HCl, *n trade names:* Diaraid, Imodium, Imodium AD, Kaopectate II, Maalox Antidiarrheal, Neo-Diaral, Pepto Diarrhea Control; *drug class:* antidiarrheal (opioid); *action:* direct action on intestinal muscles to decrease gastrointestinal peristalsis; *uses:* diarrhea (cause undetermined), chronic diarrhea, ileostomy discharge.

loracarbef, *n trade name:* Lorabid; *drug class:* antibiotic, 2nd-generation cephalosporin; *action:* inhibits bacterial cell wall synthesis, which renders cell wall osmotically unstable; *uses:* gram-negative *Haemophilus influenzae, Escherichia coli, Proteus mirabilis, Klebsiella;* gram-positive *Streptococcus pneumoniae, Staphylococcus pyogenes, Staphylococcus aureus.*

loratadine, *n trade name:* Claritin; *drug class:* antihistamine, H_1 histamine antagonist; *action:* acts on blood vessels, gastrointestinal system, respiratory system by competing with histamine for H_1-receptor site; decreases allergic response by blocking histamine; *uses:* seasonal rhinitis, allergy symptoms, idiopathic chronic urticaria.

Lorazepam, *n.pr trade name:* Ativan, Lorazepam Intensol; *drug class:* benzodiazepine antianxiety (Controlled Substance Schedule IV); *action:* depresses subcortical levels of the central nervous system, including limbic system and reticular formation; *uses:* anxiety, preoperative sedation, acute alcohol withdrawal symptoms, muscle spasm.

lordosis (lôrdō′sis), *n* an anteroposterior curvature of the spine with the convexity facing forward.

losartan potassium, *n trade name:* Cozaar; *drug class:* angiotensin II receptor antagonist; *action:* blocks the vasoconstrictor and aldosterone-secreting effects of angiotensin II; *use:* hypertension, as a single drug or in combination with other antihypertensives.

loss of bone, *n* See resorption of bone.

loss ratio, *n* the relationship between the money paid out in benefits and the amount collected in premiums.

loupe, binocular (loop) (lōōp), *n* a magnifier that consists of lenses in an optical frame; it is worn like spectacles and is used with both eyes.

lovastatin, *n trade name:* Mevacor; *drug class:* cholesterol-lowering agent; *action:* inhibits HMG-CoA reductase enzyme, which reduces cholesterol synthesis; *uses:* adjunct in primary hypercholesterolemia, mixed hyperlipidemia.

low lip line, *n* See lip line, low.

lower ridge slope, *n* See slope, lower ridge.

loxapine succinate/loxapine HCl, *n trade name:* Loxitane; *drug class:* antipsychotic; *action:* depresses cerebral cortex, hypothalamus, limbic system, all of which control activity and aggression; blocks neurotransmission produced by dopamine at synapse; *uses:* psychotic disorders.

lozenge (läz′enj), *n* a medicated, disk-shaped tablet designed to dissolve slowly in the mouth.

lubrication, *n* the application of an agent, usually an oil or grease, to diminish friction.

luciferase, *n* an enzyme present in certain luminous organisms that act to bring about the oxidation of luciferins; energy produced in the process is liberated as bioluminescence.

luciferin, *n* a chemical substance present in certain luminous organisms that, when acted upon by the enzyme luciferase, produces a glow called *bioluminescence.*

Ludwig's angina (lōōd′vigz), *n.pr* See angina, Ludwig's.

luetic (lōō-et′ik), *adj* pertaining to or affected by syphilis.

lumbosacral region, *n* that area of the back that approximates level of the lumbar and sacral vertebrae. The lower third of the back.

lumen (lōō′mən), *n* the space within a tube structure, such as a blood vessel, tube, or duct.

luminescence, *n* **1.** the emission of light by a material after excitation by some stimulus. **2.** the emission of light by intensifying screen phosphors after x-ray interaction.

lung, *n* one of a pair of light, spongy organs in the thorax, constituting the main component of the respiratory system. The lungs provide the tissue surface necessary for the exchange of gases between the environment and the blood. Oxygen is extracted from inspired air, and carbon dioxide is dispersed from the venous system back into the environment.

lung abscess, *n* a complication of an inflammation and infection of the lung, often caused by aspiration of infected material from the mouth.

lupus (lōō′pus), *n* a disease of the skin and mucous membrane.

Lupus. (Newman/Takei/Carranza, 2002)

lupus erythematosus (systemic lupus erythematosus, disseminated lupus erythematosus), *n* a chronic inflammatory disease of unknown etiology affecting skin, joints, kidneys, nervous system, serous membranes, and often other organs of the body. The classical facial "butterfly rash" facilitates diagnosis, although the rash need not be present. Other skin areas, particularly those exposed to the sun, may be involved by a scaly lesion that is referred to as *discoid lupus erythematosus.*

  lupus erythematosus, discoid, *n* a form of lupus erythematosus in which only cutaneous lesions are present. These commonly appear on the face as atrophic plaques with erythema, hyperheratosis, follicular plugging, and telangiectasia.

lupus vulgaris, *n* cutaneous tuberculosis with characteristic nodular lesions on the face, particularly about the nose and ears.

luting agents, *n.pl* agents that bond, seal, or cement particles or objects together.

luxate, *v* to be forced out of place or joint; to be displaced; to dislocate.

luxation, *n* **1.** the act of luxating or state of being luxated, as in the dislocation or displacement of a tooth or of the temporomandibular joint. **2.** the dislocation or displacement of a tooth or of the temporomandibular articulation.

Lyme disease, *n.pr* an acute, recurrent inflammatory infection transmitted by a tick-borne spirochete, *Borrelia burg-dorferi.* Knees, other large joints, and temporomandibular joints are most commonly involved, with local inflammation and swelling. Chills, fever, headache, malaise, and erythema chronicum migrans (ECM), which is an expanding annular, erythematous skin eruption, often precede the joint manifestations.

lymph, *n* a thin opalescent fluid originating in organs and tissues of the body that circulates through the lymphatic vessels and is filtered by the lymph nodes.

lymph node, n one of the many small oval structures that filter the lymph and fight infection, and in which are formed lymphocytes, monocytes, and plasma cells.

lymphadenitis, *n* **1.** an inflammation of a lymph node or nodes. **2.** an inflammation of the lymph glands, characterized chiefly by swelling, pain, and redness.

lymphadenopathy, *n* any disease process that involves a lymph node or nodes.

lymphadenopathy, generalized, n the involvement of all or several regionally separated groups of lymph nodes by a systemic disorder.

lymphadenopathy, persistent generalized (PGL), n a swelling of the lymph nodes that is associated with HIV infection and AIDS.

lymphadenopathy, regional, n the involvement of nodes draining a specific region (for example, submental nodes draining the middle of the lower lip, floor of the mouth, skin of the chin).

lymphangioma (limfanjē-ō′mə), *n* a benign neoplasm characterized by lymph vessel proliferation. A benign tumor of the lymph vessels.

Lymphangioma. (Regezi/Sciubba/Pogrel, 2000)

lymphangioma, cystic, n See hygroma, cystic.

lymphatic system, *n* a vast, complex network of capillaries, thin vessels, valves, ducts, nodes, and organs that helps to protect and maintain the internal fluid environment of the entire body by producing, filtering, and conveying lymph and by producing various blood cells.

lymphatic vessels, *n.pl* See lymphatic system.

lymphocyte(s) (lim′fōsīt), *n* a form of white blood cell originating in lymphoid tissues; possesses a single spherical nucleus and a nongranular cytoplasm. The lymphocytes constitute 25% of the white blood cells. Some lymphocytes, along with plasma cells and histiocytes, are found in clinically normal gingivae. Their numbers within the gingival connective tissue are increased in gingivitis and periodontitis. With progress of gingival inflammation to the underlying bone, lymphocytes are found within the marrow spaces of the supporting bone.

lymphocytes-B, n short-lived, non-thymus-dependent lymphocytes that synthesize antibodies for insertion into their own cytoplasmic membranes. They are the precursor of the plasma cells.

lymphocytes, in pulp tissue, n.pl a subset of white blood cells that, when present, are located near the odontoblastic layer. An increase in lymphocyte count is indicative of inflammation.

lymphocytes-T, n long-lived lymphocytes that have circulated through the thymus gland and have differentiated to become thymocytes. When exposed to an antigen, they divide rapidly and produce large numbers of new T cells sensitized to that antigen.

Some T cells are often called *killer cells,* because they secrete immunologically essential chemical compounds and assist B cells in destroying foreign protein. T cells also appear to play a significant role in the body's resistance to the proliferation of cancer cells.

lymphocytopenia (lim′fōsī′tōpē′nēə), *n* a decrease in the normal number of lymphocytes in the circulating blood. Various limits are given (for example, a total number less than 600/mm³). It may be associated with agranulocytosis, hyperadrenocorticism, leukemia, advanced Hodgkin's disease, irradiation, and acute infections with neutrophilia.

lymphocytosis (lim′fōsītō′sis), *n* an absolute or relative increase in the normal number of lymphocytes in the circulating blood. Various limits are given; for example, absolute lymphocytosis is said to be present if the total number of cells exceeds 4500/mm³, whereas relative lymphocytosis is said to be present if the percentage of lymphocytes is greater than 45% and the total number of cells is less than 4500/mm³. Lymphocytosis may be associated with infancy, exophthalmic goiter, mumps, rubella, infectious mononucleosis, sunburn, lymphatic leukemia, pertussis, and pyogenic infections in childhood.

lymphoepithelial lesion, benign (lim′fō-ep′ithē′lē-əl), *n* See disease, Mikulicz's.

lymphoepithelioma (lim′fō-ep′ithē′lē-ō′mə), *n* a malignant neoplasm arising from the epithelium and lymphoid tissue of the nasopharynx and characterized by cells of both tissues; may occur in the palate.

lymphokines, *n.pl* soluble substances, released by sensitized lymphocytes on contact with specific antigens, that help effect cellular immunity by stimulating activity of monocytes and macrophages.

lymphoma (limfō′mə), *n* any neoplasm made up of lymphoid tissue.

lymphoma, B-cell, *n* a group of heterogenous lymphoid tumors generally expressing one or more B-cell antigens or representing malignant transformations of B-lymphocytes.

lymphoma, non-Hodgkins, *n* any of a group of malignant tumors of a lymphoid tissue that differ from Hodgkin's disease, being more heterogeneous with respect to malignant cell lineage, clinical course, prognosis, and therapy. The only feature shared by these tumors is the absence of Reed-Sternberg cells, which are characteristic of Hodgkin's disease.

lymphoma, T-cell, *n* adult T-cell leukemia; an acute or subacute disease associated with a human T-cell virus, with lymphadenopathy, hepatosplenomegaly, skin lesions, peripheral blood involvement, and hypercalcemia.

lymphoreticulosis, benign inoculation (lim′fōretik′yōōlō′sis), *n* See fever, cat-scratch.

lymphosarcoma (lim′fōsärkō′mə), *n* a malignant disease of the lymphoid tissues characterized by proliferation of atypical lymphocytes and their localization in various parts of the body. The jaws may be the sites of lymphosarcomas.

lypressin, *n trade name:* Diapid; *drug class:* pituitary hormone; *action:* promotes reabsorption of water by action on collecting ducts in kidney; decreases urine excretion; *uses:* nonnephrogenic diabetes insipidus.

lysin (lī′sin), *n* See plasmin.

lysine, *n* one of the essential amino acids found in many proteins. An essential amino acid needed for proper growth in infants and for maintenance of nitrogen balance in adults. See also amino acids.

lysis (lī′sis), *n* the gradual abatement of the symptoms of a disease. The disintegration or dissolution of cells by a lysin.

lysozyme (lī′sōzīm), *n* an enzyme in major salivary secretions that may rupture bacterial cell walls and may regulate the oral flora.

mA, *n* the abbreviation for milliampere.

Macaca, *n* a genus of Old World monkeys that include the macaque and rhesus monkeys and the barbary apes. *M. mulatta,* the rhesus monkey, is used as a research animal.

macaque, *n* See *Macaca.*

macro, *pref* a prefix meaning excessively large or big.

macrochellia (mak′rok′le ə), *n* an abnormally large lip.

macrocyte, *n* a red blood cell that is unusually large; usually seen in megaloblastic anemias (e.g., B_{12} deficiency).

macrodontia (makrōdon′shē ə), *n* abnormally large teeth. One, several, or all teeth in a given individual may be involved.

macroglossia (mak′rōglôs′ē ə), *n* an enlarged tongue resulting from muscle hypertrophy, vascular or neurogenic tumor, or endocrine disturbance.

Macroglossia. (Sapp/Eversole/Wysocki, 2004)

macroglossia, amyloid, *n* See tongue, amyloid.

macrognathia (mak′rōnā′thē ə), *n* a definite overgrowth of the maxillae and mandible.

macrolides, *n* a class of antibiotics discovered in *Streptomyces,* characterized by molecules made up of large-ring lactones. An example is erythromycin.

macromolecule, *n* any substance with molecules of colloidal size, notably proteins, nucleic acids, and polysaccharides.

macrophage (mak′rəfāj), *n* any phagocytic cell of the reticuloendo-thelial system including specialized Kupffer's cells in the liver and spleen, and histiocytes in loose connective tissue. See also histiocyte.

macrophage, alveolar, *n* a dust cell, coniophage, a vigorously phagocytic macrophage on the epithelial surface of lung alveoli where it ingests inhaled particulate matter.

macroscopic, *adj* relating to macroscopy, or the examination of areas such as surfaces of teeth without magnification.

macrosomia, *n* See giantism.

macrostomia, *n* an abnormally large oral opening.

macule, *n* a lesion that is not elevated above the surface.

Oral melanotic macule. (Regezi/Sciubba/Jordan, 2003)

magaldrate, *n* (aluminum magnesium complex), *trade names:* Lowsium, Riopan, Riopan Plus; *drug class:* antacid/aluminum/magnesium hydroxide; *action:* neutralizes gastric acidity; *use:* antacid for hyperacidity.

magnesium, *n* an elemental metal with an atomic weight of 24.32. Magnesium is an essential nutritional substance. Deficiency produces irritability of the nervous system and trophic disturbances.

magnesium sulfate, *n* a salt of magnesium; also called Epsom salts, used as a therapeutic bath and as a purgative.

magnetic disk, *n* a storage device, consisting of magnetically coated disks, on the surfaces of which information is stored in the form of magnetic spots arranged in a manner to represent binary data.

magnetic fields, *n.pl* spaces in which magnetic forces are detectable; created by magnetostrictive ultrasonic scalers to cause the tips of instruments to vibrate.

M

magnetic resonance imaging (MRI), *n* also known as nuclear magnetic resonance imaging. MRI is a diagnostic technique in which the phosphorus in cellular tissues is excited by magnetic force. The distribution and alignment of these cellular elements can be captured on phosphorus nuclear magnetic resonance instruments forming a high-resolution tissue image. A higher degree of resolution of soft tissues is possible using this technique than from radiographic techniques. The word nuclear has been dropped from the term because it makes an incorrect assumption that radioactivity is involved in the imaging process.

A magnetic resonance image. (Rosenstiel/Land/Fujimoto, 2001, courtesy of Dr. J. Petrie)

magnetic tape, *n* a continuous, flexible, recording medium whose basic material is impregnated or coated with a magnetic-sensitive material ready to accept data in the form of magnetically polarized spots.

magnetostrictive instruments (mag-ne″ to-re strik′ tiv), *n.pl* See ultrasonic scalers, magnetostrictive.

mainstream smoke, *n* vaporous byproduct of burning tobacco products that is purposely taken into the lungs through the mouth.

maintenance, *n* to keep in a functional state or in the proper location.
maintenance, space, *n* See space maintainer.

maintenance phase, *n* the period following treatment for a specific condition during which the patient may undergo occasional examinations and treatments in order to regain optimal dental health.

major connector, *n* See connector, major.

major histocompatibility complex, *n* the genetic region that contains the loci of genes that determine the structure of the serologically defined (SD) and lymphocyte-defined (LD) transplantation antigens, genes that control the structure of the immune response–associated (Ia) antigens, and the immune response (Ir) genes that control the ability of an animal to respond immunologically to antigenic stimuli.

making the turn, *n* the step in the procedure of inserting and condensing foil in a Class 3 cavity preparation, at which the line of force is changed from an incisogingival direction to a gingivoincisal direction.

mal-, *pref* a prefix denoting a bad or unfavorable condition.

malaise (məlāz′), *n* a general feeling of discomfort or uneasiness, often the first indication of an infection or other disease.

malar (mā′lur), *adj* pertaining to the cheek or the zygomatic bone.
malar bone, *n* See bone, malar.

malaria, *n* a serious infectious illness caused by one or more of at least four species of the protozoan genus *Plasmodium,* characterized by chills, fever, anemia, an enlarged spleen, and a tendency to recur. The disease is transmitted from human to human by a bite from an infected *Anopheles* mosquito.

Malassez, rests of, *n.pr* See debris of Malassez.

maldevelopment, *n* an abnormal, imperfect, or deficient formation or development.

malfeasance (malfē′zəns), *n* an act that one should not do at all or the unjust performance of some act that one has no right to do.

malfunction, *n* a disorder in function or performance, which may or may not be related to a malformation of tissues, organs, or organ systems. See also dysfunction.

malice, *n* a state of mind that disregards the law and legal rights of others but that does not necessarily involve personal hate or ill will.
malice, in the law of libel and slander, *n* an evil intent arising from spite or ill will; willful and wanton disregard of the rights of the person defamed.

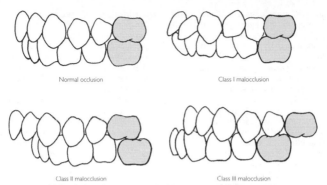

Normal occlusion

Class I malocclusion

Class II malocclusion

Class III malocclusion

Malocclusion classes as specified by Angle. (Proffit/Fields, 2000)

malignant (məlig′nənt), *adj* **1.** resistant to treatment. *adj* **2.** able to metastasize and kill the host.

malignant hypertension, n the most lethal form of hypertension. Malignant hypertension is a fulminating condition, characterized by severely elevated blood pressure that commonly damages the intima of small vessels, the brain, retina, heart, and kidneys. It affects more African Americans than white Americans and may be caused by a variety of factors such as stress, genetic predisposition, obesity, the use of tobacco, the use of oral contraceptives, high intake of sodium chloride, a sedentary lifestyle, and aging.

malignant hyperthermia, n an autosomal dominant trait characterized by often fatal hyperthermia with rigidity of muscles occurring in affected people exposed to certain anesthetic agents, particularly halothane and succinylcholine.

malingering, *n* the feigning of illness.

malleability (mal′ē əbil′itē), *n* the ability of a material to withstand permanent deformation under compressive forces without rupture.

mallet, *n* a hammer instrument.

mallet, hard, n a small hammer with a leather-, rubber-, fiber-, or metal-faced head; used to supply force or to supplement hand force for the compaction of foil or amalgam and to seat cast restorations.

malnutrition, *n* any disorder concerning nutrition. It may result from a poor diet or from impaired utilization of foods ingested.

malocclusion, *n* (relationship of teeth in occlusion), a deviation in intramaxillary and/or intermaxillary relations of teeth that presents a hazard to the individual's well-being. Often associated with other dentofacial deformities. See also Angle's classification.

malocclusion, deflective, n a type of malocclusion occurring in persons who cannot close all their teeth while holding their condyles in the rearmost position. Instead, in closure they first contact one or two pairs of poorly coupled teeth. To gain occlusal contacts of the other teeth, they must move the jaw anteriorly, laterally, or anterolaterally, as the deflectors demand in their guidance.

malposed (malpōzd′), *adj* in an abnormal position.

malposition, *n* a faulty or abnormal position of a part of the body.

malposition of jaw, n any abnormal position of the mandible.

malposition of teeth, n an improper position of teeth in relationship to the basal bone of the alveolar process, to adjacent teeth, or to opposing teeth.

malpractice, *n* in medicine and dentistry, a professional person's act or failure to act that was the proximate cause of an injury to a patient and that was below the standard of care required.

malrelation, *n* (of tooth, teeth, jaws, or facial structures), malalignment, malocclusion, and malposition are interrelated, so that one term frequently implies concurrent malrelationships of related teeth or structures.

M

maltose, *n* malt sugar, a disaccharide formed in the hydrolysis of starch and consisting of two glucose residues bound by an α(1, 4)-glycoside link.

mammotropin (mam'ōtrō'pin), *n* See hormone, lactogenic.

manage, *v* to control and direct; to administer.

managed care, *n* **I.** refers to a cost containment system that directs the utilization of health benefits by (a) restricting the type, level, and frequency of treatment; (b) limiting the access to care; and (c) controlling the level of reimbursement for services. *n* **2.** a health care system in which there is administrative control over primary health care services in a medical group practice. Patients may pay a flat fee for basic family care but may be charged additional fees for secondary care services of specialists.

management, *n* the planning, organizing, directing, and controlling of the enterprise's operation so that objectives can be achieved economically and efficiently through others.

management information system (MIS), *n* the specific type of data processing system that is designed to furnish management with information that may be of assistance in making decisions.

mandible, *n* the lower jawbone.

The mandible. (Liebgott, 2001)

mandible, inferior, *n* the border of the lower edge of the mandible. Begins anterior to the insertion of the masseter muscle at the inferior surface of the angles of the mandible and is continuous anteriorly with the incisor region.

mandible, movements of, *n.pl* See movement, mandibular.

mandible, posture of, *n* the physiologic rest position, or the rest vertical relation of the mandible.

mandibular, *adj* pertaining to the lower jaw.

mandibular angle, *n* See angle of the mandible.

mandibular axis, *n* See axis, mandibular.

mandibular border, *n* See border, mandibular.

mandibular canal, *n* See canal, mandibular.

mandibular centric relation, *n* the closing relation of the mandible with the fixed craniofacial complex as determined clinically by instruments that record jaw motion.

mandibular condyle, *n* See condyle, mandibular.

mandibular foramen, *n* See foramen, mandibular.

mandibular fracture, *n* a break in the continuity of the bone of the mandible. See also fracture.

mandibular glide, *n* See glide, mandibular.

mandibular guide prosthesis, *n* a prosthesis with an extension designed to direct a resected mandible into a functional relation with the maxillae.

mandibular hinge position, *n* See position, hinge, mandibular.

mandibular labial frenum, *n* a thin crease of mucous membrane located between the midlines of the mandibular central incisors, which connects the attached gingiva to the lower lip and safeguards against any excessive motions.

mandibular movement, *n* See movement, mandibular.

mandibular nerve, *n* the third division of the trigeminal nerve, a mixed nerve that contains the entire motor portion of the trigeminal nerve. Its principal branches are the masseteric nerve, posterior and anterior temporal nerves, medial pterygoid nerve, lateral pterygoid nerve, buccal nerve, lingual nerve, inferior alveolar nerve, and auriculotemporal nerve. See also nerve(s).

mandibular notch, *n* See notch, mandibular.

mandibular pain-dysfunction syndrome, *n* See temporomandibular joint pain-dysfunction syndrome.

mandibular rest position, *n* See position, rest, mandibular.

mandibular retraction, *n* See retraction, mandibular.

mandibulofacial dysostosis (mandib′yōōlōfā′shǝl), *n* See syndrome, Treacher Collins.

mandrel (man′drǝl), *n* a shaft that supports or holds any object to be rotated. An instrument, held in a handpiece, that holds a disk, stone, or cup used for grinding, smoothing, or polishing.

manganese (Mn), *n* a common metallic element found in trace amounts in tissues of the body, where it aids in the function of various enzymes. Its atomic number is 25 and its atomic weight is 54.9380.

mania, *n* the episode of intense euphoria found in people with bipolar disorder. Manic episodes may include rapid thought and speech, insomnia, setting unrealistic goals or engaging in risky behaviors.

manifest anxiety scale, *n* a true-false questionnaire made up of items believed to indicate anxiety, in which the subject answers verbally the statement that describes him or her.

manifestation, *n* an obvious indication or specific evidence that a disease is present; a symptom.

manikin, *n* a replica of the complete human body or its individual parts that is used for instructional purposes.

Mann-Whitney U test, *n.pr* See test, Mann-Whitney U.

mannitol, *n* a poorly metabolized sugar used as an osmotic diuretic and in kidney function tests.

mannose, *n* an aldohexose obtained from various plant sources.

manometer, *n* a device for measuring the pressure of a fluid, consisting of a tube marked with a scale and containing a relatively incompressible fluid, such as mercury. The level of the fluid in the tube varies directly with the pressure of the fluid being measured. Manometers are used to measure blood pressure.

manpower, *n* the number of persons required or needed to complete a task.

manual, *n* **1.** a book of instructions on performance of a task or the care of equipment. *adj* **2.** performed by the hand; used in the hand.

manual film processing, *n* See film processing.

manual scaling, *n* a procedure for removing bacterial plaque and calculus that utilizes a hand tool rather than a power-driven instrument.

manuscript, *n* an author's final copy of a document written by hand, typewriter, or word processor.

map, *n* a drawing or diagram, to scale, of a surface object.

maprotiline HCl, *n trade name:* Ludiomil; *drug class:* tetracyclic antidepressant; *action:* blocks reuptake of norepinephrine and serotonin into nerve endings; *uses:* depression, depression with anxiety.

marasmus (mǝraz′mus), *n* a wasting disorder of malnutrition and partial starvation which occurs in infants and young children as a result of severe protein deficiency and insufficient caloric intake. See also kwashiorkor.

Marasmus. (Thibodeau/Patton, 2002)

Marfan's syndrome, *n.pr* a hereditary disorder of connective tissue characterized by tall stature, elongated extremities, subluxation of the lens, dilatation of the ascending aorta, and "pigeon breast." Marfan's syndrome is inherited as an autosomal dominant trait.

margin, *n* **1.** the extreme edge of something. *n* **2.** the boundary of a surface. *n* **3.** in a cavity preparation for a restoration, the margin is the outside limit of the surgical preparation. See also cavosurface angle.

margin, bone, *n* the peripheral edge of a bone.

margin, enamel, *n* the part of the margin of a preparation that is laid in enamel.

margin, free gingival, *n* (free gum margin), the edge or summit of the gingival tissue immediately adjacent to the cervical portion of the crown of a natural tooth. The tissue is normally unattached to a depth of 2 to 2.5 mm.

margin, free gum, *n* See margin, free gingival.

margin, gingival, *n* **1.** the cavosurface angle of the wall of a cavity preparation closest to the apex of the root. *n* **2.** the crest or tip of the gingival tissues.

margin of safety, *n* the margin between lethal and toxic doses.

margin, thickened bone, *n* See bone, thickened margin of.

marginal ridge, *n* See ridge, marginal.

margination, *n* the adhesion of leukocytes to the luminal surface of blood vessel walls in the early stages of inflammation.

Marie's disease, *n.pr* See acromegaly.

marijuana, abuse of (mer'əwä'nə), *n* regular use of marijuana (e.g., Mary Jane, weed, pot, hemp, or grass), an example of a cannabinoid, for reasons other than recognized medical applications; may cause pupils to dilate and eyes to appear bloodshot, red, and inflamed as a result.

marital status, *n* the legal standing of a person in regard to his or her marriage state.

marketing, *n* the set of human activities directed at facilitating and consummating exchanges. The following three elements must be present to define a marketing situation: two or more parties who are potentially interested in exchange; each party possessing things of value to others; and each party capable of communication and delivery.

marking medium, *n* See medium, marking.

marsupialization (märsōō'pē-əlizā'shən), *n* to form a pouch surgically to treat a cyst when simple removal would not be effective, such as in a pancreatic or a pilonidal cyst. Under anesthesia, the cyst sac is opened and emptied. Its edges are sutured to adjacent tissues, and a drain is left in place. Over a period of several months, secretions will decrease and the sac space will be reduced until it is completely filled. See also operation, Partsch's.

MAS (MaS, mas, milliampere-second), *n* the product of the milliamperes and the exposure time in seconds (for example, 10 ma × ½ sec = 5 MAS).

mask, *n* **1.** something that conceals from view. *n* **2.** a protective covering, especially for the face. *v* **3.** to cover up.

mask, nonbreather, *n* a plastic mask worn over the mouth and nose in order to deliver additional oxygen to a patient who is able to breathe on his or her own. See also mask, oxygen.

mask, oxygen, *n* a device used during the delivery of oxygen which fits securely over the nose and mouth so that oxygen may be inhaled and carbon dioxide exhaled.

Oxygen mask. (Potter/Perry, 2001)

mask, rubber dam, *n* See pad, rubber dam.

mask, Wanscher's, *n* a mask for ether anesthesia.

mask, Yankauer's, *n* an open type of mask for administering ether.

masking, *n* an opaque covering used to camouflage the metal or other parts of a prosthesis.

Maslow's hierarchy of human needs, *n.pr* a term from sociology or social anthropology denoting the hierarchic hypothesis of Abraham Maslow of the basic needs of man. The first need is for air, food, and water; the second for safety, including protection and freedom from fear and anxiety. These are followed in order by the need to love and to be loved; the need for self-esteem; and ultimately, the need for self-actualization. The Maslow hypothesis states that the basic needs, which are those at the end of the hierarchy, cannot be fully satisfied until the lower needs are met.

masoprocol, *n trade name:* Actinex; *drug class:* antineoplastic (topical); *action:* inhibits lipoxygenase; *use:* actinic keratosis.

mass media, *n.pl* the print and broadcast enterprises used to inform the general public.

mass number (A), *n* the number of nucleons (protons and neutrons) in the nucleus of an atom.

mass screening, *n* the examination of large samples or populations to determine the presence or absence of some trait, condition, or behavior.

mass storage, *n* a storage medium in which data may be organized and maintained both sequentially and nonsequentially. Usually used for storage of files.

massage, *n/v* the manipulation of tissues for remedial or hygiene purposes (as by rubbing, stroking, kneading, or tapping) with the hand or other instrument.

massage, cardiac, n a systematic, rhythmic application of pressure to the heart to cause significant blood flow in the treatment of a cardiac arrest; may be an open- or closed-chest procedure.

massage, gingival, n the massage of the gingival tissues for cleansing purposes, increasing tissue tone, increasing the circulation of blood through the tissues, and increasing the keratinization of the surface epithelium.

mast cell, *n* a connective tissue cell whose specific physiologic function remains unknown; capable of elaborating basophilic, metachromatic, cytoplasmic granules that contain histamine.

mastalgia (mastal′jē-ə), *n* pain, tenderness, or pressure in the breast. It is one of several physical symptoms of premenstrual syndrome.

master, *n* one having authority; one who directs, instructs, or superintends; an employer.

master file, n a file of semipermanent information that is usually updated periodically.

masticate, *v* **1.** to grind or crush food with the teeth to prepare it for swallowing and digestion. *v* **2.** to chew.

masticating apparatus, *n* See apparatus, masticating.

masticating cycle, *n* See cycle, masticating.

mastication, *n* **1.** the process of chewing food in preparation for swallowing and digestion. *n* **2.** the act of chewing accomplished by the coordinated activity of the tongue, mandible, mandibular musculature, and structural components of the temporomandibular joints, and controlled by the neuromuscular mechanism.

mastication, components of, n.pl the various jaw movements made during the act of mastication as determined by the neuromuscular system, temporomandibular articulations, teeth, and food being chewed. For purposes of analysis or description, the components of mastication may be categorized as opening, closing, left lateral, right lateral, or anteroposterior jaw movements.

mastication, forces of, n.pl See force, masticatory.

mastication, insufficiency of, n inefficiency or inadequacy of the chewing act.

mastication, organ of, n See system, stomatognathic.

mastication, physiology of, n the movements of the mandible during the chewing cycle, which are controlled by neuromuscular action and are correlated with the structural attributes of the temporomandibular joints and the proprioceptive sense of the periodontal membranes. There are three phases in the physiology of mastication: the incision of food, the mastication of the bolus, and the act of swallowing. Accessory activity by the tongue and facial musculature facilitates the masticatory actions.

mastication, saliva in, *n* an increase in salivation, which serves to wet and lubricate the food to facilitate deglutition.

mastication, tongue in, *n* the muscular organ in the floor of the mouth whose function in the masticatory process consists of crushing some food by pressing it against the hard palate, forming it into a compact bolus, and assisting in placing it on the occlusal platform for tooth action.

masticatory force (mas′tikətôrē), *n* See force, masticatory.

masticatory movements, *n.pl* See movements, mandibular, masticatory.

masticatory muscles, *n.pl* See muscles, masticatory.

Mastigophora **(mas′tigof′ôrə),** *n* a subphylum of sarcomastigophora consisting of parasitic protozoa, also called flagellates. Causes diseases such as enteritis, urethritis, vaginitis, and Chagas' disease by drinking contaminated water, contact with vaginal discharge, and through bug bite.

mastoid, *n* **1.** the protuberance of the temporal bone located directly behind the external ear. *adj* **2.** breast-shaped.

mastoidale, *n* the lowest point on the contour of the mastoid process.

materia alba, *n* a soft white deposit around the necks of the teeth, usually associated with poor oral hygiene; composed of food debris, dead tissue elements, and purulent matter; serves as a medium for bacterial growth.

materia medica, *n* the study of drugs and other substances used in medicine, their origins, preparation, uses, and effects.

material(s), *n* substance(s).

material, duplicating, *n.pl* the materials used to copy casts and models; usually hydrocolloids.

material, silicone rubber impression, *n* a dimethyl polysiloxane material whose polymerization is affected by an organ-metal compound and some type of alkyl silicate.

material testing, *n* the determination of the properties of a substance in comparison with a standard or specification.

materials, dental, *n.pl* all the substances used to assist in rendering dental service.

materials, filling, *n* gutta-percha, silver cones, paste mixtures, or other substances used to fill root canals.

materials, impression, *n* any substance or combination of substances used for making a negative reproduction or impression.

materials, impression, elastomer, *n* See elastomer.

materials, provisional, *n* cements or resins used temporarily to protect soft, hard, or pulpal tissues, stabilize a tooth, allow the delivery of medications, provide the ability to chew, or encourage the comfort of the patient. See also filling, treatment.

materials, rigid impression, *n* inflexible substances (e.g., zinc oxide-eugenol, plaster, or compound) used to create casts and models for prosthodontic, orthodontic, and pedodontic appliances, or the construction of dentures.

maternal age, *n* the age of the mother at the period of conception.

matrix (mā′triks), *n* **1.** an intergranular substance that acts somewhat as a cementing material for other particles; for example, zinc phosphate cement is made of undissolved zinc oxide particles, surrounded and held or cemented together by phosphate compounds. The phosphate compounds make up the matrix *n* **2.** a mechanical or artificial wall that completes the mold into which plastic material is inserted. *n* **3.** a mold into which something is formed. See also bone; splint.

matrix, amalgam, *n* a metal form, usually of stainless steel, about 0.0015 to 0.002 inch thick, adapted to a prepared cavity to supply the missing wall so that the plastic amalgam will be confined when it is condensed into the cavity.

matrix, celluloid, *n* a strip of celluloid used to mold cement into the desired shape. See also strip, plastic.

matrix, custom, *n* a matrix made especially for a given location, tooth, or preparation.

matrix, fibrous, of alveolar bone, *n* collagen fibers in the alveolar bone, calcified by the accumulation of hydroxyapatite, a calcium salt.

matrix, fibrous, of bone, *n* a component of bone tissue consisting of collagen fibers.

matrix, fibrous, of periodontal ligament, *n* major component consisting of collagen and oxytalan fibers whose function is to provide support to the tooth.

matrix holder, n See retainer, matrix.

matrix, intermicrobial (in′turmĭkrō′bē-əl), n an intercellular substance found in plaque which is made from derivatives of saliva, gingival fluids, and microorganisms.

matrix, mechanical, n (proprietary matrix), a patented or manufactured type of matrix.

matrix, plastic, n a matrix of resin or plastic for use with cold-curing resin or cement.

matrix, platinum, n a matrix of wrought platinum foil, usually 0.001 inch or thinner, adapted to a die of a preparation for a fired porcelain restoration; serves as a vehicle to carry and maintain the applications of porcelain when they are placed in a furnace for firing.

matrix, proprietary, n See matrix, mechanical.

matrix retainer, n a mechanical device used to secure the ends of metal or plastic bands around a tooth to provide a form into which a restorative material can be condensed to replace a portion of tooth substance removed in cavity preparation. See also retainer, matrix.

matrix, T-band, n matrix material cut with a T-shaped projection at one end; the lugs are bent over to engage the band as it encircles the tooth.

maturation (mach′ərā′shən), n the process through which an organism or body structure arrives at a state of complete development. In dentistry, this is the point at which an individual's teeth have reached their full adult form, size, and function.

maxilla (maksil′ə), n the irregularly shaped bone forming half of the upper jaw. The upper jaw is made up of the two maxillae.

The maxilla. (Liebgott, 2001)

maxillary (mak′siler′ē), adj pertaining to the superior jaw.

maxillary arch, n the upper dental arch and its supporting bone.

maxillary artery, n (internal maxillary artery), arises from the external carotid artery just below the level of the mandibular neck in the substance of the parotid gland. Its many branches include the middle meningeal, lower alveolar, temporal, pterygoid, masseteric, and buccal arteries, and the posterior superior alveolar and infraorbital arteries.

maxillary diseases, n.pl inflammatory, infectious, and neoplastic diseases of the midface, maxillary alveolar process, and palatal areas.

maxillary fracture, n a break in one or both of the maxillary bones; frequently sustained in automobile accidents and contact sports injuries.

maxillary labial frenum, n a thin crease of mucous membrane located between the midlines of the maxillary central incisors, which connects the attached gingiva to the upper lip and safeguards against any excessive motions.

maxillary nerve, n the second division of the trigeminal nerve consists of three major branches; the pterygopalatine, infraorbital, and zygomatic nerves. See also nerve(s).

maxillary retrusion, n See retrusion, maxillary.

maxillary sinus, n See sinus, maxillary.

maxillary sinusitis, n an inflammation of the mucosa lining the air sac in the maxillary bone.

maxillary tuberosity, n See tuberosity, maxillary.

maxillary vein, n path of drainage for the pterygoid plexus of veins in the upper neck region. It is posterior to the mandibular condyle and merges with the superficial temporal vein in the parotid gland to form the retromandibular vein.

maxillofacial (maksil′ōfā′shəl), adj pertaining to the jaws and face.

maxillofacial injuries, n.pl wounds to the mid-face area involving the premaxillary, maxillary, malar, lacrimal, nasal, and vomer bones and the tissues overlying these skeletal structures.

maxillofacial pain, n any pain in the region of the jaws or face. Usually coupled with oral pain; that is, oral and maxillofacial pain may be present together. Maxillofacial pain frequently is associated with functional disorders of the temporomandibular joint and the muscles of mastication, which in turn may arise from structural problems in the occlusion of the teeth. Determining the cause of maxillofacial pain may require comprehensive study of many possible factors or agents.

maxillofacial prosthetics, n.pl See prosthetics, maxillofacial.

maxillomandibular relation (maksil′ōmandib′yōōlur), *n* See relation, maxillomandibular.

maxillotomy (mak′silot′əmē), *n* the surgical sectioning of the maxilla to allow movement of all or a part of the maxilla into the desired portion.

maximum allowance, *n* as specified in a fee schedule or table of allowances, the maximum dollar amount a dental plan will pay toward the cost of a dental service.

maximum benefit, *n* the maximum dollar amount a dental plan will pay toward the cost of dental care incurred by an individual or family in a specified policy year.

maximum fee schedule, *n* a compensation arrangement in which a participating dentist agrees to accept a prescribed sum as the total fee for one or more covered services.

maximum recommended dose (MRD), *n* the highest amount of an anesthetic that can be given safely and without complication to a patient while maintaining its efficacy. MDRs can also be adjusted to consider the patient's overall health and any mitigating medical factors that could hamper the patient's recovery.

mazindol, *n trade names:* Mazanor, Sanorex; *drug class:* imidazoisoindole anorexiant (Controlled Substance Schedule IV); *action:* has amphetamine-like activity and may have an effect on satiety center of the hypothalamus; *use:* exogenous obesity.

Mazzini's test (məzē′nēz, mot-sē′nēz), *n.pr* See test, Mazzini's.

MCH, *n* See mean corpuscular hemoglobin.

MCHC, *n* See mean corpuscular hemoglobin concentration.

MCV, *n* See mean corpuscular volume.

MDR, *n* the abbreviation for minimum daily requirement, specifically the Minimum Daily Requirements for Specific Nutrients compiled by the United States Food and Drug Administration.

MDS, *n* See temporomandibular pain-dysfunction syndrome.

mean (x), *n* a measure of central tendency that is the calculated arithmetic average of a series of scores.

mean (x) corpuscular hemoglobin, n a measure of the weight of hemoglobin in a single red blood cell. The value is obtained by multiplying the hemoglobin value by 10 and dividing by the number of red blood cells. The normal range is between 27 and 31.

mean (x) corpuscular hemoglobin concentration (MCHC), n a measure of red blood cells useful in identifying the type of anemia. The MCHC is obtained by multiplying the value of hemoglobin by 100 and dividing by the value of the hematocrit. The normal range is between 31.5 and 35.5.

mean (x) corpuscular volume (MCV), n indicates the size of the red blood cells. The MCV is obtained by multiplying the hematocrit value by 10 and dividing by the number of red blood cells. The normal range is between 82 and 98.

mean (x) life, n See average life.

measles (mē′zəlz), *n* an infectious disease caused by a virus. There are two types: rubeola and rubella (German measles). Both have oral manifestations.

Koplik's spots with measles. (Sapp/Eversole/Wysocki, 2004, courtesy Dr. Robert J. Achterberg)

measles, German, *n.pr* See rubella.

measles, three-day, *n* See rubella.

mebendazole (məben′dəzōl), *n* an anthelmintic agent that acts against pathogenic roundworms by inhibiting their glucose intake and secretory processes.

mecamylamine HCl, *n trade name:* Inversine; *drug class:* antihypertensive, ganglionic blocker; *action:* occupies receptor site, prevents acetylcholine from attaching to postsynaptic nerve endings in autonomic ganglia; *uses:* moderate-to-severe hypertension, malignant hypertension.

mechanical toothbrush, *n* See automatic toothbrush.

mechanism, *n* a structure of working parts functioning together to produce an effect.

mechanism, cough, *n* a short inspiration, closure of the glottis, forcible expiratory effort, and then release of the glottis, with a rush of air at a flow rate of 3,000 to 4,000 cc/sec. A cough is essentially used or regarded as a process for removing foreign material from the lungs. It involves two phases. In the first, the combined action of the cilia and bronchiolar peristalsis moves the material up to the main bronchi and the bifurcation of the trachea. Further movement out of the respiratory system depends on the cough mechanism. In all medical conditions in which this mechanism is abolished or reduced, secretions and foreign material accumulate in the alveoli, with a resultant reduction in the aerating surface and a predisposition to infection. Since ventilation of the lungs depends on a patent airway, the cough mechanism should always be used by patients whose inadequate ventilation of lungs may be related to obstruction of the airway.

mechanism, inhibitory-excitatory, *n* a mechanism that provides coordinated and continuous stimuli to the lower motor neuron for smooth, facile, and rapidly adjustable muscle contraction. This mechanism operates on every level of the central nervous system, from the final common pathway back up the spinal cord to the cerebrum. The excitatory phase of stimulation is transmitted directly to the nerve. Inhibition, however, is effected not by stimulating the motor output directly, as is done in the parasympathetic nerves, but rather by the interaction of inhibitory mechanisms on the excitatory impulses.

mechanism, respiratory control, *n* the mechanism by which the respiratory functions are controlled. Three major factors in the control of respiration concern the dentist: neurogenic control of respiration, chemical regulation of respiration, and mechanical events leading to pulmonary ventilation. These three factors are significant in practice procedures because the dentist influences each of these factors in routine dental care, for example, the patency of the airways is always subject to alteration by instrumentation, dental prostheses, and the use of pharmacologic agents, and the physically induced responses modify the rate and magnitude of the respiratory mechanism.

mechanism, self-cleansing, *n* any of the structures within the oral cavity (e.g., teeth, saliva, gingiva, cheeks, and tongue) that remove substances entering the mouth that may affect the cleanliness of the cavity and promote the production of deposits.

mechanism, suspensory, *n* the hammock-like arrangement of the structures comprising the attachment apparatus.

mechanoreceptor, *n* any sensory nerve ending that responds to mechanical stimuli, such as touch, pressure, sound, and muscular contraction.

meclizine HCl, *n trade names:* Antivert, Bonine, Dramamine II; *drug class:* antihistamine nonspecific antiemetic; *action:* a nonspecific central nervous system depressant with anticholinergic and antihistaminic activity; *uses:* dizziness, motion sickness.

meclofenamate, *n* trade name: Meclofen, Meclomen; *drug class:* nonsteroidal antiinflammatory; *action:* inhibits prostaglandin synthesis by interfering with cyclooxygenase needed for biosynthesis; possesses analgesic, antiinflammatory, antipyretic properties; *uses:* mild-to-moderate pain, osteoarthritis, rheumatoid arthritis.

media (mē′dē ə), *n.pl* the plural form of medium.

medial (me′de-əl), *adj* located in or directed toward the middle; closer to the body's midline.

median (me′dē ən), *adj* 1. pertaining to the middle. *n* 2. a measure of central tendency attained by a calculation or count that separates all cases in a ranked distribution into halves. The median may be used as an average score.

median lethal dose, n See dose, lethal, median.

median line, n See line, median.

median mandibular point, n See point, median mandibular.

median nerve, n one of the terminal branches of the brachial plexus that extends along the radial portions of the forearm and the hand and supplies various muscles and the skin of these parts.

median palatine suture, n See suture, intermaxillary.

median retruded relation, n See relation, centric.

median rhomboid glossitis, n a patch of papillae-free mucosa located in the center of the tongue immediately behind the circumvallate papillae. The area appears as a red, smooth, depressed area that is rhomboidal in shape. Generally the lesion is asymptomatic and was thought formerly to result from a fault in embryonic development of the tongue, but it is now viewed as a candidal infection because it can occur later in life after being absent in infancy. Some pathologists refer to this condition as *central papillary atrophy of the tongue.*

median sagittal plane, n See plane, median sagittal.

mediastinitis, *n* an inflammation of the mediastinum.

mediastinum, *n* a portion of the thoracic cavity in the middle of the thorax between the pleural sacs containing the two lungs. It extends from the sternum to the vertebral column and contains all the thoracic viscera except the lungs.

mediation intervention, *n* the act of a third person who interferes between two contending parties to reconcile them or to persuade them to adjust or settle their differences.

Medicaid, *n.pr* a federal assistance program established as Title XIX under the Social Security Amendments of 1965, which provides payment for medical care for certain low-income individuals and families. The program is funded jointly by the state and federal governments and administered by the states.

medical alert warning, *n* ADA, a coding of the patient's medical or dental record to indicate the presence of a serious medical condition that requires treatment planning consideration before treatment of any kind is initiated; usually a pressure-sensitive red warning label containing a notation as to the exact nature of the compromising condition is placed on the record jacket.

medical illustrator, *n* an artist qualified by special training to prepare illustrations of organs, tissues, and medical phenomena in normal and abnormal states.

medical informatics, *n* the field of information science concerned with the analysis and dissemination of medical data through the application of computers to various aspects of health care and medicine.

medical record, *n* the portion of a client's health record that is made by physicians and is a written or transcribed history of various illnesses or injuries requiring medical care, including inoculations, allergies, treatments, prognoses, and frequently health information about immediate family, occupation, and military service.

medical staff, *n* physicians and dentists who are approved and given privileges to provide health care to patients in a hospital or other health care facility.

medical waste, *n* any discarded biologic product, such as blood or tissues, removed from operating rooms, morgues, laboratories, or other medical facilities. The term may also be applied to bedding, bandages, syringes, and similar materials that have been used in treating patients, as well as animal carcasses or body parts used in research.

medical waste disposal, n the safe and proper handling of medical waste, prescribed by statute and institutional policy and designed to prevent cross contamination, reinfection, and transmission of disease.

medically necessary care, *n* the reasonable and appropriate diagnosis, treatment, and follow-up care (including supplies, appliances, and devices) as determined and prescribed by qualified appropriate health care providers in treating any condition, illness, disease, injury, or birth developmental malformation. Care is medically necessary for the purpose of controlling or eliminating infection, pain, and disease and restoring facial configuration or function necessary for speech, swallowing, or chewing.

Medicare, *n.pr* a federal insurance program enacted in 1965 as Title XVIII of the Social Security Amendments that provides certain inpatient hospital services and physician services for all persons age 65 and older and eligible disabled individuals. The program is administered by the Health Care Financing Administration.

Medicare Part A, *n* provides hospital insurance to all qualified beneficiaries under the Medicare criteria.

Medicare Part B, *n* provides medical insurance coverage for services such as physician's services, outpatient services, and home health care. Participation under Part B is voluntary, and beneficiaries pay monthly premiums. Part B is also called Supplementary Medical Insurance.

medication (med′ikā′shən), *n* **I.** a drug or other substance that is used as a medicine. *n* **2.** the administration of a medicine.

medication, antiretroviral, during pregnancy, *n.pl* substances used to treat RNA viruses (including HIV). The effects on fetal development are not known; however, antiretroviral medications are generally still administered to infected mothers.

medication, complete, *n* the combination of synergistic drugs used to sedate children undergoing prolonged or difficult dental procedures; the patient is in a state of sleep or light anesthesia.

medication, intracanal, *n* a drug used in the root canal system during the course of therapy.

medication, official, *n* See drug, official.

medication, officinal, *n* See drug, officinal.

medication, repository, *n* slowly soluble drug mixtures intended for parenteral injection and gradual absorption into the blood and hence into other tissues of the body.

medication, sustained release, *n* oral dosage forms designed to be absorbed at various levels in the gastrointestinal tract, thus prolonging action.

medication, transdermal, *n* See transdermal delivery system.

medicine (med′isin), *n* **I.** a remedy. *n* **2.** the art of healing.

medicine, oral, *n* the discipline of dentistry that deals with the significance and relationship of oral and systemic disease.

medicine, practice of, *n* a pursuit that includes the application and use of medicines and drugs for the purpose of curing or alleviating bodily diseases; surgery is usually limited to manual operations generally performed by means of surgical instruments or appliances.

mediostrusive, *n* nonfunctional side tooth contacts during lateral jaw movements.

mediotrusion, *n* a thrusting of the mandibular condyle inward (toward the median plane). When the right condyle is thrust outward (in laterotrusion) before it is rotated, the left condyle is thrust inward before it is orbited and is thus said to be in precurrent mediotrusion. If the left condyle is thrust outward before it is rotated, the right condyle is in precurrent mediotrusion.

Mediterranean anemia, *n* See thalassemia major.

medium (mē′dē um), *n* an interposed agent or material; a carrier; a material serving as an environment for the growth of microorganisms.

medium, computer, *n* the material on which data are recorded (for example, punched cards, magnetic tape, disks, diskettes).

medium, marking, *n* **I.** any of several agents, such as carbon paper or inked ribbon, used to indicate an occlusal interference. *n* **2.** any of several agents, such as stencil correction fluid, rouge and alcohol, or pressure indicator paste, used to determine ar-

M

eas of interference or pressure related to a removable prosthesis.

medium, radiopaque, *n* a substance that may be injected into a cavity or region to increase its density in x-ray examination and thereby aid in diagnosis. Lipiodol, Iodochloral, Parabodril, and Ioduron are examples of such materials.

medium, Sabouraud's, *n.pr* a nutrient agar used to grow fungi. It is especially useful for the growth and identification of *Candida albicans,* the causative agent of thrush.

medium, separating, *n* any coating that is used on a surface and serves to prevent another surface or material from adhering to the first (for example, tinfoil, cellophane, or alginate, all of which are used to protect an acrylic resin from the moisture in the gypsum mold).

MEDLARS, *n.pr* the abbreviation for Medical Literature Analysis and Retrieval System, which is a computerized literature retrieval service offered by the National Library of Medicine in Bethesda, Maryland. MEDLARS contains more than 4.5 million references to medical and dental articles in professional journals and books published since 1966. The references are made available online to more than 1,000 hospitals, universities, medical centers, and government agencies.

MEDLINE, *n.pr* a National Library of Medicine computer data base of current references published during the past 2 years. The files duplicate the contents of the Unabridged Index Medicus, which contains medical and dental reports from 3,000 professional journals from more than 70 countries.

medroxyprogesterone acetate, *n* *trade names:* Amen, Curretab, Cycrin; *drug class:* progestogen; *action:* inhibits secretion of pituitary gonadotropins, which prevents follicular maturation and ovulation; stimulates growth of mammary tissue; antineoplastic action against endometrial cancer; *uses:* abnormal uterine bleeding, secondary amenorrhea, endometrial cancer, metastatic renal cancer, contraceptive, with estrogens to reduce incidence of endometrial cancer.

medulla oblongata (mədul′ə oblôngä′tə), *n* the direct upward extension of the spinal cord that lies at the junction between the cerebrum and the spinal cord and is considered to be in a group with the pons and midbrain because the nuclei of all the cranial nerves except one are situated within this structural group. The medullary functions are associated with the nuclei of the glossopharyngeal, vagal, spinal accessory, and hypoglossal nerves. The medulla controls the reflex actions of the pharynx, larynx, and tongue, which are related to deglutition, mastication, and speech, as well as the visceral reflexes of coughing, sneezing, sucking, vomiting, and salivating, and other secretory functions.

mefenamic acid, *n* *trade name:* Ponstel; *drug class:* nonsteroidal antiinflammatory; *action:* inhibits prostaglandin synthesis by interfering with cyclooxygenase needed for biosynthesis; possesses analgesic, antiinflammatory, antipyretic properties; *uses:* mild-to-moderate pain, dysmenorrhea, inflammatory disease.

megacolon, *n* an abnormal dilation of the colon that may be congenital, toxic, or acquired.

megacolon, acquired, *n* a result of a chronic refusal to defecate, usually occurring in children who are psychotic or mentally retarded.

megacolon, congenital, *n* caused by the absence of autonomic ganglia in the smooth muscle wall of the colon.

megacolon, toxic, *n* a serious complication of ulcerative colitis that may result in perforation of the colon, septicemia, and death.

megadontismus (megədontiz′mus), *n* See macrodontia.

megestrol acetate, *n* *trade name:* Megace; *drug class:* antineoplastic (progestin); *action:* affects endometrium by antiluteinizing effect; *uses:* breast, endometrial cancer, renal cell cancer.

meiosis (mi-o′sis), *n* a type of cell division peculiar to maturing sex cells which ensures that each daughter cell contains the necessary complement of chromosomes for future embryonic development.

Second meiotic division. (Moore/Persaud, 2003)

Meissner's corpuscles (mīs′nurz), *n.pr* See corpuscle, Meissner's.

melanin (mel′ənin), *n* the dark amorphous pigment of melanotic tumors, skin, hair, choroid coat of the eye, and substantia nigra of the brain.

melanocytes (mel′ənəsīts), *n.pl* dendritic cells of the gingival epithelium that, when functional, cause pigmentation regardless of race.

melanoma (mel′ənō′mə), *n* a malignant neoplasm characterized by pigment-producing cells. It usually is dark in color but may be amelanotic, that is, free of pigment.

melanosis (mel′ənō′sis), *n* the condition in which melanin pigments appear in the tissues. Melanosis is normal in the gingivae of most dark-skinned individuals and occasionally in those with light skin.

melatonin, *n* the only hormone secreted into the bloodstream by the pineal gland. The hormone appears to inhibit numerous endocrine functions, including the gonadotropic hormones, and to decrease the pigmentation of the skin.

melena (melē′nə), *n* the passage of dark or black stools; the color is produced by altered blood and blood pigments.

melituria (mel′itōō′rē ə), *n* the presence of any sugar in the urine (e.g., glucose, lactose, pentose, fructose, maltose, galactose, or sucrose).

melphalan, *n trade name:* Alkeran; *drug class:* antineoplastic; *action:* responsible for cross-linking DNA strands, which leads to cell death; *uses:* palliative treatment of multiple myeloma and nonresectable epithelial carcinoma of the ovary.

melting range, *n* See range, melting.

member, *n* an individual enrolled in a dental benefits program. See also beneficiary.

membrane, *n* a thin layer of tissue that covers a surface or divides a space or organ.

membrane, basement, *n* the delicate, PAS-positive, noncellular membrane on which the epithelium is seated.

membrane bone, *n* See bone, membrane.

membrane, intramembranous (in′trəmem′brənus), *n* formed by differentiation of mesenchymal cells into osteoblasts and bone matrix. See also bone, membrane and bone, membrane, formation.

membrane, mucous, *n* See mucosa.

membrane, Nasmyth's, *n.pr* See cuticle, primary.

membrane, oropharyngeal, *n* a layer of tissue on the cephalic end of the embryo in the region where the mouth will later be formed. Previously called *buccopharyngeal membrane.* See also oropharynx.

membrane, periodontal, *n* See ligament, periodontal.

membrane, subimplant, *n* the fibrous connective tissue that regenerates from the periosteum and that forms between the inner surface of the implant framework and the bone surface.

memory, *n* **1.** the ability to recall events, experiences, information, and skills. *n* **2.** a general term for a device that stores data in binary code on electronic or magnetic media in computers. *n* **3.** the ability of the immune system to greatly speed up the response to pathogens that have previously been encountered.

M

memory cycle, n the time it takes to access a character in memory.

memory location, n a place in the memory where a unit of data may be stored or retrieved.

memory, long-term, n the ability to recall events, experiences, information, or skills that occurred or were acquired in the distant past.

memory register, n a register in storage of a computer, in contrast with a register in one of the other units of the computer.

memory, short-term, n the ability to retain and recall recent events or experiences.

menadiol/menadiol sodium diphosphate (vitamin K$_4$), n *trade name:* Synkavite; *drug class:* synthetic vitamin K; *action:* needed for adequate blood clotting (factors II, VII, IX, X); *uses:* vitamin K malabsorption, hypoprothrombinemia, oral anticoagulant toxicity.

menarche, the beginning of the menstrual function.

Mendelian inheritance, *n.pr* better known as Mendel's laws or mendelian laws, which are the basic principles of genetics based on the experiments of Gregor Mendel in the nineteenth century. Two basic genetic principles were established: the law of segregation and the law of independent assortment. According to the law of segregation, the genetic characteristics of a species are represented in the somatic cells by a pair of units called genes that separate during meiosis so that each gamete receives only one gene for each trait. According to the law of independent assortment, the members of a gene pair on different chromosomes segregate independently from other pairs during meiosis, so that the gametes offer all possible combinations of factors.

Meniere's disease, *n.pr* a chronic disease of the inner ear characterized by recurrent episodes of vertigo, which is progressive sensorineural hearing loss. It may occur bilaterally and may include tinnitus.

meninges, *n.pl* the three membranes enclosing the brain and the spinal cord, comprising the dura mater, the pia mater, and the arachnoid.

meningioma, n a mesenchymal fibroblastic tumor of the membranes enveloping the brain and spinal cord. Meningiomas grow slowly, are usually vascular, and occur most commonly near the superior longitudinal, transverse, and cavernous sinuses of the dura mater of the brain.

meningism, n an abnormal condition characterized by irritation of the brain and spinal cord and by symptoms that mimic those of meningitis. In meningism, however, there is no actual inflammation of the meninges.

meningitis, n any infection or inflammation of the membranes covering the brain and spinal cord. It usually is a purulent infection and involves the fluid of the subarachnoid space. The most common causes in adults are bacterial infection with *Streptococcus pneumoniae, Neisseria meningitidis,* or *Haemophilus influenzae.* Aseptic meningitis may be caused by chemical irritation, neoplasms, or viruses.

meningocele, n a saclike protrusion of either the cerebral or spinal meninges through a congenital defect in the skull or the vertebral column.

meningoencephalitis, n an inflammation of both the brain and the meninges, usually caused by a bacterial infection.

meningomyelocele, n a saclike cyst containing brain tissue, cerebrospinal fluid, and the meninges that protrudes through a congenital defect in the skull.

meniscectomy (men'isek'təmē), n the surgical removal of the meniscus or condylar disc, also referred to as *discectomy.* A popular treatment of dysfunctional maxillofacial pain in the 1950s, it is somewhat discredited today.

meniscus, n the cartilaginous intracapsular disc interposed between the mandibular condyle and the glenoid fossa of the temporal bone.

menopause, n the cessation of menstruation in the human female occurring variably from approximately 45 to 50 years of age. Menopause is accompanied by diminution of estrogen formation, often with atrophic changes occurring in the oral mucous membranes and gingivae.

menopause, hot flashes, n sudden surges of heat and perspiration encompassing the entire body which may occur day or night as the result of hormonal fluctuations during menopause.

menopause, oral symptoms of, n a burning sensation and dryness of the mouth; salty taste; edematous, reddened, atrophic-appearing, tender mucosa; glossitis; and often desquamative gingivitis.

menorrhagia, n abnormally heavy or long menstrual periods. Menorrhagia is a relatively common complication of benign uterine fibromyoma; it may be so severe, or intractable, as to require hysterectomy.

menstrual cycle, n a recurring cycle of change in the endometrium during which the decidual layer of the endometrium is shed, then regrows, proliferates, is maintained for several days, and is shed again at menstruation. The average length of the cycle is 28 days.

menstruation, n the shedding of the necrotic mucosa of the endometrium and associated bleeding that occurs in the final phase of the menstrual cycle. The average duration of menstruation is 5 days, in which approximately 30 ml of blood is lost.

mental disorder, n any disturbance of emotional equilibrium as manifested in maladaptive behavior and impaired functioning, caused by genetic, physical, chemical, biologic, psychologic, or social and cultural factors. Also called *emotional illness, mental illness, psychiatric disorder.*

mental foramen, n See foramen, mental.

mental health, n a relative state of mind in which a person who is healthy is able to cope with and adjust to the recurrent stresses of everyday living in an acceptable way.

mental health service, n any one of a group of government, professional, or lay organizations operating at a community, state, national, or international level to aid in the prevention and treatment of mental disorders.

mental protuberance, n an obvious projection or eminence of the chin near the mesioanterior surface of the mandible. See also menton.

mental retardate, n an individual who is intellectually inadequate in society.

mental retardation, n a disorder of general intellectual function impairing the ability to learn and adapt socially.

menthol, n a topical antipruritic with a cooling effect that relieves itching. It is an ingredient in many topical creams and ointments.

menton, n the most inferior point on the chin in the lateral view; a cephalometric landmark.

mentor, n an older, trusted, more experienced advisor or counselor who offers helpful guidance to younger, less experienced colleagues.

mepenzolate bromide, n *trade name:* Cantil; *drug class:* gastrointestinal (GI) anticholinergic; *action:* inhibits muscarinic actions of acetylcholine at postganglionic parasympathetic neuroeffector sites; *uses:* treatment of peptic ulcer disease, irritable bowel syndrome in combination with other drugs, other GI disorders.

meperidine HCl, n *trade name:* Demerol; *drug class:* synthetic narcotic analgesic (Controlled Substance Schedule II); *action:* interacts with opioid receptors in the central nervous system to alter pain perception; *uses:* moderate-to-severe pain, preoperative administration in sedation techniques.

mephenesin (mefen′isin), n an antispasmodic drug, 3 ortho-toloxyl, 2 propanediol. Used for the preparation of apprehensive patients for dental and periodontal procedures because of its ability to produce muscular relaxation and euphoria. Usual dosage for an adult is 1 gm in either tablet or elixir form, 20 minutes before the dental procedure.

mephenytoin, n *trade name:* Mesantoin; *drug class:* hydantoin anticonvulsant; *action:* reduces electrical discharges in motor cortex, reducing seizures; *uses:* generalized tonic-clonic seizures, single or complex-partial seizures.

mephobarbital, n *trade name:* Mebaral; *drug class:* barbiturate anticonvulsant (Controlled Substance Schedule IV); *action:* a nonspecific depressant of the central nervous system; may enhance GABA activity in the brain; *uses:* generalized tonic-clonic (grand mal) or absence (petit mal) seizures.

mepivacaine HCl (local), *n trade names:* Isocaine, Polocaine; *drug class:* amide local anesthetic; *action:* inhibits ion fluxes across membranes, particularly sodium transport across cell membranes; decreases rise of depolarization phase of action potential; blocks nerve action potential; *uses:* local dental anesthesia, nerve block, caudal anesthesia, epidural pain relief, paracervical block, transvaginal block or infiltration.

meprobamate, *n trade names:* Equanil, Miltown, Probate, Trancot; *drug class:* sedative-hypnotic, anxiolytic (Controlled Substance Schedule IV); *action:* nonspecific central nervous system depressant; acts in thalamus, limbic system, and spinal cord; *use:* anxiety disorders.

merbromin (murbrō′min), *n* a mercury-bromine compound used as a germicide for disinfection of the skin, mucous membrane, and wounds. Used in 10% alcoholic solution (Scott-Wilson reagent) in the treatment of moniliasis.

mercaptan (murkap′tən), *n* the basic ingredient of the polysulfide polymer employed in rubber base impression materials. See also Thiokol.

mercaptopurine (6-MP), *n trade name:* Purinethol; *drug class:* antineoplastic-antimetabolite; *action:* inhibits purine metabolism at multiple sites, which inhibits DNA and RNA synthesis; *uses:* chronic myelocytic leukemia, acute lymphoblastic leukemia in children, acute myelogenous leukemia.

mercurial (murkyōō′rē əl), *adj* a compound that owes its activity to the mercury it contains.

mercurial line, n See line, mercurial.

mercurialism, *n* (mercury poisoning), **1.** poisoning resulting from the ingestion of pure mercury, its salts, or its vapor. Manifestations of acute intoxication include nausea, vomiting, abdominal cramps, oral and pharyngeal pain, uremia, dehydration, diarrhea, and shock. Manifestations of chronic poisoning include hypersalivation, diarrhea, vertigo, depression, intention tremor, and stomatitis. See also acrodynia and stomatitis, mercurial. *n* **2.** poisoning by ingestion or absorption of mercury compounds. See also line, mercurial.

mercuric chloride, *n* mercury bichloride or perchloride; a corrosive, highly toxic sublimate used as a topical antiseptic and disinfectant for inanimate objects.

Mercurochrome, *n* the trade name for merbromin.

mercury, a metallic element. Its atomic number is 80 and its atomic weight is 200.6. It is the only common metal that is liquid at room temperature, and it occurs in nature almost entirely in the form of its sulfide, cinnabar. It is used in dental amalgams, thermometers, barometers, and other measuring instruments. It forms many poisonous compounds. The major toxic forms are mercury vapor, mercuric salts, and organic mercurials. Elemental mercury is only mildly toxic when ingested because it is poorly absorbed.

mercury poisoning, n a toxic condition caused by the ingestion or inhalation of mercury or a mercury compound. The chronic form, resulting from inhalation of the vapors or dust of mercurial compounds, is characterized by irritability, excessive saliva, loosened teeth, gum disorders, slurred speech, tremors, and staggering. Symptoms of acute mercury poisoning usually appear no later than 30 minutes after exposure and include a metallic taste in the mouth, thirst, nausea, vomiting, severe abdominal pain, bloody diarrhea, and renal failure that may result in death. The presence of mercury in the body is determined by a urine test.

merge, *v* to produce a single sequence of items, ordered according to some rule, from two or more sequences previously ordered according to the same rule. Merging does not change the items in size, structure, or total number.

Merrifield's knife, *n.pr* See knife, Merrifield's.

mes- (meso-), *pref* in the middle; intermediate as in position, size, type, and time degree.

mesalamine, *n* trade names: Asacol, Pentasa, Rowasa; *drug class:* antiin-flammatory; *action:* unknown, may inhibit prostaglandin synthesis; *uses:* inflammatory bowel disease, ulcerative colitis.

mescaline, abuse of (mes'kəlēn, -lin), *n* regular use of mescaline (e.g., mesc, big chief, or buttons), an example of a hallucinogen, for reasons other than recognized medical applications.

mesenchyme (mes'engkīm), *n* an embryonic connective tissue that migrates from the primitive epidermal and hypodermal layers and later produces the mesodermal layer. It is in this layer that embryonic tooth buds begin to form.

mesial (mē'zē əl), *adj* situated in the middle; median, toward the middle line of the body or toward the center line of the dental arch.

mesial migration, n the drifting of teeth toward the midline or forward in the dental arch.

mesial, unilateral, adj mesiocclusion on one side.

mesiocclusion, *n* an occlusal relationship in which the lower teeth are positioned mesially, similar to the relationship in an Angle Class III malocclusion. See also distoclusion.

mesiodens (mē'zē ədenz), *n* a supernumerary tooth appearing in an erupted or unerupted state between the two maxillary central incisors.

mesioversion (mēzē ōvur'zhən), *n* when applied to a tooth, a term indicating that the tooth is closer than normal to the median plane or midline. When applied to the maxillae or mandible, it means that the jaw is anterior to its normal position.

meso-, *pref* See mes-.

mesocephalic (mes'ōsefal'ik), *adj* a descriptive term applied to a head size between dolichocephalic and brachycephalic (cephalic index 76 to 81).

mesoderm, *n* the middle of the three cell layers of the developing embryo. It lies between the ectoderm and the endoderm. Bone, connective tissue, muscle, blood, vascular and lymphatic tissue, and the pleurae of the pericardium and peritoneum are all derived from the mesoderm.

mesodontia (mes'ōdon'shē ə), *n.pl* medium-size teeth.

mesognathic (mes'ōnāth'ik), *adj* having an average relationship of jaws to head.

mesonephros, *n* the second type of excretory organ to develop in the vertebrate embryo. The organ is the permanent kidney in lower animals, but in humans and various other mammals it is functional only during early embryonic development.

mesoridazine besylate, *n* trade name: Serentil; *drug class:* phenothiazine antipsychotic; *action:* blocks neurotransmission at dopaminergic synapses in the cerebral cortex, hypothalamus, and limbic system; mechanism for antipsychotic effects is unclear; *uses:* psychotic disorders, schizophrenia, anxiety, alcoholism, behavioral problems in mental deficiency, chronic brain syndrome.

mesostomia (mes'ōstō'mē ə), *n* an oral fissure of medium size.

mesostructure conjunction bar, *n* a connecting bar joining implant abutment copings together. Bar and copings together make up the mesostructure.

mesothelioma, *n* a rare malignant tumor of the mesothelium of the pleura or peritoneum associated with exposure to asbestos.

metaanalysis, *n* a quantitative method of combining the results of independent studies (usually drawn from the published literature) and synthesizing summaries and conclusions that may be used to evaluate therapeutic effectiveness and plan new studies, with application chiefly in the areas of research and medicine and dentistry.

metabolic disease, *n* any disorder that causes dysfunction of the metabolic action of the body, resulting in loss of control of homeostasis.

metabolism (metab'ōlizəm), *n* the sum of chemical changes involved in the function of nutrition. There are two phases: anabolism (constructive or assimilative changes) and catabolism (destructive or retrograde changes).

metabolism, basal, n See basal metabolic rate.

metabolism, bone, n the continual complex of anabolism and catabo-

M

lism taking place in bone when it is in physiologic equilibrium. Bone is a highly labile substance that reflects the adequacy of general body metabolism. See also bone, alveolar, metabolism.

metabolism, cell, n the complexity of anabolic and catabolic processes occurring within cellular structures.

metabolism, energy, n the transformation of energy in living tissues, consisting of anabolism (storage of energy) and catabolism (the dissipation of energy).

metabolism, substance, n the sum of all the physical and chemical processes by which living organized tissues are produced and maintained.

metacarpus, n the five bones of the hand between the carpus (wrist) and the phalanges (fingers).

metal, n an element possessing luster, malleability, ductility, and conductivity of electricity and heat.

metal, base, n an archaic term referring to nonprecious metals or alloys such as iron, lead, copper, nickel, chromium, and zinc. In dentistry, the term usually refers to the stainless steel and chrome-cobalt-nickel alloys.

metal ceramic alloys, n the fusion of ceramics (porcelain) to an alloy of two or more metals for use in restorative and prosthodontic dentistry. Examples of metal alloys employed include cobalt-chromium, gold-palladium, gold-platinum-palladium, and nickel-based alloys.

metal, fusion of, n the blending of metals by melting together.

metal insert teeth, n.pl See tooth, metal insert.

metal, noble, n a precious metal, usually one that does not readily oxidize, such as gold or platinum.

metal, solidification of, n the change of metal from the molten to the solid state.

metal, wrought, n a cast metal that has been cold-worked in any manner.

metallic salts, n.pl compounds such as potassium oxalate or strontium chloride used by dental professionals to help desensitize teeth. They work by forming a gritty film which blocks the dentin tubules.

metalloid (met′əloid), n a nonmetallic element that behaves as a metal under certain conditions. Carbon, silicon, and boron are three examples. These elements may be alloyed with metals.

metalloprotein, n a protein with a tightly bound metal ion or ions, such as hemoglobin.

metallothioneins (MTs) (mətal′ōthī′-ōnēn), n.pl proteins and polypeptides containing very high levels of metal and sulfur. MTs are most common in the functional tissue of an organ and are considered useful in controlling the intracellular fixation and the free ion concentration of the trace elements zinc and copper, as well as defending the body against stress and toxic substances.

metallurgy, n the study of metals and their properties, including separating metals from their ores, the making and compounding of alloys, and the technology and science of working and heat-treating metals to alter their physical characteristics.

metanephrine, n one of the two principal urinary metabolites of epinephrine and norepinephrine in the urine, the other being vanillylmandelic acid.

metaphen, tincture of (met′əfen), n the trade name for tincture of nitromersol.

metaphysis (mətaf′isis), n the line of junction of the epiphysis with the diaphysis of a long bone.

metaplasia (met′əplā′zhə), n a change in the type of adult cells in a tissue to a form that is not normal for that tissue.

metaproterenol sulfate, n *trade names:* Arm-A-Med, Metaprel, Prometa; *drug class:* selective β_2-agonist; *action:* relaxes bronchial smooth muscle by direct action on β_2-adrenergic receptors; *uses:* bronchial asthma, bronchospasm.

metastasis (mətas′təsis), n the transfer of a disease by blood vessels, lymph vessels, or the respiratory tract (through aspiration) from one organ or region to another not directly contiguous with it. Usually used in reference to malignant tumor cells, but bacteria can also metastasize (for example, in focal infection).

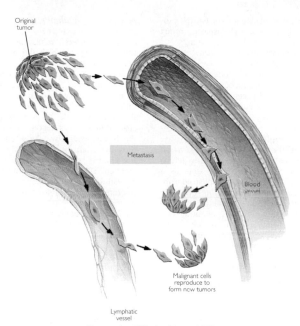

Original tumor

Metastasis

Blood vessel

Malignant cells reproduce to form new tumors

Lymphatic vessel

Metastasis. (Thibodeau/Patton, 2002)

M

meteorologic factors, *n.pl* variables of the atmosphere or weather that affect behavior, or mental or physical state.

meter, dose rate, *n* any instrument that measures radiation dose rate.

meter, integrating dose rate, *n* the ionization chamber and measuring system designed for determining the total accumulated radiation administered during an exposure.

meter, radiation, *n* an instrument for the measurement of exposure to radiation.

meter, radiation dosimeter, *n* an instrument used to detect and measure an accumulated exposure to radiation, commonly a pencil-size ionization chamber with built-in self-reading electrometer used in personnel radiation monitoring.

metformin HCl, *n trade name:* Glucophage; *drug class:* oral hypoglycemic, biguanide derivative; *action* exact mechanism unknown, requires insulin secretion to function properly; *use:* type II diabetes mellitus.

methacrylate, *n* an ester of meth-

acrylic acid used as a pit and fissure sealant. See also methyl methacrylate.

methadone HCl, *n trade names:* Dolophine, Methadone; *drug class:* synthetic narcotic analgesic (Controlled Substance Schedule II); *action:* interacts with opioid receptors in the central nervous system to alter pain perception; *uses:* severe pain, opioid withdrawal program.

methamphetamine HCl, *n trade name:* Desoxyn Gradumet; *drug class:* amphetamine (Controlled Substance Schedule II); *action:* increases release of norepinephrine and dopamine in cerebral cortex to reticular activating system; *uses:* exogenous obesity, minimal brain dysfunction, attention deficit disorder with hyperactivity.

methantheline bromide, *n trade name:* Banthine; *drug class:* synthetic anticholinergic; *action:* inhibits muscarinic actions of acetylcholine at postganglionic parasympathetic neuroeffector sites; *uses:* treatment of peptic ulcer disease, irritable bowel syndrome, pancreatitis, gastritis, biliary dyskinesia, pylorospasm, reflex neurogenic bladder in children.

methazolamide, *n* *trade name:* Neptazane; *drug class:* carbonic anhydrase inhibitor; *action:* decreases production of aqueous humor in the eye, which lowers intraocular pressure; *uses:* open-angle glaucoma or preoperatively in narrow-angle glaucoma.

methemoglobinemia (met′hēməglō′binē′mē ə), *n* an abnormality of hemoglobin in which the iron is in the ferric state as a result of exposure to industrial substances or the ingestion of toxic agents such as phenacetin, sulfonamides, aniline nitrates, or nitrates. A rare congenital form is seen most commonly in persons with Greek heritage. Symptoms include generalized cyanosis, headache, drowsiness, and confusion. Methemoglobin does not carry oxygen.

methenamine salts, *n trade names:* Hiprex, Urex; *drug class:* urinary antiinfective; *action:* in acid urine, it is hydrolyzed to ammonia and formaldehyde, which are bactericidal; *uses:* prophylaxis and treatment of uncomplicated urinary tract infections.

methicillin sodium, *n* a semisynthetic penicillin salt for parenteral administration. Restriction of its use to infections caused by penicillin G-resistant staphylococci is recommended.

methimazole, *n trade name:* Tapazole; *drug class:* thyroid hormone antagonist; *action:* inhibits synthesis of thyroid hormones by decreasing iodine use in manufacture of thyroglobulin and iodothyronine; *uses:* hyperthyroidism, preparation for thyroidectomy, thyrotoxic crisis, thyroid storm.

methionine, *n* one of the essential amino acids. See also amino acid.

methocarbamol, *n trade name:* Carbacot, Delaxin, Robamol, Skelex; *drug class:* skeletal muscle relaxant; *action:* depresses multisynaptic pathways in the spinal cord; *uses:* adjunct for relief of spasm and pain in musculoskeletal conditions.

method, *n* a manner of performing an act or operation; a technique.

method, Callahan's, *n.pr* See method, chloropercha.

method, Charters', *n.pr* a method of toothbrushing in which the brush is held horizontally, with the bristles lying against the teeth and gingivae and pointed in a coronal direction at 45 degrees so that the bristles lie half on the teeth and half on the gingivae. A vibratory cycle of a very constricted diameter is negotiated so that the brush head moves in a circular movement but the brush bristles remain fairly stationary while being agitated. The circular vibration loosens debris and pumps the bristles into interproximal areas to massage the tissues.

method, chloropercha, *n* (Callahan's method, Johnston's method), the method of filling root canals in which gutta-percha cones are dissolved in a chloroform-rosin solution in the root canal. The canal is flooded with the chloroform solution. A preselected gutta-percha cone is then pumped carefully into and out of the canal. As the cone dissolves, the material is forced into the apex as a plastic mass. Other cones and occasionally additional chloroform solution are added until the canal is sealed.

method, Collis, *n* a variation of toothbrushing that employs short, repetitive strokes with a Collis curved brush. Collis's brush design allows for brushing three surfaces of the tooth simultaneously. A 45-degree angle is used when brushing in and around the gum line. Favored by special needs patients, as well as parents and caretakers who perform the task of brushing for others. Also called *simultaneous sulcular.*

method, Fones', *n.pr* (Fones' technique), a toothbrushing technique in which, with the teeth occluded and with the brush at more or less right angles to the teeth, large sweeping, scrubbing circles are described. With the jaws parted, the palatal and lingual surfaces of the teeth are scrubbed using smaller circles. Occlusal surfaces are brushed in an anteroposterior direction.

method, Hirschfeld's, *n.pr* a toothbrushing method in which the bristles are placed against the axial surfaces of the teeth, with slight incisal or occlusal inclination from a right-angled application, in simultaneous contact with teeth and gingivae, and then rotated in a circle of exceedingly small diameter. Occlusal surfaces are brushed energetically.

method, Howard's, *n.pr* a method of artificial respiration. The patient is placed on the back, with the hands under the head, and a cushion is placed so that the head is lower than the abdomen. The physician applies rhythmical pressure upward and in ward with the hands against the lower lateral parts of the patient's chest.

method, Howe's silver precipitation, *n.pr* a method of depositing silver in enamel and dentin by the application of ammoniacal silver nitrate solution and its reduction with formalin or eugenol.

method, indirect restorative, *n* the technique of fabrication of a restoration on a cast or model of the original (for example, the indirect method of inlay construction, in which a die of amalgam or other material is made from an impression of the prepared tooth, a wax pattern is formed, and the cast inlay is fitted and finished on the die and then cemented to the tooth).

method, Johnston's, *n.pr* See method, chloropercha.

method, lateral condensation, *n* the method in which a preselected gutta-percha cone is sealed into the apex of the root. The balance of the space is filled with other gutta-percha cones forced laterally with a spreader.

method, Leonard, *n.pr* a method of teeth cleaning that advocates a vigorous drawing of the toothbrush up and down across the teeth. The teeth are held apart, so that each section is brushed separately: upper, lower, mandibular, and maxillary. Also known as *vertical toothbrushing.*

method, modified Stillman, *n.pr* a toothbrushing technique characterized by the placement of the toothbrush head against the gingiva, vibrating it, then rolling the bristles over the rest of the tooth's surface. Each stroke is repeated five times for each section of the mouth.

Modified Stillman method. (Daniel/Harfst, 2002)

method, prebook, *n* a method of scheduling appointments in which the patient schedules the next appointment while checking out from the current one. A reminder card is filled out at this time, to be mailed later.

method, rolling stroke, *n* a simple, introductory toothbrushing technique that does not include brushing of the gingival sulcus. Often taught to children as a precursor to the modified Stillman method, or as a preliminary framework for a more advanced technique incorporating vibration of the brush.

method, segmentation, *n* the method in which a preselected gutta percha cone is cut into segments. The tip section is sealed into the apex of the root. The other segments are usually warmed and condensed against the first piece with a plugger. Additional pieces are then used until the space is obliterated.

method, silver cone, *n* the method in which a prefitted silver cone is sealed into the apex of the root canal. The space not sealed with the cone is obliterated with gutta-percha or sealer.

method, Smith's, *n.pr* a toothbrushing technique referred to as physiologic, in which the brush strokes mimic the path taken by food when it is chewed.

method, SOAP (subjective, objective, assessment, plan), *n* a widely accepted method for making notes to the problem-oriented record in which S stands for subjective data obtained from the patient or family; O refers to objective data acquired by observation, inspection, or testing; A relates to the assessment of the patient's current situation and progress made throughout the course of treatment; and P represents the actual patient care plan.

method, split cast, *n* **1.** a procedure for checking the ability of an articulator to receive or to be adjusted to a maxillomandibular relation record. *n* **2.** a procedure for indexing casts on an articulator to facilitate their removal and replacement on the instrument.

method, Stillman's, *n.pr* a toothbrushing technique that incorporates gingival stimulation and dental cleansing, in which the toothbrush is held against both the gingival and the dental surfaces and manually vibrated.

method, sulcal (sul′kəl), *n* a toothbrushing technique for controlling plaque involving placement of the bristles in the sulcus at an angle of 45 degrees to the tooth's long axis and vibrating the bristles in a quick manner from side to side. It may also be called the *Bass method.*

methohexital sodium, *n* an intravenous barbiturate prescribed for the induction of anesthesia in short surgical procedures as a supplement to other anesthetics.

methotrexate/methotrexate sodium, *n trade names:* Folex, Mexate, Rheumatrex; *drug class:* folic acid antagonist, antineoplastic; *action:* inhibits an enzyme that reduces folic acid, which is needed for nucleic acid synthesis in all cells; *uses:* acute lymphocytic leukemia; in combination for breast, lung, head, neck cancer; lymphosarcoma, psoriasis; gestational choriocarcinoma, hydatid mole.

methoxamine HCl, *n* an adrenergic that acts as a vasoconstrictor and is prescribed for use during anesthesia to maintain blood pressure and in the treatment of paroxysmal supraventricular tachycardia.

methsuximide, *n trade name:* Celontin; *drug class:* anticonvulsant; *action:* inhibits spike wave formation in absence seizures (petit mal); decreases amplitude, frequency, duration, spread of discharge in minor motor seizures; *use:* refractory absence seizures (petit mal).

methyl methacrylate (meth′il methak′rilāt), *n* an acrylic resin, $CH_2 = C(CH_3)COOCH_3$, derived from

methyl acrylic acid. Monomer is the single molecule and polymer is the polymerization product.

methylation, *n* **1.** the introduction of a methyl group, CH_3, to a chemical compound. *n* **2.** the addition of methyl alcohol and naphtha to ethanol to produce denatured alcohol.

methyldopa/methyldopate, *n trade name:* Aldomet; *drug class:* centrally acting antihypertensive; *action:* stimulates central inhibitory α-adrenergic receptors or acts as a false transmitter, resulting in reduction of arterial pressure; *use:* hypertension.

methylene blue, *n* a bluish-green crystalline substance used as a histologic stain and as a laboratory indicator. It is also used in the treatment of cyanide poisoning and methemoglobinemia.

methylmalonicacidemia, *n* a genetic disorder of amino acid metabolism in which methylmalonic acid accumulates in the blood and urine at abnormally high levels. It may respond to a low-protein diet and the administration of synthetic amino acids. Also called *methylmalonicaciduria,* especially if the concentration is limited to or greatest in the urine.

methylphenidate HCl, *n trade names:* Methidate, Ritalin; *drug class:* central nervous system stimulant, related to amphetamines (Controlled Substance Schedule II); *action:* increases release of norepinephrine, dopamine in cerebral cortex to reticular activating system; exact mode of action not known; *uses:* attention deficit disorder with hyperactivity, narcolepsy.

methylprednisolone / methylprednisolone acetate/methylprednisolone sodium succinate, *n trade names:* Medrol, Meprolone; *drug class:* immediate acting glucocorticoid; *action:* decreases inflammation by suppressing macrophage and leukocyte migration; reduces capillary permeability and inhibits lysosomal enzymes and phagocytosis; *uses:* severe inflammation, shock, adrenal insufficiency, collagen disorders.

methylxanthine (meth′ilzan′thēn), *n* diuretic agent (e.g., aminophylline, caffeine, or theophylline) that serves as a smooth muscle relaxant and cardiac muscle and CNS stimulant.

Clinically, it is employed as a bronchodilator.

methysergide maleate, *n trade name:* Sansert; *drug class:* serotonin antagonist; *action:* competitively blocks serotonin HT receptors in central nervous system and periphery; *uses:* prophylaxis for migraine and other vascular headaches.

Meticorten, *n* the trade name for prednisone.

metoclopramide HCl, *n trade name:* Clopra, Maxolon, Reglan; *drug class:* central dopamine receptor antagonist; *action:* enhances response to acetylcholine of tissue in upper GI tract, which causes contraction of gastric muscle, relaxes pyloric and duodenal segments, increases peristalsis without stimulating secretions; antiemetic action occurs centrally; *uses:* prevention of nausea, vomiting induced by chemotherapy, radiation, delayed gastric emptying, gastroesophageal reflux.

metolazone, *n trade names:* Diulo, Mykrox, Zaroxolyn; *drug class:* diuretic with thiazidelike effects; *action:* acts on distal tubule by increasing excretion of water, sodium, chloride, and potassium; *uses:* edema, hypertension, CHF.

metoprolol tartrate, *n trade name:* Nu Metop; *drug class:* antihypertensive selective β_1-blocker; *action:* produces fall in blood pressure without reflex tachycardia or significant reduction in heart rate; *uses:* mild-to-moderate hypertension, acute myocardial infarction to reduce cardiovascular mortality, angina pectoris.

metric system, *n* See system, metric.

metronidazole, *n* a generic synthetic antibacterial compound available for both oral and intravenous use. Metronidazole is indicated in the treatment of serious infections caused by susceptible anaerobic bacteria. In dentistry, metronidazole is used in the treatment of HIV, gingivitis, and HIV periodontitis.

metronidazole HCl, *n trade name:* Flagyl, Metro IV, Protostat; *drug class:* trichomonacide, amebicide, antiinfective; *action:* direct-acting amebicide/trichomonacide binds, degrades DNA in organisms; *uses:* intestinal amebiasis, amebic abscess, trichomoniasis, refractory trichomoniasis, bacterial anaerobic infections.

MeV, *n* one million electron volts.

mexiletine HCl, *n trade name:* Mexitil; *drug class:* antidysrhythmic (Class IB, lidocaine analog); *action:* blocks sodium channel in His-Purkinje system, which decreases the effective refractory period and shortens the duration of the action potential; *use:* documented life-threatening ventricular dysrhythmias.

micelle (mĭsel′), *n* any one of the spaces formed by the brush structure of fibrils in colloidal gels. The spaces are occupied by water in hydrocolloid impressions.

miconazole, *n trade names:* Monistat, Monistat IV; *drug class:* antifungal; *action:* alters cell membranes and inhibits fungal enzymes; *uses:* coccidioidomycosis, candidiasis, cryptococcosis, paracoccidioidomycosis, fungal meningitis; IV used for severe infections only.

miconazole nitrate (topical), *n trade names:* Micatin, Monistat-7; *drug class:* antifungal; *action:* interferes with fungal cell membrane, which increases permeability, leaking of nutrients; *uses:* tinea pedis, tinea cruris, tinea corporis, tinea versicolor, vaginal or vulvar *Candida albicans*.

microbiology, *n* the branch of biology concerned with the study of microorganisms, including algae, bacteria, viruses, protozoa, fungi, and rickettsiae.

microbiota, *n* the microscopic organisms living within a particular region.

microcephalus (mī′krōsef′əlus), *n* an abnormally small head.

microchemistry, *n* the branch of chemistry concerned with the study of chemical processes at the cellular and subcellular levels.

microcirculation, *n* the flow of blood throughout the system of smaller vessels of the body, particularly the capillaries.

microcomputer, *n* a complete, multiuse, electronic, digital computer system consisting of a central processing unit, storage facilities, I/O ports, and a chip with megabytes of high-speed internal storage; it usually has only one user for personal, home, or office use.

microcurie, *n* one millionth of a curie.

microcyte, *n* an unusually small red blood cell associated with iron deficiency anemia.

M

microcytosis, hereditary (mī´krōsī-tō´sis), *n* See thalassemia; thalassemia major.

microdialysis, *n* a technique for measuring extracellular concentrations of substances in tissues, usually in vivo, by means of a small probe equipped with a semipermeable membrane. Substances may also be introduced into the extracellular space through the membrane.

microdontia (mī´krōdon´shē ə), *n.pl* abnormally small teeth. The term may apply to one, several, or all the teeth of a given individual.

Microdontia. (Sapp/Eversole/Wysocki, 2004)

microelectrode, *n* an electrode of very fine caliber consisting usually of a fine wire or a glass tube of capillary diameter drawn to a fine point and filled with saline or a metal used in physiologic experiments to stimulate or record action currents of extracellular or intracellular origin.

microfilaments, *n.pl* any of the submicroscopic cellular filaments, such as the tonofibrils, found in the cytoplasm of most cells, that function primarily as a supportive system.

microgenia (mī´krōjē´nē ə), *n* an abnormal smallness of the chin.

microglossia (mī´krōglôs´ē ə), *n* an abnormally small tongue.

micrognathia (mī´krōnāth´ē ə), *n* an abnormally small jaw such as that seen in brachygnathia. See also brachygnathia; retrognathism.

microleakage, *n* the seepage of fluids, debris, and microorganisms along the interface between a restoration and the walls of a cavity preparation.

micrometer (mī´krōmēter), *n* a millionth of a meter (10^{-6} meter).

micron, *n* See micrometer.

micronutrient, *n* an organic compound such as a vitamin, or a chemical element such as zinc or iodine, that is essential only in minute amounts for the normal physiologic processes of the body.

microorganism (mī´krō ōr´gənizəm), *n* a minute living organism, such as a bacterium, virus, rickettsia, yeast, or fungus. These organisms may exist as part of the normal flora of the oral cavity without producing disease. With disturbance of the more or less balanced interrelationship between the organisms or between the organisms and host resistance, individual forms of microorganisms may overgrow and induce disease in the host's tissues. Of course, organisms foreign to the individual may invade and produce pathologic processes.

Three basic shapes. (Stepp/Woods, 1998)

microphthalmos, *n* a developmental anomaly characterized by abnormal smallness of one or both eyes.

micropore, *n* **1.** microscopic pores created by enamel etching in order to increase sealant adhesion. *n* **2.** an organelle in certain protozoa that develops at the site of a damaged membrane.

microradiography, *n* a process by which a radiograph of a small or very thin object is produced on fine-grained photographic film under conditions that permit subsequent microscopic examination or enlargement of the radiograph within the resolution limits of the photographic emulsion, which approaches 1,000 lines per millimeter.

microscope, *n* an instrument containing a powerful lens system for magnifying and viewing near objects.

Microscope, Confocal Laser Scanning (CLSM), *n.pr* a microscope equipped with a laser beam light source, electronic image detector, and computer for image storage and processing that is used in the laboratory to perform high-resolution, three-dimensional microscopy.

microscope, dark-field, *n* a microscope that has a special condenser and objective with a diaphragm or stop by which light is scattered from the object with the result that the object appears bright and the background dark.

microscope, electron, *n* a microsope in which electron beams with wavelengths shorter than those of visible light are used in place of visible light, allowing much greater resolution and magnification of the object.

microscope, electron, scanning, *n* an electron microscope capable of reflecting electrons from the specimen surface, resulting in a three-dimensional image of the surface that provides both high resolution and a great depth of focus view of the object.

microscope, interference, *n* a microscope designed to split entering light into two beams that pass through the specimen and are recombined in the image plane, allowing visualization of refractile object details that are not possible with a single beam.

microscope, phase-contrast, *n* a spe-cially constructed microscope that has a special condenser and objective containing a phase-shifting mechanism whereby small differences in refraction can be made visible to intensity or contrast in the images. The phase-contrast microscope is particularly helpful in examining living or unstained cells and tissues. This microscope is an excellent aid in the education and motivation of patients in the understanding and control of dental plaque.

microscopy, *n* a technique for observing minute materials using a microscope.

microscopy, digital epiluminescence (dij'itəl ep'iloo'mines'əns mīkros'kəpē), *n* computer-aided technique that employs a binocular surface microscope to examine pigmented skin lesions.

Microsporum, *n* a genus of dermatophytes of the family Moniliaceae.

microstomia (mī'krōstō'mē ə), *n* **1.** a small oral fissure. *n* **2.** the condition of having an abnormally small mouth.

microsurgery, *n* surgery that involves microdissection and micromanipulation of tissues, usually accomplished with the aid of a binocular microscopic instrument.

microtia (mīkrō'shē ə), *n* aplasia or hypoplasia of the pinna of the ear, with a closed or missing external auditory meatus.

microtubule, *n* a hollow cylindrical structure that occurs widely within plant and animal cells. Microtubules increase in number during cell division and are associated with the movement of DNA material.

microvilli, *n.pl* tiny hairlike processes that extend from the surface of many cells. They are usually so small as to be visible only with an electron microscope.

midazolam HCl, *n trade name:* Versed; *drug class:* benzodiazepine general anesthetic, anesthesia adjunct (Controlled Substance Schedule IV); *action:* depresses subcortical levels in central nervous system; may act on limbic system, reticular formation; may potentiate γ-aminobutyric acid (GABA) by binding to specific benzodiazepine receptors; *uses:* conscious sedation, general anesthesia induction, sedation for diagnostic en-

M

M

doscopic procedures, intubation, pre-operative sedation.

midbrain (mid'brān), *n* the portion of the brain located superior to the pons and medulla and containing the motor nuclei of the ocular motor and trochlear nerves. It also contains the major pathways and decussations of fibers from the cerebrum and cerebellum.

middle age, *n* the period between young adult and elderly, usually 35 to 55 years of age; a period of great productivity. Also called *middle adult.*

midface, *n* that portion of the face comprising the nasal, maxillary, and zygomatic bones and the soft tissues covering these bones.

midline, *n* the line equidistant from bilateral features of the head.

midwife, *n* **1.** in traditional use, a (female) person who assists women in childbirth. **2.** a nurse practitioner trained and experienced in assisting women in childbirth.

migraine, *n* See headache, migraine.

migration, pathological, *n* See tooth, migration of.

migration, tooth, *n* See tooth, drifting.

migratory glossitis, *n* also known as *geographic tongue.* See also tongue, geographic.

migratory polyarthritis, *n* a temporary form of arthritis caused by rheumatic fever.

milliammeter, *n* an element on an x-ray machine used in dental procedures which controls the amount of current during an x-ray emission.

milliamperage control, *n* a crucial element in the operation of x-ray machinery used in dental procedures which regulates amperes and governs the current that flows toward the patient.

milliampere (mil'ē am'pir), *n* in radiography, milliamperage signifies the amount of current flowing in the tube circuit. With time (seconds), it is an indication of roentgen-ray quantity.

millicurie, *n* one thousandth of a curie.

milliliter (ml) (mil'ilē'tur), *n* the preferred unit of volume used in prescription writing. It is based on the fundamental unit, the liter. One liter equals 1,000 milliliters. In pre-scriptions the abbreviations ml and cc are often used interchangeably because they are so nearly equal.

milling-in, *n* the procedure of refining or perfecting the occlusion of removable partial or complete dentures by placing abrasives between their occluding surfaces while the dentures make contact in various excursions on the articulator.

millirad, (mr) *n* one-thousandth of a rad. Normal background radiation in this country varies from about 50 to 200 mr per year, depending on geographic location.

milliroentgen (mil'irent'gən), *n* a submultiple of the roentgen, equal to one thousandth of a roentgen.

Milwaukee brace, *n.pr* an orthotic device that helps immobilize the torso and the neck of a patient in the treatment or correction of scoliosis, lordosis, or kyphosis. Prolonged use may induce or complicate a malocclusion unless the teeth and jaws are supported with retaining appliances.

mineral oil, *n* See oil, mineral.

mineralization, *n* the bioprecipitation of an inorganic substance.

mineralized deposit, *n* calcified bacterial plaque, which may develop above or below the gingiva, on teeth, replacement teeth, or rehabilitative oral equipment.

mineralocorticoids (min'əral'ōkôr'tikoidz), *n.pl* (proinflammatory hormones), adrenal corticosteroids that are active in the retention of salt and in the maintenance of life of adrenalectomized animals. Typical are deoxycorticosterone and aldosterone. Aldosterone is a natural hormone for salt retention but also has some regulatory effect on carbohydrate metabolism.

minim (min'im), *n* a unit of volume in the traditional apothecary system. One minim equals 0.06 ml. A drop is sometimes used as a crude approximation of the minim.

minocycline HCl, *n trade names:* Dyancin, Minocin; *drug class:* tetracycline antiinfective; *action:* inhibits protein synthesis, phosphorylation in microorganisms by binding 30S ribosomal subunits, reversibly binding to 50S ribosomal subunits; bacteriostatic; *uses:* syphilis, *Chlamydia trachomatis* infection, gonorrhea, lymphogranuloma venereum, rickettsial infections, inflammatory acne. Also used in the treatment of some periodontal infections, generally in conjunction with mechanical therapy.

minor, *n* **1.** a person of either sex under the age of majority, that is, one who has not attained the age at which full civil rights are granted. *adj* **2.** describing a procedure or treatment that is non- or minimally invasive; describing an illness or condition that is temporary and minimally debilitating.

minor connector, n See connector, minor.

minoxidil, *n trade names:* Loniten, Rogaine (topical); *drug class:* antihypertensive; *action:* directly relaxes arteriolar smooth muscle, reducing peripheral resistance; *uses:* severe hypertension not responsive to other therapy (used with a diuretic); topically to treat alopecia (mechanism unknown).

miosis, *n* **1.** the contraction of the sphincter muscle of the iris, causing the pupil to become smaller. *n* **2.** an abnormal condition characterized by excessive constriction of the sphincter muscle of the iris, resulting in very small, pinpoint pupils.

miotic (mē ot′ik), *n* a drug that constricts the pupil.

mirror, *n* a reflective device.

mirror, mouth, n a reflective device used to examine structures within the oral cavity and prevent the lips, cheeks, and tongue from obstructing the assessment.

misappropriation, *n* the act of benefitting financially by using someone's name or likeness without permission; for example, using a dental patient's x-rays in an article without obtaining his or her permission.

miscible (mis′ ĭ-bəl), *adj* may be blended or combined; mixable.

misconduct, *n* a deviation from duty by one employed in a professional capacity; a transgression of an established rule.

misfeasance (misfē′zens), *n* the improper performance of some act that one may lawfully do.

misoprostol, *n trade name:* Cytotec; *drug class:* gastric mucosa protectant; *action:* a prostaglandin E_1 analog that inhibits gastric acid secre-

tion; *uses:* prevention of nonsteroidal antiinflammatory drug-induced gastric ulcers.

misrepresentation, *n* an intentionally false statement regarding a matter of fact.

MIST, *n.pr* an acronym for Medical Information Service via Telephone. MIST is a consultation service offered by some state-operated university medical centers.

mistake, *n* an unintentional act, omission, or error resulting from ignorance, surprise, or misplaced confidence.

mitigation (mit′igā′shən), *n* alleviation; abatement or diminution of a penalty imposed by law.

mitigation of damages, n a reduction of damages based on facts showing that the plaintiff's course of action does not entitle the plaintiff to as large an amount as the evidence would otherwise justify the jury in allowing.

mitochondria, *n.pl* small, rodlike, threadlike, or granular organelles within the cytoplasm that function in cellular metabolism and respiration and occur in varying numbers in all living cells except bacteria, viruses, blue-green algae, and mature erythrocytes.

mitogen, *n* an agent that triggers mitosis.

mitosis, *n* a type of cell division that occurs in somatic cells and results in the formation of two genetically identical daughter cells containing the diploid number of chromosomes characteristic of the species.

mitotane, *n trade name:* Lysodren; *drug class:* antineoplastic; *action:* acts on adrenal cortex to suppress activity and adrenal steroid production; *use:* adrenocortical carcinoma.

mitotic index, *n* the number of cells per unit undergoing mitosis during a given time. The ratio is used primarily as an estimation of the rate of tissue growth.

mitral valve, *n* a bicuspid valve situated between the left atrium and the left ventricle; the only valve with two, rather than three, cusps. The mitral valve allows blood to flow from the left atrium into the left ventricle but prevents blood from flowing back into the atrium.

mitral valve prolapse (MVP), *n* the protrusion of one or both cusps of the mitral valve back into the left atrium during ventricular systole, resulting in incomplete closure of the valve and mitral insufficiency.

mix, *v* to form by combining ingredients.

mixed dentition, *n* See dentition, mixed.

mixing, vacuum, *n* a method of mixing materials, such as gypsum products and water, in a vacuum.

MLD, *n* See dose, lethal, minimum.

MLT, *n* See time, median lethal.

MO cavity, *n* a cavity on the mesial and occlusal surfaces of a tooth. See also DO cavity, Class 2.

mobility, *n* the loosening of a tooth or teeth. Mobility is an important diagnostic sign that may result not only from a decrease in root attachment or changes in the periodontal ligament but also from destruction of the gingival fiber apparatus and transseptal fibers.

mobility of tooth, *n* See tooth mobility.

MOD cavity, *n* a cavity on the mesial, occlusal, and distal surfaces of a tooth. See also cavity, Class 2.

mode (mo), *n* a measure of central tendency that is the most frequently occurring score or value in a group of scores. The mode may be used as an average score.

model, *n* **1.** a replica, usually in miniature *n* **2.** a positive replica of the dentition and surrounding or adjoining structures used as a diagnostic aid and base for construction of orthodontic and prosthetic appliances. See also cast.

model, casting, *n* See cast, refractory.

model, implant, *n* See cast, implant.

model, of prepared cavity, *n* See die.

model, study, *n* See cast, diagnostic.

modeling compound, *n* See compound.

models, biologic, *n.pl* the use of the analog of a disease of man in some other animal species to study or compare the response or treatment of the disease before testing with humans.

models, statistical, *n.pl* statistical formulations or analyses which, when applied to data and found to fit the data, are used to verify the assumptions and parameters used in the analysis. Some examples of statistical models include the linear model, binomial model, polynomial model, and two-parameter model.

modem, *n* (modulator/demodulator), a device that converts data from a form compatible with computer manipulation to a form compatible with transmission equipment and vice versa.

moderator, *n* a chairman; one who presides over an assembly, group, or panel.

modiolus (mōdē′ōlus), *n* a point distal to the corner of the mouth where several muscles of facial expression converge.

modulus, *n* a constant that numerically indicates the amount in which a certain property is possessed by any object.

modulus of elasticity, *n* See elasticity, modulus of.

modulus of resilience, *n* See resilience, modulus of.

modulus of rigidity, *n* See rigidity.

modulus, Young's, *n.pr* See elasticity, modulus of.

moexipril hydrochloride, *n* *trade name:* Univasc; *drug class:* angiotensin-converting enzyme (ACE) inhibitor; *action:* selectively suppresses renin-angiotensin-aldosterone system; inhibits ACE; prevents conversion of angiotensin I to angiotensin II; results in dilation of arterial, venous vessels; *use:* hypertension as a single drug or in combination with a thiazide diuretic.

Mohs scale, *n.pr* See hardness, Mohs.

Mohs surgery, *n.pr* a surgical technique used primarily in the treatment of skin neoplasms, especially basal cell or squamous cell carcinoma of the skin. This procedure is a microscopically controlled excision of cutaneous tumors either after fixation in vivo or after freezing the tissue. Serial examinations of fresh tissue specimens are most frequently done to ensure complete excision of the lesion.

molar, *n* **1.** a reference solution in which the concentration is stated with regard to the number of gram molecular weights per liter of solution. **2.** a tooth adapted for grinding by having a broad, somewhat ridged surface. In humans, the molar is one of the 12 teeth located in the posterior aspect of the upper and lower jaws.

molar, mulberry, n a malformed first molar with a crown, suggesting the appearance of a mulberry. It may be a manifestation of congenital syphilis, although other diseases affecting the enamel organ during morphodifferentiation may produce a similar lesion.

molar sheath, n a rectangular metallic tube soldered or welded to the molar bands.

mold (mould), n a form in which an object is cast or shaped. The process of shaping a material into an object. The term is used to specify the shape of an artificial tooth or teeth.

molding, n shaping.

molding, border, n See border molding.

molding, compression, n the act of pressing or squeezing together to form a shape in a mold.

molding, injection, n the adaptation of a plastic material to the negative form of a closed mold by forcing the material into the mold through appropriate gateways. See also molding, compression.

molding, tissue, n See border molding.

mole, n a pigmented nevus.

molecular biology, n the study of biology from the viewpoint of the physical and chemical interactions of molecules involved in life functions.

molecular weight, n See weight, molecular.

molecule, n a unit of matter that is the smallest particle of an element or chemical combination of atoms (as a compound) capable of retaining chemical identity with the substance in mass.

molimina, menstrual (molim'inə), n circulatory symptoms, psychic tension, irritable behavior, belligerence, and other personality alterations before or during menstruation. The cause is unknown.

molindone HCl, n *trade name:* Moban, Moban Concentrate; *drug class:* antipsychotic; *action:* depresses cerebral cortex, hypothalamus, limbic system, which control activity, aggression; blocks neurotransmission produced by dopamine at synapse; mechanism for antipsychotic effects is unclear; *use:* psychotic disorders.

molluscum contagiosum, n a disease of the skin and mucous membranes, caused by a poxvirus and found all over the world. It is characterized by scattered flesh-toned papules. The disease most frequently occurs in children and in adults with an impaired immune response. It is transmitted from person to person by direct or indirect contact and lasts up to 3 years.

molluscum fibrosum, n See neurofibromatosis.

Molt's mouth gag, n.pr See mouth prop, ratchet type.

molybdenum (Mo), n a grayish metallic element with an atomic number of 42 and an atomic weight of 95.94. Molybdenum is poisonous if ingested in large quantities.

momentum, n quantity of motion, expressed as the product of mass and velocity.

money, n the general term for the representation of value, currency, or cash.

money market fund, n a mutual fund that invests only in high-yielding, short-term money market instruments (U.S. Treasury bills, bank certificates of deposit, and commercial paper).

mongolism (mon'gōlizəm), n discredited term for Down syndrome.

moniliasis (mō'nilī'əsis), n infection by a fungus of the genus *Candida,* usually *C. albicans.* May involve the mouth (thrush), female genitalia, skin, hands, nails, and/or lungs. *Oral moniliasis* refers to thrush or to mycotic stomatitis. The latter term is sometimes applied to erythematous patches that are not typical of the usual white patches of thrush. See also thrush.

monitor, n to observe and evaluate a function of the body closely and constantly over a period of time for diagnostic purposes.

monitoring, n the periodic or continuous determination of the dose rate in an occupied area by a person.

monitoring, ambulatory, n to observe and evaluate a patient while engaged in normal routine behaviors.

monitoring, area, n routine monitoring of the level of radiation of any particular area, building, room, equipment, or outdoor space.

monitoring, personal, n monitoring of any part of an individual (for example, breath or excretions or any part of the clothing).

monitoring, personnel, n a systematic, periodic check of the radiation dose each person receives during working hours.

monitoring, physiologic, n the observation and evaluation of physiologic functions, usually with an electronic device with surface electrodes attached to specific areas of the body.

monkey, n a vernacular term applied to a lower primate animal that is often used for experimental purposes in medicine and stomatology. Its dental and oral structures are morphologically and functionally similar to those of human beings, permitting an associated correlation of experimental findings. See also *Macaca.*

monoamine oxidase, n an enzyme that catalyzes the oxidation of amines.

monoamine oxidase inhibitor (MAOI), n an agent that blocks the oxidation and deamination of monoamines. The action of the inhibitor may increase the presence of catecholamines, which have antidepressant properties.

monobloc, n See activator.

monocyte (mon′ o-sīt), n a large mononuclear leukocyte with an ovoid or kidney-shaped nucleus, containing chromatin material with a lacy pattern and abundant gray-blue cytoplasm filled with fine, reddish, and azurophilic granules.

monocytosis (mon′ōsītō′sis), n an increase in the number of monocytes in the peripheral bloodstream. Various limits are given (for example, a total number in excess of 800/mm^3, regardless of the percentage, or a total greater than 8% with the total number less than 800). In both cases, the presence of monocytosis is indicated. Monocytosis may be associated with chronic pyogenic infections, subacute bacterial endocarditis, infectious hepatitis, monocytic leukemia, rickettsial disease, and protozoan infections.

monomer (mon′ōmur), n a single molecule. In commercial resin products, the term applies to the liquid, which is usually a mixture of monomers.

monomer, residual, n the unpolymerized monomer remaining in the appliance or restoration after processing.

mononucleosis, infectious (mon′ōnōō′klē ō′sis), n (acute benign lymphadenosis, "kissing disease," "student's disease"), an acute infectious viral disease most commonly affecting young adults and older children. Manifestations include fever, sore throat, cervical lymphadenopathy, petechial hemorrhages of the soft palate, and, at times, purpura with thrombocytopenia. Early leukopenia and relative lymphocytosis occur, with later increases in the number of large leukocytoid lymphocytes. The heterophil (usually sheep cell) antibody titer is significantly increased in most instances.

monostotic, n affecting a single bone.

Monotremata, n the lowest order of mammals, including animals that lay eggs similar to those of reptiles, and nourish their young by a mammary gland that has no nipple, in a shallow pouch developed during lactation. The only living representatives are the spiny anteater and the duck-billed platypus.

Monson curve, n.pr See curve, Monson.

moot, adj **1.** subject to argument, undecided. adj **2.** in law, in a moot case one seeks to determine that an abstract question does not arise on existing facts or rights.

moral, adj relating to the conscience or moral sense or to the general principles of correct conduct.

morale, n the mental state or condition as related to cheerfulness, confidence, and zeal.

morbidity, n the state of being diseased. Can be used as an outcome measure such as number of decayed, missing, and filled teeth.

moricizine, n *trade name:* Ethmozine; *drug class:* antidysrhythmic, type I; *action:* decreased rate of rise of action potential, which prolongs the refractory period and shortens the action potential duration; *use:* documented life-threatening dysrhythmias.

morphine (môr′fēn), *n* an effective prescription analgesic narcotic, usually administered intravascularly in the form of a salt (morphine sulfate) in the United States (morphine hydrochloride is preferred in Germany and England). Street names include *M, white stuff, Miss Emma, hocus,* and *monkey.* Constricted pupils may be a sign of abuse.

morphine sulfate, *n trade names:* Duramorph PF, MS Contin, Roxanol; *drug class:* narcotic analgesic (Controlled Substance Schedule II); *action:* depresses pain impulse transmission at the central nervous system by interacting with opioid receptors; *use:* severe pain.

morphogenesis, *n* the development and differentiation of the structures and the form of an organism, specifically the changes that occur in the cells and tissue during embryonic development.

morphology, *n* the branch of biology that deals with the form and structure of an organism or part, without regard to function.

morphology, determinants of occlusal, n.pl variable factors that determine the forms given to the crowns of teeth restored in metals, such as mandibular centricity; the intercondylar distance; the distance of teeth from the sagittal plane; the character of lateral and protrusive paths of the condylar axes; and the overlaps of the anterior teeth and wear.

mortality, *n* the death rate.

mortgage, *n* a right given to the creditor over the property of the debtor for the security of the debt; invests the creditor with the power to have the property seized and sold in default of payment.

mortgage, chattel, n a mortgage of goods or personal property.

mortgagee, *n* the person who takes or receives a mortgage.

motion, *n* envelope of, the three-dimensional space circumscribed by border movements and by occlusal contacts of a given point of the mandible. Also called *movement space.* See also movement, border, posterior.

motivation, *n* the stimulus, incentive, or inducement to act or react in a certain way. Purposeful human behavior is motivated behavior, which means that either physiologic or social stimuli activate or motivate a person to do something.

motivation, external, n incentive that accrues as a result of influence from outside sources; inducement to act or change based on the expectations and examples of other people.

motivation, internal, n incentive that accrues from within an individual; inducement to act or change based on an inherent or intrinsic desire.

motor, *n* pertaining to a muscle, nerve, or center that produces or affects movement.

motor neuron, n one of the various efferent nerve cells that transmit nerve impulses from the brain or from the spinal cord to muscular or glandular tissue.

motor neuron disease, n a progressive disease that tends to affect middle-age men with degeneration of anterior horn cells, motor cranial nerve nuclei, and pyramidal tracts. Amyotrophic lateral sclerosis is a motor neuron disease.

motor output, n the activity that results from the integrative phenomena associated with brain activity. It is expressed in function as muscle contraction of the smooth and striated muscle and as secretion of the exocrine and endocrine glands, and, in effect, represents the total behavioral activity of human life. Whereas sensory phenomena have many avenues that feed into the brain, motor activity is expressed in terms of the simple, direct state of muscle contraction and glandular secretion. Thus, muscle activity is expressed in terms of locomotion, hand-learned skills, speaking, mastication, and all forms of human activity that involve motion.

motor pathway, n all reflex actions of muscle are achieved by the passage of nerve impulses through the final common pathway–the muscle fibers. The lower motor neuron (the motor route of the cranial nerve) is the final pathway for the structures that are innervated by the cranial nerves. Impulses traverse these nerves to their respective muscles

M

from every level of the spinal cord, hindbrain, midbrain, and cerebral cortex. The cranial motor neurons collate these multiple stimuli and transmit sequences of stimuli to the motor end-plate, which in the normal muscle effects a smooth, continuous, controlled contraction.

motor skill, n the ability to make the purposeful movements that are necessary to complete or master a prescribed task.

motor unit, n the entity consisting of the lower motor neuron, motor end-plate, and muscle fibers supplied by the end-plate. The final motor activity resulting from a sequence of stimulations to the lower motor neuron is considered a function of the motor unit. The proportion of nerve fibers to the muscle fibers in motor units is designated as the innervation ratio. Motor units may have ratios ranging from 1:4 to 1:150. The closer the ratio approximates unity, the greater the finesse of specificity of the muscular action. The eye muscles have the highest ratio of striated muscles, and the tongue, facial, masticatory, and pharyngeal muscles succeed in that order.

mottled enamel, n See fluorosis, chronic endemic dental.

moulage, n a model of a part or a lesion (for example, a model of the face). It may be of wax or plaster and usually is colored by painting.

mould, n See mold.

mount, x-ray, n a windowed, stiff material on which radiographs are arranged in a specific order to correspond with the charts of the teeth.

mounting, n the laboratory procedure of attaching the maxillary or mandibular cast to an articulator or similar instrument.

mounting board, n a jig used in mounting the maxillary cast on the top articulator frame. The mounting board enables the dentist to determine the patient's axis so that the maxillary cast can be positioned accurately.

mounting, split cast, n a cast with the margins of its base or capital beveled or grooved to permit accurate remounting on an articulator. Split remounting metal plates may be

used instead of beveling or grooving in the casts.

mouth, n the oral cavity.

mouth breathing, n See breathing, mouth.

mouth, denture-sore, n traumatization and inflammation of the oral mucous membranes produced by ill-fitting dentures, hypersensitivity to the chemical components of the denture, or proliferation of *Candida albicans* with subsequent monilial infection.

mouth, floor of, n area within the oral cavity located beneath the ventral surface of the tongue.

mouth guard, n See guard, mouth.

mouth hygiene, n See hygiene, oral.

mouth preparation, n See preparation, mouth.

mouth rehabilitation, n See rehabilitation, mouth.

mouth, trench, n See gingivitis, necrotizing ulcerative.

mouthrinse, n See mouthwash.

mouthwash, n a mouth rinse possessing cleansing, germicidal, or palliative properties.

mouthwash, alcohol in, n a key ingredient in commercial oral rinses; helps oil-based ingredients blend into product. Typically constitutes from 15 to 30% of the solution. Serves to decrease surface tension while increasing the rinse's astringent properties.

mouthwash, deodorants in, n any number of active ingredients including chlorophyll; added to oral rinses to decrease unpleasant smells that are the result of unbrushed teeth.

mouthwash, flavoring agents in, n an additive in oral rinses designed to enhance the product's taste. Agents are typically derived from aromatic waters and essential oils.

mouthwash, sodium benzoate, n a solution used prior to brushing teeth for the purpose of freshening the mouth. Long-term studies have not proved this to be effective in reducing gingivitis.

movement(s), n any change of place or of position of a body.

movement, Bennett, n.pr the bodily lateral movement or lateral shift of the mandible resulting from the movements of the condyles along the lateral inclines of the mandibular fossae during lateral jaw movement.

movement, bodily, *n* movement of a tooth so that the crown and root apex move the same amount in the same direction, thus maintaining the same axial inclination; opposed to tipping movement.

movement, border, *n* any extreme muscular movement limited by bone, ligaments, or other soft tissues.

movement, free mandibular, *n* mandibular movement made without tooth interference. An uninhibited movement of the mandible.

movement, hinge, *n* an opening or closing movement of the mandible on the hinge axis. A movement around a single axis.

movement, lateral, *n* a movement of a body to one side of its established position.

movement, mandibular, *n* any movement of the lower jaw.

movement, mandibular gliding, *n* side-to-side, protrusive, and intermediate movement of the mandible, occurring when the teeth or other occluding surfaces are in contact.

movement, nonfunctional mandibular, *n* movement of the mandible for other than the accepted range of functional movements; that is, movements dictated by tension, emotion, or aggression. Also, mandibular movements may be misused to hold objects in either indulgent or work habits. These nonfunctional movements may result in a variety of pathologic manifestations.

movement, opening mandibular, *n* the movement of the mandible executed during jaw separation.

movement, posterior border, *n* any movement of the mandible occurring while the mandible is in its most posterior relation to the maxillae. This movement occurs in the vertical plane from the level of occlusal contact to the level of maximal opening of the jaws.

movement, tipping, *n* the movement of a tooth in any direction while its apex remains in almost the original position.

movement, tooth, *n* temporary or permanent deviation of a tooth from its normally fixed position in the dental arch. Also, mobility of teeth. When teeth exhibit mobility patterns, movement may be buccolingual, mesiodistal, occlusoapical, or rotational. Movement of teeth into different positions in the dental arch may be produced by repositioning them mesially, distally, buccally, lingually, or occlusally.

movement, translatory, *n* the motion of a body at any instant when all points within the body are moving at the same velocity and in the same direction.

movements, functional mandibular, *n* all natural, proper, or characteristic movements of the mandible made during speaking, chewing, yawning, swallowing, and other associated movements.

movements, intermediary (intermediate movement), *n* all mandibular movements between the extremes of mandibular excursions.

movements, jaw, *n* all changes in position of which the mandible is capable.

movements, masticatory mandibular, *n* the translatory and rotary movements of the mandible that are used in the course of chewing food.

moxibustion, *n* a method of producing analgesia or altering the function of a system of the body by igniting moxa, wormwood, or some other combustible, slow-burning substance and holding it as near the point on the skin as possible without causing pain or burning. It is also sometimes used in conjunction with acupuncture.

MPD, *n* See dose, maximum permissible.

MSH, *n* See hormone, melanocyte-stimulating.

mucin, *n* a mucopolysaccharide, the chief ingredient of mucus. Mucin is present in most glands that secrete mucus and is the lubricant that protects body surfaces from friction or erosion.

mucobuccal fold, *n* See fold, mucobuccal.

mucocele (myōō′kōsēl), *n* See cyst, mucous.

mucoepidermoid tumor, *n* a malignant neoplasm of glandular tissues, especially the ducts of the salivary glands. The tumor contains mucinous and epidermoid squamous cells.

mucolabial fold, *n* See fold, mucolabial.

mucopolysaccharides, *n.pl* a generic term for a group of compounds composed of protein and complex sugars (polysaccharides), many of which are found in blood group substances.

mucopolysaccharidosis (MPS), *n* a genetic disorder involving mucopolysaccharide metabolism and leading to excess storage of the material in the tissues. Forms include MPS I, II, III, IV, V, and VI. Eponymic designations are Hurler, Hunter, Sanfilippo, Morquio, Scheie, and Maroteaux-Lamy syndromes.

mucosa (myōōkō′sə), *n* (mucous membrane), a membrane, composed of epithelium and lamina propria, that lines the oral cavity and other canals and cavities of the body that communicate with external air.

mucosa, alveolar, n the covering on the alveolar process loosely attached to bone that extends from the mucogingival junction to the vestibular epithelium and from the lower jaw to the sublingual sulcus.

mucosa, lining, n a primary protective mucous membrane that lines the oral cavity. It covers the movable tissues of the soft palate, labial and buccal mucosa, ventral surface of the tongue, and the floor of the mouth. It comprises connective tissue and non-keratinized stratified squamous epithelium.

mucosa, masticatory, n a mucous membrane comprising the connective tissue and keratinized, stratified squamous epithelium within the oral cavity that protects the areas frequently utilized for the chewing of food (e.g., hard palate and gingiva). See also mucosa, oral.

mucosa, nonkeratinized, n mucosa in which the cells of the stratified squamous epithelium maintain their cytoplasm and nuclei. It is associated with lining mucosa. See also mucosa, oral.

mucosa, oral, n the lining of the oral cavity, composed of stratified squamous epithelium and the underlying lamina propria.

mucosa, palatine, n the mucous membrane covering the palate.

mucoserous acinus (mu″ ko-se′rəs as′ ĭ-nəs), *n* a group of secretory cells of the salivary glands from which both mucous and serous salivary products are produced.

mucositis (myōō′kōsī′tis), *n* an inflammation of the mucous membrane.

mucositis, chronic atrophic senile, n mucosal inflammation characterized by atrophy and found primarily in elderly women.

mucositis, fusospirochetal, n mucosal inflammation associated with fusiform and spirochetal microorganisms.

mucostatic, *adj* **1.** pertaining to the normal, relaxed condition of mucosal tissues covering the jaws. *adj* **2.** an agent that arrests the secretion of mucus.

mucous acinus, *n* a group of secretory cells of the salivary glands from which mucous salivary products are produced.

mucous membrane, *n* See mucosa.

mucous membrane pemphigoid, *n* See pemphigoid, benign mucous membrane.

mucous patch, *n* See patch, mucous.

mucoviscidosis (myōō′kōvis′idō′sis), *n* See disease, fibrocystic.

mucus, *n* the viscous, slippery secretions of mucous membranes and glands, containing mucin, white blood cells, water, inorganic salts, and exfoliated cells.

mulberry molars, *n.pl* first permanent molars in which the occlusal surface is composed of an aggregate of enamel nodules. All four molars are involved, usually as the result of congenital syphilis.

mulling (mul′ing), *n* the final step of mixing dental amalgam; a kneading of the triturated mass to complete the amalgamation.

multiculturalism, *n* a philosophy that recognizes ethnic diversity within a society and that encourages others to be enlightened by worthwhile contributions to society by those of diverse ethnic backgrounds.

multifactorial, *adj* related to or produced by a number of elements or causes.

multilocular (mul″ tĭ-lok′ u-lər), *adj* containing several cells, units, or spaces.

multiple sclerosis, *n* a progressive disease characterized by disseminated demyelination of nerve fibers of the brain and spinal cord. It begins slowly, usually in young adulthood, and continues throughout life with periods of exacerbation and remission. The first signs are paresthesias, or abnormal sensations in the extremities or on one side of the face. Other early signs are muscle weakness, vertigo, and visual disturbances.

multiple sclerosis, primary progressive, n form of multiple sclerosis in which the symptoms become progressively and steadily worse over time.

multiple sclerosis, progressive relapsing, n a very rare form of multiple sclerosis in which the symptoms become progressively worse over time, but in which the patient also experiences periods of accelerated deterioration.

multiple sclerosis, relapsing-remitting, n a form of multiple sclerosis in which the patient experiences periods of acute deterioration but is relatively stable between such periods.

multiple sclerosis, secondary progressive, n a form of multiple sclerosis in which the symptoms become progressively and steadily worse over time. May include periods of acute deterioration in patients with relapsing-remitting multiple sclerosis.

multiple trauma, *n* a number of injuries sustained during the same accident or assault.

multiprocessing, *n* the use of two or more processors in a system configuration. One processor controls the system, and the others are subordinate to it.

multiprogramming, *n* a technique for permitting more than one program to time-share machine components. This technique permits the concurrent handling of numerous programs by one computer.

multivariate analysis, *n* a set of techniques used when variation in several variables has to be studied simultaneously. In statistics, multivariate analysis is interpreted as any analytic method that allows simulta-

neous study of two or more dependent variables.

mumps, *n* (parotitis), a contagious parotitis caused by the mumps virus (paramyxovirus) and characterized by swelling of the parotid gland and sometimes swelling of the pancreas, ovaries, and testicles. The incubation period is 12 to 20 days; transmission is by droplet spread and direct contact; communicability begins about 2 days before the appearance of symptoms and lasts until swelling of the glands has abated. See also parotitis.

Mumps. (Zitelli/Davis, 2002, courtesy of GDW McKendrick)

mumps, iodide, n (iodine mumps), an enlargement of the thyroid gland resulting from iodides.

mumps, iodine, n See mumps, iodide.

mupirocin/mupirocin calcium, *trade name:* Bactroban; *drug class:* topical antiinfective, pseudomonic acid A; *action:* inhibits bacterial protein synthesis; *uses:* impetigo caused by *Staphylococcus aureus,* β-hemolytic *Streptococcus, Staphylococcus pyogenes;* nasal membranes: *S. aureus.*

murmur, *n* a humming or blowing sound heard on auscultation.

murmur, aortic, a murmur resulting from insufficiency of the aortic valve secondary to involvement by rheumatic fever or tertiary syphilis.

murmur, apical diastolic, n a murmur heard over the apex of the heart and caused by mitral stenosis, relative mitral stenosis, or aortic insufficiency.

murmur, apical systolic, n a murmur heard at the apex of the heart in systole and caused by mitral insufficiency, which may result from rheumatic heart disease, or by relative mitral insufficiency, which may result from congestive heart failure associated with arteriosclerosis or hypertension. The murmur may also have a functional basis.

murmur, basal diastolic, n a murmur heard over the base of the heart and caused by aortic insufficiency resulting from rheumatic heart disease or syphilis, relative aortic insufficiency associated with diastolic hypertension, or a patent ductus arteriosus.

murmur, basal systolic, n a murmur heard over the base of the heart and caused by aortic stenosis resulting from rheumatic heart disease or by relative stenosis of the aortic valve resulting from aortic dilation secondary to arteriosclerosis or hypertension. The murmur may also be functional or may result from congenital heart or vascular defects.

murmur, cardiac, n (heart murmur), an abnormal sound heard in the region of the heart at any time during the heart's cycle. Murmurs may be named according to the area of generation (mitral, aortic, pulmonary, or tricuspid) and according to the period of the cycle (diastolic or systolic).

murmur, functional, n (innocent murmur, inorganic murmur), a murmur resulting from the position of the body, severe anemia, or polycythemia. Not related to structural changes in the heart.

murmur, heart, n See murmur, cardiac.

murmur, innocent, n See murmur, functional.

murmur, inorganic, n See murmur, functional.

murmur, mitral, n a heart murmur produced by a defect in the mitral valve. It is the most common form of murmur in rheumatic heart disease.

murmur, organic, n a murmur resulting from structural changes in the heart or in the great vessels of the heart.

muscle(s), n an organ that, by cellular contraction, produces the movements of life. The two varieties of muscle structure are striated, which includes all the muscles in which contraction is voluntary and the heart muscle (in which contraction is involuntary), and unstriated, smooth, or organic, which includes all the involuntary muscles (except the heart), such as the muscular layer of the intestines, bladder, and blood vessels.

muscle, ciliary, n a tiny smooth muscle at the junction of the cornea and sclera, consisting of two groups of fibers: circular fibers, which exert parasympathetic control through the oculomotor nerve and the ciliary ganglion, and radial fibers, which exert sympathetic control. Ciliary muscles are responsible for accommodation for far vision through flattening of the lens.

muscle, concentric, contraction, n See contraction, muscle, concentric.

muscle contraction, n See contraction, muscle.

muscle, digastric (dīgas′trik), n suprahyoid muscle that helps activate the jaw for mastication and swallowing. It has both an anterior and a posterior belly. See also deglutition; mastication; muscle, hyoid.

muscle, eccentric, contraction, n See contraction, muscle, eccentric.

muscle, elasticity of, physical, n the physical quality of being elastic, of yielding to passive physical stretch.

muscle, elasticity of, physiologic, n the biologic quality, unique for muscle, of being able to change and resume size under neuromuscular control.

muscle fatigue, n the depletion of the metabolites necessary to sustain or repeat a muscle contraction.

muscle fiber, n the cell of muscle tissue. The three types of muscle fibers are striated (voluntary), cardiac, and smooth (involuntary).

muscle, functional changes of, n.pl asymmetric modifications in length, diameter, and bulk of muscle fibers as a result of variations in function. Muscle responds to normal function by maintenance of bulk. An increase in bulk is caused by an increase in the number of capillaries and in the mean diameter of individual muscle fibers. The response to function accounts for the asymmetry of the musculature, which is frequently found when the growth patterns have been influenced by a traumatogenic agent such as disease, injury, or surgery, and also by the functional processes of the body itself, such as posture and habit. Asymmetry is not necessarily pathologic; that is, it may be the result of differences in habits of chewing, incision, speech sounds, and facial gestures.

muscle, genioglossus (jē′nē-ōglōs′us), *n* an extrinsic tongue muscle that originates from the genial tubercles of the mandible and extends inside the tongue. It aids in tongue extension and prevents respiratory obstruction.

muscle, geniohyoid (jē′nē-ōhī′-oid), *n* suprahyoid muscle attached to the superior surface of the hyoid bone. This muscle, which is used for mastication and swallowing, originates on the genial tubercles of the mandible and extends along the floor of the mouth. See also deglutition; mastication; muscle, hyoid.

muscle, hyoglossus (hī′-ōglōs′əs), *n* an extrinsic tongue muscle that originates from the hyoid bone and extends on the lateral surface of the body of the tongue. It depresses the tongue during mastication and speech.

muscle, hypertenseness, n an increased muscular tension that is not easily released but that does not prevent normal lengthening of the muscle. Hypertenseness is found in patients with general nervousness.

muscle, innervation of, reciprocal, n a phenomenon of antagonistic muscles demonstrated during a concentric contraction such as that of the temporal muscle. Innervation of the antagonist, the external pterygoid muscle, is partially inhibited, so that freedom of action in flexing the temporomandibular joint is possible. This phenomenon demonstrates inhibition of antagonistic skeletal muscles in a reflex arc brought about automatically by a reduction of the motor discharges from the central nervous system. One of the two muscles in the reflex arc is activated, and the activity of the other is depressed.

muscle, isometric, contraction, n See contraction, muscle, isometric.

muscle, isotonic, contraction, n See contraction, muscle, isotonic.

muscle, masseter, n one of the four muscles of mastication. The thick rectangular muscle in the cheek that functions to close the jaw. The masseter muscle arises from the zygomatic arch and inserts into the mandible at the corner of the jaw.

Palpation of the masseter muscle.
(Rosenstiel/Land/Fujimoto, 2001)

muscle memory, n a kinesthetic phenomenon by which a muscle or set of muscles may involuntarily produce movement that follows a pattern that has become established by frequent repetition over a long period of time.

muscle, mylohyoid, n suprahyoid muscle originating from the mandible. It helps to raise the tongue and lower the mandible for mastication and swallowing and also forms the floor of the mouth. See also deglutition; mastication; muscles, hyoid.

muscle, omohyoid (ō′mōhī′-oid), *n* infrahyoid muscle with both inferior and superior bellies. It is used for chewing and swallowing. See also muscles, hyoid.

muscle, physical characteristics of primary, elasticity, n.pl a muscle is an elastic body. Its individual fibers follow Hooke's law of elastic bodies: that is, the amount of elongation is proportional to the stretching force. The muscle organs contain tissue other than muscle fibers and thus deviate slightly from this law. The human muscle fiber can contract to about half its total length.

M

muscle, regeneration of reproduction or repair of muscle fiber, n a sequela to many types of muscle damage. Reparation is always associated with the proliferation of sarcolemmic nuclei. Connective tissue elements do not participate in this process except to bridge the gap and offer support for the regenerative fibers. The regenerative process takes place in two forms: regeneration by budding from the surviving parts of the muscle fibers, which occurs when segments of the muscle fiber and its sheath are destroyed, and regeneration by proliferation of cellular bands, which occurs when the sarcolemmic nuclei are spared and can form a sarcoplasmic band by linkage of the cytoplasmic processes.

muscle relaxation, n the resting state of a muscle fiber or a group of muscle fibers.

muscle reposition, n surgical replacement of a muscle attachment into a more acceptable functional position.

muscle, sequence of, development, n the pattern of embryologic muscular development. The muscles of the neck and trunk are the first to develop; they are followed by the lingual and facial musculature and then by the distal and proximal appendicular musculature.

muscle, smooth, n the simplest of the three types of muscle (smooth, striated, and cardiac). It is the muscle of the lining of the digestive tract, ducts of glands, and viscera associated with the gut. It also supplies the muscles for the genitourinary tract, structures of the blood vessels, connective tissues of the mucous membranes, and skin with its appendages. A typical smooth muscle fiber is a slender, spindle-shaped body averaging a few tenths of a millimeter in length. There is a single, centrally striated nucleus. The cytoplasm appears homogeneous. The cells are arranged in bands, or bundles, with interspersed connective tissue fibers uniting them into an effective common mass. Smooth muscle fibers are innervated in part by nerve fibers and in part by the contraction of adjacent muscle tissues. The digestive tract, particularly, demonstrates waves of contraction that pass along a band of smooth muscle.

muscle, spasticity of, n increased muscular tension of antagonists that prevents normal movement; caused by an inability to relax (a loss of reciprocal inhibition) resulting from a lesion of the upper motor neuron.

muscle, sternothyroid (stur´nōthī´roid), n infrahyoid muscle that runs from the sternum to the thyroid cartilage and depresses the larynx and the thyroid cartilage for mastication and swallowing. See also deglutition; mastication; muscle, hyoid.

muscle, striated, n skeletal muscles forming the bulk of the body; the voluntary muscles derived from the myotomes of the embryo. Generally, they are organized as formed muscles that attach to and move the skeletal structures. The cells are large, elongated, and cylindric, with lengths ranging from 1 mm to several centimeters. The cells have multiple nuclei that are peripherally situated and scattered along the length of the fiber. The fiber contains a large number of elongated fibers that, under the microscope, appear as the alternating light and dark bands that give the characteristic striated appearance of striated muscle. The dimensional relationships between these light and dark bands are altered during contraction of the muscle fiber. The potential interaction between these bands permits the wide range of selective purposeful and rapid activity of the skeletal muscles.

muscle striations (strī ā´shənz), n.pl the transverse alternating light and dark bands of skeletal muscles that result from differences in light absorption. The light bands contain actin and are called "I" bands because they are isotropic to polarized light. The dark areas contain myosin filaments and are called "A" bands because they are anisotropic to polarized light.

muscle, styloglossus (stī´lōglôs´us), n an extrinsic tongue muscle that originates from the styloid process and inserts on the lateral surface of the tongue. It is used to retract the tongue.

muscle, stylohyoid, n suprahyoid muscle that extends from the styloid process to the hyoid bone and is used for mastication and swallowing. See also deglutition; mastication; muscles, hyoid.

muscle, thyrohyoid, n infrahyoid muscle that extends from the thyroid cartilage to the hyoid bone and is used for mastication and swallowing. See also deglutition; mastication; muscles, hyoid.

muscle tonus, n the steady reflex contraction that resides in the muscles concerned in maintaining erect posture. Tonus has its basis in the positional interactions of the muscle and its accompanying nerve structure; for example, a muscle holds the body (mandible) in a given position, and the awareness of this position is constantly being relayed by the sensory approaches to the cortex. Any change in position or contractility of the muscle that affects its tonus is immediately relayed by the sensory apparatus for readjustment. Also called tone.

muscle tonus, facial (tŏ'nus), *n* the tone of the facial musculature, which is a major factor in providing the esthetic values of the human face. The configurations of the face, which are maintained by good muscle tonus, are the modiolus, philtrum, nasolabial sulcus, and mentolabial sulcus. These functional contours are present when the nerve tissue is intact. They are altered by the loss of teeth or impaired nerve function. Their presence is an indication of a good state of health of the nerve and possibly of the dental arch.

muscle trimming, n See border molding and impression, correctable.

muscles, cervical, n.pl large, paired muscles used to turn or lower the head or to shrug the shoulders. This group includes the sternocleidomastoid and trapezius muscles.

muscles, facial, n.pl the muscles of expression, frequently called the mimetic muscles. They are quite variable in contour, are widely distributed over the scalp and face, and tend to be especially concentrated around the orbits, outer ear, and lips. It is the mobility of the lips that has extended the usefulness of the facial muscles

in expressing emotion, speech, and intelligence. The facial muscles, as a group, have only one bony origin in the facial skeleton. The muscles form a circular rim around the perimeter of the facial bones and extend anteriorly as a tube of tissue in which the lumen narrows and terminates in the orbicularis oris. The structure of the facial muscles may be regarded as a truncated cone in which the base rests on the skeleton (origin) in a fixed position, whereas the truncated top of the cone (insertion in the orbicularis oris) is variable in diameter and height. The lips are thus extensible and retractable and can constrict like a purse string.

muscles, hyoid (hī'-oid), *n.pl* a group of muscles used in mastication and swallowing. These muscles are attached to the hyoid bone, which is suspended on the neck and forms the base of the tongue and larynx. The muscles are divided into *suprahyoid* (superior) or *infrahyoid* (inferior) groups relative to the bone.

muscles, masticatory (mas'tikətôrē), *n.pl* the powerful muscles that elevate and rotate the mandible so that the opposing teeth may occlude for mastication.

muscles, mimetic (mimet'ik), *n.pl* the facial muscles by which emotion and intelligence are expressed. The facial nerve provides neurologic control over the muscles of the face.

muscles, ocular, function of, n.pl the action of the eye muscles in moving the eyeballs. The eyes are in a position of rest (their primary position) when their direction is maintained simply by the tone of the ocular muscles. This condition prevails when the gaze is straight ahead into distance and not directed to any particular point in space. The visual axes are then parallel. When the eyes view some distant definite object, they are turned by contraction of the ocular muscles and converge so that the visual axes meet at the observed object, and an almost identical image of the object falls on a corresponding point on each fovea, the centralis of the retina. The adjustment of the eye movements for acute observation is called fixation, and the point where the visual axes meet is the fixation point. Thus, the interplay of the ocular muscles permits rapid, reciprocally controlled movement of the eyeballs for fixation.

muscles, orofacial, *n.pl* the muscles of facial expression.

muscles, suprahyoid and infrahyoid (sŏŏ'prəhī'-oid), *n.pl* the muscles grouped around the hyoid bone. They aid in depressing and fixing the mandible, hyoid bone, and larynx in the performance of their several respective functions.

muscles, tongue, extrinsic, *n.pl* the muscles of the tongue that provide a scaffolding by which the intrinsic muscles can be moved around in the oral cavity while the latter are continuously modifying their dimension and contour. The extrinsic muscles are paired and originate from both sides of the cranial skeleton, mandible, and hyoid bone to radiate medially and insert into the body of the tongue, which consists principally of the intrinsic muscles.

muscles, tongue, intrinsic, *n.pl* the muscles of the tongue that have no attachments in bone, terminating either within each other or in the extrinsic muscle group. The fibers of the intrinsic muscles also lie in all three planes of space and are called *longitudinal, vertical,* and *transverse fibers* to describe their distribution. They are capable of assuming an infinite variety of shapes. They depend, however, on the activity of the extrinsic muscles to be moved bodily through space.

muscular dystrophy (mus'kyŏŏlur dis'trōfē), *n* a group of genetically transmitted diseases characterized by progressive atrophy of symmetric groups of skeletal muscles without evidence of involvement or degeneration of neural tissue. In all forms of muscular dystrophy there is an insidious loss of strength with increasing disability and deformity. Serum creatine phosphokinase is increased in affected individuals and acts as a diagnostic aid. Diagnosis is confirmed by muscle biopsy, electromyography, and genetic pedigree.

muscular dystrophy, Duchenne (dōōshen'), *n.pr* a genetic myopathic condition distinguished by the enlarged size of specific muscles (e.g., calves), noticeable indications of lordosis accompanied by a swelling of the abdominal region, diminished capacity to stand, walk and maintain balance, a progressive deterioration of the muscles, and limited intellectual development.

muscular dystrophy, facioscapulohumeral (fā'shē-ōskap'yŏŏlōhyŏŏ'mərəl), *n* a genetic myopathic condition involving the facial muscles and distinguished by prominent scapula, weak muscles of the shoulders, and marked difficulty in lifting the arms and completely shutting the eyes.

musculature (mus'kyŏŏləchur), *n* any part of the muscular apparatus of the body; the source of power for the movement of the body or its parts.

musculature, cheek, *n* the muscles giving support, form, and function to the cheeks. Should disequilibrium exist between the functional forces exerted on the dentition by the tongue and cheek musculature, deviations in tooth alignment may occur.

musculature, lip, *n* the muscles that perform the physiologic or functional activities of the lips. The primary muscles include the orbicularis oris, quadratus labii superioris, risorius, and buccinators. If the tongue and the musculature of the lips do not exert equivalent forces against the teeth, movement of the teeth may occur.

musculoskeletal system (mus'kyŏŏlōskel'ətəl), *n* all the muscles, bones, joints, and related structures, such as the tendons and connective tissue, that function in the stability and movement of the parts and organs of the body. See also system, musculoskeletal.

mushbite, *n* an obsolete type of maxillomandibular record made by introducing a mass of soft wax into the patient's mouth and instructing the patient to bite into it to the desired degree. Not a generally accepted procedure. See also record, maxillomandibular.

mutagen, *n* any chemical or physical environmental agent that induces a genetic mutation or increases the mutation rate.

mutagenesis, *n* the induction or occurrence of a genetic mutation.

mutant, *n* an individual showing a mutation.

mutation (myōōtā′shən), *n* a departure from the parent type, as when an organism differs from its parents in one or more heritable characteristics; caused by genetic change.

mutation, gene, *n* a sudden and permanent change in a gene. The term mutation is sometimes used in a broader sense to include chromosome aberrations.

mutation, lethal, *n* a mutation leading to death of the offspring at any stage.

mutism (myōōtizəm), *n* a condition in which the patient is physically unable to speak or has emotional barriers to speaking. Sometimes accompanies deafness.

mutism, elective, *n* a continual refusal to speak in children who have a confirmed capacity to articulate.

mutual, *adj* interchangeable; reciprocal; joint.

myalgia, *n* pain in the muscles.

myasthenia gravis (mī′asthē′nē-ə grā′vis), *n* an autoimmune disease resulting in incomplete communication between the nerves, thereby causing fatigue and weakness of the muscles. This is especially important for dental personnel, as the facial muscles are usually among the first affected.

myasthenic crisis, *n* a lack of acetylcholine, usually caused by insufficient medication, which results in an inability to speak, breathe, or swallow in patients with myasthenia gravis.

mycelium (mīsē′lē um), *n* the filamentous network of hyphae of a fungus.

Mycobacterium, *n* a genus of rod-shaped, acid-fast bacteria having two significant pathogenic species: *Mycobacterium leprae,* causing leprosy; and *Mycobacterium tuberculosis,* causing tuberculosis.

Mycobacterium bovis, *n* a species that is the primary cause of tuberculosis in cattle. It is transmissible to man and other cattle.

Mycobacterium phlei, *n* Timothy hay bacillus, a species found in soil, in dust, and on plants.

Mycobacterium tuberculosis, *n* (Koch's bacillus), the microorganism responsible for tuberculosis, generally a respiratory infection in man; nonrespiratory tuberculosis is considered an indicator disease for AIDS.

mycology, *n* that branch of microbiology that deals with yeasts and fungi.

mycophenolate mofetil, *n* *trade name:* CellCept; *drug class:* immunosuppressant; *action:* selective inhibitor of inosine monophosphate dehydrogenase, thereby preventing the synthesis of guanosine nucleotide and resulting in cytostatic effect on T and B lymphocytes; *uses:* prophylaxis of organ rejection in patients receiving allogenic renal transplants (in combination with cyclosporine and corticosteroids).

Mycoplasma, *n* a genus of ultramicroscopic organisms lacking rigid cell walls and considered to be the smallest free-living organisms

Mycoplasma pneumoniae, *n* a species of *Mycoplasma* causing mycoplasma pneumonia, which is characterized by symptoms of an upper respiratory infection with a dry cough and fever.

mycosis, *n* any disease caused by a yeast or fungus.

mycosis fungoides, *n* a rare, chronic, lymphomatous skin malignancy resembling eczema or a cutaneous tumor that is followed by microabscesses in the epidermis and lesions simulating those of Hodgkin's disease in lymph nodes and viscera.

mydriasis, *n* an abnormal condition of the eye characterized by contraction of the dilator muscle, resulting in widely dilated pupils.

mydriatic (mid′rē at′ik), *n* a drug that dilates the pupil.

myelin (mī′ əlin), *n* a fatlike substance forming a sheath around certain nerve fibers. It is associated with volitional nervous system fibers and is believed to be related to the capacity of nerve structures for rapid transmission of nerve impulses. Various diseases, such as multiple sclerosis, can destroy these myelin wrappings.

myelocyte (mi′ ə-lo-sīt), *n* a young white blood cell found in the bone marrow.

myeloma (mī′ əlō′mə), *n* a neoplasm characterized by cells normally found in the bone marrow.

myeloma, multiple, n a primary malignant neoplasm of bone marrow characterized by proliferation of cells resembling plasma cells. Circumscribed radiolucencies are seen within the bones, and Bence Jones protein is usually found in the urine.

Multiple myeloma. (Regezi, Sciubba, Jordan, 2003)

myeloma, plasma cell, n a malignant neoplasm characterized by plasma cells. Solitary lesions may appear as radiolucencies in the bone and are sometimes considered benign, although most authorities believe that even these lesions become multiple and terminate fatally.

myeloma, solitary plasma cell, n an incompletely understood monostotic neoplasm of bone that is histologically identical with multiple myeloma. Laboratory findings, positive in multiple myeloma, are usually negative in solitary plasma cell myeloma. Although usually benign, solitary plasma cell myelomas may be malignant.

myelomeningocele (mī´-əlōməning´gōsēl), n a condition in which part of the spinal cord protrudes from between the bones of the vertebrae. The condition can result in paralysis.

Myelomeningocele. (Moore/Persaud, 2003, courtesy AE Chudley)

myelophthisis (mī´ əlŏfthī´sis), n a displacement of bone marrow by fibrous tissue, carcinoma, or leukemia.

mylohyoid ridge, cantilevered, n a condition in which a major undercut occurs inferior to a broad mylohyoid ridge; creating a vertical groove into such an area often causes perforation of the medial cortical plate.

myoblastoma (mī´ ōblastō´mə), n a benign neoplasm characterized by large polyhedral cells resembling young muscle cells. Occurs most frequently in the tongue.

myoblastoma, granular cell, n a benign soft tissue tumor of disputed origin. The tumor cells are large and have a granular eosinophilic cytoplasm and a small nucleus.

myocardial infarction, n an occlusion or blockage of arteries supplying the muscles of the heart, resulting in injury or necrosis of the heart muscle (heart attack).

myocardial ischemia, n a loss of oxygen to the heart muscle caused by blockage of the coronary arteries or their branches.

myocardium, n the thick, contractile middle layer of uniquely constructed and arranged muscle cells (cardiac muscle) that form the bulk of the heart wall.

myoclonus, n a spasm of muscle or group of muscles.

myoepithelial cell (mi″ o-ep″ ĭ-the´ le-əl), n a contractile muscle cell found on the surface of some acini of the salivary glands, which is believed to aid in the secretion of fluids from the gland.

myofascial pain, n pain associated with inflammation or irritation of muscle or of the fascia surrounding the muscle.

myofascial pain dysfunction syndrome (MPD), n a subset of the TMJ pain dysfunction syndrome that presents with the triad of symptoms of unilateral pain in the muscles of mastication, clicking of the joint, and limitation of movement but without clinical or radiographic evidence of organic changes in the joint and a lack of tenderness in the joint when palpated from the external auditory meatus.

myolipoma (mī´ ōlipō´mə), n a myxoma containing fatty tissue.

myoma (mī ō′mə), *n* a neoplasm characterized by muscle cells.

myopathy (mī-op′əthē), *n* weakness or degeneration of skeletal muscles associated with the many forms of muscular dystrophy. This should be distinguished from neuromuscular disorders.

myopia (mī ō′pē ə), *n* a form of defective vision resulting from excessive refractive power of the eye. In this condition, commonly called *nearsightedness,* or *shortsightedness,* light rays coming from an object beyond a certain distance are focused in front of the retina.

myosin, *n* a cardiac and skeletal muscle protein that makes up close to one half of the proteins that occur in muscle tissue. The interaction of myosin and actin is essential for muscle contraction.

myosin fibrils, *n.pl* strands of protein found in muscle tissue which are among the components necessary for muscle contraction.

myositis, *n* an inflammation of muscle tissue, usually of the voluntary muscles. Causes of myositis include infection, trauma, and infestation by parasites.

myotomy (mī ot′əmē), *n* cutting or resection of a muscle.

myotonia (mī″ o-tō′ne-ə), *n* a condition in which muscles remain tense or do not quickly relax after contraction.

myxedema (mīksədē′mə), *n* a condition associated with hypothyroidism (primary myxedema) or hypopituitarism (secondary or pituitary myxedema). Characteristics include dry hair and skin; thickened skin of the lips; puffy eyelids; thinning of the eyebrows, especially the lateral half; slow, low-pitched, and hoarse speech; and slowness of thinking.

myxofibroma (mik′sōfibrō′mə), *n* a benign neoplasm characterized by mucous and fibroblastic tissues.

myxoma (miksō′mə), *n* a benign tumor composed of fibroblastic cells that have reverted to embryonic growth and produce a mucoid matrix containing widely dispersed stellate cells that have multipolar processes.
myxoma, **odontogenic,** *n* a new growth of soft tissue, gelatinous in appearance, originating from the

mesenchymal tissue of the tooth. The growth may invade tissues surrounding the region, and it does not metastasize or provide any bodily function.

myxosarcoma (mik′sōsärkō′mə), *n* a sarcoma containing myxomatous tissue.

N (n), *n* in statistics, the number of cases or observations.

N2, *n* a single visit endodontic technique better known as the *Sargenti technique,* in which paraformaldehyde (a toxic chemical that can cause permanent tissue damage if not confined to the pulp chamber or root canal) is the principal ingredient in the endodontic paste. The technique is not approved by the Council on Dental Therapeutics, and it is not taught at any accredited dental school in the United States.

nabumetone, *n trade name:* Relafen; *drug class:* nonsteroidal antiinflammatory; *action:* inhibits prostaglandin synthesis by interfering with cyclooxygenase needed for biosynthesis; possesses analgesic, antiinflammatory, and antipyretic properties; *uses:* osteoarthritis, rheumatoid arthritis.

nadolol, *n trade name:* Corgard; *drug class:* nonselective β-adrenergic blocker; *action:* competitively blocks stimulation of β-adrenergic receptors within the heart; produces negative chronotropic and inotropic activity, slows conduction of AV node, decreases heart rate, which decreases oxygen consumption in myocardium; also decreases activity of the renin-aldosterone-angiotensin system; *uses:* chronic stable angina pectoris, mild-to-moderate hypertension.

nafcillin, *n* a semisynthetic penicillin designed as an antistaphylococcal penicillin. Also effective in the treatment of infections caused by pneumococci and Group A β-hemolytic streptococci.

naftifine HCl, *n trade name:* Naftin; *drug class:* topical antifungal; *action:* interferes with cell membrane permeability in fungi; *uses:* tinea cruris, tinea corporis.

nalidixic acid, *n* an antibacterial prescribed in the treatment of urinary tract infections.

nalmefene HCl, *n trade name:* Revex; *drug class:* opioid antagonist; *action:* reverses the effects of opioids by competitive antagonism of opioid receptors; *uses:* management of opioid overdose and complete or partial reversal of opioid drug effects, including respiratory depression.

naloxone HCl, *n trade name:* Narcan; *drug class:* narcotic antagonist; *action:* competes with narcotics at narcotic receptor sites; *uses:* respiratory depression induced by narcotics, to reverse postoperative opioid depression.

naltrexone HCl, *n trade names:* ReVia, Trexan; *drug class:* narcotic antagonist; *action:* competes with opioids at opioid receptor sites; *uses:* treatment of opioid addiction following detoxification.

name, *n* a word or combination of words by which a person, object, or idea, or a group of persons, objects, or ideas is regularly known or designated.

name, generic, *n* a name that is usually descriptive of the substance. Strictly speaking, it is a name used to designate a class relationship. Often used synonymously with *nonproprietary name.*

name, nonproprietary, *n* a drug name that is not restricted by a trademark. Nonproprietary names are now selected in the United States by the United States Adopted Name (USAN) Council.

name, official, *n* the title under which a drug is listed in the *United States Pharmacopeia* (USP) or the *National Formulary* (NF).

name, proprietary, *n* a name assigned by the manufacturer that is restricted by trademark. A drug made by several companies may have more than one proprietary name.

Name, United States Adopted (USAN), *n* a name selected by the USAN Council (jointly sponsored by the American Medical Association, American Pharmaceutical Association, and United States Pharmacopeial Convention, Inc.) when a new drug is placed on the market. A nonproprietary or generic name.

Nance analysis of arch length, *n.pr* a method of determining whether there is sufficient arch length to accommodate the permanent dentition.

nandrolone deconate, *n* an androgen prescribed in the treatment of testosterone deficiency, osteoporosis, and female breast cancer, and to stimulate growth, weight gain, and the production of red blood cells.

nanometer (nm), *n* a billionth of a meter (10^{-9} meter). This term is now preferred over millimicron.

naphazoline HCl, *n trade names:* AK-Con Ophthalmic, Allerest, Clear Eyes, VasoClear, Vasocon; *drug class:* ophthalmic vasoconstrictor; *action:* vasoconstriction of eye arterioles; decreases eye engorgement by stimulation of α-adrenergic receptors; *uses:* relieves hyperemia, irritation of superficial corneal vascularity.

naproxen/naproxen sodium, *n trade names:* Naprosyn, Anaprox, Aleve; *drug class:* nonsteroidal antiinflammatory; *action:* inhibits prostaglandin synthesis by interfering with cyclooxygenase needed for biosynthesis; possesses analgesic, antiinflammatory, antipyretic properties; *uses:* mild-to-moderate pain, osteoarthritis, rheumatoid, gouty arthritis, primary dysmenorrhea.

narcissism (när′səsizəm), *n* a personality disorder in which a person is so self-absorbed that the needs and feelings of others do not matter.

narcolepsy (när′kōlepsē), *n* a disease in which the patient is unable to stay awake.

narcoma, coma or stupor from narcotics.

narcosis (närkō′sis), *n* drug-induced unconsciousness.

narcotic (närkot′ik), *n/adj* a drug, usually with strong analgesic action

N

and an addiction potential, that may be synthesized or derived from natural sources. Especially one of the opium alkaloids.

narcotism (när′kōtizəm), *n* a state of stupor induced by a narcotic.

narcotize (när′kōtīz), *v* to render unconscious by use of narcotics.

naris (nares), *n* one of two external openings into the nasal cavity; nostril.

nasal cavity, *n* See cavity, nasal.

nasal conchae, inferior, *n* the set of paired facial bones that project off the maxilla and form the lateral walls of the nasal cavity.

nasal lavage fluid, *n* a liquid, usually a saline-based water solution, used to cleanse the nasal passages.

nasal mucosa, *n* See mucosa.

nasal obstruction, *n* a narrowing of the nasal cavity, which reduces breathing capacity. Caused by an irregular septum, nasal polyps, foreign bodies, or enlarged turbinates.

nasal septum, *n* the partition dividing the nostrils. It is composed of bone and cartilage covered by mucous membrane.

nasality, *n* the quality of speech sounds when the nasal cavity is used as a resonator, especially when there is too much nasal resonance.

nascent (nas′ənt, nā′sənt), *adj* literal meaning: recently born. Also, just released from chemical combination.

nasion (nā′zē on), *n* the point at the root of the nose that is intersected by the median sagittal plane. The root of the nose corresponds to the nasofrontal suture, which is not necessarily the lowest point on its dorsum and which can usually be located with the finger.

Nasmyth′s membrane (nas′miths), *n.pr* See cuticle, primary.

nasoalveolar cyst (nā′zō alvē′ōlur), *n* an intraosseous cyst. A form of globulomaxillary cyst in which the epithelial inclusion is in the soft tissue fusion line.

nasolabial angle, *n* the angle formed by the labial surface of the upper lip at the midline and the inferior border of the nose. It is a measure of the relative protrusion of the upper lip.

nasolacrimal duct, *n* a tubular channel that carries tears from the lacrimal sac to the nasal cavity.

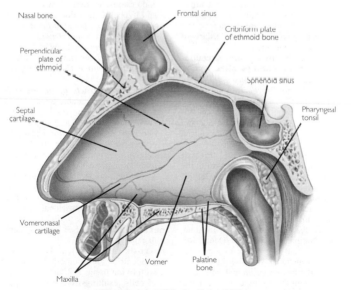

Nasal septum. (Thibodeau/Patton, 2003)

Nasal bone

Frontal sinus

Cribriform plate of ethmoid bone

Perpendicular plate of ethmoid

Sphenoid sinus

Septal cartilage

Pharyngeal tonsil

Vomeronasal cartilage

Maxilla

Vomer

Palatine bone

nasopharynx, *n* the uppermost of the three regions of the throat, or pharynx, situated behind the nose and extending from the posterior nares to the level of the soft palate.

natal teeth, *n* the presence of teeth in the mouth at birth, usually caused by the premature eruption of primary teeth but may be an extra or supernumerary tooth. The presence of natal teeth may cause discomfort to the nursing mother.

National Bureau of Standards (NBS), *n.pr* a federal agency in the Department of Commerce that sets accurate measurement standards for commerce, industry, and science in the United States.

National Formulary (NF), *n.pr* a publication containing the official standards for the preparation of various pharmaceuticals not listed in the *United States Pharmacopoeia.* It is revised every 5 years.

National Health Service Corps (NHSC), *n.pr* a program of the United States Public Health Service (USPHS) in which health care personnel are placed in areas that are underserved. Physicians, dentists, and nurses serve in rural and urban areas of need, usually as employees of local health care agencies. The USPHS pays most of the salary of each corps member.

National Institute for Occupational Safety and Health, *n.pr* an institute of the Centers for Disease Control and Prevention that is responsible for assuring safe and healthful working conditions and for developing standards of safety and health. Research activities are carried out pertinent to these goals.

National Institutes of Health (NIH), *n.pr* an agency within the United States Public Health Service comprising several institutes and constituent divisions, including the Bureau of Health Manpower Education, the National Library of Medicine, the National Cancer Institute, the National Institute for Dental Research, and a number of other research institutes and divisions.

natural bristles, *n* animal hair (usually from hogs) used in all types of brushes, including toothbrushes. They are not as durable or effective as synthetic bristles because individual hair thickness and length is not uniform, the porous nature of the bristles makes contamination more probable, and their absorbency makes rapid wear and deterioration more likely.

nausea, *n* a sensation often leading to the urge to vomit. Common causes are motion sickness, early pregnancy, intense pain, emotional stress, gallbladder disease, food poisoning, and various enteroviruses.

near-death experience, *n* the subjective observation of someone who has either been close to clinical death or who may have recovered after having been declared dead. Many claim to have witnessed similar episodes of passing through a tunnel toward a bright light and encountering people who have preceded them in death.

Necator, *n* a genus of nematode hookworms.

Necator americanus, *n* the so-called "New World" hookworm. The adults of this species attach to villi in the small intestine and suck blood, causing abdominal discomfort, diarrhea and cramps, anorexia, loss of weight, and hypochromic microcytic anemia.

necatoriasis, *n* hookworm disease. See also *Necator americanus.*

necessary, *n/adj* anything indispensable or useful for the sustenance of human life, such as food, shelter, and clothing.

necessary contracts of infants (minors), *n* things suitable to each child according to the child's circumstances.

necessary treatment, *n* a dental procedure or service determined by a dentist to be necessary to establish or maintain a patient's oral health. Such determinations are based on the professional diagnostic judgment of the dentist and the standards of care that prevail in the professional community.

neck of condyle, See process, neck of condyloid.

necrosis (nekrō′sis), *n* **1.** the death of a cell or group of cells in contact with living tissue. *n* **2.** the local death of cells resulting from, for example, loss of blood supply, bacterial toxins, or physical or chemical agents.

necrosis, caseous **(kā′sē us),** *n* a change commonly associated with tuberculosis and characterized by dry, soft, and cheesy tissue.

necrosis, exanthematous, *n* an acute necrotizing process involving the gingivae, jawbones, and contiguous soft tissues. It is of unknown cause, primarily affects children, and resembles noma. It differs from noma, however, in that it has a slight odor, tendency for self-limitation, low mortality rate, and normal leukocyte count. See also noma.

necrosis, gingival, *n* death and degeneration of the cells and other structural elements of the gingivae (for example, necrotizing ulcerative gingivitis).

necrosis, interdental, *n* a progressive disease that destroys the tissue of the papillae and creates interdental craters. Advanced interdental necrosis leads to a loss of periodontal attachment.

necrosis, ischemic, *n* death and disintegration of a tissue resulting from interference with its blood supply, thus depriving the tissues of access to substances necessary for metabolic sustenance. It may occur in the periodontal membrane as a result of occlusal trauma.

necrosis of epithelial attachment, *n* the death of cells composing the epithelial attachment. In a specific periodontitis produced by organisms similar to *Actinomyces,* necrosis of the epithelial attachment may exist, permitting a rapid apical shift of the base of the pocket.

necrosis, periodontal membrane, *n* necrosis of a portion of the periodontal membrane, usually resulting from traumatic injury (for example, in occlusal traumatism). Much of this necrotic change is the result of ischemia.

necrosis, radiation, *n* the death of tissue caused by radiation.

necrotic zone, *n* one of the four microscopically identified layers of a necrotizing ulcerative gingivitis (NUG) lesion. The necrotic zone comprises decomposed tissue and bacteria, including many spirochetes.

necrotizing stomatitis, *n* an inflammatory disease of the mouth charac-

terized by the destruction of epithelium, connective tissue, and papillae. The disease may cause a loss of periodontal attachment and the destruction of bone tissue. In advanced stages, it may lead to cancrum oris (noma).

necrotizing ulcerative periodontitis (NUP), *n* an acute periodontal disease characterized by erythema of the gingival and alveolar mucosa, ulcerated interdental papillae, interdental craters of the soft tissue and bone, and loss of periodontal attachment. See also gingivitis, necrotizing ulcerative (NUG)

nedocromil sodium, *n trade name:* Tilade; *drug class:* antiasthmatic, mast cell stabilizer; *action:* stabilizes the membrane of the sensitized mast cell, preventing release of chemical mediators after an antigen-IgE interaction; *use:* prophylaxis only in reversible obstructive airway diseases such as asthma.

needle, *n* a sharp, metal shaft that is available in a variety of forms for penetrating tissue (for example, in carrying sutures or injecting solutions).

needle biopsy, *n* the removal of a segment of living tissue for microscopic examination by inserting a hollow needle through the skin or the external surface of an organ or tumor and rotating it within the underlying cellular layers to retrieve a tissue specimen for examination.

needle, Gillmore, *n pr* an instrument used in a penetration type of test for measuring the setting time of materials such as plaster or stone. A ¼-pound needle is used for determining the initial set, and a 1-pound needle is used for defining the final set.

needle holder, *n* a forceps used to hold and pass the needle through the tissue while suturing with a suture forceps.

needle point tracer, See tracer, needle point.

needle stick injuries, *n* accidental skin punctures resulting from contact with hypodermic syringe needles. Such injuries can be dangerous, particularly if the needle has been used in treatment of a patient with a severe blood-borne infection, such as hepatitis or AIDS. A strict federal protocol for the use and disposal of needles is required for all health care facilities and personnel engaged in direct patient care.

needle, suture, *n* a small, sterile, stainless steel implement used during and after surgery to sew stitches into various types of human tissue.

needle, swaged end of (swājd), *n* the opposite end of the sharp tip of a sterile, stainless steel implement, where the thread had been attached directly to it, so that threading is not necessary.

needle, tapered suture, *n* the pointed tip of a surgical mending tool.

needle, Vicat, *n.pr* an instrument used for measuring setting time by means of a penetration test.

nefazodone HCl, *trade name:* Serzone; *drug class:* antidepressant; *action:* inhibits neuronal uptake of serotonin and norepinephrine; *uses:* major depressive disorders.

neglect, *n/v* the failure to do something that one is bound to do; lack of due care.

negligence, *n* the failure to observe, for the protection of another person, the degree of care and vigilance that the circumstances demand, whereby such other person suffers injury.

negligence, contributory, *n* negligence by an injured party that combines as a proximate cause with the negligence of the injurer in producing the injury. May bar recovery or mitigate damages.

negligence, imputed, *n* the principle that places the responsibility for negligence on a person other than the one that was directly negligent. This transfer of responsibility is based on some special relationship of the parties, such as parent and child or principal and agent (for example, a dentist may be responsible for the negligence of a dental assistant or other dental employee).

negotiate, *v* to deal or bargain with another or others to bring about an agreement or settlement.

Negri bodies, *n.pl* intracytoplasmic inclusion bodies found in the brain and central nervous system cells of rabies victims.

neighborhood, *n* an adjoining or sur-rounding district; an immediate vicinity.

Neisseria, *n* a genus of aerobic to facultatively anaerobic bacteria containing gram-negative cocci that occur in pairs with the adjacent sides flattened.

Neisseria gonorrhoeae, *n Gonococcus,* a species that causes gonorrhea.

Neisseria meningitidis, *n* a species found in the nasopharynx of man but not in other animals. The causative agent of meningococcal meningitis.

neisseriacae, *n* a vernacular term used to refer to any member of the genus *Neisseria.*

Neivert whittler, *n.pr* an instrument used to sharpen the cutting edges of blades. The sharpening end consists of tungsten carbide steel, and the handle is stainless steel. The Neivert whittler is particularly effective on curved scalers or curets.

nematodes (nē′mətōdz), *n* parasitic roundworms, such as hookworm and pinworm, that cause disease in humans.

Nematodes. (Thibodeau/Patton, 2002)

Nembutal, *n.pr* the trade name for pentobarbital.

Neo-Synephrine, *n.pr* the brand name for phenylephrine, a vasoconstrictor and pressor drug chemically related to epinephrine and ephedrine. Commonly used as a decongestant. Contraindicated for prolonged use or in patients with severe hypertension.

neodymium (Nd), *n* a rare earth element with an atomic number of 60 and an atomic weight of 144.24.

neomycin (nē′ōmī″sin), *n* an antibiotic secured from cultures of *Streptomyces fradiae,* used for preoperative sterilization. It is a constituent of topically applied ointments, solutions, and troches because of its antibacterial action against gram-negative organisms.

neomycin sulfate (topical), *n trade name:* Myciguent; *drug class:* local antibacterial; *action:* interferes with bacterial protein synthesis; *use:* skin infections.

neonatal, *adj* pertaining to a newborn child.

neonatal cytomegalovirus infection, *n* a disease caused by any of the viruses in the Cytomegalovirus family (part of the Herpesvirus family). It is transmitted to a newborn child through the birth process or contact with bodily fluids.

neonatal teeth, *n* the presence of teeth within 1 month of birth. See also natal teeth.

neoplasia (nē'ōplā'zhə), *n* the disease process responsible for neoplasm formation.

neoplasm, *n* (tumor), an abnormal mass of tissue, the growth of which exceeds and is uncoordinated with that of the normal tissues. It persists in the same excessive manner after cessation of the stimuli that evoked the change. Benign and malignant forms are recognized. See also tumor.

neoprene, *n* an oil-resistant synthetic rubber.

neostigmine bromide/neostigmine methylsulfate, *n trade names:* Prostigmin Bromide/Prostigmin; *drug class:* cholinesterase inhibitor; *action:* inhibits destruction of acetylcholine, which facilitates transmission of impulses across myoneural junction; *uses:* myasthenia gravis, nondepolarizing neuromuscular blocker antagonist, bladder distention, postoperative ileus.

nephrocalcinosis, *n* an abnormal condition of the kidneys in which deposits of calcium form in the parenchyma at the site of previous inflammation or degenerative change. Infection, hematuria, anal colic, and decreased function of the kidney may occur.

nephrology, *n* the study of the anatomy, physiology, and pathology of the kidney.

nephropathy (nə-frop'ə-the), *n* kidney disease.

nerve, *n* a cordlike structure that conveys impulses between a part of the central nervous system and some part of the body and consists of an outer connective tissue sheath and bundles of nerve fibers.

nerve, abducent (VI), *n* the sixth cranial nerve; a small, completely motor nerve arising in the pons, supplying the lateral rectus muscle of the eye.

nerve, accessory, *n* See nerve, spinal accessory.

nerve, acoustic (VIII), *n* the eighth cranial nerve; the vestibulocochlear nerve; a sensory nerve consisting of a vestibular portion and an auditory (or cochlear) portion.

nerves, afferent, in pulp, *n* any nerve that originates as a terminal free nerve ending in the dental pulp tissue and travels to the second and third divisions of the cranial trigeminal nerve.

nerve, alveolar, *n* afferent nerves that convey impulses from the pulp tissue and periodontium of the maxillary teeth to the maxillary division of the cranial trigeminal nerve.

nerve, anterior superior alveolar, *n* alveolar nerve that conveys impulses from the pulp tissue and periodontium of the maxillary anterior teeth to the infraorbital nerve.

nerve, auriculotemporal, *n* a nerve that transmits feeling from the external ear, scalp, and parotid salivary gland to the mandibular division of the cranial trigeminal nerve.

nerve, branchial, *n* one of five cranial nerves that supply the derivatives of the branchial arches: trigeminal (V), facial (VII), glossopharyngeal (IX), vagus (X), and spinal accessory (XI). Each branchial nerve may have a variety of functions, including visceral motor and visceral and somatic sensory functions.

nerve, buccal (long), *n* afferent nerve that conveys impulses from the facial periodontium of the mandibular molars and gingiva to the mandibular division of the cranial trigeminal nerve.

nerve, chiasma, optic, *n* the decussation, or crossing, of optic nerve fibers from the medial side of the retina on one side to the opposite side of the brain.

N

nerve, chorda tympani, n a parasympathetic and special sensory branch of the facial nerve supplying the submandibular and sublingual glands and the anterior two thirds of the tongue (taste).

nerve, cochlear, n one of the two major branches of the eighth cranial nerve; a special sensory nerve for the sense of hearing that transmits impulses from the organ of Corti to the brain.

nerve, cranial, n any one of 12 paired nerves, classified in three sets, arising directly in the brain and supplying various tissues of the head and neck. The cranial nerves are the special somatic sensory nerves: olfactory (I), optic (II), and acoustic (VIII); the somatic motor nerves: oculomotor (III), trochlear (IV), abducent (VI), and hypoglossal (XI); and the branchial nerves: trigeminal (V), facial (VII), glossopharyngeal (IX), vagus (X), and spinal accessory (XI).

nerve degeneration, n the reversion to a less organized and functioning state, usually detected by the loss of ability to conduct or transmit nerve impulses. Advanced degeneration might show cellular decomposition.

nerve ending, n the terminal of a nerve fiber, usually in synapse with another fiber or in a sensory organ.

nerve, facial (VII), n the seventh cranial nerve; a mixed nerve supplying motor fibers to the facial muscles, the stapedius, and posterior body of the digastric; sensory fibers from the taste buds in the anterior two thirds of the tongue (via the chorda tympani); and general visceral autonomic fibers for the submandibular and sublingual salivary glands. It travels unilaterally over the face and at one point is located in the parotid salivary gland, which it does not serve. However, pain in the parotid gland indicates a glandular malignancy, and complications with an inferior nerve block can also result from its location there.

The cranial nerves. (Thibodeau/Patton, 2002)

nerve fiber, *n* a slender process of a neuron, usually the axon. Each fiber is classified as myelinated or unmyelinated.

nerve, frontal, *n* afferent nerve from the union of the superorbital and supratrochlear nerves that carries information from the forehead, scalp, nose, and upper eyelids to the ophthalmic division of the cranial trigeminal nerve.

nerve, glossopharyngeal (IX), *n* the ninth cranial nerve; a mixed motor and sensory nerve arising in the medulla and supplying motor efferents to stylopharyngeal muscles and other pharyngeal muscles, visceral motor efferents to the otic ganglion for the parotid gland; special visceral afferents from the taste buds in the posterior third of the tongue; and general sensory afferents from the pharynx and posterior aspects of the oral cavity.

nerve, greater petrosal (petrō'səl), *n* one of the two nerves that branch off of the facial nerve and help control the muscles used in facial expression; this nerve also carries impulses to the lacrimal gland and the nasal cavity, and to and from the palate. The nerve has both afferent and efferent fibers.

nerve, hypoglossal (XII), *n* the twelfth cranial nerve; a motor nerve that arises in the medulla and supplies extrinsic and intrinsic muscles of the tongue.

nerve, incisive, *n* afferent nerve that merges with the mental nerve to later create the inferior alveolar nerve in the mandibular canal. This nerve transmits feeling from the pulp tissue and facial periodontium of the mandibular anterior teeth and premolars to the mandibular division of the cranial trigeminal nerve.

nerve, inferior alveolar, *n* a motor and general sensory branch of the mandibular nerve, with mylohyoid, inferior dental, mental, and inferior gingival branches.

nerve, infraorbital, *n* afferent nerve that enters through the infraorbital foramen and canal to merge with the maxillary branch of the cranial trigeminal nerve.

nerve, intermediate, *n* the parasympathetic and special sensory division

of the facial nerve with chorda tympani and greater petrosal branches.

nerve, lacrimal, *n* afferent nerve that is part of the ophthalmic division of the cranial trigeminal nerve and controls secretions in the upper eyelid, lacrimal gland, and the conjunctiva.

nerve, lingual, *n* a general sensory branch of the mandibular nerve having sublingual and lingual branches and connections with the hypoglossal nerve and chorda tympani.

nerve, mandibular, *n* the mandibular division of the trigeminal nerve, arising in the trigeminal ganglion and supplying general sensory and motor fibers via mesenteric, pterygoid, buccal, auriculotemporal, deep temporal, lingual, inferior alveolar, and meningeal branches.

nerve, maxillary, *n* the maxillary division of the trigeminal nerve arising in the trigeminal ganglion and supplying general sensory fibers via zygomatic, posterosuperior alveolar, infraorbital, pterygopalatine, and nasopalatine branches.

nerve, mental, *n* afferent nerve that transmits impulses from the facial periodontium of the mandibular anterior teeth, chin, and lower lip to later merge with the incisive nerve after it enters the mental foramen.

nerve, middle superior alveolar, *n* alveolar nerve that conveys impulses from the pulp tissue and periodontium of the gingiva and the maxillary premolar teeth to the infraorbital nerve. This nerve is not always present in all persons. If not present, the premolars are innervated by the posterior superior alveolar nerve.

nerve, mylohyoid, *n* a branch of the mandibular division of the cranial trigeminal nerve that serves the mylohyoid and digastric muscles of the mouth. It is thought to be a possible alternative innervation for the pulp tissues of the mandibular first molar in some cases.

nerve, nasociliary (nā'zōsil'ē-er̄ē), *n* one of three branches of the cranial trigeminal nerve that controls parts of the eyes, nasal cavity, and paranasal sinuses.

nerve, nasopalatine (nā'zōpal'ətīn), *n* afferent nerve that conveys impulses from the lingual periodontium of the maxillary anterior teeth bilaterally and the anterior hard palate to the maxillary division of the cranial trigeminal nerve.

nerve, oculomotor (III), *n* the third cranial nerve; primarily a motor nerve arising from the midbrain and supplying motor efferents to the superior rectus, medial rectus, inferior rectus, and inferior oblique eye muscles, as well as autonomic fibers via the ciliary ganglion to the ciliary body and the iris.

nerve, olfactory (I), *n* the first cranial nerve; a special sensory nerve for the sense of smell.

nerve, ophthalmic, *n* the ophthalmic division of the trigeminal nerve, arising in the trigeminal ganglion and supplying general sensory fibers via the frontal, lacrimal, and nasociliary branches.

nerve, optic (II), *n* the second cranial nerve; a special sensory nerve for vision passing from the retina of the eye to the optic chiasma.

nerve, palatine, *n* the two afferent nerves of the maxillary division of the cranial trigeminal nerve. The greater palatine nerve innervates the posterior hard palate and lingual periodontium of the maxillary molar teeth, while the lesser palatine nerve innervates the soft palate and palatine tonsillar tissue.

nerve, posterior superior alveolar, *n* alveolar nerve that conveys impulses from the maxillary sinus, gingiva, pulp tissue, and periodontium of the maxillary molar teeth to the infraorbital nerve or to the maxillary nerve directly.

nerve regeneration, *n* the reconstruction and renewal of cell structure and function; generally restricted to myelinated nerve fibers.

nerve, somatic motor, *n* (cranial), the somatic motor nerves—oculomotor (III), trochlear (IV), abducent (VI), and hypoglossal (XII)—largely comparable to the ventral motor roots of the spinal nerves. They are composed almost entirely of somatic motor fibers that emerge ventrally from the brainstem. Their arrangement is closely correlated with the distribution of the myotomes in the head. The oculomotor, trochlear, and abducent nerves, which supply the eye musculature, have the same myotomic origin and arrangement as the somatic muscles of the trunk and extremities.

nerve, special somatic sensory, *n* the structural arrangements from typical sensory nerves by which the three main sense organs, nose, eyes, and ears, are innervated. The sensory nerves are the olfactory (I), optic (II), and acoustic nerves (VIII).

nerve, spinal, *n* any one of 31 pairs of mixed peripheral nerves (8 cervical, 12 thoracic, 5 lumbar, 5 sacral, and 1 coccygeal) that are connected segmentally with the spinal cord, dorsal sensory trunk, and ventral motor root.

    nerve, spinal accessory (XI), *n* the eleventh cranial nerve; a motor nerve that derives its origin in part from the medulla and in part from the cervical spinal cord. Its internal ramus joins with the vagus nerve to supply some of the muscles of the larynx. Its external ramus joins with the spinal nerves to supply the sternocleidomastoid and trapezius muscles. The nerve and its relationship to head posture is important in maintaining stable occlusal relationships of vertical dimension and centric relation.

nerve, tensor tympani, *n* a small motor branch of the mandibular nerve.

nerve, trigeminal (V), *n* the fifth cranial nerve; a mixed motor and sensory nerve connected with the pons through three roots (motor, proprioceptive, and large sensory), the latter root expanding into the trigeminal ganglion, from which arise the ophthalmic, masseteric, and mandibular divisions.

nerve, trochlear (IV), *n* the fourth cranial nerve; a small motor nerve arising ventrally in the midbrain and supplying the inferior oblique muscle of the eye.

nerve trunk, *n* a particularly sizeable bundle of axons or nerve fibers.

nerve, vagus (X), *n* the tenth cranial nerve; a mixed parasympathetic, visceral, afferent, motor, and general sensory nerve with laryngeal, pharyngeal, bronchial, esophageal, gastric, and many other branches.

nerve, vestibular (VIII), *n* one of the two major branches of the eighth cranial nerve; a special sensory nerve for the sense of balance and the transmission of space-orientation impulses from the semicircular canals to the brain.

nerve, vestibulocochlear (VII), *n* the seventh cranial nerve; acoustic nerve; a sensory nerve consisting of a vestibular portion and an auditory, or cochlear, portion.

nerve, zygomatic (zī'gōmat'ik), *n* the afferent nerve of the maxillary division of the cranial trigeminal nerve that serves the skin of the cheek and temple. It also innervates the lacrimal gland.

nerves, dentinal, *n* any of the afferent or sensory neurons associated with the odontoblastic processes in the dentinal tubules and the attached cell body of the odontoblasts within the pulp tissue. These nerves may allow for an awareness of pain due to their monitoring of environmental changes within the dentin. There is some controversy about their overall location in the dentin tubule (full length, partial, or not at all).

nerves, periodontal ligament, *n* sympathetic fibers of the autonomic nervous system with enclosed nerve endings that control blood flow within the vessels and register pressure changes. Sensory or afferent fibers with free nerve endings cause an awareness of pain.

nerves, pulp, *n* sympathetic fibers of the autonomic nervous system located within the tissue that control blood flow within the vessels. Sensory or afferent fibers with free nerve endings in close proximity to the odontoblasts may cause an awareness of pain.

nerve block, *n* **1.** the reversible interruption of conduction along a nerve trunk or its branches because of the absorption of a suitable agent. *n* **2.** a regional anesthesia secured by extraneural or paraneural injection in close proximity to the nerve whose conductivity is to be cut. See also anesthesia, block.

nerve block, anterior middle superior alveolar, *n* an injection delivered by digital syringe into the palate that is used to anesthetize the pulp, facial and lingual periodontal tissues of the ipsilateral maxillary anterior teeth and premolars. It does not cause lip or facial muscle anesthesia.

nerve block, anterior superior alveolar, *n* an injection delivered by traditional syringe that is used to anesthetize the pulp tissue and facial periodontium of the maxillary anterior teeth.

nerve block, buccal, *n* an injection using a traditional syringe that causes anesthesia of the facial periodontium of the ipsilateral mandibular molars.

Buccal nerve block. (Daniel/Harfst, 2002, courtesy of the OHSU Department of Dental Hygiene)

nerve block, greater palatine (pal'ətin), *n* an injection delivered into the palatal tissues that is used to anesthetize the lingual periodontium of the ipsilateral maxillary posterior teeth.

nerve block, infraorbital (in'trə-ôr'bitəl), *n* an injection anesthetizing the pulp tissue and periodontium of the ipsilateral maxillary anterior teeth and premolars, including the first molar and its mesiobuccal root in some cases. One side of the nose, the upper lip, and lower eyelid may also be anesthetized.

nerve block, mandibular (inferior alveolar), *n* an injection used to anesthetize the anterior two-thirds portion of the tongue, the pulp tissue of the mandibular teeth, the floor of the mouth, the facial periodontium of the mandibular first premolar and anterior teeth, the lingual periodontium of all mandibular teeth, the skin on the chin, and the lower portion of the lip.

nerve block, middle superior alveolar, *n* an injection used to anesthetize pulp tissue and facial periodontium of the maxillary premolars and the mesiobuccal root of the first molar in some cases.

nerve block, nasopalatine, *n* an injection used to bilaterally anesthetize the lingual periodontium of the maxillary anterior teeth.

nerve block, posterior superior alveolar, *n* an injection used to anesthetize pulp tissue and facial periodontium of the ipsilateral maxillary molars. It does not always anesthetize the mesiobuccal root of the first molar.

Posterior superior alveolar nerve block. (Daniel/Harfst, 2002, courtesy of the OHSU Department of Dental Hygiene)

nervous system, *n* the extensive, intricate network of structures that activates, coordinates, and controls all the functions of the body. The nervous system is divided into the central nervous system, composed of the brain and spinal cord, and the peripheral nervous system, which includes the cranial nerves and the spinal nerves.

net, *adj* devoid of anything extraneous; free from all deductions, such as charges, expenses, taxes; remaining after expenses.

net protein utilization (NPU), *n* a comparison between the amount of nitrogen taken into the body and the amount retained, which results in a percentage value; includes a determination of whether the protein containing the nitrogen is capable of being digested in the first place.

netilmicin sulfate, *n* a parenteral aminoglycoside antibiotic used for short-term treatment of serious or life-threatening bacterial infections.

neural crest, *n* the band of ectodermally derived cells that lies along the outer surface of each side of the neural tube in the early stages of embryonic development. The cells migrate laterally throughout the embryo and give rise to certain spinal, cranial, and sympathetic ganglia.

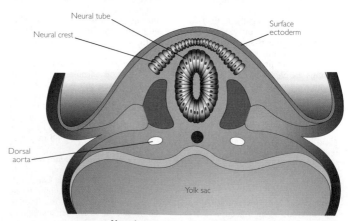

Neural crest. (Moore/Persaud, 2003)

neuralgia (nyōōral'jē ə), *n* pain associated with a nerve or nerves (for example, trigeminal and glossopharyngeal neuralgia).

neuralgia, atypical facial, n (cluster headache, lower-half headache, sphenopalatine neuralgia), severe unilateral pain behind the eye that spreads to the temple and behind the ear. It lasts 30 minutes to 3 hours and occurs once to several times a day and in cycles or clusters lasting several weeks. The clusters may be separated by several months or years. No trigger zones exist.

neuralgia, auriculotemporal, n (auriculotemporal causalgia neuralgia), sharp pain in the distribution of the auriculotemporal nerve.

neuralgia, buccal, n a throbbing, burning, and boring type of pain involving the cheeks, lips, gingivae, nose, and jaws. It may last a few minutes or several days. No trigger zones are present, although the pain may be initiated by chewing or thermal changes.

neuralgia, causalgia, n neuralgia characterized by an intense, diffuse burning sensation in a limited area.

neuralgia, facial, n See neuralgia, trigeminal.

neuralgia, glossopharyngeal, n pain in the nerves of the tongue, pharynx, ear, and neck precipitated by swallowing, sneezing, coughing, talking, or blowing the nose.

neuralgia, Sluder's irritation of the sphenopalatine ganglion, n.pr diffuse pain may affect the eye, root of the nose, teeth, and ear. Also, slight anesthesia and paralysis of the soft palate and palatine arch on the affected side may be present.

neuralgia, sphenopalatine, n See neuralgia, atypical, facial.

neuralgia, trifacial, n See neuralgia, trigeminal.

neuralgia, trigeminal, n (facial neuralgia, tic douloureux, trifacial neuralgia), an excruciating paroxysmal, stabbing, searing, or lancinating pain, usually occurring on the right side of the face and involving the distribution of the three divisions of the trigeminal nerve. It may last for a few seconds followed by additional episodes spontaneously or from stimulation of trigger zones. Intervals between attacks vary from a few hours to months or years.

neurasthenia (nyōō'rəsthē'nē ə), *n* a neurotic reaction characterized by chronic physical fatigue, listlessness, mental sluggishness, and, often, phobias.

neurectomy (nyōōrek'təmē), *n* the surgical excision of a nerve, or the more traumatic tearing away of nervous tissue from its anatomic position.

neurilemma (nyōō'rilem'ə), *n* the thin membranous outer covering surrounding the myelin sheath of a medullated nerve fiber or the axis cylinder of a nonmedullated nerve fiber. Neurilemma is associated with the booster mechanisms for the rapid transmission of impulses. Also called *sheath of Schwann.*

neurilemoma (nyōō'rilemō'mə), *n* (neurinoma, perineural fibroblastoma, schwannoma), a benign tumor of the neurilemma of disputed origin (Schwann cell vs. fibroblasts). May occur in soft tissue arid bone. Contains Verocay bodies. A malignant form occurs. See also body, Verocay and tissue.

neurinoma (nyōō'rinō'mə), *n* See neurilemoma.

neuritis (nyōōrī'tis), *n* the inflammation of a nerve, accompanied by pain and tenderness over the nerves, anesthesia, disturbance of sensation, paralysis, wasting, and disappearance of reflexes.

neuritis, endemic multiple, n See beriberi.

neuroaminidase, *n* an enzyme that is used in histochemistry to selectively remove sialomucins from bronchial mucous glands and the small intestine.

neuroanatomy, *n* the gross and microscopic structure over the nervous system.

neuroblastoma (nyōō'rōblastō'mə), *n* a malignant neoplasm characterized by proliferating nerve cells.

neuroectoderm (noor" o-ek' to-dərm), *n* specialized ectoderm cells in the embryo from which the central and peripheral nervous systems develop.

neurofibroma (nyōō'rōfibrō'mə),

n (neurogenic fibroma, perineural fibroblastoma), **1.** a benign neoplasm characterized by the various cells of a peripheral nerve (axon cylinders, Schwann cells, fibroblasts). *n* **2.** a connective tissue tumor of the nerve fiber fasciculi. Formed by the proliferation of the perineurium and endoneurium. See also neurilemoma.

Neurofibroma. (Regezi/Sciubba/Jordan, 2003)

neurofibromatosis (nyōō′rōfĭ′brōmətō′sis), *n* (molluscum fibrosum, multiple neuroma, von Recklinghausen's disease of skin), a disease characterized by multiple neurofibromas. Most frequently affects the skin but possibly involves the oral mucosa.

neurokinin (A), *n* a mammalian deca-peptide tachykinin found in the central nervous system. The compound has bronchoconstrictor, smooth muscle constrictor, and hypotensive effects and also activates the micturition reflex.

neuroleptanalgesia, *n* a form of analgesia achieved by the concurrent administration of a neuroleptic and an analgesic. Anxiety, motor activity, and sensitivity to painful stimuli are reduced; the person is quiet and indifferent to the environment and surroundings. If nitrous oxide with oxygen is also administered, neuroleptanalgesia can be converted to neuroleptanesthesia.

neurology, *n* the field of medicine that deals with the nervous system and its disorders.

neuroma (nyōōrō′mə), *n* technically, a benign neoplasm of nerve cells. As used in oral disease, the term usually refers to a traumatic neuroma, which is not a true tumor but an overgrowth of nerves associated with injury. The mental foramina and extraction scars are possible oral sites of this painful lesion.

neuroma, amputation, *n* See neuroma, traumatic.

neuroma, multiple, *n* See neurofibromatosis.

neuroma, traumatic, *n* (amputation neuroma), hyperplasia of nerve fibers and their supporting tissues in an exuberant attempt at repair after damage to, or the severing of, a nerve.

Traumatic neuroma. (Regezi/Sciubba/Jordan, 2003)

neuromuscular junction, *n* the area of contact between the ends of a large myelinated nerve fiber and a fiber of skeletal muscle. Also called *myoneural junction.*

neuron (nyōō′ron), *n* a nerve cell; the basic structural unit of the nervous system. There is a wide variation in the shape of nerve cells, but they all have the same basic structures: cell body, protoplasmic processes, axons, and dendrites. The neuron is the only body cell whose principal function is the conduction of impulses. It cannot regenerate when the cell body is destroyed; however, cell processes such as axons and dendrites can often regenerate.

A, motor neuron. B, sensory neuron. (Liebgott, 2001)

neuron, afferent, *n* a neuron that carries an impulse toward the central nervous system. See also afferent impulse.

neuron, efferent, *n* a neuron that carries an impulse toward the periphery, such as a motor neuron. See also efferent impulse.

neuron, sensory, *n* See neuron, afferent.

neuropathy, *n* an abnormal condition characterized by inflammation and degeneration of peripheral nerves.

neuropeptide, *n* any of a variety of peptides found in neural tissues, such as endorphins and enkephalins.

neurosis, *n* a diffusely defined term referring to a mental disorder for which professional help may be needed but that is milder than a psychosis; generally, a functional disorder in which there is no gross personality disorganization but there is an inability to cope effectively with some routine frustrations, anxieties, and daily problems. Somatic conditions may be factors in the cause and may be symptoms in a neurosis; however, the use of the term to describe a dysfunction of the nervous system is obsolete. Also called *psychoneurosis.*

neurostomatosis (nyōō′rōstō′mətō′sis), *n* an oral condition associated with psychosomatic or other psychological factors; for example, lichen planus and benign migratory glossitis may be considered types of neurostomatoses.

neurosurgery, *n* any surgery involving the brain, spinal cord, or peripheral nerves.

neurosyphilis, paretic (nyōō′rōsi′filis), *n* See paresis.

neurotensin, *n* a 13-amino acid peptide neurotransmitter found in synapsomes in the hypothalamus, amygdala, basal ganglia, and dorsal gray matter of the spinal cord; it plays a role in pain perception. It also affects pituitary hormone release and gastrointestinal function.

neurotomy (nyōō′rōtˈəmē), *n* the severance of a nerve process.

neurotransmitter, *n* any one of numerous chemicals that modify or result in the transmission of nerve impulses between synapses. Neurotransmitters are released from synaptic knobs into synaptic clefts and bridge the gap between presynaptic and postsynaptic neurons.

neutral, *n* a solution that has a pH level of 7. Equal numbers of hydrogen and hydroxyl ions are formed on dissociation.

neutral zone, *n* See zone, neutral.

neutralization, *n* the reaction of an acid with a base.

neutrocclusion, *n* normal mesiodistal occlusal relationships of the buccal teeth, similar to Angle class I.

neutron (nōō′tron), *n* an elementary particle with approximately the mass of a hydrogen atom but without any electrical charge; one of the constituents of the atomic nucleus.

neutron activation analysis, *n* an activation analysis in which the specimen is bombarded with neutrons. Identification is made by measuring the resulting radioisotopes.

neutron ray, *n* See ray, neutron.

neutropenia (nōō′trōpē′nē ə), *n* a relative or absolute decrease in the normal number of neutrophils in the circulating blood. Various limits are given; for example, absolute neutropenia may exist when the total is less than 1700 cells/mm³ regardless of the percentage, whereas relative neutropenia may exist when the total percentage of neutrophils is less than 38% and the total number is not less than 1500/mm³. Neutropenia may be associated with viral infections, pernicious anemia, sprue, aplastic anemia, bone marrow, neoplasms, chronic intoxication with drugs or heavy metals, malnutrition, and nonpyogenic and overwhelming infections.

neutropenia, cyclic, *n* a condition in which there is a depression in the number of circulating white cells, especially the neutrophils, at intervals of about 21 days. The neutropenia lasts for approximately 10 days; during this time, gingival inflammation and aphthous ulcer occur.

neutrophil, *n* a polymorphonuclear granular leukocyte. Neutrophils are the circulating white blood cells essential for phagocytosis and proteolysis.

neutrophilia (nōō′trōfil′ē ə), *n* an absolute or relative increase in the normal number of neutrophils in the circulating blood. Various limits are given; for example, an absolute neutrophilia may exist, regardless of percentage, if the total number of neutrophils exceeds 7000/mm³, whereas a relative neutrophilia may exist if the percentage of neutrophils is greater than 70% and the total number of neutrophils is less than 7000/mm³. May be associated with acute infections, chronic granulocytic leukemia, erythemia, therapy with adrenocorticotropic hormone (ACTH) or cortisone, uremia, ketosis, hemolysis, drug or heavy metal intoxication, or malignancy, or it may follow severe hemorrhage.

nevus (nē′vus), *n* a circumscribed new growth of congenital origin that may be vascular (resulting from hypertrophy of blood or lymph vessels) or nonvascular (with epidermal and connective tissue predominating).

nevus, blue, *n* a benign neoplasm characterized by heavily pigmented spindle cells deep in the corium; appears clinically as a dark mole.

Blue nevus. (Sapp/Eversole/Wysocki, 2004)

Cyclic neutropenia. (Sams/Lynch, 1996)

nevus, cellular pigmented, n a nevus composed of melanin-producing "nevus" cells.

nevus, compound, n a nevus in which the melanin-producing nevus cells are found in the epidermis and dermis: the intradermal nevus plus the junctional nevus.

nevus, intradermal, n a nevus in which the melanin-producing nevus cells are found only in the dermis.

nevus, junctional, n a nevus in which the melanin-producing nevus cells are found within the epidermis at the junction with the dermis.

nevus, pigmented, n a dark-colored, benign neoplasm characterized by nevus cells. Junctional, intradermal, and compound types are recognized. Melanomas (malignant neoplasms) may develop from junctional or compound nevi.

nevus, spongiosus albus mucosa, n (white folded gingivostomatitis, white sponge nevus), an inherited disease of the oral mucosa characterized by generalized white mucosal surfaces with a spongelike appearance.

White sponge nevus. (Regezi/Sciubba/Pogrel, 2000)

new attachment, n a connection formed between epithelium or connective tissue and a root surface that has lost its original attachment; this new connection may involve new cementum, epithelial adhesion, and connective adaptation.

Ney surveyor, n.pr See surveyor, Ney.

NF, n.pr the National Formulary.

niacin (vitamin B₃), n trade name: generic niacin (nicotinic acid); *drug class:* vitamin B₃; *action:* needed for conversion of fats, protein, carbohydrates by oxidation-reduction; acts directly on vascular smooth muscle, causing vasodilation; *uses:* pellagra, hyperlipidemias, peripheral vascular disease.

nib, n the part of a condensing instrument corresponding to the blade of a cutting instrument. The end is called the *face* of the condenser.

nicardipine HCl, n trade name: Cardene; *drug class:* calcium channel blocker; *action:* inhibits calcium ion influx across cell membrane during cardiac depolarization; produces relaxation of coronary vascular smooth muscle, peripheral vascular smooth muscle; dilates coronary vascular arteries; decreases sinoatrial/atrioventricular (SA/AV) node conduction; *uses:* chronic stable angina pectoris, hypertension.

nickel, n a silvery-white metallic element. Its atomic number is 28 and its atomic weight is 58.69. Large numbers of people are allergic to nickel. Nickel causes more cases of allergic contact dermatitis than all other metals combined. Many cases of allergic contact dermatitis occur from exposure to the nickel content of jewelry, coins, buckles, and snaps, and from continued use of "carbonless" business forms.

nickel-chromium alloy, n See alloy, nickel-chromium.

niclosamide (niklō′səmīd), n an anthelmintic agent that acts against pinworms and most tapeworms by inhibiting oxidative phosphorylation in the mitochondria.

nicotine, n a poisonous alkaloid found in tobacco and responsible for many of the effects of tobacco. It is first a stimulant (small doses) and then a depressant (larger doses).

nicotine gum, n an over-the-counter chewable product containing the chemical nicotine. Used by individuals who wish to quit smoking, it aids in the effort to lessen nicotine use over a period of time.

nicotine inhaler, n an inhalation device consisting of a mouthpiece into which a cartridge is inserted to deliver nicotine in gradually diminishing doses over time as a substitute for tobacco products; intended to curb nicotine cravings and to reduce the withdrawal symptoms associated with smoking cessation.

nicotine lozenge, n a dissoluble tablet intended for short-term use as a substitute source of nicotine by persons who are trying to quit smoking; as the tablet dissolves, it releases nicotine, which helps to ease cravings and relieves many of the withdrawal symptoms associated with smoking cessation.

nicotine nasal spray, n a nicotine-containing liquid that the user self-administers through the nose. Used by individuals who wish to quit smoking. Aids in the effort to lessen nicotine use over a period of time.

nicotine patch, n a press-on patch which releases the chemical nicotine slowly into the body through the skin. Used by individuals who wish to quit smoking.

nicotine polacrilex, n *trade name:* Nicorette; *drug class:* smoking deterrent; *action:* agonist at nicotinic receptors in the peripheral and central nervous systems; acts at sympathetic ganglia; on chemoreceptors of the aorta and carotid bodies; also affects adrenal-releasing catecholamines; *use:* deters cigarette smoking when combined with a program of smoking cessation.

nicotine replacement therapy, n a smoking cessation method intended to reduce nicotine cravings and ease the symptoms of withdrawal by substituting another source of nicotine, such as a specially-formulated lozenge, gum, nasal spray, inhalant, or skin patch for tobacco products.

nicotine transdermal system, n *trade names:* Habitrol, Nicoderm, Nicotrol, ProStep; *drug class:* smoking deterrent; *action:* binds to acetylcholine receptors at autonomic ganglia in the adrenal medulla, at neuromuscular junctions, and in the brain; *use:* cigarette smoking cessation program.

nicotinic stomatitis, n See stomatitis, nicotinic.

nidus (nī´dus), n the focal point; an originating position or nucleus.

Niemann-Pick disease (nē´mon pik´), n.pr See disease, Niemann-Pick.

nifedipine, n *trade names:* Procardia, Procardia XL; *drug class:* calcium channel blocker; *action:* inhibits calcium ion influx across cell membrane during cardiac depolarization; pro-

duces relaxation of coronary vascular smooth muscle, dilates coronary arteries; increases myocardial oxygen delivery in patients with vasospastic angina; dilates peripheral arteries; *uses:* chronic stable angina pectoris, vasospastic angina, hypertension.

night guard, n See guard, night.

night-grinding, n See bruxism.

Nikolsky's sign (nikol´skēz), n.pr See sign, Nikolsky's.

niobium (Nb), n the chemical element with an atomic number of 41 and an atomic weight of 92.9064. It was formerly known as *columbium.*

nitric acid, n a colorless, highly corrosive liquid that may give off suffocating brown fumes of nitrogen dioxide on exposure to air. Commercially prepared nitric acid is a powerful oxidizing agent used in photoengraving and metallurgy.

nitrofurantoin/nitrofurantoin macrocrystals, n *trade names:* Furadantin, Furalan, Macrobid, Macrodantin; *drug class:* urinary tract antiinfective; *action:* appears to inhibit bacterial enzymes; *uses:* urinary tract infections caused by *Escherichia coli, Klebsiella, Pseudomonas, Proteus vulgaris, Proteus morganii, Citrobacter,* and *Staphylococcus aureus.*

nitrogen (N), n a gaseous, nonmetallic element. Its atomic number is 7 and its atomic weight is 14.0067. Nitrogen constitutes approximately 78% of the atmosphere and is a component of all proteins and a major component of most organic substances.

nitrogen monoxide, n See nitrous oxide.

nitrogen monoxidum, n See nitrous oxide.

nitrogen, nonprotein, n See nonprotein nitrogen.

nitrogen balance, n a determination made about the body's ability to meet its nitrogen needs which is reached by comparing the amount of nitrogen taken in with the amount discharged via urine, hair, skin, or perspiration.

nitrogen balance, negative, n a condition in which nitrogen output exceeds nitrogen intake, resulting in the body's need to draw on its own stores of protein for energy; may be caused

N

by dietary imbalances, illness, infection, anxiety, or stress.

nitrogen balance, positive, n a body condition in which nitrogen intake exceeds nitrogen output; a normal state for children, pregnant women, or individuals recovering from illness or surgery, whose bodies require extra protein in order to build tissue.

nitroglycerin, *n trade names:* Nitrogard, Nitro-Bid, Nitrostat; *drug class:* inorganic nitrate, vasodilator; *action:* decreases preload/afterload, which is responsible for decreasing left ventricular end-diastolic pressure, systemic vascular resistance; arterial and venous dilation; *uses:* chronic stable angina pectoris, prophylaxis of angina pain, congestive heart failure associated with acute myocardial infarction, controlled hypotension in surgical procedures.

nitromersol, tincture (nītrōmur'sol), *n* a solution used in 1:200 strength as a topically applied antiseptic to temporarily minimize the bacterial count on an area of tissue.

nitrosamine (nītrō'səmēn), *n* compound present in tobacco that is linked to the development of cancer.

nitrous acid, HNO_2, a standard chemical reagent used in biologic and clinical laboratories.

nitrous oxide (N_2O), *n* (laughing gas, nitrogen monoxide, nitrogen monoxidum), a gas with a sweet odor and taste used with oxygen as an analgesic and sedative agent for the performance of minor operations. It is sometimes called *laughing gas* because it may excite a hilarious delirium preceding insensibility.

nizatidine, *n trade name:* Axid; *drug class:* H_2-histamine receptor antagonist; *action:* inhibits histamine at H_2-receptor site in parietal cells, which inhibits gastric acid secretion; *uses:* duodenal ulcer, Zollinger-Ellison syndrome, gastric ulcers, hypersecretory conditions, gastroesophageal reflux disease, stress ulcers.

NMR (nuclear magnetic resonance), *n* See magnetic resonance imaging.

noble, *adj* an archaic term referring to inert gases and precious metals.

noble metal, n See metal, noble.

Nocardia, n a genus of aerobic nonmotile actinomycetes, which are transitional between bacteria and fungi. They are primarily saprophytic but may cause disease in man and other animals.

nocardiosis (nōkär'dē ō'sis), *n* any of the pathologic entities that may follow infection with the bacterium *Nocardia.*

nociceptor, *n* somatic and visceral free nerve endings of thinly myelinated and unmyelinated fibers. They usually react to tissue injury but also may be excited by endogenous chemical substances.

node (nōd), *n* a swelling or protuberance.

node, brown, of hyperparathyroidism, n a central giant cell lesion of the bone seen in hyperparathyroidism. Its microscopic appearance is similar to giant cell reparative granuloma and giant cell tumor.

node of Ranvier gaps, n.pl nodes distributed at regularly spaced intervals along a myelinated nerve fiber. The intervals are 1 mm or more in length, and they function essentially as relay stations to facilitate the passage of an impulse.

nodule(s), *n* a small solid mass or knot that can be easily felt.

Bohn's nodules. (Zitelli/Davis, 2002)

nodule, pulp (nod'yōōl), n See denticle.

nodules, Bohn's, n.pl (Epstein's pearls), multiple white, ricelike lesions of the mucous membrane seen in newborn infants. Microscopically, each lesion shows a keratin-filled cyst that lies close to the mucosal surface. It disappears spontaneously in 2 to 3 months.

noma (nō'mə), *n* a progressive necrotizing process originating in the cheek with secondary involvement of the gingiva and jawbone. Occurs primarily in debilitated children, and the mortality rate is high. There is a strong, foul odor; marked surrounding edema; absence of a specific erythematous halo; marked changes in the white blood cell count; and a high temperature. See also necrosis, exanthematous and stomatitis, gangrenous.

nomenclature (nō'menklā'chur), *n* the formally adopted terminology of a science, art, or discipline; the system of names or terms used in a particular branch of science.

nomenclature, anatomical, *n* a naming system which is used to identify and classify the structures and organs of the body.

non-Hodgkin's lymphoma, *n* a form of lymphoma associated with AIDS. One of the indicator diseases of AIDS. See also lymphoma.

nonblisterform oral lesions, *n* solid wound with a firm texture located within the mouth that does not contain any fluid; may be a nodule, papule, plaque, or tumor.

noncohesive, *adj* lacking the property of sticking together, or cohesion.

noncontributory plan, *n* a method of payment for group insurance coverage in which the entire premium is paid by the employer or the union. Also referred to as *noncontributory program.*

nonduplication of benefits, *n* this term may apply if a subscriber is eligible for benefits under more than one plan. A dental benefits contract provision that relieves the third-party payer of liability for cost of services if the services are covered under another program. Distinct from a coordination of benefits provision because reimbursement would be limited to the greater level allowed by the two plans rather than a total of 100% of the charges. Also referred to as *less-benefit* or *carve-out.*

nonfeasance (nonfē'zəns), *n* the failure of a person to do some act that should be done.

nongonococcal urethritis, *n* an infection of the reproductive system caused by the bacterium *Chlamydia trachomatis.* Transmitted through sexual contact and can lead to infertility in women. See also *Chlamydia trachomatis.*

nonnutritive sucking, *n* a behavior of infants and toddlers that includes sucking on objects (fingers, pacifiers, etc.) out of habit or for psychological comfort.

nonocclusion, *n* a situation in which the tooth or teeth in one arch fail to make contact with the tooth or teeth of the other arch.

nonparticipating dentist, *n* 1. any dentist with whom the underwriter (insurer) does not have an agreement to render dental care to members of the plan. *n* 2. any dentist who does not have a contractual agreement with a dental benefits organization to render dental care to members of a dental benefits program.

nonprofit insurers, *n.pl* service corporations organized under nonprofit laws for the purpose of providing dental care insurance.

nonprotein nitrogen (NPN), *n* the nitrogen of whole blood or serum exclusive of that of the proteins. The concentration of nonprotein nitrogen is a gross measure of renal function. The upper limit of normal is 35 mg/100 ml.

nonsuccedaneous (non" suk" sə-da' ne-əs), *adj* pertaining to those permanent teeth that are not preceded by a primary form (i.e., the molars).

nonsuit, *n* a failure on the part of a plaintiff to continue the prosecution of the suit; abandonment of a suit.

nor-, *comb* a prefix that indicates lack of a methyl group.

norepinephrine (nôr'epinef'rin), *n* the neurohormonal transmitter for neuroeffector junctions of adrenergic nerve fibers. Its official drug name in the United States is levarterenol. See also levarterenol.

norethindrone acetate, *n trade names:* Aygestin, Micronor, Norlutate, Norlutin, Nor-QD; *drug class:* progesterone derivative; *action:* inhibits secretion of pituitary gonadotropins, which prevents follicular maturation, ovulation; *uses:* abnormal uterine bleeding, amenorrhea, endometriosis, contraceptive.

norfloxacin, *n trade name:* Noroxin; *drug class:* fluoroquinolone antiinfective; *action:* a broad-spectrum bactericidal agent that inhibits the enzyme DNA gyrase needed for replication of DNA; *uses:* adult urinary tract infections.

norgestrel, *n trade name:* Ovrette;

drug class: progesterone derivative; *action:* inhibits secretion of pituitary gonadotropins, which prevents follicular maturation, ovulation; *use:* oral contraception.

norm, *n* **1.** a statistical unit representative of the human species as a whole. *n* **2.** the numerical or statistical measures of the usual observed performance when related to health care provided to a given number of patients over time; often used in the building of profiles; can be the average or median or some other cutoff point in a series.

normal distribution, *n* a curve representing the frequency with which the values of a variable are obtained or observed when the number is infinite and variation is subject only to chance factors. The curve is a symmetrical, bell-shaped curve with the highest frequency occurring in the middle and gradually tapering toward the extremes. In a normal distribution, 68.2% of all scores cluster around the mean within approximately 1 standard deviation, 95.4% within approximately 2 standard deviations, and 99.7% within approximately 3 standard deviations. Also called *normal curve, Gauss' curve.*

normality, *n* a reference solution in which the concentration is stated with regard to the number of gram-equivalent weights present per liter of solution.

normalization, *n* the act of creating a lifestyle as similar as possible to that of a nonchallenged person for a person with disabilities.

normoblast (nôr′mōblast), *n* a nucleated red blood cell found in the peripheral bloodstream in severe pernicious anemia and in some leukemias.

normotensive (nôr′mōten′siv), *adj* having or dealing with having normal blood pressure.

nortriptyline HCl, *n trade names:* Aventyl, Pamelor; *drug class:* tricyclic antidepressant; *action:* blocks reuptake of norepinephrine, serotonin into nerve endings, which increases action of norepinephrine, serotonin in nerve cells; *use:* major depression.

Norwalk virus (nôr′wôlk), *n.pr* causative agent of acute gastrointestinal infection transmitted to humans through fecal-oral contact. Symptoms include cramping, fatigue, nausea, vomiting, and diarrhea.

nose, *n* the structure that protrudes from the anterior portion of the midface and serves as a passageway for air to and from the lungs. The nose filters, warms, and moistens the air on its passage into the lungs. The nose contains the end organs of smell.

nose, bones of, n the set of paired facial bones that together shape the nasal bridge, the edges of which join with the frontal bone at the top and the upper cheek bones at the sides.

nosebleed, *n* See epistaxis.

nosocomial (nos′əkō′mē-əl), *adj* related to a hospital; a condition described as nosocomial is one which occurs as a direct result of hospital treatment.

nostrum, *n* a remedy not substantiated by scientific evidence or broadly accepted by the scientific community. Some herbal supplements may fall under this category.

not-for-profit third parties, *n.pl* service corporations or dental benefits organizations established under not-for-profit state statutes for the purpose of providing health care coverage (for example, Delta Dental and Blue Cross, Blue Shield Plans).

notch, *n* an indentation.

notch, buccal, n the notch in the flange of a denture that accommodates the buccal frenum.

notch, coronoid (kôr′ənoid), *n* greatest concavity on the anterior border of the ramus of the mandible.

notch, hamular, n See notch, pterygomaxillary.

notch, labial, n the notch in the labial flange of an upper or lower denture that accommodates the labial frenum.

notch, mandibular, n a semicircular depression located on the mandible between the condyle and the coronoid process. Fibers arise from the anterior edge of the temporalis to form a distinct muscle, the temporalis minor, that inserts onto the mandibular notch.

notch, pterygomaxillary, n (hamular notch), the notch or fissure formed at the junction of the maxilla and the hamular, or pterygoid, process of the sphenoid bone.

notch, sigmoid, *n* the concavity on the superior surface of the ramus of the mandible lying between the coronoid and condyloid processes.

note, promissory, *n* a written promise to pay to another, at a specified time, a stated amount of money or other articles of value.

notice, *n* **1.** knowledge; information; awareness of facts. *v* **2.** the knowledge of facts that would naturally lead an honest and prudent person to make inquiry constitutes "notice" of everything that such inquiry pursued in good faith would disclose. *v* **3.** to observe.

notochord, *n* an elongated strip of mesodermal tissue that originates from the primitive node and extends along the dorsal surface of the developing embryo beneath the neural tube, forming the primary longitudinal skeletal axis of the body of all chordates.

Novocain, *n* the trade name for procaine hydrochloride, an ester, which is no longer used in the United States as an injectable. It is also the lay term for all types of dental local anesthesia.

noxious (nok′shus), *adj* hurtful; not wholesome.

NPN, *n* See nonprotein nitrogen.

NSAIDs, *n.pl* the acronym for nonsteroidal antiinflammatory drugs. See also naproxen.

nuclear family, *n* a family unit consisting of the biologic parents and their offspring. The nuclear family is less inclusive than the extended family. Although the nuclear family is a relatively recent product of Western society, it is threatened by the increasing dissolution of marriage.

nuclear magnetic resonance, *n* See magnetic resonance imaging.

nuclear medicine imaging, *n* the diagnostic imaging field that evaluates organ function by injecting isotopes into a structure and documenting the amount of radiation emanating from the tissues.

nucleic acid, *n* a family of macromolecules found in the chromosomes, nucleoli, mitochondria, and cytoplasm of all cells. In complexes with proteins, they are called *nucleoproteins.*

nucleic acid probes, *n* nucleic acid that complements a specific RNA or DNA molecule or fragment; used for hybridization studies to identify microorganisms and for genetic studies.

Nucleopolyhedrovirus, *n* (nuclear polyhedrosis virus), a genus of the family *Baculoviridae,* characterized by the formation of crystalline, polyhedral occlusion bodies in the host cell nucleus.

nucleoprotein (nōō′klē ōprō′tēn), *n* any one of a special group of protein substances in combination with nucleic acid. The essential component is the phosphoric acid radical. The nucleoproteins are generally confined to the nucleus of the cell and are intimately associated with chromosome and gene function.

nucleoside, *n* purine or pyrimidine bases attached to a ribose or deoxyribose.

nucleus (nōō′klē us), *n* **1.** the small, central part of an atom in which the positive electric charge and most of the mass (protons and neutrons) are concentrated. *n* **2.** an easily recognized structural component of most cells, surrounded by a membrane and containing chromosomes and nucleolus.

Nuhn's gland (nōōnz), *n.pr* the anterior lingual gland embedded in the substance of the tongue near the apex and the midline on the inferior surface of the tongue. See also gland, Blandin and Nuhn's.

nuisance, *n/adj* that which endangers life or health, offends the senses, violates the laws of decency, or obstructs reasonable and comfortable use of property.

null cell, *n* a lymphocyte that develops in the bone marrow and lacks the characteristic surface markers of the B and T lymphocytes. Null cells stimulated by the presence of antibody can directly attack certain cellular targets and are known as "natural killers" or "killer cells."

null hypothesis, *n* a statistical hypothesis that predicts that no difference or relationship exists among the variables studied that could not have occurred by chance alone.

N

number, Brinell hardness (BHN), *n.pr* a numerical expression of the hardness of a material, determined by measuring the diameter of a dent made by forcing a hard steel or tungsten carbide ball of standard dimension into the material under specified load in a Brinell machine, which was devised by J.A. Brinell, a Swedish engineer. The larger the indentation, the smaller the Brinell hardness number. See also test, Brinell hardness.

number, Vickers hardness, *n.pr* hardness as measured by the Vickers hardness test. See also test, Vickers hardness.

nurse, *n* **1.** a person educated and licensed in the practice of nursing; one who is concerned with the diagnosis and treatment of human responses to actual or potential health problems. *v* **2.** to breastfeed an infant.

nurse anesthetist, *n* a registered nurse qualified by advanced training in an accredited program in the specialty of nurse anesthesia to manage the care of the patient during the administration of anesthesia in selected surgical situations.

nurse midwife, *n* See midwife.

nurse practitioner, *n* a nurse who, by advanced education and clinical experience in a specialized area of nursing practice, has acquired expert knowledge and skill in a special branch of practice. The nurse practitioner acts as a nurse clinician, functioning independently within standing orders or protocols and collaborating with associates to implement a plan of care. The services of nurse practitioners are increasingly in demand under managed care programs and in large group practice settings.

nurse's aide, *n* a person who is employed to carry out basic nonspecialized tasks in the care of a patient, such as bathing and feeding, making beds, and transporting patients under the supervision and direction of a registered nurse.

nursing, *n* **1.** the performance of those activities that contribute to the health or recovery of a patient (or to a peaceful death). *n* **2.** the application of prescribed therapies and the management of the patient and environment to assist in healing.

nursing bottle caries, *n* dental caries of the maxillary primary teeth caused by the oral retention of milk or formula in the mouth.

nursing home, *n* a convalescent facility for the care of individuals who do not require hospitalization but who cannot be cared for at home. Preferred nomenclature: extended care facility.

nutrient, *n* the beneficial chemical in foods and beverages. Classified as carbohydrates, fats, proteins, water, vitamins, and minerals.

nutrient canal (nōō′trē ənt), *n* See canal, interdental.

nutrient dense, *adj* describes the ratio of beneficial chemicals to the number of calories in food when nutrient content is greater.

nutrient, essential, *n* See nutrient.

nutrition, *n* the process of assimilation and use of essential food elements from the diet (for example, carbohydrates, fats, proteins, vitamins, mineral elements).

nutrition survey, *n* usually a questionnaire regarding dietary habits, but may include an objective evaluation of nutritional status through the administration of physical examinations and laboratory tests of metabolism of a target population.

nutritional requirements, *n* the food and liquids necessary for normal physiologic function.

nutritional status, *n* the assessment of the state of nourishment of a patient or subject.

nutritional support, *n* the supply of foods and liquids necessary to advance healing and support health.

nutriture (nōō′trichur), *n* the nutritional status of a patient.

Nuva-lite, *n.pr* the brand name for an ultraviolet light used as a catalyst in the polymerization of Nuva-seal, a bonding agent used as a pit and fissure sealant.

Nuva-seal, *n.pr* the brand name of a bonding agent used as a pit and fissure sealant.

nyctalopia (nik′tələ͞o′pē-ə), *n* an inability to see in low-light conditions. It may be genetic or the result of a vitamin deficiency.

N

nylidrin HCl, *n trade name:* Arlidin; *drug class:* peripheral vasodilator, β-adrenergic agonist; *action:* acts on β-adrenergic receptors to dilate arterioles in skeletal muscles; increases cardiac output; may have direct vasodilatory effect on vascular smooth muscle; *uses:* arteriosclerosis obliterans, thromboangiitis obliterans, diabetic vascular disease, night leg cramps, Raynaud's disease, ischemic ulcer, frostbite, primary cochlear cell ischemia.

nystagmus (nīstag′mus), *n* the state of oscillatory movements of an organ or part, especially the eyeballs; irregular jerking movement of the eyes. Each movement of the cycle consists of a slow component in one direction and a rapid component in the opposite direction.

nystatin, *n trade names:* Mycostatin, Nystex, O-V Statin; *drug class:* antifungal; *action:* interferes with fungal DNA replication; *uses:* Candida species causing oral, vaginal, and intestinal infections.

oath, *n* an affirmation of the truth of a statement that renders one who is willfully asserting untrue statements punishable for perjury.

obesity (ōbēs′itē), *n* a bodily condition marked by excessive generalized deposition and storage of fat.

obesity, adrenocortical, *n* one of the symptoms characteristic of Cushing's syndrome; an obesity that is confined chiefly to the trunk, face, and neck. Also called *buffalo obesity.*

obesity, buffalo, *n* See obesity, adrenocortical.

object-film distance, *n* See distance, object-film.

obligation, *n* an assumed or assigned duty imposed by promise, law, contract, or society; the binding power of a vow, promise, oath, or contract.

observer variation, *n* the failure by the observer to measure or identify a phenomenon accurately, which results in an error. The observer may miss an abnormality or use faulty techniques, such as incorrect measurement or misinterpretation of the data. Two types are interobserver variation (the amount observers vary from one another when reporting on the same material) and intraobserver variation (the amount one observer varies between observations when reporting more than once on the same material).

obsessive-compulsive disorder (OCD), *n* the abnormal behavior of a person who tends to perform repetitive acts or rituals, usually as a means of releasing tension or relieving anxiety.

obstetrician, *n* a physician whose practice of medicine focuses on the care of women during pregnancy, through childbirth, and immediately following delivery. Often informally known as *OB-Gyn (obstetrician-gynecologist).*

obstetrics, *n* the branch of medicine concerned with pregnancy and childbirth, including the study of the physiologic and pathologic function of the female reproductive tract and the care of the mother and fetus throughout pregnancy, childbirth, and the immediate postpartum period.

obtain, *v* to acquire.

obtund (obtund′), *v* to diminish the ability to perceive pain and/or touch.

obtundent (obtun′dent), *n* an agent that has the property to diminish the perception of pain and/or touch.

obturation (ob′tōōrā′shən), *n* the act of closing or occluding.

obturation, retrograde, *n* See filling, retrograde.

obturation, root canal filling technique, *n* the procedure used for filling and sealing the root canal.

obturator (ob′tōōrātur), *n* a prosthesis used to close a congenital or acquired opening in the palate. See also aid, prosthetic speech.

obturator, hollow, *n* that portion of an obturator made hollow to minimize its weight.

occipital anchorage (oksip′itəl), *n* See anchorage, occipital.

occipital lymph nodes, *n* rounded masses of lymphoid tissue located near the occipital bone.

occlude, *v* to close together. To bring together; to shut. To bring the mandibular teeth into contact with the maxillary teeth.

occluder, *n* a name given to some articulators. See also articulator.

occlusal, *adj* pertaining to the contacting surfaces of opposing occlusal units (teeth or occlusion rims). Pertaining to the masticating surfaces of the posterior teeth.

occlusal adjustment, n See adjustment, occlusal.

occlusal analysis, n See analysis, occlusal.

occlusal balance, n See balanced occlusion.

occlusal contacts, n.pl See contacts, deflective occusal and contact, interceptive occlusal.

occlusal contouring, n See contouring, occlusal.

occlusal correction, n See correction, occlusal.

occlusal curvature, n See curve of occlusion.

occlusal disharmony, n See disharmony, occlusal.

occlusal disturbances, n.pl See disturbances, occlusal.

occlusal embrasure, n See embrasure, occlusal.

occlusal equilibration, n See equilibration, occlusal.

occlusal force, n See force, occlusal.

occlusal form, n See form, occlusal.

occlusal function, n See function, heavy.

occlusal glide, See glide, occlusion.

occlusal guard, n See occlusal splint.

occlusal harmony, n See harmony, occlusal.

occlusal load, n See load, occlusal.

occlusal path, n See path, occlusal.
  occlusal path registration, n See path, occlusal.

occlusal pattern, n See pattern, occlusal.

occlusal perception, See perception, occlusal.

occlusal pivot, n See pivot, occlusal.

occlusal plane, n See plane, occlusal.

occlusal position, See position, occlusal.

occlusal pressure, n See pressure, occlusal.

occlusal recontouring, n See contouring, occlusal.

occlusal rest, n See position, rest.

occlusal splint, n (occlusal guard) a bite plane designed and fabricated for patients with some types of functional temporomandibular joint disorders. Provides a stable occlusal platform from which to reconstruct a functional occlusion. See also splint.

Occlusal splint. (Christensen, 2002)

occlusal stop, n See rest, occlusal.

occlusal surface, n See surface, occlusal.

occlusal system, n See system, occlusal.

occlusal table, n See table, occlusal.

occlusal template, n See template, occlusal.

occlusal therapy, n a treatment to establish and maintain a comfortable, stable, and functional occlusion for patients with one of several types of occlusal problems. Treatment may be limited to the teeth, the neuromuscular mechanisms of chewing, or a combination of both.

occlusal trauma, n See trauma, occlusal.

occlusal unit, n one of two kinds of cusps: (1) a stamp cusp coupled with a fossa, and (2) a shear cusp. The occlusal edges of the shear cusp are coupled with the edges of a stamp cusp, by which it passes closely without sliding contacts.

occlusal wear, n See wear, occlusal.

occlusion, *n* **1.** the act of closure or state of being closed. *n* **2.** any contact between the incising or masticating surfaces of the upper and lower teeth.

occlusion, acentric, n See occlusion, eccentric.

occlusion, adjustment, n See adjustment occlusion.

occlusion, anatomic, n the ideal relation of the mandibular and maxillary teeth when closed.

occlusion, anterior determinants of cusp, n.pl the characteristics of the anterior teeth, that is, occlusion, alignment, overlaps, and capacity to disclude conjointly with the trajectories given the condyles, that determine the cusp elevations and the fossa depressions of the postcanine teeth.

occlusion, attritional, n an occlusion in which each tooth of the dentition wears occlusally and proximally as it erupts.

occlusion, balanced, n 1. an occlusion of the teeth that presents a harmonious relation of the occluding surfaces in centric and eccentric positions within the functional range of mandibular positions and tooth size. n 2. the simultaneous contacting of the upper and lower teeth on both sides and in the anterior and posterior occlusal areas of the jaws. This occlusion is developed to prevent a tipping or rotating of the denture base in relation to the supporting structures. This term is used primarily in connection with the mouth, but it may be used in relation to teeth on an articulator.

occlusion, bilateral balanced, n the closure suitable for worn dentitions that are cuspless or have flat-sided cusps; it permits an increase of the amount of surface contact in centric closure and provides as much closure contact as possible for horizontal chewing. This kind of occlusion is a therapeutic form designed to keep dentures seated when fine-textured foods are chewed horizontally. It is not found in young, unworn natural dentitions.

occlusion, canine protected, n lateral mandibular movements guided by the canine teeth.

occlusion, central, n See occlusion, centric.

occlusion, centric, n the relation of opposing occlusal surfaces that provides the maximum planned contact and/or intercuspation. It should exist when the mandible is in centric relation to the maxilla. Also called *central occlusion.*

occlusion, centrically balanced, n a centrically related centric occlusion in which the teeth close with even pressures on both sides of the mouth but have no occlusion of the postcanine teeth in attempted eccentric closures.

occlusion, components of, n.pl the various factors involved in occlusion (for example, temporomandibular joint, associated neuromusculature, and teeth). In denture prosthetics, also the denture-supporting structures.

occlusion, convenience, n the assumed position of maximum intercuspation when there is occlusal interference in the centric path of closure. The convenience occlusion may be anterior, lateral, or anterolateral to the true centric occlusion. Also called *convenience jaw relation* and *convenience relationship of teeth.*

occlusion, coronary, n a coronary thrombosis resulting in closure of the coronary artery.

occlusion, cross-bite, n an occlusion in which the lower teeth overlap the upper teeth.

occlusion, determinants of, n.pl the classifiable factors in the gnathic organ that influence occlusion. These factors are divided into two groups: those that are fixed and those that can be modified by reshaping or repositioning the teeth. The fixed factors most mentioned are the intercondylar distance; anatomy, which influences the paths of the mandibular axes; mandibular centricity; and the mating of the jaws. The changeable factors most mentioned are tooth shape, tooth position, vertical dimension, height of cusps, and depth of fossae.

occlusion, eccentric, n any occlusion other than centric occlusion.

occlusion, edge-to-edge, n an occlusion in which the anterior teeth of both jaws meet along their incisal edges when the teeth are in centric occlusion.

occlusion, end-to-end, n See occlusion, edge-to-edge.

occlusion, faulty centric, n a condition in which centric occlusion does not correspond to a patient's centric jaw relationship, resulting in premature or interceptive or deflective tooth contacts in the centric path of closure.

occlusion, functional, n **1.** occlusion in which attention is directed specifically to performance and is differentiated from structure and appearance. *n* **2.** any tooth contacts made within the functional range (according to the size) of the opposing tooth surfaces. An occlusion that occurs during function.

occlusion, gliding, n used in the sense of designating contacts of teeth in motion. A substitute for the term articulation.

occlusion, ideal, n **1.** the relationship existing when all the teeth are perfectly placed in the arches of jaws and have a normal anatomic relationship to each other. When the teeth are brought into contact, the cusp-fossa relationship is considered the most perfect anatomic relationship that can be attained. *n* **2.** the normal relationships of the inclines of the cusps of opposing teeth to each other in occlusion, when the alignment, proximal contacts, and axial positions of the teeth in both arches have resulted from normal growth and development in relation to all associated tissues and parts of the head.

occlusion, lateral, n right or left lateral movement of the mandible until the canines on the respective sides are in a cusp-to-cusp relationship. See also cross-bite.

occlusion, locked, n an occlusal relationship of such nature that lateral and protrusive mandibular movements are limited.

occlusion, malfunctional, n a disturbance in the normal or proper action of the masticatory apparatus produced by such factors as missing teeth or tilting and drifting of teeth.

occlusion, mechanically balanced, n an occlusion balanced without reference to physiologic considerations (for example, on an articulator).

occlusion, normal, n See occlusion, ideal.

occlusion, pathogenic, n an occlusal relationship capable of producing pathologic changes in the teeth, supporting tissues, and/or other components of the stomatognathic system.

occlusion, physiologic, n **1.** an occlusion in harmony with functions of the masticatory system. *n* **2.** an occlusion that operates in harmony and presents no pathologic manifestation in the supporting structures of the teeth; the stresses placed on the teeth are dissipated normally, with a balance existing between the stresses and adaptive capacity of the supporting tissues. *n* **3.** an acceptable occlusion found in a healthy gnathic system.

occlusion, physiologically balanced, n a balanced occlusion in harmony with the temporomandibular joints and the neuromuscular system. See also occlusion, balanced.

occlusion, plane of, n See plane, occlusal.

occlusion, protrusive, n an occlusion of the teeth existing when the mandible is protruded forward from a centric position. See also position, rest, physiologic.

occlusion, rim, n See rim, occlusion.

occlusion, spherical form of, n an arrangement of teeth that places their occlusal surfaces on the surface of an imaginary sphere (usually 8 inches [20 cm] in diameter) with its center above the level of the teeth, as suggested by Monson.

occlusion, static, n See occlusion, ideal.

occlusion table, n See table, occlusal.

occlusion, terminal, n the relation of opposing occlusal surfaces that provides the maximum natural or planned contact and/or intercuspation.

occlusion, traumatic, n an occlusion that results in overstrain and injury to teeth, periodontal tissues, or the residual ridge or other oral structures.

occlusion, traumatogenic, n See occlusion, traumatic.

occlusion, working, n the occlusal contacts of teeth on the side toward which the mandible is moved. From the mesial or distal view, the buccal and lingual cusps of the upper teeth appear to be end-to-end with the buccal and lingual cusps of the lower teeth, respectively. Viewed from the side, each upper cusp is distal to the corresponding lower cusp. The mesial incline of each upper cusp makes contact with the distal incline of the opposing cusp in front of it, and the distal incline of each upper cusp makes contact with the mesial incline of the opposing cusp distal to it.

occupational disease, *n* a disease that results from a particular employment, usually from the effects of long-term exposure to specific substances or from the continuous or repetitive physical acts.

occupational exposure, *n* working in an environment with one or more risk factors present.

occupational hazard, *n* See occupational risk.

occupational health, *n* the ability of a worker to function at an optimum level of well-being at a worksite as reflected in terms of productivity, work attendance, disability compensation claims, and employment longevity.

occupational risk, *n* a hazard found or likely to occur in the workplace. The number and types of hazards a health care worker may encounter in the routine conduct of health care delivery.

Occupational Safety and Health Administration (OSHA), *n.pr* a federal agency charged with establishing guidelines and regulations regarding worker safety. These guidelines include storage and disposal of toxic chemicals and hazardous materials and the safety and proper use of clinical and office equipment.

OSHA coordinator, *n* the person within an organization, agency, or healthcare facility who is the designated "expert" on OSHA standards. As the person most knowledgeable about federal and state safety requirements, he or she should be consulted whenever operating procedures are developed or revised to ensure compliance with the law.

ocular herpes (ok′yōōlur), *n* HSV-1 or HSV-2 infection of the eye, resulting in lesions on the eye. The infection can be transmitted by contaminated saliva contacting the eye.

odontalgia (ō′dontal′jə), *n* pain in a tooth; toothache.

odontalgia, phantom, *n* pain in the area from which a tooth has been removed. Also called *ghost pain.*

odontectomy (ō′dontek′təmē), *n* the removal of a tooth.

odontoblasts (ōdon′tōblasts), *n.pl*

the cells that form the dentin of the tooth.

odontoclasts, *n.pl* the cells specifically responsible for the resorption of cementum and dentin.

odontodysplasia, *n* a developmental anomaly characterized by deficient tooth development. Deficiencies are noted in enamel and dentin formation. Also called *ghost teeth.* See also tooth, shell.

Odontodysplasia. (Regezi/Sciubba/Jordan, 2003)

odontogenesis (ōdon′tōjen′əsis), *n* the process of tooth formation.

odontogenesis imperfecta, *n* a generic term that includes simultaneous defects in epithelial and mesenchymal tissue involved in tooth development.

odontogenic cysts, *n.pl* See cysts.

odontogenic myxoma (ōdon′tōjen′ik miksō′mə), *n* a deep lesion in a mandibular or maxillary tooth germ's mesenchyme. It occurs equally in males and females between the ages of 10 and 30. The tumor may displace teeth and spread to other locations.

odontogenic tumors, *n.pl* See tumors.

odontoid process, *n* the toothlike projection that rises perpendicularly from the upper surface of the body of the second cervical vertebra or axis, which serves as a pivot point for the rotation of the atlas, or first cervical vertebra, enabling the head to turn in a horizontal plane.

odontolysis (o-don-tol′ĭ-sis), *n* See resorption, root.

odontoma (ō′dontō′mə), *n* an anomaly of the teeth resembling a tumor of hard tissue (e.g., dens in dente, enamel pearl, complex or composite odontoma). It is composed of enamel, dentin, cementum, and pulp tissue that may be arranged in the form of teeth. Also called *gestant anomaly.*

Odontoma. (Regezi/Sciubba/Jordan, 2003)

odontoma, ameloblastic **(əmel′ōblas′tik),** *n* an odontogenic tumor characterized by the occurrence of an ameloblastoma within an odontoma. See also ameloblastoma; odontoma.

odontoma, composite **(kəmpoz′it),** *n* complex odontoma; an odontogenic tumor characterized by the formation of calcified enamel and dentin in an abnormal arrangement because of lack of morphodifferentiation. Compound odontoma: a tumor of enamel and dentin arranged in the form of anomalous miniature teeth. Several small abnormal teeth surrounded by a fibrous sac.

odontoma, cystic, *n* an odontoma associated with a follicular cyst.

odontoma, gestant, *n* See dens in dente.

odor, *n* a scent or smell. The sense of smell is activated when airborne molecules stimulate receptors of the first cranial nerve.

office hours, *n.pl* See business hours.

office management, *n* the oversight of the business aspects of professional practice.

office planning, *n* the physical arrangement of the rooms available within the limitations of space designed to enable the dentist to practice.

office routine, *n* See routine, office.

office visit, *n* a patient encounter with a health care provider in an office, clinic, or ambulatory care facility as an outpatient.

offline, *adj/adv* pertaining to the operation of input/output devices or auxiliary equipment not under direct control of the central processor.

offset, *n* a deduction; a counterclaim; a contrary claim or demand by which a given claim may be lessened or cancelled.

offset blade, *n* a blade that is set at an angle to the shank rather than perpendicular to it; in an area-specific curet, an offset blade is set at a 70-degree angle to the shank.

ofloxacin, *n trade names:* Floxin, Floxin IV; *drug class:* fluoroquinolone antiinfective; *action:* broad-spectrum bactericidal agent that inhibits the enzyme DNA-gyrase needed for replication of DNA; *uses:* treatment of lower respiratory tract infections, genitourinary infections, skin and skin structure infections.

ofloxacin (optic), *n trade name:* Ocuflox; *drug class:* fluoroquinolone antiinfective, topical; *action:* broad-spectrum bactericidal agent that inhibits the enzyme DNA-gyrase needed for replication of DNA; *uses:* treatment of bacterial conjunctivitis caused by susceptible organisms.

oil, *n* an unctuous, combustible substance that is liquid, or easily liquefiable on warming, and soluble in ether but insoluble in water.

oil, essential, *n* a volatile, nonfatty liquid of vegetable origin having a distinct aroma and flavor, often pleasant. Also called *volatile oil.*

oil, fixed, *n* a nonvolatile oil consisting chiefly of glycerides.

oil, mineral, *n* any one of the various grades of liquid petrolatum.

oil, volatile, *n* See oil, essential.

ointment (oint′ment), *n* a soft, bland, smooth, semisolid mixture that is used as a lubricant and as a vehicle for external medication.

ointment, hydrophilic, *n* an ointment that is miscible with water.

olfactory bulb, *n* the area of the forebrain where the olfactory nerves terminate and the olfactory tracts arise.

olfactory nerve, *n* one of a pair of nerves associated with the sense of smell. The olfactory nerve is the first cranial nerve. The olfactory sensory endings are modified epithelial cells and the least specialized of the special senses.

oligodendroglioma, *n* a relatively rare, moderately well-differentiated, relatively slow-growing glioma that occurs most frequently in the cerebrum of adults. It is grossly homogeneous, fairly well-circumscribed, moderately firm, and somewhat gritty in consistency, with interstitial calcification sufficiently dense to allow detection by x-ray imaging of the skull.

oligodontia (ol'igōdon'shē ə), *n* See partial anodontia.

oligodynamic (ol'igōdīnam'ik), *adj* effective in extremely small quantities.

oligomenorrhea (ol'igōmen'ərē'ə), *n* a condition in which a woman experiences fewer menstrual cycles than normal because each cycle lasts longer than 45 days.

oligonucleotide, *n* a compound made up of the condensation of a small number of nucleotides.

oligosaccharides (ol'igōsak'ərīdz), *n.pl* carbohydrates that are formed by combining as few as two or as many as six monosaccharides.

oliguria (ol'igyōō'rē ə), *n* a decreased output of urine (usually less than 500 ml/day), possibly associated with dehydration from diarrhea or excessive sweating, low fluid intake, lower nephron nephrosis resulting from burns, heavy metal poisoning, terminal renal disease, or an increase in extracellular fluid volume in untreated renal, cardiac, or hepatic disease.

olsalazine sodium, *n trade name:* Dipentum; *drug class:* antiinflammatory, salicylate derivative; *action:* bioconverted to 5-amino-salicylic acid, which decreases inflammation in the colon; *uses:* maintenance of remission of ulcerative colitis in patients intolerant to sulfasalazine.

omeprazole, *n trade name:* Prilosec; *drug class:* antisecretory compound; *action:* suppresses gastric secretion by inhibiting hydrogen/potassium ATPase enzyme system in the gastric parietal cell; *uses:* gastroesophageal reflux disease (GERD), severe erosive esophagitis, pathologic hypersecretory conditions (Zollinger-Ellison syndrome, mastocytosis, multiple endocrine adenomas).

omission, *n* a phoneme left out at a place where it should occur.

on account, *adv* in partial payment; in partial satisfaction of an amount owed.

on or about, *adv* a phrase used in stating the date of an occurrence or conveyance to avoid being bound by the statement of an exact or certain date.

Onchocerca, *n* a genus of elongated filariform nematodes that inhabit the connective tissue of their hosts, usually within firm nodules in which these parasites are coiled and entangled.

Onchocerca volvulus, *n* the blinding nodular nematode that causes dermatologic lesions and ocular complications that lead to blindness.

oncocytoma (ong'kōsītō'mə), *n* a rare, benign tumor usually occurring in the parotid glands in older patients. The lesion is encapsulated and composed of sheets and cords of large eosinophilic cells with small nuclei. Also called *acidophilic adenoma, oxyphilic adenoma.*

Oncocytoma. (Regezi/Sciubba/Jordan, 2003)

oncogene, *n* a potentially cancer-inducing gene.

oncology (ongkol'əjē), *n* the scientific study which focuses on tumors and malignancy; the science of cancer.

ondansetron HCl, *n trade name:* Zofran; *drug class:* antiemetic; *action:* selective 5-HT3 antagonist; *uses:* prevention of nausea and vomiting associated with cancer chemotherapy.

ondontoplasty, *n* cosmetic or rehabilitative rebuilding of a tooth.

One Stage Oratronics Weis Standard Blade Implant System, *n.pr* an ADA-acceptable endosseous dental implant system.

onlay, *n* **1.** a cast type of restoration that is retained by frictional and mechanical factors in the preparation of the tooth and restores one or more cusps and adjoining occlusal surfaces of the tooth. *n* **2.** an occlusal rest portion of a removable partial denture that is extended to cover the entire occlusal surface of the tooth.

onlay bone, *n* See graft, onlay bone.

online, *adj/adv* a system of data processing under control of the central processing unit. Data reflecting current activity are introduced into the processing system as soon as they occur.

ontogeny (ontoj'əne), *n* the natural life cycle of an individual as contrasted with the natural life cycle of the race (phylogeny).

opacification (ōpas'ifikā'shən), *n* **1.** the process of making something opaque. *n* **2.** the formation of opacities.

opalescent (ō'pəles'ent), *adj* resembling an opal in the display of various colors, as in opalescent dentin.

opalescent teeth, *n.pl* a translucent or opal-like appearance of teeth, usually associated with a genetic defect in odontogenesis.

opaque, *adj* relatively impenetrable to light. See also opacity, optical.

open bite, *n* See bite, open.

open contacts, *n* regions in which an interval between adjacent teeth exists due to the abnormal position or absence of the teeth, oral disease, dental habits, or the overdevelopment of the frena.

open enrollment, *n* the annual period in which employees can select from a choice of benefits programs.

open panel, *n* a dental benefits plan characterized by three features: (1) any licensed dentist may elect to participate, (2) the beneficiary may receive dental treatment from among all licensed dentists with the corresponding benefits payable to the beneficiary or the dentist, and (3) the dentist may accept or refuse any beneficiary. See also panel, open.

open scaling, *n* procedure for working on the subgingival surface that has been made accessible by the removal of or laying aside of the enclosing tissue.

open-end contract, *n* See contract, open-end.

opening movement, *n* See movement, mandibular, opening.

opening, vertical, *n* See dimension, vertical.

operate, *v* to work on the body with the hands or by means of cutting or other instruments to correct a deformity, remove an anatomic part, or remove pathologic processes and/or tissues.

operating field, *n* See field, operating.

operating light, *n* See light, operating.

operating procedure, *n* See procedure, operating.

operation, *n* **1.** any surgical procedure. *n* **2.** the action of a drug or other remedy. *n* **3.** an act or series of acts performed on the body of a patient for relief or cure.

operation, Abbé-Estlander, *n.pr* the transfer of a full thickness section of one lip of the oral cavity to the other lip, using an arterial pedicle to ensure survival of the graft.

operation, blind, *n* a procedure in which the surgeon operates by using the sense of touch and knowledge of surgical anatomy without making a significant mucous membrane or cutaneous incision.

operation, computer, *n* the program step undertaken or executed by a computer (for example, addition, multiplication, comparison, and data movement). The operation is usually specified by a functional command in the software used.

operation, exploratory, *n* a surgical procedure used to establish a diagnosis.

operation, Gillies', *n.pr* a technique for reducing fractures of the zygoma and the zygomatic arch through an incision in the temporal hairline.

operation, Kazanjian's, *n.pr* a technique of surgical extension of the vestibular sulcus for improved prosthetic foundation of edentulous ridges. Also known as *Kazanjian's procedure.* See also extension, ridge.

operation, modified flap, *n* a variation of the flap procedure in oral and periodontal surgery. In this variation the vertical incisions of the flap procedure are not made, but the labial and/or lingual gingival walls are distended as far as possible to ensure sufficient access and an unobstructed view for instrumentation.

operation, open, *n* a procedure in which the surgeon operates with full view of the structures through mucous membrane or cutaneous incisions.

operation, Partsch's, *n.pr* the name applied to a technique of marsupialization.

operation, pedicle flap, *n* a procedure in mucogingival surgery designed to relocate or slide gingival tissue from a donor site in close proximity to an isolated defect, usually a tooth surface denuded of attached gingiva.

operation, Sorrin's, *n.pr* a type of flap approach in the treatment of a periodontal abscess; especially suitable when the marginal gingiva appears well adapted and gives no access to the abscess area. A semilunar incision is made below the involved area in the attached gingiva, leaving the gingival margin undisturbed; a flap is raised, allowing access to the abscessed area for curettage. Suturing follows.

operation system (OS), *n* an integrated set of software modules that provide the framework for orderly assignment of a computer's resources to perform a variety of tasks. It is usually written in the assembler language of the computer.

operative dentistry, *n* the branch of dentistry that deals with the esthetic and functional restoration of the hard tissues of individual teeth.

operatory (op'ərətôrē), *n* the room or rooms in which the dentist performs professional services.

operculectomy (ōpur'kyōōlek'təmē), *n* the surgical removal of the mucosal flap partially or completely covering an unerupted tooth.

operculitis (ōpur'kyōōlī'tis), *n* See pericoronitis.

operculum (ōpur'kyōōləm), *n* flap of tissue over a partially erupted tooth, particularly a third molar in periocoronitis. See also periocoronitis.

operon, *n* a segment of DNA consisting of an operator gene and one or more structural genes with related functions controlled by the operator gene in conjunction with a regulator gene.

ophthalmology, *n* the branch of medicine concerned with the study of the physiology, anatomy, and pathology of the eye and the diagnosis and treatment of disorders of the eye.

ophthalmoscope, *n* a device for examining the interior of the eye. It includes a light, a mirror with a single hole through which the examiner may look, and a dial holding several lenses of varying strengths. The lenses are selected to allow clear visualization of the structures of the eye at any depth.

opiate (ō'pē ət), *n* **1.** a remedy containing or derived from opium. *n* **2.** any drug that induces sleep.

opinion, *n* in the law of evidence, an inference or conclusion drawn by a witness from information known to him or her or assumed.

opioids, abuse of (ō'pē-oidz), *n* a regular use of heroin, codeine, or morphine for reasons other than recognized medical applications.

opisthion (ōpis'thē ôn), *n* the hindmost point on the posterior margin of the foramen magnum.

opisthocranion (ōpis'thōkrā'nē-on), *n* the point in the midline of the cranium that projects farthest backward.

opium, *n* concrete juice of the poppy, *Papaver somniferum.* It contains morphine, codeine, nicotine, narceine, and many other alkaloids.

opportunistic infection, *n* an infection by a microbial organism to which the patient is usually resistant; however, because of reduced vitality or through suppression of the immune system, the patient has become infected.

opsin, *n* a visual pigment protein found in the retinal rods.

optic chiasm, *n* a point near the thalamus and hypothalamus at which portions of each optic nerve cross over.

optic nerve, *n* either of a pair of the second cranial nerves responsible for sight, consisting mainly of coarse, myelinated fibers that arise in the retinal ganglionic layer of the eye, traverse the thalamus, and connect with the visual cortex of the brain.

optics, *n* the science concerned with the properties of light, its refraction and absorption, and the properties of the media of the eye that refract and absorb light.

optimal (op′timəl), *adj* the best or most favorable.

optimism, *n* the tendency to look on the bright or happy side of everything, to believe that there is good in everything.

optometry, *n* the professional discipline devoted to testing the eyes for visual acuity, prescribing corrective lenses, and recommending eye exercises and other health practices to preserve sight.

Orabase, *n* the brand name of a topical dental paste containing an adrenocorticoid. The base consists of gelatin, pectin, mineral oil, and sodium carboxymethylcellulose in a hydrocarbon gel. The adrenocorticoid is hydrocortisone acetate. Orabase is used for temporary relief of symptoms associated with oral inflammation and ulcerative lesions.

oral, *adj* pertaining to the mouth.

oral contraceptives, *n.pl trade names:* Demulen, Loestrin, Lo/Ovral, Nordett; *drug class:* estrogen/progestin combinations; *action:* prevents ovulation by suppressing follicle-stimulating and luteinizing hormones; *uses:* pregnancy prevention, endometriosis, hypermenorrhea, hypogonadism. Also called *estrogens, mestranol androgens, ethinyl estradiol, levonorgestrel.*

oral environment, *n* See environment, oral.

oral evacuator, *n* a suction apparatus used to remove fluids and debris from an operating field. Also called *vacuum.*

oral hairy leukoplakia, *n* a filamentous, white plaque found on the lateral borders of the tongue that can spread across the entire dorsum of the tongue and onto the buccal mucosa. The Epstein-Barr virus has been identified in biopsy specimens of these lesions. An indicator disease for AIDS. See also leukoplakia.

oral health diet score, *n* a motivational aid to good nutrition. Merit points are earned by an adequate intake of foods from the recommended food groups. Demerits are given for frequent intake of foods high in sugars. The difference is the oral health diet score. The technique

is applicable to children with a high incidence of dental caries.

oral health index, *n* a statistical measure that quantifies one or more aspects of a person's or group's oral health status.

oral hygiene, *n* See hygiene, oral.

oral manifestation, *n* the presence of the signs, symptoms, and lesions of a systemic disease in and around the oral cavity.

oral medicine, *n* See medicine, oral.

oral mucosa, *n* See mucosa, oral.

oral physiology, *n* See physiology, oral.

oral self-examination, *n* procedure taught to dental patients in order to look for indications of cancer. The patient monitors the tissues of his or her oral cavity, as well as those of the head and neck, reporting any changes to a qualified dental health care professional.

oral surgery, *n* See surgery, oral.

oral warts, *n.pl* warts caused by human papillomavirus that may be scattered throughout the mouth or localized in one area. They frequently recur. Oral warts are associated with AIDS infection.

orangewood, *n* the wood of choice for the working tips of porte polishers, due to its resistance to splitting and its ability to carry polishing agents. See porte polisher.

Orangewood. (Rosenstiel/Land/Fujimoto, 2001)

orbital (ôr′bitəl), *adj* pertaining to the orbit.

orbital exenteration, *n* the surgical removal of the entire contents of the orbit.

orbital marker, *n* a projecting part of a face-bow that marks the location of the orbitale. Used in the orientation of casts on an articulator in relation to cranial planes.

orbital plane, *n* See plane, orbital.

orbitale (ôr′bital′ē), *n* the lowest point in the margin of the orbit (directly below the pupil when the eye is open and the patient is looking straight ahead) that may readily be felt under the skin. The eye-ear plane passes through the orbitale and tragion.

orders, *n.pl* written or verbal directions of a physician or dentist to a nurse or other assistant detailing the care to be given to a patient.

organ transplantation, *n* the replacement of a diseased organ with a healthy organ from a donor with a compatible tissue type. Organs such as a kidney may be donated by living donors or harvested from brain-dead organ donors.

organelle, *n* any one of various particles of living substance within most cells, which include mitochondria, the Golgi complex, the endoplasmic reticulum, the lysosomes, and the centrioles.

organism(s) (ôr′gənizəm), *n* any organized body of living organisms.

organism(s), Vincent's, *n.pr* the fusospirochetal organisms associated with the initiation of necrotizing ulcerative gingivitis, necrotizing ulcerative stomatitis, or Vincent's angina.

organization, *n* an arrangement of distinct but mutually dependent parts, persons, or tasks to create, enhance, or improve a functioning unit.

organogenesis (ôr′gənōjen′əsis), *n* the formation of organs within an embryo. Organogenesis occurs within the first trimester.

orientation, *n* the ability to correctly place oneself in time, space, and relationship to others and one's work and environment.

orifice (ôr′ifis), *n* the entrance or outlet of any body cavity; any foramen, meatus, or opening.

orlistat (ôr′listat), *n* a prescription drug which produces weight loss by interfering with the body's ability to digest fat. Persons taking this drug may experience up to a 30% reduction in fat absorption.

ornithine, *n* an amino acid, not a constituent of proteins, that is produced as an important intermediate substance in the urea cycle.

ornithine carbamoyltransferase, *n* an enzyme in the blood that increases in patients with liver and other diseases.

oroantral fistula, *n* an abnormal tract that connects the oral cavity with the maxillary sinus.

orodigitofacial dysostosis (OFD syndrome), *n* a syndrome characterized by abnormal development of the jaws and tongue, cleft lip and palate, hypoplasia of bones of the skull with ocular hypertelorism, nasal alar deformity, malformation of digits (frequently manifested as brachydactyly and syndactyly), mental retardation, granular skin, and alopecia of the scalp.

orofacial abnormality, *n* a structural and functional disorder of the mouth and face, usually arising from genetic or congenital defects.

orofacial pain, *n* pain within the structures of the mouth and face, usually of a diffuse pattern.

oronasal, *adj* pertaining to the mouth and nose.

oropharynx (ôr′ōfer′ingks), *n* the portion of the pharynx associated with the mouth; usually described as bounded above by the uvula, below by the epiglottis, in front by the tongue, and behind by the posterior pharyngeal wall.

orosomucoid, *n* a subgroup of the α_1-globulin fraction of the blood.

orphenadrine citrate, *n* *trade names:* Banflex, Flexoject, Norflex, Orflagen; *drug class:* skeletal muscle relaxant, central acting; *action:* acts centrally to depress polysynaptic pathways to relax skeletal muscle, inhibit muscle spasm; *uses:* pain in musculoskeletal conditions.

ortho-, *comb* straight or correct.

orthodontic, *adj* pertaining to the orthopedic correction of abnormal dental relationships, including related abnormalities in facial structures.

orthodontic appliances, *n.pl* See appliance.

orthodontic appliances, functional, *n.pl* See appliances, removable.

orthodontic appliances, removable, *n.pl* See appliances, removable.

orthodontic bracket, *n* See bracket.

orthodontic retainer, *n* See appliance, retaining orthodontic.

orthodontic toothbrush, *n* See bilevel orthodontic toothbrush.

orthodontic wire, *n* See wire.

orthodontics, *n* the area of dentistry concerned with the supervision, guidance, and correction of the growing and mature dentofacial structures. This includes conditions that require movement of the teeth or correction of malrelationships and malformations of related structures by the adjustment of relationships between and among teeth and facial bones by the application of forces or the stimulation and redirection of functional forces within the craniofacial complex. Major responsibilities of orthodontic practice include (1) the diagnosis, prevention, interception, and treatment of all forms of malocclusion of the teeth and associated alterations in their surrounding structures; (2) design, application, and control of functional and corrective appliances; and (3) guidance of the dentition and its supporting structures to attain and maintain optimum occlusal relations in physiologic and esthetic harmony among facial and cranial structures. Also called *dentofacial orthopedics.*

orthodontist, *n* a dental specialist who has completed an approved, advanced course of at least 2 years in the special area of orthodontics.

orthognathic (ôr′thognā′thik), *adj* pertaining to the normal relationships of the jaws.

orthognathic surgery, *n* surgery to alter relationships of dental arches and/or supporting bones, usually accomplished with orthodontic therapy.

orthognathous (ôr′thognāth′us), *adj* pertaining to straight jaws; no projection of the lower part of the face. The facial angle is 85 to 90 degrees.

Orthomyxoviridae **(ôr′thomik′sō-vir′idā),** *n.pl* one of the major RNA virus families, to which the influenza virus belongs. Viruses in this family have a single-stranded, eight-segmented, linear molecular structure with helical symmetry.

orthopantograph (ôr′thōpan′tōgraf), *n* a panoramic radiographic device (Panorex) that permits visualization of the entire dentition, alveolar bone, and other contiguous structures on a single extraoral film.

orthopantomograph (ôr′thōpan′tōmōgraf), *n* a radiographic system (manufactured by Siemens) that uses three axes of rotation to obtain a panoramic radiograph of the dental arches and their associated structures.

orthopedic (ôr′thōpē′dik), *adj* pertaining to the correction of abnormal form or relationship of bone structures. May be accomplished surgically (orthopedic surgery) or by the application of appliances to stimulate changes in the bone structure by natural physiologic response (orthopedic therapy). Orthodontic therapy is orthopedic therapy applied through the teeth.

orthopnea (ôr′thopnē′ə), *n* an inability to breathe except in an upright position.

orthotic, *n* an orthopedic brace used to repair or support a joint or muscle in the body. Also called *orthosis.*

OSAP, *n.pr* Organization for Safety and Asepsis Procedures, a nonprofit organization that consists of dental and healthcare professionals and others interested in promoting infection control and effective health and safety practices. OSAP also supports a research and development foundation.

Osler-Weber disease, *n.pr* See telangiectasia, hereditary hemorrhagic.

osmium (Os), *n* a hard, grayish, pungent-smelling metallic element. Its atomic number is 76 and its atomic weight is 190.2. It is used to produce alloys of extreme hardness and is highly toxic.

osmosis, *n* the passage of pure solvent from the lesser to the greater concentration when two solutions are separated by a membrane that selectively prevents the passage of solute molecules but is permeable to the solvent. The principles of osmosis and the selective permeability of the cell membrane help to regulate the transfer of fluids and metabolites to and from the cells. Thus, they also maintain the stability of the salt/ion concentration in the extracellular and intracellular fluids.

osmotic, *adj* pertaining to osmosis.

osmotic pressure, *n* See pressure, osmotic.

osseointegration (os″ e-o-in″ tə-gra′ shən), *n* **1.** the growth action of bone tissue, as it assimilates surgically implanted devices or prostheses to be used as either replacement parts or anchors. *n* **2.** a specific endosseous dental implant technique involving very slow and precise bone drilling to minimize heat production; the procedure makes use of biocompatible metal and a defined healing environment. Also known as the *Branemark technique.*

ossification (os″ ĭ-fĭ-ka′ shən), *n* the process of creating bone.

ossification, intracartilaginous endochondral, *n* development of bone from cartilage rods, as in the development of arm or leg bones.

ossification, intramembranous, *n* development of bone from tissue or membrane, as in the formation of the skull.

ostectomy (ostek′tōmē), *n* the excision of a bone or portion of a bone.

ostectomy, periodontal, *n* the removal of alveolar bone from around the tooth root to eliminate an adjacent pocket and secure physiologic osseous and gingival form.

osteitis (os′tē ī′tis), *n* an inflammation of the bone; an inflammation of the haversian spaces, canals, and their branches but generally not of the medullary cavity. The disease is characterized by tenderness and a dull, aching pain. Enlargement of the bone may occur. Osteitis of the alveolar process after tooth extraction is commonly referred to as dry socket.

Osteitis. (Regezi/Sciubba/Jordan, 2003)

osteitis, alveolar localized, *n* See socket, dry.

osteitis, condensing, *n* a chronic inflammation associated with some nonvital teeth or located in the site of extraction of such teeth, resulting in abnormally dense bone.

osteitis deformans, *n* **1.** a bone disease of unknown cause, characterized by enlargement of the cranial bones and often of the maxillae or the mandible. On x-rays it is characterized by a cotton-wool appearance. *n* **2.** a localized or generalized bone disease of unknown origin, characterized by the replacement of normal bone with soft, poorly mineralized osteoid tissue. In later stages, affected bone is replaced by densely sclerotic bone. Bony enlargement, deformities, and sometimes fractures occur. *n* **3.** a generalized disease of bone characterized by the concurrent destruction and formation of bone. The etiology is unknown. *n* **4.** a bone disease characterized by thickening and bowing of the long bones and enlargement of the skull and maxillae. It is represented radiographically by a cotton-wool appearance of the bone and microscopically by a mosaic bone pattern. Hypercementosis and loosening of the teeth may be significant manifestations. Also known as *Paget's disease.*

Osteitis deformans. (Regezi/Sciubba/Jordan, 2003)

osteitis fibrosa cystica, generalized, (von Recklinghausen's disease of bone), *n* **1.** a disease caused by parathyroid adenomas and characterized by cystlike radiolucencies in the bones (including the jaws), loosening of teeth, localized swellings, giant cell lesions, increased blood calcium and phosphatase levels, and lowered blood phosphorus levels. The term von Recklinghausen's disease (of skin) is also used as a synonym for neurofibromatosis. *n* **2.** increased resorption and destruction of bone caused by primary and secondary hyperparathyroidism.

osteoarthritis (ostē ō ärthrī′tis), *n* chronic degeneration and destruction of the articular cartilage leading to bony spurs, pain, stiffness, limitation of motion, and change in the size of joints. Considered to result from chronic traumatic injury and wear and tear. Heberden's nodes occur in a special form of the disease. Symptoms may be associated with hormonal, vascular, and/or nutritional disorders. The structural changes of advanced osteoarthritis may involve erosion of the articular cartilages or the subchondral bone. Osteoarthritis rarely affects the temporomandibular joint beyond the "creaking" state.

osteoarthropathy, hypertrophic pulmonary (os′tē ō ärthrop′əthē), *n* a clubbing of the fingers and toes resulting from deposition of calcium in the subperiosteal tissues around the joint. Related to chronic pulmonary disease and occasionally to circulatory and digestive disease.

osteoblast (os′tē ōblast), *n* the cell associated with the growth and development of bone; cuboidal in shape. In active growth, osteoblasts form a continuous layer on old bone like a sheet of epithelial cells; when the bone growth is arrested, the cells assume an elongated appearance like fibroblasts.

osteocalcin, *n* vitamin K-dependent calcium-binding protein synthesized by osteoblasts and found primarily in bone. Serum osteocalcin measurements provide a noninvasive specific marker of bone metabolism.

osteocementum (os′tē ōsēmen′tum), *n* secondary cementum; the hard, bonelike cementum deposited after root formation is completed. See also atrophy of disuse.

osteochondritis, *n* a disease of the epiphyses, or bone-forming centers of the skeleton, beginning with necrosis and fragmentation of the tissue and followed by repair and regeneration.

osteoclasia, traumatic (os′tē ōklā′zhə), *n* See cementoma; fibroma, periapical.

osteoclast (os′tēōklast), *n* **I.** a large, multinucleated giant cell associated with the resorption of bone; the nuclei resemble the nuclei of the osteoblasts and osteocytes; the cytoplasm is often foamy, and the cell frequently has branching processes. Osteoclasts may arise from stromal cells of the bone marrow. They may represent fused osteoblasts or may include fused osteocytes liberated from resorbing bone. They are usually found in close relationship to the resorption of bone and frequently lie in grooves (Howship's lacunae). *n* **2.** a large, multinucleated cell associated with the resorption of bone. Seen in irregular concavities within marginal areas of bone undergoing resorption.

osteoclastoma, *n* See granuloma, giant cell reparative, peripheral.

osteocyte (os′tē ōsīt), *n* an osteoblast that has been surrounded by a calcified interstitial substance; the cells are enclosed within lacunae, and the cytoplasmic processes extend through apertures of the lacunae into canaliculi in the bone. Like the osteoblast, the osteocyte may undergo transformations and assume the form of an osteoclast or reticular cell.

osteocyte osteodystrophy **(os′tē ōdis′trəfē),** *n* a condition marked by defective or deficient bone formation.

osteocyte, renal, *n* a form of dwarfism associated with osteoporosis produced by renal insufficiency during childhood. Periodontal changes include widening of the periodontal membrane space and marked osteoporosis of the mandibular and maxillary bones. Similar to renal rickets. See also rickets, renal.

osteofibroma (os′tē ōfibrō′mə), *n* **I.** a benign neoplasm characterized by bone developing in a connective tissue mass. *n* **2.** a benign neoplasm that develops in the spongiosa of the bone through proliferation of fibroblasts. *n* **3.** a benign neoplasm of the bone characterized by unilateral swelling and fibroblastic and osteoclastic activity in marrow spaces. Also called *calcifying fibroma, ossifying fibroma.* See also dysplasia, fibrous and dysplasia, osseous.

osteogenesis, *n* the origin and development of bone tissue.

osteogenesis imperfecta
(os'tē ōjen'əsis), *n* a congenital disease of unknown cause characterized by fragile, brittle, and easily fractured bones; presumed to stem from a failure in the formation of bone matrix. Variants are often hereditary or familial and include manifestations such as blue sclerae, dentinogenesis imperfecta, and otosclerosis. Also known as *brittle bone disease, fragilitas ossium, Lobstein's disease, osteopsathyrosis idiopathica.*

osteoid (os'tē oid), *n* the mucopolysaccharide-protein complex laid down by the osteoblasts. It is later calcified, with inclusion of osteoblasts as osteocytes within lacunae, into bone.

osteolysis (os'tē ol'əsis), *n* a process of bone resorption whereby the bone salts can be withdrawn by a humoral mechanism and returned to the tissue fluids, leaving behind a decalcified bone matrix. Also called *halisteresis.*

osteoma (os'tē ō'mə), *n* a benign neoplasm of bone or bone tissue.

osteomalacia (os'tē ōməlā'shē, ə, -shə), *n* a systemic disorder of bone characterized by decreased mineralization of bone matrix possibly resulting from vitamin D deficiency, inadequate calcium in the diet, renal disease, and/or steatorrhea. Manifestations include incomplete fractures and gradual resorption of cortical and cancellous bone.

osteomyelitis (os'tē ōmī' əlī'tis), *n* an inflammation of the bone marrow or of the bone, marrow, and endosteum.

Osteomyelitis. (Regezi/Sciubba/Jordan, 2003)

osteon (os'tē on), *n* the three-dimensional reconstruction of concentric lamellae arranged circumferentially about the course of a central blood vessel.

osteonecrosis, *n* the destruction and death of bone tissue. It may stem from ischemia, infection, malignant neoplastic disease, or trauma.

osteonectin, *n* noncollagenous, calcium-binding glycoprotein of developing bone. It links collagen to mineral in the bone matrix.

osteopenia (os'tē-ōpē'n-ə), *n* the deterioration of bone density, decrease of calcification, or insufficient synthesis of uncalcified bone material.

osteopetrosis (ostē ōpetrō'sis), *n* osteosclerosis of unknown origin that obliterates the bone marrow regions, with resultant anemia. Delayed tooth eruption and severe osteomyelitis or necrosis after dental infection may be associated with the disease. Also known as *Albers-Schönberg disease, marble bone.*

Osteopetrosis. (Regezi/Sciubba/Jordan, 2003)

osteoplasty (os'tē ōplastē), *n* a surgical procedure to modify or change the configuration of a bone.

osteoporosis (os'tē ōpôrō'sis), *n* an enlargement of the soft marrow and haversian spaces resulting from a decreased rate of formation of the hard bone matrix. With the exception of immobilized parts, it is a systemic disorder that occurs in advanced age (senile osteoporosis), during ACTH and cortisone therapy, during and after menopause, in limited physical activity, in Cushing's syndrome, during malnutrition, and in other disorders of matrix formation such as hyperadrenalism, hyperthyroidism, vitamin C deficiencies, and excessive use of androgenic steroids. See also atrophy, bone and bone rarefaction.

osteoradionecrosis (os'tē ōrā'dē-ōnekrō'sis), *n* bone necrosis secondary to irradiation and superimposed infection.

Osteoradionecrosis. (Regezı/Sciubba/Jordan, 2003)

osteosarcoma (os'tē ōsärkō'mə), *n* a malignant neoplasm of the bone-forming tissues.

Osteosarcoma. (Regezi/Sciubba/Jordan, 2003)

osteosclerosis (os'tē ōsklərō'sis), *n* an increased bone formation resulting in reduced marrow spaces and increased radiopacity.

osteosynthesis (os'tē-ōsin'thəsis), *n* See osseointegration.

osteosynthesis, miniplate, *n* an internal procedure for repairing fractures to the mandible by using titanium or stainless steel plates and screws to stabilize the bone fragments in proper alignment.

osteotomy (os'tē ot'əmē), *n* the surgical cutting or transection of a bone.

otalgia dentalis (ōtal'jē ə), *n* a reflex pain in the ear resulting from dental disease; usually propagated along the auriculotemporal nerve.

otic ganglion, *n* See ganglion, otic.

otitis, *n* an inflammation or infection of the ear.

otitis externa, *n* an inflammation or infection of the external canal or the auricle of the external ear. Major causes are allergy, bacteria, fungi, viruses, and trauma.

otitis media (ōtī'tis mē'dē ə), *n* an inflammation of the middle ear that may be marked by pain, fever, abnormalities of hearing, deafness, tinnitus, and vertigo. It may originate in the pharynx and be transmitted by the eustachian tubes.

otolaryngologist (o" to-lar" ing-gol' ə-jist), *n* a physician whose practice of medicine focuses on diagnosing and treating diseases of the ears, nose, and throat.

otolaryngology, *n* the branch or specialty of medicine that deals with diseases of the ear, nose, and throat.

otologist (ōtol'əjist), *n* a doctor who specializes in conditions and diseases of the ear.

otology (ōtol'əjē), *n* division of medicine concerning diseases of the ear.

otosclerosis (ō'tōsklərō'sis), *n* a disorder of the middle ear that generally results in hardening and fusion of the ossicles of the ear, with resultant immobilization so that sound waves cannot be conducted along their paths.

otoscope, *n* an instrument used to examine the external ear, the eardrum, and, through the eardrum, the ossicles of the middle ear. It consists of a light, a magnifying lens, and a device for insufflation.

otoscopy, *n* viewing or inspecting the tympanic membrane and other parts of the outer ear with an otoscope.

outline form, *n* See form, outline.

outpatient, *n* a patient, not hospitalized or housed in an extended care facility, who is being treated in an office, clinic, or other ambulatory care facility.

output, *n* the transfer or exit of processed or in-process information from a computer to printers, video terminals, and other peripheral devices.

ovalocytosis (ō'vəlōsītō'sis), *n* See elliptocytosis.

ovariectomy, *n* the surgical removal of one or both ovaries.

ovary, *n* one of the pair of female gonads found on each side of the lower abdomen, beside the uterus, in a fold of the broad ligament.

overbilling, *n* a nondisclosure of waiver of patient copayment.

overbite, *n* a vertical overlapping of upper teeth over lower teeth, usually measured perpendicular to the occlusal plane. See also overjet and overlap, vertical.

overclosure, *n* the raising of the mandible too far before the teeth make contact; loss of occlusal vertical dimension is the cause. See also distance, large interarch.

overcoding, *n* reporting a more complex and/or higher cost procedure than was actually performed.

overcontour, *n* a process in which the normal anatomy of the restored tooth is altered by using too much restorative material. Overcontouring can destroy the natural cleaning processes present in the periodontium.

overdenture, *n* a complete or partial removable denture supported by retained roots that is intended to provide improved support, stability, and tactile and pro- prioceptive sensation and to reduce ridge resorption. See also root retention and root submersion.

overdose (OD), *n* an excessive use of a drug, resulting in adverse reactions ranging from mania or hysteria to coma or death.

overextended, *adj* **1.** the situation occurring when any prosthetic appliance is inadvertently constructed in such a way that part of the oral mucosa is injured by the appliance. *adj* **2.** pertaining to any extrusion beyond the apical opening into the periapical area. May be with instrumentation, medication, or root canal filling.

overfilled, *adj* See overextended.

overhang, *n* an excess filling material projecting beyond cavity margins.

overhead, *n* production costs required to be expended by the dentist to practice the profession (for example, rent, utilities, salaries, laundry). Costs include any involved with management, supplies, equipment, salaries (taxes), and maintenance. Amounts deducted from the gross receipts of a dental practice before the dentist's net income (take-home pay) is received.

overjet, *n* the horizontal projection of upper teeth beyond the lower teeth, usually measured parallel to the occlusal plane. When not otherwise specified, the term is generally assumed to refer to central incisors and is measured from the labial surface of the lower central incisors to the labial surface of the upper central incisors at the level of the upper incisor edge. Unique conditions may sometimes require other measuring techniques. See also overlap, horizontal.

overlap, deep vertical, *n* an excessive vertical overlap of the anterior teeth. Also called *closed bite, deep bite, deep overbite.*

overlap, horizontal, *n* projection of the anterior or posterior teeth of one arch beyond their antagonists in a horizontal direction. Also called *overjet, overjut.*

overlap, vertical, *n* an extension of the upper teeth over the lower teeth in a vertical direction when the opposing posterior teeth are in contact in centric occlusion. This term is used especially to designate the distance that the upper incisal edges drop below the level of the lower ones, but it may also be used to describe the vertical relations of opposing cusps of posterior teeth. Also called *overbite.*

overlay, *n* See onlay.

overlay, computer, *n* a technique for bringing routines into memory from magnetic storage during processing so that several routines will occupy the same storage locations at different times. Overlay techniques are used when the total storage requirements for instructions exceed the available storage in memory.

overshooting accident, *n* the result of seating an endosteal implant beyond its normal host site (through the inferior mandibular border, into the mandibular canal or nasal or antral floor).

ovoid arch, *n* See arch, ovoid.

ovolacto vegetarian diet (ō′vōl-ak′tō), *n* a modified vegetarian diet which prohibits consumption of meat, poultry, and fish, but which permits some animal products such as eggs, milk, and cheese. The diet provides important proteins, but care must be taken to ensure adequate iron intake.

ovum, *n* (*pl* **ova**) a female germ cell containing 23 chromosomes.

owner, *n* the person holding ownership, dominion, or title of property.

ownership, *n* the legal right of possession.

Owren's disease, *n.pr* See parahemophilia.

oxacillin sodium, *n trade names:* Bactocill, Prostaphlin; *drug class:* penicillinase-resistant penicillin; *action:* interferes with cell wall replication of susceptible organisms; the cell wall, rendered osmotically unstable, swells and bursts from osmotic pressure; *uses:* effective for gram-positive cocci, infections caused by penicillinase-producing *Staphylococcus.*

oxalate, *n* any salt of oxalic acid.

oxandrolone, *n trade name:* Oxandrin; *drug class:* androgenic anabolic steroid (Controlled Substance Schedule III); *action:* reverses catabolic tissue processes; promotes build-up of protein; increases erythropoietin production; *uses:* treating catabolic or tissue-wasting processes, such as extensive surgery, burns, infection, or trauma; HIV wasting syndrome; Turner's syndrome.

oxaprozin, *n trade name:* Daypro; *drug class:* nonsteroidal antiinflammatory; *action:* inhibits prostaglandin synthesis by interfering with cyclooxygenase needed for biosynthesis; possesses analgesic, antiinflammatory, antipyretic properties; *uses:* rheumatoid arthritis, osteoarthritis, and ankylosing spondylitis.

oxazepam, *n trade name:* Serax; *drug class:* benzodiazepine (Controlled Substance Schedule IV); *action:* produces central nervous system depression by interacting with a benzodiazepine receptor to facilitate the action of the inhibitory neurotransmitter λ-aminobutyric acid (GABA); *uses:* anxiety, alcohol withdrawal.

oxidant, *n* the substance that is reduced in an oxidation/reduction reaction, thereby oxidizing the other component.

oxidation, *n* the combination of oxygen with other elements to form oxides. The process in which an element gains electrons.

oxidation, beta, *n* a metabolic process in which complex fatty acids are broken down into simple compounds.

oxidation, of metal, *n* the formation of a surface oxide during the casting or soldering of a metal or during subsequent use by the patient.

oxidative, *adj* having the ability or property to oxidize.

oxidative phosphorylation and electron transport, *n* the metabolic process which creates adenosine triphosphate (ATP), the compound needed to store energy in muscles.

oxide, *n* a compound of oxygen with another element or radical such as iron.

oxide divinyl, *n* See ether, divinyl.

oxidized cellulose, *n trade name:* Surgicel; *drug class:* cellulose hemostatic; *action:* mechanism unclear; may act physically to absorb blood and promote an artificial clot; *uses:* hemostasis in surgery, oral surgery, exodontia.

oximetry, *n* the measurement of the oxygen saturation of hemoglobin in a sample of blood with the use of an oximeter.

oxtriphylline, *n trade names:* Choledyl, Choledyl SA; *drug class:* choline salt of theophylline, a bronchodilator; *action:* relaxes smooth muscle of respiratory system by blocking phosphodiesterase; *uses:* acute bronchial asthma, reversible bronchospasm in chronic bronchitis and COPD.

oxybutynin chloride, *n trade name:* Ditropan; *drug class:* antispasmodic; *action:* relaxes smooth muscles in urinary tract; *use:* antispasmodic for neurogenic bladder.

oxycephaly (ok'sesef'ale), *n,* a high conical crown resulting from early closure of sutures and disturbed cranial development. Also called *steeple head.*

oxycodone, *n trade name:* Roxicodone; *drug class:* synthetic opioid analgesic (Controlled Substance Schedule II); *action:* attaches to opiate receptors in the central nervous system; *uses:* moderate-to-severe pain, normally used in combination with aspirin or acetaminophen, the opioid found in Percodan, Percocet, and Tylox.

oxygen (O), *n* a tasteless, odorless, colorless gas essential for human respiration. Its atomic number is 8 and its atomic weight is 15.9994.

oxygen, E-cylinder tank, *n* the gas cylinder size most commonly used in the United States to store oxygen for individual patient delivery; the cylinder is color-coded green for quick recognition as oxygen.

oxygenate (ok′sijēnāt), *v* to saturate with oxygen.

oxyhemoglobin (ok′sēhē′mōglō′bin), *n* a compound of hemoglobin with two atoms of oxygen.

oxymetazoline HCl, *n trade names:* Afrin, Afrin Children's Nose Drops, Dristan Long-Lasting, Neo-Synephrine Nasal Decongestant, Sinarest 12-Hour, Vicks Sinex 12-Hour; *drug class:* nasal decongestant, sympathomimetic amine; *action:* produces vasoconstriction of arterioles, thereby decreasing fluid exudation and mucosal engorgement; *use:* nasal congestion.

oxymetholone, *n trade name:* Anadrol-50; *drug class:* androgenic anabolic steroid (Controlled Substance Schedule III); *action:* reverses catabolic tissue processes; promotes build-up of protein, increased erythropoietin production; *uses:* anemia associated with bone marrow failure and red cell production deficiencies, aplastic anemia, myelofibrosis, and anemia caused by myelotoxic drugs.

oxytetracycline, *n* a tetracycline antibiotic prescribed in the treatment of bacterial and rickettsial infections.

oxytocin (ok′sētō′sin), *n* a hormone of the posterior pituitary gland that is the principal uterus-contracting hormone. Used in obstetrics to induce uterine contractions.

PA skull, *n* See *examination, radiographic; examination, extraoral;* and *examination, posteroanterior.*

PAB, PABA, *n* an abbreviation for **paraaminobenzoic acid.**

PAC, *n* See *aspirin, phenacetin, caffeine.*

pacemaker, *n* an electrical device used to maintain a normal sinus rhythm in heart muscle contraction. Pacemakers can be permanent in-

dwelling appliances. The use of electronic devices on patients with pacemakers is now considered permissible because of modern shields. Also called *cardiac pacemaker.*

pachymucosa alba (pak′i-myōō-kō′sə al′bə), *n* an appearance of the buccal mucosa that has a white surface and resembles elephant hide.

Pacini's corpuscle (pä-chē′nēz), *n.pr* See *corpuscle, Pacini's.*

pack, *n* a material used to protect tissue, fill space, or prevent hemorrhage.

pack, periodontal, n a surgical dressing applied to the necks of teeth and the adjacent tissue to cover and protect the surgical wound.

packing, *n* the act of filling a mold.

paclitaxel, *n trade name:* Taxol; *drug class:* antineoplastic; *action:* obtained from Western Yew tree, unique action inhibits microtubule network reorganization essential for cell division; *use:* metastatic ovarian cancer.

pad, Passavant's (pas′ə-vänts), *n.pr* (Passavant's bar, Passavant's ridge), the bulging "transverse roll" of the posterior pharyngeal wall produced by the upper portion of the superior pharyngeal constrictor muscle during the act of swallowing or during vocal effort; an objectionable term. See also *pharynx, activities of posterior and lateral pharyngeal wall.*

pad, retromolar, *n* a mass of soft tissue, frequently pear shaped, which is located at the distal termination of the mandibular residual ridge. It is made up of fibers of the buccinator muscle, the pterygomandibular raphe, the superior constrictor muscle, the temporal tendon, and the mucous glands.

pad, rubber dam, (rubber dam mask), *n* an absorbent piece of flannelette, bird's-eye, or gauze of suitable shape to interpose between a rubber dam and the face to protect the face from contact with both the rubber and the clips of the dam holder.

Paget's disease (paj′əts), *n.pr* See *osteitis deformans.*

pain, *n* an unpleasant sensation created by a noxious stimulus mediated along specific nerve pathways to the central nervous system, where it is interpreted as such. The sensation of pain is a protective mechanism that warns of danger without giving too much information about the specific nature of the danger. It initiates nociceptive reflexes.

pain and suffering, *n* an element in a claim for damages in a liability lawsuit. It requests compensation to an individual for mental and physical pain and discomfort as a result of an injury.

pain, assessment, *n* an evaluation of the reported pain and the factors that alleviate or exacerbate a patient's pain; used as an aid in the diagnosis and the treatment of disease and trauma.

pain, chest, *n* pain that occurs in the chest region because of disorders of the heart (e.g., angina pectoris, myocardial infarction, or pericarditis), pulmonary artery (pulmonary embolism or hypertension), lungs (pleuritis), esophagus ("heartburn"), abdominal organs (aerophagia, biliary tract disease, splenic infarction, or gaseous distention in the splenic flexure), or the chest wall (neoplasia, costochondral strains, trauma, hyperventilation, or muscular tension).

pain, clinic, *n* a multidisciplinary association of healthcare professionals devoted to the diagnosis and treatment of patients with acute and chronic pain.

pain, deep, *n* dull, aching, or boring pain originating in muscles, tendons, and joints. It is poorly localized and tends to radiate.

pain dysfunction syndrome, *n* a phrase used in dentistry to describe a condition in patients who appear to have a psychophysiologic basis for stress overload on the temporomandibular joint. The preferred term is *mandibular stress syndrome.*

pain, ghost, *n* see *odontalgia, phantom.*

pain, mechanism, *n* the network that communicates unpleasant sensations and the perceptions of noxious stimuli throughout the body in association with both physical disease and trauma involving tissue damage.

pain, nerve ending, *n* a receptor nerve ending that is relatively primitive and ends in an undifferentiated arborization. The nerve ending for the sensation of pain is a protective

mechanism that warns of danger without giving too much information about the specific nature of the danger. The danger stimuli give rise to nociceptive reflexes, or defensive, protective, or withdrawal movements. The nociceptive reflexes supersede other, less urgent, reflexes that are thus inhibited.

pain, projected pathologic, *n* pain erroneously perceived to arise in a peripheral region because of a stimulus from end-organs supplying the region (e.g., sciatic pain). Actually the stimulus occurred somewhere along the pain pathway from the nerve to the cortex.

pain, reaction, *n* the individual's manifestation of the unpleasant sensation.

pain, referred, *n* pain caused by an agent in one area but manifested in another (e.g., pain caused by caries in the maxillary third molar may be referred to the mandible, so the source of pain appears to be in the mandible).

pain, tactile stimuli, *n* any of a number of physical sources that may aggravate dentin hypersensitivity, such as dental instruments, toothbrush bristles, ill-fitting oral prostheses, and various personal oral habits a patient may have.

pain, thermal stimuli, *n* dentin hypersensitivity related to abrupt changes in temperature of teeth as a result of contact with very cold or very hot foods and liquids, rapid intake of air through the mouth, and during professional oral hygiene procedures requiring rapid drying of teeth.

pain threshold, *n* the point at which a stimulus causes pain. The threshold varies widely among individuals.

pair, ion, *n* See *ion.*

palatability (pal′ət-ə-bil′i-tē), *n* the quality of a food that makes it acceptable or agreeable to one's personal taste.

palatal (pal′ət-əl), *adj* relating to the palate.

palatal bar, *n* See *bar, palatal.*

palatal perforation, *n* See *perforation, palatal.*

palatal plate, *n* See *connector, major.*

palatal rugae, *n.pl* See *rugae.*

palatal seal, n See *seal, posterior palatal.*

palatal shelves, n.pl outgrowths of the embryonic upper jaw that come together during prenatal development to form the secondary palate.

palate (pal′ət), n the bone and soft tissue that closes the space encompassed by the upper alveolar arch, extending posteriorly to the pharynx. The palate forms the "roof" of the mouth and connects to the nasal septum and floor of the nose in the midline.

palate, acquired cleft, n a noncongenital defect of soft or hard tissues of the hard and soft palate.

palate, cleft, n a cleft in the palate between the two palatal processes. It can vary in involvement and can be associated with cleft lip. If both hard and soft palates are involved, it is a *uranostaphyloschisis;* if only the soft palate is divided, it is a *uranoschisis.* The term *cleft palate* is often erroneously applied to clefts between the median nasal and maxillary processes through the alveolus. The proper term for this type of cleft is *cleft jaw,* or *gnathoschisis.*

Cleft palate. (Neville/Damm/Allen/Bouquot, 2002)

palate, congenital cleft, n a congenital nonunion or inadequacy of soft and hard tissues related to the lip, nose, alveolar process, hard palate, and velum. The extent of these deformities varies among individuals. Varieties of classifications are available to identify the extent of the cleft.

palate, hard, n the anterior part of the palate, which is supported by and includes the palatal extensions of the maxillary and palatine bones.

palate, primary, n the shelf separating the oral and nasal cavities that is formed during early embryonic development from protrusions of tissue between the olfactory pits. It is also called *primitive palate.*

palate, secondary, n the final palate that is formed during embryonic development when projections from the nasal prominences come together to create portions of the upper jaw.

palate, soft, n the part of the palate lying posterior to the hard palate, composed of only soft tissues without underlying bony support.

palate, soft, redivision, n the surgical incision or removal of a V-shaped area of tissue from the soft palate to facilitate the proper placement of the pharyngeal section of a prosthetic speech aid.

palate splitting appliance, n an orthodontic appliance cemented to buccal teeth on either side, incorporating a jackscrew that is progressively extended to accomplish forceful separation of the two lateral halves of the bony palate. Similar corrections also are accomplished with removable split-palate appliances.

palatine arch (pal′ə-tin), n See *arch, palatine.*

palatine mucosa, n See *mucosa, palatine.*

palatine suture, median, n See *suture, intermaxillary.*

palato- (pal′ə-tō), comb a prefix meaning "pertaining to the palate."

palatoplasty (pal′ə-tō-plas-tē), n the surgical repair of palatal defects.

palatorrhaphy (pal′ə-tôr′ə-fē), n the surgical closure of a cleft palate using suturing.

palladium (Pd), n a hard, silvery metallic element that is highly resistant to tarnish and corrosion. Its atomic number is 46 and its atomic weight is 106.42. Palladium is used in high-grade surgical instruments and in dental inlays, bridgework, and orthodontic appliances.

palliate (pal′ē-āt), v to reduce the severity of.

palliative (pal′ē-ə-tiv), n an alleviating measure.

pallidotomy (pal′i-dot′ə-mē), n an operation in which the globus pallidus of the basal ganglia is removed to prevent the symptoms of parkinsonism.

pallor (pal′ər), n paleness; absence of skin coloration.

pallor, perioral, n paleness of soft tissues surrounding the mouth; an indication of impending syncope.

palm grasp, n See *grasp, palm-and-thumb.*

Palm grasp. (Daniel/Harfst, 2002)

Palmer's tooth notation, *n.pr* a system for designating teeth by number and quadrant. The mouth is divided into quadrants and each tooth is designated by an Arabic numeral 1 to 8, starting with the central incisor in each quadrant and continuing posteriorly to the third molar. The quadrant is indicated by a right angle symbol oriented right or left and up or down. The system was popular in the 1950s but is no longer in general use except in orthodontic practices.

palpate (pal′pāt), v to examine the soft tissues with the fingers or hands.

palpation (pal-pā′shən), n **1.** the act of feeling with the hands or fingers. n **2.** a phase of the examination procedure in which the sense of touch is used to gather data essential for diagnosis.

palpation, bilateral, n a method of examination in which both hands are used to simultaneously examine and compare symmetrical body structures on opposite sides of the body.

palpitation (pal-pi-tā′shən), n unduly rapid action of the heart that is perceptible to the patient.

palsy (pôl′zē), n a general term for *paralysis* but preferred by some to refer to certain types of paralysis.

palsy, Bell's, n.pr facial paralysis believed to result from inflammation in or around the facial nerve. One side of the face sags, the corner of the mouth droops, the eyelid does not close, and saliva dribbles from the corner of the mouth on the affected side. See also *paralysis, facial.*

Bell's palsy. (Neville/Damm/Allen/Bouquot, 2002, courtesy Dr. Bruce Brehm)

palsy, cerebral, n **1.** collective term for neurologic defects with associated disturbances of motor function. The disturbances vary in cause and anatomic type (e.g., acquired, hereditary, natal, postnatal, congenital palsy). n **2.** nonspecific term representing a group of pathologic conditions having the following common, related characteristics: agenesis, or a lesion of nervous tissue within the cranium; interference with voluntary muscular movements; disabling disorders of a chronic nature, neither acute nor progressive; and occurrence of the original lesion at the date of birth of the patient or before the development of learned human muscular function. **3.** a condition caused by damage to the motor centers of the brain, resulting in varying disturbances of motor function and often accompanied by mental subnormality.

palsy, creeping, n See *gait, spastic.*

palsy, facial, n paralysis of the muscles supplied by the seventh cranial nerve. It may be associated with peripheral lesions, neoplasms invading the temporal bone, acoustic neuromas, pontine disease, and herpes zoster involving the geniculate ganglion. Bilateral paralysis may occur in uveoparotid fever and polyneuritis.

palsy, lead, *n* weakness and paralysis of the hand, wrist, and fingers, associated with lead poisoning.

pancreatin, *n* a concentrate of pancreatic enzymes from swine or beef cattle.

pancreatitis, *n* inflammation of the pancreas that may be acute or chronic, characterized by severe abdominal pain radiating to the back, fever, anorexia, nausea, and vomiting.

pancrelipase, *n trade names:* Cotazym, Enzymase, Ilozyme, Protilase, Ultrase MT, Viokase, Zymase, others; *drug class:* digestant; *action:* pancreatic enzyme needed for proper pancreatic secretion insufficiency; *uses:* cystic fibrosis (digestive aid), steatorrhea, pancreatic enzyme deficiency.

pancuronium bromide, *n* a skeletal muscle relaxant prescribed as an adjunct to anesthesia and mechanical ventilation.

pandemic (pan-dem′ik), *adj* describing an epidemic covering a widespread area such as a country or continent. It can describe a global epidemic.

panel, open, *n* a group dental plan characterized by three features: any licensed dentist may elect to participate, the beneficiary may choose from among all licensed dentists, and the dentist may accept or refuse any beneficiary.

pangamic acid, *n* substance that is a derivative of apricot pits and contains some potentially toxic substances. No evidence that this substance is a vitamin exists. Also called *vitamin B₁₅*.

panhypopituitarism (pan-hī′pō-pi-tōō′i-tə-riz′əm), *n* a deficiency involving all the hormonal functions of the pituitary gland. See also *disease, Simmonds'*.

panic attack, *n* an episode of acute anxiety that occurs unpredictably with feelings of intense apprehension or terror, accompanied by dyspnea, dizziness, sweating, trembling, and chest pain or palpitations. The attack may last several minutes and may occur again in certain conditions.

panic disorder, *n* See *panic attack*.

panneuritis endemica (pan′nyōō-rī′tis en-dem′ik-ə), *n* See *beriberi*.

panoral, *adj* literally, "all of the oral region," a term used in diagnostic oral radiography to describe a technique that includes all of the oral structures on one film.

panoramic radiograph, *n* a tomogram of the jaws, taken with a specialized machine designed to present a panoramic view of the full circumferential length of the jaws on a single film. Also known by several trade names of machines, most of which incorporate *pan* into the name.

Panoramix, *n.pr* a radiographic system in which the source of radiation is placed inside the mouth to expose a large film placed extraorally around the face.

Panorex, *n.pr* a radiographic system (manufactured by S.S. White Co.) that uses two axes of rotation to obtain a panoramic radiograph of the dental arches and associated structures. See also *pantomography*.

pansinusitis (pan′sīn-u-sī′tis), *n* inflammation of all the sinuses, as of the facial bones.

pantograph (pan′tō-graf), *n* a figurative term given to a pair of facebows fixed to both jaws and designed to inscribe centrically related points and then arcs leading to these points on segments of planes relatable to the three craniofacial planes of space. The maxillary planes are attached to the maxillary bow, and the inscribing styluses are attached to the mandibular bow.

pantomography (pan-tə-mog′rə-fē), *n* panoramic radiography for obtaining radiographs of the maxillary and mandibular dental arches and their associated structures.

pantothenic acid (pan-tə-thēn′-ik), *n* fatty acids. See also *acid, pantothenic*.

papain, *n* an enzyme from papaya, a tropical fruit; used for enzymatic debridement of wounds and for promotion of healing.

papaverine HCl, *n trade names:* Cerespan, Genabid, Pavabid, Pavacot, Pavagen, Pavased, others; *drug class:*

peripheral vasodilator; *action:* relaxes all smooth muscle, inhibits cyclic nucleotide phosphodiesterase, which increases intracellular cAMP, causing vasodilation; *uses:* arterial spasm resulting in cerebral and peripheral ischemia; myocardial ischemia associated with vascular spasms or dysrhythmias, angina pectoris, peripheral and pulmonary embolism; visceral spasm, as in ureteral, biliary, gastrointestinal colic.

paper, articulating, *n* paper strips coated with ink or dye-containing wax, used for marking or locating occlusal interferences or deflecting occlusal contacts prior to making occlusal contacts. See also *articulating paper.*

paper point, *n* a cone of absorbent paper designed to be inserted into the length of the root canal and used to absorb fluid, carry medication into the canal, or inoculate cultures.

papilla(e) (pəp-il′ə), *n* any small, nipple-shaped elevation.

Filliform papillae

Fungiform lingual papillae

Papillae. (Bird/Robinson, 2002)

papilla, incisive, *n* the elevation of soft tissue covering the foramen of the incisive or nasopalatine canal.

papilla, interdental, *n* the part of the gingivae filling the interproximal spaces between adjacent teeth, consisting of both free and attached gingivae.

papilla, interproximal, *n* the cone-shaped projection of the gingiva filling the interdental spaces up to the contact areas when viewed from the labial, buccal, and lingual aspects. When viewed buccolingually or la-

biolingually, the crest of the interproximal papilla appears as a rounded concavity at an area below the contact point of the teeth. If recession has occurred, this concavity may become an area of pathology, and the entire papilla may require reshaping to restore health. See also *papilla, interdental.*

papillae, circumvallate (sur′kum val′āt), *n.pl* large mushroom-shaped lingual papillae that line up along the anterior side of the sulcus terminalis forming a V-shape on the tongue. This structure contains taste buds. Formerly called *vallate papillae.*

papillae, filiform (fil′i-fôrm), *n.pl* slender and thread-like protrusions that give the dorsal surface of the tongue its velvety texture and that cover the entire dorsal surface of the tongue. They are interspersed with fungiform papillae on the tongue apex and lateral surfaces.

papillae, foliate (fō′lē-āt), *n.pl* vertical ridges of lingual papillae on the lateral surface of the tongue that contain taste buds.

papillae, fungiform (fun′ji-fôrm), *n* small, mushroom-shaped dots on the dorsal surface of the tongue. They contain taste buds.

papillae, parotid, *n.pl* tiny tissue projections located inside the mouth near the maxillary second molar that protect the parotid duct.

papillae, vallate (val′āt), *n.pl* See *papillae, circumvallate.*

papillary, *adj* similar to a little, nipple-shaped elevation or projection.

papillary adenoma (pap′əl-er-ē), *n* a benign epithelial tumor in which the membrane lining the glandular tissue forms papillary processes that project into the alveoli or grow out of the surface of a cavity.

papillary-marginal-attached, *n* See *PMA.*

papilledema (pap′il-ə-dē′mə), *n* swelling of the optic disc caused by increased intracranial pressure.

papilloma (pap′il-ō′mə), *n* **1.** a benign neoplasm of epithelium, often having a warty appearance. *n* **2.** a benign, exophytic, pedunculated, cauliflower-like neoplasm of epithelium.

Oral papilloma. (Neville/Damm/Allen/
Bouquot, 2002)

papilloma, basal cell, *n* See *keratosis, seborrheic.*

**papillomatosis,   inflammatory
(pap′il-ō-mə-tō′sis),** *n* See *hyperplasia, papillary, inflammatory.*

papillomatosis, multiple, *n* See *hyperplasia, papillary, inflammatory.*

papillomaviruses, *n. pl* viruses that
cause infection of the hair, skin, and
nails known as warts, including oral
warts.

**Papillon-Lefèvre syndrome (pap′i-
yōn lə-fev′),** *n.pr* See *syndrome,
Papillon-Lefèvre.*

papoose board, *n* a board used to
stabilize the position of a pediatric
patient, or a patient with limited
psychomotor control. It comes in
various sizes and has soft flaps that
surround and hold the patient.

Papoose board. (Bird/Robinson, 2002)

Papovaviridae **(pap′ə-və-vir′i-dā),**
n.pl one of the major deoxyribonucleic acid virus families to which the
papillomavirus and polyomavirus belong. Viruses in this family have a
double-stranded, supercoiled, circular
molecular structure with icosahedral
symmetry.

papule (pap′yōōl), *n* a small, circumscribed, solid elevated lesion.
papule, split, *n* a secondary lesion of
syphilis seen at the angle of the lips,
resulting from the formation of a
papule that becomes fissured because
of its position.

paradigm (par″ ə-dīm), *n* a model
or pattern. The set of values or
concepts that represent an accepted
way of doing things within an organization or community.
paradigm shift, *n* an adjustment in
thinking that comes about as the
result of new discoveries, inventions,
or real-world experiences.

paradontosis   (per′ə-don-tō′sis), *n*
See *periodontosis.*

paraffin, *n* any of a group of hydrocarbons or hydrocarbon mixtures of
the paraffin series as indicated by the
formula $C_{11}H_{(2n+2)}$. Examples include
methane gas, kerosene, and paraffin
wax.

paraffin bath, *n* the application of
heat to a specific area of the body
through the use of paraffin wax. The
area is quickly immersed in heated
liquid wax and then withdrawn so
that the wax solidifies to form an
insulating layer. The procedure is
repeated until the layer is 5 to 10 mm
thick, and then the entire area is
wrapped in an insulating fabric. The
technique is used primarily for patients with arthritis and rheumatism
or any joint condition.

paraffin method, *n* a method used
in preparing a selected portion of
tissue for pathologic examination.
The tissue is fixed, dehydrated, and
infiltrated by and embedded in paraffin wax, forming a block that is cut
with a microtome into slices 8 mm
thick.

parafunction, *n* movements (e.g.,
bruxism, clenching, and rocking of
teeth) that are considered outside or
beyond function and that result in
worn facets.

**parahemophilia   (per′ə-hē′mō-
fil′ē-ə),** *n* (Ac globulin deficiency,
Owren's disease), a hemorrhagic disorder resulting from a deficiency of
proaccelerin. Manifestations include
mild to severe bleeding after extraction of teeth or other surgical
procedures, epistaxis, easy bruising,

monorrhagia, and hematomas. The one-stage prothrombin time is prolonged, but the bleeding time is ordinarily normal.

parainfluenza virus, *n* a myxovirus with four serotypes, causing respiratory infections in infants and young children and, less commonly, in adults.

parakeratosis (per′ə-ker-ə-tō′sis), *n* persistence of nuclei in the stratum corneum of stratified squamous epithelium.

paralgesia (per′əl-jē′zē-ə), *n* **1.** any condition marked by abnormal and painful sensations. *n* **2.** a painful paresthesia.

parallax (per′ə-laks), *n* the apparent change in position of an object when viewed from two different positions. The phenomenon is useful in determining the relative position of an object in a radiograph. Two or more radiographs are made from slightly different positions and the direction and amount of shift of the object is observed and measured.

parallel attachment, *n* See *attachment, parallel.*

parallelism, *n* the condition of two or more surfaces that, if extended to infinity, could never meet. In removable partial prosthodontics, such a condition is created on vertical tooth surfaces to act as guiding planes.

parallelometer (per′ə-lel-om′ə-tur), *n* an apparatus used to determine parallelism or a lack of parallelism or to make some part or an object parallel with some other part or object. See also *surveyor.*

paralysis (pər-al′i-sis), *n* **1.** cessation of cell function. *n* **2.** loss or impairment of the motor control or function of a part or region.

paralysis, diplegia (dīp-lē′jē-ə), *n* a loss of motor function in matching body parts (e.g., legs) on each side.

paralysis, facial, *n* paralysis of the muscles of facial expression resulting from supranuclear, nuclear, or peripheral nerve disease. With a mild case, when the face is at rest, the disorder is not readily observed.

However, during muscular contraction (e.g., wrinkling the forehead, blinking the eyes, pursing the lips, speaking), the disorder is very noticeable. Only one lid may close, and the asymmetry of the mouth is pronounced because the normal buccinator muscle contracts and is unopposed by the weakness on the paralyzed side. This imbalance produces a significant asymmetry. The affected side remains smooth, and the normal side shows contraction. See also *palsy, Bell's.*

paralysis, infantile, *n* See *poliomyelitis.*

paralysis, motor, *n* a loss of the power of skeletal muscle contraction, resulting from interruption of some part of the pathway from the cerebrum to the muscle.

paralysis, transient, *n* the sudden loss of sensation or ability to move on one side or a single part of the body, which lasts briefly and may or may not recur and is often a symptom of cerebrovascular insufficiency or other underlying serious condition.

paralysis, transient facial, *n* temporary unilateral loss of facial muscle function as a result of inadvertently injecting the parotid gland containing the facial nerve during the inferior nerve block.

parameter (pər-am′ə-tur), *n* values that refer to a population; characteristics of a population. Because a parameter is a value of a hypothetical, infinite, unknown population, it is always an estimate.

Paramyxoviridae (per′ə-mik′sō-vir′i-dā), *n* one of the major ribonucleic acid virus families, to which the measles, mumps, parainfluenza, and respiratory syncytial viruses belong. Viruses in this family have a single-stranded, nonsegmented, linear molecular structure with helical symmetry.

paranasal sinuses, *n.pl* the air cavities in various bones around the nose, such as the frontal sinus in the frontal bone and the maxillary sinus within the maxilla.

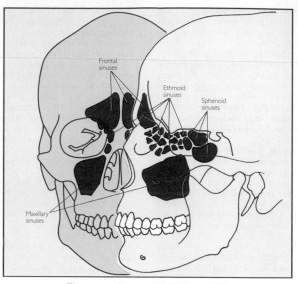

The paranasal sinuses. (Bird/Robinson, 2002)

paranesthesia (per′an-es-thē′zē ə, -zhə), *n* anesthesia of the lower part of the body and limbs.

paranoia (per′ə-noi′ə), *n* **1.** psychosis characterized by delusions and hallucinations that are well systematized. **2.** the irrational belief that one is the object of special persecution by others or by fate.

paraphilia (pər′ə-fil′ē-ə), *n* a condition in which a person derives pleasure from bizarre sexual fetishes.

paraplegia, *n* paralysis characterized by motor or sensory loss in the lower limbs and trunk. Approximately 11,000 spinal cord injuries reported each year in the United States involve paraplegia. Such events occur as a result of automobile and motorcycle accidents, sporting accidents, falls, and gunshot wounds.

parapsoriasis, *n* a group of chronic skin diseases resembling psoriasis, characterized by maculopapular, erythematous, scaly eruptions without systemic symptoms. Parapsoriasis is resistant to all treatment.

parasite, *n* an organism living in or on and obtaining nourishment from another organism.

parasympathetic (par″ə-sim″pə-thet′ ik), *adj* pertaining to the part of the autonomic nervous system that controls craniosacral activity.

parasympatholytic (per′ə-sim′pa-thō-lit′ik), *adj* See *anticholinergic.*

parasympathomimetic (per′ə-sim′pə-thō′mi-met′ik), *adj* See *cholinergic.*

Para-thor-mone (per′ə-thôr′mōn), *n.pr* trade name for parathyroid hormone.

Parathyrin (per′ə-thī′rin), *n.pr* trade name for parathyroid hormone.

parathyroidectomy, *n* the surgical removal of the parathyroid gland.

parenteral (pər-en′tər-əl), *adj* literally, "aside from the gastrointestinal tract"; not through the alimentary canal (i.e., by subcutaneous, intramuscular, intravenous, or other nongastrointestinal route of administration).

parenteral nutrition, *n* the administration of nutrients by a route other than the alimentary canal, such as subcutaneously, intravenously, intramuscularly, or intradermally. The parenteral fluid usually consists of physiologic saline with glucose, amino acids, electrolytes, vitamins, and medications, which are not nutritionally complete but maintain fluid and electrolyte balance.

paresis (pər-ī′sis), *n* a progressive psychosis associated with neurosyphilis.

paresthesia (per′es-thē′zē-ə, -zhə), *n* an altered sensation reported by the patient in an area where the sensory nerve has been afflicted by a disease or an injury. The patient may report burning, prickling, formication, or other sensations.

paresthesia, oral, n a numbness or tingling that occurs in the mucosa or tissues of the oral cavity. It may be caused by a deficiency in vitamin B_{12} (cobalamine), trauma from surgery, or local anesthesia.

parietal bone, *n* one of a pair of bones forming the sides of the cranium. Each parietal bone articulates with five bones: the opposite parietal, occipital, frontal, temporal, and sphenoid.

parity, *n* the use of a set of items, either even or odd in number, as a means for checking computer errors, such as in the transmission of information between various elements of the same computer.

parkinsonism, *n* an array of symptoms including stiffness, slow or restricted body movements, tremor, or postural problems. It has many causes, including Parkinson's disease.

paronychia, *n* an infection of the fold of skin at the margin of a fingernail or toenail.

parotid gland (pər-ot′ld), *n* one of the largest pairs of salivary glands that lie at the side of the face just below and in front of the external ear along the posterior border of the ramus of the mandible.

parotitis (per′ə-tī′tis), *n* inflammation of the parotid gland. See also *mumps.*

parotitis, endemic, n an acute viral infection characterized by unilateral or bilateral swelling of the salivary glands, especially the parotid.

parotitis, epidemic, n See *parotitis, endemic.*

parotitis, infectious, n See *parotitis, endemic.*

paroxetine, *n trade name:* Paxil; *drug class:* antidepressant; *action:* selectively inhibits the uptake of serotonin in the brain; *use:* depression.

paroxysm (per′ək-siz-əm), *n* **I.** an abrupt increase or repeated occurrence of symptoms. *n* **2.** a sudden violent attack, contraction of muscles, or convulsion.

paroxysmal (per′ək-siz′məl), *adj* recurring in paroxysms.

partial anodontia, *n* the condition of having only a few teeth. Also called *oligodontia.*

partial denture retention, *n* See *retention, partial denture.*

partial thromboplastin time (PTT), *n* a test for detecting coagulation defects of the intrinsic system by adding activated partial thromboplastin to a sample of test plasma and to a control sample of normal plasma. The time required for the formation of a clot is compared with the normal plasma. It is also used to monitor the activity of heparin in patients who are being treated for a variety of cardiovascular disorders.

participating dentist, *n* any dentist who has a contractual agreement with a dental benefits organization to render care to eligible persons.

particle, *n* a small amount of material.

particle, alpha, n (alpha ray, alpha radiation) positively charged particulate ionizing radiation consisting of helium nuclei (two protons and two neutrons) traveling at high speeds. These rays are emitted from the nucleus of an unstable element.

particle, beta, n (beta ray, beta radiation) particulate ionizing radiation consisting of either negative electrons (negatrons) or positive electrons (positrons) emitted from the nucleus of an unstable element. This phenomenon is called *beta decay.*

particulate bone grafts *n.pl* a type of autogenous bone graft that consists of small particles of cortical and cancellous bone and hematopoietic and mesenchymal marrow.

parties, *n.pl* the persons who take part in the performance of any act, who have a direct interest in any contract or conveyance, or who are actively involved in the prosecution and defense of any legal proceeding.

partnership, *n* **I.** The association of two or more persons for the purpose of carrying on business (or practice) together and dividing its profits. *n* **2.** a legal, binding contract defining the association of two or more persons in a business or professional relationship such as a dental practice.

partnership, notice of dissolution of intelligence, *n* by any of a variety of means, notice to creditors and the public that a partnership has been dissolved.

Partsch's operation, *n.pr* See *operation, Partsch's.*

parturition (pär′chōō-rish′ən), *n* the action or process of giving birth.

parulis (pər-yōō′lis), *n* an elevated nodule at the site of a fistula draining a chronic periapical abscess. These nodules occur most frequently in relation to pulpally involved deciduous teeth.

Parulis. (Neville/Damm/Allen/Bouquot, 2002)

Parvoviridae (pär′vō-vir′idā), *n* one of the major deoxyribonucleic acid virus families to which the B₁₉ virus belongs. Viruses in this family have a single-stranded linear molecular structure with icosahedral symmetry.

Passavant's bar, *n.pr* See *pad, Passavant's.*

Passavant's pad, *n.pr* See *pad, Passavant's.*

Passavant's ridge, *n.pr* See *pad, Passavant's.*

passer, foil, *n* See *foil passer.*

passive, *n* referring to an orthodontic appliance that has been adjusted to apply no effective tooth-moving force to the teeth.

passive diffusion, *n* an absorption process that occurs in the body when carbohydrates are more highly concentrated in the intestine than in the blood.

passive immunity, *n* a form of acquired immunity resulting from antibodies that are transmitted naturally through the placenta to a fetus or through the colostrum to an infant or

artificially by injection of antiserum for treatment or prophylaxis. Passive immunity is not permanent and does not last as long as active immunity.

passive reciprocation, *n* See *reciprocation, passive.*

passive smoking, *n* the inhalation by nonsmokers of the smoke from other people's cigarettes, pipes, and cigars.

passive-aggressive behavior, *n* behavior that reflects hostility or resentment through indirect nonviolent means, such as procrastination, inefficiency, forgetfulness, and stubbornness.

passive-dependent personality, *n* a personality characterized by helplessness, indecisiveness, and a tendency to cling to and seek support from others.

passivity, *n* the quality or condition of inactivity or rest assumed by the teeth, tissues, and denture when a removable denture is in place but is not under masticatory pressure.

paste, *n* a soft, smooth, semifluid mixture, often medicated.

paste, filler, *n* a semisoft mixture of materials used to fill the root canal system, unlike solid filling material such as silver or gutta-percha cones.

paste, pressure-indicating, *n* a soft mixture used to disclose areas of contact or pressure in restorations.

paste, prophylactic, *n* a substance comprising several abrasive compounds and fluoride, which cleans and polishes the teeth.

Pasteurella, *n* a genus of gram-negative bacilli or coccobacilli, including species pathogenic to humans and domestic animals. *Pasteurella* infections may be transmitted to humans by animal bites.

patch, *n* mucus, multiple gray-white patch overlying an area of ulceration and occurring on the oral mucosa as an expression of secondary syphilis; highly infectious. See also *syphilis.*

patch test, *n* a skin test for identifying allergens, especially those causing contact dermatitis.

patent, *adj* open and unblocked, such as a *patent airway.*

patent ductus arteriosus (ahr-tēr′ e-o-sis), *n* a congenital heart defect in which the passage between the aorta and the pulmonary artery is open, allowing blood to pool back into the lungs, causing the heart to work harder than necessary.

patent medicine, *n* a nonprescription drug available to the general public; usually referred to as an *over-the-counter medicine.*

paternity test, *n* a test based on genetic blood groups and used mainly to exclude the possibility that a particular man could be the father of a specific child.

path, *n* a certain course that is usually followed.

path, condyle, n See *condyle path.*

path, generated occlusal, n a registration in the mouth of the paths of movement of the occlusal surfaces of teeth on a wax, plastic, or abrasive surface attached to the opposing dental arch.

path, idling, n the path that a stamp cusp travels when the bolus is being treated on the other side of the mouth.

path, lateral, n See *condyle path, lateral.*

path, occlusal, n **1.** a gliding occlusal contact. *n* **2.** the path of movement of an occlusal surface.

path of appliance insertion and removal, n See *insertion, path of.*

path of closure, n See *closure, centric path of.*

path of insertion, n See *insertion, path of.*

path of placement, n the direction in which a removable dental restoration is positioned in relation to the planned location on its supporting structures. The restoration is removed in the opposite direction. See also *placement, choice of path of.*

path, working, n the path that the stamp cusps make when working on the bolus. At first the bolus deflects the direction of these cusps, but after the fibers of the food have been reduced enough to be almost ready for swallowing, the travel coincides directionally with the working groove.

pathfinder, *n* See *broach, smooth.*

pathogen (path′ o-jən), *n* a microorganism responsible for causing disease.

pathogen, opportunistic, n an infectious agent that can only cause disease when the host's resistance is low.

pathogenesis (path″ o-jen′ ə-sis), *n* the course of an illness or condition, from its origin to manifestation and outbreak.

pathogenic occlusion (path′ə-jen′ik), *n* See *occlusion, pathogenic.*

pathognomonic (pəth-og′nə-mon′ik), *adj* relating to a sign or symptom unique to a disease or one that distinguishes it from other diseases.

pathology (pəth-ol′ə-jē), *n* **1.** the branch of science that deals with disease in all its relations, especially with its nature and the functional and material changes it causes. *n* **2.** in medical jurisprudence, the science of disease; the part of medicine that deals with the nature of disease, its causes, and its symptoms.

pathology, experimental, n the study of disease processes induced, usually in animals; undertaken to ascertain the effect of local environmental changes or systemic disorders on particular tissues, parts, and organs of the body. This branch of medical science also attempts to correlate the interaction of local and systemic factors in the production, modification, and continuance of a disease.

pathology, oral, n the study of the characteristics, causes, and effects of diseases of the mouth, oral cavity, and associated structures.

pathology, speech, n the study and treatment of all aspects of functional and organic speech defects and disorders.

pathology, surgical, n the study of the characteristics of diseased tissues and organs removed in the process of surgery.

pathosis (pəth-ō′sis), *n* **1.** a disease entity. *n* **2.** a pathologic condition. A patient is said to have a *pathosis* rather than *pathology,* which is the study of disease.

pathway of inflammation, *n* the route of extension of chronic gingival inflammation into the subjacent structures, extending into the interdental septum from the gingivae, along the interdental vessels, or following the course of these blood vessels onto the periosteal side of the bone as well as into the bone marrow spaces.

patient, *n* a person under medical or dental care.

patient admission, *n* the formal acceptance of a patient for care into a clinic, hospital, or extended care facility.

patient, bedridden (homebound), *n* individual from any age group confined to a private home, hospital, skilled nursing facility, hospice, nursing home, or institution.

patient compliance, *n* the degree or extent to which a patient follows or completes a prescribed diagnostic, treatment, or preventive procedure.

patient education, *n* the process of informing a patient about a health matter to secure informed consent, patient cooperation, and a high level of patient compliance.

patient load, *n* the number of patients treated by a dentist or a group of dentists within a specified period.

patient satisfaction, *n* as an outcome measure of quality, refers to the perception of the patients(s) of one or more aspects of a dental care system.

patient transfer, *n* to convey the responsibility for the care of a patient from one entity to another. It may involve the discharge from one entity and the admission to another along with the patient's medical/dental records or copies.

Patient's Bill of Rights, *n.pr* a list of the patient's rights promulgated by the American Hospital Association. It offers some guidance and protection to patients by stating the responsibilities that a hospital and its staff have toward patients and their families during hospitalization, but it is not a legally binding document.

pattern, *n* a form used to make a mold, such as for a denture, an inlay, or a partial denture framework.

pattern, occlusal, *n* the form or design of the occluding surfaces of a tooth or teeth. These forms may be based on natural or modified anatomic or nonanatomic concepts of teeth.

pattern, trabecular, *p* the trabecular arrangement of alveolar bone in relation to marrow spaces; may be radiographically interpreted.

pattern, wax, *n* **I.** a wax model for making the mold in which the metal will be formed in casting. *n* **2.** a wax form of a denture that, when it is invested in a flask and the wax is eliminated, will form the mold in which the resin denture is formed.

pattern, wear, *n* the topographic attributes and distribution of areas of tooth wear (facets) resulting from attrition by food, tooth contacts during swallowing, terminal aspects of the masticatory cycle, and habits of occlusal neuroses. Wear patterns may be used to determine many of the functional and afunctional movements the mandible has been passing through in preceding years. Occlusal wear occurs with aging. The type of wear is termed the *wear pattern.*

Paul-Bunnell test, *n.pr* See *test, Paul-Bunnell.*

payable, *adj* pertaining to an obligation to pay at a future time. When used without restriction or modification, the term means that the debt is payable at once.

payback period, *n* the length of time required for the net revenues of an investment to return the cost of the investment.

payer, *n* in health care, generally refers to entities other than the patient that finance or reimburse the cost of health services. In most cases, this term refers to insurance carriers, other third-party payers, or health plan sponsors (employers or unions).

payment, *n* the performance of a duty or promise; the discharge of a debt or liability by the delivery of money or something else of value.

payment, progress, *n* interim payments by the purchaser of a dental plan contract to the carrier for use as an operating fund. A final accounting is always completed when actual costs are paid.

payroll record, *n* a printed form on which detailed records are kept of the amounts of money paid to auxiliaries. The record has columns for all the necessary tax deductions so that a detailed record is available for tax reporting and cost accounting.

PBI, *n* See *iodine, protein-bound.*

p.c. (post cibum), *n* Latin term meaning "after meals." The abbreviation may be used in writing prescriptions.

PCP, *n* an abbreviation for *Pneumocystis carinii pneumonia*, an opportunistic infection associated with acquired immune deficiency syndrome (AIDS) and used as an indicator of AIDS.

PDL, *n* See *ligament, periodontal.*

PDS, *n* See *temporomandibular pain-dysfunction syndrome.*

peak, *n* buccal, outer high point of the normal interproximal tissue that rises to a peak; connected interdentally to a lingual peak by a triangular ridge, with a depression termed a *col.*

pearl, enamel (enameloma), *n* a small focal mass of enamel formed apical to the cementoenamel junction and resembling pearls. The bifurcation of molar roots is a favorite site for this aberration in tooth development.

pearls, Epstein's, *n.pr* See *nodules, Bohn's.*

pectin (pek′tin), *n* one of several heteropolysaccharides contained in the cell walls of plants, which provides dietary fiber for digestion.

pediatric dentistry, *n* See *pedodontics.*

pediatrics, *n* a branch of medicine concerned with the development and care of children. Its specialties are the particular diseases of children and their treatment and prevention.

pedicle flap, *n* See *flap, pedicle.*

pedigree, *n* a line of descent; ancestry.

Pediwrap, *n.pr* brand name for a cloth bandage that is wrapped around a young patient from neck to ankles to stabilize the body or to minimize juvenile fidgeting. It comes in various sizes.

pedodontics (pē′də-don′tiks), *n* the branch of dentistry that includes the following: training the child to accept dentistry; restoring and maintaining the primary, mixed, and permanent dentitions; applying preventive measures for dental caries and periodontal disease; and preventing, intercepting, and correcting various problems of occlusion.

pedunculated lesion (pedung′kyōō-lā-ted), *n* a raised wound connected by a narrow stem.

peer review, *n* **I.** a retrospective consideration or an examination by one or more individuals of equal standing or rank. *n* **2.** a process established to provide for review by licensed dentists of the care by a dentist for a single patient; disputes regarding fees; cases submitted by carriers and initiated by patients or dentists; and quality of care and appropriateness of treatment.

peer review organization (PRO), *n* an organization established by an amendment of the Tax Equity and Fiscal Responsibility Act of 1982 (TEFRA) to provide for the review of medical services furnished primarily in a hospital setting or in conjunction with care provided under the Medicare and Medicaid programs. In addition to their review and monitoring functions, these entities can invoke sanctions, penalties, or other corrective actions for noncompliance in organization standards.

peer review system, *n* a professionally sponsored and operated system for the rendering of professional judgment on disagreements between or among dentists, patients, or fiscal intermediaries, respecting quality of care and related matters.

peg lateral, *n* a developmental anomaly of the maxillary lateral incisor that causes the tooth to resemble a small peg.

peg third molar, *n* a developmental anomaly of the third molar (wisdom tooth) in which the crown fails to develop fully in any one of its four quadrants.

pegs, epithelial, *n.pl* See *rete ridges.*

pellagra (pəl-ā′grə, pə-lag′rə), *n* a nutritional deficiency resulting from faulty intake or metabolism of nicotinic acid, a vitamin B complex factor. It is characterized by glossitis, dermatitis of sun-exposed surfaces, stomatitis, diarrhea, and dementia. Thiamine, riboflavin, and tryptophan deficiencies may be associated.

pellet, *n* a small, rounded mass of material.

pellet, cotton, *n* a rolled ball of cotton varying in diameter from approximately ⅜ inch to ⅛ inch. (The larger size is a cotton ball; the smaller size is a pledget.)

pellet, foil, *n* a loosely rolled piece of gold foil of various thicknesses; prepared from a portion—¹⁄₁₂₈, ¹⁄₉₆, ¹⁄₆₄, ¹⁄₄₈, ¹⁄₃₂, ¹⁄₁₆—cut from a 4-inch (10-cm) square of foil.

P

pellicle (pel'ik-əl), *n* a film or membrane.

pellicle, brown, *n* a specific name for a brownish-gray to black film formed over time on the surfaces of the teeth of 20% to 25% of the population as a result of not using an abrasive-containing dentifrice.

pellicle, salivary, *n* a thin, naturally occurring abacterial film from salivary proteins that regularly forms on teeth and other surfaces in the mouth, such as restorations or dentures. It may be brushed away, but it will reform within minutes. Also called *acquired pellicle* or *organic dental pellicle.* This serves as a base for bacterial plaque formation.

pelvis, *n* the lower portion of the trunk of the body, composed of four bones, the two innominate bones laterally and ventrally and the sacrum and coccyx posteriorly.

pemoline, *n trade name:* Cylert; *drug class:* central nervous system stimulant; Controlled Substance Schedule IV; *action:* exact mechanism unknown; may act through dopaminergic mechanisms; *use:* attention deficit disorder with hyperactivity.

pemphigoid, benign mucous membrane (pem'fi-goid), *n* a bullous disease that resembles pemphigus but is more chronic in nature. The oral mucosa, especially the gingiva where it resembles desquamative gingivitis, and conjunctiva are the sites of predilection. Skin is involved in approximately 20% of the cases.

pemphigus (pem'fi-gus, pem-fī'gus), *n* a rare, grave skin disease of unknown cause characterized by the development of bullae on the skin and mucous membrane. See also *bulla* and *sign, Nikolsky's.*

Pemphigus. (Regezi/Sciubba/Jordan, 2003)

pemphigus, acute disseminated, *n* a dread disease of unknown cause, temporarily controlled by the administration of corticosteroids. Manifested by bullous formation on the skin and mucous membranes. Desquamation of the epithelium exposes a raw, burning, oozing submucosa. Adequate nutritional status is difficult to maintain; secondary infection is common; with progressive debility, pneumonia is common and is usually the cause of death.

pen grasp, *n* See *grasp, pen.*

penbutolol, *n trade name:* Levatol; *drug class:* nonselective β-adrenergic blocker; *action:* competitively blocks stimulation of β-adrenergic receptors within the heart and decreases renin activity, all of which may play a role in reducing systolic and diastolic blood pressure; inhibits β_2 receptors in the bronchial system; *uses:* hypertension alone or with thiazide diuretics.

penetrability (pen'ə-trə-bil'i-tē), *n* the ability of a beam of x-radiation to pass through matter. The degree of penetrability is determined by kilovoltage and filtration.

penetrating (pen'ə-trā-ting), *adj* piercing; entering deeply.

penetration (pen'ə-trā'shən), *n* the ability of radiation to extend down into and go through substances. The degree of penetration is determined by the kilovoltage.

penetrometer (pen'ə-trom'ə-tur), *n* an aluminum step wedge or ladder exposed over a film to determine the quality or penetrating ability of a specific beam of x-radiation.

penicillin (pen'i-sil'in), *n* an antibiotic secured from cultures of *Penicillium notatum,* being bactericidal for gram-positive cocci, some gram-negative cocci (gonococcus and meningococcus), and clostridial and spirochetal organisms. Its topical application to the oral mucous membranes is discouraged because of the high risk of sensitization from local application of antibiotic substances.

penicillin G, *n* an acid-sensitive form of penicillin prepared as penicillin G benzathine and penicillin G procaine used for deep intramuscular administration. The penicillin is slowly released, resulting in prolonged effective blood levels of penicillin G. In dentistry, it is used prophylactically for patients predisposed to bacterial endocarditis prior to any invasive dental procedure. See also *penicillin G benzathine*.

penicillin G benzathine, n trade names: Bicillin L-A, Permapen; *drug class:* benzathine salt of natural penicillin; *action:* interferes with cell wall replication of susceptible organisms; osmotically unstable cell wall swells and bursts from osmotic pressure; *uses:* respiratory infections, scarlet fever, erysipelas, otitis media, pneumonia, skin and soft tissue infections, and yaws.

penicillin V potassium/penicillin V, n trade names: Beepen-VK, Betapen-VK, V-Cillin K, Veetids, others; *drug class:* semisynthetic penicillin; *action:* interferes with cell wall replication of susceptible organisms; the cell wall, rendered osmotically unstable, swells and bursts from osmotic pressure; *uses:* effective for gram-positive cocci and gram-negative bacilli.

pension plans, *n.pl* saving and investment programs designed to provide income at the time of retirement. These may be employer- or individual-based, in which portions of the funds may be protected from taxation at the time of earning but subject to taxation at the time of withdrawal.

pentaerythritol tetranitrate (pent′ə- er-ith′ri-tōl), *n trade names:* Duotrate, Pentylan, Peritrate, others; *drug class:* antianginal, organic nitrate; *action:* decreases preload, afterload, which is responsible for decreasing left ventricular end-diastolic pressure, systemic vascular resistance, arterial and venous dilation; *uses:* chronic stable angina pectoris, prophylaxis of angina pain.

pentamidine/pentamidine isethionate (pen-tam′i-dēn), *n trade names:* NebuPent, Pentam 300, others; *drug class:* antiprotozoal; *action:* interferes with deoxyribonucleic acid/ribonucleic acid synthesis in protozoa; *use: Pneumocystis carinii* infections in immunocompromised patients.

pentazocine HCl/pentazocine lactate (pen-taz′ō-sēn), *n trade*

names: Talwin, Talwin NX; *drug class:* synthetic opioid/mixed agonist/antagonist, Controlled Substance Schedule IV; *action:* interacts with opioid receptors in the central nervous system to alter pain perception; *uses:* moderate-to-severe pain alone or in combination with aspirin or acetaminophen.

pentobarbital/pentobarbital sodium, *n trade name:* Nembutal Sodium; *drug class:* sedative/hypnotic barbiturate, Controlled Substance Schedule II; *action:* depresses activity in brain cells, primarily in reticular activating system of brain stem; *uses:* insomnia, sedation, preoperative medication. Useful as a preoperative sedative in dentistry.

pentoxifylline, *n trade name:* Trental; *drug class:* hemorrheologic agent; *action:* decreased blood viscosity, stimulates prostacyclin formation, increases blood flow by increasing flexibility of red blood cells (RBCs), decreased RBC hyperaggregation, reduces platelet aggregation, decreases fibrinogen concentration; *uses:* intermittent claudication related to chronic occlusive vascular disease.

penumbra, geometric (pən-um′brə), *n* partial or imperfect shadow about the umbra, or true shadow, of an object. In radiography, it is influenced by the size of the focal spot, focal-film distance, and object-film distance. See also *geometric unsharpness*.

peptic ulcer (pep′tik), *n* a sharply circumscribed lesion of the mucous membrane of the stomach or small intestine or any part of the gastrointestinal system exposed to gastric acid and pepsin.

peptide, *n* a compound of two or more amino acids in which the α-carboxyl group of one is united with the α-amino group of another, with the elimination of a molecule of water, creating a peptide bond —CO—NH—.

Peptostreptococcus, n a genus of nonmotile, anaerobic, chemoorganotrophic bacteria found in the oral cavity and intestinal tracts of normal humans. They may be pathogenic and may be found in pyogenic infections, putrefactive war wounds, and appendicitis.

percentile, *n* the number in a frequency distribution below which a certain percentage of fees will fall. For example, the 90th percentile is the number that divides the distribution of fees into the lower 90% and the upper 10%, or that fee level at which 90% of dentists charge that amount or less and 10% charge more.

perception, occlusal, *n* the patient's cognizance of occlusal patterns and disharmonies, mediated by the proprioceptive sense of the nerve fibers of the periodontal membrane.

Percodan, *n.pr* brand name for oxycodone, a semisynthetic narcotic analgesic oxycodone. Percodan is a controlled substance.

percolation, *n* extraction of the soluble parts of a drug by causing a liquid solvent to flow slowly through it.

percussion (per-kush′ən), *n* the act of striking an area, a structure, or an organ as an aid in diagnosing a diseased condition by the sensations reported by the patient and by the sounds heard by the examiner.

percutaneous route (pur′kyōō-tā′nē-us), *n* a path of entry via the skin.

perforation, palatal (pur′fôr-ā′shən), *n* a perforation that exists in the palatal area after the surgical repair of a cleft.

perforation, radicular, *n* an artificial opening or hole made by boring or cutting through the lateral aspect of the root; also occurs as the result of internal or external resorption.

perforation, sublabial, *n* a perforation existing in the upper labial sulcus after surgical repair of the area. The perforation communicates between the oral and nasal cavities.

performance, *n* fulfillment of a promise, contract, or other obligation.

perfringens poisoning, *n* an infection of the gastrointestinal tract caused by the bacterium *Clostridium perfringens,* which is usually self limiting. Symptoms include nausea, vomiting, and diarrhea.

perfusion, *n* a therapeutic measure whereby a drug intended for an isolated part of the body is introduced via the bloodstream.

periadenitis mucosa necrotica recurrens (per′ē-ad′ən-ī′tis), *n* involvement of the oral mucosa with deep-seated aphthouslike ulcers that tend to heal with scars. It may be impossible to differentiate the disease from Behçet's syndrome in the absence of a diagnosis of cyclic neutropenia. Also called *recurrent scarring aphtha, Sutton's disease.* See also *disease, Miculicz'.*

perialveolar wiring, See *wiring, perialveolar.*

periapex (per′ē-ā′peks), *n* that area of tissue that immediately surrounds the root apex.

periapical (per′ē-ā′pikəl), *adj* enclosing or surrounding the apical area of a tooth root.

periapical abscess, *n* an acute or chronic inflammation of the periapical tissues characterized by a localized accumulation of pus at the apex of a tooth. It is generally a sequela of pulp death of the tooth.

periapical granuloma, *n* an accumulation of mononuclear inflammatory cells with an encircling aggregation of fibroblasts and collagen at the apex of the root of a tooth caused by chronic inflammation. Also called *chronic apical periodontitis.*

periapical radiograph, *n* a radiograph demonstrating tooth apices and surrounding structures in a particular intraoral area.

periapical radiographic survey, *n* a series of intraoral radiographs depicting periapical areas of interest. A complete mouth radiographic survey may consist of 17 or more intraoral radiographs that depict all areas of the oral cavity.

periapical tissue, *n* tissue located at the root end of a tooth. Usually connective tissue forming an attachment between the root and the alveolar bone.

periauricular (per′ē-ôr-ik′yōō-lur), *adj* surrounding the external ear.

pericarditis, *n* an inflammation of the pericardium associated with trauma, malignant neoplastic disease, infection, uremia, myocardial infarction, collagen disease, or idiopathic causes.

pericardium, *n* a fibroserous sac that surrounds the heart and the roots of the great vessels.

pericementitis (per′ē-sē′men-tī′tis), *n* See *periodontitis.*

pericoronitis (per′ē-kôr′ə-nī′tis), *n* inflammation of the operculum or tissue flap over a partially erupted tooth, particularly a third molar. Inflammation around a crown, particularly the inflammation of a partially erupted tooth.

Pericoronitis. (Neville/Damm/Allen/Bouquot, 2002)

periimplant space, *n* the space between an implant and its investing tissues.

periimplantitis (per″ē-lm′plan ti″tis), *n* inflammation in and around the area of a dental implant that may also affect abutment areas.

Periimplantitis. (Daniel/Harfst, 2002)

perikymata (per″ ĭ-ki′ mə-tə), *n* wavy ridges on the surface of a permanent tooth, which signify overlaps in the enamel structure and that may disappear as the enamel wears over time.

perimenopause, *n* the premenopausal period of approximately 3 to 6 years during which menstrual cycles become erratic and estrogen levels fall, ending with the cessation of menstruation.

perimolysis, *n* a wearing down of the tooth enamel by mechanical or chemical means, sometimes a result of repeated vomiting in those with eating disorders.

perinatal, *adj* related to the time surrounding the birth process.

perineum, *n* the part of the body situated dorsal to the pubic arch and the arcuate ligaments, ventral to the tip of the coccyx, and lateral to the inferior rami of the pubis and the ischium and sacrotuberous ligaments. The perineum supports and surrounds the distal portions of the urogenital and gastrointestinal tracts of the body.

period, latent, *n* the area of delay between the time of exposure of an organism to radiation and the manifestation of the changes produced by that radiation. This delay depends on many factors but particularly on the magnitude of the dose. The larger the dose, the earlier the appearance of the injury. In some instances the latent period for some effects may be as long as 25 years or more.

periodicity, *n* events that tend to repeat at predictable intervals.

periodontal (per′ē-ō-don′təl), *adj* relating to the periodontium.

periodontal abscess, *n* a localized area of acute or chronic inflammation found in the gingival corium, infrabony pockets, or periodontal membrane. If it is located at the apex of the tooth, it is known as a *periapical abscess.* If located between the apex and the alveolar crest, it is known as a *lateral abscess.*

periodontal atrophy, *n* See *atrophy, periodontal.*

periodontal attachment loss, *n* a reduction in the connective tissue attaching the root of the tooth to the alveolar bone, usually caused by persistent inflammation of the gingival and periodontal tissues.

periodontal disease, *n* any of a group of inflammatory and infectious diseases affecting the gums and supporting tissues of the teeth.

periodontal disease, aggressive, *n* marked by the early onset of periodontal disease that affects the gingiva and periodontal tissues. If untreated, it may result in loss of teeth.

Aggressive periodontal disease. (Newman/Takei/Carranza, 2002)

P

periodontal dressing, *n* a protective obtundent covering of the gum and periodontal tissues used after periodontal surgery.

periodontal index, *n* a method for rating or ranking the severity of periodontal disease. An early index was the PMA, which ranked the number of *p*apillary, *m*arginal, and *a*ttached gingiva affected by gingivitis. A more contemporary index is the Russell Periodontal Index (PI), which is based on a 0-to-8 score system: from negative to advanced destruction.

periodontal ligament, *n* a system of collagenous connective tissue fibers that connect the root of a tooth to its alveolus. It contains blood vessels, lymph vessels, and nerves. The ligament consists of four groups of fibers: alveolar crestal, horizontal, oblique, and apical.

periodontal pack, *n* See *pack, periodontal.*

periodontal pocket, *n* See *pocket, periodontal.*

periodontal probe, *n* See *probe, periodontal.*

periodontal prosthesis, *n* See *prosthesis, periodontal.*

Periodontal Screening and Recording (PSR), *n.pr* a proprietary method of briefly examining all of a patient's teeth, and recording the highest score in each of six regions of the mouth (mid-, mesio-, and distofacial and corresponding lingual areas). The process utilizes a blunt-tipped probe instrument and is intended to take only 2 to 3 minutes.

periodontal therapy, *n* See *therapy, periodontal.*

periodontal treatment planning, *n* the sequential arrangement of therapeutic procedures required to obtain a healthy gingival attachment and an intact, functioning attachment apparatus. Periodontal therapy cannot be performed on an empiric basis but relies on an integrated knowledge of the theory and practice of periodontology.

periodontal surgery, *n* an operative procedure used to treat disease or repair abnormalities in the tissues of the teeth and surrounding areas. See also *surgery.*

periodontia (per′ē-ō-don′shē-ə), *n* See *periodontics.*

periodontics (per′ē-ō-don′tiks), *n* the art and science of examination, diagnosis, and treatment of diseases affecting the periodontium; a study of the supporting structures of the teeth, including not only the normal anatomy and physiology of these structures but also the deviations from normal.

periodontics, concept of cure in, *n* the idea that a successful result in periodontal therapy consists of restoring any tooth or collection of teeth to functional capability, regardless of whether they are able to function alone or require stabilization to survive.

periodontitis (per′ē-ō-don-tī′tis), *n* **1.** the alterations occurring in the periodontium with inflammation. Gingival changes are those of gingivitis, with the clinical signs associated with gingivitis. Periodontitis has histologic characteristics, such as ulceration of the sulcular epithelium, epithelial hyperplasia, proliferation of epithelial rete pegs into the gingival corium, apical migration of the epithelial attachment after lysis of the gingival fiber apparatus, cellular and exudative infiltrate into tissues, and increased capillarity. Resorption of bone in an apical direction results in the loss of attachment of the periodontal fibers to the bone. A transseptal band of reconstituted periodontal fibers walls off the gingival inflammation from the underlying bone. *n* **2.** a chronic, progressive disease of the periodontium.

Periodontitis. (Neville/Damm/Allen/ Bouquot, 2002, courtesy Dr. Samuel Jasper)

periodontitis, acute, n a sharply localized, acute inflammatory process involving the interproximal and marginal areas of two or more adjacent teeth, characterized by severe pain, purulent exudate from edematous inflamed gingivae, general malaise, fever, and sequestration of the crestal aspects of the alveolar process.

periodontitis, aggressive, n a bacterial disease of the teeth and gingiva that manifests before age 35, often in prepubescent children. It is caused primarily by the bacterium *Actinobacillus actinomycetemcomitans,* leading to rapid tissue deterioration. See also *periodontitis, juvenile* and *periodontitis, early-onset (EOP).*

periodontitis, chronic periapical, n periapical inflammation characterized by dental granuloma formation.

periodontitis, early-onset (EOP), n the term given to periodontal disease affecting children, teens, and young adults, which, if left untreated, may cause premature tooth loss. Used to be considered *prepubertal periodontitis* and is now considered *aggressive periodontitis.*

periodontitis in children, n See *periodontitis, juvenile.*

periodontitis, juvenile, n periodontal disease present in children or adolescents, with radiographic and clinical findings similar to those observed in the adult, including gingivitis, periodontal pocket formation, and bone resorption but only in specific areas *(localized)* or throughout the oral cavity *(generalized).* Used to be called the outdated term *periodontosis* and now is considered *aggressive periodontosis.*

periodontitis, marginal, n the sequela to gingivitis in which the inflammatory process has spread apically to involve the alveolar process. It involves an inflammation of the marginal periodontium with resorption of the crest of alveolar bone. Apical migration of the epithelial attachment occurs with suprabony or infrabony pocket formation and cuplike resorptions and marginal translucence of the alveolar crest. In children the process may be more rapid and destructive than in adults.

periodontium (per′ē-ō-don′shē-um), n the tissues that invest (or help to invest) and support the teeth (e.g., the gingivae, cementum of the tooth, periodontal ligament, and alveolar and supporting bone).

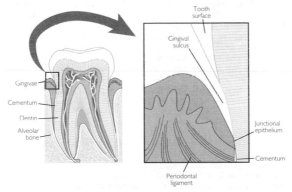

Structures of the periodontium. (Bird/Robinson, 2002)

periodontology, *n* See *periodontics.*

periodontometer (per′ē-ō-don-tom′ə-tur), *n* a device used to measure the amount of tooth movement.

periodontopathic (per″e-o-don-to′ path′ ik), *n* a substance capable of starting diseases in the surrounding tissue and supporting structures of the teeth.

periodontosis (per′ē-ō-don-tō′sis), *n* See *periodontitis, aggressive.*

perioral structures, *n.pl* the anatomic elements around the mouth, generally the lips and muscles of facial expression within the lips.

periorbital, *adj* surrounding the eyes. The periorbital soft tissues are easily contused and produce marked inflammatory responses to trauma.

periosteal elevator (per′ē-os′tē-əl), *n* See *elevator, periosteal.*

periosteum (per′ē-os′tē-um), *n* the layer of connective tissue that varies considerably in thickness in the different areas of bone. It is thick over the surfaces that do not serve as areas of muscle attachment, especially on surfaces that are covered only by skin and subcutaneous tissue. In these areas the periosteum connects loosely with the bone itself and is easily lifted from it. Muscles are attached to bones directly, or they end on the periosteum. When muscles or tendons are attached to the bone, connective tissue extends into the bone as Sharpey's fibers. In such areas a periosteum may be lacking. When muscles are attached to the periosteum and thus are indirectly attached to the bone, the periosteum is relatively thin but is strongly fixed to the bone. The periosteum consists of two layers: an outer layer, which is rich in blood vessels and nerves and shows a dense arrangement of collagenous fibers, and an inner layer, the cambium, in which the fibers are loosely arranged, the cells numerous, and the blood vessels relatively sparse. During active growth, this layer of osteoblasts covers the periosteal surface of the bone. In the quiescent state in the adult, the periosteum primarily provides support. However, the inner layer retains its osteogenetic potencies and in fractures is activated to form osteoblasts and new bone.

periostitis (per′ē-os-tī′tis), *n* an inflammation of the periosteum in which the membrane may become detached from the underlying bone, resulting from exudates produced by inflammation or infection.

Periostitis. (Neville/Damm/Allen/Bouquot, 2002)

peripheral circulation (pər-if′ər-əl), *n* See *circulation, peripheral.*

peripheral nervous system, *n* the motor and sensory nerves and ganglia outside of the brain and spinal cord.

periphery (pər-if′er-ē), *n* See *border, denture.*

periradicular (per″ ĭ-rə-dik′ u-lər), *adj* pertaining to the area immediately outside of or around the root of the tooth.

peritoneal cavity, *p* the potential space between the parietal and the visceral layers of the peritoneum.

peritonitis, *n* an inflammation of the peritoneum produced by bacteria or irritating substances introduced into the abdominal cavity by a penetrating wound or perforation of an organ in the gastrointestinal (GI) tract or the reproductive tract. Peritonitis is caused most commonly by rupture of the vermiform appendix.

peritonsillar, *adj* surrounding the tonsils. Generally used in reference to the pharyngeal tonsils.

peritonsillar abscess, *n* an infection of tissue between the tonsil and pharynx, usually after acute follicular tonsillitis.

perlèche (per-lesh′), *adj* a general term applied to superficial fissures occurring at the angles of the mouth. Lesions may result from a variety of causes but most often can be related to deep labial commissures, with associated drooling, licking of the lips, unhygienic conditions, and the overgrowth of bacteria, yeast, or fungi. The term has also been applied to angular cheilosis resulting from riboflavin deficiency but not to the split papule of syphilis or to herpetic lesions.

permanent, *adj* of a lasting or durable nature (opposite of temporary).

permanent dentition, n See *dentition, permanent.*

permeability, *n* the degree to which one substance allows another substance to pass through it.

permissible dose, n See *dose, maximum permissible.*

permucosal (biologic) seal (per′mu-ko′ səl), *n* permucosal tissue present between a dental implant and the soft tissue, the function of which is to prevent bacteria and inflammatory agents from entering the tissues.

permucosal route (pur-myōō-kō′səl), *n* a path of entry via the mucous membranes.

peroral, *adj* through or about the mouth.

peroxidase horseradish, *n* an enzyme used in immunohistochemistry to label the antigen-antibody complex.

peroxidases, *n.pl* hydrogen-peroxide–reducing enzymes, occurring in animal and plant tissues, that catalyze the dehydrogenation (oxidation) of various substances in the presence of hydrogen peroxide.

peroxide, n See *hydrogen peroxide.*

perphenazine, *n trade name:* Trilafon; *drug class:* phenothiazine antipsychotic; *action:* blocks neurotransmission at dopaminergic synapses in the cerebral cortex, hypothalamus, and limbic system; mechanism for antipsychotic effects unclear; *uses:* psychotic disorders, schizophrenia, alcoholism, nausea, vomiting.

personal, *adj* belonging to an individual; limited to the person; having the nature of the qualities of human beings or of movable property.

personal representative, n a person designated to make health care decisions on another person's behalf. See also *guardian.*

personal supervision, n necessary for certain procedures in which the dentist, while personally giving treatment to a patient, requires the hygienist to perform a supplementary or supportive procedure simultaneously.

personality, *n* **1.** the sum total of a patient's ideas, emotions, and behavior, including the rational and irrational, the conscious and unconscious, and the defensive and learned behavior patterns. Personality develops from both genetic factors and environmental factors. Thus the patient brings to a dental office an individual personality syndrome. It may be a well-adjusted, stable personality; a depressed, anxious, neurotic personality; or a manic, schizophrenic, psychotic personality. Patients have a broad spectrum of healthy and disordered personalities. *n* **2.** the characteristics of a person by which other people evaluate him or her.

personality assessment, n See *personality test.*

personality disorder, n a disruption in relatedness manifested in any of a large group of mental disorders characterized by rigid, inflexible, and maladaptive behavior patterns that impair a person's ability to function in society.

personality test, n any of a variety of standardized tests used in the evaluation of various facets of personality structure, emotional status, and behavioral traits.

personnel, *n* the sum of persons employed in an enterprise. In dentistry it refers to the staff employed by the dentist.

personnel monitoring, n See *monitoring, personnel.*

pertussis (pur-tus′is), *n* a disease caused by *bordetella pertussis* in which the patient suffers from a cough that makes a "whooping" sound. Also called *whooping cough.*

pervasive, *adj* indicates that a condition permeates the entire development of the individual.

pesticide poisoning, *n* a toxic condition caused by the ingestion or inhalation of a substance used for the eradication of insects, fungi, and other pests.

petazocine, *n* an analgesic approximately equivalent in analgesic effect to codeine; *brand name:* Talwin.

petechiae (pə-tē′kē-ā), *n.pl* capillary hemorrhages producing small red or purplish pinhead-sized discolorations of the mucous membrane and skin. Petechiae are typical of

P

blood dyscrasias, vitamin C deficiency, positive Rumpel-Leede test, liver disease, and subacute bacterial endocarditis.

Petechiae. (Regezi/Sciubba/Jordan, 2003)

petri plate, *n* a shallow dish with a loose cover that is used in the laboratory for growing microorganisms.

petrolatum (pet′rə-lā′tum), *n* a mixture of hydrocarbons obtained from petroleum. In its semisolid form it is used as a protective covering to prevent gingival dehydration and inflammation during mouth breathing. Other uses include a lubricant and a protective covering for burns.

Peutz-Jeghers syndrome (poits′je-g′urz), *n.pr* See *syndrome, Peutz-Jeghers.*

pH, *n* the concentration of hydrogen ions expressed as the negative logarithm of base 10.

  pH, critical, n the point at which the minerals in a substance begin to decrease. For enamel, critical pH is between 4.5 and 5.5 moles per liter; radical (root) critical pH is 6.0 to 6.7 moles per liter.

phagocyte (fag′ə-sīt), *n* any cell that ingests microorganisms, cells, or other substances.

phagocytosis (fag′ə-sī-tō′sis), *n* the engulfing of microorganisms, cells, and other substances by phagocytes. See also *phagocyte.*

phantom (fan′tum), *n* a device that absorbs and scatters x-radiation in approximately the same way as the tissues of the body.

pharmacist, *n* a person prepared to formulate and dispense drugs or medications through completion of an accredited university program in pharmacy. Licensure is required upon completion of the program and prior to serving the public as a pharmacist.

pharmacodynamics (fär′mə-kō-dī-nam′iks), *n* the science of drug action.

pharmacology (fär′mə-kol′ə-jē), *n* the total science of drugs, including their use in therapeutics.

pharmacotherapy (fär′mə-kō-ther′ə-pē), *n* treatment based on the use of drugs or pharmaceuticals.

pharmacy (fär′mə-sē), *n* **I.** the art and science of preparing and dispensing drugs. *n* **2.** place where drugs are dispensed.

pharyngeal arch (fər-in′jē-əl), *n* See *arch, pharyngeal.*

pharyngeal flap, *n* a pedicle flap usually raised on the posterior pharyngeal wall and attached to the soft palate to reduce the size of the velopharyngeal gap.

pharyngeal pouches, *n.pl* saclike projections of the pharynx walls that lie between the branchial arches in a developing embryo.

pharyngitis (fer′in-jī′tis), *n* inflammation of the pharynx.

  pharyngitis, gonococcal, n a throat infection caused by the same infectious microorganism that causes gonorrhea; spread by direct contact with an infected person or with fluids containing the infectious agent.

pharyngoplasty (fər-ing′gō-plas-tē), *n* reconstructive operation to alter the size and shape of the nasopharyngeal orifice.

pharyngospasm (fər-ing′gō-spaz-əm), *n* spasm of the pharyngeal muscles.

pharyngotomy, *n* any cutting operation upon the pharynx, either from without or from within.

pharynx (fer′inks), *n* a funnel-shaped tube of muscle tissue between the mouth and nares and the esophagus, which is the common pathway for food and air. The nasopharynx lies above the level of the soft palate. The oropharynx lies between the upper edge of the epiglottis and the soft palate, whereas the laryngopharynx extends from the upper edge of the epiglottis to the superior end of the esophagus behind the larynx.

  pharynx, activities of posterior and lateral pharyngeal wall, n.pl the bulging of the posterior and lateral pharyngeal wall produced by the superior pharyngeal constrictors and palatopharyngeus during the acts of swallowing and phonation; seen in individuals with a congenitally short soft palate, operated soft palate, or unoperated cleft of the soft palate. These activities are rarely present in the individual with the normal soft palate.

pharynx, implant surgical, n first stage: a major oral operation in which the mucoperiosteum is elevated, exposing the oral surface of the jawbone; the surgical jaw relations are established, and an impression is made of the exposed bone surfaces. Second stage: a major oral surgical operation in which the mucoperiosteum is reelevated, the prepared implant is placed on the bone surface, and the mucoperiosteum is coapted and sutured about the posts of the protruding implant abutments.

phase-contrast microscope, *n* a microscope with a special condenser and objective, which contains a phase-shifting ring by which small differences in the index of refraction become visible. The use of phase-contrast capabilities allows for direct viewing of transparent live cells and tissues. Phase-contrast microscopes are useful in educating patients about the oral flora associated with dental plaque and caries and periodontal disease.

phenacetin, caffeine, aspirin (fen-as'ə-tin), *n* See *aspirin, phenacetin, caffeine.*

phenazopyridine HCl, *n* trade names: Azo-Standard, Baridium, Eridium, Pyridiate, Urogesic, others, *drug class:* urinary tract analgesic; *action:* exerts analgesic anesthetic action on the urinary tract mucosa; exact mechanism of action is unknown; *use:* urinary tract irritation/infection.

phencyclidine, *n* an approved veterinary anesthetic. Illicitly, it is used as a hallucinogen. Also called *PCP, hog,* or *peace pill.*

phendimetrazine tartrate, *n* trade names: Adipost, Anorex SR, Appecon, Obalan, others; *drug class:* anorexiant, amphetamine-like Controlled Substance Schedule III; *action:* exact mechanism of action of appetite suppression is unknown but may have an effect on the satiety center of the

hypothalamus; *use:* exogenous obesity.

phenelzine sulfate, *trade name:* Nardil; *drug class:* antidepressant, monoamine antioxidase inhibitor; *action:* increases concentrations of endogenous epinephrine, norepinephrine, serotonin, dopamine in storage sites in central nervous system; *use:* depression when uncontrolled by other means.

phenobarbital/phenobarbital sodium, *n* trade names: Ancalixor, Barbita, Luminal Sodium, Solfoton; *drug class:* barbiturate, anticonvulsant, Controlled Substance Schedule IV; *action:* a nonspecific depressant of the central nervous system; may enhance gamma aminobutyric acid activity in the brain; *uses:* all forms of epilepsy, status epilepticus, febrile seizures in children, sedation, insomnia.

phenol (fē'nôl), *n* an organic compound in which one or more hydroxyl groups are attached to a carbon atom in an aromatic ring that contains conjugated double bonds.

phenol coefficient, n a basis of comparison in determining the relative effectiveness of antiseptics. Phenol is the standard for comparison with other agents for their ability to kill a well-dispersed suspension of *Salmonella* or *Staphylococcus.* It has little practical value.

phenolic, synthetic, *n* a form of a chemical agent used as a surface disinfectant that kills a wide range of microbes. It provides a residual level of treatment after initial application.

phenotype (fē'nō-tīp), *n* term referring to the expression of genotypes that can be directly distinguished (e.g., by clinical observation of external appearance or serologic tests).

phenoxybenzamine HCl, *n* trade name: Dibenzyline; *drug class:* antihypertensive; *action:* α-adrenergic blocker that binds to α-adrenergic receptors, dilating peripheral blood vessels; lowers peripheral resistance, lowers blood pressure; *use:* hypertensive episodes associated with pheochromocytoma.

phenprocoumon, *n* a long-acting, orally effective anticoagulant.

phensuximide, *n trade name:* Milontin; *drug class:* anticonvulsant, suc-

P

cinimide; *action:* suppresses spike wave formation in absence seizures (petit mal); decreases amplitude, frequency, duration, spread of discharge in minor motor seizures; *use:* absence (petit mal) seizures.

phentermine HCl/phentermine resin, *n trade name:* Adipex-P, Fastin, Ionamin, Obe-Mar, Panshape M, T-Diet, others; *drug class:* sympathomimetic, anorexiant, Controlled Substance Schedule IV; *action:* exact mechanism of action of appetite suppression unknown but may have an effect on satiety center of hypothalamus; *use:* exogenous obesity.

phentolamine mesylate, *n trade name:* Regitine; *drug class:* antihypertensive; *action:* α-adrenergic blocker; binds to α-adrenergic receptors, dilating peripheral blood vessels, lowering peripheral resistance, lowering blood pressure; *uses:* hypertension, pheochromocytoma, prevention and treatment of dermal necrosis following extravasation of norepinephrine or dopamine.

phenylalanine (fen′il-al′ə-nēn), *n* one of the essential amino acids. See also *amino acid.*

phenylephrine HCl (fen′il-ef′rin), *n trade names:* Neo-Synephrine, Vick's Sinex, others; *drug class:* nasal decongestant, sympathomimetic; *action:* produces rapid and long-acting vasoconstriction of arterioles; *use:* temporary relief of nasal congestion.

phenylketonuria (PKU) (fen′il-kē′tō-nyōō′rē-ə), *n* a condition in which metabolism is severely compromised because of the absence of a phenylaline-processing enzyme resulting in mental retardation, although a prescribed diet can minimize its severity.

phenytoin sodium/phenytoin sodium extended/phenytoin sodium prompt, *n trade names:* Dilantin, Diphenylan, Phenytex, others; *drug class:* hydantoin anticonvulsant; *action:* inhibits spread of seizure activity in motor cortex; *uses:* generalized tonic-clonic (grand mal) seizures, status epilepticus, nonepileptic seizures, trigeminal neuralgia, cardiac dysrhythmias caused by digitalis-type drugs.

pheochromocytoma, *n* a vascular tumor of chromaffin tissue of the adrenal medulla or sympathetic paraganglia, characterized by hypersecretion of epinephrine and norepinephrine, causing persistent or intermittent hypertension.

PHI, *n* See *health information, protected.*

philtrum (fil′ trəm), *n* vertical groove in the midline of the upper lip.

phlebectasia (fleb′ek-tā′zē-ə), *n* dilation of a vein.

phlebitis (flə-bī′tis), *n* inflammation of a vein. See also *thrombophlebitis.*

phlebolith (fleb′ō-lith), *n* a calcified thrombus in a vein.

phlegmon (fleg′mon), *n* **1.** an intense inflammation spreading through tissue spaces over a large area and without definite limits. *n* **2.** clinically, a hard, boardlike swelling without gross pus. See also *cellulitis.*

phobia (fō′bē-ə), *n* a specific hysterical fear.

phobia, social, *n* an anxiety disorder in which a person is afraid of social situations for fear of being judged unworthy by others.

phonation (fō-nā′shən), *n* the production of voiced sound by means of vocal cord vibrations.

phonation, speech, *n* modification by the vocal folds of the airstream as it leaves the lungs and passes through the larynx, for the purpose of producing the various sounds that are the basis of speech. By opposing each other with different degrees of tension and space, the vocal folds create a slitlike aperture of varying size and contour; and by creating resistance to the stream of air, they set up a sequence of laryngeal sound waves with characteristic pitch and intensity.

phoneme (fō′nēm), *n* a group or family of closely related speech sounds, all of which have the same distinctive acoustic characteristics despite their differences; often used in place of the term *speech sound.*

phonetic values, *n.pl* See *values, phonetic.*

phonetics (fō-net′iks), *n* the study of the production and perception of speech sounds, including individual and group variations and their use in speech.

phosphatase(s) (fos′fə-tās), *n* a

group of enzymes that are distributed throughout most cells and body fluids and are characterized by their ability to hydrolyze a wide variety of monophosphate esters to alcohols and inorganic phosphate.

phosphatase, acid, n a group of phosphatases (e.g., serum, liver, prostate) with optimal activity below a pH level of 7. Elevated serum levels have been observed in metastatic breast and prostatic cancer; Paget's, Gaucher's, and Niemann-Pick diseases and in myelocytic leukemia.

phosphatase, alkaline, n a group of phosphatases (e.g., serum, liver, bone) whose optimal activity ranges near a pH level of 9.8. Elevated blood levels occur in Paget's disease and pregnancy, whereas low levels are characteristic of dwarfism and a generalized nutritional protein deficiency.

phosphates (fos'fāts), *n.pl* the organic compounds of phosphorus. The blood phosphate level is normally 2.5 mg to 5 mg/100 mL. It is low in rickets and early hyperparathyroidism and high in tetany and nephritis.

phospholipase, *n* an enzyme that catalyzes the hydrolysis of a phospholipid.

phospholipase C, n an enzyme removing choline phosphate from a phosphatidylcholine.

phospholipid, *n* one of a class of compounds, widely distributed in living cells, containing phosphoric acid, fatty acids, and a nitrogenous base.

phosphoprotein, *n* a protein containing phosphoric groups attached to the side chains of some of its amino acids, usually serine, casein, and vitellin.

phosphorescence (fos" fo-res' əns), *adj* the seeming ability to glow in the dark; occurs in substances that continue to emit light following exposure to and subsequent removal of a radiation source.

phosphoric acid, *n* a clear, colorless, odorless liquid that is irritating to the skin and eyes and moderately toxic, if ingested. It is used in the production of fertilizers, soaps, detergents, animal feeds, and certain drugs.

phosphorus (P) (fos'fər-us), *n* a nonmetallic element; atomic weight, 30.98. It is essential, as is the phos-

phate, for the mineralization of the organic matrix of teeth and bone. It is also essential in the intermediary metabolism of carbohydrates as a vital constituent of the various intermediary compounds (e.g., glucose 6-phosphate) and of the enzyme systems (e.g., adenosine triphosphate [ATP]).

phosphorylation, *n* the addition of phosphate to an organic compound.

phosphotungstic acid (PTA), *n* a mixture of phosphoric and tungstic acids used with hematoxylin for staining muscle tissue and cell nuclei. It is also used as a negative stain of collagen in electron microscopy.

phossy jaw (fos'sē), *n* See *poisoning, phosphorus.*

phosvitin, *n* a phosphated protein with anticoagulant properties that is found in the egg yolk.

photogrammetry, *n* the process of making maps or surveys by the use of photographs.

photography, *n* the process of making images on a chemically sensitive plate or film, using the energy of light or other radiant source.

photometry, *n* the measurement of the intensity of light, usually in foot-candles.

photon (fō'ton), *n* a bullet or quantum of electromagnetic radiant energy emitted and propagated from various types of radiation sources. The term should not be used alone but should be qualified by terms that will clarify the type of energy (e.g., light photon, x-ray photon).

phylogeny, *n* the evolution or developmental history of a type of plant or animal.

physical, *adj* relating to the body, as distinguished from the mind.

physical examination, n a diagnostic inspection of the body to determine its state of health, using palpation, auscultation, percussion, and smell.

physical fitness, n the ability to carry out daily tasks with alertness and vigor, without undue fatigue, and with enough energy reserve to meet emergencies or to enjoy leisure time.

physical medicine, n the use of physical therapy techniques to return physically diseased or injured patients to a useful life.

physical plant, n the entire architectural and decorated suite of offices in which the dentist operates.

physical therapy, n the treatment of disorders with physical agents and methods, such as massage, manipulation, therapeutic exercises, cold, heat (including shortwave, microwave, and ultrasonic diathermy), hydrotherapy, electric stimulation, and light to assist in rehabilitating patients and in restoring normal function after an illness or injury. Also called *physiotherapy.*

physician, n a practitioner of medicine; one lawfully engaged in the practice of medicine.

Physician's Desk Reference (PDR), n a comprehensive reference book detailing the composition and accepted applications of pharmaceuticals from major manufacturers. A supplemental edition, which covers the effective use of herbal and botanical products, is available.

physics, n the study of material and energy, particularly as related to motion, force, heat, and light.

physiognomy, facial features.

physiologic occlusion, n See *occlusion, physiologic.*

physiologic rest position, n See *position, rest, physiologic.*

physiology (fiz′ē-ol′ə-jē), n study of tissue and organism behavior. The physiologic process is a dynamic state of tissue as compared with the static state of descriptive morphology (anatomy). Physiology is differentiated from descriptive morphology by the following qualifying properties: rate, direction, and magnitude. Physiologic processes are thus morphologic alterations in the three dimensions of space associated with a temporary (time) sequence. Physiologic processes relate to a wide spectrum of life activities on three levels: biochemical and biophysical activity of a subcellular nature, the activity of cells and tissues aggregated into organ systems, and multiorgan system activity as expressed in human behavior.

physiology, oral, n physiology related to clinical manifestations in the normal and abnormal behavior of oral structures. The principal clinical functions in which the oral structures participate are deglutition, mastication, respiration, speech, and head posture.

physioprints (fiz′ē-ō-prints), *n.pl* photographs obtained by projecting a grid on the subject's face and superimposing two exposures. The resultant picture gives a three-dimensional approach for the diagnosis of facial contours and swelling.

physiotherapy, oral (fiz′ē-ō-ther′ə-pē), n the collective procedures properly performed for the maintenance of personal hygiene of the mouth; those procedures necessary for cleanliness, tissue stimulation, tone, and preservation of the dentition. See also *aid in physiotherapy.*

physostigmine, n a cholinergic actylcholinesterase inhibitor prescribed in the treatment of some forms of glaucoma and to reverse effects of neuromuscular blocking agents.

phytic acid (fī′tik), n a component of some high-fiber foods, including many cereal grains that may, in excessive amounts, cause constipation or interfere with the body's ability to absorb minerals.

phytonadione, n (vitamin K_1) *trade names:* AquaMEPHYTON, Konakion, Mephyton; *drug class:* vitamin K_1, fat-soluble vitamin; *action:* needed for adequate blood clotting (factors II, VII, IX, X); *uses:* vitamin K malabsorption, hypoprothrombinemia, prevention of hypoprothrombinemia caused by oral anticoagulants.

pica (pī′kə), n a persistent, pathologic desire to eat nonfood items such as paper or dirt.

Pick's disease, *n.pr* See *disease, Niemann-Pick.*

pickling, n the process of cleansing from metallic surfaces the products of oxidation and other impurities by immersion in acid.

pickup impression, n See *impression, pickup.*

PICO, n acronym for diagnostic questions based on these four areas of knowledge and action: **P**atient or problem; **I**ntervention, cause, or prognosis; **C**omparison or control; and **O**utcome. This evidence-based method is designed to make a valid, successful decision based on the skills and knowledge of the clinician, the values of the patient, and the best available evidence.

Picornaviridae (pī-kôr′nə-vir′i-dā), *n* one of the major ribonucleic acid virus families, to which the polio-, rhino-, entero-, and hepatitis A viruses belong. Viruses in this family have a single-stranded, nonsegmented, linear molecular structure with icosahedral symmetry.

pie graph, *n* a circular diagram, sectioned by radial lines, used to represent distributions within a whole.

pier (pir), *n* an intermediate retaining or supporting abutment for a prosthesis. See also *abutment.*

Pierre Robin syndrome (pyer′ rō-ban′), *n.pr* See *retrognathism* and *syndrome, Pierre Robin.*

piezoelectric instruments (pī-ē′zō-ə-lek′trik), *n.pl* See *ultrasonic scalers, magnetostrictive.*

pigmentation, gingival, *n* See *gingival pigmentation.*

pigmentation, melanin, *n* the discoloration of tissues produced by the deposition of melanin. Seen normally in the oral mucous membranes (especially gingivae) of dark-complexioned individuals and abnormally in such conditions as adrenal hypofunction (Addison's disease).

pigtail explorer, *n* See *explorer, cowhorn.*

pilocarpine (pi″ lo-kahr′ pēn), *n* an alkaloid that causes parasympathetic effects (e.g., secretion of salivary, bronchial, and gastrointestinal glands). It stimulates the sweat glands and also causes vasodilation and cardiac inhibition.

pilocarpine HCl/pilocarpine nitrate (optic), *n trade names:* Adsorbocarpine, Akarpine, Isopto Carpine, Pilocar, Liquifilm, others *drug class:* miotic, cholinergic agonist; *action:* acts directly on cholinergic receptor sites; induces miosis, spasm of accommodation, fall in intraocular pressure; *uses:* primary glaucoma, early stages of wide-angle glaucoma; also used to neutralize mydriatics used during eye examination. Also taken internally for nondrug-induced xerostomia such as Sjögren's syndrome and head and neck cancer patients.

pilot program, *n* an experimental program designed to test administrative and operational procedures and to collect information on service demands and costs that will serve as a basis for operating programs efficiently.

pimozide, *n trade name:* Orap; *drug class:* antipsychotic, antidyskinetic; *action:* blocks dopamine effects on central nervous system; *uses:* motor and phonic tics in Giles de la Tourette's syndrome.

pin, *n* a small cylindrical piece of metal.

pin, cemented, n a metal rod cemented into a hole drilled into dentin to enhance retention of a restoration.

pin, friction-retained, n a metal rod driven or forced into a hole to enhance retention. It is retained solely by elasticity of dentin.

pin, incisal guide, n a metal rod that is attached to the upper member of an articulator and that touches the incisal guide table. It maintains the established vertical separation of the upper and lower arms of the articulator.

pin, retention, n the frictional grip of small metal projections extending from a metal casting into the dentin of the tooth.

pin, self-threading, n a pin screwed into a hole prepared in dentin to enhance retention.

pin, sprue, n **1.** a solid or hollow length of metal used to attach a pattern to the crucible former. *n* **2.** a metal pin used to form the hole that provides the pathway through the refractory investment to permit the entry of metal into a mold.

pin, Steinmann, n.pr a firm metal pin that is sharpened on one end; used for the fixation of fractures. It is sometimes passed through the maxilla or mandible to provide external points for attachment of upward-supporting devices.

pinch, *n* a small amount of chewing tobacco (snuff) an individual takes to use the substance for its desired effect. A "pinch" is called a *quid* in Britain.

pindolol, *n trade name:* Visken; *drug class:* nonselective β-adrenergic blocker; *action:* competitively blocks stimulation of β-adrenergic receptors within the heart and decreases renin activity, both of which may play a role in reducing systolic and diastolic blood pressure; *use:* mild-to-moderate hypertension.

pinna, *n* the external ear.

pinocytosis (pī″nō-sī-tō′sis), *n* See *phagocytosis.*

pipe tobacco, *n* dried tobacco leaves that come loosely packed in small, foldable bags for use in a handheld smoking implement that features a bowl on one end and a small cylinder for drawing in smoke on the other.

piperacillin sodium, *n* a semisynthetic extended spectrum penicillin active against a wide variety of grampositive and gram-negative bacteria.

piperazine (pi-per′ə-zēn), *n* an anthelmintic agent that acts against the roundworm *Ascaris lumbricoides* and the pinworm *Enterobius vermicularis* by interfering with their nerve transmissions, thereby causing paralysis.

pipette (pi-pet′), *n* a glass tube, usually graduated, which is used in the laboratory to measure and move liquids.

pirbuterol acetate, *n trade name:* Maxair; *drug class:* bronchodilator; *action:* causes bronchodilation with little effect on heart rate by acting on β-receptors, causing increased cAMP and relaxation of smooth muscle; *uses:* reversible bronchospasms (prevention, treatment), including asthma, may be given with theophylline or steroids.

piroxicam, *n trade name:* Feldene; *drug class:* nonsteroidal antiinflammatory; *action:* inhibits prostaglandin synthesis by interfering with cyclooxygenase needed for biosynthesis; possesses analgesic, antiinflammatory, antipyretic properties; *uses:* osteoarthritis, rheumatoid arthritis.

pit, *n* **1.** a small depression in enamel, usually located in a developmental groove where two or more enamel lobes are joined. *n* **2.** a depression in a restoration resulting from nonuniform density.

pit and fissure cavity, *n* See *cavity, pit and fissure.*

pit and fissure sealant, *n* See *sealant, pit and fissure.*

pituitary gland, *n* an endocrine gland suspended beneath the brain in the pituitary fossa of the sphenoid bone. It produces a number of hormones essential for growth, metabolism, reproduction, and vascular control.

pituitary hormones, *n.pl* the hormones of the anterior lobe of the pituitary gland controlled by hypothalamic releasing factors; they include growth hormone (somatotropin) prolactin, thyroid-luteinizing hormone, adrenocorticotropic hormone, and melanocyte-stimulating hormone. The posterior lobe is the source of vasopressin, which inhibits diuresis and raises blood pressure, and oxytocin, which stimulates the contraction of smooth muscle, especially in the uterus.

Pituitrin (pi-tōō′ə-trin), *n.pr* trade name for an extract of the posterior lobe of the pituitary gland.

pityriasis rosea (pit-ə-rī′ ə-sis rō′zē-ə), *n* a noncontagious skin disease with reddish, scaly patches and moderate fever.

pivot, adjustable occlusal, *n* an occlusal pivot that may be adjusted vertically by means of a screw or by other means.

pivot, occlusal, *n* an elevation artificially developed on the occlusal surface, usually in the molar region, and designed to induce sagittal mandibular rotation.

pK_a, *n* a mathematical function analogous to the calculation of pH. It is the negative log (p) of the constant of acid dissociation (K_a). When the pK_a of a buffering agent equals the pH of the solution to be buffered, the buffering system is most effective. According to the Henderson Hasselbach equation, pK_a = pH + log ([HOAc]/[OAc-]).

placebo (plə-sē-bō), *n* a substance that resembles medicine superficially and is believed by the patient to be medicine but that has no intrinsic drug activity.

placebo effect, *n* the real or imagined effect of a placebo, which may actually be the same effect ordinarily associated with the administration of a therapeutically active agent.

placement, *n* the act of placing an object (i.e., removable denture in its planned location on the dental arch).

placement, choice of path of, *n* determination of the direction of placement and removal of a removable partial denture on its supporting oral structures, which can be varied by altering the plane to which the guiding abutment surfaces are made parallel. The choice is a compromise to best fulfill five demands: to subject abutment teeth to a minimum or no torquing force, to encounter the least interference, to provide needed retention, to establish adequate guidingplane surfaces, and to provide acceptable aesthetics.

Placenta. (Moore/Persaud, 2003)

placenta, *n* the organ of metabolic interchange between the fetus and the mother.

placenta abruptio **(ə-brup'shē-ō),** *n* a condition in which a typically positioned placenta detaches from the uterine wall prior to delivery, which may threaten viability of both baby and mother.

placenta previa **(plə-sen'tə prē'vē-ə),** *n* atypical placental positioning and attachment within the lower third of uterus, which may cover the cervix in part or fully.

placodes (plak' ōds), *n.pl* thick, flat sections of embryonic ectoderm from which the sense organs develop.

plagiarism, *n* appropriation of the work, ideas, or words of another without proper acknowledgment.

plague, *n* **1.** any disease of wide prevalence or of excessive mortality. *n* **2.** the vernacular term for bubonic plague, marked by inflammatory enlargement of the lymphatic glands, particularly in the axillae and groins.

plaintiff, *n* the party who sues in a personal legal action and who is so designated on the record.

plan, *n* program of action.

plan, bank, *n* See *bank plan.*

plan, preventive care, *n* a long-term strategy designed to preclude the development of a disease and promote overall health. See also *preventive dentistry* and *preventive orthodontic treatment.*

plan, provisional treatment, *n* tentative treatment plan that may be modified or continued upon reevaluation of periodontal status after initial therapeutic procedures.

plan, treatment, *n* the intended sequence of procedures for the treatment of a patient.

plane, *n* an ideal flat surface that intersects solid bodies, extends uniformly in various directions (horizontally, vertically, laterally, or any relative combination thereof), and is determined by the position in space of three points.

Body in anatomical position with the median, sagittal, horizontal, and frontal planes noted. (Fehrenbach/Herring, 2002)

plane, axial, n a hypothetical plane parallel to the long axis of an object.

   plane, axial, of teeth, n term that applies to the mesiodistal or the buccolingual plane.

   plane, axial wall, n an instrument used to plane and true the axial wall of a Class 3 preparation.

plane, axiobuccolingual, of teeth, n See *plane of teeth, buccolingual.*

plane, axiomesiodistal, of teeth, n See *plane of teeth, mesiodistal.*

plane, bite, n an appliance that covers the palate. It has an inclined or flat plane at its anterior border that offers resistance to the mandibular incisors when they come into contact with it. Also called *bite plate.*

plane, Bolton-nasion, n.pr imaginary surface passing through the nasion and the postcondylar notch, used in cephalometric analysis. See also *point, Bolton.*

plane, Broca's (Brōk-əz), n.pr a plane extending from the tip of the interalveolar septum between the upper central incisors to the lowermost point of the occipital condyle.

plane, brushing, n the top uniform edge of the bristles on the head of a toothbrush; forms the surface that comes in contact with teeth and gingival margin when brushing. The plane comes in a variety of designs that assist the user to remove plaque and clean the gingiva. Also called *trim.*

plane, buccolingual, of teeth, *n* a plane that passes through the tooth buccolingually parallel with its long axis. In incisors and canines, this is the labiolingual plane. Also called *axiobuccolingual plane.*

plane, Camper's, *n.pr* a plane extending from the inferior border of the ala of the nose to the superior border of the tragus of the ear.

plane, coronal, *n* in anatomy, the imaginary, flat vertical surface used to divide the body into anterior (frontal) and posterior (back) regions. Also called the *frontal plane.*

plane, eye-ear, *n* See *plane, Frankfort horizontal.*

plane, flush terminal, *n* a relationship between primary teeth in which the buccal surfaces of the opposing second molars are aligned when occlusion is centric.

plane, Frankfort horizontal, *n.pr* a craniometric plane determined by the inferior borders of the bony orbits and the upper margin of the auditory meatus. It passes through the two orbitales and the two tragions.

plane, guide, *n* **1.** a mechanical device, part of an orthodontic appliance, having an established inclined plane that, when in use, causes a change in the occlusal relation of the maxillary and mandibular teeth and permits their movement to a normal position. *n* **2.** a plane developed in the occlusal surfaces of occlusion rims to position the mandible in centric relation. *n* **3.** two or more vertically parallel surfaces of abutment teeth shaped to direct the path of placement and removal of a remarkable partial denture. Also called *guiding plane.*

plane, guiding, *n* See *plane, guide.*

plane, Hamy's, *n.pr* a plane extending from the glabella to the lambda.

plane, His's, *n.pr* a plane extending from the anterior nasal spine to the opisthion.

plane, horizontal, *n* a plane that is parallel to the horizon and perpendicular to the vertical plane.

plane, horizontal, of teeth, *n* a plane that is perpendicular to the long axis of the tooth and may be supposed to cut through the crown at any point in its length.

plane, Huxley's, *n.pr* a plane extending from the nasion to the basion. Also called the *basicranial axis.*

plane, mandibular, *n* See *border, mandibular.*

plane, Martin's, *n.pr* a plane extending from the nasion to the inion.

plane, mean foundation, *n* the mean of the inclination of the denture-supporting (basal seat) tissues. The tissues constituting the denture foundation are irregular in form and consistency, and force may be applied from only one direction if it is to comply with the law of statics, which requires the exertion of force at a right angle to maintain support. Therefore the mean foundation plane forms a right angle with the most favorable direction of force. The ideal condition for denture stability exists when the mean foundation plane is almost at a right angle to the direction of force.

plane, mean occlusal, *n* the flat or horizontal plane or position and area between the cutting edge of the teeth.

plane, median, *n* See *plane, midsagittal.*

plane, median sagittal, *n* a plane passing through the median raphe of the palate at right angles to the Frankfort horizontal plane.

plane, median-raphe, *n* the median plane of the head.

plane, mesiodistal, of teeth, *n* a plane that passes through the tooth mesiodistally parallel with its long axis. Also called *axiomesiodistal plane.*

plane, midsagittal (mid-saj′ə-təl), *n* in anatomy, the imaginary, flat vertical surface that bisects the midline of the body used to divide the body into right and left regions. Also called the *median plane.*

plane, Montague's, *n.pr* the plane extending from the nasion to the porion.

plane, occlusal, *n* **1.** an imaginary surface that is related anatomically to the cranium and that theoretically touches the incisal edges of the incisors and tips of the occluding surfaces of the posterior teeth. It is not a plane in the true sense of the word but represents the mean of the curvature of the surface. *n* **2.** a line drawn between points representing one half of the incisal overbite (vertical overlap) in front and one-half of the cusp height of the last molars in back. See also curve of occlusion.

plane of reference, n a plane that acts as a guide to the location of other planes.

plane of teeth, n for descriptive purposes, three planes are considered in the teeth proper: buccolingual, horizontal, and mesiodistal.

plane, orbital, n **I.** a plane perpendicular to the eye-ear plane and passing through the orbitale. *n* **2.** the plane that passes through the visual axis of each eye.

plane, sagittal, n any anteroposterior plane of the body parallel to the median sagittal plane.

plane, Schwalbe's **(shvӓl'bez),** *n.pr* a plane that extends from the glabella to the inion.

plane, vertical, of teeth, n an upright plane that is perpendicular to the horizon.

plane, von Ihring's, n.pr a plane extending from the orbitale to the center of the bony external auditory meatus.

plaque (plak), *n* a flat plate or tablet.

plaque, cocci in **(kok'sī),** *n.pl* the gram-positive microorganisms occurring in early-developing plaque that are later replaced with filaments as the plaque matures.

plaque, epithelium-associated, n loosely-attached bacterial plaque found in the epithelium of the periodontal pocket that consists of gram-negative microorganisms and white blood cells.

plaque, fissure, n bacterial plaque that develops in the crevices of a tooth.

plaque, mucin, n a sticky substance that accumulates on the teeth. It is composed of mucin derived from the saliva and of bacteria and their products, and is often responsible for the inception of caries and for gingival inflammation.

plaque, pigmented dental, n similar to calculus in that bacteria thrive within it. It is not related to the development of gingivitis and is often found in mouths that are almost plaque free. The condition may be controlled by diligent plaque removal, but reoccurrence is possible. Also called *black line stain.*

plaque, subgingival, n a thick, noncalcified mass of bacteria situated inferior to the gingival margin. It may or may not be attached to the epithelium or tooth and may cover subgingival calculus. It cannot be removed with flow of saliva or water.

plaque, supragingival **(sōō'prə-jin-ji'vəl),** *n* a thick, noncalcified mass of bacteria superior to the gingival margin. It cannot be removed with flow of saliva or water.

Supragingival plaque. (Newman/Takei/Carranza, 2002)

plaque, tooth-surface-attached, n a type of plaque that uses selective attachment factors and is located in the subgingival area. This type of plaque is implicated in the formation of caries in the root calculus, and eventual breakdown of the root (resorption).

plasma (plaz'mə), *n* the fluid portion of the blood that, after centrifugation, contains all the stable components except the cells. It is obtained from centrifuged whole blood that has been prevented from clotting by the addition of anticoagulants such as citrate, oxalate, or heparin.

plasma accelerator globulin, n See *proaccelerin* and *accelerator, prothrombin conversion, I.*

plasma cell, n a lymphoid or lymphocyte-like cell found in the bone marrow, connective tissue, and sometimes the blood. Plasma cells are involved in the immunologic mechanism.

plasma, normal human, n pooled sterile plasma from a number of persons to which a preservative has

P

been added. It is stored under refrigeration or desiccated for later use as a substitute for whole blood.

plasma proteolytic enzyme, *n* See *plasmin.*

plasma thromboplastin antecedent, *n* a factor required for the development of thromboplastic activity in plasma. Also called *antihemophilic factor C, factor XI, PTA,* and *plasma thromboplastin factor C.*

plasma thromboplastin component, *n* a clotting factor in normal blood necessary for the development of thromboplastic activity in plasma. A deficiency results in Christmas disease. Also called *antihemophilic factor B, autoprothrombin II, Christmas factor, factor IX, platelet cofactor II,* and *PTC.* See also factor IX.

plasmacytoma (plaz'məsītō'mə), *n* the primary soft tissue plasma cell tumors of the oral, pharyngeal, and nasal mucous membranes. The lesion consists of typical and atypical plasma cells, and its behavior is unpredictable. See also myeloma, solitary plasma cell and dyscrasia.

plasmacytoma, soft tissue, *n* a primary plasma cell tumor of the nasal, pharyngeal, and oral mucosa that has no apparent primary bone involvement. The lesions are sessile or polypoid sessile masses in the mucous membrane. The majority remain localized, but metastases have been reported.

plasmid, *n* any type of intracellular inclusion considered to have a genetic function.

plasmin (plaz'min), *n* collective term for one or more proteolytic enzymes found in the blood. The proteolytic enzymes are capable of digesting fibrin, fibrinogen, and proaccelerin. Plasminogen, the inactive form, may become active spontaneously in shed blood. An activator, fibrinokinase (fibrinolysokinase), is found in many animal tissues. Also called *fibrinolysin, lysin, plasma proteolytic enzyme,* and *tryptase.*

plasminogen (plaz-min'ō-jen), *n* the precursor of plasmin found in plasma. It is probably activated by a tissue factor or by a blood activator, which first must be activated by a blood or tissue fibrinolysokinase. Formerly called *profibrinolysin.*

plaster (plas'tur), *n* colloquial term applied to dental plaster of paris.

plaster headcap, *n* See *headcap, plaster.*

plaster, impression, *n* plaster used for making impressions. Sets rapidly and is characterized by low-setting expansion and strength.

plaster, model, *n* plaster used for diagnostic casts and as an investing material.

plaster of paris, *n* the hemihydrate of calcium sulfate that, when mixed with water, forms a paste that subsequently sets into a hard mass. See also *beta-hemihydrate.*

plastic, *n* **1.** a restorative material (e.g., amalgam, cement, gutta-percha, resin) that is soft at the time of insertion and may then be shaped or molded, after which it will harden or set. *adj* **2.** malleable; capable of being molded.

plastic base, *n* See *base, plastic.*

plastic closure, *n* suturing of tissues that involves their displacement by sliding or rotation to create a surgical closure.

plastic strip, *n* a clear plastic strip of celluloid or acrylic resin used as a matrix when silicate cement or acrylic is inserted into proximal prepared cavities in anterior teeth.

plastic surgery, *n* branch of medicine that deals with the surgical alteration, replacement, restoration, or reconstruction of a visible part of the body to correct a structural or cosmetic defect.

plasticity (plas-tis'i-tē), *n* **1.** the quality of being moldable or workable. *n* **2.** the degree of permanent deformation resulting from stress application, usually associated with substances that are classed as solids or semirigid liquids.

plate, lingual, *n* See *connector, linguoplate major.*

plate, metal, *n* a titanium or stainless steel plate that is fastened to the bone by screws to bridge a fracture line and stabilizes bone fragments.

plate, palatal, See *connector, major.*

platelet (plāt'let), *n* a disk found in the blood of mammals that is concerned in the coagulation and clotting of blood.

platelet ac-globulin, *n* See *factor, platelet, 1.*

P

platelet activating factor, n 1-0-alkyl-2-sn-glycero-3-phosphocholine. A phospholipid derivative formed by platelets, basophils, neutrophils, monocytes, and macrophages. It is a potent platelet aggregating agent and inducer of systemic anaphylactic symptoms, including hypotension, thrombocytopenia, neutropenia, and bronchoconstriction.

platelet aggregation, n a clumping together of platelets in vitro, and likely in vivo, by a number of agents, such as adenosine diphosphate, thrombin, and collagen, as part of a sequential mechanism leading to the initiation and formation of a thrombus or hemostatic plug.

platelet aggregation inhibitors, n.pl drugs or agents that antagonize or impair any mechanism leading to blood platelet aggregation.

platelet cofactor I, n See *factor VIII.*

platelet cofactor II, n See *factor IX* and *plasma thromboplastin component.*

platelet count, n the number of platelets found in 1 mm^3 of blood; the normal range is between 200,000 and 300,000 platelets.

platelet disorder, n See *disorder, platelet.*

platelet transfusion, n **1.** the transfer of blood platelets from a donor to a recipient or reinfusion to the donor. n **2.** a treatment modality used in treating hemophilia and other conditions of impaired blood coagulation.

platinum (Pt), n a silvery-white, soft metallic element. Its atomic number is 78 and atomic weight is 195.09. Platinum is used in dentistry, jewelry, and the manufacture of chemical apparatuses that must withstand high temperatures.

platinum matrix, n See *matrix, platinum.*

Platyhelminthes (plat´ē-hel-min´thēz), n. pl parasitic flatworms, such as tapeworms and flukes, that cause disease in humans.

pleadings, n.pl written allegations of what is affirmed on the one side or denied on the other, disclosing the real matter to the court or jury having to try the case.

pledget (plej´ət), n a minute pellet of absorbent cotton used for accurately controlled placement of medication or base. See also *cotton, absorbent.*

pleomorphic adenoma (plē´ō-môr´fik ad´ən-ō´mə), n a benign tumor of the salivary gland containing varying proportions of epithelial and mesenchymal elements. The intermediate type of epithelial cells is in sheets, cords, and acini. The mesenchymal tissue varies from myxomatous to cartilaginous to densely hyalinized connective tissue. The marked variations in histologic pattern are responsible for the designation of pleomorphic. Also called *mixed salivary gland tumor.*

Pleomorphic adenoma. (Sapp/Eversole/Wysocki, 2004)

pleomorphism, n the ability to change shape or form

plethora (pleth´ər-ə), n a nonspecific increase in blood bulk. Clinically, the patient is flushed and has a feeling of tenseness in the head; the blood vessels are full, and the pulse is firm.

pleura, n a delicate serous membrane enclosing the lung, composed of a single layer of flattened mesothelial cells resting on a delicate membrane of connective tissue.

pleurisy (plur´əs-ē), n an inflammation of the pleura, with exudation into its cavity and on its surface.

plexus (plek´sus), n a network or tangle, especially of nerves, lymphatics, or veins.

plexus, Haller's, n.pr a nerve plexus of sympathetic filaments and branches of the external laryngeal nerve on the surface of the inferior constrictor muscle of the larynx.

plexus, intermediate, n a middle zone of the periodontal membrane situated between the cemental group of fibers attached to the root of the tooth and the alveolar group of fibers attached to the alveolar bone. The three groups of fibers are woven together by small, thick strands of collagen fibers. The interweaving of fiber bundles of the intermediate plexus allows for tooth eruption and tooth movement between the cemental and alveolar periodontal fibers.

plica fimbriata (plī-kā fim'brē-āt-ā), *n* a fringed fold located on the ventral surface of the tongue near the location where it attaches to the floor of the mouth.

pliers, *n* a tool of pincer design with jaws of varying shapes; used for holding, bending, stretching, contouring, and cutting.

pliers, contouring, *n* pliers with jaws curved to permit developing tooth contours in banding metal.

pliers, cotton, *n* a slender, tweezer-like instrument used to hold cotton pellets or pledgets, apply medicaments, and carry small objects to and from the mouth.

pliers, stretching, *n* pliers whose jaws are designed as a hammer and anvil, with the handles sufficiently long to develop a high leverage ratio. It is used to enlarge metal bands (gold, aluminum, copper) or to thin the contact area of matrix bands.

plosive (plo'siv), *n* any speech sound made by impounding the airstream for a moment until considerable pressure has been developed and then suddenly releasing it (e.g., *b, d,* and *g*). One of two types of stop consonants, the other being affricative (e.g., *ch*).

plug, *n* a peg or any mass filling a hole or closing an orifice.

plugger, *n* an instrument used to compress the filling material in an apical and lateral direction when a root canal is being filled. See also *condenser.*

plumbism (plum'biz-əm), *n* acute or chronic intoxication resulting from the ingestion, inhalation, or skin absorption of lead. Manifestations of acute poisoning include abdominal pain, paralysis, metallic taste, and collapse. Chronic manifestations include gastrointestinal disturbances, headache, peripheral neuropathy (foot drop and wrist drop), lead in the urine and blood, basophilic granular degeneration, coproporphyrinuria, and stomatitis. Also called *lead poisoning,* and *saturnism.* See also *stomatitis, lead.*

Plummer-Vinson syndrome, *n.pr* See *syndrome, Plummer-Vinson.*

plunger cusp, *n* a stamp cusp, the tip of which is made to occlude in an embrasure; its shoulder has not been restored to occlude in a fossa.

plutonium (Pu), *n* a synthetic transuranic metallic element. Its atomic number is 94 and its atomic weight is 242. A highly toxic waste product of nuclear power plants, plutonium was used in the assembly of early nuclear weapons.

PMA (papillary-marginal-attached), *n* a system of epidemiologic scoring of periodontal disease devised by Schour and Massler in which the symbols denote the areas involved in gingival inflammation.

pneumatic condenser (nōō-mat'ik), *n* See *condenser, pneumatic.*

pneumococcal pneumonia, *n* See *Streptococcus pneumoniae.*

pneumoconiosis, any disease of the lung caused by chronic inhalation of dust, usually mineral dusts of occupational or environmental origin. The principal agents include coal, cotton, sand, and asbestos.

Pneumocystis carinii (nōō'mō-sis'tis kər-in'ē-ī), *n* an opportunistic infection found in immunocompromised patients such as those with acquired immune deficiency syndrome.

pneumocystis pneumonia, *n* See *Pneumocystis carinii.*

pneumonia, *n* an acute inflammation of the lungs, usually caused by inhaled microorganisms. The alveoli and bronchioles of the lungs become plugged with a fibrous exudate, seriously interfering with oxygen exchange.

pneumonitis (nōō'mō-nī'tis), *n* an inflammation of the lungs of an acute, localized nature.

pneumothorax (nōō'mō-thôr'aks), *n* an accumulation of air or gas in the pleural cavity. The air enters by way of an external wound, a lung perforation, a burrowing abscess, or rupture of a superficial lung cavity. Pneumothorax is accompanied by sudden, severe pain and rapidly increasing dyspnea.

P

pocket, *n* **1.** a diseased gingival attachment, characterized by gingival discoloration, retraction of gingivae from the tooth, bleeding, the presence of an exudate, and loss of the presence of stippling. *n* **2.** a space bordered on one side by the tooth and on the opposite side by ulcerated crevicular epithelium and limited at its apex by the epithelial attachment.

pocket, bleeding, *n* an occurrence that denotes ulcerations of the pocket epithelium, with hemorrhaging through the broken surface from exposed connective tissue capillaries.

pocket bottom, *n* the base of the pocket, marked or limited by the epithelial attachment to the cementum of the root (periodontal pocket) or the enamel of the crown (gingival pocket).

pocket, calculus, *n* calcified deposits that usually occupy the entire pocket. It is attached to the tooth structure, with the gingival tissues tightly adapted to the surface of the calculus.

pocket, deepening, *n* an increase of the depth of the pocket, which depends on apical proliferation of the epithelial attachment alongside the cementum, with subsequent separation from the tooth, or on hyperplasia of the gingivae resulting from inflammation.

pocket, depth of, *n* the measurement, usually expressed in millimeters, of the distance between the gingival crest and the base of the pocket.

pocket, elimination, *n* the application of therapeutic measures to obtain a healthy gingival attachment and an intact, functioning attachment apparatus. The procedures employed include curettage (root and gingival), reattachment, or new attachment operations, gingivectomy and gingivoplasty, and osseous and mucogingival surgical procedures.

pocket, gingival, *n* a pseudopocket; gingival inflammation with edema, hyperplasia, and ulceration of the sulcular epithelium but without apical proliferation of the epithelial attachment.

pocket in marginal periodontitis, *n* a condition in which the inflammatory process has progressed from the gingival tissues to the underlying alveolar process. The changes are those associated with gingivitis plus resorptive bone lesions. The base of the pocket is at the marginal point of the union of the epithelial attachment to the cementum of the root.

pocket, infrabony, *n* a periodontal pocket, the base of which is apical to the crest of the alveolar bone. Consists basically of a vertical resorptive defect in alveolar and supporting bone, overlying which are a band of transseptal fibers connecting adjacent teeth, disintegrated fibers of gingival corium, inflammatory cellular infiltrate, and hyperplastic pocket epithelium, accompanied by apical migration of the epithelial attachment. Clinical signs are those of periodontitis, associated with radiographic evidence of vertical bone resorption. The infrabony pocket has been classified according to the number of remaining osseous walls supporting it for the purpose of therapeutic rationale. Also called *infracrestal pocket, intraalveolar pocket,* and *intrabony pocket.*

pocket, infracrestal, *n* See *pocket, infrabony.*

pocket, intraalveolar, *n* See *pocket, infrabony.*

pocket, intrabony, *n* See *pocket, infrabony.*

pocket ionization chamber, *n* See *chamber, ionization.*

pocket, marking, *n* the accurate determination and delineation of pocket depth and topography as an aid to diagnosis and prognosis or to provide a guide for the gingivectomy incision.

pocket, periodontal, *n* a pathologic deepening of the gingival sulcus produced by destruction of the supporting tissues and apical proliferation of the epithelial attachment. Ulceration of the pocket epithelium lining is characteristic.

pocket surgery, *n* a generic term referring to gingivectomy and gingivoplasty. See also *gingivectomy* and *gingivoplasty.*

podiatry, *n* a health profession that deals with the diagnosis and treatment of diseases and other disorders of the feet.

pogonion (pō-gō′nē-on), *n* the most anterior point on the chin. A cephalometric landmark in the lateral view.

poikilocytosis (poi'ki-lō-sī-tō'sis), *n* the presence in the blood of irregularly shaped red blood cells.

point, *n* **1.** a small spot or a minute area. *n* **2.** a rotating instrument having a small cutting end or surface.

point A, n the deepest point in the bony concavity in the midline at the base of the anterior nasal spine, in the region of the incisor roots. A landmark on the lateral cephalometric view.

point, abrasive, rotary, n small abrasive instruments used in straight or contraangle handpieces. Also called *mounted carborundum, diamond.*

point angle, n See *angle, point.*

point B, n a mandibular point comparable to point A.

point, bleeding, n See *bleeding points.*

point, boiling, n the temperature at which the vapor pressure within a liquid equals atmospheric pressure.

point, Bolton, n the highest point of the curvature between the occipital condyle and the basilar part of the occipital bone and located behind the occipital condyle. A substitute for the basion point when it cannot be ascertained on cephalometric headplates.

point, central-bearing, n the contact point of a central-bearing device. See also *central-bearing device.*

point, condenser, n the nib of a condensing instrument. A short instrument, for condensing foil or amalgam, that is inserted into a mechanical condenser or into a cone socket handle.

point, contact, n the area of contact of approximating surfaces of two adjacent teeth. The areas of contact are located at the line of junction between the occlusal and middle thirds of the posterior teeth and the incisal and middle thirds of the anterior teeth. Also called *contact area.*

point, convenience, n a small undercut in the cavity wall convenient for placing and retaining the first portion of a filling material. It is generally one of the retention points placed in a cavity preparation that provides the best access to the operator.

point D, n the center of the body of the symphysis.

point, faulty contact, n a defective contact between the proximal surfaces of adjacent teeth, produced by wearing of the contact areas, dental caries, improper restoration, or altered tooth position.

point, gutta-percha, n See *gutta-percha points.*

point, hinge axis, n a point placed on the skin corresponding with the opening axis of the mandible.

point, Hirschfeld's silver, n.pr a calibrated silver rod used to record the clinical depth of periodontal pockets radiographically for the purpose of diagnosis.

point, incisor, n the intersection of the lower occlusal and midsagittal planes. The point at the mesioincisal angles of the two mandibular central incisors.

point, loss of contact, n the failure of contact of convex proximal surfaces of adjacent teeth; produced by tooth migration, dental caries, or improper restoration.

point, median mandibular, n a point on the anteroposterior center of the mandibular ridge in the median sagittal plane.

point of centricity, n if the point of the buccal cusp of the lower right molar, put in lateral position, arcs around the upright axis of the right condyle, it will reach a station where further muscular efforts leftward will change the cusp's direction so that it will arc around the left condyle. The station where the right arc ends and the left arc begins is a point of mandibular centricity. While the right cusp point orbits (arcs) around the near vertical axis, all other points in the jaw join in orbiting (arcing). The left condyle arcs rearward until it reaches a cranial backstop; then the muscles start rotating it and carrying it leftward, and the right condyle begins arcing forward, downward, and medially. In the right and left swings of the jaw, a condyle reciprocally alternates between being a rotator and an orbiter. The point of centricity of the mandible is demonstrated usually on a horizontal plane, but it can be demonstrated on all three planes of projection. The point of centricity is rearmost, midmost (between the arcs of motion), and uppermost. See also *face-bow* and *relation, centric.*

point, paper, n See *paper point.*

point, registration, n any point considered as fixed for a particular pattern of analysis. Also, the midpoint of a perpendicular line from the sella turcica to the Bolton-nasion plane.

point, transition, n See *Tg value.*

point, treatment, n a piece of paper point, selected for the root canal being treated, that carries or holds the medication in place.

point, trial, n a cone of filling material placed in a canal and radiographed to check on the length and fit of the filling.

point, trigger, n the point from which referred pain initiates. In the myofascial pain syndrome, usually a localized, deep tenderness in a taut bundle of muscle fibers from which pain is referred to other sites.

point, yield, n **1.** the place on the stress-strain curve where marked permanent deformation occurs. It is just beyond the proportional limit. n **2.** the point where permanent deformation starts in a metal.

pointing, n fluctuation pertaining to the area where the purulent exudate is eroding through tissues to an external surface. At this point an incision and drainage operation usually is performed.

poison, n a substance that, when ingested, inhaled, absorbed, injected into, or developed within the body, will cause damage to structures of the body and impair or destroy their function.

poisoning, n the morbid condition caused by exposure to poison.

poisoning, arsenic, n acute or chronic intoxication from the ingestion of insecticides or administration of organic arsenicals. Manifestations of acute poisoning include abdominal pain, nausea, vomiting, and collapse. Chronic manifestations include weakness, peripheral neuropathy, hyperkeratosis, skin rashes, and oral manifestations secondary to liver dysfunction and bone marrow depression. See also *stomatitis, arsenical.*

poisoning, bismuth, n See *bismuthosis.*

poisoning, chemical, n a form of poisoning caused by ingestion of a toxic chemical agent.

poisoning, iodine, n See *iodism.*

poisoning, lead, n See *plumbism.*

poisoning, mercury, n See *mercurialism.*

poisoning, metallic, n a toxic condition produced by excessive exposure to or intake of metals. In the oral cavity there may be definite signs of arsenic, bismuth, lead, phosphorus, radium, and other metals. Fluorides produce changes in developing teeth at levels far below those that are toxic for the rest of the human economy.

poisoning, phosphorus, n the result of the ingestion of phosphorus, especially yellow phosphorus. Manifestations include burning of the mouth and throat, abdominal pain, vomiting, jaundice, liver damage, and death. In chronic poisoning, necrosis of the jaws (phossy jaw) occurs.

polacrilex (pol′ə-kril′eks), n See *nicotine, polacrilex.*

police power, n the authority of the state to enact laws to protect the public, such as a dental practice act. Police power is reserved to the states under the United States Constitution.

policy, n the document embodying the insurance contract.

policy holder, n under a group purchase plan, the employer, labor union, or trustee to whom a group contract is issued. In a plan providing for individual or family enrollment, the person to whom the contract is issued.

policy period, n the time during which an insurance contract affords protection.

policy year, n the year commencing with the effective date of the insurance contract or with an anniversary of that date.

poliomyelitis (pō′lē-ō-mī′ ə-lī′tis), n a disease produced by a small viral organism that enters the body via the alimentary tract and produces upper pharyngeal, pharyngeal, and intestinal inflammation in its mentor form. In the more severe variety, a subsequent viremia is produced, with extension of the infection to the anterior pulp horn cells and ganglia of the spinal cord, producing a flaccid paralysis. In *bulbar poliomyelitis* the viral infection involves the medulla, resulting in impairment of swallowing, respiration, and circulation. It is now recognized that three types of viruses are responsible for the non-paralytic, paralytic, and bulbar varieties of poliomyelitis. Excellent immunization procedures have been provided by use of killed viruses (Salk) and attenuated mutant vaccines (Sabin).

polishing, *n* the process of making a surface smooth and glossy or giving luster to a surface, usually by friction.

polishing brush, n See *brush, polishing.*

polishing, coronal, n the removal of mucinous film, superficial stain, or deposits to provide a smooth enamel surface that will be more resistant to future accumulation of foreign substances such as materia alba, calculus, and mucinous plaque.

polishing cup, n the working end of a powered rotary tooth-polishing tool. Attached in various ways including mounted, threaded, or slip-on and is made from synthetic or natural rubber.

polishing disk, n See *disk, polishing.*

polishing, prophy jet, n an alternative to traditional rubber cup polishing that uses a pressurized spray of water mixed with a baking soda paste to clean plaque from teeth and polish them. The pressurized water removes plaque, while the baking soda acts as a combination stain remover and acid neutralizer.

polishing, selective, n a method of rubber cup polishing in which selected teeth are targeted for stain removal. This method helps minimize the loss of enamel on natural teeth and decreases the possibility of damage to restorations, such as porcelain crowns, or to exposed root surfaces.

politics, *n* the art and science of governance, particularly in a democracy or collegial body.

pollakiuria (pol′ə-kē-yōō′rē-ə), *n* unduly frequent urination. It may result from partial obstruction, such as prostatic enlargement, or it may be of nervous origin.

pollen, *n* a fertilizing element of plants that travels in the air and produces seasonal allergic responses such as hay fever or asthma in sensitive individuals.

polyamines, *n.pl* many amines; polymers of amine, many of which normally occur in body constituents of wide distribution and are essential growth factors for microorganisms.

polyantibiotic (pol′ē-an′ti-bī-ot′ik), *n* a combination of two or more antibiotics used to eliminate bacteria from a root canal.

polycarboxylate cement, *n* See *cement.*

polychlorinated biphenyls, *n.pl* more than 30 isomers and compounds used in plastics, insulation, and flame retardants and varying in physical form from oily liquid to crystals and resins. All are potentially toxic and carcinogenic. Mild exposure may cause chloracne; severe exposure may result in hepatic damage.

polychromatophilla (pol′ē-krō-mat′ō-fil′ē-ə), *n* an irregular staining of cells, particularly red blood cells.

Polycillin (pol′ē-sil′in), *n.pr* the trade name for ampicillin, an acid-stable semisynthetic penicillin effective against some gram-negative and gram-positive organisms.

polycythemia (pol′ē-sī-thē′mē-ə), *n* an increase in blood volume as a result of an increase in the number of red blood cells, the erythrocytes. It may result from a blood-forming disease that increases cell production, or it may be a physiologic response to an increased need for oxygenation in high altitudes, cardiac disease, or respiratory disorders.

polycythemia, phlebotomy for, n the drawing of blood to check for an overabundance of red blood cells.

polycythemia, primary, n See *erythremia.*

polycythemia, relative, n an overabundance of red blood cells due to plasma loss.

polycythemia rubra, n See *erythremia.*

polycythemia, secondary, n See *erythrocytosis.*

polycythemia vera, n See *erythremia.*

polydactyly (pol′ē-dak′tilē), *n* a congenital anomaly characterized by the presence of more than the normal number of fingers or toes. It may be a part of a complex genetic syndrome. Early surgical treatment is generally used to correct the problem.

Polydactyly. (Moore/Persaud, 2003, courtesy of AE Chudley)

polydipsia (pol'ē-dip'sē-ə), *n* abnormally increased thirst.

polyglycolic acid, *n* a polymer of glycolic acid, used in absorbable surgical sutures.

polygon frequency (pol'ē-gon), *n* a type of graph using lines to display uninterrupted data.

polymer (pol'e-mur), *n* a long-chain hydrocarbon. In dentistry, the polymer is supplied as a powder to be mixed with the monomer for fabrication of appliances and restorations.

polymerase chain reaction (PCR), *n* a process whereby a strand of deoxyribonucleic acid can be cloned millions of times within a few hours. The process can be used to make prenatal diagnoses of genetic diseases and to identify an individual by analysis of a single tissue cell.

polymerization (pol'i-mər'i-zā'shən), *n* the chaining together of similar molecules to form a compound of high molecular weight.

polymerization, addition, *n* a compound formed by a combination of simple molecules without the formation of any new products; for example, methylmethacrylate.

polymerization, condensation, *n* the combination of simple, dissimilar molecules, with the formation of byproducts such as water or ammonia (e.g., vulcanite).

polymerization, cross, *n* (cross linkage, cross-linked polymerization), the formation of chemical bonds between linear molecules, resulting in a three-dimensional network. Used for artificial teeth and denture bases because of superior craze resistance.

polymerization, cross-linked, *n* See *polymerization, cross.*

polymerization, photo, *n* process in which a light source is used for polymerization

polymorphonuclear leukocytes (pol'ē-môr'fō-nōō'klē-ər lōō'kō-sīts), *n.pl* white blood cells with nuclei of varied forms.

polymyxin (pol'ē-mik'sin), *n* an antibiotic substance derived from cultures of *Bacillus polymyxa.* Used topically, in troche form, in combination with bacitracin and neomycin in the treatment of various oral infections. Not used systemically; therefore sensitization is minimized. Systemic use may be attended by renal dysfunction and toxicity.

polymyxin B sulfate, *n trade names:* Aerosporin; *drug class:* ophthalmic antiinfective; *action:* inhibits cell wall permeability in susceptible organism; *use:* superficial external ocular infections.

polyneuritis, endemic (pol'ē-nyōōr-ī'tis), *n* See *beriberi.*

polyols (pol'ē-ôlz), *n.pl* substances made up of two or more alcohols. See also *sugar alcohols.*

polyostotic (pol'ē-os-tot'ik), *adj* affecting more than one bone.

polyp (pol'ip), *n* a smooth, pedunculated growth from a mucous surface such as from the nose, bladder, or rectum.

polyp, pulp, *n* See *pulpitis, hypertrophic.*

polyphagia (pol'ē-fā'jē-ə), *n* disproportionate appetite or eating.

polypharmacy, *n* the prescription or dispensation of unnecessarily numerous or complex medicines.

polypnea (pol'ip-nē'ə), *n* a rapid or panting respiration.

polyposis, multiple (pol'ip-ō'sis), *n* See *syndrome, Peutz-Jeghers.*

polysaccharide, *n* a complex carbohydrate containing a large number of saccharide groups such as starch.

polystyrene (pol'ē-stī'rēn), *n* a polymer of styrene, which is a derivative of ethylene; often one of the resins present in materials designed for denture construction by the injection molding technique.

polysulfide polymer (pol′ē-sul′fīd pol′imur), *n* a rubber base impression material that makes use of a mercaptan bondage. It is prepared by mixing a base material (mercaptan) with either an inorganic catalyst (lead peroxide) or an organic catalyst (benzoyl peroxide).

polythiazide, *n trade name:* Renese; *drug class:* thiazide diuretic; *action:* acts on distal tubule by increasing excretion of water, sodium, chloride, potassium; *uses:* edema, hypertension, diuresis.

polyuria (pol′ē-yuor′ē-ə), *n* the passage of an abnormally increased volume of urine. It may result from increased intake of fluids, inadequate renal function, uncontrolled diabetes mellitus or diabetes insipidus, diuresis of edema fluid, or ascites.

polyvinyl alcohol, *n* a complex alcohol that is soluble in water and is used as an emulsifier and adhesive.

polyvinyl chloride, *n* a common synthetic thermoplastic material that releases hydrochloric acid when burned and that may contain carcinogenic vinyl chloride molecules as a contaminant.

pons (ponz), *n* a structure dorsal to the medulla and intimately related to the pathways to the cerebrum. The cranial nerves whose nuclei lie in the pons are the trigeminal, abducens, and facial nerves, and part of the acoustic nerve. The pons is intimately related to the medulla, has the same blood vessel supply, and is involved in many lesions that affect the medulla. It is especially involved with the cerebellar manifestations of disease and may cause serious muscular incoordination in motor function of the head, neck, and facial structures.

pontic (pon′tik), *n* the suspended member of a fixed partial denture; an artificial tooth on a fixed partial denture or an isolated tooth on a removable partial denture. It replaces a lost natural tooth, restores its function, and usually occupies the space previously occupied by the natural crown.

Pontic. (Rosenstiel/Land/Fujimoto, 2001)

population, *n* all instances about which a statement is made; all events, organisms, and items of a stated kind occurring or in existence in a specified time. In statistics, a hypothetical infinite supply or universe of events or objects like those being studied and from which a sample was drawn.

population, at-risk, *n* all individuals belonging to a certain group or community who have the potential to contract a medical condition.

porcelain, *n* a material formed by the fusion of feldspar, silica, and other minor ingredients. Most dental porcelains are glasses and are used in the manufacture of artificial teeth, facings, jackets, and occasionally denture bases and inlays.

porcelain, baked, *n* See *porcelain, dental.*

porcelain, dental, *n* (baked porcelain, fired porcelain), a fused mixture that is glasslike and more or less transparent. Classification of the type of porcelain employed in inlays and crowns is based on the fusion temperature of the porcelain: high fusing, 2350° to 2500° F (1287.5° to 1371° C); medium fusing, 2000° to 2300° F (1093.5° to 1260° C); and low fusing, 1600° to 2000° F (871° to 1093.5° C).

porcelain, fired, *n* See *porcelain, dental.*

porcelain, synthetic, *n* See *cement, silicate.*

porion (pō′rē-on), *n* the superior surface of the external auditory meatus. In craniometry, porion is identified as the margin of the bony canal on the skull. In cephalometrics it may be identified from the earpost of the cephalostat (machine porion) or from bony landmarks on the film (anatomic porion).

P

porosity (pōr-os′i-tē), *n* the presence of pores or voids within a structure.

porosity, back-pressure, *n* porosity produced in castings resulting from the inability of gases in the mold to escape through the investment.

porosity, occluded gas, *n* porosity produced by improper use of the blowpipe (that is, heating the metal in the oxidizing portion of the flame).

porosity, shrink-spot, *n* an area of porosity in cast metal that is caused by shrinkage of a portion of the metal as it solidifies from the molten state without flow of additional molten metal from surrounding areas.

porosity, solidification, *n* porosity that may be produced by improper spruing or improper heating of the metal or the investment.

porotic dentin (pôr-ot′ik), *n* a condition in which the dentin of a tooth become porous. It may occur in conjunction with vitamin C deficiency.

porphyria, congenital (pôr-fir′ē-ə), *n* See *porphyria, erythropoietic.*

porphyria, erythropoietic, *n* (congenital porphyria, photosensitive porphyria), an inborn error of metabolism (porphyrin synthesis) characterized clinically by skin photosensitivity, hypertrichosis, and reddish brown staining of the primary teeth.

Porphyria. (Zitelli/Davis, 2002)

porphyria, photosensitive, *n* See *porphyria, erythropoietic.*

porphyrin, *n* any iron or magnesium-free pyrrole derivative occurring in many plant and animal tissues. Normal findings of porphyrins in urine are 60 mg to 200 mg/24-hour period.

Porphyromonas gingivalis, *n* a species of gram-negative, anaerobic, rod-shaped bacteria originally classified within the *Bacteroides* genus. This bacterium produces a cell-bound, oxygen-sensitive collagenase and is isolated from the human mouth.

port, *n* the opening through which x-ray photons or the useful beam of radiation exits from the head of a dental x-ray machine.

porte polisher (port pol′i-shur), *n* a manual dental polishing device featuring an orangewood tip attached at a contra-angle. Considered beneficial to gingival health, it is nonthreatening to patients wary of powered equipment.

portfolio, *n* a list of stocks, bonds, and other commercial paper owned by an investor or holding company. In dentistry, it generally refers to the personal retirement investment package of the dentist or professional corporation created by the dentist.

position, *n* the placement or location of body parts to each other or the relationship of the body and its parts to other objects in space.

position, anatomic, *n* the upright, forward-facing stance used to reference the physical location of a body part. Arms are held down at the sides with palms, toes, and eyes all directed anteriorly.

position, border, posterior, *n* the most posterior position of the mandible at any specific vertical relation of the maxillae.

position, centric, *n* **1.** the position of the mandible in its most retruded relation to the maxillae at the established vertical relation. *n* **2.** the constant position into which the patient will close the jaws; this relationship may be a convenience relationship or a true centric relationship.

position, condylar hinge, *n* **1.** mandibular joints at which a hinge movement of the mandible is possible. *n* **2.** the maxillomandibular relation from which a consciously stimulated true hinge movement can be executed.

position, eccentric, *n* (eccentric jaw position), any position of the mandible other than that in centric relation. See also *relation, jaw, eccentric.*

position, eccentric jaw, *n* See *position, eccentric* and *relation, eccentric jaw.*

position, finger, *n* See *finger positions.*

position, gingival, *n* See *gingival position.*

position, hinge, *n* the orientation of parts in a manner permitting hinge movements between them.

position, intercuspal, *n* the term applied to the cuspal contacts of teeth when the mandible is in centric relation. Also called *centric occlusion.*

position, mandibular hinge, *n* any position of the mandible that exists when the condyles are so situated in the temporomandibular joints that opening or closing movements can be made on the hinge axis. See also *axis, hinge.*

position, neutral, *n* a relaxed and level arrangement of specific parts of the body so as to minimize stress or strain on the joints, nerves, or spine. The neutral position is usually defined by the horizontal plane of the adjacent part(s).

position, physiologic rest, *n* the habitual postural position of the mandible when the patient is resting comfortably in the upright position and the condyles are in a neutral, unstrained position in the glenoid fossae. The mandibular musculature is in a state of minimum tonic contraction to maintain posture and to overcome its force of gravity. See also *relation, rest jaw.*

position, protrusive, *n* occlusion of the teeth as the mandible and lower central incisors are moved straight forward toward the incisal edges of the upper central incisors; the normal anterocclusal relationship; the forward end position, with the upper and lower incisors in edge-to-edge contact.

position, rest, *n* **1.** the position of the mandible when the jaws are in rest relation. See also *position, physiologic rest,* and *relation, rest jaw.* *n* **2.** the position that the mandible passively assumes when the mandibular musculature is relaxed.

position, semi-upright, *n* a way to position a patient suffering from respiratory or cardiovascular ailments.

position, terminal hinge, *n* the mandibular hinge position from which further opening of the mandible would produce translatory rather than hinge movement. See also *position, hinge.*

position, tooth, *n* the placement or location of the tooth in the dental arch in relation to the bone of the alveolar process, its adjacent teeth, and the opposing dentition.

position, Trendelenburg, *n.pr* a position in which the patient is on his back with the head and chest lowered and the legs elevated.

positioner, *n* a removable elastic orthodontic appliance molded to fit the teeth in a "setup" made by repositioning the teeth from a plaster cast. The material may be rubber or elastomeric plastic. It is typically used to achieve fine adjustments and retain corrected positions in the finishing stages of treatment.

positioning, surgical, *n* the surgical repositioning or tilting of a tooth without injuring its blood supply.

positions at the chair, *n.pl* the posture and relative location of a dentist or chairside assistant in respect to the dental chair and patient. Classified as standing or sitting and as right side behind, right side in front, left side behind, left side in front, and directly behind. The position used should permit the most efficient performance of the current procedure and also keep paramount the health and comfort of the dentist and the patient.

positive reinforcement, *n* a technique used to encourage a desirable behavior. Also called *positive feedback,* in which the patient or subject receives encouraging and favorable communication from another person.

positron emission tomography (PET), *n* a computerized radiographic technique that employs radioactive substances to examine the metabolic activity of various body structures. Researchers and clinicians use PET to study blood flow and the metabolism of the heart and blood vessels.

possession, *n* the control or custody of anything that may be the subject of property as owner or as one who has a qualified right in it.

P

post cibum (pōst sī′bum), *adv* See *p.c.*

post, implant, *n* See *substructure, implant, neck.*

post-absorptive state, *n* the condition necessary for accurate measurement of the basal metabolic rate (BMR) in which the ambient temperature must be between 68° and 77° F (20° and 25° C) and the individual being tested must be fully awake, relaxed, and not ovulating.

postcondensation, *n* (aftercondensation), the procedure of completing the condensation of the surface of a gold-foil restoration after all the gold has been placed.

postdam area, *n* See *area, posterior palatal seal.*

posterior, *adj* situated behind.

posterior nasal spine, *n* See *spine, posterior nasal.*

posterior palatal bar, *n* See *connector, major, posterior palatal.*

posterior palatal seal, *n* See *seal, posterior palatal.*

posterior palatal seal area, *n* See *area, posterior palatal seal.*

posteroanterior extraoral radiographic examination, *n* See *examination, posteroanterior extraoral radiographic.*

postictal phase, *n* the period during which a patient recovers after an epileptic seizure. Also known as the *postconvulsion phase.*

postmortem changes, *n.pl* changes that occur after death.

postoperative care, *n* care after surgery or other invasive procedures, usually of a supportive nature.

postoperative complications, *n.pl* unexpected problems that arise following surgery. The most frequent are bleeding, infection, and protracted pain.

postoperative hemorrhage, *n* unexpected and abnormal (excessive) bleeding following surgery.

postpalatal seal, *n* See *seal, posterior palatal.*

postpalatal seal, area, *n* See *area, posterior palatal seal.*

postpartum, *adj* relating to or occurring during the period after birth.

postprandial (pōst-pran′ de-əl), *adj* after having eaten.

posttreatment review, *n* See *audit.*

posture, normal, *n* the configuration of the body in the upright position, which varies considerably among individuals. However, normal posture can be described as follows: the shoulder, pelvis, and eyes are level; the sagittal plane is between the feet, and the line of gravity passes through the center of gravity at the lumbosacral joint. When observed from the following positions, the line of gravity intersects the following structures: lateral position—anterior border of the ear, and the shoulder, hip, knee, and ankle joints; anterior position—nose, symphysis pubis, and between the knees and feet; posterior position—occiput, spinous processes, gluteal crease, and between the knees and feet.

potassium, *n* an alkali metal element, the seventh most abundant element in the earth's crust. Its atomic number is 19 and its atomic weight is 39.1. Potassium in the body constitutes the predominant intracellular cation, helping to regulate neuromuscular excitability and muscle contraction. The average adequate daily intake of potassium for most adults is 2 to 4 grams.

potassium bicarbonate/potassium acetate/potassium chloride/potassium gluconate/potassium phosphate, *n* *trade name:* Effer-K, K-Lyte, Kapon-CL, K-Dur, Micro-K, K-G Elixir; *drug class:* potassium electrolyte; *action:* needed for adequate transmission of nerve impulses and cardiac contraction, renal function, intracellular ion maintenance; *uses:* prevention and treatment of hypokalemia.

potassium chloride, *n* a white crystalline salt used as a substitute for table salt in the diet of persons with cardiovascular disorders.

potassium dichromate, *n* a compound of potassium used as an external astringent, antiseptic, and caustic.

potassium oxalate **(pō-tas′ē-um ok′sə-lāt),** *n* a dentin desensitizing agent that occludes the openings of the dentinal tubules and blocks the hydrodynamics that initiate the pain response. *Brand name:* Protect.

potassium sulfate **(pō-tas′ē-um sul′fāt),** *n* an accelerator used to speed the setting of gypsum products. Hydrocolloid impressions are fixed in a 2% solution of potassium sulfate.

potency (pō′ten-sē), *n* power.

potential, action, *n* See *action potential.*

potentiation (pō-ten'shē-ā'shən), *n* **1.** an increase in the action of a drug by the addition of another drug that does not necessarily possess similar properties. *n* **2.** the enhancement of action (for example, of a drug).

Pott's disease, *n.pr* See *disease, Pott's.*

Potter-Bucky grid, *n.pr* See *grid, Potter-Bucky.*

pour hole, *n* an aperture in a refractory investment or another mold material leading to the pattern space into which prosthetic material is deposited.

poverty, *n* a lack of material wealth needed to maintain existence.

povidone, *n* a polymerized form of vinylpyrolidone, which is a white hygroscopic powder that is easily soluble in water and used as a dispersing and suspending agent in drugs.

povidone iodine (pōv-i-dōn ī'ōdīn), *n trade names:* ACU-dyne, Aerodine, Betadine; *drug class:* iodophor disinfectant; *action:* destroys a wide variety of microorganisms by local irritation and germicidal action; *uses:* cleansing wounds, disinfection, preoperative skin preparation; *dental use:* to irrigate periodontal pockets before debridement to control bleeding and pain

powdered gold, *n* See *gold, powdered.*

power stroke, *n* See *stroke, power.*

Poxviridae (poks-vir'id-ā), *n* one of the major deoxyribonucleic acid virus families, to which the smallpox and vaccinia viruses belong. Viruses have a double-stranded, linear molecular structure with complex symmetry.

PPCF, *n* See *factor V.*

ppm (parts per million), *n* standardized measurement used to describe the level of fluoride in products that contain it (e.g., toothpaste, mouthrinse, and water).

practice, *v* **1.** to follow or work at, as a profession, trade, or art. *n* **2.** the business operated by a medical professional.

practice administration, *n* the organization, operation, and supervision of the business and professional aspects of a dental practice.

practice building, *n* increasing the number of patients and the number of services without sacrificing quality, by means of observing the principles of constantly improving professional care and maintaining effective human relations with patients.

practice goal, *n* the planning of the objectives of a dental practice and the method of reaching those objectives. To be ascertained by the dental practitioner before or immediately on entering dental practice.

practice, group, *n* a large partnership formed for the purpose of practicing dentistry; may or may not include the services of the recognized specialties in dentistry.

practice guidelines, *n* a detailed description of a process of maintenance of health status or to slow the decline in health status in certain chronic clinical conditions. Practice guidelines are established to assist in the delivery of effective and efficient health care that preserves the resources of the provider, the patient, and the funding entity.

practice management, dental, *n* the administrative organization of a dental office, including but not limited to the supervision and control of patient flow, staff assignment and evaluation, record keeping, and financial overseeing.

practice, private, *n* the business and profession in which dental services are administered for a fee.

Prader-Willi syndrome, *n.pr* a metabolic condition characterized by congenital hypotonia, hyperphagia, obesity, and mental retardation. The syndrome is associated with a less-than-normal secretion of gonadotropic hormones by the pituitary gland.

pravastatin, *n trade name:* Pravachol; *drug class:* antihyperlipidemic; *action:* inhibits HMG-CoA reductase enzyme, which reduces cholesterol synthesis; *use:* as an adjunct in primary hypercholesterolemia (types IIa, IIb).

prazepam, *n trade name:* Centrax; *drug class:* benzodiazepine, antianxiety (Controlled Substance Schedule IV); *action:* produces central nervous system depression by interacting with a benzodiazepine receptor to facilitate the action of inhibitory neurotransmitter γ-aminobutyric acid (GABA); *use:* anxiety.

praziquantel (prä″zē-kwän′tel), *n* an anthelmintic agent that acts against a variety of parasitic worms by causing paralysis, thereby forcing the worms to be displaced from the intestine.

prazosin HCl, *n trade name:* Minipress; *drug class:* antihypertensive, α-adrenergic blocker; *action:* reduction in blood pressure results from blockage of α-adrenergic receptors and reduced peripheral resistance; *use:* hypertension.

preameloblast (pre″ ə-mel′ o-blast″), *n* a cell within the enamel organ from which an ameloblast develops.

preanesthetic (prē′an-es-thet′ik), *n* a medicine for producing preliminary anesthesia (e.g., Avertin). See also premedication.

preauricular lymph nodes (prē′ôr-ik′yōō-lur), *n* rounded masses of lymphoid tissue anterior to the auricle of the ear.

preauthorization, *n* **1.** the approval of or concurrence with the treatment plan proposed by a participating dentist before the provision of service. Under some plans, preauthorization by the carrier is required before certain services can be provided. *n* **2.** a statement by a third-party payer indicating that proposed treatment will be covered under the terms of the dental benefits contract. See also *precertification* and *predetermination.*

precancerous, *adj* a stage of abnormal tissue growth that is likely or predisposed to develop into a malignant tumor.

precautions, universal, *n* See *universal precautions.*

preceptorship, *n* the position of teacher or instructor to a new or recent graduate.

precertification, *n* confirmation by a third-party payer of a patient's eligibility for coverage under a dental benefits program. See also *preauthorization* and *predetermination.*

precipitate (prē-sip′i-tāt), *n* an insoluble solid substance that forms from chemical reactions between solutions.

precipitating factor, *n* an element that causes or contributes to the occurrence of a disorder or problem.

precision attachment, *n* See *attachment, intracoronal.*

precision rest, *n* See *rest, precision.*

precordial, *adj* pertaining to the region over the heart or stomach: the epigastrium and lower thorax.

precursor, fifth plasma thromboplastin, *n* See *factor XII.*

precursors, *n.pl* particles or compounds that precede something. In biochemistry, carbohydrates may serve as precursors for structural and functional molecules. The -blast suffix indicates the precursor cell of a structure, such as in the term odontoblast.

predentin (pre-den′ tin), *n* soft material that makes up the inner layer of the dentin.

predetermination, *n* an administrative procedure whereby a dentist submits a treatment plan to the carrier before treatment is initiated. Then the carrier returns the treatment plan, indicating the patient' s eligibility, covered service amounts payable, application of appropriate deductibles, copayment factors, and maximums. Under some programs, predetermination by the carrier is required when covered charges are expected to exceed a certain amount, commonly $100. Also known as *preauthorization, precertification, preestimate of cost,* and *pretreatment estimate.*

predisposition, *n* increased vulnerability to a particular disease based on genetic factors or the existence of certain underlying conditions not yet active or revealed.

prednicarbate, *n trade name:* Dermatop Emollient Cream; *drug class:* topical corticosteroid, group III potency; *action:* possesses antipruritic, antiinflammatory actions; *uses:* relief of inflammatory and pruritic manifestations of corticosteroid-responsive dermatoses.

prednisolone/prednisolone acetate/prednisolone sodium phosphate/prednisolone tebutate, *n trade names:* Delta-Cortef, Prelone, Pedaject-50, Hydeltra TBA; *drug class:* immediate acting glucocorticoid; *action:* decreases inflammation by suppressing macrophage and leukocyte migration; reduces capillary permeability and inhibits lysosomal enzymes and phagocytosis; *uses:* severe inflammation, immunosuppression, neoplasms, adrenal insufficiency.

prednisone (pred′ni-sōn), *n trade names:* Deltasone, Sterapred; *drug class:* intermediate acting glucocorticoid; *action:* decreases inflammation by suppressing macrophage and leukocyte migration, reduces capillary permeability and inhibits lysosomal enzymes and phagocytosis; *uses:* severe inflammation, immunosuppression, neoplasms, multiple sclerosis, collagen disorders, dermatologic disorders.

preexisting condition, *n* the oral health condition of an enrollee that existed before his or her enrollment in a dental program.

preextraction cast, *n* See *cast, diagnostic* and *cast, preextraction.*

preextraction record, *n* See *record, preoperative.*

preferred provider organization (PPO), *n* a formal agreement between a purchaser of a dental benefits program and a defined group of dentists for the delivery of dental services to a specific patient population as an adjunct to a traditional plan, using discounted fees for cost savings.

prefiling of fees, *n* the submission of a participating dentist's usual fees to a service corporation for the purpose of establishing, in advance, that dentist's usual fees and the customary ranges of fees in a geographic area to determine benefits under a usual, customary, and reasonable dental benefits program.

pregnancy, *n* the gestational process, comprising the growth and development within a woman of a new individual from conception through the embryonic and fetal periods to birth. Pregnancy lasts approximately 266 days from the day of fertilization, but is clinically considered to last 280 days (40 weeks, or 10 lunar months) from the first day of the last menstrual period.

pregnancy gingivitis, *n* an enlargement or hyperplasia of the gingivae caused by hormonal imbalance during pregnancy. It is usually limited to the interdental papillae. Incomplete cleaning of the interproximal space with dental floss is the initiating factor. The hormonal change is a precipitating factor.

pregnancy tumor, *n* See *granuloma, pregnancy; granuloma, pyogenic.*

Pregnancy tumor. (Daniel/Harfst, 2002)

preicteric phase of hepatitis A (prē′ik-ter′ik), *n* the initial flu-like symptoms a patient experiences when infected with hepatitis A.

prekallikrein, *n* a plasma protein that is the precursor of kallikrein. Plasma that is deficient in prekallikrein has been found to be abnormal in thromboplastin formation, kinin generation, evolution of a permeability globulin, and plasmin formation. Prekallikrein deficiency leads to Fletcher factor deficiency, a congenital disease.

premature birth, *n* a birth in which the child is delivered before it has reached the full period of gestation (37 weeks).

prematurities, *n.pl* See *contact, deflective occlusal* and *contact, interceptive occlusal.*

premaxilla, floating, *n* See *premaxilla, loose.*

premaxilla, loose, *n* **1.** (floating premaxilla) the nonunion of the premaxillary process with the lateral maxillary segments, so that the premaxilla is loose, or floating. The position of the loose premaxilla in relation to the lateral maxillary segments varies among patients. *n* **2.** the administration of a tranquilizing drug, a drug that influences blood clotting time or any other drug that produces a preplanned set of conditions and is administered preceding any dental procedures.

premedication, *n* **1.** any sedative,

P

tranquilizer, hypnotic, or anticholinergic medication administered before anesthesia. *n* **2.** the administration of medication before anesthesia or an invasive procedure.

premedication, antibiotic, *n* the administration of an antibiotic prior to an invasive procedure that prevents a dangerous infection from occurring as a result of transient bacteria produced in the course of the procedure.

premium, *n* the amount charged by a dental benefits organization for coverage of a level of benefits for a specified time.

premium, earned, *n* that portion of a policy's premium payment for which the protection of the policy has already been given.

premium rate, *n* the price per unit of insurance.

premium tax, *n* an assessment levied by a state government, usually on the net premium income collected in that state by insurance companies.

premium, unearned, *n* that part of the premium applicable to the unexpired part of the policy period.

premolar, *n* (bicuspid), one of the eight teeth in humans, four in each jaw, between the canines and first molars; usually has two cusps; replaces the molars of the deciduous dentition.

prenatal care, *n* the health care provided the mother and fetus before childbirth.

preoperative cast, *n* See *cast, diagnostic.*

preoperative record, *n* See *record, preoperative.*

prepaid dental plan, *n* a method of financing the cost of dental care for a defined population in advance of receipt of services.

prepaid group practice, *n* See *closed panel.*

preparation, *n* the selected form given to a natural tooth when it is reduced by instrumentation to receive a prosthesis (for example, an artificial crown or a retainer for a fixed or removable prosthesis). The selection of the form is guided by clinical circumstances and physical properties of the materials that make up the prosthesis. See also *preparation, mouth.*

preparation, cavity, *n* one of the

various operations in which carious material is removed from teeth and biomechanically correct forms are established in the teeth to receive and retain restorations. A constant requirement is provision for prevention of failure of the restoration through recurrence of decay or inadequate resistance to applied stresses.

preparation, initial, *n* one of a number of procedures aimed at preparing the patient for final treatment. The objectives consist of eliminating or reducing all local causal factors and environmental influences before the operative procedures and establishing a sequence of therapy for the patient.

preparation, mouth, *n* one of the various necessary procedures applied to the oral structures preparatory to the making of a final impression for a prosthesis.

preparation, slice, *n* a type of cavity preparation for Class 2 cast restorations. The proximal portion is formed by removing a sufficient slice of the proximal convexity of the tooth to achieve cleansable margins and a line of draw; a tapered keyway or two keyed grooves or channels in the proximal surface provide retention form.

preparation, surgical, *n* any modification using surgical procedures that may be required for preparing the oral structures for prosthodontic treatment.

prepubertal (prē-pyōō′bur-təl), *adj* before the onset of puberty.

presbyopia (prez′bĭ-o′pē-ə), *n* a form of optical distortion affecting the vision of patients, particularly those of advancing age. It depends on diminution of the power of the accommodation of the lens as a result of loss of elasticity of the crystalline lens, causing the near point of distinct vision to be removed farther from the eye.

prescription (prē-skrip′shən), *n* a written direction for the preparation and use of medicine or an appliance; a medical recipe; a prescribed remedy. Also used in dentistry to describe the treatment plan.

prescription, extemporaneous, *n* **1.** (magistral prescription) a prescription for a nonofficial drug. *n* **2.** a prescription that directs the pharmacist to compound the specified medication, as contrasted with a prescription that specifics medication available in precompounded form.

prescription, magistral, n See *prescription, extemporaneous.*

prescription, official, n a prescription for an official drug.

preservation, *n* a neurologic phenomenon such as the involuntary repetition of motor response or the continuation of a sensation after the adequate external stimulus has ceased.

preservative, *n* a substance added to prevent deterioration.

pressoreceptor, *n* a nerve ending that is sensitive to changes in blood pressure.

pressure, *n* a stress or strain that may occur by compression, pull, or thrust; an applied force.

pressure area, n See *area, pressure.*

pressure atrophy, n See *atrophy, pressure.*

pressure, biting, n the actual or potential power used in bringing the teeth into contact. See also *pressure, occlusal.*

pressure, blood, n the pressure exerted on arterial walls by the blood when the heart is in systole (systolic pressure), and the pressure maintained by the elasticity of the arteries when the heart is in diastole (diastolic pressure). A consistent arterial pressure greater than 140/90 is considered abnormally high and suggestive of hypertensive vascular disease.

pressure, blood, stage, n any of the three stages of hypertension marked by elevated blood pressure. Stage I is 140-159 over 90-99; Stage II is 160-179 over 100-109; Stage III is 180-209 over 110-119.

pressure, deeper, n any pressure to the body—in excess of that which stimulates Meissner's corpuscles, Merkel's disks, or the hair receptors of light touch—that stimulates the deeper receptors such as Pacini's corpuscles. These latter deep-pressure perception organs lie in the inner layers of the dermis and in the muscle and tendon groups.

pressure, diastolic blood, n the pressure in the bloodstream when the heart relaxes and dilates, filling with blood. See also *pressure, blood, stage* and *diastole.*

pressure, equalization of, n the act of distributing pressure evenly.

pressure, hand, n force applied by an instrument held in the hand.

pressure, hydraulic, n pressure transmitted by a liquid trapped between the tooth and a restoration being cemented.

pressure, hydrostatic, n the pressure in the circulatory system exerted by the volume of blood when it is confined in a blood vessel. The hydrostatic pressure, coupled with the osmotic pressure within a capillary is opposed by the hydrostatic and osmotic pressure of the surrounding tissues. Fluids flow from the higher pressure areas to the lower pressure areas.

pressure, intrapleural, n pressure within the pleura.

pressure, occlusal, n any force exerted on the occlusal surfaces of teeth. See also *force, occlusal* and *load, occlusal.*

pressure, osmotic, n the stress that develops when solutions containing different concentrations of solute in a common solvent are separated by a membrane that is permeable to the solvent but not the solute.

pressure, partial, n the pressure exerted by each of the constituents of a mixture of gases.

pressure, pulse, n the difference between systolic and diastolic pressure.

pressure sensibility, n the ability to detect light touch and deep pressure. See also *corpuscle, Meissner's; corpuscle, Merkel's;* and *corpuscle, Pacini's.*

pressure sore, n a decubitus ulcer caused when the bony protuberances of the body are subjected to chronic pressure from the weight of the body without breaks.

pressure, systolic blood, n the pressure exerted on the bloodstream by the heart when it contracts, forcing blood from the ventricles of the heart into the pulmonary artery and the aorta. See also *pressure, blood, stage* and *systole.*

presumption, *n* an inference as to the existence of some fact, drawn from the existence of some other fact; an inference that common sense draws from circumstances usually occurring in such cases.

presurgical impression, *n* an overextended impression of the intact mandible before the first surgical stage. The cast made for this impression is altered so that the surgical tray may be fabricated on it.

pretreatment, *n* before treatment; refers to the protocols required before beginning therapy, usually of a diagnostic nature.

pretreatment estimate, *n* See *predetermination.*

prevailing fee, *n* the term used by some dental benefits organizations to refer to the fee most commonly charged for a dental service in a given area.

prevalence, *adj* in epidemiology, all of the new and old cases of a disease or occurrence of an event during a particular period. Prevalence is expressed as a ratio in which the number of events is the numerator and the population at risk is the denominator.

prevent, *v* to keep from happening or existing, especially by precautionary measures.

preventive, *adj* avoiding occurrence.

preventive dentistry, *n* the procedures in dental practice and health programs that prevent the occurrence of oral diseases.

preventive maintenance, *n* a manner of warding off future potential dental diseases or oral problems by practicing good oral hygiene on a regular basis.

preventive medicine, *n* the branch of medicine that is concerned with the prevention of disease and methods for increasing the power of the patient and community to resist disease and prolong life.

preventive orthodontic treatment, *n* dental services intended to prevent the development of a malocclusion by maintaining the integrity of an otherwise normally developing dentition. Typical services include dental restorations, temporary prostheses (space maintainers) to replace prematurely lost deciduous teeth, and removal of deciduous teeth that fail to shed normally to allow the permanent successors to erupt satisfactorily.

Prevotella, *n* a genus of gram-negative, anaerobic, nonspore-forming,

nonmotile rods. Organisms of this genus were originally classified as members of the *Bacteroides* genus but overwhelming biochemical and chemical findings in 1990 indicated the need to separate them from other *Bacteroides* species; hence, this new genus was established.

Prevotella intermedia **(pre″ vo-tel′ə in″ tər me′ de-ə),** *n* a species of gram-negative anaerobic bacilli found in gingival crevices that is believed to be responsible for gingivitis, chronic periodontitis, and other infections of the mouth.

prilocaine hydrochloride (local), *n* *trade name:* Citanest; *drug class:* amide local anesthetic; *action:* inhibits ion fluxes across membranes, particularly sodium transport across cell membrane; decreases rise of depolarization phase of action potential; blocks nerve action potential; *use:* local dental anesthesia.

prima facie (prī′mə fā′shē), *adv* on the face of it; so far as can be judged from the first appearance; presumably.

primaquine phosphate, *n* *trade name:* generic; *drug class:* antiprotozoal; *action:* unknown; thought to destroy exoerythrocytic forms by gametocidal action; *use:* malaria caused by *Prevotella vivax.*

primary, *n* first in time; first in order in any series.

primary beam, *n* See *radiation, primary.*

primary care, *n* the first contact with a healthcare provider in a given episode of illness that leads to a decision regarding a course of action to resolve the health problem presented by the patient.

primary deficiency, *n* the insufficient intake of dietary nutrients that may be due to such factors as illness, ignorance, economic status, fad diets, food preferences, overuse of convenience foods, or poor oral health.

primary dentin, *n* the dentin produced after a tooth takes its position in the mouth, but before roots are completely developed.

primary dentition, *n* See *dentition, primary.*

primary fixation, *n* the immediate postoperative fastening of an implant to bone by means of wires, screws, or a superstructure until, through natural healing and adhesion, final fixation occurs.

primary health care, *n* a basic level of health care that includes programs directed at the promotion of health, early diagnosis of disease or disability, and prevention of disease.

primary intention healing, *n* the healing of a wound directly at the incision site.

primary lymphoma of the brain, *n* a secondary neoplasm associated with acquired immune deficiency syndrome.

primary prevention, *n* action performed to preclude the development of a disease. See also *primary health care* and *secondary prevention.*

primary radiation, *n* See *radiation, primary.*

primate (prī'māt), *n* a member of the biologic order of animals of the chordate class Mammalia. The primate order includes lemurs, monkeys, apes, and humans.

primate space, *n* the space that occurs between the canine and first premolar teeth in adult primates but that is normally absent in humans. However, spacing between the primary canine and primary first molar normally occurs in the anterior primary dentition in children.

primitive streak, *n* a furrowed, rod-shaped thickening in the middle embryonic disk that appears during the early formation of neural tissues and the mesoderm.

primodone, *n trade name:* Myidone, Mysoline; *drug class:* anticonvulsant, barbiturate derivative; *action:* raises seizure threshold by unknown mechanism; may be related to facilitation of γ-aminobutyric acid; metabolized to phenobarbital; *uses:* tonic-clonic (grand mal), complex-partial psychomotor seizures.

primordium (pri-mor' de-əm), *n* the first evidence of an organ in a developing embryo.

principal, *adj* the chief; highest in rank; the source of authority.

principal in law of agency, *n* the employer; the person who gives authority to an agent to act for him.

prior authorization, *n* See *predetermination.*

privacy, *n* a culturally specific concept defining the degree of one's personal responsibility to others in regulating behavior that is regarded as intrusive.

private practice, *n* to engage in one's profession as an independent provider rather than as an employee.

privileges, *n* the authority granted to a physician or dentist by a hospital governing board to provide patient care in the hospital. Clinical privileges are limited to the individual's license, experience, and competence.

p.r.n, *adv* See *pro re nata.*

pro forma, *adj* pertaining to financial statement that shows the way that the actual statement will look if certain specified assumptions are realized. Pro forma statements are usually a future projection.

pro re nata (prō rē nē'tə), *adv* (p.r.n.), a Latin phrase meaning "occasionally as needed" or "according to circumstances."

pro-SPCA, *n* See *proconvertin.*

proaccelerin (prō'ak-sel'ər-in), *n* (factor V, labile factor, plasma accelerator globulin, plasma ac-globulin, proprothrombinase, prothrombin conversion accelerator I), an unstable protein found in the blood; the precursor of accelerin.

proandrogens (prō-an'drō-jenz), *n.pl* compounds that are not androgenic when applied locally but that have androgenic activity when metabolized in the organism. Included are cortisone and cortisol, which may be converted within the organism to androgens such as adrenosterone, 11-ketoandrosterone, and 11-hydroxyandrosterone.

probability, *n* **1.** a measure of the increased likelihood that something will occur. *n* **2.** a mathematic ratio of the number of times something will occur to the total number of possible occurrences.

probative (prō'bə-tiv), *adj* in the law of evidence, tending to prove or actually proving.

probe, *n* **1.** a slender, flexible instrument designed for introduction into a wound or cavity for purposes of exploration. *v* **2.** to use such an instrument.

probe, automated, *n* an automatically controlled instrument used to assess the severity of periodontal disease. It may provide more consistent readings than manual probes. Also called *controlled force probes*.

probe, automatic, *n* a device used to explore a cavity or a wound with minimal manual operation.

probe, depth, *n* the amount of space from the position of the tip of the periodontal probe to the gingival margin.

probe, furcation, *n* a hand-activated, blunt-tipped probing tool that is used to measure bone loss in teeth with multiple roots. See also *probe, Nabers furcation.*

probe, Hu-Friedy, *n.pr* a thin, rounded and tapered handheld tool that is used to measure periodontal pocket depth. The millimeter marks are color-coded for easier assessment.

probe, lacrimal, *n* an instrument useful in probing the lumen of duct structures, such as the nasolacrimal or salivary gland ducts.

probe, Marquis, *n.pr* the probe is color-coded by alternately colored or black and silver bands that mark 3, 6, 9, and 12 millimeters.

Marquis color coded probe. (Daniel/Harfst, 2002)

probe, Michigan O, *n.pr* a slender, round, conical-shaped device with a thin diameter used to assess the progression and extent of disease within the tissues of the oral cavity. The probe is marked at 3, 6, and 8 millimeters.

probe, Nabers furcation, *n.pr* an adapted device used to examine the

layout and extent of an advanced furcation. See also *furcation.*

Nabers probe. (Daniel/Harfst, 2002)

probe, periodontal, *n* a fine calibrated instrument designed and used for measuring the depth and topography of gingival and periodontal pockets. Also used to determine the degree of attachment and adaptation of the gingival tissues to the tooth.

probe, Williams, *n.pr* a round, conical-shaped device used to assess the progression and extent of disease within the tissues of the oral cavity. The probe has markings at 1, 2, 3, 5, 7, 8, 9, and 10 millimeters. The probe may be available with color coding.

Williams probe. (Daniel/Harfst, 2002)

probenecid, *n trade names:* Benemid, Probalan; *drug class:* uricosuric; *action:* inhibits tubular reabsorption of urates, with increased excretion of uric acids; *uses:* hyperuricemia in gout, gouty arthritis, adjunct to cephalosporin or penicillin treatment by reducing excretion and maintaining high blood levels of medication.

probucol, *n trade names:* Bifenabid, Lesterol, Lorelco, Lurselle, Superlipid; *drug class:* antihyperlipidemic; *action:* increases bile acid excretion, catabolism of low-density lipoprotein (LDL)-cholesterol; may block oxidation of LDL-cholesterol; *use:* severe hypercholesterolemia when other treatment is unsuccessful.

procabazine HCl, *n trade name:* Natulane; *drug class:* antineoplastic, miscellaneous; *action:* inhibits deoxyribonucleic acid, ribonucleic acid, protein synthesis; has multiple sites of action; a nonvesicant; also inhibits monoamine oxidase enzymes; *uses:* lymphoma, Hodgkin's disease, cancers resistant to other therapy.

procainamide HCl, *n trade names:* Procan SR, Promine, Pronestyl; *drug class:* antidysrhythmic (Class IA); *action:* depresses excitability of cardiac muscle to electrical stimulation and slows conduction in atrium, bundle of His, and ventricle; *uses:* premature ventricular contraction, atrial fibrillation, paroxysmal atrial tachycardia, atrial dysrhythmias, ventricular tachycardia.

procaine hydrochloride (prū-kān hī′drō-klôr′īd), *n* an ester local anesthetic agent; 2-diethylaminoethyl 4-aminobenzoate hydrochloride, which is no longer available in the United States as an injectable. *Trade name:* Novocain.

procedure (prō-sē′jur), *n* a series of steps followed in a regular, orderly, definite way, by which a desired result is accomplished.

procedure, dental prosthetic laboratory, n the steps in the fabrication of a dental prosthesis that do not require the presence of the patient for their accomplishment.

procedure, invasive, n an operation that causes bleeding or the possibility of bleeding.

procedure, Kazanjian's (kə-zan′jē-ən), n.pr See *operation, Kazanjian's.*

procedure, operating, n the technique or method of conducting or performing an operation or form of treatment.

procedure, order of, n the sequence of steps made in performing an operation or following through a technique. In cavity preparation the sequence is as follows: (1) obtain the required outline form, (2) obtain the required resistance form, (3) obtain the required retention form, (4) retain the required convenience form, (5) remove any remaining carious dentin, (6) finish the enamel walls, and (7) make the debridement.

procedure, orthodontic, n therapeutic measures employed to correct malalignment and malposition of the teeth and to immobilize and stabilize periodontally involved or previously moved teeth.

procedure, restorative, n a method or mode of action that reestablishes or reforms a tooth or teeth or portions thereof to anatomic or functional form and health.

process (pros′es, prō′ses), *n* in anatomy, a marked prominence or projection of a bone. In dentistry, a series of operations that convert a wax pattern, such as that of a denture base, into a solid denture base of another material. See also *denture curing.*

process, alveolar, n the portion of the maxillae or mandible that forms the dental arch and serves as a bony investment for the teeth. Its cortical covering is continuous with the compact bone of the body of the maxillae or mandible, whereas its trabecular portion is continuous with the spongiosa of the body of the jaws. See also *ridge, alveolar.*

process, condyloid (kon′di-loid), n a projection of the mandible arising on the posterosuperior aspect of the mandibular ramus. It consists of a neck and an elliptically shaped head or condyle that enters into the formation of the temporomandibular joint in conjunction with the articular disk and the glenoid fossa of the temporal bone.

process, coronoid, n the thin, triangular, rounded eminence originating from the anterosuperior surface of the ramus of the mandible. Provides insertion for the various fiber bundles of the temporal muscle.

process, dehiscence of alveolar, n See *dehiscence.*

process, fenestration of alveolar, n a circumscribed hole, located in the cortical plate over the root, that does not communicate with the crestal margin.

process, hamular, n (pterygoid process) the pterygoid process of the sphenoid bone; appears as a vertical projection distal to the maxillary tuberosity.

process, horizontal resorptive, n the pattern of bone resorption, occurring with periodontal disease, in which the resultant level of bone is more or less flat or level in nature.

process, mandibular, n the stage of embryonic development during which two sections of the first branchial arch come together to create the lower jaw.

process, maxillary, n the stage of embryonic development during which a prominence of the first branchial arch unites with the corresponding median nasal prominence to form the upper jaw.

process, medial nasal, n protrusion of tissue located midline to the olfactory pits during embryonic development from which the tip of the nose and philtrum of the lip develop.

process, neck of condyloid, n the part of the condyloid process that connects the condyle to the main part of the ramus.

process, odontoblastic, n a structure of the tooth formed during dentogenesis. It becomes encased by predentin that eventually calcifies.

process, pterygoid, n See *process, hamular.*

process, Tomes', n a narrow extension of the ameloblast from which the enamel matrix is secreted.

process of care, n See *plan, treatment.*

processing (pros'es-ing), n the term that usually refers to the procedure of bringing about polymerization of appliances; processing of dentures. See also *film processing.*

processing, denture, n the conversion of a wax pattern of a denture or trial denture into a denture with a base made of another material, such as acrylic resin. See also *process.*

processing tank, n See *tank, processing.*

prochlorperazine   edisylate/ prochlorperazine   maleate, n *trade name:* Compazine; *drug class:* phenothiazine antipsychotic; *action:* blocks neurotransmission at dopaminergic synapses in the cerebral cortex, hypothalamus, and limbic system; *uses:* antipsychotic; for nausea, vomiting.

proconvertin (prō'kən-vur'tin), n (autoprothrombin I, cofactor V, cothromboplastin, factor VII, precursor of serum prothrombin conversion accelerator [pro-SPCA], stable factor), variously described as the inactive precursor of convertin. Recently proconvertin has been considered as a collective term for pro-SPCA and Stuart factor.

proconvertin-convertin, n See *thromboplastin, extrinsic.*

proctitis, n an inflammation of the rectum and anus caused by infection, trauma, drugs, allergy, or radiation injury.

procumbency (prō-kum'ben-sē), n excessive labioaxial inclination of the incisor teeth.

procyclidine HCl, n *trade name:* Kemadrin; *drug class:* anticholinergic, antidyskinetic; *action:* blockage of central acetylcholine receptors; *uses:* Parkinson symptoms, extrapyramidal symptoms associated with neuroleptic drugs.

prodrome (prō'drōm), n a symptom, often noted prior to monitoring and diagnosis that may signal the beginning of a disease.

production, n the amount of work that can be accomplished in a specific length of time.

products, fission, n.pl See *fission products.*

profession, n a calling; vocation; a means of livelihood or gain.

professional autonomy, n the right and privilege provided by a governmental entity to a class of professionals, and to each qualified licensed caregiver within that profession, to provide services independent of supervision.

professional ethics, n the rules governing the conduct, transactions, and relationships within a profession and among its publics.

professional ethics liability, n **1.** the obligation of all professionals to their clients to do no harm. n **2.** the legal obligation of healthcare professionals, or their insurers, to compensate patients for injury or suffering caused by acts of omission or commission by the professionals.

professional ethics liability insurance, n insurance covering the insured against claims arising from injury, damage, or loss sustained by a patient during the course of professional services.

Professional Ethics Standards Review Organization (PSRO), n a federal agency, established by Public Law 92-603, to determine the quality and appropriateness of healthcare services paid for, in whole or part, under the Social Security Act. Such determinations are to be made by local committees of providers.

profibrin (prō-fī′brin), n See *fibrinogen.*

profile, n an outline or contour, especially one representing a side view of a human head.

profile, extraoral radiographic examination, n See *examination, profile extraoral radiographic.*

profile, facial, n the sagittal outline form of the face.

profile, hematologic, n a thorough study of the blood and all its components that is used to diagnose diseases of the blood and to aid in the assessment of an individual's overall health condition. The results are compared with established normal blood values.

profile, mesognathic, n side view of the face showing the forward position of the jaw where the forehead and the chin appear to be relatively equal. See also *profile, facial.*

profile record, n See *record, profile.*

profit sharing, n a mechanism for funding a retirement plan for employees or members of a professional association. Members are eligible for a percentage of the net income based on predetermined formulae. Such plans, properly executed, are legal and ethical and are to be differentiated from fee-splitting, which is illegal and unethical, in which a referring professional shares in the fee-for-service income of another professional.

progeria (prō-jir′ē-ə), n See *syndrome, Hutchinson-Gilford.*

progesterone (prō-jes′tə-rōn), n the ovarian hormone produced by the corpus luteum and responsible for preparing the endometrium for nidation and nourishment of the ovum. It also suppresses the production of the pituitary luteinizing hormone, estrus, and ovulation and stimulates the mammary glands.

progestin (prō-jes′tin), n a hormone that suppresses the release of luteinizing hormone and thereby inhibits the onset of menstruation. Synthetically produced progestin and estrogen are used in combination as an effective contraception.

progestogen (prō-jes′tō-jen), n an agent capable of producing effects similar to progesterone, used to correct abnormalities of the menstrual cycle.

prognathic (prog-nath′ik), adj pertaining to a forward relationship of the jaws to the head (anterior to the skull); denoting a protrusive lower face.

prognathism (prog′nəth-iz-əm), n facial disharmony in which one or both jaws project forward. Prognathism may be real or imaginary. Mandibular prognathism may exist when both the maxillae and the mandible increase in length or when the maxillae are of normal length but the mandible increases in length. Prognathism may be imaginary when the maxillae are underdeveloped and short and the mandible is of normal length or when the maxillary and mandibular dental relationships are normal but there is an increase in the mental prominence of the mandible.

prognathous (prog-nath′əs), n the condition of having a marked projection of the mandible, usually resulting in a horizontal overlap of the lower anterior teeth in relation to the maxillary anterior teeth

prognosis (prog-nō′sis), n **1.** the foretelling of the probable course of a disease; a forecast of the outcome of a disease. n **2.** a forecast of the probable result of a regimen of treatment.

P

program, *n* instructions coded in a computer language to solve a problem.

programmer, *n* a person who writes applications in a computer language. It is usually the programmer (not the machine) who should be held responsible for satisfactory and efficient solution of the problem.

programming, *n* the process of describing in a computer language a problem or its method of solution. Programming includes planning, designing, writing, and debugging of programs.

projection, *n* orthographic, a projection made on the assumption that the projection lines from the object to the plane of projection are at right angles to the plane.

projection, gnathic planes of orthographic, n.pl the three planes of projection to which gnathologically mounted casts are oriented: the horizontal, vertical, (frontal), and profile planes. The horizontal plane is the axis-orbital plane. The hinge axis is the line of intersection for both the horizontal and frontal planes. The profile plane is the mechanical midsagittal plane of the articulator.

prolactin, *n* See *hormone, lactogenic.*

prolapse, *v* the falling, sinking, or sliding of an organ from its normal position or location in the body.

proliferation (prō-lif′ər-ā′shən), *n* growth by reproduction of similar cells.

proliferation, epithelial, n a characteristic finding in inflammatory lesions affecting the gingival tissues; consists of hyperplasia of the pocket epithelium, with extension and elongation of epithelial rete pegs into the submucosa. Accompanying the hyperplastic changes in the crevicular epithelium, it is noticed that the epithelial attachment proliferates onto and alongside the cementum. Also, the multiplication of epithelial cells resulting either in increased thickness or new epithelial covering of a wound or an ulcer.

proline, *n* a nonessential amino acid found in many proteins of the body, particularly collagen.

promazine HCl, *n trade names:* Primazine, Prozine, Sparine; *drug class:* phenothiazine antipsychotic; *action:* blocks neurotransmission at dopaminergic synapses in the cerebral cortex, hypothalamus, and limbic system; mechanism for antipsychotic effects is unclear; *uses:* psychotic disorders, schizophrenia, nausea, vomiting, alcohol withdrawal.

promethazine HCl, *n trade names:* Phenameth, Phenazine; *drug class:* antihistamine, H_1-receptor antagonist; *action:* acts on blood vessels, gastrointestinal and respiratory systems by competing with histamine for H_1-receptor site; decreases allergic response by blocking histamine; *uses:* motion sickness, rhinitis, allergy symptoms, sedation, nausea, preoperative or postoperative sedation.

promissory (prom′is-ôr-ē), *n* a promise; stipulation for a future act or course of conduct.

promotion, *n* the gaining and retaining of acceptance by others of the views, products, or services of the originator of the message. Components of promotion: personal selling, advertising, sales promotion, and publicity.

promotion, sales, n sales promotion includes those marketing activities, other than personal selling, advertising, and publicity, that stimulate consumer purchasing and dealer effectiveness. They include point-of-purchase displays, shows and exhibit demonstrations, and other nonrecurrent selling efforts.

pronasion (prō-nā′zē-on), *n* the most prominent point on the tip of the nose when the head is placed in the eye-ear (horizontal) plane.

prone, *adj* lying flat with face down.

proof, *n* the establishment of a fact by evidence; to find the truth.

proof beyond a reasonable doubt, n in criminal law, such proof as precludes every reasonable hypothesis except that which it tends to support and is wholly consistent with the defendant's guilt and inconsistent with any other rational conclusions.

proof of loss, n the contractual right of the carrier or service corporation to request verification of services rendered (expenses incurred) by the submission of claim forms, radiographs, study models, or other diagnostic material.

prop, *n* a device inserted between the jaws to maintain an open position of the mandible.

prop, ratchet type, n a device placed in one side of the mouth that is used to keep the mouth of a patient open while work is performed on the other side. It can be set to various positions.

propafenone, *n trade name:* Rythmol; *drug class:* antidysrhythmic (Class IC); *action:* able to slow conduction velocity; reduces cardiac muscle membrane responsiveness; inhibits automaticity; increases ratio of effective refractory period to action potential duration; β-blocking activity; *use:* documented life-threatening dysrhythmias.

propagation (prop′ə-gā′shən), *n* the reproduction or continuance of an impulse along a nerve fiber in an afferent or efferent direction.

propantheline bromide, *n trade name:* Pro-Banthine; *drug class:* anticholinergic; *action:* inhibits muscarinic actions of acetylcholine at postganglionic parasympathetic neuroeffector sites; *uses:* treatment of peptic ulcer disease, irritable bowel syndrome, duodenography, urinary incontinence.

property, *n* rightful ownership; the exclusive right to a thing.

prophylactic (prō′fi-lak′tik), *adj* preventing disease; relating to prophylaxis.

prophylaxis (prō′fi-lak′sis), *n* the prevention of disease.

prophylaxis, dental, n a series of procedures whereby calculus, stain, and other accretions are removed from the clinical crowns of the teeth, and the clinical crowns of the teeth are polished.

propofol, *n trade name:* Diprivan; *drug class:* general anesthetic; *action:* produces dose-dependent central nervous system depression; mechanism of action is unknown; *use:* induction or maintenance of anesthesia as part of a balanced anesthetic technique.

proportional limit, *n* See *limit, elastic.*

propoxyphene napsylate/propoxyphene HCl, *n trade name:* Cotanal-65, Darvon, PP-Cap; *drug class:* synthetic opioid narcotic analgesic

(Controlled Substance Schedule IV); *action:* depresses pain impulse transmission in the central nervous system by interacting with opioid receptors; *use:* mild-to-moderate pain.

propranolol HCl, *n trade name:* Inderal; *drug class:* nonselective β-adrenergic blocker; *action:* competitively blocks stimulation of β-adrenergic receptors within the heart and decreases renin activity, all of which may play a role in the reduction of systolic and diastolic blood pressure; *uses:* chronic stable angina pectoris, hypertension, supraventricular dysrhythmias, migraine, myocardial infarction prophylaxis, pheochromocytoma, essential tremor, hypertrophic cardiomyopathy, anxiety.

proprietary (prō-prī′ ə-ter-ē), *adj* controlled by a private interest; protected by patent, trademark, or copyright.

proprietary name, n a brand name registered with the U.S. Patent Office under which the manufacturer markets his product. Also known as *trade name.*

proprioceptive influence, *n* the influence of the muscle sense (kinesthetic sense) in guiding the jaw to close in such a way as not to be injurious to the teeth.

proprioceptors (prō′pre-ō-sep′turz), *n.pl* sensory nerve receptors situated in the muscles, tendons, and joints that furnish information to the central nervous system concerning the movements and positions of the limbs, trunk, head, and neck, and, more specifically for the dentist, the mandible and its associated oral structures.

proptosis (prop-tō′sis), *n* the forward displacement or protrusion of the eyeball. See also *exophthalmos.*

propylthiouracil (PTU), *n trade name:* generic; *drug class:* thyroid hormone antagonist; *action:* blocks synthesis of thyroid hormones T_3 (triiodothyronine), T_4 (thyroxine); *uses:* preparation for thyroidectomy, thyrotoxic crisis, hyperthyroidism, thyroid storm.

prorating, *n* a clause in a contract with participating dentists wherein they agree to accept a percentage reduction in their billings to offset the amount by which the total cost of services provided exceeds the total premium received. Prorating is a method of spreading a "loss" equitably among participating dentists.

prospective review, *n* prior assessment by a payer or payer's agent that proposed services are appropriate for a particular patient, or the patient and the categories of service are covered by a benefits plan. See also *preauthorization; precertification predetermination;* and *second-opinion program.*

prospective study, *n* a study designed to determine the relationship between a condition and a characteristic shared by some members of a group. The population selected is healthy at the beginning of the study. Some of the members share a particular characteristic, such as cigarette smoking, while others do not. The study follows the population groups over a long period, noting the rate at which a condition, such as lung cancer, occurs in the smokers and in the nonsmokers.

prostaglandins (pros′tə-glan′dinz), *n.pl* a group of potent hormonelike substances that produce a wide range of body responses such as changing capillary permeability, smooth muscle tone, clumping of platelets, and endocrine and exocrine functions. They may be used in some instances to terminate a pregnancy.

prostate, *n* a gland in men that surrounds the neck of the bladder and the urethra and produces a secretion that liquefies coagulated semen.

prostate cancer, n a slowly progressive adenocarcinoma of the prostate gland that affects an increasing proportion of American males after the age of 50. It is the third leading cause of cancer deaths with more than 120,000 new cases reported in the United States each year.

prostatitis, *n* acute or chronic inflammation of the prostate gland, usually the result of infection.

prosthesis (pros-thē′sis), *n* the replacement of an absent part of the human body by an artificial part.

prosthesis, cleft palate, n a restoration to correct congenital or acquired defects in the palate and related structures if they are involved.

prosthesis, complete denture, n See *denture, complete.*

prosthesis, cranial, n an artificial material (alloplast) used to replace a portion of the skull.

prosthesis, definitive, n a permanent type of substitute for missing tissue.

prosthesis, dental, n an artificial replacement for one or more natural teeth or associated structures.

Dental prosthesis. (Rosenstiel/Land/ Fujimoto, 2001)

prosthesis, expansion, n a prosthesis used to expand the lateral segment of the maxilla in unilateral or bilateral cleft of the soft and hard palates and alveolar processes.

prosthesis, feeding, n a prosthesis worn by a young infant with a cleft palate to increase sucking power and to eliminate the escape of food through the nose.

prosthesis, fixed expansion, n a prosthesis that cannot be readily removed and stays in position for the required length of treatment.

prosthesis, partial denture, n See *denture, partial.*

prosthesis, pediatric speech aid, n a device temporarily used to replace lost tissue in the palate of a child to remedy inarticulate speech. The device may be used to close an opening caused by a developmental defect or surgery.

prosthesis, periodontal, n any restorative and replacement device that, by its intent and nature, is used as a therapeutic aid in the treatment of periodontal disease; it is an adjunct to other forms of periodontal therapy and does not cure periodontal disease by itself.

prosthesis, postsurgical, n an artificial replacement for a missing part or parts after surgical intervention.

prosthesis, removable expansion, n a prosthesis that can be removed from the mouth and replaced when indicated.

prosthesis, surgical, n an appliance prepared to assist in surgical procedures and placed at the time of surgery.

prosthesis, temporary, n a fixed or removable restoration for which a more permanent appliance is planned within a short period.

prosthetic appliance (prosthet'ik), *n* See *appliance, prosthetic.*

prosthetic restoration, *n* See *prosthesis.*

prosthetic speech aid, *n* See *aid, speech therapy.*

prosthetic valve endocarditis, *n* See *endocarditis, infective.*

prosthetics (pros-thet'iks), *n* the art and science of supplying, fitting, and servicing artificial replacements for missing parts of the human body.

prosthetics, complete denture, n **1.** the restoration of the natural teeth and their associated parts in the dental arch by artificial replacements. *n* **2.** the phase of dental prosthetics dealing with the restoration of function when one or both dental arches have been rendered edentulous.

prosthetics, dental, n See *prosthodontics.*

prosthetics, full denture, n See *prosthetics, complete denture.*

prosthetics, maxillofacial, n the branch of prosthodontics concerned with the restoration of stomatognathic and associated facial structures that have been affected by disease, injury, surgery, or congenital defect.

prosthetics, partial denture, n the dental service that, by replacing one or more but less than all the teeth of a dental arch, avoids the degenerative changes resulting from tooth movement and may thus achieve preventive measures of maximum benefit toward the maintenance of optimal oral health as well as reasonable restoration of dental functions.

prosthetist (pros'thǝ-tist), *n* the principal responsible individual involved in the construction of an artificial replacement for any part of the human body.

prosthion (pros'thē-on), *n* the point of the upper alveolar process that projects most anteriorly in the midline.

prosthodontia (pros'thō-don'shē-ǝ), *n* See *prosthodontics.*

prosthodontics (pros'thō-don'tiks), *n* the part of dentistry pertaining to the restoration and maintenance of oral function, comfort, appearance, and health of the patient by the replacement of missing teeth and contiguous tissues with artificial substitutes. Prosthodontics has three main branches: removable prosthodontics, fixed prosthodontics, and maxillofacial prosthetics.

prosthodontics, fixed, n the branch of prosthodontics concerned with the replacement or restoration of teeth by artificial substitutes that are not readily removable.

prosthodontist (pros'thō-don'tist), *n* a dentist engaged in the practice of prosthodontics. A specialist in the practice of prosthodontics.

protective apron, *n* See *apron, lead.*

protective clothing, *n* clothing required to shield or guard the wearer from infectious, toxic, or harmful substances while engaged in employment. Federal and state statutes govern the use of such apparel.

protective devices, *n.pl* articles designed to guard or shield an employee from harm, which include but are not limited to helmets, protective eye glasses, noise-dampening ear protectors, railings, and knife and saw guards. Federal and state statutes govern the use and placement of safety measures.

protective eyewear, *n* See *eyewear, protective.*

protein (prō'tēn), *n* any one of a group of complex organic nitrogenous compounds; the principal constituent of cell protoplasm. Polymers of amino acids that are joined by peptide or amide bonds.

protein, anabolic, n See *steroid, C-19 cortico.*

protein, Bence Jones, n.pr a special protein found in the blood and urine of patients with multiple myeloma and occasionally other diseases involving bone marrow, such as sarcoma and leukemia.

protein, C-reactive, n a mucoprotein whose presence in serum is always abnormal. It may be present in a variety of inflammatory or necrotic disease processes. It is almost always present in the serum in acute rheumatic fever.

protein chemical score (CS), n the result of a comparison between the amount of essential amino acid in a dietary protein and the amount in a reference protein.

protein, complementary, n any protein that is incomplete on its own but may become complete when combined with other proteins to provide all of the amino acids necessary for normal metabolism.

protein, complete, n protein that contains ample amounts of all the amino acids necessary for normal metabolism; animal proteins.

protein, deficiency, n See *deficiency, protein.*

protein efficiency ratio (PER), n a calculation designed to assess an individual protein's ability to sustain growth.

protein incomplete, n a protein that is missing one or more of the amino acids necessary for normal metabolism; vegetable protein.

protein kinase, n a protein that catalyzes the transfer of a phosphate group from adenosine triphosphate to produce a phosphoprotein.

protein, plasma, n blood serum contains 6.5 to 8 grams percent of a complex mixture of proteins, including albumin, globulin, and fibrinogen.

protein, reference, n a protein, usually egg, against which other proteins may be measured to evaluate their capability for supporting synthesis.

protein, spare, n one of several roles a carbohydrate food may play in a well-balanced diet. Many foods that are technically classified as carbohydrates, including some whole grains and beans, contain relatively significant amounts of protein that may, therefore, be referred to as spare.

protein specificity, n the arrangement of protein molecules in numerous spatial configurations to suit the special needs of the physical and chemical activities of the cell. The wide degree of variability of protein structures permits a high degree of specificity of tissue within one body. This characteristic of protein specificity is of great significance in blood

transfusions, tissue grafts, and many allergic manifestations.

protein, thromboplastic, n See *factor III.*

proteinuria (prō′tēn-yōō′rē-ə), n the presence of protein in the urine. Proteinuria is an indication of kidney disease.

proteinuria, orthostatic, n (postural proteinuria) proteinuria that occurs during daily activities but does not occur when the individual is recumbent.

proteinuria, physiologic, n See *proteinuria, transient.*

proteinuria, postural, n See *proteinuria, orthostatic.*

proteinuria, transient, n (physiologic proteinuria) proteinuria that occurs in normal persons after a high-protein meal, violent exercise, severe emotional stress, or syncope. It may occur after an epileptic seizure or during pregnancy. It disappears after the cause subsides.

proteoglycans, n.pl mucopolysaccharides bound to protein chains occurring in the extracellular matrix of connective tissue.

proteolytic (pro″ te-o-lit′ ik), adj pertaining to substances that aid in the breakdown and assimilation of proteins.

Proteus, n a genus of motile, gram-negative bacilli often associated with nosocomial infections and normally found in feces, water, and soil. *Proteus* may cause urinary tract infections, pyelonephritis, wound infections, diarrhea, bacteremia, and endotoxic shock.

prothrombase (prō-throm′bās), n See *factor II* and *prothrombin.*

prothrombin (prō-throm′bin), n a glycoprotein precursor of thrombin that is produced in the liver and is necessary for the coagulation of blood. A prothrombin deficiency is uncommon but may occur in liver disease. Vitamin K is essential for the synthesis of prothrombin.

prothrombin, B, n See *factor II.*

prothrombin, component A of, n See *factor V.*

prothrombin, component B of, n See *factor VII.*

prothrombin time, n a one-stage test for detecting certain plasma coagulation defects caused by a deficiency of factors V, VII, or X. Thromboplastin and calcium are added to a sample of the patient's plasma and, simultaneously, to a sample from a normal control. The amount of time required for clot formation in both samples is observed. A prolonged prothrombin time indicates deficiency in one of the factors. Normal findings of prothrombin time are 11 to 12.5 seconds.

prothrombinase (prō-throm′bi-nās), *n* (complete thromboplastin, direct activator of prothrombin, extrinsic prothrombin activator), an inferred direct activator of prothrombin common to tissue and plasma coagulation systems. See also *factor V.*

prothromboklnase (prō-throm′bō-kin′ās), *n* See *factor VIII.*

prothromboplastin, beta (prō-throm′bō plas′tin), *n* See *factor IX.*

proton (prō′ton), *n* an elementary particle having a positive charge equivalent to the negative charge of the electron but possessing a mass approximately 1845 times as great; the proton is a nuclear particle, whereas the electron is extranuclear.

protoplasm (prō′tō-plaz-əm), *n* a living substance; composed mainly of five basic materials: carbohydrates, electrolytes, lipids, proteins, and water and having the properties of both a complex solution and a heterogeneous colloid. The cell nucleus and cytoplasm are two major subdivisions of protoplasm.

protraction (prō-trak′shən), *n* a condition in which teeth or other maxillary or mandibular structures are situated anterior to their normal position.

protriptyline HCl, *n trade names:* Vivactil; *drug class:* tricyclic antidepressant; *action:* inhibits both norepinephrine and serotonin (5-HT) uptake in the brain; *use:* depression.

protrusion (prō-trōō′zhən), *n* the teeth or jaws protrude farther forward than normal.

protrusion, bimaxillary, n a relatively forward position, or prognathism, of the maxillary and mandibular teeth, alveolar processes, or jaws.

protrusion, double, n a definite labioversion of the maxillary and mandibular anterior teeth.

protrusion, forward, n a protrusion forward from the centric position.

protrusion, mandibular, n an abnormal protrusion of the mandible, as in a Class III malocclusion.

protrusion, maxillary, n an abnormal protrusion of the maxillae.

protrusive checkbite, *n* See *record, interocclusal, protrusive.*

protrusive occlusion, *n* See *occlusion, protrusive.*

protrusive position, *n* See *position, protrusive.*

protrusive record, *n* See *record, protrusive.*

protrusive relation, *n* See *relation, jaw, protrusive.*

Providencia (prov′i-den′sē-ə), *n* a genus of gram-negative, rod-shaped, facultative anaerobic bacteria, associated with urinary tract and secondary tissue infections.

provider, *n* a governmental term used to denote healthcare institutions; sometimes used as a synonym for *practitioner.*

provirus (prō-vī′rus), *n* a type of virus incorporated into a host cell's genetic material that transmits from one generation of cells to the next via cell replication without triggering the separation or decomposition of the cell.

provisional prosthesis, *n* an interim prosthesis worn for varying periods.

provisional splint, *n* See *splint, provisional.*

provitamin (prō-vī′tə-min), *n* any substance in food that may be transformed into a vitamin within the body; a potential vitamin.

proximal surface, *n* See *surface, proximal.*

proximate cause, *n* one that directly produces an effect; that which in ordinary, natural sequence produces a specific result with no agencies intervening.

pruritus (prōō-rī′tus), *n* itching.

Prussian blue, *n.pr* a chemical stain used on microscopic preparations. It demonstrates the presence of copper by developing a bright blue color.

pseudo pocket, *n* a pocket formed by gingival hyperplasia and edema without apical migration of the epithelial attachment. See also *pocket, gingival.*

pseudarthrosis (sōō′där-thrō′sis), *n* a false joint; sometimes seen after a fracture.

P

pseudoephedrine HCl/pseudoephedrine sulfate, *n trade name:* Balminil, Benylin, Cenafed, Sudafed, Sufedrin; *drug class:* α-adrenergic agonist; *action:* acts primarily on α-receptors, causing vasoconstriction in blood vessels; has more β activity and, to a lesser degree, central nervous system stimulant effects.

pseudoepitheliomatous hyperplasia (PEH) (sōō′dō-ep′i-thēl-ēō-mət-us hī′pur-plā′zē-ə, -zhə), *n* a type of epithelial hyperplasia associated with chronic inflammatory response; distinguished from squamous cell carcinoma by the lack of dysplastic cytologic characteristics.

pseudohemophilia (sōō′dō-hē′mō-fil′ē-ə), *n* the term used to describe several hemorrhagic states: (1) von Willebrand's disease, pseudohemophilia type B, vascular hemophilia; (2) a hereditary disease in which prolonged bleeding is the only consistent abnormality detected by currently available tests. See also *purpura, thrombocytopenic.*

pseudohypertropic muscular dystrophy (sōō′dō-hī′pur-trof′ik), *n* See *muscular dystrophy.*

pseudomembrane, *n* a loosely adherent, grayish false membrane typical of intracellular coagulation necrosis. It is formed by necrotic epithelium embedded in fibrin, leukocytes, and erythrocytes. It is seen in necrotizing ulcerative periodontal disease (acute necrotizing ulcerative gingivitis or periodontitis), aphthous ulcers, and diphtheria. Removal leaves a raw, bleeding surface.

Pseudomonas, *n* a genus of gramnegative bacteria that includes several free-living species of soil and water and some opportunistic pathogens isolated from wounds, burns, and infections of the urinary tract.

pseudopod, *n* a temporary protoplasmic limblike process of an amoeba that can be extended to propel itself or to engulf food.

p.s.i, *n* pounds per square inch (lb/in^2); measurement describing the amount of pneumatic or hydraulic pressure in tanks and equipment used in pressurized dental procedures.

psoriasis (sôr-ī′ ə-sis), *n* a papulosquamous inflammatory skin disease of unknown cause. Rare oral lesions consist of red patches with white, scaly surfaces.

Psoriasis. (Zitelli/Davis, 2002)

PSP test, *n* See *test, phenolsulfonphthalein.*

psychiatry, *n* the branch of medical science that deals with the causes, treatment, and prevention of mental, emotional, and behavioral disorders.

psychic, *adj* of or relating to the mind or the soul.

psychologic age, *n* age determined by a person's emotions and outlook on life rather than physiology or chronology.

psychologic dependence, *n* mental state in which an individual considers a drug to be necessary for preserving health.

psychology, *n* **1.** the study of behavior and the functions and processes of the mind, especially as related to the social and physical environment. *n* **2.** a profession that involves the practical applications of knowledge, skills, and techniques in the understanding of, prevention of, or solution to individual or social problems, especially in regard to the interaction between the individual and the physical and social environment.

psychomotor, *adj* pertaining to or causing voluntary movements usually associated with neural activity.

psychomotor development, *n* the progressive attainment (by a child) of skills that involve both mental and muscular activity.

psychomotor domain, *n* the area of observable performance of skills that requires some degree of neuromuscular coordination.

psychoneurosis (sī′kō-nyōō-rō′sis), *n* **1.** an abnormal reaction to the environment, including anxieties, phobias, hysteria, and hypochondria. *n* 2. a term that includes neurasthenia, hysteria, psychasthenia, and mental disorders short of insanity.

psychopathology, *n* 1. the study of the causes, processes, and manifestations of mental disorders. *n* 2. the behavioral manifestation of any mental disorder.

psychopharmacology, *n* the scientific study of the effects of drugs on behavior and normal and abnormal mental functions.

psychosedative (sī'kō-sed'ə-tiv), *n* a calming agent that reduces anxiety and tension without depressing mental or motor functions.

psychosis (sī-kō'sis), *n* a functional or organic kind of mental derangement marked by a severe disturbance of personality involving autistic thinking, loss of contact with reality, delusions or hallucinations.

psychosis, manic-depressive, n (cyclothymia) a psychosis characterized by varying periods of depression and excitement. One state may predominate (for example, manic-depressive reaction, manic type).

psychosomatic (sī-kō-sō-mat'ik), *adj* 1. pertaining to the expression of an emotional conflict through physical symptoms. *adj* 2. pertaining to the mind-body relationship; having bodily symptoms of a psychic, emotional, or mental origin. See also *disease, psychosomatic.*

psychosomatic factors, n See *factor, psychosomatic.*

psychosomatic, medicine, n the branch of medicine concerned with the interrelationships between mental and emotional reactions and somatic processes, in particular the manner in which intrapsychic conflicts influence physical symptoms.

psychotherapy, *n* any of a large number of related methods of treating mental or emotional disorders by psychologic techniques rather than by physical means.

PTA, *n* See *plasma thromboplastin antecedent.*

PTC, *n* See *plasma thromboplastic component.*

pterygoid lateralis (ter'i-goid), *n* one of the four muscles of mastication that functions to open the jaws, protrude the mandible, and move the mandible from side to side. Also called the *external pterygoid muscle.*

pterygoid, medialis, *n* one of the four muscles of mastication. It lies medial to the ramus of the mandible and functions with the temporalis and masseter muscles to close the mandible. Also called the *internal pterygoid.*

pterygoid plexus of veins, *n* the collection of veins that unite with the retromandibular and facial veins to carry blood from the face and brain back to the heart. It can play a role in spreading dental infection.

pterygoid process, *n* See *process, hamular.*

pterygomandibular fold (raphe) (ter″ĭ-go-man-dib′ u lər, ra-fə), *n* a fibrous strip of tissue posterior to the most distal mandibular tooth, that spans the area between the mandible and the point at which the hard and soft palates meet, from the hamulus to the posterior end of the mylohyoid line.

pterygomandibular space (triangle), *n* the space between the medial area of the mandible and the medial pterygoid muscle, a target area for administering local anesthesia to the inferior alveolar nerve.

pterygomaxillary fissure (ter'i-gō-mak'səl-er-ē), *n* See *fissure, pterygomaxillary.*

pterygomaxillary notch, *n* See *notch, pterygomaxillary.*

PTF, *n* See *factor, plasma thromboplastin.*

PTF-A (plasma thromboplastin factor A), *n* See *factor VIII.*

PTF-B (plasma thromboplastin factor B), *n* See *factor IX.*

PTF-C (plasma thromboplastin factor C), *n* See *factor XI.*

ptosis, *n* a drooping of the upper eyelid.

PTT, *n* See *partial prothrombin time.*

ptyalectasis (tī'əl-ek'tə-sis), *n* See *sialoangiectasis.*

ptyalin, *n* a salivary enzyme that changes starch into sugars.

ptyalism (tī' əl-iz-əm), *n* See *sialorrhea.*

puberty (pyōō'bur-tē), *n* the age at which the reproductive system becomes functional, with concurrent development of secondary sex characteristics. Marked by increased estrogenic activity in the female and rise of androgenic activity in the male.

pubescence (pyōō-bes'əns), *n* the age of sexual maturity.

public health, *n* a field of medicine that deals with the physical and mental health of the community, particularly in such areas as water supply, waste disposal, air pollution, and food safety.

public health authority, *n* a governmental agency responsible for matters of public health.

public health dentistry, *n* See *community dentistry.*

public opinion, *n* the pooled judgment or attitude of the public in regard to a specific issue. Public opinion is generally determined by polling a sample of the population, using statistical tools. Elections are formal public opinion polls by which registered voter citizens register their choice of candidates and referenda.

public relations, *n* the art and science of promoting good will within the public by a corporation or governmental agency.

puerperal (pyōō-er'pər-əl), *adj* relating to or occurring during childbirth or the period immediately following. See also *postpartum.*

pulmonary edema, *n* the accumulation of extravascular fluid in lung tissues and alveoli, caused most commonly by congestive heart failure.

pulmonary embolism, *n* the blockage of a pulmonary artery by foreign matter such as fat, air, tumor tissue, or a thrombus that usually arises from a peripheral vein. Pulmonary embolism is difficult to distinguish from myocardial infarction and pneumonia.

pulp (pulp), *n* (dental pulp, tooth pulp) the organ, made up of blood vessels, nerves, and cellular elements, including odontoblasts, that forms dentin. It normally occupies the central portion of teeth.

pulp amputation, *n* See *pulpotomy.*

pulp, anachoresis of, *n* the localization of microbes from the bloodstream in a damaged pulp.

pulp canal, *n* See *canal, pulp.*

pulp capping, *n* See *capping, pulp.*

pulp cavity, *n* See *cavity, pulp.*

pulp chamber, *n* See *chamber, pulp.*

pulp, dental, *n* See *pulp.*

pulp extirpation, *n* See *pulpectomy.*

pulp horn, *n* See *horn, pulp.*

pulp involvement, *n* See *involvement, pulp.*

pulp, mummification of, *n* dry gangrene of the dental pulp in which the pulp dries and shrivels.

pulp removal, *n* See *pulpectomy.*

pulp stone, *n* See *denticle.*

pulp test, *n* the application of a physical stimulus (electrical, heat, or cold) to determine the degree of vitality of the pulp tissue.

pulp test, thermal, *n* a method of applying a hot or cold stimulus to any tooth to assess the amount and degree of vitality of the structure. The clinician may use warm water, cold drinks, ice sticks, or blasts of air.

pulp tester, *n* (vitalometer) an electric instrument of high or low frequency designed to determine the response of a pulp to an electrical stimulus.

pulp, tooth, *n* See *pulp.*

pulp vitality, *n* the health status of the pulp. When the pulp tissue of a tooth has undergone complete degeneration or has been removed, the tooth is termed pulpless or nonvital.

pulpal (pul'pəl), *adj* relating to the pulp or the pulp cavity.

pulpalgia (pul-pal'jē-ə), *n* the sensitivity of the pulp to pain.

pulpectomy (pulp-ek'tə-mē), *n* (pulp extirpation, pulp removal), the complete removal of a pulp from the pulp chamber and root canal.

pulpectomy, complete, *n* the surgical removal of the pulp to the dentinocemental junction at the apex of the root.

pulpectomy, partial, *n* the surgical removal of only a part of the contents of the canal(s).

pulpitis (pulp-ī'tis), *n* an inflammation of the pulpal tissue of a tooth.

pulpitis, hypertrophic, *n* (pulp polyp) the formation and proliferation of granulation tissue from the surface of an exposed pulp.

pulpless (pulp'les), *adj* having a nonfunctioning pulp (untreated), or a pulp that has been replaced with an inert material (treated).

pulpless tooth, *n* See *tooth, pulpless.*

pulpotomy (pulp-ot'ə-mē), *n* (pulp amputation), the surgical amputation of the dental pulp coronal to the dentinocemental junction.

pulpotomy, partial, n the surgical removal of only a part of the tissue in the pulpal chamber.

pulpotomy, total or complete, n the surgical removal of the entire contents of the pulpal chamber at the entrance of the root canal(s).

pulse (pls) (puls), *n* the rhythmic expansion and contraction of arteries resulting from the surges of blood through the arteries. The pulse can be felt by the fingers in arteries that are close to the skin.

pulse, arterial, n the pulsation of an artery produced by the rise and fall in blood pressure as the heart goes into systole and diastole and observed clinically by palpation of the radial artery. The pulse rate at birth is approximately 130 beats/min and diminishes to approximately 70 beats/min in the healthy adult. The range of normalcy is around 60 to 80 beats/min.

pulse pressure, n See *pressure, pulse.*

pulse, venous, n pulsation of a vein, most easily felt in the right jugular vein.

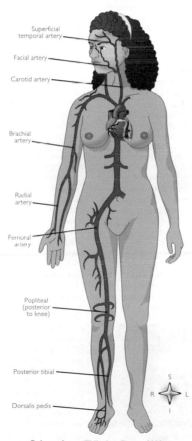

Pulse points. (Thibodeau/Patton, 2003)

pumice (pum'is), *n* a type of volcanic glass used as an abrasive. Pumice is prepared in various grits and is used for finishing and polishing in dentistry. It is also used in the polishing of natural teeth during a prophylaxis but is being replaced by less abrasive synthetic particles in some polishing pastes.

punch biopsy, *n* the removal of tissue for diagnostic purposes using a sharp, cylindrical, hollow instrument placed over the tissue to be excised and rotated with slight pressure until an incision of proper depth is achieved. The tissue within the incision is lifted, and the base is excised with a scissor or scalpel blade.

punch, rubber dam, *n* an instrument used to punch holes of varying sizes in a rubber dam so that it may be applied to the teeth.

punctate (pungk'tāt), *n* indicated with dots or points distinguished from the adjacent region by elevation, texture, or color.·

pupil, Argyll Robertson, *n.pr* pupillary abnormalities associated with tabes dorsalis (neurosyphilis), manifested by miosis, the absence of a ciliospinal reflex, and a reaction to accommodation but not to light.

purchaser, *n* a program sponsor, often an employer or union, that contracts with the dental benefits organization to provide dental benefits to an enrolled population.

purchasing cooperative, *n* a group of dentists pooling their financial resources to purchase large quantities of supplies and equipment for the purpose of obtaining a discount.

purging (purj'ing), *n* an effort to rid the body of food by vomiting or taking laxatives or diuretics.

Purpura. (Neville/Damm/Allen/Bouquot, 2002)

purpura (pur'pyōōr-ə), *n* extravasation of blood into the tissues, resulting in blue to black lesions of the skin or mucosa (petechiae and ecchymoses).

purpura, allergic, *n* (anaphylactoid purpura) any thrombocytopenic or nonthrombocytopenic purpura related to an allergic reaction. Manifestations other than ecchymoses and petechiae associated with erythema and inflammation include the common symptoms of allergy.

purpura, anaphylactoid, *n* See *purpura, allergic.*

purpura, essential, *n* See *purpura, thrombocytopenic, idiopathic.*

purpura hemorrhagica, *n* See *purpura, thrombocytopenic* and *purpura, thrombocytopenic, idiopathic.*

purpura, idiopathic thrombocytopenic, *n* (essential purpura, land scurvy, primary purpura, purpura hemorrhagica) a thrombocytopenic purpura of unknown cause.

purpura, nonthrombocytopenic, *n* purpura usually related to increased capillary permeability. Included are allergic purpuras and those resulting from vitamin C deficiency, bacterial toxins (scarlet fever, typhoid), drug intoxications, and metabolic toxins (nephritis, liver disease).

purpura, primary, *n* See *purpura, thrombocytopenic, idiopathic.*

purpura, secondary, *n* See *purpura, thrombocytopenic, symptomatic.*

purpura, symptomatic thrombocytopenic, *n* (secondary purpura) purpura resulting from the effects of chemical, physical, vegetable, or animal agents or infections or related blood disorders.

purpura, thrombocytopathic, *n* bleeding associated with qualitative abnormalities of the platelets.

purpura, thrombocytopenic, *n* (essential thrombopenia, pseudohemophilia, hemorrhagica, Werlhof's disease) severe ecchymoses and petechiae associated with marked reduction in the numbers of blood platelets. There is prolonged bleeding time and poor clot retraction, but the coagulation and prothrombin times are normal. Hemorrhage may occur spontaneously from any area of the oral mucosa. This disease may be acute and fatal, whereas in other instances it may run a chronic course with intermittent attacks.

purpura, thrombotic thrombocytopenic, *n* a febrile disease of unknown cause characterized by hemolytic anemia, neurologic symptoms, hemorrhage into the skin and mucous membranes, icterus, hepatosplenomegaly, low platelet count, and platelet thrombi occluding capillaries and arterioles.

purulent discharge (pyoor'yŏŏ-lent), *n* See *pus.*

pus (pus), *n* an inflammatory exudate formed within the tissues consisting of polymorphonuclear leukocytes, degenerated and liquefied tissue elements, microorganisms, and tissue fluids. It may form within the tissues in periodontitis and escape via the ulcerated pocket epithelium into the oral environment. The suppurative material may be retained within the tissues when the orifice of the periodontal pocket is blocked, thus creating a favorable circumstance for the formation of a periodontal abscess.

pustule (pus'chŏŏl), *n* a vesicular lesion containing pus rather than clear fluid.

putrefaction (pyŏŏ'trə-fak'shən), *n* the rotting of matter through the use of enzymes, producing substances such as ammonia, mercaptans, and hydrogen sulfide.

putrescine, *n* a foul-smelling toxic ptomaine produced by the decomposition of the amino acid ornithine during the decay of animal tissues, bacillus cultures, and fecal bacteria.

putty powder, *n* See *tin oxide.*

PVE, *n* prosthetic valve endocarditis. See *endocarditis, infective.*

pyknic (pik'nik), *adj* characterized by a short, squat appearance especially of body structures.

pyknosis (piknō'sis), *n* increased basophilia and shrinkage of the nucleus of a dying cell.

pyogenic (pī'ə-jen'ik), *adj* pus-producing.

pyorrhea (pī'ə-rē' ə), *n* an antiquated term used to designate periodontal disease. Generally, it means "flow of pus," which previously was a feature of periodontal disease. Before the use of the term *pyorrhea,* periodontitis was designated as *Riggs' disease* and *Fauchard's dis-*

ease. Still retained in some communities as a lay term for *periodontal disease.*

pyramidal (pĭ-ram' ĭ-dəl), *adj* having the shape that is peculiar to a pyramid (i.e., a solid with polygonal base and triangular faces that meet at a common point).

pyrazinamide, *n trade name:* generic; *drug class:* antitubercular; *action:* bactericidal interference with lipid, nucleic acid biosynthesis; *use:* tuberculosis, as an adjunct with other drugs.

pyrexia (pī-rek'sē-ə), *n* See *fever.*

pyridostigmine bromide, *n trade names:* Mestinon, Regonol; *drug class:* cholinergic; *action:* inhibits destruction of acetylcholine, which increases concentration at sites where acetylcholine is released. This facilitates transmission of impulses across myoneural junction; *uses:* nondepolarizing muscle relaxant antagonist, myasthenia gravis.

pyridoxine deficiency, *n* a lack of a required level of pyridoxine, which causes irritability and may lead to convulsions and peripheral neuritis.

pyridoxine HCl (pir'idok'sēn), *n* (vitamin B_6), *trade names:* Beesix, Nestrex; *drug class:* vitamin B_6, water soluble; *action:* needed for fat, protein, and carbohydrate metabolism as a coenzyme; *uses:* vitamin B_6 deficiency associated with inborn errors of metabolism, inadequate diet. See also *vitamin B_6.*

pyrimethamine (pir'meth'ə-mēn), *n* a folic acid inhibitor that acts against *Toxoplasma gondii* and *Plasmodium spp.,* which cause toxoplasmosis and malaria.

pyrolysis (pī-rol'i-sis), *n* the breaking down of a substance through the application of heat.

pyromania (pī'rō-mā'nē-ə), *n* an abnormal desire to start fires or an obsession with fire in general.

pyrometer (pī-rom'ə-tur), *n* an instrument for measuring temperature by the change of electrical resistance within a thermocouple. It is a millivoltometer calibrated in degrees of temperature.

pyrophosphatase, *n* any enzyme that cleaves an inorganic pyrophosphate from adenosyl triphosphate, leaving adenosine monophosphate.

pyrophosphate (pī'rō-fos'fāt), *n*

P

compound found in parotid saliva that helps delay calcification of bacteria plaque. It is also the active ingredient of commercial tarter-control oral hygiene products.

pyruvate kinase, *n* an enzyme essential for anaerobic glycolysis in red blood cells.

pyuria (pī-yōō′rē-ə), *n* abnormal numbers of white blood cells in the urine. Without proteinuria, it suggests infection of the urinary tract. With proteinuria, it suggests infection of the kidney (pyelonephritis).

q.4.h. (quaque quarta hora), *adv* a Latin phrase used in prescription writing meaning "every 4 hours."

q.i.d. (quater in die), *adv* a Latin phrase used in prescription writing meaning "four times a day."

q.s. (quantum satis, quantum sufficit), *adv* a Latin phrase used in prescription writing meaning "a sufficient quantity."

quack, *n* one who professes to have medical or dental skill that is not possessed; one who practices medicine or dentistry without adequate preparation or proper qualification.

quad helix appliance, *n* a fixed, spring-loaded orthodontic appliance using four helix springs; used primarily to expand the maxillary dental arch.

quadrant, *n* one quarter of a circle; also used to describe one fourth of the combined dental arches. One half of the maxillary dental arch is one quadrant of the combined dental arches.

quadriplegia, *n* an abnormal condition characterized by paralysis of both arms and legs and the trunk of the body below the level of the associated injury to the spinal cord. This disorder is usually caused by a spinal cord injury in the area of the fifth to seventh cervical vertebrae. Automobile accidents and sporting mishaps are common causes.

qualified, *adj* having the required ability; fitted; entitled.

quality, *n* in reference to the voice, the acoustic characteristics of vowels resulting from their overtone structure or the relative intensities of their frequency component.

quality assessment, *n* **1.** the measurement of quality; generally includes the selection of an aspect of dental care or the dental care system to be evaluated; establishing criteria and standards for quality dental care and comparing treatment with these criteria and standards. *n* **2.** the measure of the quality of care provided in a particular setting.

quality assurance, *n* **1.** procedures for checking the quality of dental care provided by participating dentists and correcting any irregularities. Also called *quality control* or *quality evaluation.* *n* **2.** the assessment or measurement of the quality of care and the implementation of any necessary changes to maintain or improve the quality of care rendered.

   quality assurance system, *n* a formally organized sequence of activities in dentistry that combines assessment of the existing situation, judgments about necessary changes, development of plans to effect such changes, implementation of these plans, and reassessment to determine that the desired changes have taken place.

quality of life, *n* a measure of the optimal energy or force that endows a person with the power to cope successfully with the full range of challenges encountered in the real world.

quality of radiation, *n* See *radiation quality.*

quality review committee, *n* a committee established by a professional organization or institution to assess and ensure quality. Unlike a peer review committee, it can function on its own initiative with regard to a broad range of topics.

quantum, *n* a discrete unit of electromagnetic energy or of an x-ray. A quantity becomes quantized when its magnitude is restricted to a discrete set of values as opposed to a continuous set of values.

   quantum theory, *n* See *theory, quantum.*

quarantine, *n* the isolation or confinement of a person or persons with a known or possible contagious disease.

quartz, *n* See *silica.*

quartz, fused, *n* a form of silica that is amorphous and exhibits no inversion at any temperature below its fusion point; of little use in dentistry.

quasi contract, *n* an obligation similar to a contract that arises not from an agreement of parties but from some relation between them or from a voluntary act of one of them.

quaternary (kwä´turn-er-ē), *adj* having four elements. Widely used in medicine, quaternary ammonium salts are molecules containing four alkyl or aryl groups attached to a nitrogen atom.

quazepam, *n* trade name: Doral; *drug class:* benzodiazepine, sedative-hypnotic, Controlled Substance Schedule IV; *action:* produces central nervous system depression by interacting with abenzodiazepine receptor to facilitate the action of the inhibitory neurotransmitter γ-aminobutyric acid; *use:* insomnia.

quench, *v* to cool a hot object rapidly by plunging it into water or oil.

question, hypothetical, *n* a combination of assumed or proven facts and circumstances, stated so as to constitute a coherent and specific situation or state of facts, on which the opinion of an expert is asked by way of evidence at a trial.

questionnaire, *n* a form usually filled out by patients that provides data concerning their dental and general health.

questionnaire, health, *n* a list of key questions answered by the patient that permits the diagnostician to interpret the general and oral health of the patient.

quick-cure resin, *n* See *resin, autopolymer.*

quid, *n* See *pinch.*

quinacrine (kwin´ə-krēn, -krin), *n* an anthelmintic and antiprotozoal agent used to treat giardiasis and tapeworm infections. It is not effective in treating malaria.

quinapril, *n* trade name: Accupril; *drug class:* angiotensin-converting enzyme; *action:* selectively suppresses renin-angiotensin-aldosterone system; inhibits angiotensin-converting enzyme; prevents conversion of angiotensin I to angiotensin II; results in dilation of arterial and venous vessels; *use:* hypertension, alone or in combination with thiazide diuretics.

Quincke's disease (kwing´kēz), *n.pr* See *edema, angioneurotic.*

quinidine gluconate/quinidine polygalacturonate/quinidine sulfate (kwin´i-dēn, -din), *n* trade names: Cardioquin, CinQuin, Duraquin, Quinidex Extentabs, Quinora; *drug class:* antidysrhythmic (class IA); *action:* prolongs effective refractory period; decreases myocardial excitability, conduction velocity, and contractility; *uses:* premature ventricular contractions, atrial flutter and fibrillation, paroxysmal atrial tachycardia, ventricular tachycardia.

quinine, *n* an alkaloid derived from cinchona that is effective against malaria. It is also used as an antipyretic, analgesic, sclerosing agent, and stomachic and in the treatment of atrial fibrillation and myotonia congenita.

quinine sulfate, *n* trade names: Legatrin, M-Kya, Quinamm, Q-Vel, *drug class:* antimalarial; *action:* schizonticidal, but mechanism is unclear; increases refractory period in skeletal muscles; *uses:* Plasmodium falciparum malaria, nocturnal leg cramps.

quinolone, *n* any of a class of antibiotics that act by interrupting the replication of deoxyribonucleic acid molecules in bacteria.

quinsy, *n* a peritonsillar abscess.

quintuplet, *n* any one of five offspring born in the same gestation period during a single pregnancy.

quotient, *n* the number of times one amount is contained in another.

rabies, *n* an acute, usually fatal viral disease of the central nervous system of animals. It is transmitted from animals to humans by infected blood, tissue, or most commonly, saliva.

racemic (rās-ē´mik), *adj* referring to a mixture of equal quantities of the dextro- and levo-isomers of a compound.

rad (r), *n* a unit of absorbed dose of radiation: 1 r equals 100 ergs/Gm. See also *rem.*

radial keratotomy, *n* a surgical procedure in which a series of tiny, shallow incisions are made on the cornea, causing it to bulge slightly to correct for nearsightedness. The operation is performed using local anesthesia and requires only a few minutes. Hospitalization is not necessary. Radial keratotomy usually corrects mild to moderate myopia.

radial pulse, *n* the pulse of the radial artery palpated at the wrist over the radius. The radial pulse is the one most often taken and recorded because of the ease with which it is located and palpated.

radiate (rā′dē-āt), *v* **1.** to diverge or spread from a common point; to arrange in a radiating manner. *v* **2.** to expose to radiation, as x-radiation.

radiation (rā′dē-ā′shən), *n* **1.** the process of emitting radiant energy in the form of waves or particles. *n* **2.** the combined processes of emission, transmission, and absorption of radiant energy.

Radiation. (Bird/Robinson, 2002)

radiation, actinic, *n* radiation capable of producing chemical change (for example, effect of light and x-rays on photographic emulsions).

radiation, background, *n* radiation arising from radioactive material other than the one directly under consideration. Background radiation resulting from cosmic rays and natural radioactivity is always present. Background radiation may also exist because of radioactive substances in other parts of a building (for example, building material).

radiation, backscatter, *n* radiation that deflects off its target at an angle of deflection greater than 90 degrees, possibly affecting those who may be off to the side of or behind the main beam. See also *radiation, scattered.*

radiation, biologic effectiveness of, *n* the ability of a particular type of ionizing radiation to produce biologic effects on an organism with small absorbed doses. See *relative biologic effectiveness.*

radiation, bremsstrahlung (bremsshträ′lōōng), *n* (white), describes the distribution of x-rays from extremely low energy photons to x-rays originating from the highest kilovoltage applied to an x-ray tube. *Bremsstrahlung* translates to "braking radiation," referring to the sudden slowing of electrons that occurs when they encounter nuclei with a high positive charge.

radiation caries, *n* a type of tooth decay caused by the reduction in saliva that may result from the use of ionizing radiation in the treatment of oral and facial malignancies. Radiation caries is an unfortunate side effect of a necessary radical procedure to cure or prevent the spread of cancer.

radiation cataract, *n* a cataract that is caused by extended exposure of the eye to ionizing radiation in the course of treating facial cancers.

radiation, characteristic, *n* radiation that originates from an atom after removal of an electron or excitation of the nucleus. The wavelength of the emitted radiation is specific, depending only on the element concerned and on the particular energy levels involved. Also refers to the specific type of secondary radiation resulting when rays from a radio ray tube strike another substance, such as copper.

radiation, coherent scattering, *n* See *coherent scattering.*

radiation, Compton scatter, n See *Compton scatter radiation.*

radiation, corpuscular, n subatomic particles, such as electrons, protons, neutrons, or alpha particles, that travel in streams at various velocities. All the particles have definite masses and travel at various speeds. The properties are in opposition to electromagnetic radiations, which have no mass and travel in wave forms at the speed of light. See also *radiation, electromagnetic.*

radiation, cosmic, n See *ray, cosmic.*

radiation, cumulative effect of, n reactions vary depending on the dosage; if the radiation received is in several smaller doses, the reaction is not as severe as if the same amount of radiation is received all at once. Unless a tissue is completely destroyed by the radiation, some or all of it will be repaired, although cumulative damage may cause some irreparable conditions.

radiation, dermatitis, n See *dermatitis, radiation.*

radiation detector, n any device for converting radiant energy to a form more suitable for observation and recording. Examples include x-ray films and radiometers.

radiation, direct, n (primary radiation), radiation emanating from a tube aperture and comprising the useful beam, as compared with any stray radiation, such as that which comes from the tube container.

radiation, electromagnetic, n forms of energy propagated by wave motion, such as photons or discrete quanta. The radiations have no matter associated with them, as opposed to corpuscular radiations, which have definite masses. They differ widely in wavelength, frequency, and photon energy and have strikingly different properties. Covering an enormous range of wavelengths (from 10^{-6} to 10^{17} Å), they include radio waves, infrared waves, visible light, ultraviolet radiation, gamma rays, and cosmic radiation. See also *radiation, corpuscular.*

radiation exposure, n a measure of the ionization produced in air by x-rays or gamma rays. It is the sum of the electric charges on all ions of one sign that are produced when all electrons liberated by photons in a volume of air are completely stopped, divided by the mass of air in the volume element. The unit of exposure is the roentgen.

radiation field, n See *x-ray beam, field size.*

radiation, gamma, n See *ray, gamma.*

radiation, genetic effects of, n See *genetic effects of radiation.*

radiation, grenz, n See *ray, grenz.*

radiation, hard, radiation consisting of the short wavelengths (higher kilovolt peak equals greater penetration).

radiation hazard, n See *hazard, radiation.*

radiation, heterogeneous, n a beam or "bundle" of radiation containing photons of many wavelengths.

radiation, homogeneous, n a beam of radiation consisting of photons that all have the same wavelength.

radiation hygiene, n See *hygiene, radiation.*

radiation intensity, n See *intensity, radiation.*

radiation, ionizing, n electomagnetic radiation such as x-rays and gamma rays; particulate radiation such as alpha particles, beta particles, protons, and neutrons; all other types of radiations that produce ionization directly or indirectly.

radiation leakage, n (stray radiation), the escape of radiation through the protective shielding of the x-ray unit tube head. This radiation is detected at the sides, top, bottom, or back of the tube head; it does not include the useful beam.

radiation, monochromatic, n See *radiation, homogeneous.*

radiation necrosis, n See *necrosis, radiation.*

radiation, neutron, n See *ray, neutron.*

radiation oncology, n the study of the treatment of cancer using ionizing radiation

radiation, primary, n all radiation produced directly from the target in an x-ray tube. See also *radiation, direct.*

radiation protection, n provision designed to reduce human exposure to radiation. For external radiation, this provision consists of using protective barriers of radiation-absorbing mate-

R

rial, ensuring adequate distances from the radiation sources, reducing exposure time, and combinations of these measures. For internal radiation, it involves measures to restrict inhalation, ingestion, or other modes of entry of radioactive material into the body.

radiation quality, n the ability of a beam of x-rays to allow the production of diagnostically useful radiographs. Usually measured in half-value layers of aluminum and controlled by the kilovolt peak.

radiation quantity, n amount of radiation. The amount of exposure is expressed in roentgens (R), whereas quantity of dose is expressed in rads.

radiation, relative biologic effectiveness of (RBE), n a comparison between various types of ionizing radiation with respect to the ability to produce biologic effects with small doses.

radiation, remnant, n the radiation passing through an object or part being examined that is available either for recording on a radiographic film or for measurement.

radiation, scattered, n (backscatter radiation), radiation whose direction has been altered. It may include secondary and stray radiation.

radiation, secondary, n the new radiation created by primary radiation acting on or passing through matter.

radiation shield, n See *shield, radiation.*

radiation sickness, n a self-limited syndrome characterized by varying degrees of nausea, vomiting, diarrhea, and psychic depression after exposure to very large doses of ionizing radiation, particularly doses to the abdominal region. Its mechanism is not completely understood. It usually occurs a few hours after treatment and may subside within a day. It may be sufficiently severe to necessitate interrupting the treatment series, or it may incapacitate the patient.

radiation, soft, n radiation consisting of the long wavelengths (lower kilovolt peak results in less penetration).

radiation, speed of, n the speed of light, or approximately 186,000 miles per second.

radiation, stray, n See *radiation leakage.*

radiation survey, n See *survey, radiation.*

radiation therapy, n See *therapy, radiation.*

radiation, total body, n the exposure of the entire body to penetrating radiation. In theory, all cells in the body receive the same overall dose.

radiation treatment, n a cancer treatment method that uses x-rays to modify or destroy cancer cells; dental patients who are undergoing radiation therapy may exhibit an increased need for certain nutrients. See also *therapy, radiation.*

radiation, useful, n the part of the primary radiation that is permitted to pass from the tube housing through the tube head port, aperture, or collimating device. See *beam, useful.*

radical, n **1.** a group of atoms that acts together and forms a component of a compound. The group tends to remain bound together when a chemical reaction removes it from one compound and attaches it to another compound. A radical does not exist freely in nature. *adj* **2.** a drastic measure to cure or prevent the spread of a serious disease, such as the surgical removal of an organ, limb, or other body part.

radical neck dissection, n dissection and removal of all lymph nodes and removable tissues under the skin of the neck, performed to prevent the spread of malignant tumors of the head and neck that have a reasonable chance of being controlled by such aggressive treatment.

radicular (ra-dik′yōō-lur), *adj* pertaining to the root. In restorative dentistry, the location at which the form of the preparation and restoration for the coronal portion of the natural tooth extends into the treated root canal of the pulpless tooth (e.g., radicular preparation, radicular restoration [dowel crown]).

radicular cyst, n See *cyst, radicular.*

radio-, *comb* denotes radiation from any source.

radioactive decay, n See *decay, radioactive.*

radioactive isotope, n See *radioisotope.*

radioactive tracer, *n* a molecule to which a radioactive atom has been attached so that it can be followed through a physiologic system with radiation detectors.

radioactivity (rā′dē-ō ak-tiv′i-tē), *n* spontaneous nuclear disintegration with emission of corpuscular or electromagnetic radiations. The principal types of radioactivity are alpha disintegration, beta decay (negatron emission, positron emission, and electron capture), and isometric transition. Double beta decay is another type of radioactivity that has been postulated, and spontaneous fission and the spontaneous transformations of mesons are sometimes considered to be types of radioactivity. To be considered radioactive, a process must have a measurable lifetime between approximately 1 and 10 seconds and 10^{17} years, according to present experimental techniques. Radiations emitted within a time too short for measurement are called *prompt;* however, prompt radiations, including gamma rays, characteristic x-rays, conversion and auger electrons, delayed neutrons, and annihilation radiation, are often associated with radioactive disintegrations because their emission may follow the primary radioactive process.

radioallergosorbent test (RAST), *n* a test to determine whether an atopic allergy to a substance exists. A radioimmunoassay is used to identify and quantify IgE in serum that has been mixed with any of 45 known allergens. This is an in vitro method of demonstrating allergic reactions, as opposed to the patch test, which is the common in vivo method of determining allergens.

radiobiology, *n* the branch of the natural sciences dealing with the effects of radiation on biologic systems.

radiogram (rā′dē-ō-gram), *n* See *radiograph.*

radiograph(s) (rā′dē-ō-graf), *n* an image or picture produced on a radiation-sensitive film emulsion by exposure to ionizing radiation directed through an area, region, or substance of interest, followed by chemical processing of the film. It basically depends on the differen-

tial absorption of radiation directed through heterogeneous media.

radiograph, bite-wing, *n* a form of dental radiograph that reveals approximately the coronal halves of the maxillary and mandibular teeth and portions of the interdental alveolar septa on the same film. Bite-wings can be used at any point in the dental arch.

radiograph, body-section, *n* radiograph produced by rotation of the film and x-ray source around the region of interest in opposite directions during exposure, so as to blur interposed anatomic structures outside the region of interest.

radiograph, cephalometric, *n* extraoral radiographs produced under conditions ensuring maximal dimensional accuracy and reproducible film-object-beam relationship for purposes of cephalometric study

Cephalometric radiograph. (Bird/Robinson, 2002)

radiograph, composite, *n* radiograph made by superimposing a radiograph of osseous tissue whose exposed border has been cut away on a radiograph of soft tissue for the purpose of detecting radiographic information concerning both the soft tissues and the osseous tissues of the head and face from a single radiographic view.

radiograph, contrast media, *n* radiograph that records the shadow images of the secretory apparatus of any of the salivary glands, body cavities, or fistulous tracts after the injection of a liquid radiopaque solution.

radiograph, extraoral, *n* radiograph produced on a film placed extraorally.

radiograph, follow-up, *n* radiographs made during and after therapy to follow the progress or regress of a disease, determine the course of healing, or ascertain the results of treatment.

radiograph, high kilovoltage, *n* an x-ray photo taken using a higher kilovoltage than normal. This method provides a lower contrast film with more interpretive details and can be developed in a shorter time, but it subjects the surrounding areas to more radiation.

radiograph, intraoral, *n* radiograph produced by placing a radiographic film within the oral cavity.

radiograph, microscopic examination, *n* See *microradiography.*

radiograph, occlusal, *n* a special type of intraoral radiograph made with the film held between the occluded teeth.

radiograph, oral, *n* radiographic representation of shadow images of all the tissues, structures, and regions of the oral cavity and its adjacent areas and associated parts.

radiograph, panoramic, *n* a large radiograph depicting the curvatures of the maxillae, mandible, and associated structures.

radiograph, reference, *n* a training tool in which ideal dental x-ray films are compared with recently taken films to study, compare, and improve interpretation and investigative skills in dental office employees.

radiograph, salivary gland, *n* See *sialography.*

radiograph, stereoscopic, *n* a pair of radiographs of a structure made by shifting the position of the x-ray tube a few centimeters between each of two exposures. Such pairs provide a three-dimensional, or stereoscopic, presentation of the recorded images.

radiograph, Towne's projection, *n.pr* radiographic view of the mandibular condyles and the midfacial skeleton.

radiographer (rā′dē-og′rə-fur), *n* a specialist or technician in radiography.

radiographer anatomy, *n* See *anatomy, radiographic.*

radiographer contrast, *n* See *contrast, radiographic.*

radiographer density, *n* See *density, radiographic.*

radiographer diagnosis, *n* See *diagnosis, radiographic.*

radiographer examination, *n* See *examination, radiographic.*

radiographer grid, *n* a clear plastic device with the horizontal and vertical wires crossing each other at intervals of 1 mm; used in x-ray techniques for the purpose of measurement.

radiographer interpretation, *n* See *interpretation, radiographic.*

radiographer localization, *n* See *localization, radiographic.*

radiographer, oral, *n* a specialist or technician in oral radiography.

radiographer survey, *n* See *survey, radiographic.*

radiographic (rā′dē-ō-graf′ik), *adj* relating to the process of radiography, the finished product, or its use.

radiographic film, air bubbles on, *n* See *film fault, white spots.*

radiographic film sizes, *n* nonscreen films (e.g., No. 0, 22 × 35 mm; No. 1, 24 × 40 mm, No. 2, 31 × 41 mm; No. 3, 27 × 54 mm; and No. 4, 57 × 76 mm) or (e.g., 5 × 7 in, 5 × 12 in, and 8 × 10 in) used to produce radiographic images.

radiographic film storage methods, *n* an appropriate method of safekeeping to maintain the integrity of the materials (e.g., the placement of items in regions that will prevent exposure to radiation, heat, vapors from chemical substances, and moisture), as well as the creation of a filing system that ensures the oldest product is used first.

radiography (rā′dē-og′rə-fē), *n* the making of shadow images on photographic emulsion by the action of ionizing radiation. The image is the result of the differential attenuation of the radiation in its passage through the object being radiographed. *Roentgenography* refers to production of film by the use of x-rays only.

radiography, bone in, *n* radiography of bone and marrow tissue. Translucencies and opacities in bone in radiographs depend on the different densities that bone and marrow spaces present to the x-rays. The configuration of bone tissue represents the topography and arrangement of bone trabeculae, which register as opaque in contrast to the translucency of the marrow spaces.

radiography, computerized digital, n an x-ray machine using computer technology to produce a digital image instead of using film; a digital sensor is placed in a disposable sheath inside the patient's mouth, then the sensor is exposed to radiation as in a traditional x-ray, except that the sensor produces an immediately accessible digital image that can be viewed on a computer screen.

radiography, digital subtraction, n a technique for eliminating unnecessary anatomic structures on a radiographic image by storing the pre- and postprocedure images in a computer and then combining them together digitally to display the final subtracted image, which emphasizes the differences between the two original films.

radiography, oral, n the specialized operative and technical procedures and practices for making successful radiographic surveys, with the understanding that it involves the selection of the dental x-ray unit and its adjustments as well as the generation and application of x-rays to all phases of interest to the dental profession. It also takes into consideration all the processes necessary for the production of finished radiographs of the teeth and their supporting tissues, adjacent regions, and associated parts.

radiography, subtraction, n the digital or photographic manipulation of a radiograph in which background images are eliminated to highlight areas for pre- and postoperative comparison.

radioisotope (rā′dē-ō-ī′sō-tōp), n a chemical element that has been made radioactive through bombardment of neutrons in a cyclotron or atomic pile or found in a natural state.

radioisotope scan, n a two-dimensional representation of the gamma rays emitted by a radioisotope, show-

ing its concentration in a body site such as the thyroid gland, brain, or kidney. Radioisotopes used in diagnostic scanning may be administered intravenously or orally.

radiologist (rā′dē-ol′ə-jist), n a person who has special experience in the science of radiant energy and radiant substances (including roentgen rays); especially a person engaged in the branch of medical science that deals with the use of radiant energy in the diagnosis and treatment of disease.

radiologist, oral, n a specialist in the art and science of oral radiology.

radiology (rā′dē-ol′ə-jē), n **1.** the branch of medicine dealing with the diagnostic and therapeutic applications of ionizing radiation. n **2.** the science of radiant energy, its use toward the extension of present knowledge, and its diverse applications for the benefit of humankind.

radiology, oral, n all phases of the science and art of radiology that are of interest to the dental profession. Oral radiology involves the generation and application of x-rays for the purpose of recording shadow images of teeth and their supporting tissues, adjacent regions, and associated parts. It also includes the interpretation of the radiographic findings.

radiolucence (rā′dē-ō-lōō′sens), n relative term indicating the comparatively low attenuation of an x ray beam produced by materials of relatively low atomic number. (The image on a radiograph of such materials is relatively dark because of the greater amount of radiation that penetrates to reach the film.)

radiolucency (rā′dē-ō-lōō′sens-ē), n a radiographic representation of decreased density of hard and soft tissue structures.

radiolucent (rā′dē-ō-lōō′sent), adj permitting the passage of radiant energy, with relatively little attenuation by absorption. The image of radiolucent materials on a radiograph ranges from shades of gray to black.

radiolysis of water (rādē-ol′is-is), n a separation of water via radioactive activity. The end result is the production of hydrogen peroxide.

radionuclide (rā′dē-ō-nōō′klīd), n an unstable or radioactive type of atom characterized by the constitu-

R

tion of its nucleus and capable of existing for a measurable time. The nuclear constitution is specified by the number of protons *(A)*, number of neutrons *(N)*, and energy content, or alternatively by the atomic number *(Z)*, mass number *(A − N + Z)*, and atomic mass.

radiopacity (rā'dē-ō-pas'i-tē), *n* relative term referring to the considerable attenuation of an x-ray beam produced by materials of relatively high atomic number. The image on a radiograph of such materials is relatively light because less radiation passes through, which prevents the exposure of the film in that area.

radiopaque (rā'dē-ō-pāk'), *adj* permitting the passage of radiant energy, but only with considerable or extreme attenuation of the radiation by absorption. The image of radiopaque materials on a radiograph ranges from light gray to total white or clarity on the film. See also *medium, radiopaque.*

radioparent (rā'dē-ō-per'ent), *adj* made visible by means of roentgen rays or other means of radiation. Permitting the passage of x-rays or other radiation.

radiopharmacy, *n* a facility for the preparation and dispensing of radioactive drugs and the storage of radioactive materials, inventory records, and prescriptions of radioactive substances. The radiopharmacy is usually the correlation point for radioactive wastes, the unit responsible for waste disposal or storage and the center for clinical investigations using radioactive tracers.

radioresistance (rā'dē-ō-rē-zis'təns), *n* the relative resistance of cells, tissues, organs, or organisms to the injurious effects of ionizing radiation. See also *radiosensitivity.*

radiosensitivity (rā'dē-ō-sen'si-tiv'i-tē), *n* relative susceptibility of cells, tissues, organs, organisms, and other substances to the injurious action of radiation.

radiotherapy, *n* the treatment of neoplastic disease by using x-rays or gamma rays to prevent or slow the proliferation of malignant cells by decreasing the rate of mitosis or impairing deoxyribonucleic acid synthesis. See *therapy, radiation.*

radium (Ra), *n* a radioactive metallic element of the alkaline earth groups. Its atomic number is 88. Four radium isotopes occur naturally and have different atomic weights: 223, 224, 226, and 228.

radium emanation, *n* radon. An element, used in radiotherapy, produced when radium disintegrates.

radon, *n* A byproduct of radium decomposition used in radiotherapy.

radon seed (rā'don), *n* a small sealed container or tube for carrying radon. It is made of gold or glass, is inserted into the tissues for the treatment of certain disease entities, and is visible radiographically.

rale (rāl), *n* **1.** abnormal sound that originates from the trachea, bronchi, or lungs. *v* **2.** to make such a sound.

Ramfjord teeth index (ram'fyurd), *n.pr* See *index, periodontal.*

ramify (ram'ə-fī), *v* to branch; to diverge in various directions; to traverse in branches.

ramipril, *n trade name:* Altace; *drug class:* angiotensin-converting enzyme (ACE) inhibitor; *action:* selectively suppresses renin-angiotensin-aldosterone system; inhibits ACE; prevents conversion of angiotensin I to angiotensin II; results in dilation of arterial and venous vessels; *uses:* hypertension, alone or in combination with thiazide diuretics; congestive heart failure immediately after myocardial infarction.

ramus (rā'məs), *n* **1.** a branch of an artery, nerve, or vein. In the *Basle Nomina Anatomica* terminology, the term ramus is given to a primary division of a nerve or blood vessel. *n* **2.** any constant branch of a fissure, or sulcus, of the brain.

ramus, mandibular, *n* the bilateral, upturned, angled bony process of the mandible that extends upward and backward from the horseshoe-shaped body and terminates in two processes: the articular condyloid process and the coronoid process.

random controlled trial, *n* a study plan for a proposed new treatment in which subjects are assigned on a random basis to participate in either an experimental group receiving the new treatment or a control group that does not.

R

random-access memory (RAM), *n* the part of a computer's memory available to execute programs and temporarily store data. The memory to which the operator has random access can usually be used for both reading and writing. Unless the file has been saved, RAM data are automatically erased when the computer is turned off.

range, *n* a crude measure of disper sion in a distribution; range is computed as the distance from the highest score to the lowest score plus one unit.

range, melting, *n* the temperature range from the time an alloy begins to melt until it is completely molten. It varies from 100° to 200° F (38° to 70° C), in gold-platinum-palladium alloys.

range of motion, *n* the maximum extent to which the parts of a joint can move in extension and flexion as measured in degrees of a circle.

ranitidine, *n trade name:* Zantac, Zantac EFFERdose, Zantac GEL-dose, Zantac 75; *drug class:* H_2 histamine receptor antagonist; *action:* inhibits histamine at H_2-receptor sites in parietal cells, which inhibit gastric acid secretion; *uses:* duodenal ulcers, gastric ulcers, hypersecretory conditions, gastroesophageal reflux disease.

Rankine scale, *n.pr* an absolute temperature scale calculated in degrees Fahrenheit. Absolute zero on the Rankine scale is −460° F, equivalent to −273° C.

ranula (ran′yōō-lə), *n* a large mucocele in the floor of the mouth. It usually results from obstruction of the ducts of the sublingual salivary glands. Less frequently, it results from obstruction of the ducts of the submandibular salivary glands.

Ranula. (Neville/Damm/Allen/Bouquot, 2002)

Ranvier, nodes of (rän′vē-ā′), *n.pr* See *node of Ranvier.*

raphae, midpalatine (rā′fē), *n* the ridge of mucous membrane that marks the median line of the hard palate.

raphe (ra′ fə), *n* (*pl* **raphae**) a crease or ridge that divides an organ in half.

rapport, *n* a sense of mutuality and understanding; harmony, accord, confidence, and respect underlying a relationship between two persons; an essential bond between a therapist and patient.

rare earth, *n* metallic elements used in intensifying screens. Also refers to fast exposure x-ray screen film.

rare earth screen, *n* a fluorescent material such as calcium tungstate used as the basis of x-ray intensifying screens. In recent years, new materials, including the rare earths yttrium and gadolinium, have also found application in such devices. These rare earths enable lower radiation doses to be used while producing acceptable film densities.

rarefaction, bone, *n* See *bone rarefaction.*

rash, wandering, *n* See *tongue, geographic.*

rat, Sprague-Dawley, *n.pr* an inbred strain of albino rat commonly used in laboratory research. There are 12 strains of inbred rats listed under "Medical Subject Headings," a supplement to *Index Medicus.* The Wistar rat is an equally popular inbred strain of albino rat used in laboratory research.

ratchet wrench, *n* a wrench activated by its handle through a hinged catch (pawl) that causes the wrench to rotate in one direction only (may be adjusted for either direction).

rate, *n* measurement of a thing by its ratio or given in relation to some standard.

rate, basal metabolic, *n* See *basal metabolic rate.*

rate, DEF, *n* an expression of dental caries experience in deciduous teeth. The DEF rate is calculated by adding the number of decayed primary teeth requiring filling (D), decayed primary teeth requiring extraction (E), and primary teeth successfully filled (F). Missing primary teeth are not included in the count because whether

R

they were extracted because of caries or exfoliated normally is frequently impossible to determine.

rate, DMF index, n a method of classifying the condition of the teeth based on the number of teeth in a given mouth that are decayed, missing, or indicated for removal and of those filled or bearing restorations.

rate, erythrocyte sedimentation, n the rate of settling of erythrocytes by gravity under conditions in which all factors affecting the rate are corrected, standardized, or eliminated except for alterations in the physicochemical properties of the plasma proteins. These alterations are the basis for interpretation of the rate. There is an increase in the rate in most infections. Sedimentation velocity is useful in prognosis to determine recovery from infection. Normal values vary with the method used in the determination.

rate, heart, n the rate of the heartbeat, expressed as the number of beats per minute. The heart rate is reflected in the pulse rate. The cardiac rate of contraction is described as normal (70 beats/min), rapid (more than 100 beats/min), or slow (less than 55 beats/min). Disturbances in heart rate and rhythm may be paroxysmal or persistent. Descriptive terms are *tachycardia* (increased, shallow heart rate to compensate for inadequate cardiac output) and *bradycardia* (slow, firm heart rate caused by cardiac sinus mechanisms and the vagal effect over the sympathetic innervation of the heart).

ratification (rat′i-fi-kā′shən), *n* confirmation of a previous act.

ratio, *n* proportion; comparison.

ratio, A:G, n the ratio of the protein albumin to globulin in the blood serum. On the basis of differential solubility with neutral salt solution, the normal values are 3.5 to 5 Gm% for albumin and 2.5 to 4 Gm% for globulin.

ratio, clinical crown: clinical root, n the proportion of the length of the portion of the tooth lying coronal to the epithelial attachment to the length of the portion of the root lying apical to the epithelial attachment. Radiographically the clinical crown is the portion of the tooth coronal to the al-

veolar crest; the clinical root is the part of the root apical to the alveolar crest. The radiographic crown: root ratio is useful in the evaluation and prognosis of periodontal disease.

ratio, grid, n the relation of the height of the lead strips to the width of the nonopaque material between them. Common grid ratios are 2:8, 2:12, and 2:16.

ratio, water:powder, n relative amounts of water and powder (usually gypsum products) in a mixture.

rationale (rash′ən-al′), *n* the fundamental reasons used as the basis for a decision or action.

ray(s), *n* a line of light, heat, or other form of radiant energy. A ray is a more or less distinct or isolated portion of radiant energy, whereas the word *rays* is a very general term for any form of radiant energy, whether vibratory or particulate.

ray, alpha, n See *particle, alpha.*

ray, beta, n See *particle, beta.*

ray, cathode, n See *electron stream.*

ray, central, n the center of an x-ray beam.

ray, cosmic, n radiation that originates outside the earth's atmosphere. Cosmic rays have extremely short wavelengths. They are able to produce ionization as they pass through the air and other matter and are capable of penetrating many feet of material such as lead and rock. The primary cosmic rays probably consist of atomic nuclei (mainly protons), some of which may have energies of the order of 10^{10} to 10^{15} eV. Secondary cosmic rays are produced when the primary cosmic rays interact with nuclei and electrons (for example, in the earth's atmosphere). Secondary cosmic rays consist mainly of mesons, protons, neutrons, electrons, and photons that have less energy than the primary rays. Practically all the primary cosmic rays are absorbed in the upper atmosphere. Almost all cosmic radiation observed at the earth's surface is of the secondary type.

ray, gamma, n photons with a shorter wavelength than those ordinarily used in diagnostic medical and dental radiography and that originate in the nuclei of atoms. A quantum of electromagnetic radiation emitted by

R

a nucleus as a result of a quantum transition between two energy levels of the nucleus; for example, as a radioisotope decays, it gives off energy, some of which may be in the form of gamma radiation.

ray, grenz **(grents),** *n* roentgen rays that are greater in length than 1 Å; used in radiography of soft tissues, insects, flowers, and microscopic sections of teeth and surrounding tissues. These rays are the result of using approximately 10 to 20 kV in a specially constructed radiation-generating device. They have a wavelength of about 2 Å.

ray, neutron, *n* particulate ionizing radiation consisting of neutrons. On impact with nuclei or atoms, neutrons possess enough kinetic energy to set the nuclei or atoms in motion with sufficient velocity to ionize matter or enter into nuclear reactions that result in the emission of ionizing radiation. The former variety is usually called the fast neutron, and the latter the thermoneutron, with gradations of epithermal and slow neutrons between them.

ray, roentgen (r) **(rent'gən),** *n* an international unit based on the ability of radiation to ionize air. The exposure to x or gamma radiation such that the associated corpuscular emission per 0.001293 Gm of air produces in air, ions carrying 1 esu of quantity of electricity of either sign (2.083 billion ion pairs).

Raynaud's phenomenon, *n* spasm of the digital arteries with blanching and numbness of the extremities, induced by chilling, emotional states, or other diseases.

RBC, *n* See *red blood cell count.*

RBE, *n* See *radiation, biologic effectiveness of, relative.*

RDA, *n.pr* the **Recommended Dietary Allowances** of the Food and Nutrition Board of the National Research Council.

RDH, *n* stands for **registered dental hygienist.**

reaction (rē-ak'shən), *n* opposite action, or counteraction; the response of a part to stimulation; a chemical process in which one substance is transformed into another substance or substances.

reaction, acute dystonic (dis-ton'ik), *n* extreme contraction of the jaw muscles, which can result in dislocation of the jaw bones and difficulty in opening the mouth. These symptoms may be caused by an adverse reaction to an antipsychotic drug.

reaction, alarm, *n* the first stage of the general adaptation syndrome of Hans Selye; occurs in response to severe physical and psychologic distress. Complete mobilization of body resources occurs in association with activity of the pituitary and adrenal glands and the sympathetic nervous system. See also *syndrome, general adaptation.*

reaction, anaphylactoid, *n* a reaction that resembles anaphylactic shock; probably caused by the liberation of histamine, serotonin, or other substances as a consequence of the injection of colloids or finely suspended material.

reaction, Arthus', *n pr* See *anaphylactic hypersensitivity.*

reaction, heterophil, *n* a heterophil agglutination test that measures the agglutination of the red blood cells of sheep by the serum of patients with infectious mononucleosis.

reaction, -id, secondary skin eruptions occurring at a distance from the primary lesion (for example, tuberculid).

reaction, immune, *n* altered reactivity of the tissues to a foreign substance that was previously introduced into the body or in contact with it.

reaction, leukemoid, *n* an increase in normal or abnormal white blood cells in nonleukemic conditions; simulates myelogenous, lymphatic, and rarely, monocytic leukemia.

reaction, Shwartzman, *n.pr* an antigen AB local tissue response that occurs when an intravenous injection or challenge of a bacterial endotoxin that had previously been inoculated intradermally results in a hemorrhagic, often necrotic inflammatory lesion.

reaction, tissue, *n* the response of tissues to altered conditions.

reactor (rē-ak'tur), *n* an apparatus in which nuclear fission may be sustained in a self-supporting reaction at a controlled rate.

read-only memory (ROM), *n* the portion of a computer's memory in which information is permanently stored. The operator has random access to the memory but only for purposes of reading the contents. Special equipment is required to write or erase a read-only memory.

reading, lip, *n* a method of communication in which the motions of the mouth and face are "read" as a person is speaking. The British term is *speech reading.*

reagent, *n* a chemical substance known to react in a specific way.

reagin(s) (rē′ ā-jin), *n* noncommittal term used for antibodies or antibody-like substances that differ in several respects from ordinary antibodies. It refers to the antibodies of allergic conditions (atopy) and to the antibody (reagin) concerned with the flocculation and complement fixation tests for syphilis.

real time, *n* an application of computerized equipment allowing data to be processed with relation to ongoing external events so that the operators can make immediate decisions based on the current data output. Ultrasound scanning uses real time control systems, making results available almost simultaneously with the generation of the input data.

reamer (rē′mur), *n* an instrument with a tapered metal shaft, more loosely spiraled than a file; used to enlarge and clean root canals.

reasonable and customary (R&C) plan, *n* a dental benefits plan that determines benefits based only on "reasonable and customary" fee criteria. See also *usual fee; customary fee; reasonable fee.*

reasonable fee, *n* the fee charged by a dentist for a specific dental procedure that has been modified by the nature and severity of the condition being treated and by any medical or dental complications or unusual circumstances; therefore may differ from the dentist's "usual" fee or the benefit administrator's "customary" fee.

reasonably prudent person doctrine, *n* the concept that a person of ordinary sense will use ordinary care and skill in meeting the healthcare needs of a patient.

reattachment, *n* in dentistry the reattachment of the gingival epithelium to the surface of the tooth.

rebase, *v* a process of refitting a denture by replacing the denture base material without changing the occlusal relations of the teeth.

rebound (rē′bownd), *n/v* **l.** a recovery from illness. *n* **2.** an outbreak of fresh reflex activity after withdrawal of a stimulus

rebreathing, *n* breathing into a closed system. Exhaled gas mixes with the gas in the closed system, and some of this mixture is then reinhaled. Rebreathing is used as part of a general anesthesia technique in which a rebreathing bag functions as a reservoir for anesthetic gases and oxygen. The bag may be squeezed or pumped to assist in proper respiration while the patient is under deep anesthesia.

recall, *n* the procedure of advising or reminding a patient to have his oral health reviewed or reexamined; an important phase of preventive dentistry. Term is being replaced by *preventive maintenance appointment.*

receipt, *n* a written acknowledgment by one person of having received money or something of value from another.

receipt book, *n* the book in which the dentist or one of the auxiliaries fills out forms verifying that a specific amount of money has been paid to the account.

reception room, *n* the area within the physical plant of the dental establishment through which patients enter the office. This is also the room in which patients await the attentions of the dentist or receptionist. Replaces the term *waiting room.*

receptor(s) (rē-sep′tur), *n* a site or location within a cell or its membrane that combines with a haptophore group of a toxin, drug, enzyme, hormone, or other substance and that may elicit a specific or general response; a sensory nerve terminal that responds to stimuli of various kinds.

receptor, sensory, *n* receptor system built on the theory that receptor organs are specialized and respond to the law of specific nerve energies; that is, each type of end-organ, no

R

matter what stimulus is applied, will respond (if it responds) with only a single appropriate type of sensation. Common experience shows this to be true; for example, when a person receives a blow to the eye, light is experienced as a consequence of the blow. Another factor is that the impulse will travel in only one direction, from the receptor organ back to the central nervous system. The receptor system is thus the summation in the brain of all the sensory stimuli that come from the special senses, general senses, mucous membrane, skin, and deeper tissues and is the basis for instruction sent to the musculoskeletal system for action, as in the masticatory phenomenon.

receptors, adrenergic, n alpha and beta "units" associated with sympathetic neuroeffectors that react with sympathomimetic drugs to elicit the response of the effector cells.

recession (rē-sesh′ən), *n* a moving back or withdrawal.

recession, bone, n apical progression of the level of the alveolar crest associated with inflammatory and dystrophic periodontal disease; a bone resorption process that results in decreased osseous support for the tooth.

recession, gingival, n atrophy of the gingival margin associated with inflammation, apical migration (proliferation) of the epithelial attachment, and resorption of the alveolar crest.

recidivism, *n* **1.** the tendency for an ill person to relapse or return to the hospital. *n* **2.** the return to a life of crime after a conviction and sentence.

recipient, *n* the person who receives a blood transfusion, tissue graft, or organ; also, a person who has received an honor, award, or grant.

recipient site, *n* the site into which a graft or transplant material is placed. See also *donor site.*

reciprocal arm, *n* See *arm, reciprocal.*

reciprocal forces, *n.pl* the typical method of applying corrective orthodontic forces; each applied force is balanced by a reciprocal force elsewhere in the dentition or surrounding structures.

reciprocating action device, *n* a hand-held, power-driven finishing tool with interchangeable tips that is used to shape, smooth, recontour, and polish restorations.

reciprocation (rē-sip′rō-kā′shən), *n* the means by which one part of a removable partial denture framework is made to counter the effect created by another part of the framework.

reciprocation, active, n reciprocation in a clasp unit achieved by the use of two opposing and balanced retentive clasp arms. Reciprocation cannot be achieved unless a similar and balanced arrangement on the opposite side of the dental arch occurs.

reciprocation, passive, n reciprocation in a clasp unit achieved by the use of a rigid part of the clasp, located on or above the height of contour line or on a guiding plane and opposite to the retentive arm. However, reciprocation cannot be achieved by a single clasp alone—a similar action must occur by another component of the removable partial denture located across the arch.

reciprocity, *n* a mutual agreement to exchange privileges, dependence, or relationships, as in an agreement between two governing bodies to accept the credentials of a physician, dentist, or other health professional licensed in either jurisdiction.

Recklinghausen's disease (rek′ling-how-zen), *n pr* See *neurofibromatosis; osteitis fibrosa cystica.*

recombinant DNA hepatitis B vaccine, *n* a vaccine against hepatitis B that is cultured in yeast.

reconstructive surgery, *n* surgery to rebuild a structure for functional or esthetic reasons.

recontour, *n* a reshaping process that uses instruments, such as power-driven finishing tools, to remove excess restorative material and restore natural anatomic form.

recontouring, occlusal, *n* the reshaping of an occlusal surface of a natural or artificial tooth.

record, *n* information committed to and preserved in writing or electronically.

record base, n See *baseplate.*

record, centric interocclusal, n a record of the centric jaw position (relation).

R

record, eccentric interocclusal, n a record of a jaw relation other than the centric relation; a record of a lateral eccentric jaw position.

Eccentric interocclusal record.
(Rosenstiel/Land/Fujimoto, 2001)

record, face-bow, n registration, by means of a face-bow, of the position of the mandibular axis or the condyles. The face-bow record is used to orient the maxillary cast to the opening and closing axis of the articulator.

record, functional chew-in, n **1.** a record of the natural chewing movement of the mandible made on an occlusion rim by teeth or scribing studs. *n* **2.** a record of the movements of the mandible made on the occluding surface of the opposing occlusion rim by teeth or scribing studs and produced by simulated chewing movements.

record, interocclusal, n a record of the positional relation of the teeth or jaws to each other; made on occlusal surfaces of occlusal rims or teeth in a plastic material that hardens, such as plaster of paris, wax, zinc oxide-eugenol paste, or acrylic resin.

record, jaw relation, n a registration of any positional relationship of the mandible in reference to the maxillae. The record may be of any of the many vertical, horizontal, or orientation relations.

record, maxillomandibular relationship, n See *record, interocclusal.*

record, occluding centric relation, n a registration of centric relation made at the vertical dimension at which the teeth make contact or are to make contact.

record, patient, legal aspects of, n.pl record must include proper identification of patient, signed consent forms, a complete medical and dental history, progress notes, and clinical observations from patient examinations. Improper record-keeping is grounds for malpractice. Records are also strictly confidential—unauthorized or inappropriate disclosure is an invasion of privacy and liable for legal action.

record, plaque control, n document used to measure and assist the progress of a patient undertaking a more purposeful approach to controlling bacterial plaque.

record, preoperative, n any record or records made for the purpose of study, diagnosis, or use in treatment planning or for comparison of treatment results with the pretreatment status of the patient.

record, profile, n a registration or record of the profile of a patient's face.

record, protrusive, n a registration of the relation of the mandible to the maxillae when the mandible is anterior to its centric relation with the maxillae.

record, protrusive interocclusal, n a record of a protruded eccentric jaw position.

record rim, n See *rim, occlusion.*

record, terminal jaw relation, n a record of the relationship of the mandible to the maxillae made at the vertical relation of the occlusion and at the centric position.

record, three-dimensional, n a maxillomandibular interocclusal record.

recording, *n* the act of making a written or electronic record of the data collected during examination.

recovery, *n* in a lawsuit, the obtaining or restoration of a right to something by a verdict, decree, or judgment of court.

recrystallization, *n* the return of a wrought metal to crystalline form because of excessive cold working or excessive application of heat.

rectification (rek′ti-fi-kā′shən), *n* conversion of electric current from alternating to direct (unidirectional).

rectifier (rek′ti-fi-ur), *n* a device used for converting an alternating current to a direct current; it also prevents or limits the flow of current in the opposite direction.

rectifier, full-wave, n an apparatus for rectifying the entire wave of an alternating current in an x-ray machine by means of a mechanical rectifier or valve tube.

rectifier, half-wave, n an apparatus used in the rectifying of half of the sine wave in an x-ray unit.

recumbent, *adj* to be lying down, leaning backward, or reclining.

recuperation, n the process of recovering health, strength, and mental and emotional vigor.

recurrence, n the reappearance of a sign or symptom of a disease after a period of remission.

red blood cell count, n the number of red blood cells (erthrocytes) in 1 mm³ of blood; a useful diagnostic tool in the determination of several kinds of anemia. See also *mean corpuscular hemoglobin.*

red marrow, n the red vascular substance consisting of connective tissue and blood vessels, containing primitive blood cells, macrophages, megakaryocytes, and fat cells. Red marrow is found in the cavities of many bones. It manufactures and releases leukocytes and erythrocytes into the bloodstream.

redressment (rē-dres′ment), n replacement of a part or correction of a deformity.

reduced fee plan, n a program in which the fees established for some or all services are lower than those usually charged by dentists in the community. In some industrial plans, employers make lower fees possible by partially subsidizing the cost of providing care (for example, furnishing rent-free facilities and paying costs of utilities). In welfare plans with limited funds, dentists may in effect subsidize the programs by accepting lower fees than they usually charge.

reducer, n a solution used to remove some silver from the image on a radiograph and thereby produce a less intense image; an oxidizing agent used to remove excess density.

reduction in area, n a test to assess the ductility of a metal or an alloy, whereby the cross-sectional area of the fractured end of a wire or rod is compared with the original area. A tensile test is used to break the wire.

refereed journal, n a professional or literary journal or publication in which articles or papers are selected for publication by a panel of readers or referees who are experts in the field.

referral, n the recommendation of another health professional to a patient for a specified reason.

referred pain, n pain felt at a site different from that of an injured or diseased organ or part of the body. Angina pain is frequently felt at a site distant from the heart, such as arm or shoulder.

reflection, n the act of elevating and folding back the mucoperiosteum, thereby exposing the underlying bone.

reflection, mucobuccal, n See *fold, mucobuccal.*

reflex(es) (rē′fleks), n a reflected action or movement; the sum total of any specific involuntary activity.

reflex, arc, n See *arc, reflex.*

reflex, Breuer, n.pr See *reflex, Hering-Breuer.*

reflex, Cheyne-Stokes, n.pr See *respiration, Cheyne-Stokes.*

reflex emesis, n gagging or vomiting induced by touching the mucous membrane of the throat or as a result of other noxious stimuli. Also called *gag reflex.*

reflex, Hering-Breuer, n.pr the nervous mechanism that tends to limit the respiratory excursions. Stimuli from the sensory endings in the lungs (and perhaps in other parts) pass up the vagi and tend to limit both inspiration and expiration during ordinary breathing.

reflex, jaw, n an extension-flexion reflex that is initiated by tapping the mandible downward. The masseter and other elevators of the mandible are the first stretched; then the reflex flexion-contraction elevates the mandible by flexion of elevator muscles while simultaneous stretching (extension) of the depressor muscles of the mandible occurs.

reflex, pharyngeal, n contraction of the constrictor muscles of the pharynx, elicited by touching the back of the pharynx.

reflex, stretch, n one of the most important features of tonic contraction of muscle. It is the reflex contraction of a healthy muscle that results from a pull. It has been found that stretching a muscle by as little as 0.8% of its original length is suffi-

R

cient to evoke a reflex response. A stretch of constant degree causes a maintained steady contraction, muscle spindles and stretch receptors in the tendons show very slow adaptation, and the reflex ceases immediately on withdrawal of the stretching force. The stretch reflex is obtained predominantly from those muscles maintaining body posture, among which are the masticating muscles that maintain the position of the mandible and the neck muscles holding the head erect. Together the masticating muscles and neck muscles are responsible for the maintenance of the air and food passages.

reflex, vagovagal, n a reflex in which the afferent and efferent impulses travel via the vagus nerve. The afferent impulses travel centrally via the sensory nucleus of the vagus. The efferent impulses travel via the motor fibers of the vagus nerve.

reflexes, allied, n.pl reflexes that join to effect a common purpose, such as mastication. They may arise from diverse stimuli, such as smell, taste of food, and texture, shape, and resistance of the food bolus. Collectively, they encourage salivation and a sequence of masticatory closures of the mandible, followed by deglutition.

reflexes, antagonistic, n.pl reflexes that cannot occupy the final pathway simultaneously. The weaker of these reflexes will give way to the stronger, especially if the latter is a protected reflex (for example, a hot or nauseating food causes involuntary retching or even vomiting rather than the pleasurable gustatory experience associated with chewing and swallowing tasty food).

reflexes, flexion-extension, n.pl the reflexes based on the principle of reciprocal innervation. When a voluntary or reflex contraction of a muscle occurs, it is accompanied by the simultaneous relaxation of its antagonist. For example, when the jaw reflex is initiated by tapping the mandible downward, the masseter and other elevators of the mandible are stretched. Then, reflex flexion-contraction of the elevators takes place, the mandible is elevated, and the depressor muscles of the mandible are stretched. Many combinations

exist, not only between the agonists and the antagonists of a given joint but also between reflexes that cross over to muscle groups of contralateral extremities, joints, and muscles.

reflexes, pathologic, n.pl reflexes observed in the abnormal or inappropriate motor responses of controlled stimuli initiated in the sensory organ that is appropriate to the reflex arc. They may be initiated in the superficial reflexes of the skin and mucous membrane; in the deep myotatic reflexes of the joints, tendons, and muscles; and in the visceral reflexes of the viscera and other organs of the body. The pathologic reflexes are thus syndromes of abnormal responses to otherwise normal stimuli.

reflux, *n* the reverse flow of a liquid.

refractory (rē-frak′tər-ē), *adj* pertaining to the ability to withstand the high temperatures used in certain dental laboratory procedures. See also *cast, refractory.*

refractory periodontitis (per′ē-ō-don-tī′tis), *n* a progressive inflammatory destruction of the periodontal attachment that resists conventional mechanical treatment.

refusal, informed, *n* decision by the patient to forego a professional recommendation for dental care.

regeneration (rē-jen′ər-ā′shən), *n* the renewal or repair of lost tissue or parts.

regeneration, muscle, n repair of muscle tissue. When surgical intervention or inflammatory disease of dental structures injures the facial and masticatory muscles, two types of repair take place: repair by budding and repair by proliferation.

regeneration, muscle, by budding, n regeneration that takes place in destructive lesions of muscle, traumatic necrosis, hemorrhage, infarction, and suppurative myositis. The buds consist of undifferentiated plasmodial masses and certain sarcolemma nuclei. The rebuilt architecture is not classic and has bizarre and sometimes fibrous extensions that look like scarred defects.

regeneration, muscle, by proliferation, n regeneration in degenerating muscles by proliferation of bands of sarcoplasm in which the sarcolemma and its nuclei are preserved.

R

region, mylohyoid (mī′lō-hī′oid), *n* the region on the lingual surface of the mandible marked by the mylohyoid ridge and the attachment of the mylohyoid muscle; a part of the alveololingual sulcus.

regional, *adj* pertaining to a region or regions.

registered dietitian, *n* See *dietitian, registered.*

registered nurse (RN), *n* a professional nurse who has completed a course of study at an approved and accredited school of nursing and who has passed the National Council of Licensure Examination. RNs are licensed to practice by individual states.

registered record administrator (RRA), *n* a medical record administrator (Health Information Manager) who has successfully completed the prescribed curriculum and the credentialing examination conducted by the American Medical Record Association.

registration, *n* the record of desired jaw relations that is made to transfer casts having these same relations to an articulator.

registration of functional form, *n* See *impression, functional.*

registration, tissue, *n* the accurate record of the shape of tissues under any condition by means of suitable material.

regression analysis, *n* a method of correlation for computing the most probable value of one variable, *y,* from the known value of another variable, *x;* a method for computing the amount of change in one variable for a unit change in another. It is spoken of as the regression of *x* on *y* and notated r_{xy}.

regulated waste, *n* refuse material made up of or contaminated by saliva, blood, or tissue (including teeth). Such waste includes contaminated sharp instruments as well as any solid waste materials that have been soaked or covered by the contaminants. Also called *infectious waste.*

regulator, *n* the mechanical part of a gas delivery system that controls gas pressure that allows a manageable flow of drug vapor to escape.

regurgitation (rē-gur′ji-tā′shən), *n* a backward flowing (for example, casting up of undigested food, backward flowing of blood into the heart or between the chambers of the heart).

regurgitation, heart valve, *n* blood flow in the wrong direction (from a ventricle to an atrium or into the heart from an artery) through a valve that has failed to close completely. See also *heart valves.*

rehabilitation (rē′hə-bil′i-tā′shən), *n* restoration of form and function.

rehabilitation, mouth, *n* (oral rehabilitation), restoration of the form and function of the masticatory apparatus condition to as near normal as possible.

rehalation, *n* rebreathing.

reimbursement, *n* payment made by a third party to a beneficiary or dentist on behalf of the beneficiary toward repayment of expenses incurred for a service covered by the contractual arrangement.

reimplant, *v* to replace a lost or extracted tooth back into its alveolus.

reimplantation, *n* See *replantation.*

reinforcement, *n* the increasing of force or strength.

reinsurance, *n* insurance for third-party payers to spread their risk for losses (claims paid) over a specified dollar amount.

reintubation (rē′in-tōō-bā′shən), *n* intubation performed a second time.

Reiter's syndrome (rī′terz, -turz), *n.pr* See *syndrome, Reiter's.*

relapse, *v* to slip or fall back into a former state.

relation(s), *n* the designation of the position of one object as oriented to another (for example, centric relation of the mandible to the maxillae).

relation, acentric, *n* See *relation, jaw, eccentric.*

relation, acquired centric, *n* See *relation, jaw, eccentric, acquired.*

relation, acquired eccentric jaw, *n* an eccentric relation that is assumed by habit to bring the teeth into a convenient occlusion.

relation, centric, *n* (centric jaw relation), the relation of the mandible to the maxillae when the condyles are in their most posterosuperior unstrained positions in the glenoid fossae, from which lateral movements can be made at the occluding vertical relation normal for the individual. Centric relation is a relation that can

R

exist at any degree of jaw separation.

relation, centric jaw, *n* See *relation, centric.*

relation, cusp-fossa, *n* See *cusp-fossa relations.*

relation, dynamic, *n* relations of two objects involving the element of relative movement of one object to another (relationship of the mandible to the maxillae).

relation, eccentric, *n* See *relation, jaw, eccentric.*

relation, eccentric jaw, *n* (convenience relationship, eccentric relation, eccentric jaw position), any jaw relation other than centric relation.

relation, intermaxillary, *n* the relation between the right and left maxilla. See also *relation, maxillomandibular.*

relation, jaw, *n* Any relation of the mandible to the maxillae.

relation, lateral, *n* the relation of the mandible to the maxillae when the lower jaw is in a position on either side of centric relation.

relation, maxillomandibular **(mak-sil′o-man-dib′yōō-lur),** *n* any one of the many relations of the mandible to the maxillae, such as the centric maxillomandibular relation or eccentric maxillomandibular relation.

relation, median, *n* See *relation, centric.*

relation, median jaw, *n* any jaw relation existing when the mandible is in the median sagittal plane.

relation, median retruded, *n* See *relation, centric.*

relation, occluding, *n* the jaw relation at which the opposing teeth contact or occlude.

relation, posterior border jaw, *n* the most posterior relation of the mandible to the maxillae at any specific vertical dimension.

relation, protrusive, *n* See *relation, jaw, protrusive; position, rest, physiologic.*

relation, protrusive jaw, *n* (protrusive relation), a jaw relation resulting from a protrusion of the mandible.

relation, rest, *n* See *position, physiologic rest.*

relation, rest jaw, *n* (rest), the postural relation of the mandible to the maxillae when the patient is resting comfortably in the upright position, the condyles are in a neutral unstrained position in the glenoid fos-

sae, and the mandibular musculature is in a state of minimum tonic contraction to maintain posture.

relation, ridge, *n* the positional relation of the mandibular ridge to the maxillary ridges.

relation, static, *n* the relationship between two parts that are not in motion.

relation, unstrained jaw, *n* the relation of the mandible to the skull when a state of balanced tonus exists between all the muscles involved.

relation, vertical, *n* the relative position of the mandible in a vertical direction; one of the basic jaw relations.

relationship, *n* the condition of being associated or interconnected.

relationship, abnormal occlusal, *n* occlusal relationships that deviate from the regular and established type to produce esthetic disharmonies, interference with mastication, occlusal traumatism, and speech difficulties.

relationship, buccolingual **(buk′ō-ling′gwəl),** *n* the position of a space or tooth in relation to the tongue and cheek.

relationship, convenience, of teeth, *n* See *occlusion, convenience.*

relationship, normal, *n* a relationship in which structures conjoin as they should.

relationship, occlusal, *n* the individual and collective relationships of the mandibular teeth to the maxillary teeth and the relationship of the adjacent teeth in the same dental arch.

relationship, structure-activity (SAR), *n* the relationship between the chemical structure of a drug and its activity.

relationship, tissue-base, *n* the relationship of the base of a removable prosthesis to the structures subjacent to it. Three possibilities exist: the base may be entirely tissue borne, it may be completely tooth borne, or support may be shared by both the tissue subjacent to its base and the abutment that bounds the edentulous space at one terminus.

relative value system, *n* coded listing of professional services with unit values to indicate relative complexity as measured by time, skill, and overhead costs. Third-party payers typically assign a dollar value per unit to calculate provider reimbursement.

relaxant (rē-lak′sənt), *n* an antispasmodic; a drug that relaxes spasms of smooth or skeletal muscle; a drug used to eliminate muscle spasms, thus facilitating the establishment of centric relation, centric occlusion, rest position, and so on. Also used in the treatment of painful muscle spasms associated with occlusal traumatism. Examples are mephenesin, the meprobamates, and methocarbamol (Robaxin).

relaxant, muscle, *n* a drug that specifically aids in lessening muscle tension.

relaxation training, *n* a stress-reduction technique that uses a sequence of progressive exercises under the direction of a therapist to lower the level of anxiety and its neuromotor manifestations.

release, *v* to give up as a legal claim; to discharge or relinquish a right.

release, sustained, *adj* See *medication, sustained release.*

reliability, *n* **1.** in research, the reproducibility of an experimental result; the extent to which an experiment, test, or measuring procedure yields the same result during independent, repeated trials. *n* **2.** the ability of two or more observers to examine the same data and arrive at a similar judgment within predefined bounds concerning the quality of care.

relicensure, *n* being licensed to practice for a specific period with the license either being renewed at the end of that period or being forfeited. In some instances, evidence of continued competency must be submitted.

relief, *n* **1.** the mitigation or removal of pain or distress. *n* **2.** the reduction or elimination of pressure from a specific area under a denture base.

relief chamber, *n* See *chamber, relief.*

relief, gingival, *n* relief given to removable partial denture units at all gingival crossings to avoid impingement.

relief space, *n* See *space, relief.*

relieve, *v* **1.** to mitigate or remove pain or distress. *v* **2.** the procedure of placing hard wax in strategic areas.

reline, *v* to resurface the tissue side (basal surface) of a denture with new base material so that it will fit more accurately. See also *rebase.*

rem (roentgen-equivalent-man), *n* a unit of absorbed radiation dose adjusted for biologic effects equivalent to 1 rad of 250 kV x-rays (dental and cephalometric x-rays require less than 100 kV).

remedial (rə-mē′dē-əl), *adj* curative; acting as a remedy.

remineralization (rē′min′ər-əl-i-zā′shən), *n* the reintroduction of complex mineral salts into bone, enamel, dentin, or cementum.

remission, *n* the partial or complete disappearance of the clinical and subjective characteristics of a chronic or malignant disease.

remit, *v* to send; to relinquish.

removable lingual arch, *n* See *arch, removable lingual.*

removable partial denture, *n* See *denture, partial, removable.*

removal, pulp, *n* See *pulpectomy.*

remuneration, *n* pay; recompense; salary.

Rendu-Osler-Weber disease, *n.pr* See *telangiectasia, hereditary hemorrhagic.*

rent, *n* a payment made by a tenant to an owner for the use of land or a building.

rental, *n/adj* the fee paid by the dentist for the use of space in a building owned by someone else. Equipment may also be obtained under a rental or lease agreement.

reovirus, *n* any one of three ubiquitous, double-stranded ribonucleic acid viruses found in the respiratory and alimentary tracts in healthy and sick people. Reoviruses have been implicated in some cases of upper respiratory tract disease and infantile gastroenteritis.

reoxidation (rē-ok′si-dā′shən), *n* the act of taking up oxygen again, as the hemoglobin of the blood.

repair, *n* **1.** the process of reuniting or replacing broken parts of a denture; a means for extending the usefulness of a denture. *v* **2.** to make sound; to mend; restoration to former condition. *n* **3.** formation of new tissues by processes such as fibroplasia, osteogenesis, and endothelioplasia to replace tissues damaged by disease or injury.

repair, cemental, *n* repair of areas of cemental resorption and cemental tears by apposition of cementum.

R

Repair may be by formation of either cellular or acellular cementum.

replacement, prosthetic, *n* See *prosthesis.*

replantation, *n* (reimplantation), replacement of a tooth (or teeth) that has been removed from the alveolus either intentionally or unintentionally, as in an accident.

replenisher, *n* a concentrated developing solution designed to maintain the active strength of developer through periodic addition to maintain original volume.

report generator, *n* a computer program for producing complete data processing reports giving only a description of the desired content and format of the output reports, as well as certain information concerning the input file.

reportable diseases, *n.pl* contagious diseases that must be reported by the physician to public health authorities. They include but are not limited to malaria, influenza, poliomyelitis, relapsing fever, typhus, yellow fever, cholera, and bubonic plague.

repositioning, jaw, *n* the changing of any relative position of the mandible to the maxillae, usually by altering the occlusion of the natural or artificial teeth.

repository, *n* long-acting drugs, usually administered intramuscularly. See also *medication, repository.*

repository, rapid, n mixtures of rapid-acting and slow-acting drugs, usually administered intramuscularly.

representative group, *n* a group whose members represent all the various sectors of a community or population under study.

reputation, *n* a person's credit, honor, and character; esteem in which one is held.

request for proposal (RFP), *n* a solicitation by a funding agency for proposals to accomplish a particular goal. The RFP lists the requirements a project must meet to receive funding.

require arch length, *n* the circumference of the dental arch sufficient to accommodate the sum of the mesiodistal widths of all the natural teeth in the dental arch.

res ipsa loquitur (rās′ ip′sə lō′kwi-toor), *adj* a Latin phrase meaning "the thing speaks for itself." Used in actions for injury by negligence in which the happening itself is accepted as proof.

res judicata (rās′ jōō′di-kä′tə), *adj* decided or determined by judicial power; a thing judicially decided.

research, *v/n* the diligent inquiry or examination of data, reports, and observations in a search for facts or principles. Generally a disciplined protocol is followed to ensure objectivity and reproducibility. Most research employs the scientific method or a similar model.

research, analytical epidemiologic, n a method of investigation used to establish a disease origin or the existence of an contributory relationship between a cause and a disease.

research, convenience sample, n a method of investigation used when measuring an entire population is not possible. Participants are numbered as they enroll, then they are randomly assigned to either the control or experimental group.

research, epidemiologic, n a method of investigation (e.g., descriptive, analytical, and experimental) used to study the rate of occurrence, method of transmission, and control of a disease within a population.

research, epidemiologic survey, n a method of data collection from target population samples to establish factors causing or contributing to a disease and to develop potential methods for prevention.

research, experimental, n See *controlled clinical trial.*

research, experimental epidemiologic, n a method of investigation used after the establishment of a disease origin to determine the result of altering at least one cause.

resection, *n* excision of a considerable portion of an organ.

resection, root, n See *amputation, root.*

reserpine, *n trade names:* Serpalan, Serpasil; *drug class:* antiadrenergic agent, antihypertensive; *action:* depletes catecholamine stores in central nervous system and adrenergic nerve endings; *use:* hypertension.

reserve, *n* something kept in store for future use.

reserve, alkali, n See *reserve, alkaline.*

reserve, alkaline, *n* (alkali reserve), **1.** the amount of buffer compounds (for example, sodium bicarbonate, dipotassium phosphate, proteins) in the blood capable of neutralizing acids; one of the buffer systems of the blood that can neutralize the acid valences formed in the body. It is made up of the base of weak acid salts and is usually measured by determining the bicarbonate concentration of the plasma. *n* **2.** the concentration of bicarbonate ions (HCO_3^-) in the blood. These ions serve as a reserve in that they may be displaced by anions (for example, Cl^-, $SO_4^{-?}$, PO_4^{-3}). Displacement of bicarbonate ions occurs mainly by means of the chloride shift. The role of the buffer system is such that a large influx of acid or base ions from either metabolic function or ingestion can be neutralized by the alkaline reserves from the mineral and protein salts in the blood and tissue fluids. A strong acid is transformed into a weak base. Consequently, the pH level of the blood fluctuates very little, and the tissue cells are constantly bathed in a continuously buffered solution.

reserve, cardiac, *n* the reserve strength or pumping ability of the heart, which may be called on in an emergency.

reservoir bag, *n* a repository for excess gas that is attached to an anesthesia machine. It may be used as a source of gas during manual ventilation or to gauge the patient's respiratory rate and depth while under anesthesia.

resident, *n* a graduate and licensed dentist or physician who has completed an internship and is serving in the hospital while pursuing advanced didactic and clinical studies in special disciplines of knowledge.

residual, *adj* pertaining to the portion of something that remains after an activity that removes the bulk of the substance; usually refers to the amount of air remaining in the lungs at the end of a maximum expiration.

residual ridge, *n* See *ridge, residual.*

residue, *n* remainder; that which remains after the removal of other substances.

resilience (rē-zil'yəns), *n* **1.** an act of springing back. *n* **2.** capability of a strained body to recover its size and shape after deformation. *n* **3.** the recoverable potential energy of an elastic solid body or stricture resulting from its having been subjected to stress not exceeding the elastic limit.

resilience, modulus of, *n* the amount of energy stored up by a body when one unit volume is stressed to its proportional limit.

resin (rez'in), *n* broad term used to indicate organic substances that are usually translucent or transparent and are soluble in ether, acetone, and similar substances but not in water. They are named according to their chemical composition, physical structure, and means for activation or curing. Examples are acrylic resin, autopolymer resin (cold-curing resin), synthetic resin, styrene resin, and vinyl resin. See also methyl methacrylate; varnish, cavity.

resin, acrylic, *n* **1.** general term applied to a resinous material of the various esters of acrylic acid. It is used as a denture base material and also for trays and other dental restorations. *n* **2.** An ethylene derivative that contains a vinyl group (e.g., polymethacrylate [methyl methacrylate], the principal ingredient of many plastics used in dentistry).

resin, activated, *n* See *resin, autopolymer.*

resin, autopolymer, *n* (activated resin, autopolymerizing resin, cold-curing resin, direct restorative acrylic resin, self-curing resin), any resin that can be polymerized by an activator and a catalyst without the use of external heat.

resin, composite, *n* a resin used for restorative purposes and usually formed by a reaction of an ether of bisphenol-A (an epoxy molecule) with acrylic resin monomers, initiated by a benzoyl peroxideamine system, to which is added as much as 75% inorganic filler (glass beads and rods, lithium aluminum silicate, quartz, and tricalcium phosphate).

resin, copolymer, *n* a synthetic resin that is the product of the concurrent and joint polymerization of two or more different monomers of polymers.

resin, direct restorative, *n* See *resin, autopolymer.*

R

resin, epoxy, *n* a resin molecule characterized by reactive epoxy, or ethoxyline, groups that serve as terminal polymerization points. Used in dentistry for denture bases.

resin, heat-curing, *n* any resin that requires heat to activate its polymerization.

resin, quick cure, *n* See *resin, autopolymer.*

resin, self-curing, *n* See *resin, autopolymer.*

resin, thermoplastic, *n* a synthetic resin that may be softened by heat and hardened by cooling.

resin, vinyl, *n* an ethylene-derivative copolymer of vinyl chloride and vinyl acetate; used at one time for denture bases.

resin-filled, *adj* pertaining to a resin, usually poly (methylmethacrylate), to which has been added an inert material such as glass beads or glass rods.

resistance, *n* ability of an individual to ward off the damaging effects of physical, chemical, or microbiologic injury; an immeasurable factor controlled and qualified by numerous local, systemic, and metabolic processes such as blood supply to tissues, nutritional status, age, and antibody formative ability.

resistance, cross-, *n* a state in which an organism is insensitive to several drugs of similar chemical nature.

resistance form, *n* See *form, resistance.*

resolution, *n* the discernible separation of closely adjacent radiographic image details.

resonance (rez'ən-əns), *n* the vibratory response of a body or air-filled cavity to a frequency imposed on it.

resonance, speech, *n* the resonance of the body cavities and surfaces involved in the production of speech. The sound waves produced at the vocal folds are still far from the finished product heard in speech. The resonators give the characteristic quality to the voice. The resonating structures are the air sinuses; organ surfaces; cavities such as the pharynx, oral cavity, and nasal cavity; and chest wall. The resonating structures contribute no energy to the stream of air; they act to conserve and concentrate the energy already present in the laryngeal tone rather than to let it dissipate into the tissues. However, the resonated laryngeal tone still is not speech.

resorcinol, *n* an antiseptic substance used as a keratolytic agent in dermatoses.

resorption (rē-zôrp'shən), *n* **1.** loss of substance (bone) by physiologic or pathologic means; the reduction of the volume and size of the residual alveolar portion of the mandible or maxillae. *n* **2.** the cementoclastic and dentinoclastic action that often takes place on the root of a replanted tooth.

resorption, apical root, *n* dissolution of the apex of a tooth, resulting in a shortened, blunted root.

Apical root resorption. (Rosenstiel/Land/Fujimoto, 2001)

resorption, bone, *n* **1.** destruction or solution of the elements of bone. *n* **2.** loss of bone resulting from the activity of multinucleated giant cells, the osteoclasts, which are noted in irregular concavities on the periphery of the bone (Howship's lacunae).

resorption, cemental, *n* destruction of cementum by cementoclastic action. Noted as the presence of irregular concavities in the cemental surfaces.

resorption, frontal, *n* osteoclastic resorption of alveolar bone (lamina dura) by multinucleated cells on the osseous margin adjacent to the periodontal ligament.

resorption, horizontal, *n* a pattern of bone resorption in marginal periodontitis in which the marginal crest of the alveolar bone between adjacent teeth remains level; in these instances the bases of the periodontal pockets are supracrestal; a pattern of bone loss in which the crestal margins of the alveolar bone are resorbed. A horizontal pattern, rather than vertical loss along the root, is the typical type of bone loss in periodontitis.

resorption, idiopathic, *n* resorption that is not attributable to any known disease or is without an apparent cause.

resorption, internal, *n* (idiopathic internal resorption, pink tooth), a special form of idiopathic root resorption from within the pulp cavity; granulation tissue is present within the tooth, apparently with the resorption of the dentin occurring from the inside outward. The cause is unknown.

Internal resorption. (Neville/Damm/Allen/Bouquot, 2002)

resorption, lacunar, *n* See *osteoclast.*

resorption, osteoclastic, *n* loss of bone by cellular activity; osteoclasts are large, multinucleated cells seen in irregular concavities in the margin of the bone (Howship's lacunae) and currently believed to be directly responsible for the active destruction of bone.

resorption, pressure, of bone, *n* osteoclastic destruction of bone resulting from the application of sustained, excessive force. Remodeling of bone may occur to better adapt to these forces, or destruction may continue if the stresses are repeated and excessive.

resorption, rear, *n* See *resorption, undermining.*

resorption, root, *n* destruction of the cementum or dentin by cementoclastic or osteoclastic activity.

resorption, surface root, *n* localized resorptive areas on the cemental surface of the tooth root.

resorption, undermining, *n* indirect, as opposed to frontal, removal of alveolar bone where pressure applied to a tooth has resulted in loss of vitality of localized areas of the periodontal membrane.

resorption, vertical, *n* a pattern of bone loss seen in occlusal traumatism, marginal periodontitis, periodontosis, and other conditions; a pattern of bone loss in which the alveolar bone adjacent to a tooth is destroyed without simultaneous crestal loss, so that a vertical rather than a horizontal pattern of loss is observed.

respect, *n/v* to hold in high regard; to show consideration for another. Mutual respect is the basis for a good doctor-patient relationship.

respiration (res´pi-rā´shən), *n* the gaseous exchange between cells of the body and the environment. Four stages exist: pulmonary ventilation, diffusion of gases in the alveoli, transport of gases in the blood to and from cells, and regulation of the process

respiration, artificial, *n* maintenance of respiratory movements by artificial means. When respiration has been arrested and no mechanical device is available, resuscitation by means of artificial respiration is the only practical means of ventilating the lungs.

respiration, Cheyne-Stokes **(chān´stōks´),** *n.pr* (Cheyne-Stokes reflex), a type of breathing characterized by rhythmic variations in intensity that occur in cycles: rhythmic acceleration, deepening, and stopping of breathing movements.

respiration, controlled, *n* maintenance of adequate pulmonary ventilation in apneic patients.

respiration, external, *n* ventilation of the lungs and oxygenation of the blood.

respiration in speech, *n* in normal

R

speech, the action of the respiratory apparatus during exhalation, which provides a continuous stream of air with sufficient volume and pressure (under adequate voluntary control) to initiate phonation. The stream of air is modified in its course from the lungs by the facial and oral structures, giving rise to the sound symbols that are recognized as speech.

respiration, internal, n the mechanism of gaseous exchange between blood and tissues.

respirator (res'pir-ā-tur), n an apparatus that qualifies the air breathed through it; a device for giving artificial respiration.

respiratory distress syndrome (RDS) of the newborn, n an acute lung disease of the newborn, characterized by airless alveoli, inelastic lungs, more than 60 respirations per minute, nasal flaring, intercostal and subcostal retractions, grunting on expiration, and peripheral edema. The condition occurs most often in premature babies. It is caused by a deficiency of pulmonary surfactant. The disease is self-limited; the infant either dies in 3 to 5 days or completely recovers with no aftereffects. Treatment includes measures to correct shock, acidosis, and hypoxemia and the use of continuous positive airway pressure to prevent alveolar collapse.

respiratory failure, n a condition in which the level of oxygen in the blood is too low and the level of carbon dioxide is too high. This condition may be life threatening.

respiratory rate, n the normal rate of breathing at rest, about 12 to 20 inspirations per minute.

respiratory rhythm, n a regular, oscillating cycle of inspiration and expiration, controlled by neuronal impulses transmitted between the muscles of inspiration in the chest and the respiratory centers in the brain. The respiratory rate is influenced by metabolic rate, emotional state, neurologic disorders, and obstructive disease.

respiratory therapy, n any treatment that maintains or improves the ventilatory function of the respiratory tract.

respiratory tract, n the complex of organs and structures performing the pulmonary ventilation of the body and the exchange of oxygen and carbon dioxide between the ambient air and the blood circulating through the lungs. It includes all the structures from the external nares to the alveoli of the lungs.

respirometer (res'pir-om'ə-tur), n an instrument for studying and determining the character and extent of respiration.

respondeat superior, n a legal doctrine that passes the legal responsibility for acts or omissions of an employee to the employer.

response, n action or movement resulting from the application of a stimulus.

response diagnosis, n the evaluation of previous treatment at the follow-up appointment. A method of assessing the previous treatment.

response time, n the period between the application of a stimulus and the response of a cell or tissue.

rest, n **1.** passive support. n **2.** an extension from a prosthesis that affords vertical support for a restoration.

rest area, n See *area, rest.*

rest, auxiliary, n the rest other than the one used as a component part of a primary direct retainer.

rest, finger, n See *finger rest.*

rest, incisal, n a metallic extension onto the incisal angle of an anterior tooth to supply support or indirect retention for a removable partial denture.

rest, lingual, n a metallic extension onto the lingual surface of an anterior tooth to provide support or indirect retention for a removable partial denture.

rest, occlusal, n (occlusal lug), a rest placed on the occlusal surface of a posterior tooth.

rest occlusion, n See *position, rest, physiologic.*

rest position, n See *position, rest.*

rest, precision, n a unit consisting of two closely fitted parts, the insert of which rests firmly against the gingival portion of the tubelike receptacle.

rest relation, n See *relation, jaw, rest.*

rest seat, n See *area, rest.*

R

resting potential, *n* the electrical potential across a nerve cell membrane before it is stimulated to release the charge. The resting potential for a neuron is between 50 and 100 millivolts.

restless legs syndrome, *n* a benign condition of unknown origin characterized by an irritating sensation of uneasiness, tiredness, and itching deep within the muscles of the legs, accompanied by twitching and sometimes pain. The only relief is walking or moving the legs.

restoration, *n* (prosthetic restoration), broad term applied to any filling, inlay, crown, bridge, partial denture, or complete denture that restores or replaces lost tooth structure, teeth, or oral tissues; a prosthesis.

restoration, amalgam, *n* a direct restoration made from an alloy consisting of mercury and other metals (e.g., silver, copper, or tin), which is carved and contoured after placement in the tooth; allow a minimum of 24 hours between placement and polishing.

Amalgam restoration. (Bird/Robinson, 2002)

restoration, ceramic, *n* an indirect restoration made from metal and nonmetal compounds, which is carved and contoured before placement in the tooth; closely resembles natural teeth in strength, hardness, chemical inertness, and esthetic appearance.

restoration, dental prosthetic, *n* See *prosthesis, dental.*

restoration, direct, *n* a restoration prepared for immediate application to the tooth or cavity, as opposed to one prepared on a diagnostic cast and applied later.

restoration, faulty, *n* restoration in which there are imperfections or incorrect attributes (for example, overhanging or deficient fillings, incorrect anatomy of occlusal and marginal ridge areas, faulty clasps). Such faults may be present in individual tooth restorations, fixed bridges, and removable partial dentures and are conducive to the initiation and perpetuation of inflammatory and dystrophic diseases of the teeth and periodontium.

restoration groove, *n* an opening between the restoration and the tooth structure, which results from either a broken flash or a material contraction; may also be called *ditch.*

restoration, implant, *n* the single-tooth implant crown or multiple-tooth implant, crown, or bridge that replaces a missing tooth or teeth.

restoration of cusps, *n* (preferred to tipping, capping, or shoeing cusps), reduction and inclusion of cusps within a cavity preparation and their restoration to functional occlusion with restorative material.

restoration, overcontoured, *n* a restoration containing so much excess restorative material that normal anatomic structure is altered; may cause plaque retention and open or deficient gingival margin.

restoration, porcelain, *n* an indirect restoration made from a ceramic material that is cast in a laboratory prior to insertion in the mouth and finished during placement. See also *ceramic restoration.*

Porcelain restoration. (Bird/Robinson, 2002)

R

restoration, prosthetic, n See *prosthesis.*

restoration, undercontoured, n a restoration containing too little restorative material so that a space occurs between the margin and the cavity wall; may result when either the matrix band or wedge is improperly placed.

restorative, *adj* **1.** promoting a return to health or consciousness; a remedy that aids in restoring health, vigor, or consciousness. *adj* **2.** pertaining to rebuilding, repairing, or reforming.

restorative dentistry, n the branch of dentistry that deals with the reconstruction of the hard tissues of a tooth or group of teeth injured or destroyed by trauma or disease.

restorative materials, n materials used to reconstruct the hard tissues of teeth lost through trauma or disease.

restrainer, n a chemical ingredient (potassium bromide) of photographic developing solution. Its function is to inhibit the fogging tendency of the solution. Like the activator, the restrainer also controls the rate of development.

restraint, n any one of a number of devices used in aiding the immobilization of patients, especially children in traction.

restraint of trade, n an illegal act that interferes with free competition in a commercial or business transaction so as to restrict the production of a product or the provision of a service, affect the cost of a product or service, or control the market in any way to the detriment of consumers or purchasers of the service or product.

restrictive covenant, n common clause found in a contract for the sale of a dental practice. The seller contracts that he or she will not practice dentistry within a certain time and area. A junior partner may be asked to sign such a covenant to guarantee that he or she will not compete with the partnership for a period after leaving the partnership. Also used in an employment situation.

resuscitation (rē-sus´i-tā´shən), n restoration of life or consciousness to one who appears to be dead.

resuscitator (rē-sus´i-tā-tur), n an apparatus for initiating respiration in asphyxia.

retail dentistry, n fee-for-service dentistry practiced in an exclusively retail environment (for example, shopping center, department store) and directed to the clientele of that retail center, using the marketing technique of the parent retailer.

retail store dentistry, n dental services offered within a retail, department, or drug store operation. Typically, space is leased from the store by a separate administrative group that in turn subleases to a dentist or dental group providing the actual dental services. The dental operation generally maintains the same hours of operation as the store, and appointments often are not necessary. It is considered to be a type of practice, not a dental benefits plan model.

retainer, n (retaining appliance), **1.** The part of a dental prosthesis that unites the abutment tooth with the suspended portion of the bridge. It may be an inlay, partial crown, or complete crown. n **2.** an appliance for maintaining the positions of the teeth and jaws gained by orthodontic procedures. n **3.** the portion of a fixed prosthesis attaching a pontic(s) to the abutment teeth (for example, inlay, three-quarter crown). n **4.** a form of clasp, attachment, or device used for the fixation or stabilization of a prosthetic appliance. n **5.** any orthodontic appliance, fixed or removable, used to maintain teeth in corrected positions during the period of functional adaptation following corrective treatment.

retainer, continuous bar, n a metal bar that is attached to a major connector and contacts lingual surfaces of anterior teeth, on or incisal to the cingula; it aids in the stabilization of a distal extension removable partial denture.

retainer, direct, n a clasp, attachment, or assembly applied to an abutment tooth for the purpose of maintaining a removable restoration in its planned position in relation to oral structures.

retainer, extracoronal, n **1.** a type of retainer in which the preparation and its cast restoration lie largely external to the body of the coronal portion of the tooth and complement the contour of the crown. The retention or resistance to displacement is developed between the inner surfaces of the casting and the external walls of the prepared tooth. The extracoronal retainer may be a partial crown or a complete crown. *n* **2.** a direct retainer of the clasp type that engages an abutment tooth on its external surface in such a way as to afford retention and stabilization to a removable partial denture; a direct retainer of the manufactured type, the male portion of which is attached to the external surface of a cast crown on an abutment tooth (e.g., Dalbo and Crismani attachments).

retainer, Hawley, *n.pr* a wire and acrylic resin removable appliance designed to stabilize teeth after tooth movement; serves as a basis for tooth movement by providing an anchorage for the wires and rubber dam elastics used in orthodontic tooth movement.

retainer, indirect, *n* that part of a removable partial denture that resists movement of a free end denture base away from its tissue support through lever action opposite the fulcrum line of the direct retention.

retainer, intracoronal, *n* **1.** a type of retainer in which the prepared cavity and its cast restoration lie largely within the body of the coronal portion of the tooth and within the contour of the crown (for example, inlay). The retention or resistance to displacement is developed between the casting and the internal walls of the prepared cavity. *n* **2.** the type of direct retainer used in the construction of removable partial dentures; it consists of a female portion within the coronal portion of the crown of an abutment and a fitted male portion attached to the denture proper. These retainers may be fabricated in the dental office or obtained through commercial sources.

retainer, matrix, *n* (matrix holder), a mechanical device designed to engage the ends of a matrix around the tooth.

retainer, radicular, *n* a type of retainer that lies within the body of the tooth and is usually confined to the

root portion of the tooth (for example, dowel crown). The retention or resistance to displacement and shear is developed by extending an attached dowel into the root canal of the tooth.

retardation, *n* the slowing down of any mental or physical activity or the abnormal development of intellectual abilities.

retarder, *n* a chemical added to a substance to slow a chemical reaction, prolong the set of the material, and provide more working time.

retention (rē-ten′shən), *n* **1.** power to retain; capacity for retaining; the inherent property of a restoration to maintain its position without displacement under stress; results from close adaptation of the restoration to the prepared form of the tooth, usually aided by cement. *n* **2.** term relating to the provision in cavity preparation for preventing displacement of a restoration. Retention supplements resistance form and is specifically created to resist any lateral or tipping force that may be brought against the restoration during and after its insertion. *n* **3.** resistance of a denture to removal in a direction opposite that of its insertion; the quality inherent in the denture that resists the force of gravity, adhesiveness of foods, and forces associated with the opening of the jaws. *n* **4.** the period of treatment during which the individual wears an appliance to maintain the teeth in the desired position.

retention arm, *n* See *arm, retention.*

retention, circumferential, *n* frictional resistance to displacement derived from completely veneering the exposed tooth surface.

retention, denture, *n* **1.** the means by which dentures are held in position in the mouth; the maintenance of a denture in its position in the mouth; the resistance to the movement of a denture from its basal seat in a direction opposite to that in which it was inserted. *n* **2.** the resistance of a denture to vertical movement in the occlusal direction from its basal seat.

retention, direct, *n* retention obtained in a removable partial denture by the use of attachments or clasps that resist removal from abutment teeth.

R

retention form, n See *form, retention.*

retention, indirect, n retention obtained in a removable partial denture through the use of indirect retainers.

retention, partial denture, n the fixation of a fixed partial denture by means of crowns, inlays, or other retainers.

retention, pin, n See *pin, retention.*

retention, pinhole, n one or more small holes, 2 to 3 mm in depth, placed in suitable areas of a cavity preparation parallel with the general line of draft to provide or supplement resistance and retention form.

retention, radicular, n retention derived from projections of metal into the root canals of pulpless teeth.

retention, removable partial denture, n the resistance to movement of a removable partial denture from its supporting structures, gained by the use of direct and indirect retainers or other attachments.

retention terminal, n See *clasp, circumferential arm; clasp, circumferential, arm retentive.*

rete (epithelial) ridges, *n.pl* extensions of the epithelium into the connective tissue. They occur to an excess where epithelium-lined tissues are irritated and inflamed such as the junctional epithelium during periodontal disease. Outdated term is *rete pegs.*

rete pegs (rē′tē), See *rete ridges.*

reticular fibers, connective tissue, n fibers that come together to form a net of tissue in the lymph and bone marrow. These fibers may also be found in some glands and skin layers.

reticulocyte, n an immature erythrocyte. Reticulocytes normally account for less than 2% of the circulating erythrocytes.

reticulocytosis (rē-tik′yōō-lō-sī-tō′sis), n an increase in the normal number of reticulocytes in the circulating blood. Normal values range from 0.5% to 1.5% of the red blood cells.

reticuloendotheliosis, nonlipid (rē-tik′yōō-lō-en′dō-thē′lē-ō′sis), n abnormal increase of normal cells of reticuloendothelial tissue.

retina, n a 10-layered, delicate nervous-tissue membrane of the eye, continuous with the optic nerve, that receives images of external objects and transmits visual impulses through the optic nerve to the brain.

retinal detachment, n a separation of the retina from the choroid in the back of the eye, usually resulting from a hole in the retina that allows the vitreous humor to leak between the choroid and retina. Severe trauma to the eye may be the proximate cause, but in the great majority of cases, retinal detachment is the result of internal changes in the vitreous chamber associated with aging or with inflammation of the interior of the eye.

retinitis (ret′in-ī′tis), n a condition in which the retina becomes inflamed.

retinoblastoma, n a congenital, hereditary neoplasm developing from retinal germ cells.

retinol equivalent (RE) (ret′in-ôl), n a unit of measurement used to determine the value of vitamin A in sources of vitamin A. Retinol equivalent is 3.3 IU of vitamin A. 1 retinol equivalent = 6 μg β-carotene or 1 μg retinol.

retinopathy, n any one of a number of diseases of the retina, excluding retinitis. Often named for the underlying condition which causes it, such as diabetic retinopathy.

retraction, n **1.** a drawing or shrinking back; the laying back of tissues to expose a given part. n **2.** distal movement of teeth; a distal or retrusive position of the teeth, dental arch, or jaw.

retraction, gingival, n laying back of the free gingival tissue to expose the gingival margin area of a preparation by mechanical, chemical, or electrical means.

retractor, n an instrument for retracting tissues to assist in gaining access to an area of operation or observation.

retractor, beaver-tail, n a broad-bladed periosteal elevator.

retractor, rake, n a metallic instrument with prongs set transversely for engaging and retracting soft tissues.

retractor, vein hook, n a metallic instrument ending in a rounded flange set transversely for engaging and retracting soft tissues.

retroclination, n posterior angulation (inclination) of anterior teeth.

retrofill, v obturation of the apex of a tooth root by the direct surgical approach.

retrognathic (ret′rō-nath′ik), adj **1.** the condition of a mandible that is posterior to its normal relationship with other facial structures; may be a result of small mandibular size or posteriorly positioned temporomandibular fossae. adj **2.** mandibular retrusion.

retrognathism (ret′rō-nath′iz-m), n facial disharmony in which one or both jaws (usually the mandible) are posterior to normal facial relationships. This condition may be real or imaginary.

retrognathism, bird-face, n typical facial profile associated with an underdeveloped mandible; a retrognathia and small mandible usually associated with interference of condylar growth because of trauma or infection affecting the condyles. Surgical intervention is necessary for improvement.

retrognathism, Pierre Robin, n.pr See *syndrome, Pierre Robin.*

retrograde, v to move backward, degenerate, or return to an earlier state or worse condition.

retromolar pad, n See *pad, retromolar.*

retromylohyoid eminence, n See *eminence, retromylohyoid.*

retrospective review, a posttreatment assessment of services on a case-by-case or aggregate basis after the services have been performed.

retrospective study, a study in which a search is made for a relationship between one phenomenon or condition and another that occurred in the past (e.g., the exposure to toxic agents and the rate of occurrence of disease in the exposed group compared with a control group not exposed).

retrosternal pain, n a pain behind the sternum that usually occurs on swallowing. If retrosternal pain is associated with oral or pharyngeal candidiasis, it may indicate candidiasis of the esophagus, which is an opportunistic infection indicative of acquired immune deficiency syndrome.

retroversion (ret′rō-vur′zhən), n a condition in which teeth or other maxillary and mandibular structures are located posterior to the normal or generally accepted standard.

Retrovir, n.pr brand name for zidovudine, a dideoxynucleoside used in the treatment of human immunodeficiency virus-positive patients.

retrovirus (ret′rō-vī-rus), n a virus containing ribonucleic acid rather than deoxyribonucleic acid.

retruded contact position, n A tooth-to-tooth position at centric relation, sometimes referred to as centric relation occlusion.

retrusion (rē-trōō′zhən), n teeth or jaws posterior to their normal positions.

retrusion, mandibular, n abnormal retrusion of the mandible, as in a Class II malocclusion.

retrusion, maxillary, n abnormal retrusion of the maxillae.

reversal lines, n.pl stained scalloped microscopic lines caused by the resorption in bone and cementum.

reverse curve, n See *curve, reverse.*

reverse transcriptase, n an enzyme within a retrovirus that converts its ribonucleic acid into deoxyribonucleic acid (DNA), which then penetrates the cell nucleus and joins the host's DNA.

reverse Trendelenburg, n.pr a position in which the lower extremities are lower than the body and head, which are elevated on an inclined plane.

reverse-cut suture needle, n small, curved, hand-held tool used to secure surgical stitches; characterized by three cutting surfaces; one on the outside edge of the curve of the needle, with the other two on opposite sides near the tip.

reversible, adj capable of going through a series of changes in either direction, forward or backward (for example, reversible chemical reaction).

reversible hydrocolloid, n See *hydrocolloid, reversible.*

review coordinator, n a member of the staff of a Professional Standards Review Organization or hospital who is generally responsible to a utilization review committee. Such persons perform or assist in concurrent review or audit studies, initiating or coordinating discharge planning, recording and transmitting review decisions, or acting as liaison with persons and organizations participating in and affected by the review system.

rewards, n.pl a motivation technique to improve patient compliance with

R

oral hygiene protocols, generally used with young patients.

Rh factor, *n* an antigenic substance present in the erthrocytes of 85% of humans. A person having the factor is Rh positive, and a person lacking the factor is Rh negative.

Rh incompatibility, *n* a condition in which two groups of blood cells are antigentically different because of the presence of Rh factor in one group and the absence of the Rh factor in the other. See also *Rh factor.*

rhabdomyosarcoma (rab′dō-mī-ō-sär-kō′mə), *n* a malignant tumor of striated, or voluntary, muscle.

Rhabdomyosarcoma. (Regezi/Sciubba/Jordan, 2003)

Rhabdoviridae **(rab′dō-vir′i-dā),** *n* one of the major ribonucleic acid virus families, to which the rabies virus belongs. Viruses have a single-stranded, nonsegmented, linear molecular structure with helical symmetry.

rhagades (rag′ə-dēz), *n.pl* fissures or cracks in the skin seen around body orifices and in regions subjected to frequent movement.

rheology (rē-ol′ə-jē), *n* the study of blood flow, pressure, and velocity through the vascular system.

rheostat (rē′ ō-stat), *n* a resistor for regulating a current by means of variable resistances.

Rheostat. (Bird/Robinson, 2002)

rheostat pedal, n foot pedal that controls the speed on rotary powered, variable speed dental polishing equipment.

rheumatic carditis, *n* See *rheumatic heart disease.*

rheumatic fever, *n* See *fever, rheumatic.*

rheumatic heart disease, *n* damage to heart muscle and heart valves caused by episodes of rheumatic fever. Rheumatic heart disease may result when a susceptible person acquires a group A beta-hemolytic streptococcal infection; an autoimmune reaction may occur in heart tissue, resulting in permanent deformities of heart valves or chordae tendineae.

rheumatism (rōō′mə-tiz′əm), *n* (rheumatic disease), a nonspecific term indicating any painful disorder related to joints, muscles, bone, or nerves; acute rheumatic fever; or, as used by lay persons, rheumatoid arthritis, bursitis, myositis, or degenerative joint disease.

rheumatoid arthritis, *n* a chronic, destructive, sometimes deforming collagen disease that has an autoimmune component. Rheumatoid arthritis usually first appears in early middle age, between 36 and 50 years of age and most commonly in women.

rheumatoid arthritis, juvenile, n a chronic disease affecting the immune system that occurs in children younger than age 16. Symptoms include joint inflammation in the spine, knees, and wrists, and a limited ability to open the jaw and mouth.

rheumatoid factor (RF), *n* antiglobulin antibodies often found in the serum of patients with a clinical diagnosis of rheumatoid arthritis.

rhinitis, *n* inflammation of the mucous membranes of the nose, usually accompanied by swelling of the mucosa and a nasal discharge. Rhinitis may be acute, allegic, atrophic, or vasomotor.

rhinolalia (rī′nō-lā′lē-ə), *n* nasalized speech, of which there are two types: rhinolalia clausa (closed port) and rhinolalia aperta (open port).

rhinoplasty (ri′nō-plas-tē), *n* plastic or reconstructive surgery of the nose.

rhinovirus, *n* any of about 100 serologically distinct, small ribonucleic acid viruses that cause about 40% of acute respiratory illnesses. Infection is characterized by dry, scratchy throat, nasal congestion, malaise, and headache. Fever is minimal. Nasal discharge lasts 2 or 3 days.

rhizotomy, retrogasserian (rīz-ot'ə-mē, ret'rō-gas-ser'ē-ən), *n* intracranial sectioning of the sensory root of the trigeminal nerve posterior to the semilunar ganglion; used in the treatment of severe trigeminal neural gia.

rhodium (Rh), *n* a grayish-white metallic element. Its atomic number is 45, and its atomic weight is 102.9055. Rhodium is used for providing a hard, lustrous coating on other metals and in the making of mirrors.

Rhodococcus **(rō-dō-kok'us),** *n* a genus of gram-positive, rod-shaped, aerobic bacteria, some of which are pathogenic in humans.

rhodopsin (rō-dop'sin), *n* a purple light-receptive pigment found in the retina and consisting of opsin and retinal. Rhodopsin helps the eye adjust to drastic changes in environmental lighting.

rhythm (rith'əm), *n* a measured movement; the recurrence of an action or function at regular intervals.
rhythm, heart, *n* the rhythm pattern in the sequence of heart beats, which may be altered in the presence of cardiac disease.

rhytidoplasty, *n* a procedure in reconstructive plastic surgery in which the skin of the face is tightened, wrinkles are removed, and the skin is made to appear firm and smooth.

ribavirin (rī'bə-vir'in), *n* an antiviral agent that acts against many ribonucleic acid and deoxyribonucleic acid viruses by inhibiting protein synthesis and replication. Used in the United States only for aerosol therapy for infants to treat acute lower respiratory infections resulting from respiratory syncitial virus.

riboflavin (rī'bō-flā'vin), *n* (vitamin B₂), *trade names:* many generic sources; *drug class:* vitamin B₂ water soluble; *action:* needed for normal tissue respiratory reactions; functions as a coenzyme; *uses:* vitamin B₂ deficiency.

ribonuclease (rī'bō-nōō'klē-ās), *n* an enzyme that acts as a catalyst for ribonucleic acid hydrolysis. It may also be called *RNase.*

ribonucleic acid (RNA), *n* a nucleic acid, found in both the nucleus and cytoplasm of cells, that transmits genetic instructions from the nucleus to the cytoplasm. RNA functions in the assembly of proteins.

ribose, *n* a 5-carbon sugar that occurs as a component of ribonucleic acid.

ribosomal RNA (rī'bō-sō'məl), *n* a type of protein-containing ribonucleic acid produced by the nucleolus and found connected to the endoplasmic reticulum or moving freely within the cytoplasm.

rickets (rik'əts), *n* a condition caused by deficiency of vitamin D or calcium in infants and children, with disturbance in the mineralization of osseous and dental tissues. Marked by bending and bowing of bones, nodular enlargements at the ends of bones, myalgia, delay in closure of fontanels, and other problems. See also *osteomalacia.*
rickets, adult, *n* See *osteomalacia.*
rickets, refractory, *n* See *rickets, resistant.*
rickets, renal, *n* a disturbance marked by excessive excretion of phosphorus and calcium resulting from a lowered renal threshold of excretion of these mineral elements. See also *osteodystrophy, renal.*
rickets, resistant, *n* (late rickets, refractory rickets), rickets that responds only to extremely large amounts of vitamin D.

Rickettsia, *n* a genus of microorganisms that combine aspects of both bacteria and viruses. Examples of rickettsial diseases are Rocky Mountain spotted fever and typhus.

ridge, *n* the remainder of the alveolar process after the teeth are removed.
ridge, alveolar, *n* the bony ridge of the maxillae or mandible that contains the alveoli (sockets of the teeth). See also *process, alveolar.*
ridge, alveolar, remodeling, *n* an eroding of the residual ridge that occurs as the result of wearing dentures. It may cause changes to the bone structure of the face so that dentures must be repaired or replaced to obtain a secure, comfortable fit.

R

ridge, center of, *n* the buccolingual midline of the residual ridge.

ridge, central labial, *n* a groove appearing on the buccal midline of a canine tooth that is caused by a larger than usual middle labial developmental lobe.

ridge, crest of, *n* the highest continuous surface of the ridge, but not necessarily the center of the ridge; the top of a residual or alveolar ridge.

ridge extension, *n* See *extension, ridge.*

ridge, key, *n* (zygomaxillare), the lowest point of the zygomaticomaxillary ridge.

ridge lap, *n* the part of an artificial tooth that is adjacent to the residual ridge; the part of the artificial tooth that laps the ridge.

ridge, marginal, *n* a ridge or elevation of enamel that forms the boundary of the occlusal surface of a tooth.

ridge, mental, *n* a dense ridge extending from the symphysis to the premolar area on the anterolateral aspect of the body of the mandible.

ridge, mylohyoid, *n* a dense line or ridge of bone on the medial surface of the body of the mandible that extends obliquely upward and posteriorly from the symphysis, covers the cervical portion of the third molar, and then goes upward and backward onto the vertical ramus. The mylohyoid muscle is inserted into this ridge of bone.

ridge, oblique, *n* an elevated prominence that crosses the occlusal table of a maxillary molar from the distobuccal to the mesiolingual cusp.

ridge, Passavant's, *n.pr* See *pad, Passavant's.*

ridge relation, *n* See *relation, ridge.*

ridge, residual, *n* the portion of the alveolar ridge that remains after the alveoli have disappeared from the alveolar process after extraction of the teeth.

ridge support, *n* See *area, supporting.*

ridge, transverse, *n* an elevation that connects the buccal and lingual cusps and extends crosswise over the occlusal table of mandibular and maxillary posterior teeth.

ridge, triangular, *n* an elevation on a posterior tooth that extends from

the tip of the cusp to the center of the occlusal table.

rifabutin, *n* *trade name:* Mycobutin; *drug class:* antimycobacterial agent; *action:* inhibits deoxyribonucleic acid-dependent ribonucleic acid (RNA) polymerase synthesis of bacterial RNA; *uses:* prevention of disseminated *Mycobacterium avium* complex (MAC) disease with advanced human immunodeficiency virus infection.

rifampin, *n* *trade names:* Rifadin IV, Rimactane; *drug class:* antitubercular antiinfective; *action:* inhibits deoxyribonucleic acid-dependent ribonucleic acid (RNA) polymerase synthesis of bacterial RNA; *uses:* pulmonary tuberculosis, prevention of meningococcal caries.

right of action, *n* the right to sue; a legal right to maintain an action, based on a happening or state of fact.

right-to-know laws, *n.pl* laws that require employers to inform workers regarding health effects of materials they must handle, including toxic chemicals and radioactive substances. Right-to-know statutes are administered under the authority of the U.S. Occupational Safety and Health Administration (OSHA).

rigidity, *n* the characteristic of being nonflexible, which is essential in a connector, a reciprocal arm, or an indirect retaining unit of a removable partial denture.

rigor mortis, *n* the stiffening of skeletal and cardiac muscle shortly after death.

Riley-Day syndrome, *n.pr* See *syndrome, Riley-Day.*

riluzole, *n* *trade name:* Rilutek; *drug class:* glutamate antagonist; *action:* inhibits presynaptic release of glutamic acid in central nervous system; *use:* treatment of amyotrophic lateral sclerosis (Lou Gehrig disease).

rim, *n* the outer edge; often curved or circular.

rim, occlusion, *n* (record rim), an occluding surface built on temporary or permanent denture bases for the purpose of making maxillomandibular relation records and arranging teeth.

rim, record, *n* See *rim, occlusion.*

rim, surgical occlusion, *n* a conventional occlusion rim, the base of which has been reduced until it is smaller than the surgical impression tray with which the surgical jaw relations are recorded.

rimantadine HCl, *n trade name:* Flumadine; *drug class:* antiviral; *action:* may inhibit viral uncoating; *uses:* adults, prophylaxis and treatment of illnesses caused by strains of influenza A virus; in children, prophylaxis against influenza A virus.

rimexolone, *n trade name:* Vexol; *drug class:* corticosteroid; *action:* interacts with steroid cytoplasmic receptors to induce antiinflammatory effects; *uses:* inflammation of the eye associated with ocular surgery and uveitis.

ringworm, *n* a fungal infection of the skin, nails, and hair caused primarily by dermatophytes, symptoms of which include inflammation, patching, and scaling of lesions.

rinse bath, *n* a tank or container of water used in film processing to wash residual developer from the film before placement in the fixer.

Risdon wire, *n.pr* See *wire, Risdon.*

Risdon's incision, *n.pr* See *incision, Risdon's.*

risk factors, *n.pl* elements that may contribute to or increase the risk to one's health, economic stability, or personal and professional liability.

risk management, *n* a program designed to identify, contain, reduce, or eliminate the potential for harm to patients, visitors, and employees and the potential financial loss to the facility if a compensable event occurs; usually concerned with the delivery system and site rather than practitioner performance.

risk pool, *n* a portion of provider fees or capitation payments withheld as financial reserves to cover unanticipated utilization of services in an alternative benefits plan.

risk-benefit analysis, *n* the consideration as to whether a medical or surgical procedure, particuarly a radical approach, is worth the risk to the patient compared with the possible benefits if the procedure is successful.

risorius, *n* one of the 12 muscles of facial expression. It acts to retract the angle of the mouth, as in a smile.

risperidone, *n trade name:* Risperdal; *drug class:* antipsychotic; *action:* may be related to antagonism for dopamine and serotonin receptors; also has affinity for alpha receptors and histamine (H_1) receptors; *use:* psychotic disorders.

RNA splicing, *n* the process by which base pairs that interrupt the continuity of genetic information in deoxyribonucleic acid are removed from the precursors of messenger ribonucleic acid.

RNA viruses, *n* See *viruses.*

Roach clasp, *n* See *clasp, bar.*

Rockwell test, *n.pr* See *test, Rockwell.*

Rocky Mountain spotted fever (RMSF), *n* a serious tick-borne infectious disease occurring throughout the temperate zones of North and South America, caused by *Rickettsia rickettsii,* and characterized by chills, fever, severe headache, myalgia, mental confusion, and rash.

rod, *n* a straight, slim, cylindric form of material, usually metal.

rod, analyzing, *n* the vertical part of a dental cast surveyor that is brought into contact with the surface contour of a tooth as a tangent related to a curve. It is used to determine the relative parallelism of one surface of a cast to other surfaces of the same cast. It is also used to estimate the cervical convergence of an infrabulge area of a tooth as it slopes from the contacting point of the surveying rod toward the cervical line, permitting evaluation of the retentiveness of the surface.

rod, condyle, *n* the adjustable pointers of a face-bow, which are placed over the condyles or at points on the face to mark the opening axis of the mandible.

rod, enamel, *n* a calcified column or prism, with an average diameter of 4 microns; extends in a wavy pattern through the entire thickness of the enamel and is generally perpendicular to the surface of the tooth.

rodent ulcer, *n* a slowly developing serpiginous ulceration of a basal cell carcinoma of the skin. See also *basal cell carcinoma.*

roentgen, equivalent man (rem), the dose of any ionizing radiation

R

that produces the same biologic effect as that produced by 1 roentgen of high-voltage x-radiation.

roentgen, equivalent physical (rep), *n* an unofficial unit of dose used with ionizing radiation other than x-rays or gamma rays. It is defined as the dose that produces an energy absorption of 93 ergs per Gm of tissue. For most purposes the rep can be considered equal to the rad; the latter is gradually replacing the use of rep.

roentgeno- (rent′gən-ō), *pref* denotes radiation originating only from an x-ray tube.

roentgenogram (rent′gən-ō-gram′), *n* See *radiograph.*

roentgenograph (rent′gən-ō-graf′), *n* See *radiograph.*

roentgenographer (rent′gən-og′rə-fur), *n* See *radiographer.*

roentgenographic detail, *n* See *detail, radiographic.*

roentgenography (rent′gən-og′rə-fē), *n* See *radiography.*

roentgenologist (rent′gən-ol′ō-jist), *n* See *radiologist.*

roentgenologist, oral, n See *radiologist, oral.*

roentgenolucent (rent′gən-ōl-ōō′sent), *n* See *radiolucent.*

roentgenopaque (rent′gən-ō-pāk′), *n* See *radiopaque.*

roentgenoparent (rent′gən-ō-per′ent), *n* See *radioparent.*

roentgenotherapy (rent′gən-ō-ther′ə-pē), *n* See *therapy, radiation.*

role model, *n* a person who inspires others to imitate his or her persona, values, and goals.

Romberg sign, *n.pr* an indication of loss of the sense of position in which the patient loses balance when standing erect, with feet together and eyes closed. Also called *Romberg test.*

rongeur forceps, *n* a strong and heavy cutting or biting forceps that is used for cutting bone.

root, *n* **1.** the part of a human tooth covered by cementum. *n* **2.** a nerve root; the part of a nerve adjacent to the center with which it is connected; in spinal and cranial nerves the part of the nerve between the cells of origin or termination and the ganglion.

root amputation, n See *amputation, root.*

Root amputation. (Rosenstiel/Land/Fujimoto, 2001)

root axis line (RAL), n a hypothetical vertical line that could be drawn from the crown of a tooth to the root apex.

root, bifurcated, n the root structure of a tooth divided into two segments.

root canal, accessory, n a nonprimary passage typically located near the root's apex that extends from the cementum to the pulp. It may be located at a higher point on the tooth and connect to a periodontal pocket.

root canal instrument stop, n a device placed on a root canal instrument to mark the measured depth of instrument penetration.

root, clinical, n the portion of the tooth that is below the attached periodontal tissues and not exposed to the oral cavity.

root concavity, n a longitudinal depression located on the surface of a root.

root curettage, n See *curettage, root.*

root, intraalveolar, n the portion of a tooth root enclosed in and supported by alveolar bone.

root planing, n a procedure that smooths the surface of a root by removing abnormal toxic cementum or dentin that is rough, contaminated, or permeated with calculus.

Root planing. (Newman/Takei/Carranza, 2002)

root resection, n See *apicoectomy.*

root resorption of teeth, n the destruction of the cementum or dentin by cementoclastic or osteoclastic activity. It may result in a shortening or blunting of the root. Lateral root resorption may also occur, resulting in a loss of root substance along the side or length of the root. Severe lateral resorption may result in penetration of the pulp canal. Root resorption may be caused by inflammation resulting from trauma or infection, or it may be unknown or idiopathic. See also *resorption.*

root retention, n removal of the crown of a root-canal-treated tooth, whose periodontium is not adequate to support a prosthesis but with enough retention of the root and gingival attachment to support a removable prosthesis. See also *overdenture.*

root submersion, n root retention in which the tooth structure is reduced below the level of the alveolar crest and the soft tissue is allowed to heal over it. It is believed that residual ridge resorption can be minimized by this approach. See also *root retention.*

root, trifurcated, n the root structure of a tooth divided into three segments.

root trunk, n the section of root nearest the crown from which multiple roots emerge.

Rorschach test, n.pr better known as the inkblot test, this test consists of 10 pictures of inkblots, five in black and white, three in black and red, and two multicolored, to which the subject responds by telling, in as many interpretations as is desired, what images and emotions each design evokes.

rosary, rachitic, n a beading of the ribs at the costochondral junction such as occurs in rickets.

rose fever, n a common misnomer for seasonal allergic rhinitis caused by pollen, most frequently of grasses, that is airborne when roses are in bloom.

rotary cutting instrument, n See *instrument, cutting, rotary.*

rotating anode, n See *anode, rotating.*

rotating condyle, n See *condyle, rotating.*

rotating spring, n an auxiliary wire used in conjunction with arch wire to rotate a tooth into proper position.

rotation, n **1.** the act of turning about an axis or a center. n **2.** movement of a tooth around its longitudinal axis.

rotation center, n See *center, rotation.*

rotavirus, n a double-stranded ribonucleic acid molecule that appears as a tiny wheel, with a clearly defined outer layer or rim and an inner layer of spokes. It is a cause of acute gastroenteritis with diarrhea, particularly in infants.

rouge, n See jeweler's rouge.

rounds, n a teaching conference or meeting in which the clinical problems encountered in the practice of medicine, dentistry, nursing, or other service are discussed.

roundworm, n any worm of the class Nematoda, including *Ancylostoma duodenale, Ascaris lumbricoides, Enterobius vermicularis, and Strongyloides stercoralis,* that may infect the gastrointestinal tract of humans.

routine, n **1.** a fixed pattern of procedures used in any phase of treatment. n **2.** a set of instructions arranged in proper sequence to direct the computer to perform a desired operation or series of operations.

routine, office, n a series of steps, to be followed in a carefully planned sequence, that provide a means of dealing with situations commonly encountered in dental practice.

r.p.m. (revolutions per minute), n the speed of rotary dental surface polishing equipment. High speed is classified as 100,000 to 800,000 r.p.m. and low speed as 6000 to 10,000 r.p.m.

RU486, n a drug that can end a pregnancy when administered as a 1-dose pill within the first 6 weeks after conception.

rubber dam, n See *dam, rubber.*

rubber dam clamp, n See *clamp, rubber dam.*

rubber dam clamp forceps, n an instrument used to place a clamp on a tooth, adjust a clamp, or remove it from a tooth. It engages the holes or notches of the flanges of the clamp.

rubber dam holder, n in endodontics, a rubber dam frame holder; in

R

operative dentistry, a rubber dam frame.

rubber polishing cup, *n* See *polishing cup.*

Rubber polishing cup. (Daniel/Harfst, 2002)

rubefacient, *n* a substance or agent that increases the reddish coloration of the skin.

rubella (rōō-bel′ə), *n* (German measles, 3-day measles), a highly contagious viral disease spread chiefly by direct contact that has an incubation period of about 18 days. Manifestations include pharyngitis, regional lymphadenopathy, mild constitutional symptoms, and a maculopapular rash that becomes scarlatiniform. Oral lesions are red macules. When rubella occurs in pregnant women, it may cause congenital rubella syndrome with serious malformations of the developing fetus. Children infected with rubella before birth (a condition known as *congenital rubella*) are at risk for the following: growth retardation; malformations of the heart, eyes, or brain; deafness; and liver, spleen, and bone marrow problems.

rubeola (rōō-bē-ō′lə), *n* See *measles.*

rudimentary, *adj* pertaining to something either vestigial or embryonic.

Ruffini's corpuscles (rōō-fē′nēz), *n.pr* See *corpuscle, Ruffini's.*

rugae (rōō′gē, rōō′jē), *n.pl* the irregular ridges in the mucous membrane covering the anterior part of the hard palate.

rugae area, n See *area, rugae.*

rule, Clark's, *n.pr* a formula used to estimate the dosage of a drug for individuals whose weight varies significantly from the arbitrarily selected official standard of 150 pounds (67.5 kg). The dose is calculated by dividing the weight of the patient by 150 and multiplying by the dose to determine the current dose for a patient weighing more or less than 150 pounds.

rule of confidentiality, *n* a principle that personal information about others, particularly patients, should not be revealed to anyone not authorized to receive such information.

rule, Young's, *n.pr* a mathematics expression used to determine a drug dosage for children. The correct dosage is calculated by dividing the child's age by an amount equal to the child's age plus 12 and then multiplying by the usual adult dose.

Rumpel-Leede test, *n.pr* See *test, capillary resistance.*

run, *n* one performance of a program on a computer; performance of one routine or several routines automatically linked so that they form an operating unit, during which time manual manipulation by the computer operator is usually not required.

rupture, *n* a tear or break in the continuity or configuration of an organ or body tissue, including those instances when other tissue protrudes through the opening.

Sabouraud's medium (säbōōrōz′), *n* See medium, Sabouraud's.

saccharin, *n* the chemical sweetener benzosulfimide, which is 300 to 500 times as sweet as sucrose. Tests have demonstrated that large amounts of benzosulfimide may cause cancers in experimental animals. Saccharin is no longer in general use as a low-calorie sweetener.

Saccharomyces, n a genus of yeast fungi, including brewer's and baker's yeast, as well as some pathogenic fungi, that cause such diseases as bronchitis, moniliasis, and pharyngitis.

sacroiliac joint, *n* an irregular synovial joint between the sacrum and ilium on either side of the pelvis.

saddle, *n* See base, denture.

saddle connector, n See connector, major.

saddle, metal, n See base, metal.

saddle, nose, n a sunken nasal bridge caused by injury or disease and resulting in damage to the nasal septum.

safelight, n a source of illumination in a darkroom of a color and intensity that does not fog radiographic film.

safelighting test, n a procedure used to determine whether darkroom lights are too bright. It involves bringing unprocessed film into the darkroom and placing a coin on the film. The safelight is then turned on for a short period of time, and the film is processed normally. Evidence of the coin's shape on the film will disqualify the safelight.

safety measures, n.pl actions (for example, use of glasses, face masks) taken to protect patients and office personnel from such known hazards as particles and aerosols from high-speed rotary instruments, mercury vapor, radiation exposure, anesthetic and sedative gases, falls, inadequate sterilization, cuts, puncture wounds, and laboratory accidents.

sagittal (saj′ətəl), adj shaped like or resembling an arrow; straight; situated in the direction of the sagittal suture. Said of an anteroposterior plane or section parallel to the long axis of the body.

sagittal axis, n a hypothetical line through the mandibular condyle that serves as an axis for rotation movements of the mandible.

sagittal plane, n See plane, sagittal.

sagittal splitting of mandible, n intraoral osteotomy of the ascending ramus and posterior body of the mandible in the sagittal plane for the correction of prognathism, retrognathism, or apertognathia. An alternative procedure confines the split to the body of the mandible.

Saint Vitus's dance, n.pr See chorea.

Sainton's disease, n.pr See dysostosis, cleidocranial.

salary, n **1.** a fixed, regular compensation paid for services rendered involving professional knowledge or skill; employment above the degree of mechanical labor. **2.** the amount of take-home pay received by the dentist from the practice.

salary arrangements, n.pl the clear understanding between the dentist and auxiliaries concerning the amount of money they will be paid, the increase in pay they may expect, and the time interval between pay increases.

salicylamide (sal′isilam′id), n an analgesic, antipyretic, and antiarthritic similar in action to aspirin.

salicylanilide (sal′isilan′ilīd), n an antifungal agent useful in the treatment of tinea capitis caused by *Microsporum audouinii.*

salicylates (səlis′əlāts), n.pl salts or esters of salicylic acid; salicylates are used as preservatives, antiseptics, fungicides, and keratolytic agents.

salicylism (sal′isil′izəm), n a toxic state resulting from excess ingestion of salicylates.

saline (sā′lēn), adj salty; of the nature of a salt; containing a salt or salts.

saliva (səlī′və), n the clear mucoserous secretion formed mainly in the major glands of the parotid, submandibular, and sublingual, as well as minor glands. It has lubricative, cleansing, microbial, excretory, and digestive functions and also is an aid to deglutition. While its pH level is slightly more acidic than blood—6.3 to 6.9—it is more basic than dental plaque and acts as a buffering agent within the oral cavity. Emotional disturbances affect the rate of salivary secretion either by stimulation of secretion or inhibition of activity, leading to xerostomia. A lowered rate of flow has been noted in patients suffering from depression, whereas a higher degree of salivary activity has been observed in patients with mania. However, most xerostomia is due to medications and is related to an increased caries risk.

saliva, lingual, n saliva secreted by von Ebner's glands and other serous glands of the tongue.

saliva, loss of CO_2 in, n a theory of calculus formation in which the loss of carbon dioxide (CO_2) from saliva reduces the salivary carbonic acid content and causes the calcium phosphate in solution in the saliva to become supersaturated; calcium phosphate then precipitates in areas of stasis of the saliva.

saliva, parotid, n saliva produced by the parotid gland. It is thinner and less viscous than are the other varieties and contains no mucin.

saliva, supersaturated, n saliva overladen with mineral elements associated with calculus formation. With a loss of carbon dioxide ($CO_2$2) and a rise in the pH level of saliva, precipitation of calcium, phosphates, and magnesium carbonate occur, thus providing the mineral components of salivary calculus.

saliva tests, n.pl See tests, colorimetric caries susceptibility.

salivant (sal′ivənt), adj provoking a flow of saliva.

salivary duct openings, palatal, n minute, darkened areas distributed on the soft and hard palates.

salivary glands, n.pl three pairs of exocrine glands that produce saliva and empty it into the mouth. The parotid glands produce serous fluid, the sublingual glands produce mucous fluid, and the submandibular glands produce serous and mucous secretions.

salivary glands, von Ebner's, n.pr the secretory glands located at the base of the circumvallate papillae on the posterior dorsal surface of the tongue. Also known as *Ebner's glands.*

salivary Lactobacillus count, n determination of the number of *lactobacilli* per milliliter of saliva; an indicator of caries susceptibility. High lactobacillus counts generally correlate with high caries activity.

salivary stone, n a tiny, pebble-like mass of calcified saliva that forms in the major salivary ducts or glands. Also called *sialolith.* See also calculus, dental.

salivation (sal′ivā′shən), n excessive discharge of saliva; ptyalism.

salmeterol xinafoate, n trade name: Serevent Inhalation Aerosol; *drug class:* long-acting selective β_2-agonist; *action:* relaxes bronchial smooth muscle by directly acting on β_2-adrenergic receptors; also inhibits release of mast cell mediators; *uses:* treatment of bronchospasm, maintenance treatment of asthma and exercise-induced bronchospasm.

Salmonella, n a genus of motile, gram-negative, rod-shaped bacteria that include species causing typhoid fever, paratyphoid fever, and other forms of gastroenteritis.

salmonellosis (sal′mənelō′sis), n an infection of the gastrointestinal tract caused by *Salmonella* bacteria, usually contracted by the ingestion of tainted food or drink. Symptoms include fever, bacteremia, and lesions.

salsalate, n trade names: Armigesic, Anaflex, Arthra-G, Mono-Gesic, Salflex, and Salsitab; *drug class:* salicylate, nonnarcotic analgesic; *action:* blocks formation of peripheral prostaglandins, which cause pain and inflammation; antipyretic action results from inhibition of hypothalamic heat-regulating center; does not inhibit platelet aggregation; *uses:* treatment of mild-to-moderate pain or fever, including arthritis and juvenile rheumatoid arthritis.

salt (sôlt), n a compound of a base and an acid; a compound of an acid, some of the replaceable hydrogen atoms of which have been substituted.

salt, basic, n a salt containing replaceable, or hydroxyl, groups.

salt depletion, n See depletion, salt.

salt solution, n a homemade mouthrinse consisting of one-half teaspoon salt and one-half cup of tepid water, used to decrease inflammation and promote healing.

samarium (Sm), n a rare earth, metallic element. Its atomic number is 62, and its atomic weight is 150.35.

sample, n a selected part of a population that is taken to be representative of the whole population.

sample, random, n a sample drawn by chance; a sample drawn in such a way that every item in the population has an equal and independent chance of being included in the sample.

sample, stratified, n a sample derived by dividing the population into a number of nonoverlapping classes or categories from which cases are selected at random, the number of cases selected from each category being proportional to the number therein.

sanguinaria (sang′gwiner′ē ə) (bloodroot), n *Sanguinaria canadensis* contains an isoquinoline alkaloid thought to be useful in reducing plaque and gingivitis. Although it has been marketed, test results have been equivocal, and untoward side effects have been reported. It can be highly toxic if swallowed.

sanguine, adj **1.** pertaining to an abundant and active blood circulation, ruddy complexion. n **2.** an attitude full of vitality and confidence.

sanitarium, *n* a facility for the treatment of patients suffering from chronic mental or physical diseases or for the recuperation of convalescent patients. Also called a *sanatorium.*

sanitation, *n* the science of maintaining a healthful, disease- and hazard-free environment.

saponification, *n* the production of soap.

saprophyte, *n* an organism that lives on dead organic matter.

saquinavir mesylate, *n trade name:* Invirase; *drug class:* antiviral; *action:* inhibits human immunodeficiency virus (HIV) protease important for viral replication; *use:* used in combination with nucleoside analogues, zidovudine, or zalcitabine in the treatment of acquired immunodeficiency syndrome (AIDS).

SAR, *n* See relationship, structure-activity.

Sarcina **(sär′sinə),** *n* bacterium belonging to the genus *Sarcina,* which encourages disease, dental caries, and periodontal inflammation.

sarcoadenoma, *n* a mixed tumor containing characteristics of both glandular and connective tissue.

sarcocarcinoma, *n* a mixed tumor with characteristics of both sarcomas and carcinomas.

Sarcodina **(sär′kōdī′nə, -dē′nə),** *n.pl* also called *amoebae,* a subphylum of sarcomastigophora of parasitic protozoa, which causes diseases such as dysentery and meningocephalitis by drinking, swimming, or bathing in water contaminated with feces.

sarcoidosis (sär′koidō′sis) (Besnier-Boeck-Schaumann disease, Boeck's sarcoid), *n* a chronic granulomatous disease of unknown etiology. Causes noncaseating granulomas in the skin, lymph nodes, salivary glands, eyes, lungs, and bones.

Sarcoidosis. (Regezi/Sciubba/Jordan, 2003)

sarcoma (särkō′mə), *n* **1.** a malignant neoplasm of connective tissue elements. **2.** a malignant neoplasm arising from mesenchyme or its derivatives.

sarcoma, ameloblastic, n a rare mixed tumor of odontogenic origin in which the mesenchymal component has undergone malignant transformation.

sarcoma, Ewing's, n.pr See tumor, Ewing's.

sarcoma, Kaposi's, n.pr a condition affecting blood vessels; believed to be of a neoplastic nature and of multicentric origin. Skin lesions appear as multiple red-brown nodules ranging from a few mm to 1 cm in size. Histologically, endothelial proliferation in sheets or small vessels, hemosiderin deposits, fibroblastic proliferation, and an inflammatory infiltrate of lymphocytes are seen. Associated with HIV infection.

Kaposi's sarcoma. (Regezi/Sciubba/Jordan, 2003)

sarcoma, neurogenic **(malignant schwannoma),** *n* the malignant form of neurilemoma.

sarcoma, osteoblastic **(osteogenic sarcoma),** *n* an osteosarcoma in which atypical bone formation is the most evident histopathologic feature. See also osteosarcoma.

sarcoma, osteogenic, n a malignant connective tissue tumor that produces bone.

sarcoma, reticulum cell, n a malignant tumor of reticulum cells. It may occur as a primary neoplasm in soft tissue or bone.

Sarcomastigophora **(sär′kōmas′tigof′ərə),** *n.pl* one of the four phyla of parasitic protozoa, to which the sarcodina and mastigophora subphyla belong. Capable of causing keratitis.

S

Sargenti technique, *n.pr* See N2.

satin finish, *n* See finish, satin.

satisfaction, *n* discharge of an obligation by actual payment of what is due or what is awarded by a court or other authority.

saturated, *adj* having all chemical affinities satisfied; unable to hold in solution any more of a given substance.

saturated fatty acid, *n* any of a number of glyceryl esters of certain organic acids in which all atoms are joined by single bonds. These fats are chiefly of animal origin but include cocoa butter, coconut oil, and palm oil.

saturation, *n* **1.** a condition in which a solution contains as much solute as can remain dissolved. **2.** a measure of the degree to which oxygen is bound to hemoglobin, expressed as a percentage of the possible limit. **3.** a chemical compound in which all the valency bonds have been filled.

saturation, color, n the quality of color that distinguishes the degree of vividness of hue.

saucerization **(sôs′ərizā′shən),** *n* excavation of the tissue of a wound to form a shallow, saucerlike depression.

saucerization, pericervical, n the circular bone resorption that occurs about the necks of endosteal implants shortly after their insertion and continues slowly during the time of the implant's biologic presence.

saw, *n* a cutting blade with a toothed edge used to cut material too hard to slice with a knife.

saw, Gigli's wire, n.pr a flexible wire with teeth used for osteotomy procedures; frequently used in blind operations.

saw, gold, n an instrument with a thin sawlike blade used for removing surplus metal from the contact area of gold-foil restorations.

saw, Joseph, n.pr a nasal saw often used in ramusotomy of the mandible.

saw, Koeber's, n.pr a saw consisting of a thin, replaceable blade held in a frame; used to trim gross excess from the proximal portion of a Class II foil restoration in the preliminary stages of finishing and contouring.

saw, oscillating **(Stryker-type saw),** *n* an oscillating blade in an electrical or compressed gas-driven unit; used to cut bone.

saw, rotary, n a rotary blade on a shaft in an electrical or compressed gas-driven unit; used to cut bone.

scabies, *n* a contagious disease caused by *Sarcoptes scabiei,* the itch mite, characterized by intense itching of the skin.

Scabies. (Zitelli/Davis, 2002)

scaffold, *n* a support, either natural or artificial, that maintains tissue contour.

scaler (skā′lur), *n* an instrument used to remove calculus from teeth.

scaler, sickle, n a hook-shaped instrument available in various sizes and shapes; used for the removal of tenacious supragingival deposits of calculus.

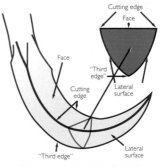

Sickle scaler. (Daniel/Harfst, 2002)

scaler, sickle, straight, n a sickle scaler that has an angled blade with a straight, flat face and two cutting edges that come to a point. Also called the *Jacquette scaler.*

scaler, sonic, *n.pl* instrument that uses compressed air delivered from dental unit handpiece line to drive rotor system to move tip about 2,500 to 7,000 cycles per second in an elliptical pattern. Although sonic scalers do not get hot, they cause tissues to heat, requiring fluid for cooling tissues. This technology is generally not capable of removing heavy, hard deposits, but it removes softer, less tenacious deposits.

scaler, ultrasonic, *n* an electronic generator that transmits high-frequency vibrations from 25,000 to 40,000 or more cycles per second to a handpiece that is used to remove all types of deposits from the surface of a tooth.

Ultrasonic scaler. (Bird/Robinson, 2002)

scaler, ultrasonic, chisel tip, n a power-scaling tip especially designed for removing calculus above the gingival margin on the posterior teeth. It may also be used to remove overhanging restorations.

scaler, ultrasonic, contra-angled, n a power-driven device with a tip that is specially curved for removal of calculus on certain hard-to-reach tooth surfaces.

scaler, ultrasonic, magnetostrictive, n an instrument that uses a pulsing magnetic field applied to a metal "stack" that flexes to move tip in an elliptical pattern. A vibrating metal stack generates heat requiring fluid for cooling handpiece and tissues.

scaler, ultrasonic, piezoelectric, n an instrument that uses pulsing voltage applied to ceramic crystals that fly and move the tip in a reciprocating pattern. Increased power increases tip amplitude for the most robust scaling but also increases patient discomfort. Although some claim that piezoelectric systems produce no heat, they cause tissues to heat, requiring fluid for cooling them.

scaler, ultrasonic, plastic tip, n a plastic cover used on the working end of an ultrasonic scaler when removing deposits from the implant surface.

scaler, ultrasonic, probe tip, n a thin, straight working end that is designed to provide access to sub-gingival calculus.

scaler, ultrasonic, straight, n a power-driven instrument that utilizes high-frequency electricity to vibrate an arched tip that is designed for use in all parts of the mouth. Also called a *universal ultrasonic scaler.*

scaling, *n* the removal of calcareous deposits from the teeth using suitable instruments.

scaling, channel, n a method of manual calculus removal in which the scaling instrument is applied in overlapping strokes across the surface of the tooth to ensure complete coverage and removal of all deposits.

scaling, coronal, n the removal of deposits of calculus, heavy stains, and materia alba from the crowns of the teeth by suitable instrumentation.

scaling, electrosurgical, n See electrosurgery and scalpel, electrosurgical.

scaling, root, n a technique of root surface cleansing designed to remove accretions of calculus and debris in the supragingival uninvested areas of a tooth.

scaling, subgingival, n the removal of accretions and debris from the surfaces of the tooth apical to the gingival margin. This process accomplishes the removal of primary irritants to the gingival tissues and permits the reduction of inflammation in these tissues.

scaling, supragingival, n the technique of meticulous cleansing of the surfaces of the teeth coronal to the gingival margin.

scalpel, *n* a delicate, razor-sharp, pointed knife, usually with a convex edge.

scalpel, electrosurgical, n a scalpel that severs tissue by means of an electrically heated wire.

scandium (Sc), *n* a grayish metallic element. Its atomic number is 21, and its atomic weight is 44.956.

scanning, *n* a technique and protocol for carefully studying an area, organ, or system of the body by recording and displaying an image of the area using radioactive substances that have affinities for specific tissues.

scanning electron microscope (SEM), *n* an instrument similar to an electron microscope in that a beam of electrons instead of visible light is used to magnify the surface of a sample. The electrons are deflected, collected, accelerated, and directed against a scintillator. The surface image produced is of less magnification than that produced by an electron microscope, but it appears three dimensional and lifelike. It is an essential research tool for the study of dental materials.

scar, *n* See cicatrix.

scar, apical, *n* the end product of wound repair. A radiolucent area characterized histologically by dense fibrous connective tissue.

scarify, *v* to make multiple superficial incisions into the skin.

scarlatina, *n* See scarlet fever.

scarlet fever, *n* an acute contagious disease of childhood caused by an erythrotoxin-producing strain of group A hemolytic *Streptococcus.* The infection is characterized by sore throat, fever, strawberry tongue, enlarged lymph nodes in the neck, prostration, and a diffuse bright red rash.

scattered radiation, *n* See radiation, scattered.

Schaumann's body, *n.pr* See body, Schaumann's.

Schaumann's disease, *n.pr* See sarcoidosis.

schedule, *n* the division of the working day into segments of time to enable the dentist to render treatment.

Schedule I, n a category of drugs not considered legitimate for medical use. Included are heroin, lysergic acid diethylamide (LSD), and marijuana.

Schedule II, n a category of drugs considered to have a strong potential for abuse or addiction but that also have legitimate medical use. Included are opium, morphine, and cocaine.

Schedule III, n a category of drugs that have less potential for abuse or addiction than Schedule I or II drugs and have a useful medical purpose. Included are short-acting barbiturates and amphetamines.

Schedule IV, n a medically useful category of drugs that have less potential for abuse or addiction than those of Schedules I, II, and III. Included are diazepam and chloral hydrate.

Schedule V, n a medically useful catiegory of drugs that have less potential for abuse or addiction than those of Schedules I through IV. Included are antidiarrheals and antitussives with opioid derivatives.

schedule of allowances, n a list of specified amounts that will be paid toward the cost of dental services rendered; the patient pays the difference between the allowance and the actual cost of service. Also called *table of allowances.*

schedule of benefits, n a listing of the services for which payment will be made by a third party without specification of the amount to be paid.

schedule plan, n a plan that bases covered expenses on a schedule of allowances.

scheme, occlusal, *n* See system, occlusal.

Schick test (shik), *n.pr* a skin test used to determine immunity to diphtheria in which diphtheria toxin is injected intradermally. A positive reaction, indicating susceptibility, is marked by redness and swelling at the site of injection; a negative reaction, indicating immunity, is marked by absence of redness and swelling.

schistometer (shis'tom'ətur), *n* an instrument for measuring the aperture between the vocal cords.

schistosomiasis (shis'tōsōmī' əsis), *n* (bilharziasis), infestation with blood flukes of the genus *Schistosoma,* which causes cystitis, chronic dysentery, hepatosplenomegaly, and esophageal varices.

schizophrenia (skit'səfrē'nē ə), *n* (dementia praecox), a functional psychosis (split personality) characterized by emotional distortion, withdrawal from reality, and disturbances of thought processes. It includes such disorders as hebephrenia, catatonia, and paranoia.

Schüller-Christian disease, *n.pr* See disease, Hand-Schüller-Christian.

Schüller's disease (shēl'ərz), *n.pr* See osteoporosis.

S

schwannoma (shwänō′mə), *n* See neurilemoma.

schwannoma, malignant, n See sarcoma, neurogenic.

sciatica, *n* an inflammation of the sciatic nerve, usually marked by pain and tenderness along the course of the nerve through the thigh and leg.

scientific method, *n* a formal style of study or research in which a problem is identified, pertinent information is assembled, a hypothesis is advanced and tested empirically, and the hypothesis is accepted or rejected.

scissors, Fox, *n.pr* delicate, fine-pointed scissors designed to gain access to interproximal areas and remove small tissue tabs or slight soft tissue deformities during gingivoplasty and gingivectomy. They also may be used to smooth the cut gingival surfaces.

scleroderma (sklerʹōdurʹmə), (dermatosclerosis, hidebound disease), *n* a collagen disease of unknown etiology; skin lesions are characterized by thickening, rigidity, and pigmentation in patches or diffuse areas. Dermal atrophy also may be seen. Periodontal lesions may simulate those of periodontosis, with widening of periodontal membrane space (verified by radiographic evidence), resulting from bone resorption, loss of architectural arrangement, and degeneration of periodontal fibers, with absence of inflammatory change in the gingivae and remaining periodontium.

Scleroderma. (Regezi/Sciubba/Jordan, 2003)

sclerosing solution, *n* a liquid containing an irritant that causes inflammation and resulting fibrosis of tissues. It may be used in cauterizing ulcers, arresting hemorrhage, and treating hemangiomas.

sclerosis (sklerō′sis), *n* hardening. As applied to the jaws, sclerosis usually indicates an increased calcification centrally, with radiopacity. Tracts of increased density in the dentin are referred to as areas of *dentinal sclerosis.* Sclerosis occurs beneath caries and with abrasion, attrition, and erosion.

sclerosis, multiple, n a remitting and relapsing disease of the central nervous system affecting principally the white matter. Manifestations include sensory and motor incoordination and paresthesias; often dementia, blindness, paraplegia, and death result.

sclerotherapy, *n* the use of sclerosing chemicals to treat such varicosities as hemorrhoids and esophageal varices.

scoliosis (skō′lē ō′sis), *n* a lateral curvature of the spine.

scope of services, *n* the number, type, and intensity or complexity of services being provided.

scopolamine (skōpol′əmēn), *n* an alkaloid found in the leaves and seeds of *Atropa belladonna* and other solanaceous plants having an action similar to atropine and used when spasmolytic or antisecretory effects are desired.

scopolamine, transdermal, trade names: Transderm-Scōp, Transderm-V; *drug class:* antiemetic, anticholinergic; *action:* competitive antagonism of acetylcholine at receptor sites in the eye, smooth muscle, cardiac muscle, glandular cells; inhibition of vestibular input to the central nervous system (CNS), resulting in inhibition of vomiting reflex; *use:* prevention of motion sickness.

scorbutic gingivitis, *n* an abnormal condition, characterized by inflamed or bleeding gums; caused by vitamin C deficiency.

scorbutus (skôrbyōō′təs), *n* See scurvy.

scratch test, *n* a skin test for identifying an allergen, performed by placing a small quantity of a solution containing a suspected allergen on a lightly scratched area of the skin. If a wheal forms within 15 minutes, allergy to the substance is indicated.

screen, intensifying, *n* a layer of fluorescent crystals (usually calcium tungstate) supported on a flat base. Used in intimate contact with light-sensitive radiographic film in a cassette. The crystals fluoresce when exposed to x radiation and subsequently expose the film with light.

screen, oral, *n* a plexiglas or acrylic resin appliance that fits into the vestibule of the mouth for the correction of mouth breathing.

screening, *n* **1.** any examination of individuals or their records to ascertain dental needs, assess treatment plans, or evaluate services rendered. Prescreening is the review by designated dentists of patients' examination records as a prerequisite to the authorization of some or all types of treatment. Postscreening is the examination by designated dentists, usually on a sample basis, of records to determine whether services have been rendered adequately and in accordance with prescribed administrative procedures. **2.** a sample survey to determine initial treatment needs of a group seeking coverage under a dental plan; used in setting the initial premium.

screw, expansion, *n* an orthodontic mechanism for achieving movement of teeth or arch segments, consisting of a threaded shaft and sleeve arrangement that permits controlled separation of elements of the appliance.

screw, implant, *n* a small screw 3 to 5 mm long that is used as a means for primary retention of the implant.

Implant screw. (Rosenstiel/Land/Fujimoto, 2001)

Screw-Vent, *n.pr* a brand name of a blade implant of solid design of pure titanium and much smaller than the companion product, the Core-Vent system, both manufactured by Core-Vent.

screwdriver, *n* See instrument, screwdriver.

scribe, *v* to write, trace, or mark by making a line or lines with a pointed instrument or carbon marker.

scrofula (skrof´yŌōlə), *n.* a primary tuberculosis complex occurring in the orocervical region and consisting of tuberculous cervical lymphadenopathy and tuberculosis of adjacent skin (lupus vulgaris), with chronic draining sinuses below the angle of the jaw and cervical region.

scurvy (skur´vē), *n.* (scorbutus), a condition resulting from an ascorbic acid deficiency that is severe enough to desaturate the tissues. The development and manifestations depend on tissue storage of ascorbic acid and factors that influence the rate at which it is used in or released from the tissues. Manifestations of frank scurvy include weakness, poor wound healing, anemia, and hemorrhage under the skin and mucous membranes. Presence or severity of gingival changes is directly related to the presence of local irritants such as calculus. In a severe form and in infantile scurvy, painful subperiosteal hemorrhages occur.

Scurvy. (Neville/Damm/Allen/Bouquot, 2002)

scurvy, infantile **(Barlow's disease, Cheadle's disease, Moeller's disease),** *n* a nutritional disease of infants caused by a deficiency of vitamin C in the diet. It has the same symptoms as scurvy does in adults.

scurvy, land, *n* See purpura, idiopathic thrombocytopenic.

seal, *n* **1.** something that firmly closes or secures. **2.** a tight and perfect closure. *v* **3.** to keep shut, enclosed, or confined.

seal, border, *n* See border seal.

seal, double, *n* a seal consisting of gutta-percha underneath another material such as temporary cement; used to close the coronal opening in a tooth during endodontic treatment.

seal, hermetic, n perfect and absolute obliteration of all space within a tooth.

seal, peripheral, n See border seal.

seal, posterior palatal, n the seal at the posterior border of a denture produced by displacing some of the soft tissue covering the palate by extra pressure developed in the impression or by scraping a groove along the posterior seal area in the cast on which the denture is to be processed.

seal, postpalatal, n See seal, posterior palatal.

sealant, n enamel or pit and fissure, a resinous material designed for application to the occlusal surfaces of posterior teeth to seal the surface irregularities and prevent ingress of oral fluids, food, and debris.

sealant, fluoride-releasing, n a type of sealant that contains fluoride for the purpose of resisting the development of caries in the tooth to which it is applied.

sealer, n a substance used to fill the space around silver or gutta-percha points in a pulp canal. Most sealers contain some combination of zinc, barium, and bismuth salts and eugenol, Canadian balsam, and eucalyptol.

seasonal affective disorder (SAD), n a mood disorder associated with the shorter days and longer nights of autumn and winter. Symptoms include lethargy, depression, social withdrawal, and work difficulties

seat, basal, n See basal seat.

seat, rest, n See area, rest.

sebaceous glands (sēbā′shəs), n.pl exocrine glands of the skin, many of which open into the hair follicles and secrete an oily substance that coats the hair and surrounding epithelium, helping to prevent evaporation of sweat and retain body heat. In the oral cavity, these glands are known as *Fordyce's granules* or *Fordyce's spots* and can be seen with the unaided eye as yellowish-white in color and are more common in older adults on the buccal and labial mucosa.

seborrhea, n any of several common skin conditions in which an overproduction of sebum results in excessive oiliness or dry scales.

seborrhea capitis, n seborrhea of the scalp frequently seen in infants. Also called *cradle cap.*

secobarbital/secobarbital sodium (sē′kōbär′bətal), n *trade names:* Novosecobarb, Seconal; *drug class:* sedative-hypnotic barbiturate, controlled substance Schedule II; *action:* nonselective depression of the central nervous system (CNS), ranging from sedation to hypnosis to anesthesia to coma depending on the dose; *uses:* treatment of insomnia, status epilepticus, and acute tetanus convulsions, sedation, preoperative medication.

second-opinion program, n an opinion about the appropriateness of a proposed treatment provided by a practitioner other than the one making the original recommendation, some benefit plans require such opinions for selected services.

secondary, adj **1.** not primary, immediately following the first position; supplemental. **2.** directly emerging or resulting from an original source or condition.

secondary bone, n a second layer of bone tissue that supersedes the original bone as part of the maturation process.

secondary cancer, n an opportunistic neoplasm imposed on a host with reduced vitality and resistance result ing from a preceding neoplasm or infection.

secondary deficiency, n an inadequacy of nutrients in the diet that is the result of the body's inability effectively to process and use the foods ingested, however healthy those foods might be; may be caused by disease, allergies, or interactions between drugs and nutrients or between two nutrients.

secondary dental caries, n.pl dental caries developing in a tooth already affected by the condition; often a new lesion formed adjacent to or beneath a restoration.

secondary dentition, n See dentition, permanent.

secondary hemorrhage, n bleeding that develops 24 hours or more after the original injury or surgery. It is often caused by an infection.

S

secondary infectious disease, n an opportunistic infection imposed on a host with reduced vitality and resistance resulting from a preceding infection by a more virulent organism.

secondary prevention, n action performed to take care of early symptoms of a disease and preclude the development of possible irreparable medical conditions. See also primary health care and primary prevention.

secondary radiation, n See radiation, secondary.

secondary sex characteristic, n any of the external physical characteristics of sexual maturity that distinguish one gender from the other, such as the distribution of hair and voice changes.

secretary-receptionist, n the auxiliary whose chief responsibilities are to receive patients into the office, handle the correspondence and bookkeeping, order supplies, supervise housekeeping, and answer the telephone.

secrete, v to discharge or empty a substance into the bloodstream or a cavity or onto the surface of the body. The substance secreted is called a *secretion.* Glands that secrete internally are *endocrine* or *ductless glands*; glands that secrete into a cavity or onto the surface are *exocrine* or *duct glands.*

section, frontal, n a segment of the skull or other part of the body that has been split into front and back sections for the purpose of examination or study.

section, midsaggital, n, a segment of the body that has been split vertically into two sections for the purpose of examination or study.

section, transverse, n a segment of the body that is at right angles to the body's longitudinal axis.

sectional arch wire, n an orthodontic wire that occupies less than a complete dental arch. It usually is attached to only a few teeth. Typically it spans one or both buccal segments of the dental arch or is limited to the anterior teeth. It facilitates the application of differential forces in effecting tooth movement.

sectional impression, n an impression made in two or more parts.

sectioning, surgical, n the action dividing a tooth to facilitate its removal. A variety of instruments, including osteotomes and power-driven burs, are used.

sedation (sēdā′shən), n the production of a sedative effect; the act or process of calming.

sedation, conscious, n a condition induced by drugs or other means in which the patient retains a minimum level of consciousness while continuing to breathe on his or her own and to respond to verbal and physical prompts.

sedation, deep, n a condition induced by drugs or other means in which the patient enters a temporary state of semiconsciousness, causing partial loss of sensory perception and the inability to respond to verbal prompts.

sedative (sed′ətiv), n **1.** production of sedation. A drug that can produce sedation. **2.** any one of the drugs that produces cortical depression of varying degrees. **3.** a remedy that allays excitement and slows down the basal metabolic rate without impairing the cerebral cortex.

sedative-hypnotic, n a drug that reversibly depresses the activity of the central nervous system, used chiefly to induce sleep and allay anxiety.

sediment, n a deposit of relatively insoluble material that settles to the bottom of a container of liquid.

sedimentation rate (SR), n the speed of settling of red blood cells in a vertical glass column of citrated plasma. It is used to monitor inflammatory or malignant disease.

seed, radon, n See radon seed.

segment, n any of the parts into which a body naturally separates or is divided, either actually or by an imaginary line.

seizure, n See epilepsy.

seizure, absence, n a seizure characterized by sudden interruption of conscious physical and mental activities and a short period of unconsciousness. Formerly known as *petit mal,* sometimes simply called *absence.*

seizure, clonic phase, n a seizure's convulsion stage.

seizure, complex partial, n a seizure stemming from a localized part of the brain indicated by the presence of a

S

state similar to a trance, varying degrees of awareness, and the manifestation of purposeless behaviors or motions. The seizure may be followed by an indeterminate period of confusion, garbled speech, poor mood, and an inability to recall the events of the episode.

seizure, generalized, n a nonfocalized, convulsive spell that has a simultaneous effect on the entire brain.

seizure, grand mal (grand mäl, grän mäl), n an outdated term for a major or generalized seizure. See seizure, generalized.

seizure, simple partial, n a type of seizure where only one part of the brain is involved. Patients experiencing this type of seizure may feel intense emotions (joy, fear) or involuntary muscle spasms, depending on the region affected.

Seldane, *n.pr* a trade name for an oral antihistamine (terfenadine).

selection, n 1. the act of choosing between or among a variety of options or alternatives. 2. the process by which various factors or mechanisms determine and modify the reproductive ability of a genotype within a specific population. Also referred to as *natural selection.*

selection, shade (**tooth color selection**), n the determination of the color (hue, brilliance, saturation, translucency) of the artificial tooth or set of teeth for a given patient.

selection, tooth, n the selection of a tooth or teeth (shape, size, color) to harmonize with the individual characteristics of a patient.

selection, tooth color, n See selection, shade.

selective grinding, n See grinding, selective.

selectivity, sensory, n the property of the specialized receptor end-organ by which it responds to one type of stimulus rather than another.

selegiline HCl, n *trade names:* Eldepryl, SD-Deprenyl; *drug class:* antiparkinson agent; *action:* increased dopaminergic activity by inhibiting monoamine oxidase (MAO) type B activity; *uses:* adjunct management of Parkinson's disease in patients being treated with carbidopa-levodopa.

selenium (Se) (sələ̄'nē um), n a trace element used in the treatment of seborrhea and dandruff of the scalp. Selenium is toxic in large amounts.

Selenomonas (sel'enōmō'nas), n a genus of gram-negative, anaerobic, rod-shaped bacteria found in the oral cavity.

self-analysis, n introspection on one's own behavior and actions in the total environment.

self-concept, n the composite of ideas, feelings, and attitudes that a person has about his or her own identity, worth, capabilities, and limitations.

self-curing resin, n See resin, autopolymerizing.

self-esteem, n the degree of worth and competence one attributes to oneself.

self-funding, n the method of providing employee benefits in which the sponsor does not purchase conventional insurance but rather elects to pay for the claims directly, generally through the services of a third-party administrator. Self-funded programs often have stop-loss insurance in place to cover abnormal risks.

self-history, n a patient's own accounting of his or her medical history, usually on a preprinted form.

self-injury, n the act of intentionally hurting oneself. One manifestation of this is known as *cutting.*

self-insurance, n the setting aside of funds by an individual or organization to meet anticipated dental care expenses or dental care claims, and accumulation of a fund to absorb fluctuations in the amount of expenses and claims. The funds set aside or accumulated are used to provide dental benefits directly instead of purchasing coverage from an insurance carrier.

self-limited disease, n a disease restricted in duration by its own pattern of characteristics and not by other influences or interventions.

self-tapping implant, n an implant that cuts its own path into bone.

self-tapping screw, n a screw that cuts its own spiral threads into bone or tooth structure.

sella turcica (S), n the pituitary fossa. The center is used as a cephalometric landmark.

S

sella turica, floor of, n lowermost point on the internal contour of the sella turcica.

semantics, *n* the study of language with special concern for the meanings of words and other symbols.

semicoma, *n* a mild coma from which the patient may be aroused.

semiconductor, *n* a solid crystalline substance the electrical conductivity of which is intermediate between that of a conductor and an insulator.

semipermeable (sem´ēpur´mē əbəl), *adj* permitting the passage of certain molecules and hindering that of others.

senescence (sənes´əns), *n* the process of growing old.

senescence, dental, n a condition of the teeth and associated structures in which deterioration results from aging or premature aging processes.

senile dental caries, *n* tooth decay occurring at an advanced age. Senile dental caries is usually characterized by cavity formation at the cemento-enamel junction or in the cemental layer covering the root.

senile psychosis, *n* an organic mental disorder of aged people resulting from a generalized atrophy of the brain with no evidence of cerebro-vascular disease.

senility (sənil´itē), *n* old age; generally used to describe the cognitive and physiologic signs of advancing age.

sensation (sensā´shən), *n* an impression conveyed by an afferent nerve to the sensorium commune.

sensation, psychologic effects of, n arousal, facilitation, and distortion of sensation by psychologic factors, the basis for which lies in the corticalization of the special senses.

sensation, referred, n a group of vaguely classified sensations that are a consequence of cortical experience. They are the sensory hallucinations, *paresthesias,* and the phenomenon called *phantom limb.* Nonspecific and poorly localized pain in the alveolar ridges, which have poor vascular supply, may be evidence of this phantom limb phenomenon associated with neurotic behavior.

sensation, specialized, n sensation that is perceived by the specialized end organs associated with special senses such as vision, hearing, and smell.

sense (sens), *n* a faculty by which the conditions or properties of things are perceived. Hunger, thirst, malaise, and pain are varieties of sense.

sense, special, n one or all of the five senses: feeling, hearing, seeing, smell, and taste.

sensitive (sen´sitiv), *adj* able to receive or transmit a sensation; capable of feeling or responding to a sensation.

sensitivity, *n* **1.** the ability to feel or experience physical stimuli. **2.** compassion or thoughtfulness toward a person or situation.

sensitivity, tactile, n a capacity to sense the transference of vibrations from the parts of the instrument (e.g., handle, shank, and working end) to the fingers of the clinician.

sensitivity test, n a laboratory method for testing antibiotic effectiveness.

sensitivity, tooth, n the state of responsiveness of teeth to external influences such as heat, sugar, and trauma. May result from occlusal trauma, especially if the anatomic relation of the apical foramen to the traumatized tissue is such that the circulation of the pulp is disturbed.

sensitivity, tooth, hydrodynamic theory, n a theory that attributes tooth sensitivity to the expansion and contraction of fluids within the dentinal tubules, thus causing the nerve endings to trigger pain responses in the tooth pulp.

sensitivity, tooth, neurophysiology theory of, n a theory that attributes tooth sensitivity to the stimulation of either A-type fibers, which cause short, sharp, localized pains, or C-type fibers, which produce dull, aching pains that may be spread across a wide area.

sensitivity training, n the use of group dynamics to experiment with and alter behavioral patterns and interpersonal reactions. Also called *T group.*

sensitization (sen´sitizā´shun), *n* the process of rendering a cell sensitive to the action of a complement by subjecting it to the action of a specific amboceptor; anaphylaxis.

sensorium (sensôr´ē um), *n* any

sensory nerve center; more frequently, the whole sensory apparatus of the body.

sensory (sen'sərē), *n* that part of the nervous system that receives and perceives sensations such as sound, touch, smell, sight, pain, heat, cold, and vibration.

sensory threshold, *n* the point at which a stimulus triggers the start of an afferent nerve impulse. Absolute threshold is the lowest point at which response to a stimulus can be perceived.

separating medium, *n* See medium, separating.

separating spring, *n* spring placed between adjacent teeth to obtain separation.

separating wire, *n* See wire, separating.

separator, *n* an instrument used to wedge teeth apart and out of normal contact by immediate separation; useful in the examination of proximal surfaces of teeth and in finishing proximal restorations. Must be used with care; it should be stabilized against the teeth with modeling compound to prevent tissue damage.

separator, Ferrier's, *n.pr* one of a set of balanced, double-bowed, adjustable separators designed by W.I. Ferrier.

separator, noninterfering, *n* See separator, True's.

separator, True's (noninterfering separator), *n.pr* a single-bowed separator designed to give greater access to the surface being operated on; designed by Harry A. True.

sepsis, oral (sep'sis), *n* a condition occurring within the mouth and adjacent areas characterized by the presence of pathogens.

septic sore throat, *n* a severe throat infection, usually caused by a *Streptococcus* strain, resulting in fever and marked exhaustion.

septicemia (sep'tisē'mē ə), *n* a condition in which pathogenic bacteria and bacterial toxins circulate in the blood. Manifestations include high temperature, leukocytosis, malaise, rapid pulse, and subsequent diffuse systemic degenerative disturbances.

septum, interdental (interdental alveolar septum), *n* the portion of the alveolar process extending between the roots of adjacent teeth.

septum, nasal, *n* the thin, vertical bony septum separating the right and left nasal cavities.

sequela, *n* any abnormal condition that follows and is the result of a disease, treatment, or injury, such as paralysis after poliomyelitis or scar formation after a laceration.

sequence, *n* order of occurrence or performance.

sequence planning, *n* a method of identifying all of the various treatments that a patient will need and putting those treatments in the most logical and effective order.

sequester, *v* to detach, separate, or isolate. A patient might be sequestered to prevent the spread of an infection or the isolation of a jury during the conduct of a trial.

sequestrum (sēkwes'trum), *n* a piece of dead bone that has become separated from vital bone.

Sequestrum. (Newman/Takei/Carranza, 2002)

serendipity, *n* the act of accidental discovery.

serial extraction, *n* a program of selective extraction of deciduous and sometimes permanent teeth over a period of time, with the objective of relieving crowding and facilitating the eruption of remaining teeth into improved positions. Close supervision of ensuing eruption is essential, because overclosure of the spaces and other sequelae may be expected in a significant number of cases. Comprehensive orthodontic treatment should almost always be initiated in the course of or after eruption for space management, control of the autonomous tipping usually induced by the procedure, and other malrelationships that commonly accompany these conditions.

serine (Ser), *n* a nonessential amino acid found in many proteins in the body. It is a precursor of the amino acids glycine and cysteine.

seroconversion (sir′ōkənvur′zhən), *n* a blood test in which the amount of time required for the blood to change from seronegative to seropositive is indicative of specific diseases.

serology tests (sērol′əjē), *n.pl* diagnostic tests of serum usually used to determine the immune or lytic properties of serum.

seronegative (sir′ōneg′ətiv), *n* serologic evidence of the lack of an antibody of a specific type in the serum; diagnostically useful in ruling out Lyme disease, syphilis, human immunodeficiency virus (HIV), serum hepatitis B, and many other viral diseases.

seropositive (sir′ōpoz′itiv), *n* serologic evidence of the presence of an antibody of a specific type in the serum; diagnostically useful in identifying many types of viral diseases.

seroprevalence rates (sir′ōprev′-ələns), *n.pl* a statistical measure of the rate of occurrence of seropositive status in a population or sample; used as a criterion of comparison between populations or samples.

serotonergic drugs (ser′ətōnur′jik), *n.pl* the prescription drugs used for weight loss that contain serotonin, a vasoconstrictor that acts as an appetite suppressant; examples are fenfluramine and dexfenfluarmine (the *fen* of Phen-fen), both of which have been removed from the U.S. market because of their links to heart valve disease, and fluoxetine, which has not been approved by the FDA for treatment of obesity.

serotonin (ser′ətō′nin), *n* (enteramine, thrombocytin), a local vasoconstrictor (5-hydroxytryptamine) and general hypotensive agent synthesized from tryptophan and found in tissues, rather than being transferred by blood to sites of action. Most serotonin in mammals is found in the gastrointestinal tract, although the kidney, liver, and brain also produce it. It is absorbed by platelets from the site of tissue damage, where it aids hemostasis locally by vasoconstriction and systemically by reducing blood pressure.

serotonin re-uptake inhibitors, selective, *n.pl.* a class of antidepressant drugs such as fluoxetine, sertraline, paroxetine, or voxamine.

serotonin serozyme (sir′ōzīm), *n* See factor VII.

serous fluid, *n* a fluid that has the characteristics of serum in color and viscosity.

serous membrane, *n* one of the many thin sheets of tissue that line closed cavities of the body, such as the pleura lining the thoracic cavity and the pericardium lining the sac enclosing the heart.

serrated (ser′ āt-ed), *adj* having a jagged or notched edge; saw-toothed.

Serratia, *n* a genus of motile, gram-negative bacilli capable of causing infection, including bacteremia, pneumonia, and urinary tract infections, in humans.

sertraline, *n trade name:* Zoloft; *drug class:* antidepressant; *action:* selectively inhibits the uptake of serotonin in the brain; *use:* treatment of major depression.

serum (sir′um), *n* the fluid component of the blood containing all stable constituents except fibrinogen. When blood is allowed to clot and stand, a clear yellowish fluid, the serum, separates.

serum accelerator globulin, *n* See accelerator, prothrombin conversion, I.

serum marker, *n* a specific indicator found in a blood test that identifies a disease.

serum protein determination, electrophoretic, *n* separation of serum protein fractions (albumin, alpha globulin, beta globulin, and gamma globulin) based on their different isoelectric points and mobility in an electric field. Electrophoretic patterns and concentrations are of value in evaluating the hyperglobulinemias. Electrophoretic evaluation of serum protein abnormalities is usually related to moving-boundary or paper-strip separation patterns.

serum prothrombin conversion accelerator (SPCA), *n* See factor VII; thromboplastin, extrinsic.

serum sickness, *n* anaphylactoid or allergic reaction after injection of foreign serum; marked by urticarial rashes, edema, adenitis, arthralgia, high fever, and prostration.

servant, *n* one who is employed to perform personal services (other than those that would be rendered in an independent calling) for an employer and who, in that service, remains entirely under the control of the employer.

servant, loaned, *n* a person whose services have been granted by an employer to another person.

service, *n* the performance of labor for the benefit of another.

service, denture, *n* diagnosis and treatment of edentulous and partially edentulous patients, including the diagnosis of existing and potential oral pathosis, planning of treatment for the preparation of the mouth for complete or partial dentures, fabrication and adjustment of the prostheses, and continuing observation of the changes in the oral conditions as the prostheses are in use.

service, gratuitous, *n* a service that does not involve a return, compensation, or consideration.

services, health, *n.pl* those services, including dentistry, that improve the general physical and mental well-being of the patient.

service of process, *n* the delivery of a writ, summons, or complaint to a defendant or witness. Service of process gives reasonable notice to allow the person to appear, testify, and be heard in court.

service, therapeutic, *n* treatment of a clinical nature deliberately performed to regulate or stop disease and sustain healthy oral tissues.

sessile lesion (ses′il), *n* a raised, wide-based lesion.

set, *n* term applied to the state of a plastic material after it has hardened or jelled by chemical action, cooling, or saponification. It is used in connection with impression materials, waxes, and gypsum materials.

set-square tooth numbering system, *n* See Palmer's tooth notation.

setoff, *n* See offset.

setting expansion, *n* See expansion, setting.

setting time, *n* See time, setting.

settlement, *n* an agreement made between parties to a suit before a judgment is rendered by a court.

setup, *n* **I.** the arrangement of teeth on a trial denture base. **2.** a labora-

tory procedure in which teeth are removed from a plaster cast and repositioned in wax. May be used as a diagnostic tool to evaluate alternatives, as when some teeth are missing; also used to produce the mold to make a positioner appliance.

sex, *n* classification of an individual as male or female on the basis of anatomic, functional, hormonal, and chromosomal characteristics.

sex, anatomic, *n* (genotype), classification of sex based on the sexual differentiation of the primary gonads.

sex, chromosomal, *n* chromosomal characteristics involving normally 44 somatic and 2 sex chromosomes, the latter designated as XX for the normal female and XY for the normal male. The presence of the Y chromosome is associated with a male phenotype and its absence with a phenotypic female.

sex chromosomes, *n* chromosomes responsible for sex classification—XX for female, XY for male.

sex, functional (phenotype), *n* designation of sex based on the state of maturation and potential for use of the external genitalia.

sex, hormonal, *n* contributory assignment of sex on the basis of adequate levels of estrogen and androgen for the development of typical phenotypic secondary sex characteristics.

sex hormones, *n.pl* See hormone(s), sex.

sex, legal, *n* that sex assigned at birth or legally by a court of law.

sex, nuclear, *n* sex determination based on the presence or absence of the hyperchromatic nucleolar satellite in squamous cells from a buccal mucosa smear or of "drumsticks" in the polymorphonuclear neutrophil. Positives are normally seen in the female.

sex-linkage, *n* See linkage, sex.

sextant (seks′ tənt), *n* one of the three sections into which each dental arch may be divided depending on its proximity to the midline of the arch.

sexual harassment, *n* in 1986, the U.S. Supreme Court adopted the definition of sexual harassment formulated by the Equal Employment Opportunity Commission as follows: unwelcome sexual advances, requests for sexual favors, and other verbal or physical conduct of a sexual nature when (1) submission to such conduct is made either explicitly or implicitly a term or condition of an individual's employment, (2) submission to or rejection of such conduct by an individual is used as a basis for employment decisions affecting such individual (both quid pro quo harassment), or (3) such conduct has the purpose or effect of unreasonably interfering with an individual's work performance or creating an intimidating, hostile, or offensive working environment (condition of work harassment).

sexually transmitted diseases, *n.pl* See venereal diseases.

shaken baby syndrome, *n* a condition of whiplash-type injuries ranging from bruises on the arms and trunk to retinal hemorrhages, coma, and convulsions, as observed in infants and children who have been violently shaken. Physicians are required by law to report cases of suspected child abuse and are granted immunity from liability for filing such reports.

shallow breathing, *n* a respiration pattern marked by slow, shallow, and generally ineffective inspirations and expirations. It is usually caused by drugs and indicates depression of the medullary respiratory centers.

shank, *n* the part of the instrument that connects the working end to the handle.

Working end

Terminal shank

Functional shank

Shank. (Daniel/Harfst, 2002)

shank flexibility, *n* the degree of rigidity that makes the shank of a hand-held instrument suited to a particular task. The thinner and more pliable the shank, the greater the tactile sensitivity of the instrument.

shank, lower, *n* the section of the working end of a dental instrument that is closest to the blade. Also called *terminal shank.*

shank, straight, *n* the linear, uncurved or unangled portion of an instrument that connects the working end to the handle. A straight shank is generally used in easily accessible areas while those with an angled shank are used in more confined areas.

shank, terminal, *n* See shank, lower.

shared services, *n.pl* administrative, clinical, or other service functions that are common to two or more hospitals or their health care facilities and used jointly or cooperatively by them.

sharpening, instrument, *n* the act establishing or restoring of a keen edge on a cutting instrument.

sharpening, instrument, automated technique, *n* a technique for sharpening the blade of a cutting instrument using a device that secures both the instrument and stone during the process.

sharpening, instrument, moving stone technique, *n* a technique for sharpening the blade of a cutting instrument, with the stone moving against the cutting edge of an instrument placed at an angle on a secure surface.

sharpening, instrument, stationary flat stone technique, *n* a technique for sharpening the blade of a cutting instrument; with the stone flat on a secure surface and the finger resting on the edge or side of the stone, the cutting edge of the instrument is drawn over the face of the stone.

Sharpey's fiber, *n.pr* See fiber, Sharpey's.

sharpness, *n* the quality of a blade that has a thin, keen cutting edge; a cutting edge is suitably sharp when it functions efficiently and safely.

sharpness, visual test of, *n* an examination of the cutting edge of a blade (usually magnified) to determined its extent of sharpness. The cutting edge is sharp when the line of its edge is too fine to reflect light. Also called *glare test.*

sharps, *n.pl* any needles, scalpels, wires, endodontic files, or other articles that could cause wounds or punctures to personnel handing them.

sharps container, *n* a container designed for the disposal of sharps required and regulated by the Occupational Safety and Health Administration (OSHA).

shave biopsy, *n* the removal of a thin layer of tissue using a dermatome knife. See also biopsy, shave.

shear, *n* See strength, shear and strength, ultimate.

shearing cusps, *n.pl* the upper buccal cusps, lower lingual cusps, upper canines, and upper incisors. Each of these cusps helps form the fossae that receive the stamp cusps. In the postcanine teeth, the triangular ridges of the shearing cusps arm the fossae with cutting ridges.

sheath of Schwann, *n.pr* See neurilemma.

shedding, *n* See exfoliation.

sheep cell test, *n* a method that mixes human blood cells with the red blood cells of sheep to determine the absence or deficiency of human T-lymphocytes.

shelf, buccal, *n* the surface of the mandible from the residual alveolar ridge or alveolar ridge to the external oblique line in the region of the lower buccal vestibule. It is covered with cortical bone.

shelf life, *n* the length of time a material may be stored without deterioration; the length of time it remains usable.

shellac base, *n* See base, shellac.

shield, radiation, *n* a body of material used to prevent or reduce the passage of particles of radiation. A shield may be designated according to what it is intended to absorb (for example, gamma ray, neutron shield) or according to the kind of protection it is intended to give (for example, background, biologic, thermal shield). The shield of a nuclear reactor is a body of material surrounding the reactor to limit the escape of neutrons and radiation into the protected area. Shields may be required to protect personnel and reduce radiation sufficiently to allow use of counting instruments for research or for locating contamination or airborne radioactivity.

shift, axis, *n* See axis shift.

shift to right or left, *n* an arbitrary description of an increase in the number per unit volume of immature (shift to left) or mature (shift to right) forms of neutrophils, in the differential counting system of Schilling.

Shigella, *n* a genus of gram-negative pathogenic bacteria that causes gastroenteritis and bacterial dysentery.

shigellosis (shig′əlō′sis), *n* an infection of the gastrointestinal tract caused by *Shigella* bacteria, usually contracted by the ingestion of tainted food or drink. Symptoms include fever, abdominal pain, and diarrhea.

shingles, *n* See herpes zoster.

shock, *n* **1.** a state of collapse of the body after injury or trauma. Shock may be either primary or secondary. The principal effects of shock are slowing of the peripheral blood flow and reduction in cardiac output. **2.** circulatory insufficiency caused by a disparity between circulating blood volume and vascular capacity.

shock, galvanic, *n* pain produced as a result of galvanic currents caused by similar or dissimilar metallic restorations.

shock, hemorrhagic, *n* an ineffectual circulating volume of blood resulting from loss of whole blood.

shock, insulin, *n* coma resulting from too much insulin or an inadequate intake of food. Symptoms include wet or moist skin, hypersalivation or drooling, normal blood pressure, tremors, dilated pupils, normal or bounding pulse, and firm eyeballs. Sugar and acetoacetic acid may be present in bladder urine but are absent in the second specimen. The blood sugar is low. See also coma, diabetic.

shock, neurogenic, *n* shock caused by loss of nervous control of peripheral vessels, resulting in an increase in the vascular capacity. Onset is usually sudden but is quickly reversible if the cause is removed and treatment is instituted immediately.

shock, primary, *n* shock that has a neurogenic basis in which pain and psychic factors affect the vascular system. Occurs immediately after an injury.

S

shock, secondary, n shock that occurs some time after the injury (6 to 24 hours later). Secondary shock is associated with changes in capillary permeability and subsequent loss of plasma into the tissue spaces. Changes in capillary permeability are probably related to histamine release associated with tissue injury.

shock, traumatic, n any shock produced by trauma, whether psychic or physical. In general usage, this term refers to shock following physical trauma, with hemorrhage, peripheral blood vessel dilation, and changes in capillary permeability.

shoeing cusps, *n.pl* See restoration of cusps.

short-bowel syndrome, n a loss of intestinal surface for absorption of nutrients caused by the surgical removal of a section of bowel.

short-cone technique, n See technique, short-cone.

shotgun therapy, n any treatment that has a wide range of effect and may be expected to correct the abnormal condition even though the particular cause is unknown.

shoulder, n **1.** the junction of the clavicle, scapula, and humerus where the arm attaches to the trunk of the body. **2.** in extracoronal cavity preparation of the ledge formed by the meeting of the gingival and axial walls at a right angle.

shoulder, linguogingival, n the portion of a prepared cavity in the proximal surface of an anterior tooth that is formed by the angular junction of the gingival and lingual walls. Developed to facilitate the dense compaction of gold in this area.

shrinkage, n **1.** reduction or decrease in extent or quantity. **2.** reduction in volume.

shrinkage, casting, n volume change (contraction) that occurs when molten metal solidifies after being cast into a pattern mold. It is compensated for in three ways: by using the indicated water:powder ratio for the refractory investment to gain the maximal setting expansion of which that investment is capable; by exposing the investment to moisture as the refractory investment sets, causing some hydroscopic expansion; and by properly heating the mold to achieve thermal expansion. The total expan-

sion must equal the contraction of the metal being cast.

shunt, arteriovenous, n (arteriovenous aneurysm, arteriovenous fistula), abnormal communication between an artery and a vein; usually caused by trauma.

shunt, ventriculoatrial (ventrik′yōōlō-ā′trē-əl), n a surgically manufactured passage made of plastic tubing between a cardiac atrium and cerebral ventricle for the treatment of hydrocephalus. See also ventriculoureterostomy.

shut, n the part of an anterior artificial tooth between the ridge lap and the shoulder. The pins for retaining the tooth in the base material are located in the shut.

sialadenitis (sī′ əlad′ənī′tis), n inflammation of the salivary glands, especially the major glands, because of such trauma as surgery or infection. Noted in mumps due to viral infection.

sialagogue (sī al′əgog), n a substance that increases the flow of saliva.

sialoadenectomy (sī′ əlō ad′ənek′təmē), n excision of a salivary gland.

sialoangiitis, n inflammation of salivary gland ducts.

sialodochoplasty (sī′ əlōdō′kōplastē), n a surgical procedure for the repair of a defect or restoration of a portion of a salivary gland duct.

sialogram (sī al′əgram), a radiograph made to determine the presence or absence of calcareous deposits in a salivary gland or its ducts.

sialography (sī əlog′rəfē), n **1.** inspection of the salivary ducts and glands by x-ray examination after injection of a radiopaque medium. **2.** production of a sialogram.

sialolith (sī al′əlith), n a salivary calculus. See also culus, dental.

Sialolith. (Regezi/Sciubba/Jordan, 2003)

sialolithiasis (sīal'əlithī' əsis), *n* presence of salivary gland or duct stones.

Sialolithiasis. (Regezi/Sciubba/Jordan, 2003)

sialolithotomy (sī aləlithôt'ōmē), *n* removal of calculus from a salivary gland or duct.

sialometaplasia, necrotizing (sī'-əlōmct'əplā'zē-ə nck'rōtīzing), *n* an oral cavity lesion due to a blood flow blockage to the region because of ischemia or trauma. The condition is indicated by localized tender swelling and pain and a well-defined ulcer, usually in the hard palate region.

Necrotizing sialometaplasia. (Sams/Lynch, 1990)

sialorrhea (sīal' ərē' ə), *n* (hypersalivation, ptyalism), excessive flow of saliva. It may be associated with acute inflammation of the mouth, mental retardation, neurologic disorders with lenticular involvement, mercurialism, pregnancy, ill-fitting dental appliances, dysautonomia, periodic diseases, cystic fibrosis of the pancreas, teething, alcoholism, and malnutrition.

sialorrhea, periodic, *n* recurrent episodes of hypersalivation; of unknown cause but probably related to recurrent parotitis and other so-called periodic diseases.

sib, *n* abbreviation for *sibling*, meaning brother or sister.

sibilant (sib'ilənt), *adj* accompanied by a hissing sound; especially a type of fricative speech sound. The phonemes /s/ and /z/ are sibilants.

sibling, *n* one of two or more children who have both parents in common.

sibutramine (sībyōō'trəmēn), *n* an FDA-approved prescription drug for weight loss containing a combination of serotonin and andronergics that has been shown to promote a feeling of fullness while apparently not influencing hunger; Meridia(r) is an example.

sickle (sik'əl), *n* See scaler, sickle.

sickle cell anemia, *n* a severe, chronic, incurable, hemoglobinopathic, anemic condition that occurs in people homozygous for hemoglobin S (Hb S).

sickle cell crisis, *n* an acute, episodic condition that occurs in children with sickle cell anemia. The crisis may be vaso-occlusive, resulting from the aggregation of misshapen erythrocytes, or anemic, resulting from bone marrow aplasia.

sickle cell trait, *n* the gene that carries sickle cell anemia. Only the presence of two genes in a person's genetic code leads to the manifestation of sickle cell anemia. See also sickle cell anemia.

sicklemia (siklē'mē ə), *n* See sickle cell anemia.

side effect, *n* an effect not sought in the case under treatment.

side-shift, *n* an imprecise term for lateral thrust of the rotating condyle.

sidestream smoke, *n* the vaporous byproduct of burning tobacco that enters the air from the smoldering part of a tobacco product, such as the lit tip of a cigarette or cigar.

SIDS, *n* abbreviation for sudden infant death syndrome.

sievert (Sv) (sē'vurt), *n* unit used for measuring the combined effects of various types of radiation, its quality and distribution, plus other relative factors.

sigh (sī), *n* an audible and prolonged inspiration followed by a shortened expiration.

sight, *n* the special sense that enables the shape, size, position, and color of

S

objects to be perceived; the sense or faculty of vision.

sigmoid (sig′moid), *adj* of or pertaining to an S shape, as in the shape of the pelvic end of the colon prior to its joining the rectum.

sigmoid notch, *n* See notch, mandibular.

sign (sīn), *n* an indication of the existence of something; any objective evidence of a disease.

sign, Battle's, *n.pr* the ecchymosis that appears near the mastoid process of the temporal bone; indicative of a fracture of the base of the skull.

sign, Bell's, *n.pr* the turning up of the eyeball on the affected side when a patient with Bell's palsy attempts to close the eyelid.

sign, Nikolsky's, *n.pr* a diagnostic feature wherein apparently normal epithelium may be rubbed off with finger pressure.

sign, Tinel's, *n.pr* a paresthesia in the area served by a sensory nerve when the site of a lesion or injury to the nerve is percussed. Indicative of partial injury of a nerve or regeneration of an injured nerve.

signa (sig′nə), *n* (signature), the portion of a prescription that contains a statement of the directions for use.

signature, *n* See signa.

signs and symptoms, diagnostic, *n.pl* the objective and subjective features of disease that are carefully evaluated to establish a diagnosis.

silex (sī′leks) (silicon dioxide), *n* a substance used in dental surface polishing due to its abrasive characteristics.

silica (sil′ikə) (quartz), *n* the purest of three major ingredients that make up dental porcelain. It imparts stiffness and hardness to the product and is the framework around which the kaolin and feldspar contract.

silicate cement (sil′ikāt), *n* See cement, silicate.

silicon (Si), *n* a nonmetallic element, second to oxygen as the most abundant of the elements. Its atomic number is 14, and its atomic weight is 28. It occurs in nature as silicon dioxide and in silicates. The silicates are used as detergents, corrosion inhibitors, adhesives, and sealants. Elemental silicon is used in metallurgy

and in transistors and other electronic components. Protracted inhalation of silica dusts may cause silicosis, which increases susceptibility to other pulmonary diseases.

silicone (sil′ikōn), *n* a compound of organic structural character in which all or some of the positions that could be occupied by carbon atoms are occupied by silicon. A plastic containing silicons.

silicophosphate cement, *n* See cement, silicophosphate.

silicosis, *n* a lung disorder caused by continued, long-term inhalation of the dust of an inorganic compound silicon dioxide, which is found in sands, quartzes, flints, and many other stones.

silk suture, *n* a braided, fine black suture material, usually used to close incisions, wounds, and cuts in the skin. It is not absorbed by the body and is removed after approximately 7 days.

silver (Ag), *n* a whitish precious metal occurring mainly as a sulfide. Its atomic number is 47, and its atomic weight is 107.88. It is quite soft and is usually alloyed with small amounts of copper to increase its durability. It is used extensively in photography, radiography, and dentistry.

silver amalgam, *n* See amalgam, silver.

silver cones, *n* an endodontic filling material used in conjunction with gutta-percha points and sealing agents to effect a seal of the pulp chamber and canal. Also known as *master cones.*

silver halide crystals, *n* See crystal, silver halide.

silver nitrate, ammoniacal **(am′ōnī′əkəl),** *n* (ammoniated silver nitrate, Howe's silver nitrate), an ammonium compound of silver nitrate, introduced by Percy R. Howe in 1917, that is more readily reduced to silver and silver proteinates than is the usual silver nitrate; formerly used to disclose carious tooth structure and immunize incipient carious lesions of the enamel. It is highly irritating to the pulp.

silver nitrate, Howe's, *n.pr* See silver nitrate, ammoniacal.

silver points, *n* See silver cones.

simian crease, *n* a single crease across the palm produced from the fusion of proximal and distal palmar creases, seen in such congenital disorders as Down syndrome.

Simmonds's disease, *n.pr* See disease, Simmonds's.

Simon's classification of malocclusion, *n* a classification of malocclusion in which tooth malpositions are related to three craniofacial planes: midsagittal, orbital, and Frankfort. Teeth too close to the midsagittal plane are in *contraction,* whereas those too far away are in *distraction.* Teeth too anterior to the orbital plane are in *protraction,* whereas those too posterior to the orbital plane are in *retraction.* Teeth too close to the Frankfort plane are in *attraction,* whereas those too distant are in *distraction.*

simple fracture, *n* an uncomplicated closed fracture in which the fractured ends of the bone do not break the skin.

simple reflex, *n* a reflex with a motor nerve component that involves only one muscle and level of the afferent and efferent nerve synapse.

simulation, *n* a mode of computer-assisted instruction in which a student receives basic information about a topic and then must interact with the computer to gain deeper understanding of the information and topic. Simulation provides the student with the opportunity to gain experience at limited cost and with reduced risk.

simvastatin, *n trade name:* Zocor, *drug class:* cholesterol-lowering agent; *action:* inhibits 3-hydroxy-3-methylglutaryl coenzyme A (HMG-CoA) reductase enzyme, which reduces cholesterol synthesis; *use:* as an adjunct in primary hypercholesterolemia types IIa and IIb.

sine curve, *n* the wave form of an alternating current characterized by a rise from zero to maximal positive potential, a descent back through zero to its maximal negative value, and then a rise back to zero.

single emulsion, *n* (film), See emulsion, single.

single-blind study, *n* an experiment in which the person collecting the data knows whether the subjects are in the control or experimental groups but the subjects do not.

single-crystal sapphire, *n* a single-crystal endosteal implant made of alpha alumina oxide with a Knoop hardness number of 1.750. The implants are threaded and supplied in three sizes: 3, 4, and 5.

sinoatrial (SA) node, *n* a cluster of hundreds of cells located in the right atrial wall of the heart near the opening of the superior vena cava. It constitutes a knot of modified heart muscle that generates impulses, which travel swiftly throughout the muscle fibers of both atria, causing them to contract.

sinus (sī′nus), *n* a cavity, recess, or hollow space.

sinus, alveolar, n a passage connecting a pathologic cavity in the alveolus with the oral or nasal cavity and penetrating the mucous membrane. See also fistula, alveolar.

sinus balloon, n See balloon, sinus.

sinus, carotid, n the dilated portion of the internal carotid artery.

sinus, coronary, n the venous sinus in the groove between the left cardiac auricle and the left ventricle.

sinus, maxillary (antrum of Highmore, maxillary antrum), n a large pyramidal cavity within the body of the maxilla. Its walls are thin and correspond to the orbital, nasal anterior, and infratemporal surfaces of the body of the maxilla. On dental radiographs the floor of the sinus is often observed approximating the root apices of the teeth and is seen to extend from the canine or premolar region posteriorly to the molar or tuberosity region.

sinus, paranasal, n accessory sinuses of the nose.

sinus tract, n See tract, sinus.

sinusitis, *n* inflammation of the sinus.

site visit, *n* a visit to an institution by designated officials to evaluate or gather information about a program, department, or institution. A site visit is a step in the accreditation of an institution and in the funding of many major research and training projects.

sitz bath, *n* a bath in which only the hips and buttocks are immersed in water or saline solution. The proce-

S

dure is used for patients who have had rectal or perineal surgery.

Sjögren's syndrome (shœ′grenz), *n.pr* See syndrome, Sjögren's.

skeletal discrepancies, *n* an orthodontic term used to describe the nature of a malocclusion as being a malrelationship of the bony base rather than merely of the teeth.

skeletal relationships, *n.pl* the orientations of bony parts to one another; usually the lower to upper jaw or to the bases with which they articulate.

skeletal system, *n* all bones and cartilage of the body that collectively provide the supporting framework for the muscles and organs.

skeleton, axial, *n* the bones that constitute the head and neck, including those that enclose the brain, face, and the neck bones. Some researchers include the entire mid-line vertebral column.

skill, *n* practical knowledge of an art, science, profession, or trade and the ability to apply it properly in practice.

skill, reasonable, *n* skill that is ordinarily possessed and exercised by persons of similar qualifications engaged in the same employment or profession.

skin, *n* the tough, supple cutaneous membrane that covers the entire surface of the body. It is the largest organ of the body and is composed of five layers of cells. See also stratum, stratum basale, stratum corneum, stratum granulosum, stratum lucidum, stratum spinosum.

slander, *n* oral defamation; the saying of false and malicious words about another, resulting in injury to his or her reputation.

slant of occlusal plane, *n* the inclination measured by the angle the occlusal plane makes when extended to intersect with the axis-orbital plane.

sleep, *n* a period of rest for the body and mind, during which volition and consciousness are in partial or complete abeyance and the bodily functions partially suspended.

sleep apnea, *n* a sleep disorder characterized by periods of an absence of attempts to breathe. The person is momentarily unable to move respira-

tory muscles or maintain airflow through the nose and mouth.

sleep, twilight, *n* (seminarcosis), a state of amnesia and analgesia produced by an injection of scopolamine and morphine.

slice, *n* in cavity preparation a straight-line (plane) cut that removes a thin layer from an axial convexity.

slim disease, *n* a constitutional disease of acquired immunodeficiency syndrome (AIDS); also called *human immunodeficiency virus (HIV) wasting syndrome.* It is characterized by fever for more than 1 month, involuntary weight loss of greater than 10%, and diarrhea persisting for more than 1 month.

slope, lower ridge, *n* the slope of the mandibular residual ridge in the second and third molar region as seen from the buccal side.

slotted attachment, *n* See attachment, intracoronal.

slough (sluf), *n* **I.** dead tissue that has been shed or discarded. *v* **2.** to remove dead tissue.

Slough. (Regezi/Sciubba/Jordan, 2003)

Sluder's neuralgia, *n.pr* See neuralgia, Sluder's.

slurry, *n* a thin mixture of insoluble material floating in liquid.

smallpox, *n* See variola.

smear, bacterial, *n* the act of taking bacteria taken from a lesion or area, spreading them on a slide, and staining them for microscopic examination.

smear layer, *n* a thin layer with minute crystalline characteristics. It appears on the surface of teeth that have undergone dental instrumentation procedures, including root planing and cutting done with a dental bur. Not easily rinsed away, it must be removed by acid etching.

Smear plug

Smear layer

2 μm

Dentinal tubule

Smear layer. (Hatrick/Eakle/Bird, 2003)

smell, *n* the special sense that enables odors to be perceived through the stimulation of the olfactory nerves.

smokeless tobacco (spit), *n* chewing tobacco or tobacco powder (snuff) that allows the nicotine to be absorbed through the mucous membrane of the mouth or digestive tract. It is related to a high risk of oral cancer.

smooth surface caries, *n* a lesion that forms on the surface of a tooth without pits, fissures, or enamel faults; usually below a contact area between two teeth.

sneeze, *n* an involuntary, sudden, violent expulsion of air through the mouth and nose; may be elicited during thiopental (Pentothal) anesthesia by corneal stimulation.

snuff, *n* See smokeless tobacco.

snuff dipper's lesion, *n* a white or discolored lesion of the oral mucosa occurring at the site at which the powdered tobacco is retained. Malignant transformations are not common but do occur, usually as low-grade verrucous carcinomas.

Snyder's test, *n.pr* See test, colorimetric caries susceptibility.

soap, *n* a salt or mixture of salts, of aliphatic acids, such as palmitic, stearic, or oleic acid, with sodium or potassium used for cleaning purposes.

soap, antimicrobial (an'tĭmĭkrō'bē-əl), *n* hand cleanser infused with ingredients against microorganisms found on the skin.

sob, *n* a short, convulsive inspiration, attended by contraction of the diaphragm and spasmodic closure of the glottis.

social functioning, *n* ability of the individual to interact in the normal or usual way in society; can be used as a measure of quality of care.

socialized medicine, *n* a system for the delivery of health care in which the expense of care is borne by a governmental agency supported by taxation rather than being paid directly by the client on a fee-for-service or contract basis.

socioeconomic status, *n* the position of an individual on a socioeconomic scale that measures such factors as education, income, type of occupation, place of residence, and in some populations, ethnicity and religion.

sociology, *n* the study of group behavior within a society.

socket, *n* **1.** the hollow part of a joint; the excavation in one bone of a joint that receives the articular end of another bone. **2.** any hollow or concavity into which another part fits, as the eyes.

socket, dry, *n* (alveolalgia, infected socket localized alveolar osteitis), an osteitis or periostitis associated with infection and disintegration of the clot after tooth extraction. Because of its painful nature, it also is called *alveolalgia.*

socket, infected, *n* See socket, dry.

socket, tooth, *n* alveolus; the cavity

S

in the alveolar process of the jaw in which the root of a tooth is fixed.

soda, *n* a compound of sodium, particularly sodium bicarbonate, sodium carbonate, or sodium hydroxide.

sodium (Na) (sō′dē əm), *n* a soft, grayish metal of the alkaline metals group. Its atomic number is 11, and its atomic weight is 22.9898. Sodium is one of the most important elements in the body. Sodium ions are involved in acid-base balance, water balance, the transmission of nerve impulses, and the contraction of muscle. The recommended daily intake of sodium is 250 to 750 mg for infants, 900 to 2,700 mg for children, and 1,100 to 3,300 mg for adults.

sodium aluminum fluoride **(flôr′ĭd, floor′ĭd),** *n* See cryolite.

sodium bicarbonate, *n* an antacid, electrolyte, and urinary alkalinizing agent.

sodium chloride, *n* common table salt.

sodium fluoride (NaF), *n* a white, odorless powder used in 2% aqueous solution and applied topically to teeth as a caries-preventing agent; used as 33% NaF in kaolin and glycerin as a desensitizing agent for hypersensitive dentin. In drinking water, one part per million of NaF is used as a caries-prophylactic substance.

sodium fluoride poisoning, *n* a chronic condition of fluorine poisoning that occurs in some communities where the fluorine concentration in the water supply exceeds one part per million. Signs of the condition include mottling of the tooth enamel and severe osteosclerosis.

sodium hypochlorite (NaOCl), *n* a popular chemical disinfectant made of a chlorine compound and usually combined with distilled water for enhanced stability. NaOCl is often used to clean dentures if they have no metal parts and to disinfect and decontaminate water lines. It is corrosive and toxic when applied directly to the skin. The chemical name for household bleach.

sodium iodide, *n* an iodine supplement to the diet, usually an additive to common table salt.

sodium monofluorophosphate, *n* a form of fluoride added to oral hygiene products at a strength of 1,500 ppm, which is considered extra-strength.

sodium perborate **(purbôr′āt),** *n* an oxygen-liberating antiseptic that has

been used in the treatment of necrotizing ulcerative gingivitis and other forms of gingival inflammation. Prolonged or indiscriminate use has produced burns of the oral mucosa and hyperplasia of the filiform papillae of the tongue (black hairy tongue). Also used to bleach pulpless teeth.

sodium pump, *n* a mechanism for transporting sodium ions across cell membranes against an opposing concentration gradient.

sodium thiosulfate **(thī′ ōsul′fāt),** *n* a powdered chemical, commonly called *hypo,* that is an ingredient of the fixing solution used in film processing. It clears the film of undeveloped silver halide crystals.

soft diet, *n* a diet that is soft in texture, low in fiber residue, easily digested, and well tolerated. It is commonly recommended for people who have gastrointestinal (GI) disturbances.

soft palate, *n* the structure composed of mucous membranes, muscular fibers, and mucous glands, suspended from the posterior border of the hard palate forming the roof of the mouth. When the soft palate rises, as in swallowing, it separates the nasal cavity and nasopharynx from the posterior part of the oral cavity and oral portion of the pharynx. In sucking the soft palate and posterior superior surface of the tongue occlude the oral cavity from the orapharynx, creating a posterior seal. Thus the soft palate prevents the escape of fluid and food up through the nose and with the tongue allows fluid and food to collect in the mouth until swallowed.

soft radiation, *n* See radiation, soft.

soft tissue, *n* all body tissue except bone, teeth, nails, hair, and cartilage.

soft tissue undercut, *n* See undercut, soft tissue.

soft water, *n* water that does not contain salts of calcium or magnesium, which precipitate soap solutions.

software, *n* various programming aids supplied by manufacturers to facilitate the user's efficient operation of computer equipment. The collection of programs, routines, and documents associated with a computer (for example, compilers, library routines).

solar radiation, *n* the emission and diffusion of actinic rays from the sun. Overexposure may result in sunburn, keratosis, skin cancer, or lesions associated with photosensitivity.

S

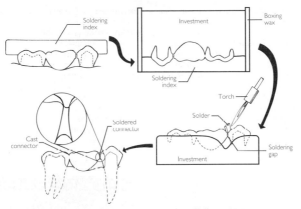

The soldering process. (Rosenstiel/Land/Fujimoto, 2001)

solder (sod´ur), *n* a fusible alloy of metals used to unite the edges or surfaces of two pieces of metal.

soldering flux, *n* See flux, soldering.

soldering investment, *n* See investment, soldering and investment, refractory

solubility (sol´yo͞obil´itē), *n* the quality or fact of being soluble; susceptible to being dissolved.

solute (sol´yo͞ot), *n* the dissolved (usually the less abundant) constituent of a solution.

solution (səlo͞o´shən), *n* the process of dissolving. In chemistry a homogeneous dispersion of two or more compounds. In pharmacy, usually a nonalcoholic solution. Solutions containing alcohol are variously called *elixirs, tinctures, spirits, essences,* or *hydroalcoholic solutions.*

solution, Carnoy's, *n.pr* a sclerosing solution; mild; does not cauterize normal oral mucosa if used judiciously. A mild hemostatic.

solution, cleansing, *n* a solution especially suited to the removal of adherent food particles by immersion of the denture to avoid damaging the denture by brushing.

solution, disclosing, *n* a topically applied dye used in aqueous solution to stain and reveal the extent of calcareous and mucinous deposition on the teeth.

solution, hardening, *n* an aqueous solution (often of 2% potassium sulfate) in which a hydrocolloid impression may be immersed to reduce or retard syneresis of the impression material.

solution, hypertonic, *n* a mixture containing a concentration of solute in excess of the concentration of the same solute in another mixture to which it is compared. When the two solutions are placed on opposite sides of a permeable membrane (either artificial or natural, as with cell membranes), the hypertonic solution attracts the solvent from the hypotonic solution, equalizing the concentration of the solute in both. See also solution, hypotonic; solution, isotonic and osmosis.

solution, hypotonic, *n* a mixture containing a concentration of solute that is lower than the concentration of the same solute in another mixture to which it is compared. When two such solutions are separated by a permeable membrane, the solvent of the hypotonic solution flows through the membrane to the hypertonic solution, equalizing the concentration of the solute in both. See also solution, hypertonic; solution, isotonic and osmosis.

solution, isotonic, *n* a mixture containing the same concentration of solute as another mixture to which it is compared. When separated by a permeable membrane, osmosis does not occur. See also solution, hypertonic; solution, hypotonic and osmosis.

S

solution, parenteral, n a sterile solution or substance prepared for injection.

solution, physiologic saline, n a salt solution containing 0.9% sodium chloride in distilled water that exhibits the same molecular concentration as blood.

solution, pickling, n a solution of acid used for removing oxides and other impurities from dental castings (for example, solutions of hydrochloric or sulfuric acid).

solution, sclerosing, n an agent that causes intense inflammation, resulting in fibrosis; used to treat subluxation of the temporomandibular joint, cauterize ulcers, arrest hemorrhage, and treat hemangiomas.

solution, Skinner's, n.pr an iodine preparation used as a disclosing agent, containing iodine crystals, potassium iodide, zinc iodide, water and glycerine. It is seldom used because of its bad taste.

solution, solid, n an alloy all of whose constituents are mutually soluble in the solid state.

solvent, n a substance capable of or used in dissolving or dispersing one or more other substances; a liquid component of a solution present in greater amount than the solute.

soma (sō′mə), n See somatic.

somatic (sōmat′ik), n derived from *soma,* meaning the body, as distinguished from the mind. Pertains to the framework of the body as distinguished from the viscera; hence the term *somatic nerves* describes the nerves associated with the musculoskeletal function of the muscles of the body.

somatotropin (sō′matōtrō′pin), n See hormone, growth.

somites (so-mīts), n.pl paired masses of mesoderm that form along the neural tube of the embryo to create the vertebral column.

somnambulism (somnam′byōōlizəm), n habitual walking in the sleep; a hypnotic state in which the subject has full possession of senses but no subsequent recollection.

somnifacient (som′nifā′shənt), adj **1.** causing sleep; hypnotic. n **2.** a medicine that induces sleep.

somniferous (somnif′ərus), adj inducing or causing sleep.

somnolence (som′nəlens), n sleepiness; also unnatural drowsiness.

somnolism (som′nəlizəm), n a state of mesmeric or hypnotic trance.

sonant (son′ant), n a speech sound that has in it a component of tone generated by laryngeal vibrations (for example, "a-a-a," "z-z-z").

sonic devices, n.pl See ultrasonics.

sonogram (son′ōgram), n the readily usable graph of the frequency bands (formants) produced by the sound spectrograph.

Sonogram. (Callen, 2000)

sonograph (son′ōgraf), n a wave analyzer that produces a permanent visual record showing the distribution of energy in both frequency and time.

soporific (sop′ərif′ik), n a sleep-producing drug.

sorbic acid, n a compound occurring naturally in berries of the mountain ash. Commercial sorbic acid is used in fungicides, food preservatives, lubricants, and plasticizers.

sordes (sôr′dēz), n unclean material consisting of food particles, debris, skin, and microorganisms that forms a crust and gathers on the oral mucosa, lips, and teeth of a feverish or dehydrated individual with a chronic incapacitating condition.

sore, canker, n (aphthous ulcer, aphthous stomatitis), colloquial term for a shallow ulcer of the oral mucosa; characterized by a grayish-yellow base and erythematous halo; the result of local minor trauma and possibly immune or microbial factors.

sore, cold, n See sore, canker and herpes labialis.

S

sore, denture, *n* See ulcer, decubitus.

sort, *v* to arrange units of information according to rules dependent on a key or field contained in or with the information.

sort generator program, *n* a generalized program that can produce many different sorting programs in accordance with control information specified by the user.

sotalol HCl, *n trade name:* Betapace; *drug class:* nonselective β-adrenergic blocker; *action:* competitively blocks stimulation of β-adrenergic receptors in the heart and decreases renin activity, all of which may play a role in reducing systolic and diastolic blood pressure; inhibits β$_2$-receptors in the bronchial system; *use:* treatment of life-threatening ventricular dysrhythmias.

source file, *n* a file containing information used as input to a computer program.

source language, *n* a language that is an input to a given translation process.

source program, *n* a program coded in other than machine language that must be translated into machine language before being executed.

source-collimator distance, *n* distance from the focal spot to the diaphragm or collimator in an x-ray tube head.

source-film distance (SFD), *n* distance from the focal spot of an x-ray tube to the radiographic film. Also known as *target-film distance.*

source-object distance (SOD), *n* distance from focal spot to object of which a radiographic image is to be obtained. Also known as *target-object distance.*

Southern blot test, *n.pr* a gene analysis method used to identify specific deoxyribonucleic acid (DNA) fragments and diagnose cancers and hemoglobinopathies.

space, *n* a delimited, three-dimensional region.

space, freeway, *n* the interocclusal distance or separation between the occlusal surfaces of the teeth when the mandible is in its physiologic rest position. *Interocclusal distance* is the preferred term. See also distance, interocclusal; clearance, interocclusal.

space, interalveolar, *n* See distance, interarch.

space, interocclusal rest, *n* See distance, interocclusal.

space, interproximal, *n* the space between adjacent teeth in a dental arch. It is divided into the *embrasure* (occlusal to the contact point) and the *septal space* (gingival to the contact point).

space, interradicular, *n* the area between the roots of a multirooted tooth; it is normally occupied by bony septum and the periodontal membrane.

space, lattice, *n* See lattice space.

space maintainer, *n* a fixed or removable appliance designed to preserve the space created by the premature loss of a tooth.

Space maintainer. (Cameron/Widmer, 2003)

space maintainer cast, *n* a space maintainer fabricated by a casting technique and cemented into place.

space maintainer, fixed, *n* a space maintainer not intended to be removable by the patient.

space maintainer, orthodontic, *n* a removable or fixed appliance fabricated to maintain space in the arch for erupting permanent teeth. The appliance may be designed to regain space needed to accommodate the erupting tooth or teeth.

space maintainer, removable, *n* a space maintainer designed for easy removal for cleaning and adjustment.

space, marrow, *n* spaces in the spongiosa of bone; in the mandible and maxilla the marrow spaces are occupied by fatty and hematogenic (blood-forming) marrow. When inflammation progresses into these

S

spaces, the marrow becomes fibrous. The spaces enlarge in atrophy of disuse because of resorption of surrounding trabeculae, and the marrow remains fatty in nature.

space obtainer, *n* an appliance used to increase the space between two teeth.

space, occupied, *n* the space that might be occupied by persons or radiation-sensitive materials and devices during the time that x-ray equipment is in operation or radiation is being emitted.

space, physiologic dead, *n* the air passages up to but not including the alveoli of the lungs; equal to about 150 cc.

space regainer, *n* a fixed or removable appliance capable of moving a displaced permanent tooth into its proper position in the dental arch.

space relief, *n* fabrication of a prosthesis so that certain predetermined, non-stress-bearing areas will not be contacted by the appliance.

spasm (spaz´əm), *n* a sudden involuntary contraction of a muscle or muscle group. It may cause a twitch or close a canal or passage, depending on its location.

spasm, muscle, *n* increased muscular tension and shortness that cannot be released voluntarily and prevents lengthening of the muscles involved. Caused by pain stimuli to the lower motor neurons.

spasmolysant (spazmol´izənt), *n* relieving or relaxing spasms; any agent that relieves spasm.

spasmolytic (spaz´mōlit´ik), *adj* pertaining to a drug that reduces spasm in smooth or skeletal muscle.

spastic (spas´tik), *adj* characterized by a more or less constant state of hypertonic contraction of a muscle or group of muscles. The condition is regarded as abnormally heightened muscular tonus present even in states of inactivity.

spasticity, *n* a form of muscular hypertonicity with increased resistance to stretch.

spatter, *n* droplets of airborne particulate matter larger than 50 μm that fall to the ground.

spatula, *n* a flat-bladed instrument without sharp edges used for mixing certain dental materials (for example,

cement, plaster of paris, impression pastes).

spatulate (spach´ōōlāt), *v* to manipulate or mix with a spatala.

spatulation (spach´ōōlā´shən), *n* manipulation of material with a spatula to mix it into a homogeneous mass.

spatulator, *n* a mechanical device that mixes ingredients to form a homogeneous mass. Also called a *mechanical spatulator.*

SPCA, *n* acronym for serum prothrombin conversion accelerator. See also factor VIII; thromboplastin, extrinsic.

Spearman's rho, *n.pr* a statistical test for correlation between two rank-ordered scales. It yields a statement of the degree of interdependence of the scores of the two scales.

specialist, *n* a health care professional who is qualified to limit practice to a narrow spectrum of health care. A specialist usually has advanced clinical training and postgraduate education in the discipline or specialty.

specialization, *n* the limiting of professional services to one isolated and distinct phase of dental practice.

specialty, *n* particular field of attention and endeavor to which a therapist's efforts are devoted.

specialty, dental, *n* organized dentistry recognizes nine specialties: endodontics, public health dentistry, oral radiology, oral surgery, oral pathology, orthodontics, pediatric dentistry, periodontics, and prosthodontics.

specific dynamic energy (SDE), *n* the amount of energy an individual body must expend in order to process and use food; equal to approximately 10% of basal metabolism rate and activity energy components. Also called *nonshivering thermogenesis.*

specific gravity, *n* See gravity, specific.

spectrum, antibacterial, *n* the range of antimicrobial activity of a drug.

spectrum, electromagnetic, *n* a family of radiant energies that travel in wave form, have neither mass nor charge, and travel at the speed of light. Radiations within the spectrum vary only in wavelength. X-ray photons and light rays are examples of electromagnetic radiation.

Spee, curve of, *n.pr* See curve of Spee.

speech, *n* **1.** communication through conventional vocal and oral symbols. **2.** a basic biologic function of the maxillofacial structures. The essential characteristic of the speech function is the production and organization of sound into symbols.

speech aid, *n* See aid, speech.

speech, delayed, *n* failure of speech to develop at the expected age, usually resulting from slow maturation, hearing impairment, brain injury, mental retardation, or emotional disturbance.

speech device, *n* a prosthesis that assists in the management of speech disorders associated with congenital or acquired defects of the palate.

speech disorder, cerebrovascular, *n* a diminished capacity to speak due to the location of traumatic brain damage and the involvement of the throat, tongue, and mouth.

speech, infantile, *n* a speech defect characterized by substitution of speech sounds similar to those used by the child who speaks normally in the early stages of speech development.

speech pathology, *n* **1.** the study of abnormalities of speech or organs of speech. **2.** the diagnosis and treatment of abnormalities of speech as practiced by a speech pathologist or speech therapist.

speech phonation, *n* See phonation, speech.

speech reading, *n* See reading, lip.

speech resonance, *n* See resonance, speech.

speech, retarded, *n* slowness in speech development in which intelligibility is severely impaired; often preceded by late or delayed emergence of speech.

speech, slurred, *n* abnormal speech in which words are not enunciated clearly or completely but are run together or partially eliminated. The most common causes are alcohol toxicity and drug abuse. It may be a sign of damage to a motor neuron or cerebellar disease.

speech therapy, *n* the application of treatments and counseling in the prevention or correction of speech and language disorders.

speech, visible, *n* audible speech patterns that have been transformed by electronic apparatus into visual patterns that may be read by people who are deaf.

speed, *n* relative rapidity of action; rate of motion.

speed, film, *n* See film speed.

speed, high, *n* relatively great rapidity of motion. In cavity preparations, rotary instruments are classified according to the number of revolutions per minute (rpm) made by the cutting tool. Designation of each speed range presently varies. In general, conventional speed is 10,000 to 60,000 rpm, high speed is 60,000 to 100,000 rpm, and ultrahigh speed is more than 100,000 rpm.

speed of light, *n* a speed of 186,300 miles/sec.

speed of radiation, *n* See radiation, speed of.

sperm, *n* cells contained in the male's semen that fertilize the female's egg during the process of conception.

Sperm. (Leonard, 2001, Courtesy Fisher Scientific Company)

sphenoid bone (sfē'noid), *n* See bone, sphenoid.

Sphenoid bone. (Liebgott, 2001)

spherocytosis, hereditary (sfir´ōsī-tō´sis), *n* See jaundice, congenital hemolytic.

sphincter, *n* a circular band of muscle fibers that constricts a passage or closes a natural opening in the body.

sphygmomanometer, *n* an instrument for indirect measurement of blood pressure.

spicule (spik´yōōl), *n* a small needle-shaped body.

spillway, *n* a channel or passageway through which food escapes from the occlusal surfaces of the teeth during mastication. The occlusal, developmental, and supplemental grooves, as well as the incisal, occlusal, labial, buccal, and lingual embrasures, become spillways during function.

spillway, axial, *n* a groove that first crosses a cusp ridge or marginal ridge and extends onto an axial (mesial or distal) surface of the tooth.

spillway, interdental, *n* a sluiceway formed by the interproximal contours of adjoining teeth and investing tissues.

spillway, occlusal, *n* a groove that crosses only a cusp ridge or marginal ridge of a tooth; numerous on marginal ridges, thus increasing masticatory function.

spina bifida, *n* a congenital neural tube defect characterized by a developmental anomaly in the posterior vertebral arch. Spina bifida is relatively common, occurring approximately 10 to 20 times per 1,000 births.

Spina bifida. (Zitelli/Davis, 2002)

spinal anesthesia, *n* a state of insensitivity to pain in the lower part of the body produced by injection of an analgesic or anesthetic drug into the subarachnoid space of the spinal cord. See anesthesia.

spinal cord, *n* a long, nearly cylindric structure lodged in the vertebral canal of the spinal column and extending from the foramen magnum at the base of the skull to the upper part of the lumbar region. It is a major component of the central nervous system. The cord conducts sensory and motor impulses to and from the brain and controls many reflexes.

spinal cord injury, *n* traumatic disruption of the spinal cord as a result of vertebral fractures and dislocations, usually associated with car accidents, sports injuries, and other violent impacts. The degree of paralysis is directly related to the level and severity of the injury. Injury below the first thoracic vertebra may produce paraplegia. Injuries above the first thoracic vertebra may cause quadriplegia.

spinal shock, *n* a reaction to a spinal cord injury in which the body's reflexes are lost, resulting in a limp paralysis below the point of injury. May last several hours.

spindle, *n* muscle, a fusiform body lying parallel to and between muscle fibers. It is composed of a conspicuously smaller modified muscle fiber that has its own motor end plate to cause it to contract and its own special sensory end organs (the flower spray ending and the anulospiral ending) that send information to the central nervous system regarding the state of contraction of the main muscle body.

spine, anterior nasal, *n* the small bony projection extending forward from the medial anterosuperior part of each maxilla. The tip of the anterior nasal spines may be seen on lateral radiographic head plates and cephalometric radiographs.

spine, posterior nasal, *n* the small, sharp, bony point projecting backward from the midline of the horizontal part of the palatine bone.

spirapril, *n trade name:* Renormax; *drug class:* angiotensin-converting enzyme (ACE) inhibitor; *action:* selectively suppresses the renin-angiotensin-aldosterone system; inhibits ACE, prevents conversion of angiotensin I to angiotensin II; results in dilation of arterial and venous vessels; *use:* treatment of hypertension.

Spirillum (spīril'um), *n* a genus of aerobic, gram-negative helix-shaped bacteria, found in fresh and salt waters.

spirit of ammonia, *n* a solution of 3% ammonium carbonate in alcohol with flavorings added. It is mixed with water for use as a stimulant and carminative.

spirochete, *n* any bacterium of the genus *Spirochaeta* that is motile and spiral shaped with flexible filaments. Spirochetes include the organisms responsible for leprosy, relapsing fever, syphilis, and yaws.

spirograph (spī'rəgraf), *n* an instrument for registering respiratory movements.

spirography (spirog'rəfē), *n* the graphic measurement of breathing, including breathing movements and breathing capacity.

spirometry, *n* laboratory evaluation of the air capacity of the lungs by means of a spirometer.

spironolactone, *n trade names:* Aldactone, Spirozide; *drug class:* potassium-sparing diuretic; *action:* competes with aldosterone at receptor sites in distal tubule, resulting in excretion of sodium chloride and water and retention of potassium and phosphate; *uses:* treatment for edema, hypertension, diuretic-induced hypokalemia, and cirrhosis of the liver with ascites.

spit tobacco, *n* See smokeless tobacco.

spleen, *n* a soft, highly vascular, roughly ovoid organ situated between the stomach and the diaphragm in the left hypochondriac region of the body. It is considered part of the lymphatic system.

splenomegaly, *n* an abnormal enlargement of the spleen, usually associated with portal hypertension, hemolytic anemia, and malaria.

splint, *n* **1.** a rigid appliance for the fixation of displaced or movable parts. **2.** a support or brace used to fasten or confine. **3.** metal, acrylic resin, or modeling compound fashioned to retain in position teeth that may have been replanted or have fractured roots.

splint, abutment, *n* adjacent tooth restorations that have been rigidly united at their proximal contact areas to form a single abutment with multiple roots.

splint, acrylic resin bite-guard, *n* an appliance, usually fabricated of resin, designed to cover the occlusal and incisal surfaces of the teeth to immobilize and stabilize the teeth and thus prevent them from being subjected to the effects of trauma from occlusal forces.

splint, bridge, *n* See splint, fixed.

splint, buccal, *n* a material such as plaster that can be placed on the buccal surfaces of assembled fixed partial denture units and onto which these components can be assembled and held in accurate relation after hardening.

splint, cap, *n* plastic or metallic fracture appliance designed to cover the crowns of the teeth; usually held in place by cementation.

splint, cast bar, *n* a provisional splint consisting of cast continuous clasps that follow the facial and lingual surfaces of the teeth at the height of contour. It is cemented onto the teeth to be splinted and simultaneously wired closed to bring the clasps into intimate contact with the teeth. May not be cemented in place to serve as a removable cast splint. Also called *Friedman splint.*

splint, continuous clasp, *n* a cast splint used for the provisional immobilization of teeth.

splint, copper band-acrylic, *n* a splint fabricated from copper bands and acrylic resin.

splint, crib, *n* an appliance used for temporary tooth stabilization; constructed of gold, acrylic resin, chrome-cobalt alloys, or combinations thereof. It consists of a continuous crib clasp covering the facial and lingual surfaces of the teeth to be splinted.

splint, cross arch bar, *n* a splint formed by a metal bar that unites one or more teeth of one side of the dental arch to one or more teeth of the opposite side. Used to stabilize weakened teeth against lateral tilting forces. See also connector, cross arch bar splint.

splint, cross arch bar, Bilson fixable-removable, n.pr type of cross arch bar splint.

splint, dental, n implement designed to hold teeth in place. It may be temporary or permanent.

splint, fixed, n a fixed (nonremovable) restorative and replacement prosthesis used as a therapeutic aid in the treatment of periodontal disease. It serves to stabilize and immobilize the teeth and replace missing teeth.

splint, Friedman, n.pr See splint, cast bar.

splint, implant surgical, n See superstructure, temporary.

splint, inlay, n an inlay casting designed to give fixation or support to one or more approximating teeth. This may be accomplished by two inlays soldered together or a single casting made for prepared cavities.

splint, interdental, n an appliance made of plastic or metallic materials that is applied to the labial and lingual aspects of the teeth to provide points for applying mandibular and maxillofacial traction and fixation.

splint, labial, n an appliance of plastic, metal, or combinations of plastic and metal made to conform to the labial aspect of the dental arch. Used in the management of mandibular and maxillofacial injuries.

splint, lingual, n an appliance similar to a labial splint but conforming to the lingual aspect of the dental arch.

splint, provisional, n a splint placed for a relatively short period. It is used to stabilize the teeth either during the healing period after accidental or deliberate tooth avulsion and replantation or in conjunction with periodontal therapy. It also may be used during a period of observation to determine the prognosis of the involved teeth.

splint, Stader, n.pr See appliance, fracture.

splinting, *n* the ligating, tying, or joining of periodontally involved teeth to one another to stabilize and immobilize the teeth, thus preventing them from being adversely affected by occlusal forces. Splinting includes acrylic resin bite guards, orthodontic band splints, wire ligation, provisional splints, and fixed prostheses.

splinting, cross arch, n the stabilizing of weakened teeth against tilting movements caused by laterally directed occlusal stress loads. This is accomplished by the use of a rigid connector that projects to the opposite side of the dental arch where attachment is made to one or more teeth, thus producing effective counterleverage.

splinting of abutments, n the joining of two or more teeth into a rigid unit by means of fixed restorations.

split cast mounting, *n* See mounting, split cast.

split ring, *n* a casting ring made of three parts and designed to take advantage of the maximal expansion of the investment.

spondylitis, *n* inflammation of any of the spinal vertebrae, usually characterized by stiffness and pain.

spongiosa, *n* bone, cancellous.

spoon, *n* an instrument with a round or ovoid working end; designed to be used for scraping or scooping.

spore, *n* 1. a reproductive unit of some genera of fungi and protozoa. 2. a form assumed by some bacteria that is resistant to heat, drying, and chemicals. Diseases caused by spore-forming bacteria include anthrax, botulism, gas gangrene, and tetanus.

spore testing, n a procedure in which test strips or receptacles containing microorganisms are checked for positive color changes or negative growth to verify that a sterilization technique is effective.

sporicide (spôr′əsīd), *n* a substance used to destroy spores.

sporotrichosis (spôr′ōtrikō′sis), *n* a fungal infection of the skin and nails caused by *Sporothrix schenckii.* Gardeners and farmers are most susceptible to the infection, which causes lesions in the tissue of the nails and extremities.

sports medicine, *n* a branch of medicine that specializes in the prevention and treatment of injuries from training and participation in athletic activities. More than one million people are treated for sports injuries each year in the United States.

spot, *n* a small circular area.

spot, café-au-lait, n brown-pigmented areas of the skin occurring particularly in neurofibromatosis.

spot, effective focal, n (prolonged focus), the apparent size and shape of the focal spot when viewed from a position in the useful beam. With the use of a suitably inclined anode face, the area from which the useful beam stems is sharply concentrated, if seen from the perspective of the useful beam. See also line, focus.

spot, focal, n the specific area of the face of the anode or target that is bombarded by the focused electron stream when an x-ray tube is in action. It is usually an insert of tungsten.

spot, Fordyce's, n.pr (Fordyce's disease, ectopic sebaceous glands), the chamois-colored, slightly raised spots on the oral mucosa or lips produced by sebaceous glands in those tissues. The term *Fordyce's disease* is sometimes erroneously applied to these spots, which are present in 70% to 80% of the population.

spot, Koplik's, n.pr oral lesion of measles (rubeola); usually occurs on the buccal mucosa opposite the molar teeth as small white or bluish-white spots surrounded by red zones.

spot, pink, n See resorption, internal.

sprain, n an injury to a joint, with possible rupture of some of the ligaments or tendons but without dislocation or fracture. See also strain.

spray, n a liquid minutely divided, as by a jet of air or steam.

spreader, n See condenser.

spring, n a piece of metal having the physical characteristic that when bent it returns to its original shape.

spring, auxiliary, n (finger spring), a short piece of wire, attached to an orthodontic appliance at one end, that serves as a lever to apply force to a tooth or teeth.

spring, coil, n a spiral winding of fine wire attached to an orthodontic appliance.

spring, finger, n See spring, auxiliary.

sprue (sprōō), n in casting the ingate through which molten metal passes into the heated mold. The waste piece of metal cast in the ingate.

sprue base, n See sprue former and crucible former.

sprue former, n a cone-shaped base made of metal or plastic to which the sprue is attached. Forms a crucible in the investment material. Also called *crucible former.*

sprue pin, n See pin, sprue.

sputum (spyōō′təm), n matter ejected from the mouth; saliva mixed with mucus and other substances from the respiratory tract.

squamous cell carcinoma (skwā′-mus), n See carcinoma, epidermoid.

squeeze-releasing technique, n a procedure for releasing an orthodontic bracket from the adhesive resin. The squeeze-releasing technique uses a small pliers to bend the bracket wings together and cause the edges of the bracket to pull away from the surface of the tooth.

SRS-A, n abbreviation for slow-reacting substance of anaphylaxis.

stabile (sta′bil), adj resistant to move ment; fixed or stationary. See also stable.

stability, n the quality of being physically or emotionally predictable, orderly, not readily moved.

stability barriers, n.pl specific conditions obstructing or interfering with the accessibility of services pertaining to oral health care, for example, limited motion and assistive devices use, involuntary or abrupt movements, involuntary or violent actions potentially causing danger to the lives of the care provider and patient, and the inability of the patient to become comfortable with the space and procedures being performed.

stability, denture, n the characteristic of a removable denture that resists forces that tend to alter the relationship between the denture base and its supporting bony foundation.

stability, dimensional, n the property of a material that retains its size and form.

stability, emotional, n state of an individual that enables him or her to have appropriate feelings about common experiences and act in a rational manner.

stabilization, n **1.** the act or process of stabilizing; the state of being stabilized. **2.** the seating or fixation of a fixed or removable denture so that it does not tilt and is not displaced under pressure. **3.** the control of induced stress loads and development of measures to counteract these forces so effectively that the tilting of the teeth or the movement of a prosthesis is minimized to a point within tissue tolerance limits.

stabilized baseplate, *n* See baseplate, stabilized.

stabilizer, *n* an instrument used in an x-ray unit to render the milliamperage output of the tube constant.

stabilizing, *n* the process of fixing movable parts; making firm and steady. The fixing of clamps, separators, or matrices to teeth by the application of tacky compound to the parts, then chilling the compound. In the case of clamps and separators, this distributes the force of operating over adjacent teeth and the one being operated on.

stabilizing circumferential clasp arm, *n* See clasp, circumferential, arm, stabilizing.

stable, *adj* term applied to a substance that has no tendency to decompose spontaneously. As applied to chemical compounds, it denotes their ability to resist chemical alterations.

stable isotope, *n* See isotope.

stack, *n* a set of metal strips that is inserted into ultrasonic and sonic instruments. A stack converts magnetic fields into vibrations that move the tip of the instrument.

Stader splint (stā′dər), *n.pr* See appliance, fracture.

staff, *n* See personnel.

stage, surgical, *n* a period or distinct phase in the course of anesthesia.

staging, *n* a method for describing the growth and rate of metastasization of a tumor, as well as its prognosis. There are four stages, each evaluated according to size, amount of metastasis, and whether or not the lymph nodes are involved. See also TNM staging system.

stain, *v* 1. to discolor with foreign matter. *n* 2. a discoloration accumulating on the surface of a denture or teeth.

stain, alexidine **(əlek′sidēn),** *n* a brownish discoloration of the teeth and exposed roots that occurs as the result of using mouthrinses containing the antiplaque agent alexidine. Stains are more frequent on tooth surfaces that are difficult to reach during normal brushing.

stain, betel leaf **(bē′təl),** *n* the thick, hard, dark brown or black deposits

left on the teeth after chewing the leaves of the betel palm; commonly seen in adults and children in the Eastern Hemisphere where betel leaves and nuts are used as stimulants; must be removed by scaling.

Betel leaf stain. (Daniel/Harfst, 2002)

stain, black line dental, *n* a fine black or dark brown line composed of gram-positive microorganisms that appears along the gingival margin in adults and children who may be predisposed to this condition. The condition is not related to oral cleanliness or the presence of periodontal disease. Also called *black stain.* See also plaque, pigmented dental.

Black line stain. (Daniel/Harfst, 2002)

stain, Gram's, *n.pr* a staining method for microorganisms that places them into two broad groups: *gram-positive,* which retains crystal violet stain, and *gram-negative,* which decolorizes but counterstains with a red dye.

stain, green dental, *n* a light to very dark green stain appearing primarily on the labial surface of the teeth due to inadequate daily removal cleaning, chromogenic bacterial deposits, or decomposed hemoglobin. It may also represent stained enamel cuticle (Nasmyth's membrane). The condition is more common in children than adults.

stain, metallic dental, n an uncommon, green, brown, yellow, or blue-green dental discoloration. Source is environmental, typically entering the individual's mouth through breathing air containing metals or metal salts.

stain, methyl violet, n a dye used to color bacteria for microscopic examination.

stain, orange dental, n tooth discoloration of the cervical third caused by chromogenic bacteria.

stain, red dental, n tooth discoloration caused by chromogenic bacteria; found at the cervical third.

stain, yellow dental, n a frequently occurring discoloration of the teeth, generally caused by poor oral hygiene.

staining, n modification of the color of the teeth or denture base to achieve a more lifelike appearance.

stainless steel, n See steel, stainless.

stamp cusp, n a cusp made to work in a fossa. The maxillary lingual cusps are stamp cusps. In tooth-to-tooth occlusion all lower buccal cusps may stamp into fossae. In tooth-to-two-tooth occlusion the stamp cusps of the lower premolars may have their tips in embrasures and have only their shoulders in tiny fossae. See also cusp-fossa relations.

standard, n that which is established by authority, custom, or general acceptance as a model; criterion.

standard deviation (SD), n a computed measure of the dispersion or variability of a distribution of scores around a given point or line. It measures the way an individual score deviates from the most representative score (mean). A small SD indicates little individual deviation or a homogeneous group, and a large SD indicates much individual deviation or a heterogeneous group.

standard error, n a measure or estimate of the sampling errors affecting a statistic; a measure of the amount the statistic may be expected to differ by chance from the true value of the statistic.

standard error of estimate, n the standard deviation of the differences between the actual values of the dependent variables (results) and the predicted values. This statistic is associated with regression analysis.

standard error of the mean, n an estimate of the amount that an obtained mean may be expected to differ by chance from the true mean.

standard of care, n a written statement describing the rules, actions, and conditions that direct patient care. Standards of care guide practice and may be used to evaluate performance.

standard operating procedure (SOP), n a method of functioning that has been established over time in order to execute a specific task or react to a specific set of circumstances.

standard orders, n.pl rules, policies, procedures, regulations, and orders for the conduct of patient care in various stipulated clinical situations.

standard score, n any derived score indicating the degree of deviation of an individual score from the mean using the standard deviation as the unit of measure.

stanine, n a unit consisting of one-ninth of the total range of the standard scores (SDs) of a normal distribution. The term is a condensation of "standard nine." The mean falls at 5, the SD at ±2. The stanine was developed by the U.S. Air Force and is used to report scores on the Dental Aptitude Test.

stannic oxide, n See tin oxide.

stannous fluoride (stan′us flôr′īd), n a fluoride salt of tin used in toothpaste and mouthrinses to reduce dental caries incidence and gingivitis and as an antiplaque agent.

stanozolol, n *trade name:* Winstrol; *drug class:* androgenic anabolic steroid, controlled substance Schedule III; *action:* reverses catabolic tissue processes, promotes buildup of protein, increases erythropoietin production; *use:* hereditary angioedema prophylaxis.

Staphcillin, n.pr See methicillin.

Staphylococcus albus **(staf′əlōkok′us al′bus) (Staphylococcus pyogenes var. albus),** n a species of spherical, gram-positive bacteria growing in grapelike clusters; of low pathogenicity, although occasional strains may be coagulase positive and produce hemolysis. Normally present as part of the oral flora and in mucosa-lined cavities such as the mouth and nasal cavity. May be isolated, along with *S. aureus,* streptococci, pneumococci, fusiform bacilli, *Borrelia vincentii,* molds, and yeasts from the gingival crevices by cultural examination.

Staphylococcus aureus (ôr′ē us) (Staphylococcus pyogenes var. aureus), *n* a pathogenic variety of staphylococci capable of producing suppurative lesions; cultured colonies are golden yellow. Produces hemolysis on blood agar, is coagulase positive, and may be resistant to commonly used antibiotics. Has been isolated with other microorganisms such as *S. albus* from the gingival crevice.

Staphylococcus epidermidis, *n* a bacterium normally present on the skin and in the mouth that causes oral infection when allowed to grow unchecked. Symptoms include inflammation of the lower jaw and parotid glands.

Staphylococcus pyogenes var. albus, *n* See *Staphylococcus albus.*

Staphylococcus pyogenes var. aureus, *n* See *Staphylococcus aureus.*

starch, *n* the principal molecule used for the storage of food in plants. Starch is a polysaccharide and is composed of long chains of glucose subunits.

starch amylopectin **(am′ilōpek′tin),** *n* a component of starch that consists of glucose residues arranged in a branched chain.

starch amylose **(am′ilōs),** *n* a component of starch that consists of glucose residues arranged in a straight chain.

starvation, *n* a condition resulting from the lack of essential nutrients over a long period and characterized by multiple physiologic and metabolic dysfunctions.

statement, *n* **1.** a printed form stating the balance of the account due the dentist. **2.** in computer programming a meaningful expression or generalized instruction in a source language.

static electricity, *n* See film fault, static electricity.

stationary grid, *n* See grid, stationary.

stationary lingual arch, *n* an orthodontic arch wire designed to fit the lingual surface of the teeth and soldered to the associated anchor bands, which are then cemented to the molar teeth.

statistic, *n* any value or number that describes a series of quantitative observations or measures; a value calculated from a sample.

statistical significance, *n* a difference of such magnitude between two statistics, computed from separate samples, that the probability of the value obtained will not occur by chance alone with significant frequency and hence can be attributed to something other than chance. In modern investigation the generally accepted value for significance must have a probability of occurrence by chance factors equal to or less than five times in 100 ($p < 0.05$). Other significance levels commonly used are as follows: less than one chance in 100 ($p > 0.01$), less than five chances in 1,000 ($p < 0.005$), and less than one chance in 1,000 ($p < 0.001$).

statistically based utilization review, *n* a system that examines the distribution of treatment procedures based on claims information and, to be reasonably reliable, the application of such claims. Analyses of specific dentists should include data on type of practice, dentist's experience, socioeconomic characteristics, and geographic location.

statistics, *n* the branch of mathematics that gathers, arranges, condenses, coordinates, and mathematically manipulates obtained facts so that the numerical relationships between those facts may be seen clearly and freed from anomalies resulting from chance factors.

statistics, descriptive, n.pl statistics used to describe only the observed group or sample from which they were derived; summary statistics such as percent, averages, and measures of variability that are computed on a particular group of individuals.

statistics, inference, n.pl inferences made regarding characteristics or general principles about an unseen population based on the characteristics of the observed sample. Statistical findings from a sample are generalized to pertain to the entire population. The process of drawing inferences, making predictions, and testing significance are examples of inferential statistics.

statistics, nonparametric, *n.pl* statistical methods used when the statistician cannot assume that the variable being studied is normally distributed in a population. Also called *distribution-free statistics.*

status (stat'us), *n* state or condition.

status asthmaticus **(stā'tus azma-t'ikus),** *n* a continual worsening of an asthmatic condition even with the use of medications for therapeutic purposes; may cause life-threatening situations; creates tremendous strain on the respiratory and circulatory systems.

status epilepticus **(stā'tus ep'ilep'tikus),** *n* a seizure lasting more than 30 minutes, or a series of seizures without pause between them. Patient often does not respond to medication.

status lymphaticus, *n* enlargement of lymphoid tissue, particularly the thymus, in children. It may lead to sudden death under inhalation anesthesia.

status thymicolymphaticus, *n* a constitutional disturbance of controversial existence believed to be responsible in some way for sudden and unexplained deaths from trivial causes such as the extraction of teeth. Enlargement of the thymus and lymphoid tissue and underdevelopment of the adrenal glands, gonads, and cardiovascular system are evident.

statute, *n* a law enacted and established by a legislative department of government.

statute of frauds, *n* a requirement that, for legal validity, contracts for conveying real property or contracts for the performance of personal services requiring a year or more to perform must be in writing.

statute of limitations, *n* a statute that sets a time limit within which legal action on certain causes of action must be brought.

statute, wrongful death, *n* a statute that provides for the recovery of damages by a party other than the party who received the fatal injuries.

statutory (in law) rape, *n* sexual intercourse with a female below the age of consent, which varies from state to state.

stavudine, *n trade name:* Zerit; *drug class:* antiviral; *action:* inhibits replication of human immunodeficiency virus (HIV); *uses:* treatment of adults with advanced HIV infection who are intolerant of other therapies or who have significant deterioration while receiving other therapies.

steady state, *n* a basic physiologic concept implying that the various forces and processes of life are in a state of homeostasis.

steam sterilization, *n* the destruction of all forms of microbial life on an object by exposing the object to moist heat (under pressure) for 15 minutes at 121° C.

steel crown, *n* See crown, stainless steel.

steel, stainless, *n* a steel that contains a minimum of 12% chromium and approximately 0.5% carbon to resist corrosion.

stellate reticulum, *n* one of the two layers between the outer and inner enamel epithelium of the enamel organ, which consists of star-shaped cells.

Stellite (stel'īt), *n.pr* **1.** any of various cobalt-chromium alloys. **2.** a very hard, noncorrosive alloy of cobalt, chromium, and sometimes tungsten used for special instruments, particularly surgical instruments.

stem, brain, *n* See brainstem.

stenosis (stenō'sis), *n* narrowing or stricture of a duct, canal, or vessel.

Stensen's duct, *n.pr* See duct, Stensen's.

stent, *n* **1.** a device used to hold a skin graft placed to maintain a body orifice, cavity, or space. An acrylic resin appliance used as a positioning guide or support. **2.** an appliance that maintains tissue (for example, to maintain a skin transplant in a predetermined position).

step, distal, *n* condition in which the mandibular second molar is in a distal position compared to the maxillary second molar, usually in reference to primary or mixed dentition. See also step, mesial.

step, mesial, *n* condition in which the mandibular second molar is in a mesial position compared to the maxillary second molar, usually in reference to primary or mixed dentition. See also step, distal.

step-up transformer, *n* See transformer, step-up.

stepwedge, *n* an aluminum device that, when exposed to x-rays, displays a range of exposure intensities on a radiograph. These "steps" are analyzed to determine the speed characteristics of the radiographic film. See also penetrometer.

stereognosis, *n* the ability to perceive and understand the form and nature of objects by the sense of touch.

stereoisomer, *n* See isomer.

stereoscope, *n* an optical instrument for viewing photographs or radiographs; it produces binocular vision, or a blending of images, so that new perspectives may be seen with an appearance of depth. It operates on the same principle as the eyes—that is, two views are registered on the retinas of the eyes, and the brain merges them into one.

stereoscopic microscope, *n* a microscope that produces three-dimensional images through the use of double eyepieces and double objectives, creating two independent light paths.

stereotype, *n* a generalization about a form of behavior, an individual, or a group.

sterile, *adj* free from viable microorganisms.

sterile field, *n* **1.** a specified area (such as within a tray or on a sterile towel) that is considered free of microorganisms. **2.** an area immediately around a patient that has been prepared for a surgical procedure.

sterilization, *n* the act or process of rendering sterile; the process of freeing from germ life.

sterilization, chemical, *n* a method of sterilization in which an object is immersed in a liquid containing sanitizing chemicals. Used for objects that cannot withstand high temperatures. Glutaraldehyde is one such sterilizer, which must be in contact with the instrument for at least 10 hours for proper sterilization. Other chemical sterilizers may require up to 24 hours of instrument contact.

sterilizer for root canal instruments, *n* a special device for heat sterilization of root canal instruments and dressings; depends on molten metal, glass beads, salt, or fine sand for the conduction of the heat.

sternocleidomastoid, *n* a muscle of the neck that is attached to the mastoid process and superior nuchal line and by separate heads to the sternum and clavicle. It functions with other muscles to turn the head from side to side and tilt the head to one side or the other.

sternum, *n* the elongated, flattened bone forming the middle portion of the thorax. It supports the clavicles and articulates directly with the first seven pairs of ribs.

steroid (ster′oid), *n* a group name for compounds that resemble cholesterol chemically and also contain a hydrogenated cyclopentanoperhydrophenanthrene ring system. Included are cholesterol, ergosterol, bile acids, vitamin D, sex hormones, adrenocortical hormones, and cardiac glycosides.

steroid, 11-oxy, *n* the C-21 corticosteroids, all of which are oxygenated at carbon 11.

steroid, 17 α-hydroxycortico- (17-OHCS), *n* term used for cortisol and other 21-carbon steroids possessing a dihydroxyacetone group at carbon 17. Serum and urinary determinations give a direct measurement of adrenocortical activity.

steroid, 17-keto- (17-KS), *n* steroidal compounds with a ketone (carbonyl) group at carbon 17. Derived from cortisol and adrenal and testicular androgen. Urinary neutral 17-ketosteroids represent the catabolic end products of the endocrine glands. Produced by the adrenal cortex and testes. Increased values occur in adrenogenital syndromes, adrenocortical carcinoma, bilateral hyperplasia of the adrenal cortex, and Leydig cell tumors. Normal adult values for a 24-hour urine sample are 10 to 20 mg for men and 5 to 15 mg for women.

steroid, adrenocortical (**adrenal corticosteroid**), *n* **1.** a hormone extracted from the adrenal cortex or a synthetic substance similar in chemical structure and biologic activity to such a hormone. **2.** the biologi-

S

cally active steroid of the adrenal cortex, which include 11-dehydrocorticosterone (compound A), corticosterone (compound B), cortisone (compound E), 17 α-hydroxycorticosterone (compound F, hydroxycortisone, or cortisol), and aldosterone. The effects of the corticosteroids include increased resorption of sodium and chloride by the renal tubules and metabolic effects on protein, carbohydrate, and fat.

steroid, C-19 cortico- **(anabolic protein, N hormone),** *n* adrenocortical hormones similar in action to the male and female sex hormones. They cause nitrogen retention and, in excessive amounts, masculinization in the female.

steroid, C-21 cortico- **(glycogenic steroid, sugar hormone),** *n* 21-carbon adrenocortical hormones that are oxygenated at carbon 11 or at both carbon 11 and 17. They affect protein, carbohydrate, and fat metabolism; for example, they elevate blood sugar, increase glyconeogenesis, decrease hepatic lipogenesis, mobilize depot fat, and increase protein metabolism.

steroid, glycogenic, *n* See steroid, C-21 cortico-.

sterols (ster'ôlz), *n.pl* steroids having one or more hydroxyl groups and no carbonyl or carboxyl groups (for example, cholesterol).

stethoscope, *n* an instrument used to assist the health professional to listen to body sounds: heart, lungs, pulse, and gastrointestinal. It consists of two earpieces connected by means of flexible tubing to a diaphragm, which is placed against the skin of the patient at a location appropriate to pick up the sound.

Stevens-Johnson syndrome, *n.pr* See syndrome, Stevens-Johnson.

stillborn, *n* an infant that is born dead.

Stillman's cleft, *n.pr* See cleft, Stillman's.

stimulant (stim'yo͞olənt), *n* an agent that causes an increase in functional activity, usually of the central nervous system.

stimulant, abused, *n* any of a number of substances—such as amphetamines (e.g., methamphetamine or "ice"), cocaine (e.g., "crack" or "coke"), nicotine products (e.g., cigars, cigarettes, or chewing tobacco), and caffeine products (e.g., tea, soft drinks, and soda)—that are misused to increase the functioning of the central nervous system.

stimulant, psychomotor **(steroid, psychomotor),** *n* a drug that increases psychic activity.

stimulation, *n* **1.** increased functioning of protoplasm induced by an extracellular substance or agent. **2.** the act of energizing or activating.

stimulus (stim'yo͞olus), *n* a chemical, thermal, electrical, or mechanical influence that changes the normal environment of irritable tissue and creates an impulse.

sting, *n* an injury caused by a sharp, painful penetration of the skin, often accompanied by exposure to an irritating chemical or the venom of an insect or other animal.

stippling (stip'ling), *n* **1.** an orange-peel appearance of the attached gingiva, believed to result from the bundles of collagen fibers that enter the connective tissue papillae. **2.** a roughening of the labial and buccal surfaces of denture bases to imitate the stippling of natural gingiva.

Stippling. (Daniel/Harfst, 2002)

stippling, basophilic, *n* See basophilia.

stippling, gingival, *n* See gingiva, stippling.

stipulation, *n* an article in an agreement; an agreement in writing to do a certain thing.

stitch, *n* See suture.

stitch, blanket, *n* See suture, blanket.

stock, *n* a security certificate that represents an equity ownership in a corporation.

stoma (sto' mə), *n* a tiny surface opening or pore. It may occur naturally or be the result of a surgical incision, as in a colostomy, or as the result of an abscess. *Stoma* is the Greek word for "mouth."

stomatitides (stō′mətit′idēz), *n.pl* the oral lesions associated with various forms of stomatitis.

stomatitis (stō′mətī′tis), *n* inflammation of the soft tissues of the mouth occurring as a result of mechanical, chemical, thermal, bacterial, viral, electrical, or radiation injury or reactions to allergens or as secondary manifestations of systemic disease.

stomatitis, acute herpetic, n (acute herpetic gingivostomatitis), the manifestations of clinically apparent primary herpes simplex characterized by regional lymphadenopathy, sore throat, and high temperature, followed by localized itching and burning, with the formation of small vesicles of an erythematous base that give way to plaques and then painful herpetic ulcers. The gingivae are swollen and erythematous, and they bleed easily. Manifestations subside in 7 to 10 days, and recovery usually occurs within 2 weeks.

stomatitis, aphthous (aphthae, canker sore), *n* refers to recurrent ulcers of the mouth that appear to be the same clinically as herpetic ulcers and for that reason have been considered to be a manifestation of recurrent herpes simplex, although the herpesvirus has never been conclusively isolated from recurrent aphthae. See also gingivostomatitis, herpetic; stomatitis.

stomatitis, arsenical, n oral manifestation of arsenic poisoning. The oral mucosa is dry, red, and painful. Ulceration, purpura, and mobility of teeth also may occur.

stomatitis, Atabrine, n.pr a stomatitis considered by some to be associated with the use of the antimalarial and anthelmintic drug quinacrine hydrochloride (Atabrine) and characterized by oral changes simulating lichen planus.

stomatitis, bismuth, n a stomatitis resulting from systemic use of bismuth compounds over prolonged periods. Sulfides of bismuth are deposited in the gingival tissue, resulting in bluish-black pigmentation known as a bismuth line. Oral manifestations of

bismuth poisoning include gingivostomatitis similar to that of Vincent's infection, a blue-black line on the inner aspect of the gingival sulcus or pigmentation of the buccal mucosa, a sore tongue, metallic taste, and a burning sensation of the mouth.

stomatitis, epidemic, n See disease, hand, foot, and mouth.

stomatitis, epizootic, n See disease, hand, foot, and mouth.

stomatitis, gangrenous (cancrum oris, noma), *n* destruction of large masses of the oral tissues, particularly the cheek. It usually is found in weakened patients with very low resistance to infection because of lowered white blood cell count or other causes. In advanced stages a large segment of the cheek may be lost, leaving the teeth visible through the defect. See also noma.

stomatitis, gonococcal, n inflammation of the oral mucosa caused by gonococci.

stomatitis, herpetic, n **1.** oral manifestation of primary herpes simplex infection. The term also is used by some for herpetiform ulcers considered to be oral manifestations of secondary or recurrent herpes simplex. See also ulcer, aphthous, recurrent. **2.** inflammation of the oral mucosa caused by herpesvirus. See also gingivostomatitis, herpetic.

stomatitis, iodine, n See iodism.

stomatitis, lead, n oral manifestation of lead poisoning. Included are a bluish line along the free gingival margin, pigmentation of the mucosa in contact with the teeth, metallic taste, excessive salivation, and swelling of the salivary glands.

stomatitis medicamentosa, n an allergic response of the oral mucosa to a systemically administered drug. Possible manifestations include asthma, skin rashes, urticaria, pruritus, leukopenia, lymphadenopathy, thrombocytopenic purpura, and oral lesions (erythema, ulcerative lesions, vesicles, bullae, and angioneurotic edema).

stomatitis, membranous, n inflammation of the oral cavity, accompanied by the formation of a false membrane.

stomatitis, mercurial, n oral manifestation of mercury poisoning, consisting of hypersalivation, metallic taste, ulceration and necrosis of the gingivae with a tendency to spread posteriorly and to the buccal mucosa and palate, glossodynia, and periodontitis with loosening of the teeth in severe cases of chronic intoxication.

stomatitis, mycotic, *n* infection of the oral mucosa by a fungus, most commonly *Candida albicans,* which produces moniliasis (thrush). See also moniliasis.

stomatitis, nicotinic, *n* an inflammation of the palatal minor salivary ducts caused by irritation by tobacco smoke or hot fluids and characterized by raised small palatal lesions with red centers and white borders. The palatal mucosa usually has a generalized keratosis accompanying the smaller lesions. Also called *stomatitis nicotina.*

Nicotinic stomatitis. (Regezi/Sciubba/Jordan, 2003)

stomatitis, recurrent, *n* recurrent manifestation of herpes simplex involving the lips and labial and buccal mucosa (fever blisters, cold sores). Considered by many to include also recurrent aphthae (canker sores). Episodes may result from fever, sunlight, menses, trauma, and gastrointestinal upset. Lesions begin as clear vesicles with an erythematous base that give way to ulcers and superficial crusts if the outer surfaces of the lips and skin are involved.

stomatitis, uremic, *n* oral manifestation of uremia, consisting of varying degrees of erythema, exudation, ulceration, pseudomembrane formation, foul breath, and burning sensations. See also gingivitis, nephritic.

stomatitis venenata, *n* inflammation of the oral mucosa as the result of contact allergy. The most common causative agents are volatile oils, iodides, dentifrices, mouthwashes, denture powders, and topical anesthetics. Possible manifestations include erythema, angioneurotic edema, burning sensations, ulcerations, and vesicles.

stomatodynia (stō′mətōdin′ē ə), *n* sore mouth.

stomatoglossitis (stō′mətōglôsī′tis), *n* inflammation involving oral and mucous membranes and the tongue. May be seen in nutritional disorders such as pellagra, beriberi, vitamin B complex deficiency, and infections.

stomatognathic system (stō′mətōnath′ik), *n* See system, stomatognathic.

stomatology (stō′mətol′əjē), *n* the study of the morphology, structure, function, and diseases of the contents and linings of the oral cavity.

stomion (stō′mē on), *n* the median point of the oral slit (orifice) when the mouth is closed.

stomodeum (sto″ mo-de′ əm), *n* a superficial depression on the ectoderm of the developing embryo that later becomes the mouth.

stone, *n* an abrading instrument or tool.

stone, Arkansas, *n.pr* a fine-grained stone, novaculite, used to make hones for the final sharpening of instruments.

stone, artificial, *n* (dental stone), a specially calcined gypsum derivative similar to plaster of paris. Because its grains are nonporous, the product is stronger than plaster of paris.

stone, Carborundum, *n.pr* **1.** a stone made of silicon carbide. **2.** an abrasive, handpiece-mounted rotary instrument of various sizes, shapes, and degrees of abrasiveness.

stone, dental, *n* (Hydrocal), **1.** α-hemihydrate of calcium sulfate. **2.** a gypsum product that, when combined with water in proper proportions, hardens in a plasterlike form. Used for making casts and dies.

stone, diamond, *n* rotary instruments containing diamond chips as the abrasive. Available in various sizes, shapes, and abrasive consistency. Used for tooth reduction in operative dentistry and crown and bridge prostheses, tooth contouring in the occlusal adjustment procedure, and os-

S

seous and gingival contouring in periodontal surgery.

stone die, n See die, stone.

stone, lathe, n (lathe wheel), a grindstone mounted on a chuck and used on a lathe.

stone, mounted point, n a small abrasive tooth of various shape and size bonded or cemented onto a shaft or mandrel.

stone, pulp, n See denticle.

stone, rotary, n the stone in a mandrel-mounted (power-driven) sharpening instrument.

stone, sharpening, n a hand stone, or a stone driven mechanically, that is used to sharpen instruments.

stones, sharpening cone, n.pl cylindrical or rounded rectangular stones used to sharpen curved blades.

stone, wheel, n a small grindstone of Carborundum or corundum of various grit, mounted on a mandrel; of various thickness, ranging in diameter from ½ to 1 inch (1.3 to 2.5 cm).

stop, n See rest.

stop, occlusal, n See rest, occlusal.

stop-loss, n a general term referring to that category of coverage that provides insurance protection (reinsurance) to an employer for a self-funded plan.

stopping, n temporary, gutta-percha mixed with zinc oxide, white wax, and coloring. Softens on heating and rehardens at room temperature. Used for temporary sealing of dressings in cavities. Lack of strength makes it ineffective in areas under occlusal stress. It has poor sealing properties.

storage, computer, n a device or portion of a device that is capable of receiving data, retaining them for an indefinite time, and supplying them on command. Also called *memory.*

strabismus, n an abnormal ocular condition in which the eyes are crossed.

straight wire fixed orthodontic appliance, n See appliance, straight wire fixed.

straightening of teeth, n See orthodontics.

strain, n 1. deformation induced by an external force. 2. deformation expressed as a pure number or ratio resulting from the application of a load. 3. a traumatic stretching or compression of such tissues as the ligaments, capsule, or musculature associated with a joint. See also sprain.

strain hardening, n See hardening, strain.

strangulation, n choking or throttling. The arrest of respiration resulting from occlusion of the air passage or arrest of the circulation in part because of compression.

stratum, n.pl (n.pl **strata**) a layer of the epidermis or the epithelium of the oral mucosa.

stratum basale, n the deepest of the five layers of the epidermis or epithelium of the oral mucosa, composed of a single layer of tall cylindrical cells or cubodial cells, respectively. This layer provides new cells by mitotic cell division. Also called the *basal layer* or *germative layer.*

stratum corneum, n the tough, outermost layer of the epidermis or epithelium of keratinized oral mucosa, composed of flat, closely packed, dead cells converted to keratin that continually flake away. Also called the *keratin layer* or *corneal layer.*

stratum granulosum, n one of the layers of the epidermis or the epithelium of the keratinized oral mucosa, situated just inferior the stratum corneum in keratinized tissues except in the palms of the hands and the soles of the feet, where it lies just inferior the stratum lucidum (transparent layer). Also called the *granular layer.*

stratum intermedium, n one of the two layers between the outer and inner enamel epithelium of the enamel organ that consists of a compressed layer of flat to cubodial cells.

stratum lucidum, n one of the layers of the epidermis situated just beneath the stratum corneum and present only in the thick skin of the palms of the hands and the soles of the feet. Also called the *transparent layer.*

stratum spinosum, n one of the layers of the epidermis or epithelium of oral mucosa, composed of several layers of polygonal cells. It lies on superior to the stratum basale. Also called the *prickle cell layer.*

stratum spongiosum, n one of the three layers of the endometrium of the uterus.

strawberry tongue, n a strawberry-like coloration of inflamed tongue papillae. It is a clinical sign of scarlet fever and also is seen in Kawasaki syndrome.

stray radiation, *n* See radiation leakage.

strength, *n* toughness; ability to withstand or apply force.

strength, biting, *n* **1.** the force available for application against food or other material placed between the teeth. See also force, masticatory. **2.** the amount of force the muscles of mastication are capable of exerting. See also force, masticatory.

strength, compressive (**crushing strength**), *n* the amount of resistance of a material to fracture under compression. See also strength, ultimate.

strength, crushing, *n* See strength, compressive.

strength, dry, *n* term generally used in conjunction with materials whose strengths vary markedly in the wet and dry states. The strength of gypsum products is usually reported in both wet and dry states.

strength, edge, *n* term indicative of the ability of fine margins to resist fracture or abrasion. No specific test is available to assess this property; it is a composite of ductility and shear, tensile, and other strength characteristics.

strength, gel, *n* usually, the ability of a material to withstand a load without rupture.

strength, impact, *n* the ability of a material to withstand a striking force.

strength, shear, *n* **1.** resistance to a tangential force. **2.** resistance to a twisting motion.

strength, tensile, *n* **1.** resistance to a pulling force. **2.** the amount of stress a material is able to withstand when being pulled lengthwise before permanent deformation results.

strength, ultimate, *n* the greatest stress that may be induced in a material or object before or during rupture; may be compressive, tensile, or shear strength. See also strength, tensile.

strength, wet, *n* compressive strength while water in excess of that required for hydration of the hemihydrate present in the specimen. Used in connection with gypsum products.

strength, yield, *n* a definite proportionality obtained by drawing a line parallel to the proportional limit line. Yield strength is reported in terms of the degree of strain.

strep throat, *n* an infection of the oral pharynx and tonsils caused by hemolytic species of *Streptococcus.* The infection is characterized by sore throat, chills, fever, swollen lymph nodes in the neck, and sometimes nausea and vomiting.

Streptococcus, **alpha hemolytic** (**strep'tōkok'us al'fa hē'mōlit'ik**), *n* a spherical, gram-positive bacterium occurring in chains of bacterial cells. Produces a zone of greenish discoloration around the colony in blood-agar medium. Part of an individual's normal oral flora; has been isolated from the gingival crevice. Capable of producing bacteremia and subsequent subacute bacterial endocarditis in patients with a history of rheumatic fever; thus prophylactic antibiotic therapy is necessary before, during, and after periodontal, operative, and surgical therapy.

Streptococcus, **beta-hemolytic,** *n* an infectious bacterium responsible for causing strep throat and scarlet fever, illnesses that are transmitted primarily through respiratory droplets spread from one person to another by direct contact. Also called *group A Streptococcus.*

Streptococcus, **group A,** *n* See *Streptococcus,* beta hemolytic.

Streptococcus mitis (**mī'tis**), *n* a bacterium found in soft tissues of the mouth that causes dental decay in animals.

Streptococcus mutans, *n* cariogenic bacteria found in dental plaque and one of two the index organisms (*Lactobacillus* is the other) used to assess caries susceptibility.

Streptococcus pneumoniae, *n* any of 70 antigenic types of pneumococci that cause pneumonia and other diseases in humans.

Streptococcus pyogenes, *n* a species of *Streptococcus* with many strains that are pathogenic to humans. It causes such suppurative disease as scarlet fever and strep throat.

Streptococcus salivarius, *n* a bacterium found in dental plaque that may cause endocarditis and dental caries.

Streptococcus sanguis, *n* a bacterium

S

found in dental plaque that may cause endocarditis and dental caries.

Streptococcus sobrinus (sōbrī′nus), *n* a mutans *Streptococcus* bacterium the role of which in dental decay is still being determined.

Streptococcus viridans (vir′idanz), *n* See *Streptococcus,* alpha hemolytic.

streptokinase, *n* a fibrinolytic activator that enhances the conversion of plasminogen to the fibrinolytic enzyme plasmin. It is used in the treatment of certain cases of pulmonary and coronary embolism.

streptokinase-streptodornase, *n.pl* two enzymes derived from a strain of *Streptococcus hemolyticus.* It is prescribed for debridement of purulent exudates, clotted blood, radiation necrosis, or fibrinous deposits resulting from trauma or infection.

Streptomyces (strep′tōmī′sēz), *n* a genus of gram-positive, fungus-like bacteria belonging to the order actinomycetales. Several antibiotics, such as tetracyclines and aminoglycosides, are produced from *Streptomyces* species.

streptomycin, *n* an antimicrobial drug often used to treat infections caused by gram-negative bacteria (such as tuberculosis). Though no human studies have been conducted, streptomycin administered during pregnancy or breastfeeding may cause damage to the ear of the fetus or infant.

streptothricosis (strep′tōthrikō′sis), *n* See actinomycosis.

stress, *n* I. a force induced by or resisting an external force; measured in terms of force per unit area. **2.** the force of energy directed against a tissue structure or against the function of tissue as the result of injury and trauma associated with fracture, burn, infection, surgical procedure, pharmacologic action, or anxiety states. The response to stress involves local metabolic function, the hormonal activity of the endocrine system regulated by the pituitary gland, and the autonomic and central nervous systems. The stress phenomenon is frequently associated with the general adaptation syndrome. **3.** in prosthetic dentistry, forcibly exerted pressure (for example, the pressure of the upper teeth against the mandibular teeth or the pressure contact of a distorted removable partial denture on the supporting teeth or ridge structures).

stress, axial, *n* excessive force applied vertically to the teeth and their attachment apparatus.

stress, bone in, *n* responses of bony structures to applied force. With application of excessive pressure stimuli to bone, adaptation may occur by the formation of thicker and more numerous trabeculae. If tissue components cannot compensate for excessive stress, bone resorption will occur.

stress, buccolingual, *n* excessive pressure exerted against teeth and their attachment apparatus from a buccal or lingual aspect.

stress, compressive, *n* the internal induced force that opposes shortening of the material in a direction parallel to the direction of the stress.

stress control, *n* See control, stress.

stress, damage to restorations by, *n* a mechanical property that pertains to the capacity of substances used for restorative and preventive applications to loosen in response to a continual pressure over a period of time. See also strain.

stress, shearing, *n* the internal induced force that opposes the sliding of one plane of the material on the adjacent plane in a direction parallel to the stress.

stress, tensile, *n* the internal induced force that opposes elongation of a material in a direction parallel to the direction of stress.

stress-bearing area, *n* See area, basal seat.

stressbreaker (stress equalizer, stress divider), *n* a device or system that is incorporated in a removable partial denture to relieve the abutment teeth of occlusal loads that may exceed their physiologic tolerance. See also connector, nonrigid.

stretch receptors, *n.pl* specialized sensory nerve endings in muscle spindles and tendons that are stimulated by stretching movements. They are active in maintaining dynamic posture.

stretch reflex, *n* See reflex, stretch.

stretching, longitudinal, *n* the vertical elongations of gutta-percha that occur because of packing forces during the filling of large root canals. The material returns to the original form when force is released.

stretching pliers, *n* See pliers, stretching.

stridor (strī'dôr), *n* a peculiar, harsh, vibrating sound produced during respiration.

stridor, inspiratory, n the sound heard in inspiration through a spasmodically closed glottis.

stridor, laryngeal, n stridor resulting from laryngeal stenosis.

strip, *n* a thin, narrow, comparatively long piece of material.

strip, abrasive (linen strip), n a ribbonlike piece of linen of varying length and width, on one side of which are bonded abrasive particles of selected grit; used for contouring and polishing proximal surfaces of restorations.

strip, boxing, n a metal or wax strip used for making an enclosure to regulate the size and form of a cast.

strip, celluloid, n See strip, plastic.

strip, lightning, n (separating strip), a strip of steel with abrasive bonded on one side; used to open rough or improper contacts of proximal restorations or begin the reduction of proximal excess of a foil restoration.

strip, linen, n See strip, abrasive.

strip, plastic, n a clear plastic strip of celluloid or acrylic resin that is used as a matrix when silicate cement or acrylic resin cement is inserted into proximal prepared cavities in anterior teeth.

strip, polishing, n a strip with a very fine abrasive, such as crocus powder.

strip, separating, n See strip, lightning.

stripping, *n* **1.** the mechanical removal of a very small amount of enamel from the mesial or distal surfaces of teeth to alleviate crowding. **2.** (electrochemical) the process of subjecting the surface of a gold casting, attached to an anode from a rectifier and transformer unit, to the dissolving action of a heated cyanide solution, the metal container for which is the cathode of the unit. A microscopic amount of the surface of the alloy is removed by reverse electrolysis. The electrochemical stripping or milling is in

contrast to electropolishing, wherein sharp edges are dissolved more rapidly than are broader areas.

stroke, *n* **1.** a single, unbroken movement made by an instrument or the mandible. **2.** common term for accident, cerebrovascular.

stroke, circular, n an unbroken spherical movement of approximately 1 to 2 mm in diameter, combined with pressure, that is used to apply paste in polishing.

stroke, circumferential, n one of the basic strokes used for root and gingival curettage; the blade of the periodontal curet is negotiated mesiodistally while it is in contact with either the root or the inner aspect of the soft tissue wall of the gingival or periodontal pocket.

stroke, exploratory, n a phase of subgingival root scaling in which the curet is held in a featherlike grasp to ascertain tactilely the amount and extent of the accretions on the root surface; the ingress stroke into the pocket area.

stroke, horizontal, n a short movement against a tooth that is made parallel to its occlusal surface.

stroke, oblique, n a single, continuous diagonal movement of an instrument over the external face of the object being worked on.

stroke, placement, n a single, continuous movement of an instrument over the surface of an object being worked on; a placement stroke positions the instrument at the intended location.

stroke, power, n the phase of the working stroke that is designed to split or dislodge calculus from the root surface. It is prefaced by the exploratory stroke and followed by the shaving stroke.

stroke, probe walking, n the technique of assessing the progression and extent of disease within the oral cavity by inserting a periodontal probe into the sulcus or pocket of the tooth and moving the device up and down between 1 to 2 mm in height while simultaneously advancing forward in 1 mm increments.

stroke, pull, n a single, continuous movement of an instrument over the surface of an object being worked on. A pull stroke is enacted to remove

S

calculus from the surface of a tooth.

stroke, push and pull, n the technique of using a subgingival explorer vertically or diagonally to assess a defect of the tooth's surface by inserting the lower shank of the instrument under the gingival margin and into the sulcus or pocket and moving the device up and down while simultaneously applying equal pressure and advancing forward.

stroke, shaving, n the phase of the working stroke of a periodontal curet that is designed to smooth or plane the root surface. It follows the power stroke, which is designed to dislodge calculus from the root surface.

stroke, vertical, n a single, continuous movement of an instrument over the external face being treated. The vertical stroke is in a direction that parallels the length of the tooth (from the root to the occlusal surface).

stroke volume, n the volume of blood put out by the heart per heartbeat. Stroke volume is directly proportional to the volume of blood filling the heart during diastole.

stroke, working, n a single, continuous movement of an instrument that achieves a task or treatment.

strontium (Sr), n a metallic element. Its atomic number is 38, and its atomic weight is 87.62. It is chemically similar to calcium and is found in bone tissue. Isotopes of strontium are used in radioisotope scanning procedures of bone.

structure, n the architectural arrangement of the component parts of a tissue, part, organ, or body. Also the individual components of the body.

structure, border, n See border structures.

structure, cored, n in metallurgy a grain structure with composition gradients resulting from the progressive freezing of the components in different proportions. Nonmetals used in dentistry (e.g., zinc phosphate, silicate cements) also are cored structures, in that they have a nucleus of undissolved powder particles surrounded by a matrix of reacted material.

structure, denture-supporting, n the tissues, including teeth and residual ridges, that serve as the foundation or basal seat for removable partial dentures.

structure, functional form of supporting, n the state of denture-supporting structures when they have been placed in such a position as to be able to begin resisting occlusal forces.

structure, histologic, n the minute structure of organic tissues.

structure, radiolucent, n the structures or substances that permit the penetration of x radiation and are thus registered as relatively dark areas on the radiograph.

structure, radiopaque, n structures of such density that x-rays cannot penetrate them, causing them to appear as light areas on the radiograph.

structure, supporting, n the tissues that maintain or assist in maintaining the teeth in position in the alveolus (e.g., gingivae, cementum of the tooth, periodontal ligament, alveolar and trabecular bone).

Stuart factor, *n.pr* See factor X.

study, n pursuance of education; analysis.

study cast, n See cast, diagnostic.

study, graduate, n baccalaureate educational efforts pursued for credit toward an advanced degree in institutions of higher learning.

study model, n See cast, diagnostic.

study, postgraduate, n postdoctoral educational endeavors that may or may not earn credits for advanced degrees.

study, time, n the technique of random sampling used for analysis of the time spent for rendering each phase of each of the various professional services performed by the dentist.

stupor, n the condition of being only partly conscious or sensible; also, a condition of insensibility.

Sturge-Weber-Dimitri disease, *n.pr* See disease, Sturge-Weber-Dimitri.

stuttering, n a speech dysfunction characterized by spasmodic enunciation of words, involving excessive hesitations, stumbling, repetition of the same syllables, and prolongation of sounds.

stylet, n a wire inserted into a soft catheter or cannula to secure rigidity;

a fine wire inserted into a hollow needle to maintain patency.

stylohyoid ligament, *n* the ligament attached to the tip of the styloid process of the temporal bone and the lesser cornu of the hyoid bone.

stylohyoideus, *n* one of the four suprahyoid muscles. It is a slender muscle that arises from the styloid process and inserts into the hyoid bone. It serves to draw the hyoid bone up and back.

stylomandibular ligament, *n* one of a pair of specialized bands of cervical fascia, forming an accessory part of the temporomandibular joint. It extends from the styloid process of the temporal bone to the ramus of the mandible.

stylus, *n* ancient writing instrument. It is still used much as it was when the Egyptians were exploring geometry with a stylus and sand sprinkled on a polished stone. It has assumed importance in gnathology because a well-pointed stylus can be slid on dust-covered glass with a minimum of friction, thereby making the jaw-writing data more accurate.

stylus, **surgical indicator,** *n* a small pointed instrument devised to mark the spot in the tissue where the intramucosal inserts will be placed. Styluses are seated in prepared depressions in the denture base and mark the mucosal tissue by puncturing it.

stylus tracer, *n* See tracer, needle point.

stylus tracing, *n* See tracing, needle point.

styptic, *n* a hemostatic astringent.

sub-, *pref* prefix signifying under, beneath, deficient, near, or almost.

subacute, *adj* less than acute.

subarachnoid hemorrhage (SAH), *n* an intracranial hemorrhage into the cerebrospinal fluid.

subclinical, *adj* pertaining to an illness or condition in its earliest stage; having no symptoms or readily discernible signs.

subconscious, *n* the state in which mental processes take place without the mind's being distinctly conscious of its own activity.

subculture, *n* an ethnic, regional, economic, or social group with characteristic patterns of behavior and ideals that distinguish it from the rest of the culture or society.

subdural, *adj* situated below the dura mater and above the arachnoid membrane.

subgingival (subjin´jivəl), *adj* at a level apical to the gingival margin.

subgingival calculus, *n* a deposit of various mineral salts that accumulate with organic matter and oral debris on the teeth below the margin of the gingiva.

subgingival curettage, *n* See curettage, subgingival.

subgingival irrigation, **preanesthetic antimicrobial,** *n* a procedure for delivering a liquid antimicrobial agent to a subgingival area before; used to destroy or inhibit the growth of microorganisms and prevent contamination or infection and to promote healing in deep pockets.

subgingival scaling, *n* a procedure for removing bacterial plaque and calculus located on enamel or cementum below the gingival margin.

subjective data collection, *n* the process in which information relating to the patient's problem is elicited from the patient.

subjects, *n.pl* the people, animals, or events selected for study to examine a particular variable or condition, such as the effects of a new medication or treatment.

sublease, *n* a lease executed by the lessee of an estate to a third person, conveying the same estate for a shorter term than that for which the lessee holds it.

subliminal, *adj* below the threshold of sensory perception or outside the range of conscious awareness.

sublingual (subling´gwəl), *adj* pertaining to the region of structures located beneath the tongue.

Sublingual. (Liebgott, 2001)

S

sublingual administration, n See administration, sublingual.

sublingual crescent, n See crescent, sublingual.

sublingual fold, n See fold, sublingual.

sublingual gland, n See salivary glands.

subluxation (sub′luksā′shən), *n* **1.** incomplete dislocation of a joint. **2.** term applied loosely to the temporomandibular joint, indicating relaxation of the capsular ligaments and improper relationship of the joint components, resulting in cracking and popping of the joint during movement.

submandibular, *adj* below the mandible.

submandibular caruncle, n See caruncle, submandibular.

submandibular fossa in image interpretation, n porous site within the region located in the body of the mandible that allows x-rays to gain a clear representation of the lingual depression of the salivary gland located within the submandibular area.

submandibular ganglion, n See ganglion, submaxillary.

submandibular gland, n one of a pair of salivary glands in the submandibular triangle. The gland secretes saliva into the oral cavity through a small duct that opens on a small papilla at the side of the lingual frenum.

submandibular lymph nodes, n filters in the lymphatic system located at the gonial angle of the mandible.

submarginal, *adj* pertaining to a deficiency of contour at the margin of a restoration or pattern.

submaxillary, *adj* situated beneath the maxilla.

submental, *adj* situated below the chin.

submental lymph nodes, n filters in the lymphatic system inferior to the chin.

submucosa (sub′myōōkō′sə), *n* the tissue layer beneath the oral mucosa. It contains connective tissues, vessels, and accessory salivary glands.

submucous cleft, *n* a congenital anomaly in which the midportion of the soft or hard palate lacks proper mesodermal development. Nonunion of bone and muscle tissues of the soft

and hard palates and concealment by the superficial intact mucoperiosteum. Also called *occult cleft.*

subnasion (sub′nā′zē on), *n* the point of the angle between the septum and the surface of the upper lip. It is sought at the point where a tangent applied to the septum meets the upper lip.

subocclusal connector, *n* See connector, subocclusal.

subpoena (sub′pē′nə), *n* the process or writ issued by the court requiring the attendance of a witness at a certain time and place for testimony. It also may order him or her to bring books, records, or other relevant items as evidence.

subpoena duces tecum, n a subpoena commanding a person to bring books, papers, records, or other items to the court.

subroutine, *n* the set of instructions necessary to direct the computer to carry out a well-defined mathematical or logical operation; a subunit of a routine.

subscriber, *n* the person, usually the employee, who represents the family unit in relation to the prepayment plan. Other family members are *dependents.* Also called *certificate holders* or *enrollees.*

subsistence, *n* the state of being supported or remaining alive with a minimum of essentials.

subspecialty, *n* a limited portion of a narrowly defined professional discipline. For example, surgery is a specialty of medicine and pediatric vascular surgery is a subspecialty.

subspinale (sub′spīnā′lē), *n* the deepest midline point on the premaxilla between the anterior nasal spine and the prosthion.

substance abuse, *n* the overindulgence in and dependence on a stimulant, depressant, or other chemical substance, leading to effects that are detrimental to the individual's physical or mental health or the welfare of others.

substance P, *n* one of several endogenous inflammatory substances thought to mediate or cause pain.

substandard, *adj* below an acceptable level of performance.

substantivity, *adj* pertaining to the capacity of an oral antimicrobial agent to continue its therapeutic activity for a prolonged period of time.

substitute, *n* one acting for or taking the place of another.

substitute, tinfoil, *n* alginate separating material painted on gypsum molds to serve as a liner in preventing both the penetration of monomers into the surrounding investing medium and the leakage of water into acrylic resin.

substitution, *n* a standard or nonstandard speech sound used for another consonant speech sound (for example, *w* for *l* [*wady* for *lady*])

substructure, *n* a structure built to serve as a base or foundation for another structure.

substructure, implant **(implant denture substructure),** *n* **1.** a skeletal frame of inert material that fits on the bone under the mucoperiosteum. **2.** the metal framework that is embedded beneath the soft tissues in contact with the bone for the purpose of supporting an implant superstructure.

substructure, implant, abutment, *n* the portion of the implant that extends from the surface of the mucosa into the oral cavity for the retention of crowns, bridges, or superstructure bearing the teeth of the denture.

substructure, implant, auxiliary rest, *n* a small metal protrusion through the mucosa connected to the labial or buccal and lingual (peripheral) frame to furnish additional support for the superstructure between the abutments.

substructure, implant, interspace, *n* any one of the spaces between the primary and secondary struts that allows infiltration of tissue.

substructure, implant, neck **(implant post, implant substructure, post),** *n* the constriction that connects the implant frame with the implant abutment.

substructure, implant, part, *n* the root section shaped in the form of a wire loop. This part of the substructure sinks into the alveolar socket or sockets after the extraction of one or two remaining anterior teeth. Newly formed bone tissue grows through the loop and firmly affixes the implant.

substructure, implant, peripheral frame, *n* the labial, buccal, lingual, and distal outline of the frame.

substructure, implant, post, *n* See substructure, implant, neck.

substructure, implant, primary struts, *n* the main traverse struts that connect the implant necks or posts with the peripheral frame.

substructure, implant, secondary struts, *n* the additional smaller transverse, diagonal, and longitudinal struts that are added when necessary to give additional strength and rigidity to the implant, increase the area of bone support, and afford additional intermeshing of the mucoperiosteal tissue.

subtle, *adj* having a low intensity; not severe and having no serious sequelae.

successional dental lamina, *n* an elongation of the primary tooth germ from which a permanent tooth will eventually take shape.

succinimides (suksin′imidz), *n* a class of drugs used in the treatment of epilepsy.

succinylcholine chloride, *n* a skeletal muscle relaxant used as an adjunct to anesthesia, to reduce muscle contractions during surgery or mechanical ventilation and to facilitate endotracheal intubation.

sucralfate, *n* trade name: Carafate; drug class: protectant, aluminum salt of sulfated sucrose; action: forms an ulcer-adherent complex that covers and protects the ulcer site; use: treatment of duodenal ulcer.

sudden infant death syndrome (SIDS), *n* the unexpected and sudden death of an apparently normal and healthy infant that occurs during sleep and with no physical or autopsic evidence of disease. It is the most common cause of death of children in the United States between 2 weeks and 1 year of age.

sudorific, *n* an agent, substance, or condition, such as heat or emotional tension, that promotes sweating.

sufentanil citrate, *n* an intravenous analgesic and anesthetic used as an adjunct to general anesthesia and as a primary anesthetic with 100% oxygen.

suffocate, *v* asphyxiate; to prevent the exchange of air into the lungs, causing death.

suffocation, *n* interference with the entrance of air into the lungs.

sugar, *n* one of a number of water-soluble carbohydrates. Sugars are divided into two major categories, *monosaccharides* and *disaccharides.* Table sugar or sucrose is the principal disaccharide; glucose or blood sugar is the principal monosaccharide.

sugar alcohols, n.pl the nutritive sweeteners found in most grains, fruits, and vegetables that undergo natural fermentation as they are broken down by oral bacteria; not directly linked to the development of dental caries but may cause diarrhea if ingested in excessive amounts.

suggestion, *n* **1.** the process by which one thought or idea leads to another, as in the association of ideas. **2.** the use of persuasion to implant an idea, thought, attitude, or belief in the mind of another as a means of influencing or altering behavior or state of mind.

suicide, *n* the intentional taking of one's own life.

suit, *n* any proceeding in court in which the plaintiff pursues a remedy that the law gives for the redress of an injury or the enforcement of a right.

sulconazole nitrate, *n trade name:* Exelderm; *drug class:* topical antifungal; *action:* interferes with fungal cell membranes, increasing permeability and leaking of nutrients; *uses:* treatment of tinea pedis, tinea corporis, tinea cruris, and tinea versicolor.

sulcus (sul′kəs), *n* **1.** a furrow, trench, or groove, as on the surface of the brain or in the folds of mucous membranes. **2.** a groove or depression on the surface of a tooth. **3.** a groove in a portion of the oral cavity.

sulcus, alveololingual, n the space between the alveolar or residual alveolar ridge and the tongue. It extends from the lingual frenum to the retromylohyoid curtain and is a part of the floor of the mouth.

sulcus, gingival, n the shallow groove between the free gingiva and the surface of a tooth and extending around its circumference.

sulcus, implant gingival, n a sulcus around the implant abutment post that resembles the sulcus around a healthy natural tooth.

sulcus, occlusal, n a groove or spillway on the occlusal surface of a tooth.

sulcus, terminalis, n V-shaped shallow groove on the surface of the tongue that separates the distal third of the tongue from the proximal two-thirds.

sulfa (sul′fə), *adj/n* a vernacular term used to describe a group of antibacterial agents. See also sulfacetamide and sulfamethizole.

sulfacetamide sodium (ophthalmic), *n trade names:* Bleph-10, Cetamide, Isopto Cetamide; *drug class:* antibacterial sulfonamide; *action:* inhibits folic acid synthesis by preventing paraaminobenzoic acid (PABA) use, which is necessary for bacterial growth; *uses:* treatment of conjunctivitis, superficial eye infections, and corneal ulcers.

sulfamethizole, *n trade name:* Thiosulfil Forte; *drug class:* sulfonamide, short acting; *action:* interferes with bacterial biosynthesis of proteins by competitive antagonism of paraaminobenzoic acid (PABA); *use:* treatment of urinary tract infections.

sulfamethoxazole, *n trade names:* Gamazole, Gantanol, Urabak; *drug class:* sulfonamide; *action:* interferes with bacterial biosynthesis of proteins by competitive antagonism of paraaminobenzoic acid (PABA); *uses:* treatment of urinary tract infections, lymphogranuloma venereum, and systemic infections.

sulfamethoxazole/trimethoprim, *n trade names:* Bactrim, Cotrim, Septra, Sulfatrim, Sulfamethoprim, Triazole, Uroplus SS; *drug class:* sulfonamide and folic acid antagonist; *action:* interferes with bacterial biosynthesis of proteins by competitive antagonism of paraaminobenzoic acid (PABA) when adequate levels are maintained; *uses:* treatment of urinary tract infections, otitis media.

sulfasalazine, *n trade name:* Asulfidine-EN-Tabs, Azulfidine; *drug class:* sulfonamide derivative with anti-inflammatory action; *action:* acts as a prodrug to deliver sulfapyridine and mesalamine (5-aminosalicylic acid) to the colon; *uses:* treatment of ulcerative colitis, Crohn's disease.

sulfhemoglobinemia
(sulfēm´əglō´binē´mē ə), *n* an abnormality of the heme moiety of the hemoglobin molecule resulting from inorganic sulfides (e.g., acetanilide).

sulfinpyrazone, *n trade name:* Anturane; *drug class:* uricosuric; *action:* inhibits tubular reabsorption of urates, with increased excretion of uric acid; inhibits prostaglandin synthesis, which decreases platelet aggregation; *use:* treatment of chronic gouty arthritis.

sulfisoxazole, *n trade name:* Gantrisin; *drug class:* sulfonamide, short-acting; antiinfective; *action:* interferes with bacterial biosynthesis of proteins by competitive antagonism of paraaminobenzoic acid (PABA); *uses:* treatment of urinary tract, systemic infections, chancroid; trachoma; toxoplasmosis, acute otitis media; lymphogranuloma venereum; eye infections.

sulfonamide (sulfon´əmīd), *n* a derivative of sulfanilamide that is effective against microorganisms.

sulfonylureas (sul´ fə-nil-u-re´ əs), *n* a class of medications used in the treatment of diabetes. They cause the pancreas to release more insulin.

sulfur (S), *n* a nonmetallic, multivalent, tasteless, odorless chemical element that occurs abundantly in yellow crystalline form or in masses, especially in volcanic areas. Its atomic number is 16, and its atomic weight is 32.064. It has wide use in industry. Sulfur has been used in the treatment of gout, rheumatism, and bronchitis and as a mild laxative.

sulfur granules, n a yellow-white particle found in actinomycosis and diagnostic of actinomycosis infection.

sulindac, *n trade name:* Clinoril; *drug class:* nonsteroidal antiinflammatory; *action:* inhibits prostaglandin synthesis by interfering with cyclo-oxygenase, an enzyme needed for biosynthesis; possesses analgesic, antiinflammatory, and antipyretic properties; *uses:* osteoarthritis, rheumatoid, acute gouty arthritis, tendinitis, bursitis, ankylosing spondylitis.

sumatriptan succinate, *n trade name:* Imitrex; *drug class:* serotonin agonist; *action:* selective agonist for the vascular 5-hydroxytryptamine (5-HT-1) (serotonin) receptor in cranial arteries, causing vasodilation with little or no effect on peripheral pressure; *use:* treatment of migraine headaches.

summary judgment, *n* a judgment requested by any party to a civil action to end the action when it is believed that no genuine issue or material fact is in dispute.

summary plan description, *n* See benefit plan summary.

summation, *n* the phenomenon in which similar actions of more than one drug result in a total action that may be expressed as the arithmetical sum of the effects of the individual drugs.

summons, *n* a writ requiring a proper officer to notify a defendant that an action has been begun against him or her in the court from which the writ was issued and that he or she is required to appear on a certain day to answer the complaint.

superficial, *adj* involving only the surface or to be minor in severity, not grave or dangerous.

superinfection, *n* an infection occurring during antimicrobial treatment for another infection.

supernumerary tooth, *n* any tooth in addition to the normal 32 teeth in the permanent dentition or the 20 teeth in the primary dentition.

superoxide, *n* a common form of oxygen that is formed when molecular oxygen gains a single electron. Superoxide radicals may attack susceptible biologic targets, including lipids, proteins, and nucleic acids.

superoxol, *n* a 30% solution of hydrogen peroxide used to bleach endodontically treated teeth.

supersaturation, *n* the addition to or presence of an ingredient in a solution in greater quantity than the solvent can permanently take up.

superstructure, *n* a structure constructed on or over another structure.

superstructure casting, n in the subperiosteal implant, a surgical alloy bar designed with clasps to telescope over the four abutments. To this casting is processed the final denture superstructure.

superstructure, implant, n (implant denture superstructure), **1.** a removable denture that fits snugly onto the protruding implant abutments. Sometimes called the *implant denture*. **2.** the denture that is retained, supported, and stabilized by the implant denture substructure.

superstructure, implant, attaching material, n the denture resin by which the superstructure teeth are attached to the superstructure frame.

superstructure, implant, attachment, n any part of the superstructure that fits onto the implant abutments. May be a precision attachment coping, a conventional clasping, or a combination of a precision attachment with clasps.

superstructure, implant, connectors, n the rigid bars that unite the superstructure attachments into one strong element.

superstructure, implant, denture, n See superstructure, implant.

superstructure, implant, frame, n the metal skeleton of the superstructure, consisting of attachments and connectors.

superstructure, temporary (**implant surgical splint**), n an acrylic resin immediate appliance with six anterior teeth; has no metal clasps, precision coping, or frame; fitted closely over the implant abutments immediately after the surgical insertion of the substructure.

supervision, n the active administering and overseeing of all the functionings of the dental practice and the auxiliaries employed therein.

supine, adj lying horizontally on the back.

supplemental tooth, n a type of supernumerary tooth that is so well formed that it mimics a fully formed tooth. A supplemental tooth usually appears distal to a lateral incisor. Its detection requires the careful counting and identification of each tooth in the dental arch.

supplements, n.pl usually, dietary substances used to augment, enhance, or enrich the nutritional status of a patient.

support, n resistance to vertical components of masticatory force in a direction toward the basal seat.

support, ridge, n See area, supporting.

supporting area, n See area, supporting.

supporting bone, n See bone, cancellous.

supportive periodontal therapy, n See periodontal therapy.

suppressant, n an agent that retards or diminishes a physical or mental activity. Commonly used to describe a drug that inhibits coughing (cough suppressant).

suppuration (sup″ u-ra′ shən), n the formation and discharge of pus. See also pyogenic.

suprabulge, n the portion of the crown of a tooth that converges toward the occlusal surface from the height of contour of survey line.

supraclavicular lymph nodes (sōō′prəklavik′yōōlur), n filters in the lymphatic system located above the collarbone.

supraclusion (sōō′prəklōō′zhən), n a position occupied by a tooth that is too high in the line of occlusion.

supragingival calculus, n a deposit composed of various mineral salts with accumulations of organic matter and oral debris that adheres to the surface of the tooth above the gingival margin.

supramentale (sōō′prəməntā′lē), n the most posterior point in the concavity between infradentale and pogonion.

supraversion (sōō′prəvur′zhən), n a condition in which teeth or other maxillary structures are situated above or below their normal vertical relationships.

suprofen, n an oral nonsteroidal antiinflammatory analgesic used in the treatment of mild-to-moderate pain and primary dysmenorrhea.

suramin sodium, n an antitrypanosomal and an antifilarial available from the Centers for Disease Control and Prevention. It is used primarily for treatment and prophylaxis of *African trypanosomiasis* and *A. onchocerciasis.*

surcharge, n a stated dollar amount paid to the dentist by the beneficiary in addition to other reimbursement received by third-party payers.

surface, n the outer portion of a mass or object.

surface, balancing occlusal, the surfaces of the teeth or denture bases that make contact to provide balancing contacts.

surface, basal, n See denture, basal surface of.

surface, buccal, n any surface adjacent to and facing the cheek.

surface, foundation, n See denture, basal surface of.

surface, implant-bearing, n the area of bone that has been selected from the surgical bone impression to be in direct contact with the implant frame.

surface, impression, n See denture, basal surface of.

surface markers, n.pl identification labels applied to the external surfaces of dentures. They may be ink or engraved and may include name, initials, social security number, national registration number, date of birth, etc.

surface, occlusal, n the anatomic superior surface of the mandibular posterior teeth and the inferior surface of the maxillary posterior teeth. These surfaces are limited mesially and distally by marginal ridges, and buccally and lingually by the buccal and lingual boundaries of the cusp eminences.

surface, proximal, n the surface of a tooth or the portion of a cavity that is nearest to the adjacent tooth; the mesial or distal surface of a tooth.

surface radiation exposure, n See exposure, entrance.

surface, smooth, n a surface of a tooth on which pits and fissures are not found normally.

surface, working occlusal, n the surface or surfaces of the teeth on which chewing can occur.

surfactant   (surfak′tənt), n a surface-active agent.

surgeon, n a person whose profession is to cure diseases or injuries by manual operation or by medication.

surgery, n work performed by a surgeon.

surgery, access flap in osseous, n a full-thickness or split-thickness flap created for the purpose of gaining access to the alveolar bone when surgical remodeling is indicated.

surgery, apically repositioned flap in mucogingival, n a surgically created flap of gingival tissue that is repositioned apically to maintain or create a functionally adequate zone of attached gingiva. In the surgical procedure the existing attached and free gingiva is detached by employing a reverse bevel incision and apically repositioning the flap.

surgery, full flap in mucogingival, n a flap in which all the soft tissue elements are raised and repositioned, as opposed to the split-thickness flap.

surgery, mucogingival, n surgical procedure designed to retain a functionally adequate zone of gingiva after surgical pocket elimination, create a functionally adequate zone of attached gingiva, alter the position of or eliminate a frenum, or deepen the vestibule.

surgery, oblique flap in mucogingival, n an increased band of attached gingiva created by preparing a narrow papillary flap (to avoid donor site radicular recession), which is then rotated 90° and sutured into the prepared recipient site.

surgery, osseous, n the therapeutic surgical measures used and designed to eliminate osseous deformities by means of ostectomy or osteoplasty or create a favorable environment by means of meticulous removal of the soft tissue contents of the infrabony osseous defect for the formation of new bone, periodontal membrane, and cementum to fill in the area of bone resorption.

surgery, pedicle flap in mucogingival, n an increased band of attached gingiva created to repair a cleft by using proximal gingiva situated mesial and distal to the cleft, because gingiva in either location alone is not wide enough to cover the cleft if repositioned. The pedicles are repositioned laterally and sutured. Also called a *double papilla procedure.*

surgical preparation, n See preparation, surgical.

surgical prosthesis, n See prosthesis, surgical.

surgical scrub, n a health care provider's first hand and arm wash of the day prior to entering a sterile surgical field. It involves a systematic routine in which a minimum of 10 minutes are spent lathering, soaking, and brushing one hand and arm, and then the other.

surgical template, n See template, surgical.

surrogate, n a substitute; a person or thing that replaces another.

survey, *n* the study and examination of an area of consideration, a diagnostic cast, or a radiograph.

survey, radiation, *n* evaluation of the radiation hazards incidental to the production, use, or existence of radioactive materials or other sources of radiation under a specific set of conditions.

survey, radiographic, *n* the production of the minimal number of radiographic examinations necessary for a radiographic interpretation.

survey, roentgenographic, *n* See survey, radiographic.

survey, vertical bitewing, *n* a series of oral x-rays in which the teeth are viewed and recorded from a series of positions: the *molar* position, where the film is positioned approximately over the center of the second molar on each side of the mouth; *premolar,* where the film is positioned over the mandibular premolar teeth on each side; *anterior,* where the film is centered between the canine and lateral teeth; and *central bitewing,* where the film is placed at the midline.

survey, x-ray, *n* See survey, radiographic.

survey line, *n* See line, survey.

surveying, *n* the procedure of studying the relative parallelism or lack of parallelism of the teeth and associated structures to select a path of placement for a restoration that will encounter the least tooth or tissue interference and provide adequate and balanced retention; locating guiding plane surfaces to direct placement and removal of the restoration and to achieve the best appearance possible.

surveyor, *n* an instrument used to determine the relative parallelism of two or more surfaces of teeth or other portions of a cast of the dental arch.

surveyor, Ney, *n.pr* the first commercially available dental cast surveyor designed to select a path of placement or insertion for a restoration.

susceptible, *adj* the opposite of immune; having little resistance to disease.

suspension (suspen′shən), *n* a mixture of two or more immiscible phases, such as a solid in a liquid or a liquid in a liquid. Suspensions differ from emulsions in that the former usually have to be shaken before each use.

sustenance, *n* the act or process of supporting or maintaining life and health.

Sutton's disease, *n.pr* See periadenitis mucosa necrotica recurrens.

suture, *n* **1.** a synarthrosis between two bones formed in a membrane, the uniting medium (which tends to disappear eventually) being a fibrous membrane continuous with the periosteum. **2.** a surgical stitch or seam. **3.** material with which body structures are sewn, as after an operation or injury. *v* **4.** to sew up a wound.

suture, absorbable, *n* a suture that becomes dissolved in body fluids and disappears (e.g., catgut).

suture, approximation, *n* a suture made to bring about apposition of the deeper tissues of an incision or laceration.

suture, blanket, *n* a suturing technique that loops each stitch over the previous one to create a succession of loops along one side and stitches across the incision. Also called *continuous lock stitch.*

suture, button, *n* a suture passed through buttonlike disks on the skin to prevent the suture cutting the soft tissue.

suture, chromic, *n* a chromatized sheepgut suture.

suture, circumferential, *n* suture completely surrounding the tooth; generally used to suspend or retain a flap.

suture, continuous, *n* a suture in which an uninterrupted length of suture material is used to close an incision or laceration.

suture, frontomalar, *n* most lateral point of the suture between the frontal and malar bones.

suture, interdental, *n* a suture that joins two sides of the gingiva by passing between the teeth.

suture, intermaxillary **(median palatine suture),** *n* the line of fusion of the two maxillae, starting between the central incisors and extending posteriorly across the palate, separating it into two nearly equal parts.

suture, interrupted, *n* individual stitches, each tied separately.

suture knot, *n* the tiny fastening

used to hold a suture in place firmly but not too tightly. The specific type is dictated by procedure, incision location, and tension required to close the wound.

suture, mattress, n a continuous suture that is applied back and forth through the tissues in the same vertical plane but at a different depth, or in the same horizontal plane but at the same depth.

suture, median palatine, n See suture, intermaxillary.

suture, monofilament, n refers to the single-strand composition of the material used to secure surgical stitches.

suture, multifilament, n refers to the multiple-strand composition of the material used to secure surgical stitches.

suture, natural, n a type of organic material used to secure surgical stitches that may react adversely with body tissue.

suture needle, conventional cut, n a suturing needle with three cutting edges, one on either side and a third located on the inside curve.

suture, nonabsorbable, n a suture that does not dissolve in body fluids (e.g., silk, tantalum, nylon).

suture, purse-string, n a horizontal mattress suture used generally about an implant cervix.

suture, shoelace, n a continuous surgical suture for depression of the tongue and retention and holding of the lingual flap out of the field of operation during the surgical impression.

suture, suspension (sling), n a type of surgical stitching used when the flap being repaired is open on the lingual or facial side; surrounds the tooth by passing between the surrounding teeth and gum tissue. The stitch is adjustable and allows for adjustment of the flap for proper healing.

Suspension suture. (Daniel/Harfst, 2002)

suture, synthetic, n new technology in surgical stitches developed to counteract the unreliable absorption rates and tissue sensitivity associated with natural stitches.

swage (swāj), v to shape metal by adapting or hammering it onto a die. Usually completed by forcing a counterdie into position on a die with the metal sheet interposed.

swager, n a laboratory instrument used for swaging.

swager, wax, n an instrument used to swage wax to a die.

swallowing, n See deglutition.

swallowing threshold, n See threshold, swallowing.

swear, v to take an oath; to become legally obligated by an oath properly administered.

sweat (swet), n perspiration. A clear liquid exuded or excreted from the sudoriferous glands. It possesses a characteristic odor, is slightly alkaline, salty to the taste, and, when mixed with sebaceous secretion, acidic. Sweating is under the control of the sympathetic nervous system, although it may be stimulated by parasympathetic drugs. Thermoregulatory sweating is influenced by the blood temperature's affecting the nervous centers and by reflexes associated with heat receptors in the skin.

sweating, gustatory, n See syndrome, auriculotemporal.

sweeteners, dietary, n any of a number of substances that provide the body with calories for energy; sources include sugars, other carbohydrates, sugar-alcohols, and nonnutritive sweeteners obtained from monosaccharides.

swelling, n one of the cardinal signs of acute inflammation; caused by the exudation of fluid from the capillary vessels into the tissue.

swelling, familial intraosseous, n See cherubism.

symbiotic relationship (sim′bī ot′ik), n in implantology, that relationship assumed by an implant and the natural teeth to which it has been splinted. The continuing existence of their relationship is based on their independence.

symbolic coding, n instructions written in nonmachine language.

symmetric, *adj* evenly balanced or uniformly developed.

sympathectomy, *n* a surgical interruption of part of the sympathetic nerve pathways, performed for the relief of chronic pain or to promote vasodilation in vascular diseases.

sympathetic (sim′pəthet′ik), *adj* pertaining to the sympathetic nervous system.

sympathetic nervous system, n See autonomic nervous system.

sympatholytic (sim′pəthōlit′ik), *adj* pertaining to a drug that blocks the effects of stimulation of the sympathetic nervous system. See also adrenolytic.

sympathomimetic (sim′pəthōmimet′ik), *adj* resembling the effect produced by stimulation of the sympathetic nervous system. See also adrenergic.

sympathy, *n* the kind understanding of a patient.

symphysis, *n* a line of union between two bony surfaces such as the pubic symphysis or symphysis of the mandible.

symptom, *n* any morbid phenomenon or departure from the normal in function, appearance, or sensation, experienced by the patient and indicative of disease.

symptom, constitutional, n symptom related to the systemic effects of a disease (e.g., fever, malaise, anorexia, weight loss).

symptoms, diagnostic signs and, n.pl See signs and symptoms, diagnostic.

symptom, prodromal, n the first observable indicator of an illness; the initial manifestation of a disease.

synapse (sin′aps), *n* the region of contact between the processes of two adjacent neurons forming the place where a nervous impulse is transmitted from the axon of one neuron to the dendrites of another. It also is called the *synaptic junction.*

synarthrosis (sinärthrō′sis), *n* a joint formed by thin intervening layers of cartilage, connective tissue, or direct contact of bone to bone. It results in a rigid union, and little movement of the bones occurs except during growth. Suture lines may be obliterated in adults, with a synarthrodial joint when the bones joined together become fused.

synchondrosis, *n* a cartilaginous joint between two immovable bones such as the union between the sphenoid and occipital bones at the base of the skull.

synchronous, *adj* having constant time intervals between events or occurrences.

synchronous device, n a term applied to a device in which the performance of a sequence of operations is controlled by equally spaced clock signals or pulses.

syncope (sing′kəpē), *n* swooning or fainting; temporary suspension of consciousness caused by cerebral anemia. See also shock.

syndactyly (sindak′təlē), *n* a congenital anomaly characterized by the fusion of fingers or toes, usually as a finding of a more complex congenital syndrome.

syndrome (sin′drōm), *n* a group of signs and symptoms that occur together and characterize a disease.

syndrome, adaptation, n See disease, adaptation; syndrome, general adaptation.

syndrome, adrenogenital, n disorder of sexual development or function associated with abnormal adrenocortical function resulting from bilateral adrenal hyperplasia, carcinoma, or adenoma. Pseudohermaphroditism occurs congenitally, and masculinization occurs later in females. Precocious sexual development and occasionally feminization occur in males.

syndrome, AHOP, n.pr **a**diposity, **h**yperthermia, **o**ligomenorrhea, and **p**arotitis appearing in females. Parotid gland enlargement begins at puberty and is followed by obesity, oligomenorrhea, and psychic disturbances.

syndrome, Albright's, n.pr a polyostotic form of fibrous dysplasia, usually associated with precocious puberty in females, endocrine disturbances influencing growth, and brown pigmentation of the skin.

syndrome, Apert's, n.pr craniostenosis characterized by oxycephaly and syndactyly of the hands and feet. Facial manifestations include exophthalmos, high prominent forehead, small nose, and malformation of the mandible and mouth. Also called *acrocephalosyndactyly.*

syndrome, Ascher, n.pr syndrome consisting of double lip, a redundance of the skin of the eyelids (blepharochalasis), and nontoxic thyroid enlargement. The sagging eyelids are obvious when the eyes are open; the double lip is seen when the patient smiles.

syndrome, auriculotemporal (**Bogarad's syndrome, Frey's syndrome, gustatory hyperhidrosis syndrome, gustatory lacrimation, gustatory sweating syndrome**), n sweating and flushing in the preauricular and temporal areas when certain foods are eaten. May be related to parotid trauma or a complication of parotidectomy.

syndrome, autoimmune, n See disease, autoimmune.

syndrome, Behçet's (**bā'sets, bekh'chets**) (**Behçet's disease**), n.pr recurrent iritis and aphthous ulcers of the mouth and genitalia. Other manifestations include arthralgia, hydrarthrosis, swelling of the salivary glands, cutaneous eruptions, and central nervous system disorders.

syndrome, Bloch-Sulzberger (**incontinentia pigmenti**), n.pr syndrome in which pigmented skin lesions, defects of the eyes and central nervous system, skeletal anomalies, and hypoplasia of the teeth occur.

syndrome, Bogarad, n.pr See syndrome, auriculotemporal.

syndrome, Böök's (**bœks**), n.pr syndrome characterized by premature graying of the hair, hyperhidrosis, and premolar hypodontia.

syndrome, Bourneville-Pringle (**epiloia**), n.pr neurocutaneous complex consisting of adenoma sebaceum, mental deficiency, and epilepsy.

syndrome, burning mouth, n a condition characterized by a burning sensation in the mouth, despite the absence of any visible irritation to the mucous membranes.

syndrome, Caffey-Silverman, n.pr See hyperostosis, infantile cortical.

syndrome, Christ-Siemens-Touraine, n.pr See hypohidrotic ectodermal dysplasia.

syndrome, Costen's, n.pr discomfort, pain, and jaw pathosis claimed by Costen to be caused by lack of posterior occlusion, loss of vertical dimension, malocclusion, trismus, or muscle tremor.

syndrome, cri-du-chat, n clinical syndrome associated with the deletion of the short arm of a B chromosome. Manifestations include mental retardation, various congenital abnormalities, and an infant cry resembling the mewing of a cat.

syndrome, crocodile tears, n a syndrome in which a spontaneous lacrimation occurs with the normal salivation of eating. It follows facial paralysis and seems to result from straying of the regenerating nerve fibers, some of those destined for the salivary glands going to the lacrimal glands.

syndrome, Crouzon's, n.pr See dysostosis, craniofacial.

syndrome, Cushing's (**Cushing's disease**), n.pr a symptom complex associated with an excess of adrenal steroids of all types resulting from hyperplasia of the adrenal cortex, malignant neoplasms, pituitary basophilia, or prolonged administration of adrenocorticotropic hormone (ACTH). Manifestations include hypertension, obesity, diabetes mellitus, osteoporosis, purple striae of the skin in areas of tension, and disorders of glucose tolerance.

syndrome, Down, n.pr See Down syndrome.

syndrome, Ehlers-Danlos, n.pr a congenital or familial disorder characterized by fragility of the skin and blood vessels, hyperlaxity of the joints, hyperelasticity of the skin, subcutaneous pseudotumors, and tendency to hemorrhage postoperatively.

syndrome, Ekman's, n.pr See osteogenesis imperfecta.

syndrome, Ellis-van Creveld, n.pr See chondroectodermal dysplasia.

syndrome, Feer's, n.pr See acrodynia.

syndrome, fetal hydantoin, n disorder developing in children who have been exposed to anticonvulsant therapy during the mother's pregnancy; indicated by mental deficiency, growth retardation, craniofacial abnormalities, cleft palate or lip, and congenital heart defects.

syndrome, Frey's, n.pr See syndrome, auriculotemporal.

syndrome, Fröhlich's (**adiposogenital dystrophy**), n.pr adiposity and genital hypoplasia resulting from hy-

S

popituitarism or hypothalamohypophysdystrophy.

syndrome, Gardner's, n.pr the development of multiple osteomas, polyposis of the large bowel, epidermoid or sebaceous cysts, and cutaneous fibromas.

syndrome, general adaptation (**adaptation syndrome, GAS**), *n* a three-stage physiologic response to physical or psychologic stress. The first stage is the alarm reaction, consisting of bodily changes typical of emotion. A second stage is resistance to stress, wherein an attempt is made to adapt to the physiologic changes. Certain hormones of the anterior pituitary gland and the adrenal cortex hypersecrete to increase resistance. Such resistance leads to diseases of adaptation, such as hypertension. Continual stress results in the third stage, exhaustion.

syndrome, Goldscheider's, n.pr dystrophic form of epidermolysis bullosa, leading to scars. The disturbance is inherited on an autosomal dominant or recessive basis. This form of epidermolysis bullosa leads to retardation of mental and physical growth. See also syndrome, Weber-Cockayne.

syndrome, Greig's, n.pr a condition manifested by ocular hypertelorism, often mental retardation, ectodermal and mesodermal abnormalities, and dental and oral anomalies.

syndrome, Gunn's, n.pr See syndrome, jaw-winking.

syndrome, gustatory hyperhidrosis, n See syndrome, auriculotemporal.

syndrome, gustatory sweating, n See syndrome, auriculotemporal.

syndrome, Heerfordt's, n.pr See fever, uveoparotid.

syndrome, Horner's, n.pr a tetrad of symptoms resulting from paralysis of the cervical sympathetic trunk: pupillary constriction, ptosis of the upper eyelid, dilation of the orbital blood vessels (redness of conjunctiva), and blushing and anhidrosis of the side of the face.

syndrome, Hunt's, n.pr herpetic inflammation of the geniculate ganglion, with herpes zoster of the soft palate, anterior faucial pillar, and auricular area.

syndrome, Hurler's (**mucopolysaccharidosis I H, gargoylism, dysostosis multiplex**), *n.pr* a heritable disorder of mucopolysaccharide metabolism in which excessive acid mucopolysaccharides—dermatan sulfate and heparitin sulfate—are made and stored in the tissues. Clinical manifestations include hypertelorism, open mouth with large-appearing tongue, thick eyelids and lips, anomalies of the teeth, and short, broad neck. The skeletal and facial deformities resemble the gargoyles of Gothic architecture. Mental retardation, corneal clouding, hepatosplenomegaly, deafness, and cardiac defects are present.

syndrome, Hutchinson-Gilford (**progeria**), *n.pr* syndrome of dwarfism, immaturity, and pseudosenility. Patient appears to be bald and elderly at an early age. Hypoplasia of the mandible occurs, and the face is small in relation to the neurocranium.

syndrome, jaw-winking (**winking-jaw syndrome**), *n* congenital unilateral ptosis and elevation of the lid on opening of the jaw or moving of the mandible to the contralateral side.

Jaw-winking syndrome. (Zitelli/Davis, 2002)

syndrome, Klinefelter's (**XXY syndrome, chromatin-positive syndrome, medullary gonadal dysgenesis**), *n.pr* presence in men of an abnormal sex-chromosome constitution. Persons with XXY constitution show the clinical signs of sterility, aspermatogenesis, variable gynecomastia, and often mental retardation. About 50% of subjects with XXXXY variant have cleft palate.

syndrome, Klippel-Feil, n.pr fusions of cervical vertebrae, short neck with limited head movement, and extension of the posterior hairline.

syndrome, Lobstein's, n.pr See osteogenesis imperfecta.

syndrome, Marfan, n.pr tall, thin stature, long, tapered fingers and toes (arachnodactyly), dislocation of the lens of the eye (ectopia lentis), and aneurysm leading to rupture of the aorta.

syndrome, Melkersson-Rosenthal, n.pr transient facial edema, especially swelling of the upper lip, facial paralysis, and lingua plicata. Plicated swelling of the mucosa of the tongue, palate, and buccal mucosa may not be present, or the paralysis may be incomplete.

syndrome, Mikulicz's, n.pr a condition characterized by swelling of the parotid, submandibular, sublingual, and lacrimal glands; associated with lymphosarcoma, leukemia, tuberculosis, sarcoidosis, and syphilis.

syndrome, Möbius's, n.pr congenital facial diplegia consisting of facial paralysis as well as lingual and masticatory muscle paralysis, inability to abduct the eyes, and anomalies of the extremities.

syndrome, Munchausen (**moon′chou-zen**), n.pr a condition in which a patient repeatedly reports to a physician or hospital for treatment of an illness, the symptoms and history of which have been entirely fabricated.

syndrome, myeloproliferative, n extramedullary myelopoiesis in adults. It may follow contact with benzol compounds or polycythemia, or it may precede leukemia.

syndrome, nephrotic (**nefrot′ik**), n syndrome that includes proteinuria, hyperlipemia, hypoproteinemia, and edema. It occurs in a variety of conditions in which increased glomerular permeability and urinary loss of protein occur.

syndrome, nonarticular pain, n one of several painful disorders that limit joint motion and affect the periarticular structures: the tendons, tendon sheaths, bursae, connective tissue, and muscles. Patients commonly call this syndrome "muscular aches and pains." The pains are chronic and nagging and may occur in acute exacerbations. The neck, shoulder, back, thighs, hands, and legs are common sites of irritation. The nonarticular disorders are associated with fibrositis, tendinitis, tenosynovitis, and periarticular muscle spasm. The precipitating agents are frequently obscure and may be associated with postural or personality disorders. When the acute symptoms of pain, stiffness, and restricted motion are reduced, the tissues resume their normal function. The common temporomandibular joint syndrome is believed to be caused by a postural occlusal imbalance associated with the muscular tension induced by psychologic stress. The combination precipitates an acute muscle spasm in the muscles associated with the protection and movement of the joint.

syndrome, Papillon-Lefèvre, n.pr extensive periodontal disease in young patients (juvenile periodontosis) accompanied by keratotic lesions of the palmar and plantar surfaces. In some patients changes similar to hereditary ectodermal dysplasia also are present.

Papillon-Lefèvre syndrome. (Neville/Damm/Allen/Bouquot, 2002, courtesy of Dr. James L. Dickson)

syndrome, paratrigeminal, n trigeminal neuralgia, sensory loss, weakness and atrophy of the masticatory muscles, miosis, and ptosis of the upper eyelid on the affected side of the face resulting from a lesion of the semilunar ganglion and fibers of the carotid plexus.

syndrome, Patau's, n.pr See trisomy-D.

syndrome, Paterson-Kelly, n.pr See syndrome, Plummer-Vinson.

syndrome, Peutz-Jeghers, n.pr generalized multiple polyposis of the intestinal tract, consistently involving the jejunum, and associated with melanin spots of the lips, buccal mucosa, and fingers; autosomal dominant inheritance.

syndrome, PHC, n See syndrome, Böök's.

syndrome, Pierre Robin, *n.pr* micrognathia of the newborn. Congenital retrognathism associated with cleft palate, glossoptosis, difficulty in swallowing, respiratory obstruction, and cyanosis. This congenital micrognathia corrects itself during the growth of the child if proper care is provided.

syndrome, Plummer-Vinson, *n.pr* a symptom complex that includes fissures at the corners of the mouth, sore tongue, dysphagia, achlorhydria, and iron-deficiency anemia. Most commonly seen in females in the fourth and fifth decades of life and associated with a predisposition to carcinoma of the oral cavity and esophagus.

syndrome, premenstrual (PMS), *n* a condition that occurs within 10 days before menstruation and ends soon after menstruation begins. The most common physical and psychological symptoms may include fatigue, heightened appetite, lack of coordination, headache, bloating or cramping of the abdomen, pain in the joints or back, pressure or pain in the breasts, depression, apprehension, and inappropriately aggressive behavior.

syndrome, Reiter's, *n.pr* a syndrome that consists of arthritis (often of the rheumatoid type), conjunctivitis, nonspecific urethritis, and occasionally aphthous ulcers of the oral mucosa.

syndrome, Rieger's, *n.pr* a syndrome the characteristics of which include hypodontia, conical crowns, enamel hypoplasia, dysgenesis of the iris and cornea, and myotonic dystrophy.

syndrome, Riley-Day (familial dysautonomia), *n.pr* disturbances of the autonomic and central nervous systems consisting of hypersalivation, defective lacrimation, excessive sweating, erythematous blotching after emotional upset, relative indifference to pain, and hyporeflexia. Normal growth and motor development are retarded.

syndrome, Robin, *n.pr* See syndrome, Pierre Robin.

syndrome, Roger's, *n.pr* continuous excessive secretion of saliva as the result of cancer of the esophagus or other esophageal irritation.

syndrome, Rosenthal, *n.pr* See hemophilia C.

syndrome, rubella, *n* enamel defects of the primary teeth attributed to prolonged effect of the rubella virus on ameloblasts during fetal life and in the postnatal period.

syndrome, Scheuthauer-Marie-Sainton, *n.pr* See cleidocranial dysostosis.

syndrome, sicca, *n* See syndrome, Sjögren's.

syndrome, Sjögren's (sicca syndrome, xerodermostecisis), *n.pr* condition related to deficient secretion of salivary, sweat, lacrimal, and mucous glands (xerostomia, keratoconjunctivitis, rhinitis, dysphagia), increased size of salivary glands, and polyarthritis.

syndrome, Smyth's, *n.pr* See hyperostosis, infantile cortical.

syndrome, Stevens-Johnson, *n.pr* an acute inflammatory disease characterized by oral, ocular, and genital lesions with severe generalized symptoms. The oral lesions are irregularly shaped, painful ulcers. See also erythema multiforme.

Stevens-Johnson syndrome. (Zitelli/Davis, 2002)

syndrome, Sturge-Weber, *n.pr* an encephalofacial angiomatosis characterized by cutaneous facial cerebral angiomatosis, ipsilateral gyriform calcifications of the brain, mental retardation, seizures (epilepsy), contralateral hemiplegia, and ocular involvement. Facial lesions (port-wine stain) may join intraoral angiomas on the buccal mucosa and gingiva.

syndrome, Swift's, n.pr See acrodynia.

syndrome, temporomandibular joint, n an acute muscle spasm in the muscles associated with the protection and movement of the joint. It is believed to be caused by a postural (occlusal) imbalance associated with the muscular tension induced by psychologic stress. The principal symptoms are pain in the region of the joint, limitation of mobility of the mandible, crepitus, clicking sounds in the joint, and frequently tinnitus.

syndrome, thalassemia (**Cooley's anemia, Mediterranean anemia, hereditary leptocytosis**), n any of a group of closely related and genetically determined disorders in which a specific decrease in one of the polypeptide chains constituting hemoglobin occurs. The defect results in hypochromic microcytic erythrocytes. Alpha, beta, and delta variants occur, as well as several subtypes based on biochemical techniques. See also thalassemia.

syndrome, Treacher Collins, n.pr an incomplete mandibulofacial dysostosis in which congenital deformities of the eyelids, mandible, and malar bones occur, as well as malocclusion, cleft lip and palate, and nasal deformities.

syndrome, Turner's (**XO syndrome, gonadal dysgenesis, genital dwarfism**), n.pr absence of one of the X chromosomes, with affected females being sterile and short of stature and having various congenital anomalies, such as webbing of the neck, low-set ears, wide set eyes, shield-like chest, absence of breasts, and cubitus valgus. Common orofacial findings are hypoplastic mandible, high palatal vault, and dental anomalies.

syndrome, Ullrich-Feichtiger, n.pr micrognathia, polydactyly, and genital malformations.

syndrome, Urbach-Wiethe, n.pr hyalinosis of the skin and mucous membranes and hoarseness. The skin is infiltrated with yellowish, waxy nodules, and the oral tissues with similar plaques beginning before puberty and becoming increasingly severe. The teeth may be hypoplastic or may fail to develop.

syndrome, vestibular disorder, n one of several syndromes involving the vestibule of the ear. The two most common syndromes of vestibular disorders are seasickness, which results from the continuous movement of the endolymph in susceptible individuals (probably related to a disturbance in the reflex control of the eyeball movements), and Meniere's syndrome, of which paroxysmal vertigo is the principal sign but other associated vascular and metabolic disorders can occur.

syndrome, Waardenburg-Klein, n.pr a syndrome consisting of congenital deafness, white forelock, increased distance between the inner canthi, the iris of the same eye or of the two eyes having different color (heterochromic iridon), and prognathism. Inherited as an autosomal dominant disorder.

syndrome, Weber-Cockayne, n.pr simple nonscarring form of epidermolysis bullosa; transmitted as an autosomal dominant trait. See also syndrome, Goldscheider's.

syndrome, Weech's, n.pr See hypohidrotic ectodermal dysplasia.

syndrome, Witkop-von Sallman, n.pr hereditary benign intraepithelial dyskeratosis with gelatinous plaques on hyperemic bulbar conjunctiva and white folds and plaques involving the oral mucosa.

syndrome, Zinsser-Engman-Cole, n.pr syndrome consisting of reticular atrophy of the skin, with pigmentation, dystrophic fingernails and toenails, and oral leukoplakia. Hyperhidrosis of the palms and soles is prevent, as well as acrocyanosis of the hands and feet.

syneresis (siner'əsis), n a process by which a fluid exudate forms on the surface of a hydrocolloid gel, even when the gel is in water or in a humid atmosphere. It is accompanied by shrinkage of the gel.

synergism (sin'urjizəm), n joint action of two drugs in such a manner that one supplements or enhances the action of the other to produce an effect greater than that which may be obtained with either one of the drugs in equivalent quantity or produce effects that could not be obtained with any safe quantity of either drug, or both. See also potentiation.

synergy, n the process in which two organs, substances, or agents work simultaneously to enhance the functions and effects of one another.

synostosis, n the joining of two bones

by the ossification of connecting tissues. It occurs normally in the fusion of cranial bones to form the adult skull.

synovial joint, *n* a freely movable joint in which contiguous bony surfaces are covered by articular cartilage and connected by ligaments lined with synovial membrane. Also called *diarthrosis.*

synovitis, *n* an inflammatory condition of the synovial membrane of a joint as the result of an aseptic wound or a traumatic injury, such as a sprain or severe strain.

syntax, *n* a property of language involving structural cues for the arrangement of words as elements in a phrase, clause, or sentence.

synthesis, *n* a putting together. The creation of a new entity or idea from elements not previously joined.

synthetic, *n* a substance that is produced by an artificial rather than a natural process or material.

synthetic porcelain, *n* See cement, silicate.

Synthodont, *n.pr* a brand name for a prefabricated ceramic implant.

syphilid (sif'ilid), *n* a cutaneous lesion of syphilis.

syphilis (sif'ilis) (lues), *n* a contagious venereal disease caused by *Treponema pallidum* and usually transmitted by direct contact. Oral lesions include primary chancre, secondary mucous patches and split papule, and tertiary gumma.

syphilis, congenital, *n* syphilis transmitted prenatally by the mother to the fetus. Congenital syphilis may lead to Hutchinson's incisors, mulberry molars, or rhagades. See also chancre; gumma; incisors, Hutchinson's; molar, mulberry; patch, mucous; and *Treponema pallidum.*

syphilis, latent, *n* a stage of syphilis in which no clinical signs or symptoms of the disease are present. It is usually discovered by serologic tests.

syphilis, primary, *n* the appearance of a small painless pustule on the skin of a mucous membrane within 10 to 90 days after exposure. The lesion may appear anywhere on the body where contact with a lesion on an infected person has occurred, but it is most often seen in the anogenital region. It quickly erodes, forming a painless, bloodless ulcer, called a *chancre,* exuding a fluid that swarms with spirochetes. The disease is highly contagious during this stage.

Primary syphilis. (Kerr/Ash/Millard, 1983)

syphilis, secondary, *n* occurs about 2 months after the primary stage. Secondary syphilis is characterized by general malaise, anorexia, nausea, fever, headache, alopecia, bone and joint pain, or the appearance of a morbilliform rash that does not itch, flat white sores in the mouth and throat, and condylomata lata papules on the moist areas of the skin. The disease is highly contagious during this stage.

Congenital syphilis. (Regezi/Sciubba/Jordan, 2003)

Secondary syphilis. (Regezi/Sciubba/Jordan, 2003)

syphilis, tertiary, n stage may not develop for 3 to 15 years after the initial infection. It is characterized by the appearance of soft, rubbery tumors, called *gummas;* the valves of the heart may be damaged, and late stages may lead to mental or physical disability and premature death.

Tertiary syphilis. (Regezi/Sciubba/Jordan, 2003)

syringe (sirinj´), *n* an apparatus of metal, glass, or plastic material consisting of a nozzle, or needle, barrel, and plunger or rubber bulb; used to inject a liquid into a cavity or under the skin.

Medical syringe. (Potter/Perry, 2001)

syringe, air, n a device by which air may be applied to a given area. An instrument supplied as part of the dental unit, consisting of a hand grip, nozzle, pressure-regulating valve, and hose connected to the compressed air supply.

syringe, aspirating, n a type of hypodermic syringe used in local anesthesia that allows the user to confirm, in advance of delivering the anesthetic agent, that the needle has not entered a blood vessel.

syringe, aspirating, breech-loading, n an aspirating syringe, used to deliver a local anesthetic, that is assembled by inserting the rubber stopper end of the anesthetic cartridge first toward the thumb ring, then the diaphragm end toward the needle opening before

setting the harpoon and attaching the needle.

syringe, combination, n a syringe that is usually part of the dental unit through which air, water, or a combination of the two may be delivered under pressure to the desired area.

syringe, hand air, n an air syringe consisting of a metal tube bent at one end, terminating in a reduced diameter, and enlarged at the other end to engage a rubber bulb. The bulb is compressed by hand to supply a controlled spurt of air to a given area.

syringe, warm air, n an air syringe equipped with an electric heating element to heat the air to any desired temperature.

syringe, water, n a device, usually part of the dental unit, permitting controlled application of water to a given area. It has a flow control, pressure regulator, and heating element.

system, *n* a set or series of organs or parts that unite in a common function.

system, acid-base buffer, n the system by which a virtually constant pH level of the blood and body fluids is maintained. The base and acid electrolytes associated with normal metabolism are continuously introduced into the bloodstream. Notwithstanding the marked amounts of base or acid or both introduced into the bloodstream during exercise, rest, hunger, or the ingestion of fluid and solid foods, the pH level of the blood remains rather constant between 7.3 and 7.5. Four means by which this relatively narrow but constant pH level is maintained are: the buffer system of the blood, tissue and cell fluids, and mineral salts of the bone matrix; excretion and retention of carbon dioxide by the lungs; excretion of an acid or alkaline urine; and the formation or excretion of ammonia and organic compounds.

system, apothecaries', n a nondecimal system of weights and measures traditionally used by druggists. See also system, avoirdupois.

system, autonomic nervous, n the part of the nervous system that regulates the reflex control of bodily functions. It controls the functioning of glands, smooth muscle, and the heart.

S

system, avoirdupois, *n* a commercial nondecimal system of weights and measures. See also system, apothecaries'.

system, central nervous (CNS), *n* the brain and spinal cord, including their nerves and end organs; controls all voluntary acts.

system, circulatory, *n* the heart and blood vessels. Three major groups of blood vessels are defined: arteries, capillaries, and veins. The system transports metabolites to and from the tissue cells.

system, computer, *n* an assembly of procedures, processes, methods, routines, techniques, and equipment united by some form of regulated interaction to form an organized whole. It is an approach to a complex problem.

system, flowchart, *n* a pictorial diagram illustrating the flow of information into, through, and out of a system of programs.

system, hematopoietic, *n* term used to describe collectively the blood, bone marrow, lymph nodes, spleen, and reticuloendothelial cells.

system, masticatory, *n* the organs and structures primarily functioning in mastication: the jaws, teeth, and their supporting structures; temporomandibular articulation; mandibular musculature; tongue; lips; cheeks; and oral mucosa and their nerve supplies.

system, metric, *n* a decimal system of weights and measures almost universally used in scientific and professional work, including the writing of prescriptions. The individual units are based on an international set of standards, notably the meter, liter, and kilogram.

system, musculoskeletal, *n* the system of body structures that provides the energy and movement necessary for the functions of life. The muscles, bones, and connective tissues of the body are grouped together into one system, and they are intimately connected in their individual and combined functions. For example, for muscle to accomplish its ultimate purpose of movement by contraction, bone, leverage, and connective tissue are required to transmit the force that the contraction generates. In the oral cavity and its related structures the musculoskeletal tissues fulfill the mechanical and structural requirements for movement of the mandible and some related visceral functions, such as respiration and digestion.

system, neurohormonal, *n* the system by which the hormone secretions of the endocrine glands function in part as the regulators of both visceral and somatic function and have intimate anatomic and functional relationships with the nervous system by the union of the pituitary gland and the hypothalamus of the cerebrum. The pituitary gland has a pars nervosa, which is an extension of the anterior part of the hypothalamus, and a pars intermedia, which is an epithelial evagination of the secretory tissue from the stomodeum of the embryo. From its position in the cranial structures in the sella turcica, the pituitary gland regulates, by its union with the nervous system, the whole endocrine system, with its many glands; these glands in turn partially regulate the viscera and somatic muscle organs.

system, occlusal (occlusal scheme), *n* the form or design and arrangement of the occlusal and incisal units of a dentition or of the teeth on a denture. See also system, masticatory.

system, parasympathetic nervous, *n* one of the motor divisions of the autonomic nervous system. It is described as the *craniosacral division* and does not have the simplified structural apparatus of the strong sympathetic adrenal axis about which to function. The parasympathetic system inhibits the heart, contracts the pupils, and, in emotional states, produces a vagus-insulin axis of activity. The several parts function rather independently. The ocular division relates to the midbrain, and the bulbar division relates to the hindbrain. The bulbar division supplies the facial, glossopharyngeal, and vagus nerves. It also supplies the secretory and vasodilator fibers of the salivary glands and mucous membranes of the mouth and pharynx. In conditions of very loud noise or unusual anxiety states, the parasympathetic system causes unaccounted-for spontaneous urination, excessive salivary and gas-

S

tric juices, and either nausea or vomiting.

system, proaccelerin-accelerin, *n*
See factor V.

system, proconvertin-convertin, *n*
See factor VII.

system, stomatognathic, *n* the combination of all the structures involved in speech and the reception, mastication, and deglutition of food. The system is composed of the teeth, jaws, muscles of mastication, epithelium, and temporomandibular joints and nerves that control these structures.

system, sympathetic nervous, *n* one of the two opposing motor systems in the autonomic nervous system that mediate the activity of the viscera. (The other is the *parasympathetic system*.) The sympathetic system is composed of 21 or 22 ganglia in chains on each side of the spinal cord. The fibers connect with the spinal cord through these ganglia. The actions of the sympathetic division of the autonomic nervous system are closely allied to the action of the medulla of the adrenal gland; thus a sympathetic-adrenal axis that functions as a unit to protect and regulate the body environment may be conceived. The sympathetic control is modified by the volitional somatic control of the patient. The volitional control, superimposed on the autonomic control, gives rise to great variations in motor patterns, as seen in the face in the presence of emotional changes, such as in the blushing of shame and pallor of fear.

system, vascular, closed tube, *n* the type of vascular system, as in humans, in which the blood circulates through the vessels (or tubes) and is not dissipated into the tissues. The closed vascular tube system offers resistance to the pumping action of the heart because the pressures are cumulative with each pumping action. The elastic walls in the arterial vessels, particularly in the aorta, absorb the additional energy and release it slowly, thus creating the possibility of maintaining a fairly steady and safe pressure head throughout the vascular system. The high-pressure point at the height of cardiac contraction is the *systole,* and the low point

before the ventricular contraction is the *diastole.*

system, vascular, open tube, *n* in some vertebrates a vascular system with an open end that causes the blood fluid to dissipate into the tissues. This system starts with a maximal head pressure that diminishes until inertia in the blood is overcome. The blood is returned to the heart by muscle function, gravity, and diffusion. The blood pressure in this system fluctuates from a maximum at the heart to a minimum at the tissue cell.

system, venous, *n* a system of interconnected blood vessels that returns blood to the heart from the tissue and capillary bed through progressively larger vessels. The following affect the return of blood to the heart: thoracic pressure, associated with respiration; gravity, associated with body posture; the valves, diameter of the lumen, and muscle structure of the veins; muscle contraction of the somatic structures; the pressures in the arteriole system and capillary bed; and the nervous and hormonal system controls that regulate cardiomuscular activity. The influences over the venous system circulation are collectively termed *venopressor mechanisms.*

systematic error, *n* a nonrandom statistical error that affects the mean of a population of data and defines the bias between the means of two populations.

systematically, *adj* done in a well-organized, carefully followed pattern of procedure.

systemic lupus erythematosus (SLE) (sistem′ik lōō′pus er′əthem′ətō′sus), *n* an autoimmune disease that can be life threatening. Patients may have a distinctive pattern of facial redness and oral lesions. Endothelial damage to heart valves similar to that caused by rheumatic fever may occur.

systole (sis′təlē), *n* the period of contraction of the heart. The term specifically designates the contraction of the ventricles, as distinguished from auricular contraction. It occurs with the first heart sound. The pressure from the systolic contractions is taken up and stored as potential energy by the elastic properties of the aorta and other great vessels of the arterial system. This storage of energy protects the smaller, more fragile vessels from undue pressure. The even flow and steady pressure of the blood are sustained by the controlled release of the potential energy stored in the arterial walls into kinetic energy for movement of the blood during the diastolic phase of heart function. The pressure recorded at the height of the ventricular contraction is the systolic pressure. In the adult the normal blood pressure is 120/80 mm Hg (systolic/diastolic). It rises with advancing age to 135/89 at 60 years of age. See also diastole; pressure, blood, stage; and pressure, systolic blood.

T cell, *n* a small, circulating lymphocyte produced in the bone marrow that matures in the thymus. T cells primarily mediate cellular immune responses, such as graft rejection and delayed hypersensitivity.

T-4 cell, *n* a thymus-derived lymphocyte of the body's immune system with a role of destroying or neutralizing cells or substances identified as "nonself." The human immunodeficiency virus (HIV) commonly targets the T-4 cells, with the result that the body's immune defenses are severely damaged and opportunistic infections are allowed to flourish.

tabes, *n* a gradual, progressive wasting of the body in any chronic disease.

tabes dorsalis **(tā′bēz dôrsal′is) (locomotor ataxia),** *n* a form of neurosyphilis in which degeneration in the posterior roots of the spinal nerves and posterior column of the spinal cord exists. Manifestations include pain and paresthesia of the trunk, hands, and feet, abdominal pain crises, ataxia, Argyll Robertson

pupil, atrophy of the optic nerve, and Charcot's joint.

table, occlusal, *n* the occlusal surfaces of the premolars and molars; the basic collective topography, including the form of the cusps, inclined planes, marginal ridges, and central fossae and grooves of the teeth.

table of allowances, *n* a list of covered services with an assigned dollar amount that represents the total obligation of the plan with respect to payment for such service but does not necessarily represent the dentist's full fee for that service. Also called *schedule of allowances* and *indemnity schedule.*

tablet, *n* a small, solid dose form of a medication. It may be compressed or molded in its manufacture, and it may be of almost any size, shape, weight, and color. Most tablets are intended to be swallowed whole.

tachycardia (tak′ikär′dē ə), *n* an excessively rapid action of the heart; the pulse rate is usually above 100 beats/min.

tachyphylaxis (tak′əfəlak′sis), *n* **1.** the rapid development of tolerance on administration of closely spaced successive doses of a drug or poison. **2.** a decreasing response that follows consecutive injections at short intervals.

tachypnea (tak′ipnē′ ə), *n* an excessively rapid respiration. A respiratory neurosis marked by quick, shallow breathing.

tacrine HCl, *n trade name:* Cognex; *drug class:* cholinesterase inhibitor; *action:* a centrally acting, reversible inhibitor of cholinesterase enzyme; *use:* treatment of mild-to-moderate cognitive defects associated with Alzheimer's disease.

tacrolimus (FK506), *n trade name:* Prograf; *drug class:* immunosuppressant; *action:* inhibits T-lymphocyte activation leading to immunosuppression; *use:* prophylaxis of organ rejection in patients receiving allogenic liver transplants.

tactile, *adj* pertaining to the sense of touch.

tailpiece, *n* See aid, speech, prosthetic, velar section.

Takahara's disease, *n.pr* See disease, Takahara's.

Talwin, *n.pr* the brand name for pentazocine lacatate, a potent analgesic, which is as effective as morphine. Talwin is a controlled substance.

tamoxifen citrate, *n trade name:* Nolvadex; *drug class:* antineoplastic, antiestrogen hormone; *action:* inhibits cell division by binding to cytoplasmic receptors, inhibits DNA synthesis; *use:* advanced breast cancer that has not responded to other ther apy.

tang, *n* See connector, minor.

tank, processing, *n* a receptacle used in the photographic or radiographic darkroom for the chemical solutions used in the processing of films.

tannic acid, a vegetable tanning agent that attaches itself to collagen by hydrogen bonds. Tannic acid is used in dentistry as a cavity conditioner before placing a restoration.

tantalum (Ta) (tan′tǝlum), *n* a silvery metallic element, its atomic number is 73, and its atomic weight is 180.9479. Tantalum is a relatively inert, noncorrosive, malleable metal used in prosthetic devices, such as skull plates and wire sutures.

tantrum, *n* a sudden outburst or violent display of rage, frustration, and bad temper, usually occurring in a maladjusted child or immature or disturbed adult.

tape, dental, *n* a ribbon of waxed nylon or silk used to aid the prophylaxis of interproximal spaces and the proximal surfaces of the teeth. The flattened, wide form of dental floss.

tapering, *n* a process of shaping a clasp arm the better to distribute flexure throughout its length, thus reducing fatigue, strain hardening, and resultant fracture.

tapering arch, *n* a dental arch that converges from the molars to the central incisors to such a degree that lines passing through the central grooves of the molars and premolars intersect within one inch anterior to the central incisors. See also arch, tapering.

tardive dyskinesia (tär′div dis′kinē′zē-ǝ, -zhǝ), *n* possible reaction to the extended use of antopsychotic medicines in which the jaw and mouth move uncontrollably.

target, *n* the small tungsten block, embedded in the face of the anode, that is bombarded by electrons from the cathode in an x-ray tube.

target cell, *n* **1.** also called *leptocyte,* an abnormal red blood cell characterized by a densely stained center surrounded by a pale, unstained ring that is encircled by a dark, irregular band. **2.** any cell having a specific receptor that reacts with a specific hormone, antigen, antibody, antibiotic, sensitized T cell, or other substance.

target group, *n* a set of persons who serve as the focal point for a particular program or service. This is a smaller sample than the target population.

target organ, *n* **1.** an organ intended to receive a therapeutic dose of irradiation. **2.** an organ intended to receive the greatest concentration of a diagnostic radioactive tracer.

target population, *n* all individuals belonging to a certain group who have a distinct set of qualities.

target symptoms, *n.pl* symptoms of an illness that are most likely to respond to a specific treatment.

target-film distance (TFD), *n* See distance, target-film; source-film distance.

target-object distance (TOD), *n* See source-object distance.

tarnish, *n* **1.** surface discoloration or loss of luster by metals. Under oral conditions, it often results from hard and soft deposits. **2.** a chemical process by which a metal surface is discolored or its luster destroyed.

tartar, *n* See calculus, dental.

taste, *n* the sense of perceiving different flavors in soluble substances that contact the tongue and trigger nerve impulses to special taste centers in the cortex and the thalamus of the brain. The four basic traditional tastes are sweet, salty, sour, and bitter.

taste bud, *n* any one of many peripheral taste organs distributed over the tongue and the roof of the mouth.

taste enhancers, *n.pl* food additives that have little or no flavor of their own but when added to food bring out the taste of certain foods. Monosodium glutamate (MSG) is the most common flavor or taste enhancer.

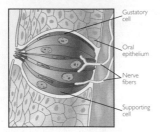

Taste bud. (Thibodeau/Patton, 2003)

tattoo, amalgam, *n* See amalgam tattoo.

taurodontism (tôr'ōdon'tizəm), *n* a tooth in which the pulp chamber is elongated and enlarged, and extends deeply into the region of the roots. A similar condition is seen in the teeth of cud-chewing animals.

Taurodontism. (Regezi/Sciubba/Jordan, 2003)

tautomer, *n* structural isomers that differ only in the position of a hydrogen atom, or proton.

tax, *n* a ratable portion of the proceeds or value of the property and labor of the citizen; any contribution imposed by government for the use and service of the state.

tax brackets, *n.pl* the income intervals of the graduated income tax law that establish the rate of tax for each level of income.

Tax Equity and Fiscal Responsibility Act of 1982 (TEFRA), *n.pr* legislation (Public Law 97-248) affecting health maintenance organizations and the Medicare and Medicaid programs. Provides regulations for the development of HMO risk contracting with the Medicare program and, through an amendment, establishes new provisions for the foundation and operation of peer review organizations.

tax planning, *n* making business and investment decisions based on estimated income and current and projected tax laws.

tax shelter investments, *n.pl* investments that reduce, remove, or defer income from state and federal income tax liability.

taxes, *n.pl* the sum of monies collected by the various branches of a government.

taxonomy, *n* a system for classifying organisms on the basis of natural relationships and assigning them appropriate names.

Tay-Sachs disease, *n.pr* an inherited, neurodegenerative disorder of lipid metabolism caused by a deficiency of the enzyme hexosaminidase A, which results in the accumulation of sphingolipids in the brain. The condition, which is transmitted as an autosomal recessive trait, occurs predominantly in families of Eastern European Jewish origin, specifically the Ashkenazic Jews.

teaching rounds, *n.pl* See rounds.

team practice, *n* professional practice by a group of complementary health care providers who collectively manage the care of a patient population.

technetium 99, *n* the radionuclide most commonly used to image the body in nuclear medicine scans. It is preferred because of its short half-life and because the emitted photon has an appropriate energy for imaging techniques.

technic (tek'nik), *n* See technique.

technical competence, *n* the ability of the practitioner, during the treatment phase of dental care and with respect to those procedures combining psychomotor and cognitive skills, consistently to provide services at a professionally acceptable level.

technical quality, *n* the degree to which the physically measurable attributes of procedures in dental care meet professionally acceptable standards.

technician, *n* a person skilled in the performance of technical procedures.

technician, dental, *n* See technician, dental laboratory.

technician, dental laboratory, *n* an individual skilled in the art of executing the dentist's prescription for the mechanical fabrication of dental appliances.

technique (teknēk´), *n* **1.** a skillful and detailed method of executing procedures to accomplish a desired result. **2.** the method of performance of manipulation in any art; the terms *technique* and *technic* are used synonymously, but the word *technique* pertains more to the artistic skill involved.

technique, aseptic, *n* task performed in a sterile environment in order to avoid contact with harmful bacteria.

technique, bisection of the angle, *n* an intraoral radiographic technique whereby an angle formed by the mean plane of the tooth and the mean plane of the film is bisected, and the central ray is directed through the tooth perpendicular to the bisection. This is the application of Cieszynski's rule of isometry. See also rule of isometry, Cieszynski's.

technique, calibrated angle, *n* an intraoral radiographic technique using a specified degree in vertical angulation from the horizontal plane. It is a variation of the bisection of the angle technique and assumed to be the correct angulation for the majority of patients.

technique, chew-in, *n* See chew-in technique.

technique, double investing, *n* a method of investing wax patterns, whereby the pattern is covered with a primary layer of investment; this core is then invested, before or after the primary investment has set, in an outer, thinner mix of the same or a different type of investing material.

technique, dual impression, *n* a technique by which the anatomic form of the teeth and immediately adjacent structures is recorded and by which the free-end denture foundation areas are registered in their functional form.

technique, Eames's, *n.pr* in dental amalgam, a procedure using mercury and alloy in approximately a 1:1 ratio, thus not having residual mercury in the plastic mix.

technique, filling, *n* the method used to obliterate the space in the root of the tooth once occupied by the dental pulp.

technique, Fones's, *n.pr* See method, Fones's.

technique, Gow-Gates (GG) anesthetic, *n* the injection of a local anesthetic that anesthetizes the mandible, along with the floor of the mouth, the anterior two-thirds of the tongue, the skin covering the zygomatic bone, and corresponding facial, buccal, and lingual tissues.

technique, hydroflow, *n* See dentistry, washed-field.

technique, impression, *n* a method and manner used in making a negative likeness. The series of operations or procedures used for making an impression.

technique, long cone, *n* the use of an extended cone distance, generally 14 inches (35 cm) or more, in oral radiography. It is generally used with, but not confined to, parallel film placement.

technique metered spray, *n* refers to a topical anesthetic dispersal technique that controls the amount and rate at which a drug is administered.

technique, Miller's radiographic localization, *n* a method of identifying the buccolingual dimension of a tooth by taking a second radiographic image at an angle of 90 degrees to the first. The technique is also useful for identifying the position of subgingival anomalies. Also called *right-angle technique; SLOB rule,* which stands for same lingual, opposite buccal. See also localization, radiographic; technique, parallel.

technique, parallel (**right-angle technique**), *n* a technique in intraoral radiography in which the film is positioned parallel to the long axes of the teeth and the central ray is directed perpendicular to both the film and the teeth.

technique, scoop, *n* office jargon for a one-handed method of needle recap and disposal in which the needle is used in an upward sweep to lift a safety cap onto the needle. The needle is then removed and discarded into a sharps container.

technique, short cone, *n* the use of a short cone distance, usually 8 inches (20 cm) or less, that is supplied by the manufacturer as short cone. It is generally used with, but not confined to, the bisection of the angle technique.

technique, telephone, *n* the friendly but businesslike conveying of ideas over the telephone.

technique, thermal expansion, *n* a casting procedure whereby compensation is made for metal shrinkage by thermal expansion of the refractory investment mold.

technique, wax expansion, *n* a casting procedure whereby compensation is made for metal shrinkage by thermal expansion of the wax pattern before setting of the investment.

teeth, *n* See tooth.

teething, *n* the eruption of primary teeth, which is preceded by increased salivation. Young children may become restless and irritable during this period. Inflammation of the gingival tissues before complete emergence of the crown may cause a temporary painful condition.

Teflon, *n.pr* trade name of a proprietary plastic material (polytetrafluoroethylene) used in reconstructive surgery of the jaw and chin.

Tegopen, *n.pr* the brand name for cloxacillin, an antistaphylococcal penicillin.

Tegretol, *n* See carbamazepine.

telangiectasia (təlan′jē ektā′zhə), *n* **1.** the dilation of the capillaries and small arteries of a region. A hereditary form (hereditary hemorrhagic telan-giectasia) may appear intraorally. **2.** a disorder characterized by cutaneous and mucosal vascular macules, nodules, and arterial spiders that tend to bleed sporadically.

telangiectasia, hereditary hemorrhagic **(Rendu-Osler-Weber disease),** *n* the dilation of small vessels and capillaries resulting from a genetic factor, with a tendency to bleed. Lesions may occur on the tongue as small, raised, red to bluish-red elevations.

Hereditary hemorrhagic telangiecta-sia. (Regezi/Sciubba/Jordan, 2003)

Telecommunication Device for the Deaf (TDD), *n* a machine that converts written text to speech, enabling the deaf to use the telephone.

Telecommunication Relay Service (TRS), *n* a system that enables the deaf and hard of hearing to use the telephone. The caller talks to a third party, who types the information so the deaf party can read it on a TDD.

telediagnosis, *n* a process whereby a disease diagnosis or prognosis is made by the electronic transmission of data between distant medical facilities. See also telemedicine.

telemedicine, *n* the use of two-way television communication by which two or more physicians can consult on a patient. The consulting physicians have access to the diagnostic information as well as the ability to view and question the patient directly before making a diagnosis or offering a professional opinion.

telemetry, *n* the electronic transmission of data between distant points.

teleradiography

(tel′ərā′dē og′rəfē), *n* Radiography at a longer distance than is usually used (6 feet, or 1.8 m).

telic (tel′ik), *adj* (teleologic), assigning purpose to functions as if they were provided by a creative planner.

temazepam, *n* *trade name:* Restoril; *drug class:* benzodiazepine, sedative-hypnotic (Controlled Substance Schedule IV); *action:* produces central nervous system (CNS) depression at limbic, thalamic, hypothalamic levels of the CNS; *uses:* sedative and hypnotic for insomnia.

temperature, *n* the degree of sensible heat or cold.

temperature, body, *n* the measurable temperature of the body. Normal range of variations, 98° to 99° F (35.5° to 37° C) orally and 99° to 100° F (37° to 38° C) rectally, with much wider ranges for skin.

temperature, body, regulation, *n* homeostasis of body temperature. Results from a balance of heat production (external heat plus heat from muscle contraction and other chemical processes) and heat loss (through lungs, sweating, surface radiation, and excretions).

temperature, casting, *n* the required degree of heat necessary to bring a metal to proper fluidity for introduction into a refractory mold.

temperature, core, *n* the temperature of the internal tissues of the body, this temperature stays stable, unlike the temperature of the outer body surfaces, which are affected by the environment.

temperature, recrystallization, *n* the lowest temperature at which the distorted grain structure of a cold worked metal is replaced by a new, strain-free grain structure during prolonged annealing. Time, purity of metal, and prior deformation are important factors.

tempering (hardening heat treatment), *n* the hardening or toughening of steels by heating. Treatment of an alloy in such a manner that solid-solid transformation occurs. Precipitation of intermetallic sub stances occurs, increasing the proportional limit and hardness of the alloy.

tempering, gold, *n* the hardening of gold alloys by cold working or by heating and then cooling slowly.

tempering, hydrocolloid, *n* storing of the material after liquefaction at a temperature that will increase the viscosity to the optimal manipulative degree of sol.

tempering, steel, *n* counteracting of the hardening heat treatment to the extent needed for the particular tool or structure. It is heated to a predetermined temperature and then quenched in water or oil.

template (tem´plət), *n* a pattern or mold forming an accurate copy of an object or shape.

template, implant, *n* an early type of subperiosteal implant that was fabricated from a cast carved to simulate the host bone. Measurements made from radiographs taken with a template or wire mold resting on the soft tissues determined the carving of the cast.

template, occlusal, *n* a stone or metal (electroformed) occlusal table made from a wax occlusal path registration of jaw movements and against which the opposing supplied teeth are occluded.

template, orthodontics, *n* a cephalometric tracing of an age- and sex-normed facial and dental profile used in the analysis of facial and dentition variations in malocclusion.

template, prosthetic, *n* a curved or flat plate used as an aid in setting denture teeth.

template, surgical, *n* a thin transparent resin base shaped to duplicate the form of the impression surface of an immediate denture and used as a guide for surgically shaping the alveolar process and its soft tissue covering to fit an immediate denture.

template, viral, *n* the process of RNA/DNA replication associated with retrovirus activity.

template, wax, *n* a wax recording of the occlusion of the teeth.

temporal arteritis, *n* a progressive inflammatory disorder of cranial blood vessels, principally the temporal artery, occurring most frequently in women over 70 years of age. The temporal artery is typically tender, swollen, and pulseless. Symptoms are intractable headache, difficulty in chewing, weakness, rheumatoid pain, and loss of vision if the central retinal artery becomes occluded.

temporal artery, *n* any one of three arteries on each side of the head: the superficial temporal artery, the middle temporal artery, and the deep temporal artery.

temporal bone, *n* one of a pair of large bones forming part of the lower cranium and containing various cavities and recesses associated with the ear. Each temporal bone consists of four portions: the mastoid, the squama, the petrous, and the tympanic.

temporal eminential angle, *n* the degree of slope between the axis-orbital plane and the discluding slope of the eminence.

temporal lobe, *n* the lateral region of the cerebrum, below the lateral fissure. It contains the center for smell, some association areas for memory and learning, and a region where choice is made of thoughts to express.

temporalis, *n* one of the four muscles of mastication. It arises in a fan-shaped pattern from the squama of the temporal bone and courses downward to insert along the anterior border of the ramus of the mandible.

It is a major closing muscle of the jaw.

temporary, *adj* pertaining to the interim treatment used to protect a patient between appointments.

temporary base, *n* See baseplate.

temporary prosthesis, *n* See prosthesis, temporary.

temporary stopping, *n* See stopping, temporary.

temporary superstructure, *n* a prosthodontic appliance (removable or fixed) that is used, often immediately postoperatively, as a transitional appliance either for cosmetics or splinting, or both.

temporomandibular articulation (tem′pərōmandib′yōōlur), *n* See articulation, temporomandibular.

temporomandibular disorder, *n* a disorder associated with one or both of the temporomandibular joints.

temporomandibular extraoral radiographic examination, *n* See examination, radiographic, extraoral, temporomandibular.

temporomandibular joint, *n* See articulation, temporomandibular.

temporomandibular joint (TMJ) arthrography, *n* a form of radiographic imaging using a compound of radioactive iodine that appears light-gray or whitish and contours soft tissues within the space between the joints.

temporomandibular ligament, *n* an oblique band of tissue that extends downward and backward from the zygomatic process to the neck of the mandible.

temporomandibular pain-dysfunction syndrome, *n* a triad of signs and symptoms consisting of pain in the muscles of mastication and jaw joints, clicking in the jaw joints, and limitation in jaw movements. Lesser findings may include dislocation and/or locking of the jaw joints and sensory changes in hearing. Also called *Costen's syndrome, mandibular pain-syndrome (MDS), TMJ pain-dysfunction syndrome (PDS),* and *myofacial pain-dysfunction syndrome (MPD).*

tenant, *n* one who has the temporary use and occupation of real property owned by another, the length and terms of the tenancy being usually fixed by a lease.

tender, legal, *n* coin or money that the law compels a creditor to accept in payment of a debt when offered by the debtor in the right amount.

tendon, *n* one of many white, glistening fibrous bands of tissue that attach muscle to bone.

tendonitis, *n* the inflammation of a tendon, usually stress or strain related.

tenosynovitis, *n* the inflammation of a tendon sheath caused by calcium deposits, repeated strain or trauma, high levels of blood cholesterol, rheumatoid arthritis, gout, or gonorrhea. Occasionally movement yields a crackling noise over the tendon.

tensile, *adj* having a degree of elasticity; having the ability to be extended or stretched.

tensile strength (ten′sil, -sīl), *n* See strength, tensile.

tension (ten′shən), *n* the state of being stretched, strained, or extended.

tension headache, *n* a pain that affects the head as the result of overwork or emotional strain, involving tension in the muscles of the neck, face, and shoulders.

tension, interfacial surface, *n* the tension or resistance to separation possessed by the film of liquid between two well-adapted surfaces (for example, the thin film of saliva between the denture base and the tissues).

tentative, *adj* not final or definite, such as an experimental or clinical finding that has not been validated.

teratogenesis, *n* the development of physical defects in the embryo.

teratogenic agents, *n.pl* See teratogens.

teratogenic effect, *n* the combined consequences of consuming a harmful substance, such as alcohol, on a developing fetus; may manifest itself as growth deficiency and/or mental retardation; fetal alcohol syndrome is an example.

teratogens (tərat′ōjens), *n.pl* agents that cause congenital malformations and developmental abnormalities if introduced during gestation.

teratology, *n* the study of the causes and effects of congenital malformations and developmental abnormalities.

teratoma (ter′ətō′mə), *n* a tumor composed of cells capable of differentiating into any of the three primary germ layers. Teratomas in the ovary are usually benign dermoidal cysts; those in the testis are generally malignant.

Teratoma. (Moore/Persaud, 2003, courtesy of AE Chudley)

terazosin HCl, *n trade name:* Hytrin; *drug class:* antihypertensive, antiadrenergic; *action:* decreases total vascular resistance, which is responsible for a decrease in blood pressure; *use:* hypertension as a single agent or in combination with diuretics or β-blockers.

terbinafine HCl, *n trade name:* Lamisil; *drug class:* antifungal; *action:* inhibits key enzyme, squalene epoxidase, involved with resultant fungal cell death; *uses:* tinea pedis, tinea cruris, tinea corporis.

terbutaline sulfate, *n trade names:* Brethaire, Brethine, Bricanyl; *drug class:* selective β_2-agonist; *action:* relaxes bronchial smooth muscle by direct action on β_2-adrenergic receptors; *uses:* bronchospasm, asthma prophylaxis, premature labor inhibitor.

terconazole, *n trade names:* Terazol 3, Terazol 7; *drug class:* local antifungal; *action:* interferes with fungal DNA replication; binds sterols in fungal cell membranes, which increases permeability, leaking of nutrients; *uses:* vaginal, vulvar, vulvovaginal candidiasis.

terfenadine, *n trade name:* Seldane; *drug class:* antihistamine; *action:* acts on blood vessels and gastrointestinal and respiratory systems by competing with histamine for peripheral H1-receptor sites; decreases allergic response by blocking histamine; *uses:* rhinitis, allergy symptoms.

term infant, *n* any neonate, regardless of birth weight, born after the end of the 37th and before the beginning of the 43rd week of gestation.

terminal, *adj* **1.** near or approaching an end, such as a terminal bronchiole or a terminal illness. *n* **2.** an input/output device that has a two-way communication capability with a computer.

terminal, computer, *n* a device in a system or communications network at which data can either enter or leave.

terminal hinge position, *n* See position, hinge, terminal.

terminal illness, *n* an advanced stage of a disease with an unfavorable prognosis and no known cure.

terminal jaw relation record, *n* See record, terminal jaw relation.

terminal plane, *n* ideal molar relationship in the primary dentition when in centric occlusion.

termination date, *n* See expiration date.

terminology, technical, *n* terms that are descriptive and meaningful to the dentist but are not a part of the patient's vocabulary.

terra alba (ter′ə al′bə), *n* gypsum added to plaster or stone to accelerate the setting reaction.

tertiary health care, *n* a specialized, highly technical level of health care that includes diagnosis and treatment of disease and disability in sophisticated large research and teaching hospitals. Specialized intensive care units, advanced diagnostic support services, and highly specialized personnel are characteristic of tertiary health care services.

tertiary syphilis, *n* the most advanced stage of syphilis, resulting in infections of the cardiovascular and neurologic systems and marked by destructive lesions involving many tissues and organs.

test(s), *n* any clinical or laboratory procedure designed to evaluate constituents or functions of the body.

test, acetone, *n* See test, ketone bodies.

test, ACTH-stimulation (**Thorn's test**), *n* a test of adrenocortical reserve based on changes in the eosinophil count and urinary levels of 17-ketosteroids and 17-hydroxycorticoids as a result of intravenous infusion or intramuscular injection of ACTH.

test, allergy, intradermal, *n* a test for allergy performed by injecting a preparation containing the suspected allergen into the dermis.

test, amylase (**am'ilās**), *n* a determination of serum amylase, which is useful in the diagnosis of acute pancreatitis and after operations in which the pancreas might have been injured. The Somogyi sarcogenic method is often used, and the results are given in *Somogyi* units, defined as the amount of amylase needed to digest 1.5 gm of starch in 8 minutes at 37° C. The normal range is 60 to 200 units/100 ml. The serum amylase is also elevated in mumps and other diseases of the salivary glands.

test, amyloid (**am'iloid**), *n* See test, Congo red.

test, antiviral antibody, *n* antibody tests in viral diseases. Included are complement-fixation tests for poliomyelitis, psittacosis, and Coxsackie infections; hemagglutination-inhibition tests for mumps, influenza, and encephalitides; and neutralization tests.

test, Aschheim-Zondek (**ash'hīm-tson'dek**), *n.pr* See test, pregnancy.

test, ascorbic acid, intradermal, *n* a test for ascorbic acid deficiency based on the decoloration of an intradermal injection of a purple dye (2,6-dichlorphenol-indophenol). Normally with a wheal of 4 mm, using a dye concentration of N/300, decoloration occurs in 10 to 15 minutes.

test, basophilic aggregation (**bā'sō-fil'ik**), *n* a test for lead poisoning based on increased stippling of erythrocytes. More than 2% stippled cells are seen in lead poisoning. See also test, lead.

test, Bell's palsy, *n.pr* simple clinical tests, such as motor function tests, in which the patient is asked to whistle, pucker the lips, smile, or wrinkle the forehead; also sensory function tests in which the patient is asked to taste sweet with sugar, sour with citric acid, bitter with quinine, and salt with sodium chloride.

test, Benedict's, *n* a nonspecific copper reduction test for glucose in the urine. Cupric sulfate in the Benedict's reagent is reduced by glucose during the reaction to cuprous oxide, a reddish-orange precipitate.

test, bilirubin (**bil'irōō'bin**), *n* qualitative, presumptive, quantitative, or specific determinations for bilirubin in the urine and blood serum. Included are Gmelin's test and van den Bergh's test.

test, bleeding time, *n* techniques for determining the time interval required for hemostasis to occur after a standardized wound has been made in the capillary bed. See also test, Duke's and test, Ivy's.

test, Brinell hardness (**brinel'**), *n.pr* a means of determining surface hardness by measuring the amount of resistance to the indentation of a steel ball. Recorded as the Brinell hardness number (BHN); the higher the number, the harder the material. Generally indicative of abrasion resistance.

test, Bromsulphalein (BSP), *n* a test of liver function based on the removal of a known quantity of Bromsulphalein from the blood in a measured period of time. Normal values are less than 5% retention at the end of 45 minutes with an intravenous dose of 5 mg/kg body weight. It is a useful test of hepatocellular disease and detoxifying ability but is not applicable in the presence of extrahepatic or intrahepatic obstructive jaundice.

test, Bunnell, *n.pr* See test, Paul-Bunnell.

test, capillary resistance (**Rumpel-Leede-Hess test, Gothlin's test**), *n* a test of capillary fragility based on the number of petechiae that develop when a standardized intraluminal positive pressure is applied to the capillaries either by a blood pressure cuff or a suction cup applied to the skin. See also test, tourniquet.

test, caries activity, n a test used to predict the probability of developing new or increased decay; may include assessments of saliva and plaque for the presence of certain designated microorganisms or studies of salivary secretion and sugar clearance.

test, CO_2 capacity (CO_2 combining power test), n a general measure of the alkalinity or acidity of the blood. Various normal adult ranges are given (for example, 23 to 30 mEq/L of serum or 55 to 70 vol/100 ml of serum). A low value is found in diabetic acidosis, hyperventilation, certain kidney diseases, and severe diarrhea. A high value is found in excessive administration of ACTH or cortisone, intake of sodium bicarbonate, and persistent vomiting.

test, CO_2 combining power, n See test, CO_2 capacity.

test, cold bends, n a mechanical test used for assessing ductility.

test, colorimetric caries susceptibility (**Snyder's test**), n a method of determining the concentration of acid-producing bacteria in the saliva by use of bromcresol green in a culture medium. The reliability of this and other salivary bacterial tests for dental caries susceptibility is questionable.

test, Congo red, n.pr a test for amyloidosis based on the more rapid disappearance (excess of 60% injected dye in 1 hour) of Congo red from the serum of affected patients than from that of normal individuals. Gingival biopsy and positive staining with methyl violet or crystal violet also indicate amyloidosis.

test, creatinine clearance (**krē at'inin**), n a renal function test of exogenous creatinine clearance. It is a convenient clinical test of glomerular filtration rate. It is calculated as the quotient of the product of urine creatinine (mg/L) and urine volume (L/24 hr) divided by the serum creatinine concentration (mg/L). The normal value for young healthy adults of average size (1.73 M^2 body surface area) is 115 to 155 L/24 hr (±15%).

test, dermal, n See test, skin.

test, Dick's (scarlet fever test), n a skin test to determine susceptibility or immunity to scarlet fever. A positive test is indicated when an area of erythema and edema measuring more than 10 mm in diameter occurs 8 to 24 hours after an intradermal injection of a standardized erythrogenic toxin.

test, Duke's, n.pr a test of bleeding time as indicated by the time that elapses before a puncture wound of the earlobe ceases to bleed. Normal range is 2 to 4½ minutes.

test, electric, n a test to determine whether a pulp is vital.

test, erythrocyte sedimentation, n a macroscopic test of the blood used to detect certain pathologic conditions, particularly inflammation. The blood cells are allowed to settle in the presence of an anticoagulant and the time (sedimentation time) determined. The greater the time or rate, the more severe the condition. Pregnancy and menstruation affect the sedimentation.

test, flow, n used in the ADA specification for dental amalgam; measured as the percentage shortening of a cylinder of the material.

test, fluorescent treponemal antibody, absorbed (FTA-APS), n a modification of the original FTA test for syphilis that employs a protein preparation from the Reiter treponeme.

test for trigeminal nerve function, n.pl three simple clinical tests for trigeminal nerve function: (1) *sensation:* apply gentle touch, pinpricks, or warm or cold objects to areas supplied by the nerve and note responses; (2) *reflex:* try the jaw jerk and eye and sneeze reflexes; (3) *motor function:* test the patient's ability to chew and work against resistance and observe contraction of the masseter and temporal muscles by visual examination and digital palpation.

test, Foshay's, n.pr a skin test for tularemia using the Foshay antigen.

test, Friedman's (frēdmənz), n.pr See test, pregnancy.

test, glare, n an examination of blade sharpness using a magnifying glass under light, which reveals dull edges as round, shiny, reflective surfaces.

test, glucose paper, *n* a test in which paper is impregnated with glucose oxidase and other reagents (TesTape, Clinistix). When the paper is moistened with fresh urine, the presence of glucose will cause a change in the color of the paper.

test, glucose tolerance (GTT), *n* a test for abnormalities of carbohydrate tolerance by glucose loading and subsequent serial measurements of the concentration of glucose in the blood. Graphic representation of the concentration and the elapsed time makes up the glucose tolerance curve. Abnormal curves occur in diabetes mellitus, thyrotoxicosis, Cushing's syndrome, acromegaly, and pheochromocytoma.

test, Gothlin's, *n.pr* See test, capillary resistance.

test, hardness, *n* See hardness, Mohs; test, Brinell hardness; test, Knoop hardness; and test, Vickers hardness.

test, Hess's, *n.pr* See test, capillary resistance.

test, histoplasmin **(his'tōplaz'min),** *n* a skin test to determine sensitization to *Histoplasma capsulatum.* A positive test indicates past or present infection (histoplasmosis).

test, infectious mononucleosis, *n* one of several tests for the diagnosis of infectious mononucleosis (for example, Paul-Bunnell test).

test, intracutaneous, *n* See test, skin.

test, intradermal, *n* See test, skin.

test, Ivy's, *n.pr* a test of bleeding time performed by making a standard wound and touching the blood with filter paper every 30 seconds until no blood appears on the paper. Normal range is 3 to 7 minutes.

test, Janet's, *n.pr* a test to differentiate between functional and organic anesthesia. With the eyes closed, patients are instructed to say "yes" or "no" as they feel or do not feel the examiner's touch. In functional anesthesia, they will say "no," whereas in organic anesthesia, they will say nothing.

test, ketone bodies **(acetone test, Rothera's test),** *n* nitroprusside reaction tests for acetone and acetoacetic acid and the ferric chloride test for

acetoacetic acid. Commercially prepared nitroprusside test tablets (Acetest) and powder (Acetone Test Denco) are available.

test, Kline's, *n.pr* a flocculation test for syphilis based on the combination of the cardiolipin antigen with reagin to form grossly visible aggregates.

test, Knoop hardness, *n.pr* a means of measuring surface hardness by resistance to the penetration of an indenting tool made of diamond. Produces an indentation that has a diamond or rhombic shape. Especially preferred for testing hardness of tooth structure.

test, laboratory, *n* investigative procedures performed in the laboratory that are useful in the diagnosis of disease, including biopsy examination of tissue specimens, determination of type and characteristics of associated microorganisms, serology, blood and urine chemistry, hemogram (red cell count, hemoglobin content, white cell count, differential white cell count), and metabolic studies (basal metabolic rate).

test, LE, *n* a test for lupus erythematosus based on the presence of a single (or multiple) homogenous basophilic inclusion(s) in polymorphonuclear leukocytes. Such LE cells have also been found in cases of rheumatoid arthritis, allergic reactions to penicillin, hydralazine toxicity, and "lupoid cirrhosis." Thus the test is not definitive for lupus only; it is one of the diagnostic tests for causation.

test, lead, *n* any of several tests used to detect clinical lead poisoning or exposure to lead (for example, coproporphyrinuria test, trace element analysis, urinary lead content test, and basophilic aggregation test).

test, Leede's, *n.pr* See test, capillary resistance.

test, Mann-Whitney U, *n.pr* a powerful nonparametric statistic test of significance between two means with unequal sample sizes.

test, Mantoux **(mäntōō'),** *n.pr* an intracutaneous tuberculin test using either old tuberculin (OT) or purified protein derivative (PPD). A positive reaction read 24 and 48 hours after injection shows erythema and edema greater than 5 mm in diameter and indicates past or present tuberculosis.

test, Mazzini's **(motsē'nēz),** *n.pr* a flocculation test for syphilis.

test, Mohs, *n.pr* See hardness, Mohs.

test, nontreponemal antigen, *n.pl* serologic tests for syphilis using nontreponemal antigens. Such tests are not absolutely specific or sensitive for syphilis. Included are the Kline, Kahn, and Kolmer tests, and the VDRL slide test.

test, one-stage, *n* See time, prothrombin.

test, patch, *n* (percutaneous test), a test for allergies that is performed by placing the suspected allergen in direct contact with the skin or mucosa. See also test, skin.

test, Paul-Bunnell, *n.pr* a test for infectious mononucleosis based on increased agglutination of sheep red blood cells resulting from heterophil antibodies in the serum. The test is considered positive if dilution of serum of 1:80 or higher agglutinates the sheep cells. Elevated agglutinin titers are more likely to be found during the second or third week of the disease, but the serum may not become positive until 7 weeks have elapsed.

test, percussion, *n* a method of examination executed by striking the tissues of the area being examined with the fingers or an instrument, listening for resulting sounds, and observing the response of the patient.

test, percutaneous **(pur'kyōōtā'nē-us),** *n* See test, patch.

test, Phelan's (fā'lənz), *n* a common test for diagnosing carpal tunnel syndrome. In a positive Phelan's test, tingling or numbness is felt within one minute when the subject's hands are held with the wrists flexed (usually at a 90° angle).

test, phenolsulfonphthalein (PSP) **(fē'nôlsul'fonthā'lēn),** *n* a renal test that roughly estimates glomerular function by measuring the rate of excretion of the dye after intravenous injection. Normally, after 15 minutes, 25% or more of the dye should be excreted in the urine.

test, plasma ketone *n* a test using nitroprusside for the detection of high levels of ketone bodies in the blood. The test is read 0 to 4 plus. A strongly positive reaction is seen in diabetic ketoacidosis.

test, prothrombin consumption **(serum prothrombin time),** *n* a convenient screening test of the first stage of blood coagulation as determined by the quantity of prothrombin remaining after coagulation. The test reflects the formation of plasma thromboplastin, provided the one-stage prothrombin time of plasma is normal. See also time, prothrombin.

test, pulp, *n* a diagnostic test to determine clinical pulp vitality and/or abnormality.

test, Reiter protein complement-fixation (RPCF) **(rī'tur),** *n.pr* treponemal antigen test for syphilis using extracts from the nonpathogenic Reiter treponeme.

test, Rockwell, *n* an indentation test for hardness of a material. A static load is placed on a steel ball or diamond point, and the depth of the indentation is measured on the instrument. The depth of the indentation is remeasured after the load is increased. The hardness number is related to the type of point used and to the depth of the indentation.

test, Rothera's, *n.pr* See test, ketone bodies.

test, routine, *n* a test or group of tests performed on most or all patients to detect relatively common disorders or to establish a base for further evaluation of a patient.

test, Rumpel-Leede-Hess, *n.pr* See test, capillary resistance.

test, scarlet fever, *n* See test, Dick's.

test, Schick, *n.pr* a skin test to demonstrate the presence or absence of an immunity to diphtheria.

test, scratch (skin test), *n* a test for allergies performed by placing a preparation containing the allergen on the skin and scratching the skin. A positive reaction is indicated by the formation of a wheal and flare.

test, serologic **(ser'əloj'ik),** *n* test of blood serum for the diagnosis of infectious diseases.

test, Snyder's, *n.pr* See test, colorimetric caries susceptibility.

test, sterilizer, *n* the periodic use of spore strip, color strip, or other microbial test to ensure that a sterilizer

T

(autoclave, oven) is killing all microbes predictably.

test strip, *n* a blood test used to check blood sugar levels in diabetics. The patient places a drop of blood on the strip, and the strip changes color according to the level of blood sugar present.

test, subcutaneous, *n* See test, skin.

test, syphilis, *n* any serologic test for syphilis based on the presence of a reagin, appearing during the second or third week of infection. Included are the Hinton, Kahn, Kline, Mazzini, Wassermann, and *Treponema pallidum* immobilization tests.

test, tension, *n* an evaluation used to determine the presence or absence of attached gingiva within the oral cavity. The tongue, cheek, and lip are retracted to apply pressure at the mucogingival junction and make the alveolar mucosa taut.

test, thermal, *n* the use of heat or cold as an aid in diagnosis (for example, the use of heat or cold in testing the pulp).

test, Thorn's, *n.pr* See test, ACTH-stimulation.

test, thromboplastin generation, *n* a test of the integrity of the first stage of blood coagulation and the nature of the defect. A patient's serum, plasma, or platelets are substituted in a system that is complete except for one of the factors to be tested for (antihemophilic factor, plasma thromboplastin antecedent, plasma thromboplastin component, or platelets), and the rate of thromboplastin generation is determined.

test, tourniquet **(tur′niket),** *n* a test for capillary fragility based on counting petechiae in a given area of the arm after application of the rubber cuff of a sphygmomanometer for 15 minutes.

test, transillumination, *n* a test for a pulpless tooth in which the use of transmitted light shows a shadow of the root when the pulp is necrotic or has been replaced by a filling (not always reliable).

test, **Treponema pallidum** *immobilization (TPI),* *n* a test to confirm syphilis by demonstrating the immobilization of *Treponema pallidum* by

specific antibodies in the serum of an infected individual; not widely used.

tests, treponemal antigen, *n.pl* tests for syphilis using *Treponema pallidum* or extracts from a treponeme as antigen. Included are *T. pallidum* immobilization (TPI), *T. pallidum* agglutination (TPA), fluorescent treponemal antibody (FTA), Reiter protein complement-fixation (RPCF), and *T. pallidum* complement-fixation (TPCF) tests.

test, tuberculin, *n* a test for past or present infection with tubercle bacilli. See also test, Mantoux.

test, tuberculin skin **(tōōbur′kyōō- lin),** *n* an intradermal injection of old tuberculin (OT) or purified protein derivative (PPD) to determine a specific sensitivity or susceptibility to tuberculosis.

test, tularemia, *n* See test, Foshay's.

test, U, Mann-Whitney, *n.pr* See test, Mann-Whitney U.

test, urea clearance, *n* a clinical test of renal function determined by the clearance of urea from the plasma by the kidney each minute. Average normal value is 75 ml/min (75% to 125% of normal).

test, urine, routine, *n* the routine examination of the urine, including amount, appearance, pH level, specific gravity, qualitative tests for sugar and protein, and microscopic examination of sediment.

test, van den Bergh's, *n.pr* a test of hepatic function by measuring serum conjugated ("direct-reacting") 1-minute bilirubin, total serum bilirubin, and, by difference, unconjugated (indirect) bilirubin. Obstructive jaundice and hemolytic jaundice give abnormal values.

test, VDRL (Venereal Disease Research Laboratory), *n.pr* a serologic nontreponemal antigen test for the detection of syphilitic reagin by means of a reaction between the reagin and a standard antigen.

test, Vickers hardness, *n.pr* a penetration type of hardness test using a square-based pyramid made of diamond.

test, vitality, *n* the procedure using thermal, electrical, or mechanical stimuli to determine the response of the pulp in a tooth.

T

test, Wassermann, *n.pr* a complement-fixation test for syphilis.

test, Zondek's, *n.pr* See test, pregnancy.

tests, liver function, *n.pl* tests to measure the severity of liver disease, aid in the differential diagnosis of the various types of disease of the hepatobiliary system, and follow the course of liver disease. Screening tests include urine bile, urine urobilinogen, Bromsulphalein (BSP) excretion, serum transaminases, thymol turbidity, cephalin-cholesterol flocculation, and van den Bergh's reaction (1 minute direct and total).

tests, pancreatic function, *n.pl* tests of enzyme levels in blood and urine (amylase, lipase), fecal fat content, trypsin activity, nitrogen content, alteration of digestive capacity, and alteration of pancreatic secretion via duodenal intubation.

tests, pregnancy (**Aschheim-Zondek test, Friedman's test**), *n.pl* biologic or chemical tests that determine pregnancy. The tests are usually based on changes in the ovaries of an animal injected with the urine of a pregnant woman. Included are the Aschheim-Zondek test (using mice or rats) and the Friedman test (using virgin rabbits). Male frogs and female and male toads are also used. A saliva test has also been used.

tests, pulmonary function, *n.pl* tests used to evaluate respiratory function (for example, tests of vital capacity, tidal volume, maximal breathing capacity, timed vital capacity, arterial blood gases).

tests, rapid reagin, *n.pl* serologic tests for syphilis that permit rapid and economic screening in the field. Included are the rapid plasma reagin (RPR) test and the unheated serum reagin (USR) test.

tests, renal function, *n.pl* quantitative tests including inulin or mannitol clearance for the glomerular filtration rate (GFR), paraaminohippurate (PAH) clearance for renal plasma flow, and the maximum rate of tubular excretion of paraaminohippurate and of reabsorption of glucose for the measurement of excretory and reabsorptive functions of the renal tubules. Clinical renal tests are used to assess the extent of renal impairment. They include blood urea nitrogen (BUN), nonprotein nitrogen (NPN), urea clearance, endogenous creatinine clearance, filtration fraction, phenolsulfonphthalein (PSP), and concentration tests.

tests, screening, *n.pl* a group of tests especially chosen to detect specific abnormalities.

tests, skin, *n.pl* tests to determine the sensitivity or susceptibility to infections by a specific agent, the presence of an allergy, or the presence of a nutritional deficiency. Included are the Mantoux, Schick, Dick, Frei, histoplasmin, and Foshay tests for infectious diseases (tests in which allergens are placed onto or into the skin) and the intradermal ascorbic acid, dermal, intradermal (intracutaneous), patch (percutaneous), scratch, and subcutaneous tests.

tests, thyroid function, *n.pl* tests for thyroid function (for example, radioactive iodine uptake, protein-bound iodine, basal metabolic rate, serum cholesterol, triiodothyronine suppression, thyroid-stimulating hormone tests).

tests, transaminase (**transam′inās**), *n.pl* tests for serum glutamic oxaloacetic trans-aminase (SGOT) and serum glutamic pyruvic transaminase (SGPT). The normal value for serum glutamic oxaloacetic transaminase is 40 units or less; that for serum glutamic pyruvic transaminase is 35 units or less. The serum glutamic oxaloacetic transaminase value in myocardial infarction is 3 to 20 times the normal.

testing stick, *n* a sterile plastic or acrylic rod that has a 3-inch length and a ¼-inch diameter and is used to determine the sharpness of an instrument.

testosterone/testosterone cypionate/testosterone enanthate/testosterone propionate, *n* *trade names:* Andro-100, Histerone-50, Testamone-100, Testaqua, Testoject-50; *drug class:* androgen, anabolic steroid (Controlled Substance Schedule III); *action:* in many tissues, testosterone is converted to dihydrotestosterone, which interacts with cytoplasmic protein receptors to increase protein production; natural hormone that functions to regulate spermatogenesis and male secondary sex characteristics; also functions as an anabolic steroid; *uses:* treatment of androgen deficiency, delayed puberty, female breast cancer, certain anemias.

tetanic contraction, *n* a condition of continuous contraction in a voluntary muscle caused by a steady stream of efferent nerve impulses.

tetanus, *n* an acute, potentially fatal infection of the central nervous system caused by tetanospasmin, which is an exotoxin, elaborated by an anaerobic bacillus, *Clostridium tetani.*

tetanus and diphtheria toxoids (Td), *n* an active immunizing agent containing detoxified tetanus and diphtheria toxoids that slowly produce an antigenic response to the diseases. Typically administered as part of the immunization series of preschool children.

tetany, *n* a disorder characterized by hyperreflexia, muscle spasms and cramps, foot and ankle spasms, choreiform convulsions, and sometimes stridor. Tetany is due to the malfunction of calcium metabolism. Possible causes are vitamin D deficiency, the ingestion of alkaline salts, hyperthyroidism, or alkalosis. There are many types of tetany, some of which are more common in animals.

tetany, hyperventilation
(hī'purven'tilā'shən tet'ənē), *n* the neuromuscular irritability and tonic carpopedal muscle spasm resulting from the alkalosis that may be caused by forced respiration over an extended length of time.

tetracaine/tetracaine HCl (topical), *n trade name:* Pontocaine Cream; *drug class:* topical anesthetic (ester group); *action:* inhibits nerve impulses from sensory nerves, which produces anesthesia; *uses:* local anesthesia of mucous membranes, pruritus, sunburn, sore throat, cold sores, oral pain, rectal pain and irritation, control of gagging.

tetracycline (te'trəsī'klēn), *n* an antibiotic produced by certain strains of *Streptomyces.* Its administration dur-

ing tooth formation may lead to enamel discoloration.

tetracycline HCl, *n trade names:* Achromycin, Achromycin V, Tetracyn; *drug class:* tetracycline, broad-spectrum antibiotic; *action:* inhibits protein synthesis and phosphorylation in microorganisms, bacteriostatic; *uses:* syphilis, gonorrhea, lymphogranuloma venereum, rickettsial infections, acne, actinomycosis, anthrax, bronchitis, GU infections, sinusitis and many other infections.

tetracycline periodontal fiber, *n trade name:* Actisite; *drug class:* tetracycline, broad-spectrum antiinfective; *action:* antimicrobial effect related to inhibition of protein synthesis; decreases incidence of postsurgical inflammation and edema; suppresses bacteria and acts as a barrier to bacterial entry; acts on cementum or fibroblasts to enhance periodontal ligament regeneration; *use:* adjunctive treatment in adult periodontitis.

tetrology of Fallot, *n* a congenital heart problem in which four defects occur at the same time: a hole between the two ventricles, a narrowing below the pulmonary valve, a misaligned aorta, and an overdeveloped cardiac muscle tone.

Tg value, *n* the transition point of glass; in dentistry, the temperature at which resin becomes soft.

thalamus (thal'əmus), *n* an ovoid mass in the brain immediately lateral to the third ventricle that serves as the principal relay and integration station for the sensory systems in the body.

thalassemia (thal'əsē'mē ə) (hereditary leptocytosis, hereditary microcytosis), *n* a hereditary, chronic, hemolytic anemia with erythroblastosis. A complex of hereditary disorders characterized by microcytosis and increased red blood cell destruction and frequently associated with abnormal hemoglobins and increased normal trace hemoglobins. These disorders are prevalent in people of Mediterranean, African, and Asian ancestry. Disorders include Cooley's anemia, Cooley's trait, hemoglobin H disease, Hb S-thalassemia, Hb C-thalassemia, and Hb E-thalassemia.

Thalassemia. (Hockenberry/Wilson/ Winkelstein/Kline, 2003, courtesy of James DeLeon, Texas Children's Hospital)

thalassemia major (**Cooley's anemia, erythroblastic anemia, familial erythroblastic anemia, hereditary microcytosis, Mediterranean anemia, Mediterranean disease**), *n* the severe homozygous form of thalassemia characterized by a marked microcytic hypochromic anemia, atypical nucleated red blood cells, marked increase in hemoglobin F, and skeletal changes (underdevelopment, mongoloid facies, anterior open bite).

thalassemia minor (**Cooley's trait**), *n* a heterozygous form of thalassemia that is a carried state with relatively mild manifestations; α_2 hemoglobin is elevated.

theophylline/theophylline sodium glycinate, *n trade names:* Aerolate Sr, Asmalix, Respbid, Slo-Bid, Theolair, Theovent, Uniphyl; others; *drug class:* xanthine; *action:* relaxes smooth muscle of respiratory system by blocking phosphodiesterase, which increases cAMP; *uses:* bronchial asthma, bronchospasm of chronic obstructive pulmonary disease, chronic bronchitis.

theorem, *n* **1.** a proposition to be proved by a chain of reasoning and analysis. **2.** a proven proposition used in the solution of a more advanced problem.

theory (thē′ ər̄ē), *n* an opinion or hypothesis not based on actual knowledge.

theory, Prothero "cone," *n.pr* See retention.

theory, quantum, *n* the theory that in emission or absorption of energy by atoms or molecules, the process is not continuous but takes place by steps, each step being the emission or absorption of an amount of energy called a *quantum.*

theory, somatotype, *n* the theory of W. H. Sheldon, suggesting that body structure is correlated with certain temperaments and predisposes to mental disorders.

therapeutic dose, *n* the amount of a medication required to produce the desired effect.

therapeutic index (ther′əpyōō′tik), *n* See index, therapeutic.

therapeutic vehicle, *n* a device used to transport and retain some agent for therapeutic purposes (for example, radium carrier).

therapeutics, *n* the art and science of treatment of disease.

therapist, *n* a person with special skills, obtained through education, training, and experience, in one or more areas of health care.

therapy (ther′əpē), *n* the treatment of disease, injury, or illness.

therapy, antibiotic, *n* the treatment of disease states by the local or systemic administration of antibodies.

therapy, antimicrobial, *n* a treatment modality that attacks the microorganisms responsible for a specific disease or condition.

therapy, chlorhexidine chip, *n* controlled delivery of the antimicrobial agent chlorhexidine in which a tiny, biodegradable dose of the drug is inserted into the periodontal pocket, where it continues to slowly release medication for approximately 7 to 10 days before disintegrating. This therapy is a means of attacking periodontal infection at its source without systemic involvement.

therapy, compromise periodontal maintenance, *n* a program of continuing periodontal treatment designed to slow disease progression in pa-

T

tients for whom surgery is not an option because of specific health concerns or economic restrictions.

therapy, doxycycline polymer, n delivery via syringe and cannula of a biodegradable liquid form of the antimicrobial agent doxycycline polymer directly into a periodontal pocket. The medication hardens upon contact with moisture, thus sealing the pocket and allowing the agent to destroy periodontal pathogens as it dissolves.

therapy, hormonal replacement, n the administration of synthetic female hormones in order to ease the negative impacts of losing these hormones due to menopause, hysterectomy, or disease.

therapy, indirect pulpal, n the application of a drug that heals the pulpal cells beneath a layer of sound or carious dentin, as in a moderately deep preparation for a restoration.

therapy, megavoltage radiation, n a form of radiation therapy used in the treatment of oral cancer. It delivers a more precise point of contact than other forms.

therapy, myofunctional (myotherapeutic exercises), n the use of muscle exercises as an adjunct to mechanical correction of malocclusion.

therapy, oxygen, n the providing of additional oxygen for patients who need it.

therapy, periodontal, n the treatment of the periodontal lesion. Such therapy has two principal objectives: the eradication or arrest of the periodontal lesion with correction or cure of the deformity created by it; and the alteration in the mouth of the periodontal climate that was conducive or contributory to the periodontal breakdown.

therapy, periodontal, maintenance phase, n the part of periodontal therapy that is necessary for the preservation of the results obtained during active therapy and for the prevention of further periodontal disease; an extension of active periodontal therapy, requiring the combined efforts of both the periodontist and the patient.

therapy, pulp canal, n See endodontology.

therapy putty, n a malleable, dough-like substance used in hand exercises to enhance the force and control of the hand muscles.

therapy, radiation (radiotherapy), n the treatment of disease with any type of radiation.

therapy, radiation, external beam, n a treatment for cancer in which a beam of high- or low-yield radiation is directed from outside of the body at the site of the cancerous tumor or lesion; may cause unnecessary radiation to normal tissues.

therapy, radiation, internal, n a treatment for cancer in which the radiation source takes the form of an interstitial implant. It is placed in the body among the affected tissues to provide a directed dose of radiation that is not possible using external methods.

therapy, radiation, orthovoltage, n a form of cancer treatment in which a beam of low-yield radiation is directed from outside the body at a superficial lesion, such as those found in the mouth or on the lips.

therapy, radiation, supervoltage, n See therapy, radioation, megavoltage.

therapy, replacement, n the administration, as a therapeutic agent, of an essential constituent in which the body is deficient (for example, insulin in diabetes mellitus).

therapy, root canal, n See endodontology.

therapy, speech, n the science that deals with the use of procedures, training, and remedies for the cure, alleviation, or prevention of speech disorders.

thermal conductivity, n See conductivity, thermal.

thermal expansion, n See expansion, thermal.

thermal sensitivity, n See sensitivity, tooth.

thermionic emission, n the release of electrons when a material is heated (for example, electron emission when the tungsten cathode filament of an x-ray tube is heated to incandescence by means of its low-voltage heating circuit).

thermistor, n an electronic device, functioning as a thermometer, for measuring minute changes in temperature. The resistance of a thermistor varies with the ambient temperature, thereby enabling accurate measurements of small temperature changes.

thermocoagulation, *n* the use of high-frequency electric currents to destroy tissue through heat coagulation. Also known as electrocautery.

thermocouple, *n* the joining of two dissimilar metals. The unequal thermal expansion of the two metals is used to indicate temperature changes.

thermography, *n* a technique for sensing and recording on film hot and cold areas of the body by means of an infrared detector that reacts to blood flow.

thermoluminescence (thur´mōlōō´mines´əns), *n* the capability of certain crystalline compounds such as lithium fluoride to release stored energy as luminescent energy when heated.

thermoluminescent dosimetry (thur´mōlōōmines´ənt dōsim´ətrē), *n* the determination of the amount of radiation to which a thermoluminescent material has been exposed. This is accomplished by heating the material in a specially designed instrument that relates the amount of luminescence emitted from the material to the amount of radiation exposure.

thermometer, *n* instrument used for taking temperature readings. Varying designs of the thermometer allow the temperature to be taken in the mouth, rectum, or externally at the axillary or groin areas.

Thermometers. (Zakus, 2001)

thermometer, external, *n* a reading from a thermometer which is taken at an external location (the armpit or groin) instead of by an internal method (the mouth or rectum).

thermometer, rectal, *n* a thermometer used to take temperature readings by insertion into the rectum of the patient.

thermoplastic (thur´mōplas´tik), *adj* the property of becoming soft with the application of heat, rigid at normal temperature, and again soft with the reapplication of heat. A reversible physical phenomenon.

thermosetting, *adj* having the property of becoming irreversibly rigid or hardened with the application of heat. In dentistry the term is used in connection with resins.

thermostat, *n* an automatic temperature control device.

thiabendazole (thī´-əben´dəzōl), *n* anthelmintic agent most effective against infection with the roundworm *Strongyloides.* Its effectiveness in treating other roundworm infections is varied.

thiamine HCl (vitamin B₁) (thī´ əmin), *n trade names:* Betalin S, Bewon, many others; *drug class:* vitamin B₁ water soluble; *action:* needed for carbohydrate metabolism; *uses:* treatment of vitamin B₁ deficiency or in prophylaxis, beriberi, and Wernicke-Korsakoff syndrome.

thiazides (thī´-əzīdz), *n.pl* See diuretics.

thiazolidinediones, *n.pl.* a class of medications used in the treatment of diabetes to make the tissues more reactive to insulin.

thickeners, *n.pl* See binder.

Thiersch's skin graft (tir´shəz), *n.pr* See graft, Thiersch's skin.

thiethylperazine maleate, *n trade name:* Torecan; *drug class:* phenothiazine, antiemetic; *action:* acts centrally by blocking chemoreceptor trigger zone, which in turns acts on vomiting center; *uses:* treatment of nausea, vomiting.

thimble, *n* See coping.

thimble, ionization chamber, *n* See chamber, ionization, thimble.

thinking, *n* **1.** the cognitive process of forming mental images or concepts. **2.** the process of cognitive problem solving through the sorting, organizing, and classification of facts and relationships.

thiocynate (thī´-ōsī´-ənāt), *n* compound present in tobacco smoke derived from hydrogen cyanide, used to confirm the use of tobacco by an individual.

T

Thiokol (thī′ ōkôl), *n.pr* trade name for polysulfide polymer using a mercaptan bond. The basic ingredient of rubber-base impression materials. See also mercaptan.

thiopental sodium, *n* a potent ultrashort-acting barbiturate used as a general anesthetic for surgical procedures that are expected to require 15 minutes or less, as an induction agent for other general anesthetics, as a hypnotic component in balanced anesthesia, and as an adjunct to regional anesthesia.

thioridazine HCl, *n trade names:* Mellaril, SK Thioridazine; *drug class:* phenothiazine antipsychotic; *action:* blocks neurotransmission at dopaminergic synapses in cerebral cortex, hypothalamus, and limbic system; exhibits strong peripheral α-adrenergic, anticholinergic blocking action; *uses:* treatment of psychotic disorders, schizophrenia, behavioral problems in children, alcohol withdrawal as adjunct, anxiety, major depressive disorders, organic brain syndrome.

thiothixene, *n trade name:* Navane; *drug class:* thioxanthene/antipsychotic; *action:* depresses the cerebral cortex, hypothalamus, and limbic system, which control activity and aggression; blocks neurotransmission produced by dopamine at the synapse; *uses:* treatment of psychotic disorders, schizophrenia, and acute agitation.

third party, *n* the party to a dental benefits contract that may collect premiums, assume financial risk, pay claims, and provide other administrative services. Also called *administrative agent carriers, insurers,* or *underwriters.*

third-party administrator (TPA), *n* claims payer who assumes responsibility for administering health benefit plans without assuming any financial risk. Some commercial insurance carriers and Blue Cross/Blue Shield plans also have TPA operations to accommodate self-funded employers seeking administrative services only (ASO) contracts.

third-party payer, *n* an organization other than the patient (first party) or health care provider (second party)

involved in the financing of personal health services.

third-party payment, *n* payment for services by someone other than the beneficiary (for example, when an employer or union makes such payment).

thixotrophic (thik′sōtrop′ik), *n* a type of gel with the ability to liquify when activated.

thoracic surgery, *n* the branch of surgery that deals with disease and injuries of the thoracic area, including the heart and major vessels and the lungs and respiratory tract.

thoracostomy, *n* an incision made into the chest wall to provide an opening for the purpose of drainage.

threat, *n* a menace; a statement of intention to harm or injure the person, property, or rights of another.

threonine (thrē′ōnīn), *n* one of the essential amino acids needed for proper growth in infants and maintenance of nitrogen balance in adults. See also amino acid.

threshold (thresh′ōld), *n* the lowest limit of stimulus capable of producing an impression on the consciousness or evoking a response in irritable tissue.

threshold dose, *n* See dose, threshold.

threshold, high pain, *n* higher than average capacity to withstand pain; exceptional pain tolerance.

threshold, low pain, *n* lower than average capacity to withstand pain; minimal pain tolerance.

threshold, swallowing, *n* the minimal stimulation required to initiate the reflex action of deglutition.

thrill, *n* **1.** a vibration felt on the chest wall over the heart. It is caused by the eddy flow of the blood, which is produced by a structural defect in the heart. **2.** palpable high-frequency vibration that may accompany cardiac murmurs or vascular disease.

throat, *n* a portion of the neck located in front of the spinal column; contains the trachea, larynx, pharynx, and upper segment of the esophagus.

thrombasthenia (throm′basthē′nē ə), *n* a hemorrhagic diathesis associated with qualitative abnormalities of the platelets.

thrombin (throm′bin), *n* a proteolytic enzyme formed from prothrombin by the action of thromboplastin, factor IV calcium (Ca^{++}), and other factors. Thrombin forms fibrin from fibrinogen, speeds up the disruption of platelets, and activates factor V.

thrombocatalysin
(throm′bōkatal′isin), *n* See factor VIII.

thrombocytes (throm′ bo-sīts), *n.pl* See platelets.

thrombocythemia
(throm′bōsīthē′mē ə), *n* an increase in the number of circulating blood platelets.

thrombocytin (throm′bōsī′tin), *n* See serotonin.

thrombocytopenia, *n* an abnormal hemotologic condition in which the number of platelets is reduced. Thrombocytopenia is the most common cause of bleeding disorders. See also purpura, thrombocytopenic.

Thrombocytopenia. (Neville/Damm/Allen/Bouquot, 2002)

thrombocytosis
(throm′bōsītō′sis), *n* unusually large numbers of platelets in the circulating blood. It may occur after surgical procedures, parturition, and injury, or with thrombocythemia.

thromboembolism, *n* a condition in which a blood vessel is blocked by an embolus carried in the bloodstream from the site of formation of the clot. The obstruction of the pulmonary artery or one of its main branches may be fatal. Emboli are diagnosed by x-ray films and other radiologic techniques.

thrombogen (throm′bōjen), *n* prothrombin. See also factor V.

thrombogene, *n* See factor V.

thrombokinase (throm′bōkin′ās), *n* See factor III.

thrombokinin (throm′bōkin′in), *n* See factor III.

thrombopenia, essential
(throm′bōpē′nē ə), *n* See purpura, thrombocytopenia.

thrombophlebitis
(throm′bōfləbī′tis), *n* an inflammation of the vein in which the vein becomes closed or occluded resulting from the development of a clot or thrombus.

thromboplastic plasma component (TPC), *n* See factor VIII.

thromboplastin
(throm′bōplas′tin), *n* a substance necessary to the coagulant activity of tissue extracts; also has been referred to as the direct activator of prothrombin and as a substance from plasma, platelets, and tissues that initiates thromboplastic activity in blood coagulation. See also thromboplastin, extrinsic.

thromboplastin, activated, n See thromboplastin, extrinsic.

thromboplastin, cofactor of, n See factor V.

thromboplastin, extrinsic, n a direct prothrombin activator formed by the interaction of brain extracts, factors V and VII, and factor IV calcium (Ca^{++}).

thromboplastin, incomplete, n tissue thromboplastin.

thromboplastin, intrinsic (plasma **thromboplastin, intrinsic prothrombin activator),** n a prothrombin activator formed from interaction of blood coagulation factors V, VIII, IX, and X and factor IV calcium (Ca^{++}) with a foreign surface.

thromboplastin, partial time (PTT), n a blood test used to determine von Willebrand's disease, hemophilia, and to monitor anticoagulant medications. Normal coagulation time is 68 to 82 seconds. An updated form of the test, activated partial thromboplastin time (APTT), is replacing PTT.

thromboplastin, tissue, n a factor in tissue extract responsible for coagulation of blood.

thromboplastinogen
(throm′bōplastin′ōjen), *n* See factor VIII.

thromboplastinogenase
(throm′bōplastin′ōjənās), *n* See factor, platelet, 3.

thrombosis (thrombō′sis), *n* presence of a clot or deposit in a blood vessel, formed in situ and remaining in place. An abnormal vascular condition in which a thrombus (blood clot) develops within a blood vessel of the body.

thrombosis, cavernous sinus, n a blood clot in the cavernous sinus occasionally arising from maxillary periapical infection. The prognosis is poor but not so grave as before antibiotic therapy.

thrombosis, coronary, n thrombosis of the coronary artery; also called *heart attack* and *coronary occlusion.*

thrombotonin, *n* See serotonin.

thrombozyme (throm'bōzīm), *n* See factor II.

thrombus (throm'bus), *n* a blood clot in a vessel or in one of the chambers of the heart that remains at the point of its formation.

thrush, *n* (candidiasis, moniliasis), a disease caused by *Candida albicans* and characterized by white patches that scrape off with some difficulty, leaving bleeding bases. This term usually is used for the intraoral disease, whereas *moniliasis* is applied to the condition in other areas of infection by the yeast, as well as in the oral cavity. See also candidiasis; moniliasis.

thumb sucking, *n* See finger sucking.

thymol, *n* a synthetic or natural thyme oil, used as an antibacterial and antifungal. It is an ingredient in some over-the-counter preparations for the treatment of acne, hemorrhoids, and tinea pedis.

thymoma, *n* a usually benign tumor of the thymus gland that may be associated with myasthenia gravis or an immune deficiency disorder.

thymus, *n* a single unpaired gland located in the mediastinum that is the primary central gland of the lymphatic system. The T cells of the cell-mediated immune response develop in this gland before migrating to the lymph nodes and spleen.

thyroid crisis (thī'roid), *n* a sudden exacerbation of symptoms of thyrotoxicosis characterized by fever, sweating, tachycardia, extreme nervous excitability, and pulmonary edema. If untreated, the crisis often is fatal. Also called *thyroid storm.*

thyroid function test, *n* one of several tests to evaluate the function of the thyroid gland. These include protein-bound iodine, butanol-extractable iodine, radioactive iodine uptake, and radioactive iodine excretion.

thyroid gland, *n* a highly vascular organ at the front of the neck, consisting of bilateral lobes connected in the middle by a narrow isthmus. The thyroid gland secretes the hormone thyroxine directly into the blood. It is essential to normal body growth in infancy and childhood. It also regulates the metabolic rate in adults.

Thyroid gland. (Thibodeau/Patton, 2002)

thyroid, lingual, *n* presence of thyroid tissue in the tongue, which is related to abnormal embryonic activity of the thyroglossal duct.

thyroid USP (desiccated), *n trade names:* Armour Thyroid, Thyroid USP Enseals, Thryo-Teric, others; *drug class:* thyroid hormone; *action:* increases metabolic rate; increases cardiac output, oxygen consumption, body temperature, blood volume, and growth and development at cellular level; *uses:* treatment of hypothyroidism, cretinism, and myxedema.

thyroiditis, *n* inflammation of the thyroid gland.

thyrotoxicosis (thī'rōtok'sikō'sis), *n* See hyperthyroidism.

thyroxine (thīrok'sin), *n* the hormone secretion of the thyroid gland, L-3,5,3′,5′-tetraiodothyronine.

tic, *n* an involuntary, purposeless movement of muscle, usually occurring under emotional stress. It is a survival in stereotyped form of a movement or muscle set once used voluntarily and purposefully.

tic douloureux, *n* spontaneous trigeminal neuralgia associated with a "trigger zone" and causing spasmodic contraction of the facial muscles. See also neuralgia, trigeminal.

ticarcillin (tĭk´ärsil´in), *n* an anti-*Pseudomonas* penicillin.

ticlopidine, *n trade name:* Ticlid; *drug class:* platelet aggregation inhibitor; *action:* inhibits first and second phases of adenosine diphosphate (ADP)-induced effects in platelet aggregation; *use:* effective in reducing the risk of stroke in high-risk patients.

t.i.d., *n* abbreviation for *ter in die,* Latin for "three times a day."

tidal volume, *n* the amount of air inhaled and exhaled during normal ventilation.

time, *n* a measure of duration.

time, clot retraction, *n* the time required for a given quantity of blood to separate in the tube in which it has been placed. For 3 mL of blood at room temperature, 1 hour is normal. It is very slow in thrombocytopenia.

time, coagulation, *n* the time required for blood clotting to begin in a capillary tube, normally 2 to 8 minutes. A coagulation time three times normal is a definite danger sign.

time, gel, *n* (gelation time), the interval of time required for a colloidal solution to become a solid or semisolid jelly or gel. Usually refers to the working time of a hydrocolloid or alginate impression material.

time, gelation, *n* See time, gel.

time limits, *n.pl* the periods of time within which a notice of claim must be filed.

time, median lethal, *n* (LD$_{50}$ time, MLT), the time required for 50% of a large group of animals or organisms to die after administration of a specified dose of radiation.

time, prothrombin, *n* (one-stage test), a gross but useful screening test of the completeness of the second and third stages of blood coagulation. Normal prothrombin time by the Quick method is 12 to 15 seconds. The time is affected by deficiencies of factor V or VII as well as of prothrombin. See also test, prothrombin consumption.

time, serum prothrombin, *n* See test, prothrombin consumption.

time, setting, *n* the length of time for a mixed preparation of materials to reach a state of hardness, measured from the start of the mixing. The end point for dental materials is usually determined by a penetration test.

time-sharing, *n* performing two or more tasks with a computer at the same time, made possible because computer speed is so much faster than operator speed that the computer can switch from one to another in brief time segments. The operators are not aware of the computer switching or any time delay.

timer, *n* radiographic timing device that functions as an automatic exposure timer and a switch to control the current to the high-tension transformer and filament transformer. The face of the timer is calibrated in seconds and fractions of seconds. The timer controls the total time that the current passes through the x ray tube and thus the time during which the x rays are emitted. The timer activates a switch or contractor that closes and opens the low-voltage circuit of the high voltage.

timer, electronic, *n* an electronic vacuum tube device, with no moving parts, that covers a time range of 1/20 to 10 seconds. It automatically sets itself, is more accurate than mechanical timers, and meets all the needs of modern high speed dental techniques.

timer, foot, *n* a timer with an attachment that permits the timing device to be activated by foot pressure. This is the preferred type of timer.

timer, hand, *n* an attachment to or part of a timer that requires thumb or finger pressure to activate the timing device.

timer, mechanical, *n* a timer using a spring mechanism for determination of length of exposure. Accuracy of timing is not assumed in exposures of less than 1 second with a mechanical timer.

timolol maleate, *n trade name:* Blocadren; *drug class:* nonselective β-adrenergic blocker; *action:* competitively blocks stimulation of β-adrenergic receptors in the heart and decreases renin activity, all of which may play a role in reducing systolic and diastolic blood pressure; inhibits β_2 receptors in the bronchial system; *uses:* treatment of mild-to-moderate hypertension, reduction of mortality after myocardial infarction (MI), and migraine prophylaxis.

timolol maleate (optic), *n trade names:* Betimol, Timoptic Solution, Timoptic-XE; *drug class:* β-adrenergic blocker; *action:* reduces production of aqueous humor by unknown mechanism; *uses:* treatment of ocular hypertension, chronic open-angle glaucoma, secondary glaucoma, and aphakic glaucoma.

tin octoate (ok′tō āt), *n* substance used to accomplish vulcanization of silicone rubber impression materials. It is not a true catalyst, because it becomes part of the final polymer.

tin oxide (SnO₂), *n* a polishing agent in the form of a purified white powder, prepared as a paste with glycerine or water.

tinfoil, *n* See foil, tin.

tinfoil substitute, *n* See substitute, tinfoil.

tincture (tink′chur), *n* an alcoholic, hydroalcoholic, or ethereal solution of a drug.

tinea, *n* a group of fungal skin diseases caused by dermatophytes of several kinds, characterized by itching, scaling, and sometimes painful lesions. *Tinea* is a general term that refers to infections of various causes, which are seen in several sites.

Tinea. (Habif, 1990)

tinea capitis, *n* a superficial fungal infection of the scalp seen most common in children.

tinea corporis, *n* a superficial fungal infection of the nonhairy skin of the body, most prevalent in hot, humid climates.

tinea cruris, *n* a superficial fungal infection of the groin.

tinea pedis, *n* a chronic superficial fungal infection of the foot, especially of the skin between the toes.

tinea unguium, *n* a superficial fungal infection of the nails.

tinea versicolor, *n* a fungal infection of the skin caused by *Malassezia furfur* and characterized by finely desquamating pale tan patches on the upper trunk and upper arms.

Tinel's sign (tinelz′), *n.pr* See sign, Tinel's.

tinnitus (tinī′tus), *n* noises or unpleasant sounds in the ears, such as ringing, buzzing, roaring, or clicking; usually high pitched. Heard by many persons with auditory impairment. Clicking tinnitus may be heard by others.

tinted denture base, *n* See base, denture, tinted.

tip frequency, *n* the measurement of the number of times the tip of an ultrasonic instrument moves back and forth to complete a cycle in one second.

tipping of cusps, *n* See restoration of cusps.

tissue (tish′ōō), *n* an aggregation of similarly specialized cells united in the performance of a particular function.

tissue adhesives, *n* agents or materials that may be used to seal two cut tissue surfaces together or cover a surgically exposed surface such as butyl cyanoacrylate, which is used to cover palatal donor sites in periodontal surgery.

tissue, compression of, *n* See tissue displaceability.

tissue conditioning, *n* a disciplined program of patient-performed plaque control measures designed for gingiva that is soft, spongy, and bleeds easily from poor oral hygiene habits, in order to improve gingival health before subgingival scaling is performed.

tissue, connective, *n* the binding and supportive tissue of the body; derived from the mesoderm; depending on its location and function, it is composed of fibroblasts, primitive mesenchymal cells, collagen fibers, and elastic fibers, with associated blood and lymphatic vessels and nerve fibers.

tissue, critical, *n* tissue that reacts most unfavorably to radiation or by its nature attracts and absorbs specific radiochemicals.

tissue displaceability, *n* the quality of oral tissues that permits them to be placed in or assume other positions than their relaxed position.

tissue displacement, *n* change in the form or position of tissues as a result of pressure.

tissue, flabby, *n* See tissue, hyperplastic.

tissue, hyperplastic, *n* in dentistry, excessively movable tissue about the mandible or maxillae resulting from increases in the number of normal cells.

tissue, interdental, *n* the gingivae, cementum of the teeth, free gingival and transseptal fibers of the periodontal membrane (ligament), and alveolar and supporting bone.

tissue molding, *n* See border molding.

tissue, peripheral, *n* See border structures.

tissue, redundant, *n* See epulis fissuratum.

tissue sloughing, *n* a surface layer of flesh peeling away. Possible causes are extensive exposure to topical anesthetic, overly abrasive toothpaste, smokeless tobacco, tissue burn, or mouthrinses. Also called *epithelial desquamation.*

tissue, subjacent, *n* the structures that underlie or are in border contact with a denture base; they may or may not have a supporting relationship to the overlying base.

tissue-borne partial denture, *n* See denture, partial, tissue-borne.

titer (tī′tur), *n* the standard amount by volume of a material required to produce a desired reaction with another material.

title, *n* evidence of the right of a person to the possession of property.

titration (tītrā′shən), *n* incremental increase in drug dosage to a level that provides the optimal therapeutic effect.

TMJ facebow, *n* See facebow, kinematic.

TMJ pain-dysfunction syndrome, *n* See temporomandibular pain-dysfunction syndrome.

TMP-SMX, *n* acronym for trimethoprim-sulfamethoxazole.

TNF, *n* an abbreviation for tumor necrosis factor, a genetic-triggered, tumor-killing agent produced by the body in small amounts to counteract neoplastic growth; an experimental agent used in the treatment of cancers.

TNM staging system, *n.pr* stands for tumor node metastasis, a recognized method used to identify and predict the course of disease of a patient diagnosed with cancer.

tobacco pipe, *n* a small, hand-held tobacco burning device that holds a burning, dried tobacco leaf in a small cup at one end, while user uses lips to draw smoke through a small cylinder attached to the side of the bowl.

tobacco use, *n* the practice of purposely using tobacco for its perceived physical and psychological benefits—for example, mental alertness, relaxation, weight control. Repeated use often leads to addiction. Product may be taken in to the body by inhaling the smoke from burning tobacco or by chewing a variety of smokeless tobacco products. Tobacco use is linked to diseases occurring in nearly every system in the human body, including but not limited to cancer, emphysema, hypertension, sudden death syndrome (SIDS), and osteoporosis.

Tobacco use. (Daniel/Harfst, 2002)

tobacco withdrawal syndrome, *n* a change in mood or performance associated with the cessation of or reduction in exposure to nicotine. Symptoms may range from lack of concentration to anxiety and temper outbursts.

tobramycin (ophthalmic), *n trade name:* Tobrax; *drug class:* antiinfective; *action:* inhibits bacterial protein synthesis; *use:* treatment of infection of the eye.

tocainide HCl, *n trade name:* Tonocard; *drug class:* antidysrhythmic (Class IB), lidocaine analog; *action:* decreases sodium and potassium conductance, which decreases myocardial excitability; *use:* treatment of documented life-threatening ventricular dysrhythmias.

Togaviridae (tō′gəvir′idā), *n* a family of enveloped, linear, nonsegmented RNA viruses with icosahedral symmetry, which includes the rubella and yellow fever viruses.

toilet of cavity, *n* See cavity, toilet.

tolazamide, *n trade name:* Tolinase; *drug class:* sulfonylurea (1st generation) oral antidiabetic; *action:* causes functioning β-cells in pancrease to release insulin, leading to drop in blood glucose levels; *use:* treatment of type II diabetes mellitus.

tolbutamide, *n trade name:* Orinase; *drug class:* sulfonylurea (1st generation) oral antidiabetic; *action:* causes functioning β-cells in pancrease to release insulin, leading to drop in blood glucose levels; *use:* treatment of type II diabetes mellitus.

tolerance (tol′ərəns), *n* the ability to endure the influence of a drug or poison, particularly acquired by continued use of the substance. See also resistance.

tolerance, acquired, n tolerance that develops with successive doses of a drug. If it develops within a short span of time, such as 24 hours, it is called *tachyphylaxis.* Slowly acquired tolerance is sometimes called *mithridatism.*

tolerance, carbohydrate, n the ability of the body to use carbohydrates. A decrease in tolerance is seen in diabetes mellitus, liver damage, and some infections and in the presence of hyperactivity of the adrenal cortex or pituitary gland.

tolerance, cross, n tolerance to a number of drugs of similar mode of action or chemical structure.

tolerance, individual, n tolerance characteristic of an individual.

tolerance, pseudo-, n a state of apparent tolerance indicated due to

failure of the drug to reach its usual receptor sites.

tolerance, species, n tolerance characteristic of a species of animal.

tolerance, tissue, n the ability of structures to endure environmental change without ill effect.

tolerance, upper intake level, n the specified limit of any given substance that an individual may consume and not suffer detrimental or toxic effects.

tolmetin sodium, *n trade name:* Tolectin; *drug class:* nonsteroidal antiinflammatory; *action:* inhibits prostaglandin synthesis by interfering with cyclooxygenase needed for biosynthesis; *uses:* treatment of osteoarthritis, rheumatoid arthritis, juvenile rheumatoid arthritis.

tolnaftate (topical), *n trade name:* Aftate, Tinactin, Ting, others; *drug class:* antifungal, topical; *action:* interferes with fungal cell membrane, which increases permeability and leaking of cell nutrients; *uses:* treatment of tinea pedis, tinea cruris, tinea corporis, tinea capitis, tinea unguium, and tinea versicolor.

toluidine blue dye (tolyōō′idēn), *n* a chemical substance used to identify potentially malignant mucosal deviations; use as a mouth rinse or apply over the affected area with a cotton swab.

Tomes's granular layer (tōmz′ əs), *n* a grainy appearing layer within dentin located in the root of the tooth beneath the dentinocemental junction.

tomogram, *n* See examination, radiographic, extraoral body section.

tomograph, *n* a radiograph produced while rotating the film and x-ray source in opposite directions around an axis located in the region of interest. This movement blurs outside structures while maintaining sharpness in the region of interest.

tomography, *n* an x-ray technique that produces a film representing a detailed cross section of tissue structures at a predetermined depth.

tongue (tung), *n* the muscular organ that is the main articulatory element in the production of speech and accounts for the clarity and fluidity of speech. Two groups of tongue muscles, the intrinsic and extrinsic, are united into one organ. Each group, however, has separate structural and functional characteristics.

Median sulcus   Filiform papillae (gray, thread-like)

Fungiform papillae (bright red, globular)

Tongue. (Liebgott, 2001)

tongue, amyloid (**amyloid macroglossia**), *n* enlargement of the tongue resulting from amyloidosis.

tongue, antibiotic, n a glossitis caused by sensitivity to an antibiotic, vitamin B complex deficiency associated with antibiotic therapy.

tongue, bald, n See glossitis, atrophic.

tongue, beefy, n erythematous or *atrophic glossitis.* See also glossitis, atrophic; glossitis, Moellcr's.

tongue, bifid (**cleft tongue**), *n* a tongue divided by a midline cleft.

tongue, black hairy, n (lingua nigra), a black appearance of the dorsal surface of the tongue; caused by elongated filiform papillae and an accumulation of dark pigments, microorganisms, and food debris.

Black hairy tongue. (Tyldesley, 1991)

tongue, cleft, n See tongue, bifid.

tongue, coated, n nonspecific term used to describe the condition of the tongue resulting from whitish or otherwise discolored accumulations of food debris, bacterial plaques, and hyperplastic filiform papillae. Reduced function, as in general illness or laryngitis, is a primary cause.

tongue, cobblestone, n hyperplasia and hyperemia of fungiform and filiform papillae of the tongue in riboflavin deficiency. Formerly used to describe syphilitic glossitis with leukoplakia.

tongue crib, n an appliance used to limit undesirable tongue movements, usually constructed to prevent its protrusion between the anterior teeth.

tongue depressor, n.pl a flat wooden stick used to position the tongue so that the back of the throat may be seen. Several may be used together as mouth props.

tongue, fissured (**furrowed tongue**), *n* a tongue traversed by clefts that may be arranged like the veins of a leaf or give the tongue a "pavement block" appearance. It is seen in 5% of all dental patients but in 13% of those older than 50 years.

tongue, flat, n paralysis of the transverse lingual muscles such that the borders of the tongue cannot be rolled. The condition results from congenital syphilis.

tongue, furrowed, n See tongue, fissured.

tongue, geographic, n (benign migratory glossitis, glossitis areata exfoliativa, glossitis migrans, wandering rash), a condition characterized by a chronic, circumscribed, more or less circinate desquamation of the superficial epithelium of the dorsum of the tongue. The spots of desquamation migrate continuously, usually passing from the region near the vallate papillae toward the tip of the tongue.

tongue, hairy, n hyperplasia of the filiform papillae of the tongue, frequently associated with oral moniliasis and the use of antibiotics or tobacco.

tongue, lobulated, n a congenital defect, with a secondary lobe of the tongue arising from its surface.

tongue, magenta, *n* the reddish-purple tongue of riboflavin deficiency.

tongue room, *n* See tongue space.

tongue, Sandwith's bald, *n.pr* a condition in which the tongue is very smooth because of a loss of fusiform papillae and is fiery red and enlarged because of severe inflammation; seen in pellagra.

tongue scraper, *n* an oral hygiene implement drawn down the tongue from the back to the front in order to reduce mouth odors and plaque-producing bacteria.

Tongue scraper. (Christensen, 2002)

tongue, smooth, *n* See glossitis, atrophic.

tongue space, *n* the space available for functioning of the tongue.

tongue, strawberry, *n* the red, inflamed tongue with prominent fungiform papillae characteristic of scarlet fever.

tongue thrust, *n* thrusting of the tongue between the anterior teeth, especially in the initial stage of swallowing. This action, often combined with a resting position also between the teeth, may inhibit normal eruption and produce an open bite.

***tongue, white hairy* (lingua alba, lingua villosa alba),** *n* hairy tongue characterized by elongation of the filiform papillae but without the dark staining seen in lingua nigra (black hairy tongue). See also tongue, black hairy.

tonguetie, *n* a condition in which a shorter-than-average lingual frenum connecting the tongue to the floor of the mouth limits tongue movement.

tonic convulsion, *n* a prolonged generalized contraction of the skeletal muscles.

tonofibril (ton′əfī′bril), *n* a fibril emanating from epithelial cells. Recent electron microscopy has shown such fibrils to be irregular formations of the cell membrane.

tonsil (ton′sil), *n* a rounded mass of tissue, usually of a lymphoid nature.

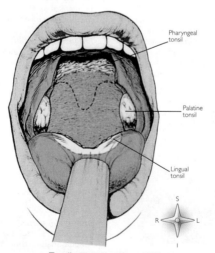

Pharyngeal tonsil

Palatine tonsil

Lingual tonsil

Tonsil. (Thibodeau/Patton, 2002)

tonsil, palatine, *n* one of two small tissue masses on opposite sides of the oropharynx, between the faucial pillars, which are believed to serve as the first line of defense against bacteria that enters the oral cavity via the mouth.

tonsillar, *adj* of or relating to the tonsils.

tonsillar recess, *n* depressed region located between the posterior and anterior faucial pillars. This is the location of the paltine tonsils.

tonsillar region, *n* area surrounding the tonsils. See also fauces.

tonsillectomy, *n* the surgical excision of the palatine tonsils, performed to prevent recurrent tonsillitis.

tonsillitis (ton′sili′tis), *n* inflammation of the tonsils.

Tonsillitis. (Neville/Damm/Allen/Bouquot, 2002)

tonsillitis, lingual, *n* a form of tonsillitis at the posterior part of the base of the tongue in the lymphoid masses (lingual tonsils) located there.

tooth (teeth), *n* one of the hard bodies or processes usually protruding from and attached to the alveolar process of the maxillae and the mandible; designed for the mastication of food.

teeth, anterior, *n.pl* the incisor or canine front teeth.

teeth, canine, *n.pl* the four canines; the third tooth located distal to the midline in any one of the four quadrants of the dentition.

teeth, deciduous, *n* See deciduous; tooth, primary.

teeth, drugs for sensitivity of, *n.pl* the medicaments used to treat hypersensitivity of the teeth. They should cause relatively little pain when applied; be easily applied, rapid in action, and permanently effective; and not discolor the teeth or unduly irritate the pulp. Substances used include 33% sodium fluoride in kaolin and glycerin, a 25% aqueous solution of strontium chloride, hot medicinal olive oil, and 0.9% solution of sodium silicofluoride.

teeth, grinding of, *n* the selective modification of tooth form and contour in the occlusal adjustment operation to eliminate occlusal interferences and establish tooth contours conducive to the health of the periodontium. See also bruxism.

teeth, hereditary brown, *n.pl* See hypoplasia, enamel, hereditary.

teeth, neonatal, *n.pl* primary teeth that erupt into the oral cavity during the neonatal period (from birth to 30 days).

teeth, permanent, *n* See dentition, permanent.

teeth, polishing of, *n* the removal of extrinsic stain, plaque, and soft deposits from the teeth by appropriate hand- or engine-driven instrumentation. Abrasive cups, wheels, and disks often are used in conjunction with such abrasive pastes as pumice and water, although less abrasive synthetic particles are replacing pumice. See also polishing, selective.

teeth, posterior, *n.pl* the maxillary and mandibular premolars and molars of the permanent dentition or the premolars and molars of prostheses.

teeth, primary, *n.pl* **1.** term used by some in preference to deciduous teeth; however, it has not received the approval of preference by the American Dental Association. **2.** as a result of a survey of the terminology used to name the teeth of the first dentition, the College Committee Report of Dentistry for Children recommended in 1942 the use of *primary teeth* in place of deciduous, first, milk, temporary, baby, or foundation teeth. The term primary was suggested as a word "which may be acceptable to the dental profession, significant in its meaning, with no connotations of impermanence, and readily understood by nonprofessional people." See also deciduous.

teeth, sensitivity of, *n* a painful pulpal response to external stimuli such as heat, cold, and sweet substances. The most common clinical finding is a hyperesthetic state of the root surface resulting from loss of a portion of the cemental covering with exposure of the dentin.

teeth, separation of, *n* the action of moving a tooth mesially or distally out of contact with its neighboring tooth.

teeth, set of, *n* usually a full complement of maxillary and mandibular artificial teeth as they are carded by the manufacturer.

teeth, slow separation of, *n* drifting apart of teeth accomplished over a long period, usually by the wedging action of a material such as gutta-percha, orthodontic wire, thread, or fibers in orthodontic therapy.

teeth, supportive mechanisms of, *n.pl* the anatomic structures that function to maintain or aid in maintaining the teeth in position in their alveoli: the gingivae, cementum of the tooth, periodontal membrane, and alveolar and supporting bone. See also structures, supporting.

teeth, vital staining of, *n* the staining of enamel and dentin of primary and permanent teeth during development with vital stains (for example, with bile pigment in Rh incompatibility or with tetracyclines).

tooth, abutment, *n* a tooth or teeth selected to support a prosthesis on the basis of the total surface areas of a healthy attachment apparatus.

tooth, accessory (akses´ə re), *n* supernumerary teeth that do not resemble normal teeth in size, shape, or location. See also distomolar; mesiodens; paramolar; tooth,

tooth, acrylic resin (əkril´ik), *n* a tooth made of acrylic resin.

tooth, anatomic, *n* an artificial tooth that closely resembles the anatomic form of a natural unabraded tooth.

tooth, ankylosed, *n* abnormal calcification of the periodontal ligament resulting in abnormal fixation of a tooth.

tooth, artificial, *n* a tooth fabricated for use as a substitute for a natural tooth in a prosthesis; usually made of porcelain or plastic.

tooth-borne, *adj* term used to describe a prosthesis or a part of a prosthesis that depends entirely on the abutment teeth for support.

  tooth-borne base, *n* the denture base restoring an edentulous area

that has abutment teeth at each end for support. The tissue it covers is not used for support of the base.

tooth buds, *n.pl* embryonic teeth formed during the fifth and sixth weeks of embryo development. See also odontogenesis.

tooth, conical (**peg-shaped tooth**), *n* failure of morphologic development of the tooth germ found in ectodermal dysplasia and other disorders and occasionally found in normal children.

tooth, cross-bite, *n.pl* posterior teeth designed to permit the modified buccal cusps of the upper teeth to be positioned in the central fossae of the lower teeth.

tooth, cuspless, *n.pl* teeth designed without cuspal prominences on the masticatory surfaces.

tooth, devital, *n* See tooth, pulpless.

tooth, drifting, *n* the migration of teeth from their normal positions in the dental arches as a result of such factors as loss of proximal support, loss of functional antagonists, occlusal traumatic tooth relationships, inflammatory and retrograde changes in the attachment apparatus, and oral habits.

tooth, embedded, *n* an unerupted tooth, usually one completely covered with bone; also spelled *imbedded.* See also tooth, impacted.

tooth eruption, *n* the process by which the tooth moves from its site of formation to its position of function.

tooth, evulsed (**avulsed tooth**), *n* a tooth that has been abnormally luxated from its alveolar support, commonly as a sequela to trauma.

tooth form, *n* See form, tooth.

tooth, fulcrum, *n* the axis of movement of a tooth when lateral forces are applied to the tooth. The fulcrum is considered to be at the middle third of the portion of the root embedded in the alveolus and thus moves apically as the bone resorbs in periodontal disease.

tooth fracture, *n* See fracture, tooth.

tooth, fused, *n.pl* two teeth united during development by the union of their tooth germs. The teeth may be joined by the enamel of their crowns, root dentin, or both. Usually consists of a single large crown.

tooth germ, *n* the earliest evidence of a tooth. It includes the dental follicla, dental papilla, and enamel organ.

tooth, geminated (jem′inātəd), *n* teeth with bifid crowns and confluent root canals resulting from the division of the enamel organ during the developmental period.

tooth, Hutchinson's, *n.pr* after Sir Jonathan Hutchinson, who reported the typical defects of the permanent incisors associated with congenital syphilis. Dental hypoplasia affects primarily the incisors, canines, and first permanent molars. The incisors have a somewhat screwdriver or peg-shaped appearance. See also triad, Hutchinson.

tooth, hypoplasia of (hī′pōplā′zhə), *n* a reduction in the amount of enamel formed, resulting in irregular pits and grooves of the enamel.

tooth, immediate separation of, *n* separation of teeth accomplished by the rapid wedging action of an appliance during restorative procedures.

tooth, impacted, *n* a condition in which the unerupted or partially erupted tooth is positioned against another tooth, bone, or soft tissue so that complete eruption is unlikely. An impacted third molar tooth may be further described according to its position: buccoangular, distoangular, or vertical. An impacted maxillary canine tooth also may be further described according to its position: palatal (maxillary canine), lingual (mandibular canine), labial, or vertical.

tooth, inclination of, *n* the angle of slope of teeth from the vertical planes of reference. A tooth may be mesially, distally, lingually, buccally, or labially inclined.

tooth, loss of, *n* the separation of a tooth from its investing and supporting structures as a result of normal exfoliation attending loss of primary dentition, exfoliation as a sequela to excessive bone resorption and periapical migration of the epithelial attachment in periodontal disease, and instrumentation for extraction necessitated by pathologic involvement of the dental pulp, periodontium, or periapical tissues.

tooth, mesial movement of, *n* migration of teeth toward the midline, occurring as a phenomenon associated with the action of the anterior component of force. Mesial migration of teeth occurs with the wear of their proximal surfaces resulting from the buccolingual movements of the teeth.

tooth, metal insert, *n* an artificial tooth, usually of acrylic resin, containing an inserted ribbon of metal, or a cutting blade, in its occlusal surface, with one edge of the blade exposed; sometimes used in removable dentures.

tooth, migration of, *n* the movement of teeth into altered positions in relationship to the basal bone of the alveolar process and adjoining and opposing teeth as a result of loss of approximating or opposing teeth, occlusal interferences, habits, or inflammatory and dystrophic disease of the attaching and supporting structures of the teeth.

tooth, missing, *n* the absence of teeth from the dentition because of congenital factors, exfoliation, or extraction.

tooth mobility, *n* the movability of a tooth resulting from loss of all or a portion of its attachment and supportive apparatus. Seen in periodontitis, occlusal traumatism, and periodontosis.

tooth morphology, *n* the anatomic topography of the teeth.

tooth movement, *n* See movement, tooth.

tooth, natal, *n.pl* primary tooth found in the oral cavity at birth.

Natal tooth. (Neville/Damm/Allen/Bouquot, 2002)

tooth, nonanatomic, *n* artificial teeth so designed that the occlusal surfaces are not copies from natural forms but

T

are given forms that in the opinion of the designer seem more nearly to fulfill the requirements of mastication and tissue tolerance.

tooth, peg-shaped, *n* See tooth, conical.

tooth, pink, *n* See resorption, internal.

tooth, plastic, *n* artificial teeth constructed of synthetic resins.

tooth position, *n* See position, tooth.

tooth, pulpless, *n* a tooth from which the dental pulp has been removed or is necrotic.

tooth, replaced, *n* See tooth, supplied.

tooth, rotated, *n* an altered position of the tooth in relation to the adjacent and opposing teeth and its basal alveolar process; in such an altered position the tooth has been turned on its long axis and is in a state of torsiversion. The result is an altered contact with adjacent teeth that produces a possible locus for food impaction between the teeth, with consequent gingival damage.

tooth selection, *n* See selection, tooth.

tooth, setting up of, *n* the arranging of teeth on a trial denture base; includes proper relation with occluding teeth.

tooth, shell, *n* a form of dentinal dysplasia characterized by large pulp chambers, meager coronal dentin, and usually no roots.

tooth size discrepancy, *n* lack of proportional harmony in the width of various teeth, causing relative spacing and crowding in different parts of the dentition.

tooth, submerged, *n* a tooth that has not erupted to the point of making contact with the opposing maxillary or mandibular tooth during mastication. Such a tooth may be immobile as a result of ankylosis to the mandible or maxilla.

tooth, succedaneous (suk′sēdā′nē-us), *n* any of the permanent teeth with primary predecessors (i.e., premolars, canines, and incisors).

tooth, supernumerary, *n* extra erupted or unerupted teeth that resemble teeth of normal shape.

Supernumerary tooth. (Regezi/Sciubba/Jordan, 2003)

tooth, supplied (**replaced teeth**), *n.pl* artificial replacements for natural teeth.

tooth surface pocket wall, *n* the portion of a narrow, infected sulcus that is adjacent to the surface of a tooth.

tooth, tube, *n.pl* artificial teeth constructed with a vertical, cylindric aperture extending from the center of the base into the body of the tooth into which a pin or cast post for the attachment of the tooth to a denture base may be placed.

tooth, Turner's, *n.pr* a permanent tooth showing hypoplasia resulting from injury or inflammation of the precedent primary tooth.

tooth wear, *n* the erosion of a tooth by chemical or mechanical processes.

tooth, zero degree, *n.pl* prosthetic teeth having no cusp angles in relation to the horizontal plane; cuspless teeth.

toothache, *n* pain located in the tooth or its surrounding supporting tissues. Dental pain may have a halo effect, making location of the precise source or location of the pain difficult. Determining the location may require several diagnostic tests.

toothbrush, *n* a manually or automatically operated device with an arrangement of bristles at one end, and a handle designed to reach effectively all exposed surfaces of the teeth and gingiva. A dentifrice is usually applied to the bristles for the purpose of cleaning the teeth and gingiva.

Toothbrush. (Daniel/Harfst, 2002)

toothbrush, automatic, *n* electric, handheld oral hygiene device. Also called *power-assisted toothbrush.*

toothbrush, bi-level orthodontic, *n* handheld oral hygiene tool specifically designed to clean orthodontic appliances. The head of the tool features soft bristles that are shorter down the center, with hedges of taller bristles on either side, allowing the brush to pass over the appliance without causing abrasion to the teeth.

toothbrush, end-tuft, *n* an oral cleaning tool that features a very small number of filaments. Handle may be angled to assist difficult-to-reach areas of both natural and replacement teeth. Also called *single-tuft* or *unituft.*

End-tuft toothbrush. (Daniel/Harfst, 2002)

toothbrush head, *n* the section of the common oral hygiene tool that comes in direct contact with the teeth and gingiva, comprising various configurations of nylon bristles (filaments). The profile, or trim, of the head depends upon the number and height of bristle rows.

toothbrushing, *n* the use of a brush of varying design to brush the teeth and gingivae for cleanliness and to massage for oral hygiene.

toothbrushing, clock system, *n* a technique where a clock or timer is observed to ensure that brushing is sustained for a predetermined amount of time.

toothbrushing, faulty, *n* the improper performance of toothbrushing, resulting in defective cleansing, inadequate stimulation of the gingival tissues, and destructive effects on the teeth and marginal gingivae resulting from overzealous brushing.

toothbrushing, horizontal, *n* a method of teeth cleaning considered more harmful than beneficial. Characterized by long, parallel weight-bearing scrubbing movements, that tend to damage teeth and gingiva, while neglecting crucial areas between teeth.

toothbrushing, vertical, *n* See method, Leonard.

toothpaste, *n* See dentifrice.

toothpick, *n* a wood sliver used to cleanse the interdental space.

toothpick, balsa wood, *n* a triangular wedge of balsa wood used to clean the teeth interproximally and stimulate the interdental gingival tissues.

topical, *adj* **1.** of or pertaining to the surface of a part of the body. **2.** of or pertaining to a drug or treatment applied to the surface of a part of the body.

topical anesthesia, *n* surface analgesia produced by application of an anesthetic in the form of a solution, gel, or ointment to the surface of the skin, mucous membrane, or cornea.

topographic anatomy, *n* the study of a specific region of a body structure, such as a lower leg, including all the systems in the part and their relationships to one another. Also referred to as *regional anatomy.*

topographic intraoral radiographic examination, *n* See examination, true occlusal topographic intraor.

topography, *n* a detailed physical representation of anatomic features within a specific region.

torque (tôrk), *n* **1.** a force that produces or tends to produce rotation in a body. Such force applied to a tooth tends to cause rotation around its long axis. **2.** force applied to a tooth to produce rotation of a tooth on a mesiodistal or buccolingual (labiolingual) axis. **3.** a rotary force applied to a denture base.

torque wire, *n* an auxiliary wire used to torque the roots of the anterior teeth.

torsemide, *n trade name:* Demadox; *drug class:* loop diuretic; *action:* acts on loop of Henle to decrease the reabsorption of chloride and sodium with resultant diuresis; *uses:* treatment of hypertension and edema associated with congestive heart failure (CHF), liver disease, and chronic renal failure.

torsion, *n* in dentistry the twisting of a tooth on its long axis. Also, the loading of a wire by twisting it along its long axis.

T

torsion, clasp, *n* the twisting of the retentive clasp arm on its long axis. A retentive clasp may be formed so that it traverses a vertical distance before encircling the abutment to increase the torsion component of the clasp opening as compared with the flexure it experiences.

torsiversion, *n* an axially rotated tooth position.

tort, *n* a legal wrong perpetrated on a person or property, independent of contract.

torticollis, *n* an abnormal condition in which the head is inclined to one side as a result of the contraction of the muscles on that side of the neck.

Torticollis. (Moore/Persaud, 2003)

torus, *n* a bulging projection of bone.

torus mandibularis, *n* a bony enlargement (hyperostosis) appearing unilaterally or bilaterally on the lingual aspect of the mandible in the canine-premolar region of about 7% of the population.

Torus mandibularis. (Regezi/Sciubba/Jordan, 2003)

torus palatinus, *n* a bony enlargement (hyperostosis) occurring in the midline of the hard palate in about 20% of the population.

Torus palatinus. (Regezi/Sciubba/Jordan, 2003)

total filtration, *n* See filtration, total.

total hip arthroplasty, *n* total hip replacement; surgical reconstruction of the hip in which the ball-and-socket joint is replaced with a prosthesis.

total parenteral nutrition (TPN), *n* the administration of a nutritionally adequate hypertonic solution consisting of glucose, protein hydrolysates, minerals, and vitamins through an indwelling catheter into the superior vena cava.

total treatment plan, *n* a listing of all of the necessary treatments and measures that dental staff must perform in order to restore full oral health to the patient.

touch, *n* the sense by which contact with an object provides evidence of its properties.

touch, light, *n* tactile sense. The principal organs of light touch are Meissner's corpuscles, which are large and oval. Each capsule receives several nerve fibers that shed their myelin sheaths and coil into a spiral complex network. Associated with Meissner's corpuscles in the perception of light touch are both Merkel's disks and a basketlike arrangement of nerve fibers around the hair follicles.

touch screen, *n* a type of screen on some video terminals that may be touched with the finger to specify the selection of an item from a displayed list.

Tourette's syndrome, *n* a condition in which the patient is unable to control numerous muscular and vocal tics, often resulting in twitching, grunting, or the making of inappropriate comments.

tourniquet, *n* a device used in controlling hemorrhage, consisting of a wide constricting band applied to the limb proximal to the site of bleeding.

toxic (tok′sik), *adj* poisonous; produced by a poison.

toxic delirium, *n* a symptom of disordered mental status as a result of poisoning.

toxic shock syndrome (TSS), *n* a severe, acute disease caused by infection with strains of *Staphylococcus aureus,* phage group I, that produce a unique toxin, enterotoxin F. It is most common in menstruating women using high-absorbency tampons but has occurred in infants, children, and men

Toxic shock syndrome. (Zitelli/Davis, 2002, courtesy Dr. George Pazin)

toxic waste, *n* refuse material that may be poisonous.

toxicity (toksis′itē), *n* the ability of a drug or poison to produce harm, especially to cause permanent injury or death. Usually distinguished from *allergenic properties.*

toxicity, acute, *n* a condition produced after short-term use of a toxic agent. See also dose, lethal, median; dose, lethal, minimum.

toxicity, chronic, *n* a condition produced after long-term use of a toxic agent.

toxicologist (tok′sikol′əjist), *n* a person versed in toxicology.

toxicology (tok′sikol′əjē), *n* the scientific study of the nature and effects of poisons, their detection, and the treatment of their effects.

toxin, *n* a poisonous protein made by specific animals, higher levels of plants, and disease-causing bacteria.

toxoids, *n.pl* toxins that have been treated to destroy their toxic properties but retain their ability to induce antibody production, thus creating an active immunity.

***Toxoplasma gondii* (tok′sōplaz′mə gon′dē-ī),** *n* a protozoa commonly found in cat feces and undercooked meat. Pregnant women should avoid coming in contact with cat litter boxes, because the protozoa can cross the placenta and cause stillbirth or other serious physical or psychomotor defects in utero. See also toxoplasmosis.

toxoplasmosis (tok′sōplazmō′sis), *n* a disease caused by protozoa in the bloodstream and body tissues.

Toxoplasmosis. (Neville/Damm/Allen/Bouquot, 2002)

toxoplasmosis, neonatal, *n* an infection passed to the fetus during pregnancy via the placenta that can cause mental retardation, blindness, or an abnormally small head. See *Toxoplasma gondii.*

TPI, *n* See test, Treponema pallidum immobilization.

trace element, *n* an element essential to nutrition or physiologic processes, found in such minute quantities that analysis yields a presence of virtually none.

tracer, *n* **1.** a mechanical device used to trace a pattern of mandibular movements. **2.** a foreign substance mixed with or attached to a given substance to enable the distribution or location of the latter to be determined subsequently. A radioactive tracer is a physical or chemical tracer having radioactivity as its distinctive property.

tracer, Gothic arch, *n* See tracer, needle point.

tracer, needle point, *n* a mechanical device consisting of a weighted or a spring-loaded needle that is attached

T

to one jaw and a coated plate attached to the other jaw. Movement of the mandible causes a tracing to be formed on the horizontally placed plate. When the needle point is in the apex of the tracing, the mandible is said to be in the horizontal position of centric relation.

trachea (trā′kē ə), *n* the windpipe; a cartilaginous and membranous tube extending from the lower end of the larynx to its division into two bronchi.

tracheo- (trā′kē ō), *comb* combining form denoting connection with or relation to the trachea.

tracheobronchial (trā′kē ōbrong′kē əl), *adj* pertaining to the trachea and a bronchus or bronchi.

tracheobronchoscopy (trā′kē ōbrongkos′kəpē), *n* inspection of the interior of the trachea and bronchus.

tracheolaryngeal (trā′kē ōlərin′jē əl), *adj* pertaining to the trachea and larynx.

tracheolaryngotomy (trā′kē ōləringot′ōmē), *n* incision into the larynx and trachea; tracheotomy and laryngotomy.

tracheoscopy (trā′kē os′kəpē), *n* inspection of the interior of the trachea by means of a laryngoscopic mirror and reflected light or inspection through a bronchoscope.

tracheostenosis (trā′kē ōstənō′sis), *n* abnormal constriction or narrowing of the trachea.

tracheostomy (trā′kē os′tōmē), *n* 1. the formation of an opening into the trachea and the suturing of the edges of the opening to an opening in the skin of the neck. 2. surgical formation of an opening into the trachea, usually through the tracheal rings below the cricoid cartilage, to give the patient an airway.

tracheotome (trā′kē ōtōm), *n* 1. a cutting instrument used in tracheotomy; a tracheotomy knife. 2. an instrument for use in creating an airway through the skin into the trachea below the cricoid cartilage.

tracheotomy (trā′kē ot′əmē), *n* the operation of cutting into the trachea to give the patient an airway.

tracing, *n* a line or lines or a pattern scribed by a pointed instrument or stylus on a tracing plate or tracing paper.

tracing, arrow point, *n* See tracing, needle point.

tracing, cephalometric, *n* a line drawing of pertinent features of a cephalometric radiograph made on a piece of transparent paper placed over the radiograph.

tracing, extraoral, *n* a tracing of mandibular movements made outside the oral cavity.

tracing, Gothic arch, *n.pr* See tracing, needle point.

tracing, intraoral, *n* a tracing of mandibular movements made within the oral cavity. A tracing made by a mechanical device consisting of a weighted or spring-loaded stylus that is attached to one jaw and contacts a coated plate attached to the other jaw. Movement of the mandible causes a tracing to be formed on the horizontally placed coated plate. When the stylus point is in the apex of the tracing, the mandible is said to be in the horizontal position of centric relation. The shape of the tracing depends on the relative location of the marking point and tracing table. The various tracing shapes have been called *Gothic arch, arrow point,* and *sea gull tracings.* The apex of a properly made tracing indicates the most retruded unstrained relation of the mandible to the maxillae (that is, the centric relation). The tracings are made by a stylus or needle point by the movement of the mandible. Unless otherwise designated, stylus tracings are made by lateral movements registered on a horizontal plate.

tracing, sea gull, *n* See tracing, needle point.

tracing, stylus, *n* See tracing, needle point.

tracings, pantographic, *n.pl* tracing of mandibular movements. A stylus is attached to the mandible traces line on vertical and horizontal plates attached to the maxilla, providing a graphic of lower jaw movements.

tract, sinus, *n* a communication between a pathologic space and an anatomic body cavity or between a pathologic space and the skin. A sinus tract may or may not be lined with epithelium.

traction, *n* the act of drawing (pulling).

traction, external, *n* a fracture reduction appliance principally used in the management of midfacial fractures. Points of fixation are located in the oral cavity and over the cranial area, and elastic or rigid connectors are placed between the cranial and oral points of fixation.

traction, intermaxillary, *n* See traction, maxillomandibular.

traction, internal, *n* a pulling force created by using one of the cranial bones above the point of fracture for anchorage.

traction, maxillomandibular (intermaxillary traction), *n* the technique for reducing fractures of the maxilla or mandible into functional relations with the opposing dental arch through the use of elastic or wire ligatures and interdental wiring or splints.

trademark, *n* a word, symbol, or device assigned to a product by its manufacturer, possibly registered, as a part of its identity.

tragion (trā′jē on), *n* the notch just above the tragus of the ear. It lies 1 to 2 mm below the spina helicis, which may be easily palpated.

tragus (trā′gus), *n* a prominence in front of the opening of the external ear.

training grant, *n* an award of money or other resources to provide training in a particular field, usually in areas of public need or demand.

trait (trāt), *n* an inherited set of mental or bodily characteristics.

trait, Cooley's, *n,pr* See thalassemia minor.

trait, sickle cell, *n* a form of sickle cell disease in which patients are asymptomatic but their erythrocytes can be caused to assume a sickle shape under certain conditions. The trait is present when one parent has the gene (heterozygous condition) for sickle cell disease. See also disease, sickle cell.

tramadol HCl, *n trade name:* Ultram; *drug class:* synthetic opioid analgesic; *action:* unknown, but it has been shown to bind to opioid receptors and inhibit the reuptake of norepinephrine and serotonin; *use:* treatment of moderate-to-severe pain.

tranquilizer (trang′kwilīzur), *n* one of a poorly defined group of drugs designed to control anxiety and reduce tension or stress. Tranquilizers tend to induce drowsiness and may cause physical and psychologic dependence. Most tranquilizers are controlled substances.

transaminase (transam′inās), *n* one of several enzymes involved in the reversible transfer of an amino (NH_2) group from an α-amino acid to an α-ketoacid, especially α-ketoglutaric acid. Characteristic high values are seen in myocardial infarction and viral hepatitis.

transamination (tranzam′inā′shən), *n* the reaction between an alpha-ketoacid and an amino acid in which the amino group moves to the alpha-ketoacid, creating a new amino acid and a new ketoacid.

transdermal delivery system, *n* a method of applying a drug to unbroken skin. The drug is absorbed through the skin and enters the body's systems. It is used particularly for the administration of nitroglycerin and in nicotine patches used to assist individuals to withdraw from the use of tobacco.

transducer (tranzdōō′sur), *n* a device that is activated by power from one system and then supplies a different form of power to a second system; used to convert electric energy into mechanical energy in ultrasonic and sonic scalers.

transfection, *n* the process by which a bacterial cell is infected with purified deoxyribonucleic acid (DNA) or ribonucleic acid (RNA) isolated from a virus or a viral vector after a specific pretreatment.

transfer agreement, *n* a written contract between two health care institutions for the transfer of patients from one to the other and for the orderly exchange of pertinent clinical information on the patients transferred.

transferase, *n* any of a group of enzymes that catalyze the transfer of a chemical group or radical from one molecule to another.

transferrin, *n* a trace protein present in the blood that is essential in the transport of iron from the intestine

T

into the bloodstream, making it available to the normoblasts in the bone marrow.

transformer, *n* an electrical device that increases or reduces the voltage of an alternating current by mutual induction between primary and secondary coils or windings.

transformer, auto-, *n* See autotransformer.

transformer, Coolidge filament, *n.pr* a step-down transformer that reduces line voltage of 110 volts to 12 volts, which in turn heats the tungsten filament of the Coolidge tube for the production of electrons.

transformer, step-down, *n* a transformer in which the secondary voltage is less than the primary voltage.

transformer, step-up, *n* a transformer in which the secondary voltage is greater than the primary voltage.

transforming growth factor (TGF), *n* a group of proteins produced by cells of a tumor that, when inoculated into a normal cell culture, causes a disorderly increase in the number of cells in the culture.

transfusion, *n* the introduction into the bloodstream of whole blood or blood components such as plasma, platelets, or packed red cells. Infused donor blood must be matched to the recipient's blood type and antigen group.

transient, *adj* pertaining to a condition that is temporary or of short duration, usually not recurring.

transillumination (tran'silōō'minā'shən), *n* 1. examination of an organ, cavity, or tissue (for example, tooth or gingival tissue) by transmitted light. A valuable aid in detecting carious lesions, disclosing carious or demineralized dentin during cavity preparation, checking the finish or gingival margins of restorations, and revealing cement, debris, or calculus subgingivally. 2. a test in which the use of transmitted light may disclose a discoloration of the coronal aspect, indicating dentinal tubular hemorrhage as a result of trauma, pulpal necrosis, or fracture. 3. examination of tissues by means of a light placed so that the region under study is between the light source and the observer.

transition point, *n* See Tg value.

transitional dentition (mixed), *n* an older term for the final phase of the transition from primary to permanent teeth, in which most primary teeth have been lost or are in the process of shedding and the permanent successors are not yet in function.

translation, *n* movement of a rigid body in which all parts move in the same direction at the same speed.

translatory movement, *n* See movement, translatory.

translocation, *n* the rearrangement of genetic material within the same chromosome or the transfer of a segment of one chromosome to another nonhomologous one.

transmission, *n* the transfer or conveyance of a thing or condition, such as an infectious or genetic disease or hereditary trait, from one person to another.

transmission, horizontal, *n* the transfer of an infection from person to person; direct transmission of a disease.

transmission, vertical, *n* the transmission of a disease from mother to child either during pregnancy, childbirth, or by breastfeeding.

transmission scanning electron microscope, *n* an instrument that transmits a highly magnified, well-resolved, three-dimensional image to a television screen, thus combining the advantages of the transmission electron and scanning electron microscopes.

transmucosal (tranz'myōōkō'səl), *adj* administration of a substance, such as a drug, through the mucous membranes.

transosteal implant jig, *n* an instrument designed to guide a bone drill from the inferior border through the alveolar ridge to create a path for the seating of a transosteal implant.

transplant, *v* 1. to remove and plant in another place, as from one body or part of a body to another. *n* 2. implantation of living or nonliving tissue or bone into another part of the body; it then serves as a scaffold in the healing process and is progressively resorbed and replaced by newly formed bone. *v* 3. to move a tooth or tissue from one site to another, often but not always autogenously.

transplantation, allogenic bone marrow (al'ōjen'ik), *n* the transfer of healthy bone marrow taken from a sibling in order to stimulate normal blood cell production.

transplantation, autogenous, *n* tooth, transplantation of a tooth from one position to another in the same individual.

transplantation, autologous bone marrow (ôtol'əgus), *n* the transfer of healthy bone marrow from one site to another in the same body in order to stimulate normal blood cell production.

transplantation, homogenous tooth, *n* transplantation of a tooth from one human to another.

transport, *n* the movement of biochemical substances from one site to another.

transport, active, *n* transport of substances through membranes or epithelium, requiring metabolic energy.

transport, passive, *n* transport along a gradient without the use of metabolic energy.

transseptal fiber, *n* See fiber, transseptal.

transudate (tran'sōōdāt), *n* any fluid substance that has passed through a membrane, possibly associated with inflammation. It is low in proteins and colloids and has a low specific gravity.

transverse, *adj* at right angles to the long axis of any common part.

transverse palatine suture, *n* the line of junction between the palatal processes of the maxillary bones and horizontal portions of the palatine bones that form the hard palate.

transverse ridge, *n* ridge formed by the joining of two triangular ridges crossing the occlusal table transversely or from the labial to the lingual outline.

transversion, *n* eruption of a tooth in the wrong position

tranylcypromine sulfate, *n* *trade name:* Parnate; *drug class:* antidepressant, monoamine oxidase inhibitor (MAOI); *action:* increases concentrations of endogenous norepinephrine, serotonin, and dopamine in central nervous system (CNS) storage sites; *use:* treatment of depression (when uncontrolled by other means).

trauma (trou'mə, trô'mə), *n* a hurt; a wound; an injury; damage; impairment; external violence producing bodily injury or degeneration.

trauma, cumulative, *n* medical condition developing in the peripheral and autonomic nervous systems and musculoskeletal system due to forceful, awkward, and repetitive bodily motions as well as exposure to cold temperatures, mechanical stress, and vibrations.

trauma, injury in occlusal, *n* the damaging effects of occlusal trauma, which are of a dystrophic nature and affect the tooth and its attachment apparatus. Lesions include wear facets on the tooth, root resorption, cemental tears, thrombosis of blood vessels of the periodontal membrane, necrosis and hyalinization of the periodontal membrane on the pressure side, and resorption of alveolar and supporting bone. Clinically, tooth mobility and migration may be evident; radiographically, evidence includes the widening of the periodontal membrane space and fraying or fuzziness of the lamina dura and formation of intrabony resorptive defects. Pocket formation is not a sequela to occlusal traumatism.

trauma, occlusal, *n* abnormal occlusal relationships of the teeth, causing injury to the periodontium.

traumatic (trômat'ik), *adj* of, pertaining to, or caused by an injury.

traumatic occlusion, *n* See occlusion, traumatic.

traumatic shock, *n* See shock, traumatic.

traumatism, *n* **1.** an injury. **2.** a wound produced by an injury; trauma.

traumatism by food, *n* impingement of the gingival margin by coarse foodstuff caused by improper contour of the tooth or faulty position of the tooth.

traumatism by food, occlusal, *n* lesions of the attachment apparatus; caused by force placed on the tooth in excess of that which the supporting structures can withstand.

traumatism by food, periodontal, *n* the application of stress to the structures constituting the attachment apparatus exceeding the adaptive capacities of the tissues, with resultant tissue destruction.

traumatism by food, primary occlusal, n force or forces caused by mandibular movement and resultant tooth percussion and capable of producing pathologic changes in the periodontium.

traumatism by food, secondary occlusal, n destruction of the attachment apparatus by factors other than those of occlusion (for example, periodontitis). In secondary occlusal traumatism, even the forces of mastication become pathologic in nature.

traumatogenic (trô'mətōjen'ik), *adj* capable of producing a wound or injury.

traumatogenic occlusion, n See occlusion, traumatic.

tray, n a receptacle or device that holds or carries.

tray, acrylic resin, n a tray made of acrylic resin.

tray, impression, n a receptacle or device that is used to carry impression material to the mouth, confine the material in apposition to the surfaces to be recorded, and control the impression material while it sets to form the impression.

tray, impression, maxillary, n a tray consisting of a body with a protruding edge and handle used to contain a material (e.g., rubber, hydrocolloid, or alginate) against the upper portion of the oral cavity for making a mold of the structures.

trazodone HCl, n *trade names:* Desyrel, Trazon, Trialodine; *drug class:* antidepressant; *action:* selectively inhibits serotonin-specific reuptake in the brain; *use:* treatment of depression.

Treacher Collins syndrome, *n.pr* See syndrome, Treacher Collins.

treatment, n the mode or course pursued for remedial ends.

treatment, atraumatic restorative (ART), n a procedure for preventing and treating dental caries using hand instruments and adhesive filling material. Does not require electricity or anesthesia and may be performed in the field by trained health care workers or nondental personnel.

treatment, hardening heat, n See tempering.

treatment, heat, n **1.** subjecting a metal to a given controlled heat, followed by controlled sudden or gradual cooling to develop the desired qualities of the metal to the maximal degree. **2.** a process of giving a metal predetermined physical properties by controlled temperature changes.

treatment, homogenizing heat, n See anneal.

treatment, indirect pulp capping, n See capping, indirect pulp.

treatment, indirect, relationship, n an association between a health care provider and an individual where the health care provided to the individual by the health care provider has been ordered by another provider.

treatment plan, n in dentistry a schedule of procedures and appointments designed to restore, step by step, the oral health of a patient.

treatment, prescription, n the formal outline of the projected treatment of a patient (for example, the blueprint from which the dentist projects treatment).

treatment, rest (**sedative treatment**), n use of a drug sealed into a root canal to relieve pain or discomfort; not used primarily for its antiseptic value.

treatment, root canal, n the techniques and pharmaceuticals used in removing pulp tissue, sterilizing the root canal, and preparing the root canal for filling.

treatment, sedative, n See treatment, rest.

treatment, softening heat, n See anneal.

trematodes (trem'ətōdz), n parasitic worms such as *Paragonimus westermani* that reside in contaminated water and can be transmitted to humans who are exposed to such water sources or who eat improperly cooked fish from the same.

tremolo (trem'əlō), n an irregular and exaggerated speech pattern that may be the symptom of an emotional disturbance or of various diseases affecting the nervous control of the organs of respiration and phonation.

tremor, n rhythmic, purposeless, quivering movements resulting from the involuntary alternating contraction and relaxation of opposing skeletal muscle groups.

trench mouth, *n* See gingivitis, acute necrotizing ulcerative.

Trendelenburg position (trendel′ənburg), *n.pr* See position, Trendelenburg.

Trendelenburg position. (Bird/Robinson, 2002)

trepanation (trephination), *n* the act of surgically cutting a round hole.

trephine (trefēn′), *n* a circle-cutting surgical instrument designed to remove a circumscribed portion of tissue. It permits the insertion of the heads of intramucosal inserts into the tissue.

Treponema **(trep′ənē′mə),** *n* a genus of schizomycetes composed of parasitic and pathogenic spiral microorganisms.

Treponema microdentium, *n* a species found in the normal oral cavity.

Treponema mucosum, *n* a species found in periodontal infections in man.

Treponema pallidum, *n* the spirochete that causes syphilis in humans.

Treponema vincentii, *n* a spirochete associated with acute necrotizing ulcerative gingivitis.

tretinoin (vitamin A acid, retinoic acid), *n trade name:* Retin-A; *drug class:* vitamin A acid; *action:* decreases cohesiveness of follicular epithelium, decreases microcomedone formation; *use:* treatment of acne vulgaris.

triad, Hutchinson (trī′ ad), *n.pr* interstitial keratitis, deafness, and Hutchinson teeth resulting from congenital syphilis. Not current.

triage, *n* **1.** (in military medicine) a classification of casualties of war and other disasters according to the gravity of injuries, urgency of treatment, and place for treatment. **2.** a process in which a group of patients is sorted according to need for care. The kind of illness or injury, severity of the problem, and facilities available govern the process, as in the emergency room of a hospital. **3.** (in disaster medicine) a process in which a large group of patients is sorted so that care may be concentrated on those who are likely to survive.

trial, *n* an examination before a competent tribunal of the facts or law in issue in a cause of action for the purpose of determining the issue.

trial base, *n* See baseplate.

triamcinolone, *n* a synthetic adrenocorticosteroid that has a potent antiinflammatory effect and is used topically in the treatment of angular cheilosis.

triamcinolone acetonide (topical), *n trade names:* Aristocort, Flutex, Kenalog, Kenlog in Orabase, Oracort, Triacet, Triderm, others; *drug class:* topical corticosteroid; *action:* interacts with steroid cytoplasmic receptors to induce antiinflammatory effects; possesses antipruritic and antiinflammatory actions; *uses:* treatment of psoriasis, eczema, contact dermatitis, pruritus; special dental paste used to treat nonviral inflammatory oral lesions, including aphthous stomatitis, lichen planus, and cicatrical pemphigoid.

triamcinolone/triamcinolone acetonide/triamcinolone diacetate/ triamcinolone hexacetonide, *n trade names:* Triamcinolone (oral), Aristocort, Atolone, Kenacort, many others; *drug class:* glucocorticoid, intermediate-acting; *action:* decreases inflammation by suppressing macrophage and leukocyte migration, reduces capillary permeability and inhibits lysosomal enzymes and phagocytosis; *uses:* treatment of severe inflammation; immunosuppression; neoplasms; collagen, respiratory, and dermatologic disorders; and seasonal and perennial allergic rhinitis.

triamterene, *n trade name:* Dyrenium; *drug class:* potassium-sparing diuretic; *action:* acts on distal tubule to inhibit reabsorption of sodium, chlorine; increases potassium retention; *uses:* treatment of edema; hypertension.

triangle, *n* a three-cornered area.

triangle, Bolton, n.pr a triangle

formed by drawing a line from the nasion to the sella turcica and from there to the Bolton point.

triangle, Bonwill, *n.pr* an equilateral triangle with 4-inch (10 cm) sides bounded by lines from the contact points of the lower central incisors (or the median line of the residual ridge of the mandible) to the condyle on either side and from one condyle to the other. It is the basis for Bonwill's theory of occlusion.

triangle, Tweed, *n.pr* a triangle formed by the mandibular plane, Frankfort plane, and long axis of the lower central incisor. Proposed as a diagnostic aid by C.H. Tweed.

triangular fossa, *n* fossa that has a triangular shape where the triangular grooves terminate.

triangular ridges, *n.pl* cusp ridges that descend from the cusp tips toward the central portion of the occlusal table.

triazolam, *n trade name:* Halcion; *drug class:* benzodiazepine, sedative-hypnotic, controlled substance schedule IV; *action:* produces central nervous system (CNS) depression by interacting with a benzodiazepine receptor to facilitate the action of the inhibitory neurotransmitter gamma-aminobutyric acid (GABA); *use:* treatment of insomnia.

Trichinella spiralis (trik′inel′ə spīral′is), *n* a round worm found in raw or undercooked pork products. The worm resides in muscle tissue and is implicated in trichinosis food poisoning. Symptoms of infection, when they occur, are similar to those of food poisoning.

trichoepithelioma (trik′ō ep′ithē′lē ō′mə), *n* See epithelioma adenoides cysticum.

Trichuris, *n* a genus of parasitic roundworms that infect the intestinal tract. Adult worms are 30 to 50 mm long and resemble whips with a threadlike anterior and a thicker posterior. Also called *whipworm.*

triclosan (trīklō′san), *n* an antibacterial agent, combined with a liquid, paste, or powder, used to clean the teeth by reducing gingivitis and bacterial plaque within the oral cavity. It can be used in combination with fluoride.

trident, *n* a tooth with three cusps. Also called *tridentate* or *tricuspid.*

tridymite (trid′imīt), *n* a physical form of silica used in combination with cristobalite to limit thermal expansion.

trifluoperazine HCl, *n trade name:* Stelazine; *drug class:* phenothiazine antipsychotic; *action:* blocks neurotransmission at dopaminergic synapses in cerebral cortex, hypothalamus, and limbic system; *uses:* treatment of psychotic disorders, nonpsychotic anxiety, and schizophrenia.

triflupromazine HCl, *n trade name:* Vesprin; *drug class:* phenothiazine, antipsychotic; *action:* blocks neurotransmission at dopaminergic synapses in the cerebral cortex, hypothalamus, and limbic system; *uses:* treatment of psychotic disorders, schizophrenia, acute agitation, nausea, and vomiting.

trifluridine (ophthalmic), *n trade name:* Viroptic ophthalmic solution; *drug class:* antiviral; *action:* inhibits viral deoxyribonucleic acid (DNA) synthesis and replication; *uses:* treatment of primary keratoconjunctivitis, recurring epithelial keratitis, and keratitis associated with herpes simplex virus types 1 and 2.

trifurcation, *n* division into three parts or branches, as the three roots of a maxillary first molar.

trigeminal nerve, *n* the fifth cranial nerve, which provides motor innervation to the muscles of mastication and sensory innervation to the face, jaws, and teeth.

trigeminal neuralgia, *n* a neurologic condition of the trigeminal nerve characterized by paroxysms of flashing, stablike, unilateral pain radiating along the course of a branch of the nerve. Any or all of the three branches may be affected. The attacks are initiated by stimuli, such as a light touch of the skin, chewing, washing the face, or brushing the teeth. In some individuals the attacks may be initiated by painless physical stimulation of specific areas that are located on the same side of the face as the pain. Also called *tic douloureux.*

trigger point, *n* See point, trigger.

trihexyphenidyl HCl, *n trade names:* Trihexane, Trihexy-5; *drug class:* antiparkinsonian, anticholinergic; *action:* block central muscarinic receptors, which decreases the severity of involuntary movements; *use:* treatment of Parkinson's disease symptoms.

triiodothyronine, *n* a hormone that helps regulate growth and development, control metabolism and body temperature, and by a negative-feedback system, inhibit the secretion of thyrotropin by the pituitary gland.

trilaminar embryonic disk, *n* a plate-like area of ectoderm, mesoderm, and endoderm within a zygote that represents the first stage of embryonic development.

trilogy of Fallot, *n* a congenital cardiac anomaly consisting of a combination of pulmonic stenosis, interatrial septal defect, and right ventricular hypertrophy.

trimeprazine tartrate, *n* *trade name:* Temaril; *drug class:* antihistamine H_1 receptor antagonist; *action:* acts by competing with histamine for H_1 receptor sites; decreases allergic response by blocking histamine effects; *use:* treatment of pruritus.

trimester, *n* one of the three periods of approximately 3 months each into which pregnancy is divided.

trimethadione, *n* *trade name:* Tridione; *drug class:* anticonvulsant; *action:* increases the threshold for seizures initiated in the cortex, decreases central nervous system (CNS) synaptic stimulation to low-frequency impulses; *use:* treatment of refractory absence (petit mal) seizures.

trimethobenzamide, *n* *trade name:* Arrestin, Bio-Gan, Stemetic, Ticon, Tigan, T-Gen, Triban, others; *drug class:* antiemetic; *action:* acts centrally by blocking the chemoreceptor trigger zone, which in turn acts on vomiting center; *uses:* treatment of nausea and vomiting and prevention of postoperative vomiting.

trimethoprim-sulfamethoxazole,
n a synthetic antibacterial combination effective in urinary tract infections; it is the drug of choice in the treatment of *Pneumocystis carinii* pneumonia, one of the opportunistic infections associated with acquired immunodeficiency syndrome (AIDS).

trimetrexate glucuronate, *n* *trade name:* Neutrexin; *drug class:* folate antagonist; *action:* inhibits the enzyme dihydrofolate reductase, which leads to interference with deoxyribonucleic acid (DNA), ribonucleic acid

(RNA), and protein synthesis in the *Pneumocystis carinii* organism; *uses:* alternative therapy for *P. carinii* pneumonia in immunocompromised patients, including patients with acquired immunodeficiency syndrome (AIDS).

trimipramine maleate, *n* *trade name:* Surmontil; *drug class:* antidepressant-tricyclic; *action:* inhibits both norepinephrine and serotonin (5-HT) uptake in the brain; *uses:* treatment of depression and of enuresis in children.

trimmer, gingival margin, *n* (margin trimmer), a binangled, double-paired, chisel-shaped, single-beveled, double-planed lateral cutting instrument. The blade is curved left or right similar to a spoon excavator; the cutting edge is straight and not perpendicular to the axis of the blade. The pair with the end of the cutting edge farthest from the shaft forming an acute angle is termed *distal* and is used to bevel a distal gingival margin or accentuate a mesial axiogingival angle; the pair with the acute angle of the cutting edge closest to the shaft is called *mesial* and is used to bevel a mesial gingival margin or accentuate a distal axiogingival angle. When one of these trimmers is used, all four must be used.

trimmer, margin, *n* See trimmer, gingival margin.

trimmer, model, *n* a device used to trim the edges of the full-scale stone or plaster reproduction of the teeth and nearby tissues. It may be a mechanical tool or plaster knife. See also cast, trimming diagnostic.

trimming, tissue, *n* See border molding.

tripelennamine HCl, *n* *trade names:* PBZ, PBZ-SR, Pelamine; *drug class:* antihistamine, H_1 receptor antagonist; *action:* acts by competing with histamine for H_1 receptor sites; *uses:* treatment of rhinitis and allergy symptoms.

triplegia (trīplē′jē-ə), *n* a condition where three out of the four limbs are paralyzed.

tripoding (trī′pōding), *n* the marking of a cast at three points in the same plane as a means of repositioning the cast in that plane during subsequent procedures.

tripodism, *n* a widely used principle to gain instant stability on uneven terrains in all landings. It is referred to as a three-point landing. Stamp cusps in well-organized occlusion have only three-point contacts with their fossa brims (none with their tips).

triprolidine HCl, *n* *trade name:* Myidil; *drug class:* antihistamine, H_1 receptor antagonist; *action:* acts by competing with histamine for H_1 receptor sites; *uses:* treatment of rhinitis and allergy symptoms.

trismus (triz′məs), *n* spasms of the muscles of mastication resulting in the inability to open the mouth; often symptomatic of pericoronitis.

trisomy (trī′səmē), *n* an additional chromosome in the normal complement, so that in each nucleus a chromosome is represented three times rather than double.

trisomy B, *n* (trisomy 13-15, Patau's syndrome) Clinical syndrome associated with an autosomal abnormality in which the extra chromosome occurs in the 13 to 15 group. Numerous anatomic defects are present, including hemangiomas, hernia, arrhinencephaly, eye anomalies, cleft lip and palate, and characteristic changes in the footprint and palm print.

trisomy syndrome, *n* any congenital condition caused by the addition of an extra member to a normal pair of homologous autosomes or to the sex chromosome or by the translocation of a portion of one chromosome to another. Trisomy 21 results in Down syndrome. See also mongolism.

trituration (trich′o͞orā′shən), *n* the process of mixing together silver alloy fillings with mercury to produce amalgam.

trituration, hand, *n* the mixing of ingredients by hand in a mortar and pestle.

trituration, mechanical, *n* the mixing of constituents in a mechanical device or amalgamator.

troche (trō′kē), *n* See lozenge.

trophoblast (trof′ o-blast), *n* the layer of peripheral embryonic cells from which the placenta is formed.

true vocal cords, *n.pl* the vocal folds of the larynx as distinguished from the vestibular folds, called the *false vocal cords.*

True's separator, *n.pr* See separator, True's.

truss arm, *n* See connector, minor.

trust, *n* a relationship in which one person or entity holds fiduciary responsibility for another's property or enterprise.

truth serum, *n* a common name for any of several sedatives administered intravenously in subjects to elicit information that may have been repressed. It has been used successfully to help identify amnesia victims.

try-in, *n* a preliminary placement of a trial denture (complete or removable partial), a partial denture casting, or a finished restoration to evaluate fit, appearance, and maxillomandibular relations.

try-in, mandibular tray, *n* the initial dry run to position a mandibular impression tray into the lower portion of the oral cavity to ensure the correct fit of a cast.

try-in, maxillary tray, *n* the initial dry run to position a maxillary impression tray into the upper portion of the oral cavity to ensure the correct fit of a cast.

trypsin, *n* a proteolytic digestive enzyme produced by the exocrine pancreas that catalyzes in the small intestine the breakdown of dietary proteins to peptones, peptides, and amino acids.

tryptase (trip′tās), *n* See plasmin.

tryptophan, *n* one of the essential amino acids. See also amino acid.

TSH, *n* See hormone, thyrotropic.

t-test, *n* an inferential statistic used to test for differences between two means (groups) only. This statistic is used for small samples (for example, N <30). Also called *t-ratio, student's t.*

tub and tray system, *n* a system of instrument and supply management in which the instruments for a particular task are prearranged on a tray and the accompanying disposables are prearranged in an accompanying tub. The prepared trays and tubs are appropriately sterilized, stored, and delivered to the dental operatory at the proper time.

tubal pregnancy, *n* an ectopic pregnancy in which the conceptus implants in the fallopian tube.

tube, *n* a hollow cylindrical structure. *tube, buccal,* *n* a section of tubing attached to the buccal side of a molar band in a horizontal position, serving as an attachment for the labial arch wire, which slides into the tube.

tube, Coolidge, *n.pr* an x-ray tube in which the gas pressure is purposely made so low that it plays no role in the operation of the tube, the operation of which depends on the emission of electrons by the heated filament of the cathode. See also x-ray tube, Coolidge.

tube, discharge, *n* any vacuum tube in which a high-voltage electric current is discharged (for example, an x-ray tube).

tube, horizontal, *n* a metal tube attachment that is placed in a horizontal position on the buccal surface of each anchor molar tooth to allow for the insertion of the labial arch wire.

tube, intubation, *n* a tube for insertion into the larynx through the mouth.

tube, line focus, *n* an x-ray tube in which the target face is about 20 inches (50 cm) from the cathode face. The focal spot is rectangular, with the length approximately three times the width. The acute angle provides an effective focal spot area approximately square and a fraction of the actual area in size.

tube, protective, housing, *n* an x-ray tube enclosure that provides radiation protection.

tube, protective, housing, diagnostic, *n* a tube housing that reduces the leakage of radiation to, at most, 0.10 r/hr at a distance of 1 mm from the tube target when the tube is operating at its maximal continuous rated voltage.

tube, protective, housing, therapeutic, *n* a tube housing that reduces the leakage of radiation to, at most, 1 r/hr at a distance of 1 m from the tube target when the tube is operating at its maximal continuous rated current for the maximal rated voltage.

tube, right-angle, *n* an x-ray tube in which the target is at right angles to the cathode.

tube tooth, *n* See tooth, tube.

tube, vertical, *n* an attachment that is usually placed on the lingual surface of the anchor band to allow for the insertion of the lingual wire.

tube, x-ray, *n* See x-ray tube.

tube feeding, *n* a method for supplying liquid nutrition through a tube that passes through the nasal passages and into the stomach. This method is utilized when ingesting food through the mouth is inadvisable or painful due to surgery or injury.

tubercle (tōō′burkəl), *n* a small rounded nodule or elevation on the surface of the skin, bone, or other tissue.

tubercle, genial **(jēnē′ əl),** *n* (geniohyoid tubercle), a small rounded elevation on the lingual surface of the mandible on either side of the midline near the inferior border of the body of the mandible, serving as a point of insertion for the geniohyoid muscles.

tubercle, geniohyoid **(jē′nē ōhī′ oid),** *n* See tubercle, genial.

tubercle, superior genial, *n* the small spines on the lingual surface of the mandible that serve as the attachment for the genioglossus muscles. On resorbed mandibles, these tubercles may be at or above the crest of the residual ridge.

tubercle, superior labial, *n* midline thickening of the superior lip.

tuberculin skin test, *n* See test, tuberculin.

tuberculum impar, *n* portion of the developing tongue located in the midline.

tuberculosis (tōōbur′kyōōlō′sis), *n* an infectious disease caused by *Mycobacterium tuberculosis* and characterized by the formation of tubercles in the tissues.

Tuberculosis of tongue. (Regezi/Sciubba/Pogrel, 2000)

tuberculous lymphadenitis, *n* an inflammation of the lymph glands caused by the presence of *Mycobacterium tuberculosis*.

tuberculosis, multidrug-resistant, *n*

tuberculosis that no longer responds to treatment due to incomplete or improper use of medication.

tuberculosis, reactivation, *n* a recurrence of tuberculosis in a patient who has been symptom free for a period of years. Reactivation tuberculosis usually responds to treatment.

tuberosity (tōōbərosʹitē), *n* a protuberance or elevation from the surface, usually of a bone.

tuberosity, maxillary, *n* the most distal aspect of the maxillary alveolar process, with its posterior border curving upward and distally.

tuberosity reduction, *n* surgical excision of excessive fibrous or bony tissue in the area of the maxillary tuberosity before the construction of prosthetic appliances.

tubule, *n* a small tube, such as one of the collecting tubules in the kidneys. The dentin of the tooth contains dentinal tubules that communicate from the pulp to the dentinoenamal interface.

tuft (toothbrush), *n* part of the toothbrush head, refers to the small, individual clusters of bristles that proceed from a single opening.

tumor, *n* a swelling. Through usage the term is now synonymous with *neoplasm.* See also neoplasm.

tumor, basaloid mixed, *n* See carcinoma, adenocystic.

tumor, Brooke's, *n.pr* See epithelioma adenoides cysticum.

tumor, brown, *n* a central giant cell tumor of the bone; associated with parathyroidism.

tumor, carotid body, *n* a tumor formed about the carotid artery.

tumor, collision, *n* a rare condition in which two neoplasms, both growing in the same general area, collide with the tumor elements and become intermingled.

tumor, Ewing's (endothelioma, Ewing's sarcoma), *n.pr* a rare malignant tumor of disputed histogenetic origin in bone. It is characterized by pain, a radiographic appearance called *onionskinning,* and a histologic picture consisting of solid sheets of small round cells that appear on the many small blood vessels present.

Ewing's sarcoma. (Regezi/Sciubba/Jordan, 2003)

tumor, giant cell, *n* a benign neoplasm of bone, producing resorption and characterized by giant cells.

tumor, hormonal, *n* localized enlargements of the gingivae that have the appearance of neoplasms and are associated with hormonal imbalance during pregnancy.

tumor, inflammatory, *n.pl* a benign tissue growth made up of inflammatory cells. The majority of oral tumors fall into this category. See also granuloma, neoplasm.

tumor, mixed, *n* **1.** one of a group of neoplasms of the salivary glands the histologic appearance of which suggests both epithelial and connective tissue origin, although they presently are considered of epithelial origin only. Benign and malignant types are possible. **2.** any tumor arising from cells derived from more than one germ layer.

tumor, mucoepidermoid, *n* a tumor of the salivary glands composed of mucous cells, epidermoid cells, and clear cells. Benign and malignant forms are recognized.

tumor, odontogenic (ōdonʹtōjenʹik), *n* **1.** a neoplasm produced from tooth-forming tissues (for example, odontogenic fibroma, odontogenic myxoma, ameloblastoma). **2.** a gingival enlargement seen during pregnancy, the microscopic examination of which reveals the features of a pyogenic granuloma. See also calcifying epithelial odontogenic tumor.

tumor, turban, *n* See carcinoma, basal cell.

tumor, Warthin's, *n.pr* See cystadenoma, papillary, lymphomatosum.

tumor necrosis factor (TNF), *n* a natural body protein with anticancer effects. It is produced in the body in response to the presence of toxic substances, such as bacterial toxins. Adverse effects are toxic shock and cachexia.

tunica intima, *n* the membrane lining an artery.

tunica media, *n* the muscular middle layer of an artery.

tunnel vision, *n* a defect in sight in which a great reduction occurs in the peripheral field of vision, as if one is looking through a hollow tube or tunnel.

turbidity, *n* a condition of light scattering in a liquid resulting from the presence of suspended particles in the fluid.

turbulence, *n* casting term used to denote irregular flow of metal into a mold. May result in porosity.

turgor, *n* the normal resiliency of the skin caused by the outward pressure of the cells and interstitial fluid. Dehydration results in a decreased skin turgor, manifested by lax skin that, when grasped and raised between two fingers, slowly returns to a position level with the adjacent tissue.

Turner's tooth, *n.pr* See tooth, Turner's.

Tweed triangle, *n.pr* See triangle, Tweed.

twilight sleep, *n* light anesthesia obtained by the parenteral administration of a mixture of morphine and scopolamine to reduce pain and obtund recall in childbirth.

twin-wire, *n* See appliance, twin-wire.

twins, *n.pl* two siblings produced in the same pregnancy and developed from one egg (identical, monozygotic) or from two eggs fertilized at the same time (fraternal, dizygotic).

twist drill, *n* **1.** a drill having one or two deep helical grooves extending from the point to the smooth portion of the shank. **2.** a spiral bone bur.

twitch, *n* **1.** the contraction of small muscle units, manifested as a quick, simple, spasmodic contraction of a muscle. **2.** a short, sudden pull or jerk.

twitching, *n* an irregular spasm of a minor extent.

twitching, **Trousseau's,** *n.pr* a twitching of the face that the patient

can exhibit at will and occurs obsessively to relieve tension.

Tylenol, *n.pr* See acetaminophen.

tympanic membrane, *n* a thin, semitransparent membrane in the middle ear that transmits sound vibrations to the internal ear by the means of the auditory ossicles. Also called the *eardrum.*

type A hepatitis, *n* See hepatitis, infectious.

type A personality, *n* a behavior pattern as associated with individuals who are highly competitive and work compulsively to meet deadlines. The condition is associated with a higher than usual incidence of coronary heart disease.

type B hepatitis, *n* See hepatitis, homologous serum.

type B personality, *n* a form of behavior associated with people who appear free of hostility and aggression and who lack a compulsion to meet deadlines, are not highly competitive at work or play, and have a lower risk of heart attack.

type E personality, *n* a term used to describe professional women who fit neither Type A nor Type B personality categories but who have a marked sense of insecurity and strive to convince themselves that they are worthwhile.

typewriter ribbon as a marking medium, *n* typewriter ribbon is more desirable than carbon paper when setting teeth because the porcelain tooth that is being adjusted will not perforate the ribbon and abrade the surface of the stone template record of jaw movement.

typhoid carrier, *n* a person without signs or symptoms of typhoid fever who carries in the body the bacteria that cause the disease but sheds the pathogens in bodily excretions.

typhoid fever, *n* a bacterial infection usually caused by *Salmonella typhi;* transmitted by contaminated milk, water, or food and characterized by headache, delirium, cough, watery diarrhea, rash, and a high fever.

typhus, *n* any of a group of acute infectious diseases caused by various species of *Rickettsia* and usually transmitted from infected rodents to humans by the bites of lice, fleas, mites, or ticks.

typical implant connective tissue, *n* the tendon-like condensed elongated avascular tissue formed in direct contact with implant infrastructure metal underlain by normal collagenous fibrous connective tissue.

typodont (tī′pōdont), *n* an artificial model containing artificial or natural teeth used for teaching technique exercises.

tyramine, *n* an amino acid synthesized in the body from the essential acid tyrosine. Tyramine stimulates the release of the catecholamines epinephrine and norepinephrine. It is important that people taking monoamine oxidase inhibitors avoid the ingestion of foods and beverages containing tyramine, particularly aged cheese, meats, bananas, yeast-containing products, and alcoholic beverages.

tyrosine (Tyr), *n* an amino acid synthesized in the body from the essential amino acid phenylalanine. Tyrosine is found in most proteins and is a precursor of melanin and several hormones, including epinephrine and thyroxine.

tyrosinemia (tī′rōsinē′mē-ə), *n* a genetic disorder of amino acid metabolism in which tyrosine acid accumulates in the blood and urine at abnormally high levels; seen primarily in infants born prematurely; may respond to a low-protein diet and the administration of synthetic amino acids.

"Ugly duckling" stage of mixed dentition. (Daniel/Harfst, 2002)

ulcer (ul′sur), *n* a loss of covering epithelium from the skin or mucous membranes, causing gradual disintegration and necrosis of the tissues.

ulcer, aphthous, recurrent (RAU) **(af′thus),** *n* periodic episodes of aphthous lesions lasting from 1 week to several months. Trauma, menses, immunologic factors, upper respiratory tract infections, and herpes simplex are suggested causes. The single or multiple discrete or confluent ulcers have a well-defined marginal erythema and a central area of necrosis with sloughing. The herpetic appearance suggests a common mechanism with herpes simplex, but no known infectious agents have been demonstrated. Also called *canker sore* and *recurrent aphthae.*

ulcer, autochthonous **(ôtok′thənus),** *n* See chancre.

ulcer, decubitus **(dēkyōō′bitus),** *n* **1.** a bedsore. **2.** loosely used to refer to a traumatic ulcer of the oral mucosa. Also called *traumatic ulcer.*

Decubitus ulcer. (Regezi/Sciubba/Jordan, 2003)

ulcer, diabetic **(dī′ əbet′ik),** *n* an ulcer, usually of the lower extremities, associated with diabetes mellitus.

ulcer, herpetic **(hurpet′ik),** *n* an ulcer that is secondary to the vesicle of herpes simplex; a shallow ulcer

ugly duckling stage, *n* a stage of dental development preceding the eruption of the permanent canines, in which the lateral incisors may be tipped laterally because of crowding by the unerupted canine crowns. This tipping may cause spacing of the incisor crowns despite the crowding of the roots. The condition may be transitory in an otherwise normal dentition. The stage was first described and named by B. H. Broadbent.

with an irregular, erythematous border and a yellow-gray base.

ulcer, Mikulicz's **(mik′yōōlichəz),** *n.pr* See periadenitis mucosa necrotica recurrens.

ulcer, pemphigoid aphthous, n a lesion located on the gingiva or mucous membranes due to a chronic disease of the autoimmune system. It is indicated by a wound with a thick wall that ruptures within 24 to 48 hours and leaves an eroded and painful surface area. It heals through the formation of a scar. See also ulcer, aphthous, recurrent (RAU).

ulcer, peptic **(pep′tik),** *n* an ulcer of the stomach or duodenum probably resulting in large part from an increased secretion of hydrochloric acid. Nervous, emotional, and endocrine factors have been implicated.

ulcer, pterygoid **(ter′igoid),** *n* See aphtha, Bednar's.

ulcer, rodent, n See carcinoma, basal cell.

ulcer, traumatic, n See ulcer, decubitus.

ulceration (ul′sərā′shən), the process of forming an ulcer or of becoming ulcerous.

ulcerative stomatitis, recurrent (ul′sərātiv, ul′sərətiv stō′mətī′tis), *n* See ulcer, aphthous, recurrent.

ultimate strength, *n* See strength, ultimate.

ultra (ul′trə), *adj* beyond; in addition; in excess of.

ultra damages, n damages beyond those paid in court.

ultracentrifuge, *n* a high-speed centrifuge with a rotation rate fast enough to produce sedimentation of viruses, even in blood plasma. Many kinds of biochemical analyses use ultracentrifuge, including such analyses as the measurement and separation of some proteins and viruses.

ultrafilrate, *n* a solution that has passed through a semipermeable membrane with very small pores. It usually contains only low-molecular-weight solutes.

ultrasonic (ul′trəson′ik), *adj* pertaining to sound frequencies so high (greater than 20 kilohertz) they cannot be perceived by the human ear.

ultrasonic cleaner, n an electronic generator that transmits high-energy and high-frequency vibrations to a fluid-filled container used to remove particulate matter from dental instruments and appliances.

ultrasonography, *n* the process of imaging deep structures of the body by measuring and recording the reflection of pulsed or continuous high-frequency sound waves. It is valuable in many medical situations, including the diagnosis of fetal abnormalities, gallstones, heart defects, and tumors. Also called *sonography.*

ultraviolet light, *n* light beyond the range of human vision, at the short end of the spectrum. It occurs naturally in sunlight; it burns and tans the skin and converts precursors in the skin to vitamin D. It is used in the treatment of psoriasis and other skin conditions. Prolonged or excessive exposure to ultraviolet light can damage the skin and increase the susceptibility of the skin to cancer.

unbundling of procedures, *n* the separating of a dental procedure into component parts with each part having a cost so that the cumulative cost of the components is greater than the total cost for the same procedure to patients who are not beneficiaries of a dental benefits plan.

uncompensated care, *n* health care services provided by a hospital, physician, dentist, or other health care professional for which no charge is made and for which no payment is expected.

unconscious (unkon′shəs), *adj* insensible; not receiving any sensory impression and not having any subjective experiences.

undecylenic acid (topical), *n trade names:* Caldesene Medicated Powder, Cruex products, Desenex Aerosol Powder, others; *drug class:* local antifungal; *action:* interferes with fungal cell membrane permeability; *uses:* tinea cruris, tinea pedis, diaper rash, minor skin irritations.

undercut, *n* **1.** the portion of a tooth that lies between its height of contour and the gingivae, only if that portion is of less circumference than the height of contour. **2.** the contour of a cross-section of a residual ridge of dental arch that would prevent the placement of a denture or other prosthesis. **3.** the contour of flasking stone that interlocks to prevent the separation of parts. **4.** the portion of a prepared cavity that creates a mechanical lock or area of retention; may be desirable in a cavity to be filled with gold foil or amalgam but is undesirable in a cavity prepared for a restoration to be cemented.

undercut gauge, n See gauge, undercut.

undercut, retentive, n an area of the abutment surface suitable for the location of a retentive clasp terminal, which in order to escape the undercut would be forced to flex and thus generate retention.

undercut, soft tissue, n an undercut in a residual ridge or soft-tissue covering of a dental arch that would prevent or influence the placement of a removable denture.

undercut, unusable, n the area of an abutment tooth or soft tissue across which a unit of the removable partial denture must pass without interference and hence must be blocked out (filled with wax or clay) before the master cast is duplicated. Use of a surveyor produces a surface that is parallel to the proposed path of a placement and removal.

underjet, n a malocclusion describing the positional relationship between the maxillary and mandibular incisors in which the maxillary incisors are measurably within the perimeter of the mandibular incisors.

undermine, v to separate surgically the skin or mucosa from its underlying stroma so that it can be stretched or moved to cover a defect or wound.

unemployment, n the state of being without a job or compensation for work, usually involuntarily.

unerupted, adj not having perforated the oral mucosa. In dentistry, used in reference to a normal developing tooth, an embedded tooth, or an impacted tooth.

unification, n the act of uniting or the condition of being united (e.g., the result of joining the components of a removable partial denture by connectors).

unilateral, adj one-sided.

union-sponsored plan, n a program of dental benefits developed through a union's initiative. May be operated directly by the union or the union may contract for provision of the benefits. Funds to finance the benefits are usually paid out of a trust fund that receives its income from employer contributions, employer and union member contributions, or union members alone.

Unipen, n.pr See nafcillin.

unit, n one of the components of a whole.

unit, Ångstrom, (Å, a.u.) (ang′strəm), n the unit of measure of wavelengths; one one-hundred-millionth of a centimeter.

unit, dental, n **1.** basically, the tooth, attachment apparatus, and gingival unit, all of which are necessary for proper masticatory activity. **2.** an article of equipment that contains an assembly of numerous items used in dental operations, such as a dental engine, cuspidor, operatory light, bracket, working table, saliva ejector, water supply, electric outlets, compressed air, or miscellaneous instruments.

unit, dentoperiodontal, n the tooth and periodontium together.

unit dosing, n a method for storing dental sealant materials and other products that lessens the risk of cross-contamination.

unit, gingival, n the tough collagenous and epithelial covering of the neck of the tooth and the underlying attachment apparatus.

unit, partial denture, n the individual elements of the partial denture, each contributing some particular function.

unit, x-ray, n a device designed to produce x-rays.

unit, x-ray, calibration, n the determination of the kilovoltage peak (KVP) value of each autotransformer tap at various milliamperages, checking these values by means of a sphere gap or a prereading voltmeter.

United States Department of Agriculture (USDA), n.pr established in 1862, USDA is responsible for the safety of meat, poultry, and egg products. It conducts ongoing research in areas from human nutrition to new crop technologies and also helps ensure open markets for U.S. agricultural products.

United States Department of Health and Human Services (USDHHS), n.pr a cabinet-level government organization comprising 12 agencies, including the Food and Drug Administration and the Centers for Disease Control.

United States dietary goals, *n.pr* the recommendation of a U.S. Senate committee in 1977 outlining the levels of consumption of complex carbohydrates, sugar, protein, fat, cholesterol, and salt for diets necessary to enhance the health status of Americans.

United States Food and Drug Administration (FDA), *n pr* a unit of the Public Health Service created to protect the health of the nation against impure and unsafe foods, drugs, and cosmetics.

United States Health Resources and Services Administration (HRSA), *n.pr* a unit of the Public Health Service created to provide leadership and direction to programs and activities designed to improve the health services for all people of the United States and to develop health care and maintenance systems that are adequately financed, comprehensive, interrelated, and responsive to the needs of all members of American society.

United States Indian Health Service, *n.pr* a unit of the Department of Health and Human Services with 51 hospitals, 99 health centers, and several hundred field health stations established to improve the health status of the American Indian and Alaskan Native.

United States Occupational Safety and Health Administration (OSHA), *n.pr* a unit of the U.S. Department of Labor, created to develop and promulgate occupational safety and health standards, develop and issue regulations, conduct investigations and inspections to determine the status of compliance with safety and health standards and regulations, and issue citations and propose penalties for noncompliance with safety and health standards and regulations.

United States Pharmacopeia (USP), *n.pr* a compendium officially recognized by the Federal Food, Drug, and Cosmetic Act that contains the descriptions, uses, strengths, and standards of purity for selected drugs.

United States Public Health Service (USPHS), *n.pr* a major division of the Department of Health and Human Services. The USPHS provides oversight of the following agencies: the Centers for Disease Control (CDC); Food and Drug Administration (FDA); Health Resources and Services Administration (HRSA); Agency for Toxic Substances and Disease Registry; National Institutes for Health (NIH); Alcohol, Drug Abuse and Mental Health Administration; Health Care Financing Administration (HCFA); Social Security Administration; Office of Child Support Enforcement; and Office of Community Services.

universal donor, *n* a person with type O, Rh factor negative red blood cells. Packed red blood cells of this type may be used for emergency transfusion with minimal risk of incompatibility.

universal precautions, *n.pl* **1.** approaches to infection control designed to prevent transmission of blood-borne diseases, such as AIDS and hepatitis B in health care settings. Universal precautions were initially developed in 1987 by the Centers for Disease Control and in 1989 by the Bureau of Communicable Disease Epidemiology in Canada. The guidelines include specific recommendations for use of gloves and masks and protective eyewear when contact with blood or bodily secretions containing blood or blood elements is anticipated. *n.pl* **2.** the protocols used to maintain an aseptic field and to prevent cross-contamination and cross-infection between health care providers, between health care providers and patients, and between patients. These include, but are not limited to, the sterilization of instruments and goods; the isolation and disinfection of the immediate clinical environment; the use of sterile disposables; scrubbing, masking, gowning, and gloving; and the proper disposal of contaminated waste.

universal recipient, *n* a person with blood type AB, who can receive a transfusion of blood of any group type without agglutination or precipitation effects.

U

universal tooth designation system, *n* a tooth numbering system in which each permanent tooth carries an Arabic numeral from 1 to 32, beginning with the maxillary right third molar and ending with the mandibular left third molar. The primary teeth are similarly numbered, preceded by a D for deciduous. The ADA numbering system is similar to the universal system, except that the primary teeth are identified by letters from A to T.

unmedullated (unmed´yōōlātəd), *adj* not possessing a medulla or medullary substance.

unpolarized, *adj* not polarized.

unsaturated fatty acid, *n* any of a number of glyceryl esters of certain organic acids in which some of the atoms are joined by double or triple valence bonds. These bonds are split easily in chemical reaction, and other substances are joined to them. Monounsaturated fatty acids have only one double or triple bond per molecule and are found in such foods as fowl, almonds, pecans, cashew nuts, peanuts, and olive oil. Polyunsaturated fatty acids have more than one double or triple bond per molecule and are found in fish, corn, walnuts, sunflower seeds, soybeans, and safflower oil.

unsaturated fatty acids, *n.pl* the double- or triple-bonded fatty acids contained primarily in vegetable oils and fish, which remain liquid at room temperature; linked to a reduction in the risk of developing heart disease.

unsharpness, geometric, *n* See geometric unsharpness.

unstable, *adj* **1.** not firm or fixed in one place; likely to move. **2.** capable of undergoing spontaneous change. A nuclide in an unstable state is called *radioactive.* An atom in an unstable state is called *excited.*

unstable angina, *n* a form of pain that is prodromal to acute myocardial infarction. It typically has a sudden onset, sudden worsening, and stuttering recurrence over days and weeks. It carries a more severe short-term prognosis than stable chronic angina. Nearly one-third of unstable angina patients experience myocardial infarction within 3 months of the first episode.

unstratified epithelium, epithelium that consists of a single layer of cells.

upcode, *n* use of a procedure code that reflects a higher-intensity service than would normally be used for the services delivered.

upright arm, *n* See connector, minor.

uprighting spring, *n* an auxiliary wire used to torque roots mesially or distally.

uranium (U), *n* a heavy, radioactive metallic element. Its atomic number is 92, and its atomic weight is 238.0289. Uranium is the heaviest of the natural elements. Isotopes of uranium are used in nuclear power plants to provide neutrons for nuclear reactions that result in release of energy.

urban health, *n* the health of a population that lives and works closely together, usually in an incorporated area, such as a city or town, with a common water supply and with similar environmental conditions.

urban population, *n* the population of an incorporated area, such as a city or town.

urea (yōōrē´-ə), *n* a water-soluble compound that is the primary constituent of urine.

Ureaplasma **(yōōrē´-əplaz´mə),** *n* gram-negative eubacteria from the family Mycoplasmataceae that serve as a hydrolitic for urea. The bacteria do not have cell walls.

urease, *n* an enzyme that divides urea into carbon dioxide and ammonia.

uremia (yōōrē´mē ə), *n* the presence of urinary components in the circulating blood and the resultant symptoms. Manifestations include weakness, headache, confusion, vomiting, and coma, and in terminal chronic renal disease, purpura and epistaxis may be present. Uremia is caused by insufficient urinary excretion for any reason. See also stomatitis, uremic.

ureteritis, *n* an inflammatory condition of a ureter caused by infection or by the mechanic irritation of a kidney stone as it passes through the ureter.

urethane, *n* ethyl carbamate used as an anesthetic agent for laboratory animals, formerly used as a hypnotic in humans.

urethritis, *n* an inflammatory condition of the urethra that is characterized by dysuria, usually the result of an infection in the bladder or kidneys.

uric acid (yoor'ik), *n* a product of protein metabolism and present in the blood and urine. See also gout.

urinalysis (yoor'inal'isis), *n* a physical, microscopic, and chemical diagnostic examination of urine. Abnormal constituents indicate disease and can include ketone bodies, protein, bacteria, blood, glucose, pus, and certain types of crystals.

urinary tract, *n* all organs and ducts involved in the secretion and elimination of urine from the body, principally the kidney, ureter, bladder, and urethra.

urinary tract infection, *n* an infection of one or more structures in the urinary tract. Gram-negative bacteria cause most of these infections.

urine, *n* the fluid excreted by the kidneys. Normal urine is clear, straw-colored, and slightly acidic, and has the characteristic odor of urea.

Urised, *n.pr* a trademark for a urinary fixed-combination drug containing an antibacterial (methenamine), an analgesic (phenyl salicylate) anticholinergics (atropine sulfate and hyoscyamine), an antifungal (benzoic acid), and an antiseptic (methylene blue).

urobilin, *n* a brown pigment formed by the oxidation of urobilinogen, normally found in feces and, in small amounts, in urine.

urokinase, *n* an enzyme produced in the kidney and found in urine that is a potent plasminogen activator of the fibrinolytic system. A pharmaceutic preparation of urokinase is administered intravenously in the treatment of pulmonary embolism.

urology, *n* the branch of medicine concerned with the study of the anatomy, physiology, and pathology of the urinary tract, with the care of the urinary tract of men and women; and with the care of the male genital tract.

ursodiol, *n trade names:* Actigall, Ursofalk; *drug class:* gallstone solubilizing agent; *action:* suppresses hepatic synthesis, secretion of cholesterol; inhibits intestinal absorption of cholesterol; *uses:* dissolution of radiolucent noncalcified gallstones of

less than 20 mm in diameter, in which surgery is not indicated.

urticaria (ur'tiker'ē ə), *n* a vascular reaction pattern of the skin marked by the transient appearance of smooth, slightly elevated patches that are more red or more pale than the surrounding skin and are accompanied by severe itching. Also called *hives.*

Urticaria. (Zitelli/Davis, 2002)

urticaria, bullosa, *n* a skin eruption in which the lesions are capped by blisters.

urticaria, giant, *n* See edema, angioneurotic.

USAN Council, *n.pr* the United States Adopted Names Council, responsible for the selection of appropriate nonproprietary names for drugs used in the United States.

USDA, *n.pr* See United States Department of Agriculture.

USDHHS, *n.pr* See United States Department of Health and Human Services.

useful beam, *n* See beam, useful.

user-friendly, *adj* simple for the unsophisticated user to master; used in reference to computer operating systems or software applications.

USP, *n.pr* See *United States Pharmacopeia.*

usual, customary and reasonable (UCR) plan, *n* a dental benefits plan that determines benefits based on usual, customary, and reasonable fee criteria. See also usual fee, customary fee, and reasonable fee.

usual fee, *n* the fee that an individual dentist most frequently charges for a given dental service. See also customary fee and reasonable fee.

ut dict., *n* abbreviation for *ut dictum,* Latin for "as directed."

utilization, *n* **1.** the extent to which a given group uses a particular service

U

in a specified period of time. Although usually expressed as the number of services used per year per 100 or per 1,000 persons eligible for the service, utilization rates may be expressed in other ratios. **2.** the extent to which the members of a covered group use a program over a stated time, specifically measured as a percentage determined by dividing the number of covered individuals who submitted one or more claims by the total number of covered individuals.

utilization management, n a set of techniques used by or on behalf of purchasers of health care benefits to manage the cost of health care before its provision by influencing patient-care decision making through case-by-case assessments of the appropriateness of care based on accepted dental practices.

utilization review (UR), n **1.** analysis of the necessity, appropriateness, and efficiency of medical and dental services, procedures, facilities, and practitioners. In a hospital, this includes review of the appropriateness of admissions, services ordered and provided, and length of stay and discharge practices, on concurrent and retrospective bases. **2.** a statistically based system that examines the distribution of treatment procedures based on claims information and, to be reasonably reliable, the application of such claims. Analyses of specific dentists should include data on type of practice, dentists' experience, socioeconomic characteristics, and geographic location.

uveitis, *n* inflammation of the uveal tract: the iris, ciliary body, and choroid of the eye.

uveoparotitis (yōō′vē ōper′ōtī′tis), *n* See fever, uveoparotid.

Uvula. (Liebgott, 2001)

uvula (yōō′vyōōlə), *n* a general term indicating a pendent fleshy mass.

uvula, bifid, n a congenital cleft resulting in a split uvula.

uvula, palatine, n a small, fleshy mass hanging from the posterior soft palate.

vaccination, *n* any injection of attenuated microorganisms, such as bacteria, viruses, or rickettsiae, administered to induce immunity or to reduce the effect of associated infectious diseases.

vaccine (vaksēn′), agent prepared to produce active immunity that usually kills microbes, attenuated live microbes, or variant strains of microbes and can induce antibody production without producing disease.

Vacudent (vak′yōōdent), *n.pr* trade name for a high-volume suction apparatus designed to remove strongly but gently any fluids and debris from an operating field.

vacuole, *n* a clear space in the substance of a cell. It may stem from a degenerative process, or it may serve the cell as a temporary cell stomach for the digestion of a foreign body inclusion.

vacuum, *n* See oral evacuator.

vacuum mixing, *n* See mixing, vacuum.

vagomimetic (vā′gōməmet′ik), *adj* pertaining to a drug with actions similar to those produced by stimulation of the vagus nerve.

Valacyclovir HCl, *n trade names:* Valtrex, Zeilirex; *class:* antiviral; *action:* converted to acyclovir, which interferes with DNA synthesis required for viral replication; *uses:* herpes zoster in immunocompetent patients.

valence, *n* **1.** in chemistry, a numeric expression of the capability of an element to combine chemically with atoms of hydrogen or their equivalent. *n* **2.** in immunology, an expression of the number of antigen-binding sites for one molecule of any given antibody or the number of antibody-binding sites for any given antigen.

validation, *n* an agreement of the listener with certain elements of the patient's communication.

validity, *n* the degree to which data or results of a study are correct or true.

valine (val'ēn), *n* one of the essential amino acids. See also amino acid.

Valium, *n.pr* See diazepam.

valproate sodium/valproate sodium-valproic acid/valproic acid, *n* *trade names:* Depakene, Myproic Acid, Depakote; *class:* anticonvulsant; *action:* increased levels of λ-aminobutyric acid (GABA) in brain; *uses:* simple, complex (petit mal), absence, mixed seizures.

value system, *n* the accepted mode of conduct and the set of norms, goals, and values binding any social group that serves as a frame of reference for the individual in reaching decisions and achieving a meaningful life.

values, normal laboratory, *n.pl* generally, statistically and biologically significant qualitative and/or quantitative measurements of cellular and clinical components of the body. The values derived from such measurements are based on averages of a survey of presumably healthy persons. The concept of individual normal values is based on an acceptable response (comparable with known evidence of health or disease) of the individual to a known alteration of cellular and/or chemical components or systems.

values, phonetic (fonet'ik), *n.pl* the characteristics of vocal sounds.

valve, *n* a structure that controls flow of the contents of a canal or passage.

valve, exhalation, *n* a valve that permits escape of exhaled gases into the atmosphere and prevents them from being rebreathed.

valvular heart disease, *n* a potentially life-threatening cardiac valve disorder, characterized by the constriction or obstruction of blood vessels, in which a valve malfunctions so that blood is forced to flow backward rather than through the vessel. The condition may be present at birth or acquired as the result of an illness, such as rheumatic fever, syphilis, or bacterial endocarditis.

van den Bergh's test, *n.pr* See test, van den Bergh's.

vancomycin HCl, *n* *trade name:* Vancocin; *class:* glucopeptide-type antiinfective; *action:* inhibits bacterial cell wall synthesis; *uses:* resistant staphylococcal infections, pseudomembranous colitis, staphylococcal enterocolitis, endocarditis prophylaxis for dental procedures.

vapor, *n* **1.** the gaseous form assumed by a solid or liquid when sufficiently heated. *n* **2.** a visible emanation of fine particles of a liquid.

Vaquez' disease (vəkāz'), *n.pr* See erythremia.

variability, *n* the degree or range of divergence of an object from a given standard or average.

variable, *adj* **1.** changing; able to vary in quantity or magnitude. *n* **2.** a characteristic that may assume several values.

variable, continuous, *n* a variable for which it is possible to find an intermediate value between any two values. Continuous variables can be refined by more precise values. Length, weight, and time, and the points on a line are continuous variables.

variable costs, *n* costs, such as dental service claims, that generally increase or decrease as the size and composition of the enrollment fluctuates.

variable, dependent, *n* a variable whose value is consequent on change in the independent variable. The dependent variable is always the response or reaction to the independent variable. Also called *criterion variable.*

variable, discrete, *n* a variable that is expressed in whole units or mutually exclusive categories. Whole numbers and category designations such as sex and marital status are examples of discrete data.

variable, independent, *n* the variable being studied that is manipulated or controlled by an experimenter. In a drug study an investigator may give several doses of a drug (independent variable) to determine the most effective, symptom-reducing (dependent variable) level.

variables, control, *n.pl* those variables not being studied that are held constant so as not to influence the experimental outcome. Environmental conditions, intelligence quotients, and social and psychologic variables are examples of variables that must be controlled.

variation (genetic), *n* deviation from the genotype in structure, form, physiology, or behavior.

varicella (ver'isel'ə), *n* (chickenpox), an acute communicable disease with an incubation period of 2 or 3 weeks and caused by herpesvirus, usually found in children. Manifestations include coryza, fever, malaise, and headache, followed in 2 or 3 days by the eruption of macular vesicles.

Varicella. (Regezi/Sciubba/Jordan, 2003)

varicosity (ver'ikos'itē), *n* an abnormal condition characterized by the presence of tortuous, abnormally dilated veins, usually in the legs or the lower trunk; may also appear in the esophagus.

Varicosity. (Neville/Damm/Allen/Bouquot, 2002)

variola (ver'ē ō'lə), *n* (smallpox), an acute, viral, contagious disease transmitted by the respiratory route and direct contact. The incubation period is 1 to 2 weeks. Manifestations include headache, chills, and temperature up to 106° F. On the third and fourth day, macules appear, which then become papules; then constitutional symptoms abate. On the sixth day the papules become vesicles. The vesicles then become pustules, with desquamation occurring in about 2 weeks.

varnish, *n* (cavity liner, cavity varnish), a clear solution of resinous material or natural gum, such as copal or rosin dissolved in acetone, ether, or chloroform, which is capable of hardening without losing its transparency. Varnish is used in cavity preparations to seal out dentinal tubules, reduce microleakage, and insulate the pulp against shock from thermal changes.

varnish, fluoride, *n* a sticky yellowish protective coating of 5% sodium fluoride in a resin base that is painted over the teeth to prevent dental caries in children and adults. It hardens on contact with saliva. It is also used to reduce root sensitivity. Its effects on enamel fluoride appear to provide a lower risk of accidental fluoride ingestion than most other topical fluoride treatments.

Varnish, fluoride. (Bird/Robinson, 2002, Courtesy Ivoclar Vivadent)

vascular diseases, *n.pl* diseases of the peripheral circulatory system.

vascular reactions, *n.pl* the responses of the blood vessels to injury or introduction of chemical agents, particularly certain chemical mediators such as histamine and bradykinin.

vascular resistance, *n* the degree to which the blood vessels impede the flow of blood. High resistance causes an increase in blood pressure, which increases the workload of the heart.

vascular spasm, *n* a sudden constriction of the blood vessels causing reduction or stoppage in blood flow. A vascular spasm in vessels of the brain can result in a stroke; in the vessels of the heart it can result in a heart attack.

vasculitis, *n* an inflammatory condition of the blood vessels that is characteristic of certain systemic diseases or is caused by an allergic reaction.

vasoconstrictor (vā′zōkənstrik′tur), *n* (vasopressor), an agent that causes a rise in blood pressure by constricting the blood vessels. In local areas, it causes constriction of the arterioles and capillaries.

vasoconstrictor, adrenergic agents as, n adrenaline-mimicking drugs that increase the duration of local anesthesia by constricting the blood vessels, thereby safely concentrating the anesthetic for an extended duration and reducing hemorrhage. Excessive amounts can cause systemic toxicity, especially in certain medical conditions or when combined with certain medications. Also used in gingival retraction cord impregnated with epinephrine.

vasodepressor (vā′zōdēpres′ur), *n* an agent that depresses circulation and causes vasomotor depression.

vasodilator (vā′zōdī′lātur), *n* **1.** an agent that causes dilation of the blood vessels. *n* **2.** a drug that relaxes the smooth muscle walls of the blood vessels and increases their diameter.

vasomotor (vā′zōmōtur), *adj* pertaining to any agent or nerve that causes expansion or contraction of the walls of blood vessels.

vasopressin (vā′zōpres′in), *n* See hormone, antidiuretic.

vasopressor (vāz′ōpres′ur), *n* See vasoconstrictor.

vault, *n* **1.** an anatomic part resembling an arched roof or dome, such as the vault of a denture. *n* **2.** a cavity or specially prepared area within the jawbone for placement of an implant magnet.

V-bends, *n* V-shaped bends placed in an orthodontic arch wire, usually mesially to the canines. The V-bends create an adjustment site at which torquing bends may be placed.

VDRL test, *n.pr* abbreviation for Ve-

nereal Disease Research Laboratory test, a serologic flocculation test for syphilis or yaws.

vector, *n* a carrier that transmits a disease from one party to another.

vegan diet (vē′gən), *n* the strictest form of vegetarian diet, which prohibits the consumption of all animal products, including dairy, eggs, meat, poultry, fish, and animal fats. Care must be taken to avoid the risk of developing calcium, iron, zinc, or vitamin B_{12} deficiencies.

vehicle (vē′hikəl), *n* a pharmaceutic ingredient, usually a liquid, employed as a medium for dissolving or dispersing the active drug in a mass suitable for its administration.

Veillonella alcalescens (vā′yənel′ə alkəles′enz), n **1.** an organism of the genus *Veillonella. n* **2.** a schizomycete that has been found in the flora of the periodontal pocket and, by association, has been implicated in the origin and perpetuation of periodontitis in human beings.

vein (vān), *n* a blood vessel that conducts blood from the capillary bed to the heart. Size may range from the venules to small veins to large veins.

vein, retromandibular (ret′rōmandib′yōōlur), *n* the vein formed posterior to the mandible by the joining of maxillary and superficial temporal veins. The posterior branch connects with the external jugular vein while the anterior branch enters the internal jugular vein.

velopharyngeal adequacy (vē′lōfərin′jē əl), *n* See closure, velopharyngeal.

velopharyngeal closure, *n* See closure, velopharyngeal.

velopharyngeal inadequacy, *n* See inadequacy, velopharyngeal.

velum (vē′lum), *n* a membranous cover that resembles a curtain or veil.

velum palatinum (vē′lum pal′ətī′num), n See soft palate.

velum platinum, n a membranous cover on the roof of the mouth.

veneer (vənir′), *n* in the construction of crowns or pontics, a layer of tooth-colored material, usually porcelain or acrylic resin, attached to the surface by direct fusion, cementation, or mechanical retention.

venereal disease (vənir′ē əl), *n* any

contagious condition acquired by sexual intercourse or genital contact. Venereal diseases include chancroid, gonorrhea, granuloma inguinale, herpes simplex type II, HIV, lymphogranuloma venereum, and syphilis. More commonly called *sexually transmitted disease.*

venipuncture (ven´əpungkchur), *n* surgical or therapeutic puncture of a vein.

venlafaxine HCl, *n trade name:* Effexor; *class:* bicyclic antidepressant; *action:* inhibits both norepinephrine and serotonin (5-HT) uptake and, to a lesser extent, dopamine uptake; *use:* depression.

venous sinus, *n* the space between two layers of tissue, which is filled with blood.

ventilate, *v* 1. to provide with fresh air. *v* 2. to provide the lungs with air from the atmosphere. *v* 3. to open, to free, as in to openly express one's feelings.

ventilation (ven´tilā´shən), *n* the constant supplying of oxygen through the lungs.

ventilation, air, *n* the process of supplying alveoli with air or oxygen.

ventilation, mouth-to-mouth, *n* a method by which a rescuer uses the air in his or her own lungs to fill the lungs of another person who has stopped breathing in order to oxygenate that person's blood. See respiration, artificial.

ventilation, respiratory, *n* the process of getting air into and out of the lungs. The air enters the mouth and nose and must go through the conduction system (the pharynx, larynx, trachea, and bronchial tree) into the lungs. This ventilating process involves many other structures as well, including the abdomen, thorax, and maxillofacial tissues. The latter structures make two significant contributions to the respiratory process: they provide the portal of entry and egress for the air to and from the lungs, and they alter the physical properties of inspired air for protection of the very sensitive lung tissues.

venting, *n* an exit passage constructed in a casting mold to allow gases to escape during the casting process.

ventral, *adj* pertaining to the anterior part of a structure, or the part opposite the anatomical back.

ventricle, *n* a small cavity, such as one of the cavities filled with cerebrospinal fluid in the brain, or the right or left ventricle of the heart.

ventricular dysfunction, *n* an abnormality in contraction and wall motion within the ventricles.

ventricular fibrillation (VF), *n* a cardiac dysrhythmia marked by rapid, disorganized depolarizations of the ventricular myocardium. The condition is characterized by a complete lack of organized electric impulse, conduction, and ventricular contraction. Blood pressure falls to zero, resulting in unconsciousness. Death may occur within 4 minutes. Defibrillation and ventilation, i.e., cardiopulmonary resuscitation (CPR), must be initiated immediately.

ventricular function, *n* the cyclic contraction and relaxation of the ventricular myocardium.

ventricular septal defect (VSD), *n* an abnormal opening in the septum separating the ventricles of the heart. It is the most common congenital heart defect. Children with small defects are usually without symptoms. Large defects can prevent proper oxygenation of the blood and may initiate congestive heart failure, if not surgically corrected.

ventriculoureterostomy, *n* a surgical procedure for directing cerebrospinal fluid into the general circulation; performed in the treatment of hydrocephalus, usually in the newborn.

venue (ven´yōō), *n* the neighborhood, place, or county in which an injury is declared to have occurred or fact is declared to have happened; also designates the county in which an action or prosecution is presented for trial.

venule (ven´yōōl), *n* the smallest of the venous blood vessels; consists of an endothelial tube enclosed in a variable amount of elastic and collagenous tissue. Smooth muscle is introduced in the media as the caliber of the vessel increases. The muscle fibers are distributed sparsely in the smaller vessels but coalesce into circumferential bands in the larger vessels.

veracity (vəras´itē), *n* legal principle that states that a health professional should be honest and give full disclosure to the patient, abstain from misrepresentation or deceit, and report known lapses of the standards of care to the proper agencies.

verapamil HCl, *n trade names:* Calan, Isoptin, Calan SR, Isoptin SR, others; *class:* calcium-channel blocker; *action:* inhibits calcium ion influx across cell membranes during cardiac depolarization; produces relaxation of coronary vascular smooth muscle, dilates coronary arteries, decreases SA/AV node conduction, and dilates peripheral arteries; *uses:* chronic stable angina pectoris, vasospastic angina, dysrhythmias, hypertension.

verbal, *adj* by word of mouth; oral, as in a verbal agreement.

verdict, *n* the formal decision or finding of a jury on the matters or questions duly submitted to them at a trial.

vermilion border, *n* the junction between the lip and the facial skin.

vermilion zone, *n* the external darkish area of the upper and lower lips, extending from the junction of the lips, with the surrounding facial skin on the exterior to the labial mucosa within the mouth.

vernier (vur′nē ur), *n* See gauge, Boley.

verruca (vəroo′kə), *n* a benign, viral, warty skin lesion with a rough, papillomatous surface. It is caused by a common contagious papovavirus.

verruca senilis **(sənil′is),** *n* See keratosis, seborrheic.

verruca vulgaris, *n* (wart), a common wart of the skin or mucosa.

Verruca vulgaris. (Sapp/Eversole/Wysocki, 2004)

verrucous carcinoma (vəroo′kus kär′sinō′mə), *n* See carcinoma, verrucous.

vertebra, *n* any one of the 33 bones of the spinal or vertebral column that comprises the 7 cervical, 12 thoracic, 5 lumbar, 5 sacral, and 4 coccygeal vertebrae.

vertical, *adj* perpendicular to the horizontal plane.

vertical angulation, *n* See angulation, vertical.

vertical bite-wing film, *n* a small, photosensitive piece of material that is used to take x-rays of the teeth at an angle that allows the viewing of any existing overhangs, root caries, crowns, furcation, and bone loss. The film is placed vertically rather than horizontally to get a more complete view of the root.

vertical bone loss, *n* an abnormal decrease in the alveolar crestal bone height indicated by a visible loss of bone on one tooth's proximal surface compared to the tooth on the adjacent side.

vertical dimension, *n* See dimension, vertical.

vertical lug, *n* See connector, minor.

vertical opening, *n* See dimension, vertical.

vertical overlap, *n* See overlap, vertical.

vertical relation, See relation, vertical.

vertical-integrated health care, a health care delivery system in which the complete spectrum of care, including financial services, is provided within a single organization, such as a health maintenance organization (HMO).

vertigo (vur′təgō), *n* **1.** a sensation described as dizziness. *n* **2.** a sensation of the room revolving about the patient or the patient revolving in space. It is a form of dizziness, but the terms are not synonymous.

very low-density lipoproteins (VLDLs), *n.pl* lipoproteins containing approximately 9% protein that transport triglycerides from the liver to tissues throughout the body.

vesicant (ves′ikənt), *n* a chemically active substance that can produce blistering on direct contact with the skin or mucous membrane.

vesicle (ves′ikəl), *n* **1.** a small, blisterlike elevation of the skin or mucous membrane resulting from an intraepithelial collection of fluid. It is a primary type of lesion and may be seen in herpes simplex, recurrent herpes, recurrent aphthae, stomatitis medicamentosa, stomatitis venenata, erythema multiforme, Reiter's syndrome, Behçet's syndrome, Stevens-Johnson syndrome, herpangina, varicella, and many others. *n* **2.** a circumscribed, elevated lesion of the skin containing fluid and having a diameter of up to 5 mm.

vessel(s), *n* an avenue through which something can travel.

vessels, afferent, n.pl vessels that carry fluids such as lymph or blood toward a structure or a part.

vessels, blood, visualization of, n any one of various methods by which the blood vessels are seen by the examiner. Direct visualization of blood vessels is possible only to a limited extent. The blood vessels in the retina can be directly visualized; the capillary loops in the fingernail can be seen by microscopy, and the blood vessels in the oral mucosa and gingivae can be visualized by infrared photography. More recently, radiography and cineradiography are used to visualize radiopaque substances. These methods can reveal the actual blood column, its width, variation in contour, and pathway. Arteriograms and venograms are useful in revealing spasms, obstructions, congenital defects, and collateral circulation of the deeper tissues.

vessels, efferent, n.pl vessels that carry fluids such as lymph or blood away from a body part.

vested, *adj* pertaining to a nonforfeitable interest of a participant in a pension plan.

vestibule, buccal, *n* the space between the alveolar ridge and teeth or between the residual ridge and the cheek distal to the buccal frenum.

vestibule, labial, *n* the space between the alveolar ridge and the teeth or the residual ridge and lips anterior to the buccal frenum.

vestibule, lower buccal, *n* the space between the mandibular alveolar ridge and teeth and the cheek; bounded anteriorly by the lower buccal frenum and posteriorly by the distobuccal end of the retromolar pad.

vestibule of the oral cavity, *n* the part of the oral cavity that lies between the teeth and gingivae and lips and cheeks or between the residual ridges and the lips and cheeks.

vestibule, upper buccal, *n* the space between the maxillary alveolar ridge and teeth or the residual ridge and the cheek; bounded anteriorly by the upper buccal frenum and posteriorly by the hamular notch.

vestibuloplasty (vestib´yōōlōplastē), *n* any of a series of surgical procedures designed to restore alveolar ridge height by lowering the muscles attached to the buccal, labial, and lingual aspects of the jaws.

Vestibuloplasty. (Genco/Goldman/Cohen, 1990)

veteran, *n* **1.** a person who has a long period of service in an occupation or profession. *n* **2.** a person who has served in the armed forces, especially one who has fought for his or her country. *n* **3.** a long-serving member of a state legislature or the U.S. Congress.

veterinarian, *n* a Doctor of Veterinary Medicine, who is educated and trained to provide medical and surgical care for domestic and exotic animals.

viable (vī´əbəl), *adj* capable of life; able to live.

Viadent, *n.pr* brand name for an anti-plaque mouthrinse containing sanguinarine, an alkaloid, as the active ingredient. See also sanguinarine.

vibrating line, *n* See line, vibrating.

vibrios, *n.pl* bacteria belonging to the genus *Vibrio* found in plaque after one to two weeks of no flossing or brushing.

Vicat needle (vēkä), *n.pr* See needle, Vicat.

Vickers hardness number, *n.pr* See number, Vickers hardness.

Vickers hardness test, *n.pr* See test, Vickers hardness.

Vicodin, *n.pr* brand name for hydrocodone, a ketone derivative of codeine that is about six times more potent than codeine. Vicodin is a controlled substance.

vidarabine, *n* (ophthalmic), *trade name:* Vira-A Ophthalmic; *class:* antiviral; *action:* inhibits DNA synthesis by blocking DNA polymerase; *use:* keratoconjunctivitis due to herpes simplex virus.

viewbox, *n* used for viewing dental radiographs consisting of a table-top box with a transparent surface through which light is transmitted. When radiographs are laid on the surface, visibility of important details is greatly increased, ensuring greater accuracy of interpretation.

Viewbox. (Bird/Robinson, 2002)

Vincent's angina, *n.pr* See angina, Vincent's.

Vincent's bacillus, *n.pr* See *Fusobacterium fusiforme.*

Vincent's gingivitis, *n.pr* See gingivitis, necrotizing ulcerative.

Vincent's infection, *n.pr* See gingivitis, necrotizing ulcerative.

vinegar (as a solvent), *n* a warm, dilute solution of household vinegar; used as a substitute for acetic acid to dissolve accumulated dental calculus from a removable dental prosthesis.

Vinethene (vin'ethēn), *n.pr* trade name for vinyl ether.

vinyl resin (vī'nil), *n* See resin, vinyl.

violation, injury, *n* encroachment; breach of right, obligation, or law.

violence, *n* severe physical force; the forceful assault of a person.

violet, gentian (vī'əlet, jen'shən), *n* a rosaniline dye, useful as a protective covering and an antiseptic in the treatment of minor lesions of the oral mucosa. It is an effective fungicide and is therefore of value in the treatment of moniliasis.

violet stain, *n* See stain, methyl violet.

viral hepatitis, *n* See hepatitis.

viral infection, *n* an infection by any of the more than 200 pathogenic viruses. A virus acts on the cell nucleus, taking over the genetic material within the nucleus and replicating itself.

viral shedding, *n* process that occurs when a virus is present in bodily fluids or open wounds and can thereby be transmitted to another person, as with herpetic lesions.

viremia (vīrē'mē-ə), *n* an elevation of virus levels occurring 2 to 4 weeks after infection with HIV.

virion (vir'ē-on, vī'rē-), *n* the whole virus, including the inner nucleus and the outer shell.

virology, *n* the scientific study of viruses and the diseases caused by viruses.

virulence, *n* the power of a microorganism to produce disease.

virus (vī'rus), *n* one of a group of heterogeneous infective agents characterized by the lack of independent metabolism or the ability to replicate outside the host cell.

virus, herpes simplex, *n* See herpes simplex.

virus replication, *n* the ability of viruses to reproduce within a host cell.

viscera, *n.pl* (*sg* **viscus**), the internal organs enclosed within a body cavity, primarily the abdominal organs.

viscerocranium (vis'ərōkrā'nē-um), *n* the category of the 14 bones of the human skull

V

that encircle the face. Also called the *facial bones.*

viscosity, *n* the ability or inability of a fluid solution to flow easily. High viscosity indicates a slow-flowing fluid.

visible light, *n* the radiant energy in the electromagnetic spectrum that is visible to the human eye. The wavelengths cover a range of approximately 390 to 780 nm.

visible-light cure, *n* system designed to control the curing time of material that hardens over a period of time; when light is withheld, the material is malleable for a longer duration; when light is applied, the material hardens rapidly.

vision (vizh′ən), *n* sight; the faculty of seeing.

vision, direct, *n* the category of sight in which an image is focused directly on the macula of the retina. Also called *central vision.*

vision, field of, *n* the portion of space that the fixed eye can see.

vision, indirect, *n* **1.** in dentistry, the capacity to see the treatment area by using a mouth mirror. *n* **2.** the category of sight in which an image is focused on an area of the retina other than the macula. Also called *peripheral vision.*

Indirect vision. (Bird/Robinson, 2002)

vision, stereoscopic, *n* vision in which the visual fields of the two eyes are unified. Sensations from a common object received by the two eyes are superimposed, and as a result of the slight differences in the fields and the superimposition of the fields, the effects of depth and shape of the object are attained.

visit, *n* a meeting between a health care professional and a patient for diagnostic, therapeutic, or consultative reasons, usually a scheduled appointment in a professional office. Also called *patient visit* or *patient encounter.*

visual acuity, *n* a measure of the resolving power of the eye, particularly its ability to distinguish letters and numbers at a given distance. See also acuity, visual.

visual analogue scale for pain (VAS), *n* a simple assessment tool consisting of a 10 cm line with 0 on one end, representing no pain, and 10 on the other, representing the worst pain ever experienced, which a patient marks to indicate the severity of his or her pain.

visual disorders, *n.pl* See disorders, visual.

visual treatment objective (VTO), *n* a diagnostic and communication aid, consisting of a cephalometric tracing, modified to show changes anticipated in the course of growth and treatment.

vital, *adj* necessary to or pertaining to life.

vital capacity, *n* a measurement of the amount of air that can be expelled at the normal rate of exhalation after a maximum inspiration, representing the greatest possible breathing capacity.

vital signs, *n.pl* the measurements of pulse rate, respiration rate, and body temperature. Although not strictly a vital sign, blood pressure is also customarily included in this category.

vital statistics, *n.pl* data relating to births (natality), deaths (mortality), marriages, health, and disease (morbidity).

vitalometer (vī′təlom′əter), *n* an electric-powered instrument for delivering and measuring an electrical stimulus to a tooth. See also pulp tester.

vitalometry (vi′təlom′ətrē), *n* the use of high-frequency pulp-testing equipment to establish the vital condition of the pulp of a tooth.

vitamin (vi′təmin), *n* one of a number of unrelated organic substances that occur in small amounts in food and are required for normal metabolic activity. The vitamins may be water soluble or fat soluble.

vitamin A, *n* (retinal, retinol, retinoic

acid), a fat-soluble substance, occurring in several chemical forms in food and function: retinal, an aldehyde; retinol, an alcohol; and retinoic acid, an acid. All three function in calcified and epithelial tissue growth. The aldehyde-alcohol (retinal-retinol) interconversion allows regeneration of rhodopsin (visual purple) in the rod cells of the retina. A deficiency results in hyperkeratinization of nonsecretory protective epithelium, deranged secretory function of the mucous membrane, dark dysadaptation (night blindness), and possibly, enamel hypoplasia. Dietary sources include liver, kidney, and lung as well as carotenes (provitamins A) from the plant kingdom.

vitamin, ascorbic acid (skôr'bik), *n* (vitamin C, antiscorbutic factor), a water-soluble vitamin resembling glucose in structure; it is found in citrus fruits, tomatoes, cabbage, and other fresh fruits and vegetables. Necessary for hydroxylation of peptide-bound lysine and proline to hydroxylysine and hydroxyproline during collagen synthesis. A deficiency leads to scurvy, in which pathologic signs are confined mainly to the connective tissues with hemorrhages, loosening of teeth, gingivitis, and poor wound healing.

vitamin B_1, *n* See vitamin, thiamine.
vitamin B_2, *n* See vitamin, riboflavin.
vitamin B_6, *n* See vitamin, pyridoxine.
vitamin B_{12}, *n* See vitamin, cobalamin.
vitamin B complex, *n* collectively, the various B vitamins: thiamine, riboflavin, nicotinic acid, pyridoxine, biotin, *para*-aminobenzoic acid, folic acid, pantothenic acid, cyanocobalamin, pteroylglutamic acid, and others that are unknown.

vitamin, biotin (bi' ətin), *n* (vitamin H, anti-egg-white factor), one of the B complex vitamins found in organ meats (e.g., liver, heart, kidney), egg yolk, cauliflower, chocolate, and mushrooms. Its synthesis by intestinal bacteria makes human deficiency states rare, unless the diet contains significant raw egg white protein (avidin), which complexes the vitamin to prevent intestinal absorption. Derma-

titis, retarded growth, and loss of hair and muscular control occur in experimental animals with deficiency. Biotin functions as a coenzyme for carboxylase enzymes that catalyze fixation of carbon dioxide (e.g., in fatty acid synthesis).

vitamin C, *n* See vitamin, ascorbic acid.
vitamin, calciferol, *n* See vitamin D.
vitamin, cholecalciferol, *n* See vitamin D.

vitamin, choline (kō'lēn), *n* not truly a vitamin, because it can be synthesized in the body if sufficient precursors are available. Prevents the accumulation of fat in the liver of certain animal species. Occurs as a constituent of lecithin, sphingomyelin, and acetylcholine.

vitamin, cobalamin (kōbal'əmin), *n* (antipernicious factor, vitamin B_{12}, cyanocobalamin, erythrocyte maturing factor [EMF], extrinsic factor), a vitamin that contains cobalt and is essential for the maturation of erythrocytes. Inability of the body to produce intrinsic factor, which is necessary for vitamin B_{12} absorption, results in pernicious anemia. Liver, kidney, muscle, and milk are good sources.

vitamin D (antirachitic factor, calciferol, cholecalciferol, ergosterol, ergocalciferol), *n* the group of lipid-soluble sterol compounds capable of preventing rickets. Of primary importance are D_2, or ergosterol, from plants and D_3, or cholecalciferol, from animal sources, especially fish liver oils. The latter is also formed in the skin from 7-dehydrocholesterol on exposure to ultraviolet light. Liver mitochondria further activate vitamin D to 25-(OH)-D, which in turn is metabolized to 1,25-$(OH)_2$-D by the kidney. The dihydroxy metabolites significantly increase dietary calcium absorption and bone resorption to maintain proper blood calcium and phosphorus levels. A primary vitamin D deficiency results from inadequate exposure to sunlight and low dietary intake. Secondary deficiencies occur from abnormalities of intestinal resorption and interference with vitamin D hydroxylation. The manifestations of rickets include enamel hypoplasia, poorly calcified bones,

V

bowed legs, and a deformed rib cage with beadlike swellings of the ribs (rachitic rosary) in infants and children and osteomalacia in adults. Vitamin D intake in excess is toxic.

vitamin E, *n* (tocopherol, tocotrienol antisterility factor), the tocopherol and tocotrienols have varying degrees of vitamin E activity but α-tocopherol is the most active. These fat-soluble compounds are found in eggs, muscle meats, liver, fish, chicken, oatmeal, and the oils of corn, soya, and cottonseed. In rats, the lack of vitamin E leads to fetus resorption in the female and atrophy of spermatogenic tissue with permanent sterility in the male. Vitamin E deficiency in humans is correlated with increased hemolysis of erythrocytes. The tocopherols prevent peroxidation of unsaturated fatty acids, and vitamin E requirements appear to be directly related to the dietary intake of unsaturated fatty acids. Although animals develop symptoms of muscular dystrophy on deficient diets, the vitamin has no effect on the human disease.

vitamin, ergocalciferol, *n* See vitamin D.

vitamin, folacin, *n* (adermine, folic acid, citrovorum factor, pteroylglutamic acid, vitamin M, vitamin B_c), occurs in many tissues as the free acid or is conjugated with one to seven glutamic acid molecules. Green, leafy vegetables, kidney, liver, and yeast are good sources, and bacterial synthesis in humans occurs readily. As a coenzyme, the vitamin serves as a carrier of one-carbon units (formyl, hydroxymethyl, formimino groups), especially in the synthesis of nucleoproteins. Inadequate folate levels produce a variety of species-dependent symptoms that include megaloblastic anemia in humans.

vitamin G, *n* See vitamin, riboflavin.

vitamin H, *n* See vitamin, biotin.

vitamin, inositol **(inō′sətôl),** *n* (*myo*-inositol, *meso*-inositol), a six-carbon alcohol closely related to the hexoses. Inositol is not truly a vitamin because the body can synthesize significant amounts from glucose. Its biologic role is not established, but it is essential to the growth of liver and bone marrow cells and helps alleviate fatty livers.

vitamin K, *n* (phytonadione, antihemorrhagic factor), one of the many fat-soluble naphthoquinone compounds with vitamin D activity. Vitamin K_1 is found primarily in leafy vegetables, K_2 is synthesized by human intestinal bacteria, and K_3 (menadione, N.F.) is a synthetic compound. Vitamin K is essential for the synthesis of prothrombin by the liver. A dietary deficiency of vitamin K is rare, however. The vitamin has been used in conjunction with extensive oral antibiotic therapy to treat hemorrhagic disease of the newborn, hemorrhage of obstructive jaundice, and sprue, and during anticoagulant therapy. Prothrombin, Stuart factor, Christmas factor, and serum prothrombin conversion accelerator require vitamin K for their synthesis.

vitamin, niacin **(nī′ əsin),** *n* (nicotinic acid, nicotinamide, niacinamide, pellagra-preventive factor), a deficiency of niacin or its amide derivative, niacinamide, results in acute pellagra that is characterized by dermatitis, diarrhea, dementia, stomatitis, and glossitis. Dietary sources include liver, kidney, lean meats, wheat germ, yeast, soybeans, and peanuts. There is some intestinal synthesis by bacteria. Although the amino acid tryptophan contributes to the body supply of niacin, sufficient vitamin B_6 must be present for its metabolism. Niacin and niacinamide are interconvertible in the body, and the latter functions as a constituent of two coenzymes, NAD and NADP, which operate as hydrogen and electron transfer agents by virtue of their reversible oxidation and reduction in several enzyme systems.

vitamin, pantothenic acid **(pan′təthen′ik),** *n* (pantothen, panthenol), this vitamin is a component of coenzyme A and thereby functions in the metabolism of lipids, carbohydrates, and proteins. A deficiency is unusual because of its wide distribution, but a "burning feet syndrome" has been reported in people suffering from acute malnutrition.

vitamin, pyridoxine **(pir′ədok′sēn),** *n* (vitamin B_6, pyridoxal, pyridoxol, pyridoxamine), part of the B complex vitamins, the group includes three chemically related substances: pyridoxol, pyridoxal, and pyridoxamine, all of which serve as substrate in the formation of pyridoxal phosphate, the prosthetic group for several enzymes that decarboxylate, deaminate, transaminate, or desulfurate specific amino acids. It further functions in porphyrin, fatty acids, and cholesterol metabolism. Deficiency signs include an acrodynia-like syndrome, convulsive seizures, arteriosclerotic-like lesions, hypochromic microcytic anemia, and impaired antibody formation. Dietary sources include wheat, corn, liver, milk, eggs, and green, leafy vegetables.

vitamin, retinal, n See vitamin A.

vitamin, retinoic acid, n See vitamin A

vitamin, retinol, n See vitamin A.

vitamin, riboflavin (rī'bōflāvin), n (vitamin B_2, vitamin G, lactoflavin), a heat-stable B complex vitamin that functions as a component of FAD and FMN for the reversible transfer of hydrogen and electrons in several enzyme systems. It is found in green, leafy vegetables, whole grains, eggs, liver, milk, and legumes; small amounts are synthesized in the intestinal tract by microorganisms. Signs of ariboflavinosis include angular stomatitis, seborrheic dermatitis of the face, and glossitis (magenta tongue).

vitamin, thiamine (thī'əmin), n (vitamin B_1, aneurine, antiberiberi factor, antineuritic factor), a B complex vitamin found primarily in plants, especially legumes, whole grains, and green, leafy vegetables; it is also synthesized by bacteria in the large intestine, which is not a reliable source. Thiamine pyrophosphate (TPP, cocarboxylase) is a coenzyme in the oxidative decarboxylation of pyruvate and α-ketoglutarate, in the transketolase reaction of glucose metabolism and in the metabolism of branched chained amino acids. A deficiency results in beriberi.

vitamin, tocopherol, n See vitamin E.

vitamin, tocotrienol, n See vitamin E.

vitiate (vish'ē āt), v to weaken; to make void or voidable.

vitiligo (vit'ilē'gō, vit'ilī'gō), n a skin condition characterized by spotty areas of depigmentation.

vitrification (vit'rifikā'shən), n the act, instance, art, or process of converting dental porcelain (frit) to a glassy substance; the process of becoming vitreous by heat and fusion.

VLDL, *n.pl* abbreviation for very-low-density lipids.

vocabulary, n **1.** the stock or range of words possessed by an individual or a culture used for self-expression or communication. n **2.** the sum of the distinct words related to a discipline or profession.

vocal cords, *n.pl* See cords, vocal.

voice, n sound produced primarily by the vibration of the vocal bands.

void, n **1.** empty or unfilled space. n **2.** space not filled with anything solid. *adj* **3.** ineffectual; having no legal, binding effect

volatile (vol'ətil), *adj* having a tendency to evaporate rapidly.

volatile oil, n See oil, essential.

volatile sulfur compounds (VSCs), *n.pl* bad-smelling substances such as hydrogen sulfide, methyl mercaptan, dimethyl sulfide, and dimethyl disulfide that are produced by the metabolism of a microscopic organism.

Volkmann's canal, *n.pr* a passage distinct from a Haversian canal that carries nutrients through bone.

volt (V), n the unit of electromotive force or electrical pressure; the force necessary to cause 1 ampere of current to flow against 1 ohm of resistance. A volt is the unit that is used to measure the tendency of a charge to move from one place to another.

volt, electron (eV), n the kinetic energy gained by an electron by falling through a potential difference of 1 volt. 1 eV is equivalent to 1.6×10^{-12} ergs. 1,000 eV is referred to as 1 kilo electron volt, or keV, and 1,000,000 eV are referred to as 1 mega electron volt, or MeV.

voltage, n the potential of electromotive force of an electric charge, measured in volts.

volume, n measure of the quantity of space occupied by a substance, such as air.

volume, blood, n the total amount of blood in the body.

volume, expiratory reserve, n (re-

V

serve air, supplemental air, supplemental volume), the maximum volume that can be expired from the resting expiratory level.

volume, index of blood, n See blood, volume index of.

volume, inspiratory reserve, n (complemental air), the maximum volume that can be inspired from the end of tidal inspiration

volume, packed-cell, n See hematocrit.

volume, residual, n the volume of air in the lungs at the end of maximum expiration.

volume, stroke, n See stroke volume.

volume, supplemental, n See volume, expiratory reserve.

volume, tidal, n the volume of gas inspired or expired during each respiratory cycle.

vomer, n the bone forming the posterior and inferior part of the nasal septum and having two surfaces and four borders.

vomiting, n the forcible voluntary or involuntary emptying of the stomach contents through the mouth.

von Recklinghausen's disease of bone, *n.pr* See hyperparathyroidism and osteitis fibrosa cystica, generalized.

von Recklinghausen's disease of skin, *n.pr* See neurofibromatosis.

voucher, n a receipt or release that may serve as notice of payment of a debt or may prove the accuracy of accounts.

vowel, n a conventional vocal sound in the production of which the speech organs offer little obstruction to the airstream and form a series of resonators above the level of the larynx.

vs, *prep* abbreviation for *versus* (against); commonly used in legal proceedings, particularly in designating the title of cases.

vulcanite (vul′kənīt), n a hard material with a form of rubber as the base; formerly used for denture bases.

vulcanization, n the process of treating crude rubber to improve such qualities as strength and hardness. This process usually involves heating the rubber with sulfur in the presence of moisture, the sulfur uniting with the rubber to produce saturated double bonds.

vulcanize, v to produce flexible or hard rubber, as desired, by subjecting caoutchouc, in the presence of sulfur, to heat and high-steam pressure in a vulcanizer.

VZ virus, n varicella zoster virus, which causes chickenpox in humans.

wages, n the compensation to an employee, agreed on by the employee and employer, for work completed by the employee.

waiting period, n the period of time between employment or enrollment in a dental program and the date when an insured person becomes eligible for benefits.

waiver (wā′vur), n **1.** repudiation, abandonment, or surrender of a claim, right, or privilege. n **2.** the intentional relinquishment of a known right.

walker, n an extremely light, movable apparatus, about waist-high, made of metal tubing, used to assist a patient in walking. It has four widely placed, sturdy legs. The patient holds onto the walker, takes a step, then moves the walker forward, and takes another step.

wall, n the outside layer of material surrounding an object or space; a paries.

wall, cavity, n one of the enclosing sides of a prepared cavity. It takes the name of the surface of the tooth adjoining the surface involved and toward which it is placed. Parts of a surrounding or peripheral wall are the cavosurface angle, the enamel wall, the dentinoenamel junction, and the dentin wall.

wall, enamel, n the portion of the wall of a prepared cavity that consists of enamel.

wall, finish of enamel, n the planing of the enamel in finishing a cavity preparation; includes the treatment of the cavosurface angle.

wall, gingival cavity, n the peripheral wall that most closely approximates the apical end of the tooth.

wall, incisal, *n* the wall of a prepared cavity in an anterior tooth that is closest to or in direct relation to the incisal edge of the tooth.

wall, peripheral cavity, *n* See wall, surrounding cavity.

wall, surrounding cavity, *n* one of the external, bounding side walls of a cavity; one side forms a part of the cavosurface angle of the preparation. Also called *peripheral cavity wall.*

Walter Reed staging system, *n.pr* an alternative classification system used to describe various stages of HIV infection. See Centers for Disease Control classification.

wandering rash, *n* See geographic tongue.

Wanscher's mask (vän'shuz), *n.pr* See mask, Wanscher's.

ward, *n* a person, especially a minor, placed by authority of law under the care of a guardian.

Ward's Wonderpack, *n.pr* trade name for a type of periodontal dressing used to cover and protect a surgical site; the basic components include tannic acid, zinc oxide, and powdered rosin.

warfarin sodium, *n trade names:* Coumadin, Panwarfin, Sofarin; *drug class:* oral anticoagulant; *action:* interferes with blood clotting by indirect means; depresses hepatic synthesis of vitamin K-dependent coagulation factors (II, VII, IX, and X); *uses:* pulmonary emboli, deep vein thrombosis, MI, atrial dysrhythmias.

warp, *n* uncontrolled torsional change of shape or outline, such as that which may occur in swaging sheet metal, in denture material, or in other materials exposed to varying temperatures.

wart, *n* See verruca vulgaris.

Warthin's tumor, *n.pr* See cystadenoma, papillary and lymphomatosum.

Wassermann test, *n.pr* See test, Wassermann.

waste disposal, *n* a removal of all potentially contaminated objects (e.g., objects soaked with saliva or blood) and placement in a secure site to prevent or decrease the risk of infection. See also sharps container.

waste management, *n* protocol for the safe disposal of waste products, such as needles, tissue specimens, and instruments used in dental procedures.

waste products, *n.pl* the products of metabolic activity after oxygen and nutrients have been supplied to a cell. These include primarily carbon dioxide and water, along with sodium chloride and soluble nitrogenous salts, which are excreted in feces, urine, and exhaled air.

waste products, biohazard, *n* unusable biological materials that can carry infection, which could then be transmitted to other organisms.

waste products, contaminated, *n.pl* **1.** instruments that have become nonsterile after coming into contact with blood, saliva, urine, or any other bodily fluids. *n.pl* **2.** the fluids or substances that contain the byproducts of metabolic activity. See also waste products.

waste products, infectious, *n* contaminated waste that may potentially cause infectious disease.

wasting, *n* a process of deterioration marked by weight loss and decreased physical vigor, appetite, and mental activity.

water, *n* a tasteless, odorless, colorless compound made of hydrogen and oxygen (H_2O), which freezes at 32° F (0° C) and boils at 212° F (100° C). The autonomic nervous system regulates water balance in the body.

water depletion, *n* cellular dehydration through decreased water intake, dysphagia, excessive sweating, and diuresis.

water, distilled, *n* a type of purified water that has undergone evaporation and recondensation prior to bottling.

water need, *n* the amount of water needed to maintain metabolism, approximately 1000 ml/day.

water syringe, *n* See syringe, water.

water:powder ratio, *n* See ratio, water:powder.

Waters extraoral radiographic examination, *n.pr* See examination, Waters extraoral radiographic.

Waters view, *n.pr* See examination, Waters extraoral radiographic.

Watson-Crick helix, *n.pr* a model of the DNA molecule proposed by Watson and Crick as two right-handed polynucleotide chains coiled around the same axis as a double helix.

watt (W), *n* the unit of electric power or work; 1 watt of power is dissipated when a current of 1 ampere (A)

flows across a difference in potential of 1 volt (V).

wave, electromagnetic, *n* energy manifested by movements in an advancing series of alternate elevations and depressions.

wavelength, *n* the distance between the peaks of waves in any wave form, such as light, x-rays, and other electromotive forms. In electromagnetic radiation, the wavelength is equal to the velocity of light divided by the frequency of the wave.

wavelength, effective, *n* the wavelength that would produce the same penetration as an average of the various wavelengths in a heterogeneous bundle of x-rays.

wax, *n* one of several esters of fatty acids with higher alcohols, usually monohydric alcohols. Dental waxes are combinations of various types of waxes compounded to provide the desired physical properties.

wax, baseplate, *n* a hard, pink wax used for making occlusion rims and baseplates for occlusion rims.

wax, bone, *n* a plastic mixture that may contain antiseptic and hemostatic drugs, designed for temporary application to freshly cut bone to prevent hemorrhage and infection.

wax, boxing, *n* a soft wax used for boxing impressions.

wax burnout, *n* See burnout, inlay and wax elimination.

wax, carnauba (kärnô′bə, -nou′bə), *n* a hard, high-melting wax used for control of the melting range of dental waxes.

wax, casting, *n* a composition containing various waxes with controlled properties of thermal expansion and contraction; used in making patterns to determine the shape of metal castings.

Wax casting. (Rosenstiel/Land/Fujimoto, 2001)

wax elimination, *n* the procedure of removing the wax from a wax pattern invested in a mold preparatory to the introduction of another material into the resulting cavity. This may be done by dry heat alone or by irrigation with boiling water followed by use of dry heat. Also called *wax burnout.*

wax expansion, *n* the enlargement of wax patterns to compensate for the shrinkage of gold during the casting process.

wax, fluid, *n* a series of waxes, each having different physical properties, used for making a correctable impression of the foundation structures that are to support a denture base. The term indicates that the wax is applied in fluid form as required.

wax inlay, *n* See wax casting.

wax out, *n* See blockout.

wax pattern, *n* See pattern, wax.

wax template, *n* See template, wax.

wax-bite, *n* See record, interocclusal.

waxing, *n* the contouring of a wax pattern or the wax base of a trial denture into the desired form. Also called *waxing up.*

WBC, *n* stands for white blood cell. See also leukocyte and white blood cell count.

weaning, *n* the process of withdrawing an infant from breast milk or formula and instituting nourishment with other food.

wear, *n* a loss of substance or a diminishing through use, friction, or other destructive factors.

wear, abnormal occlusal, *n* wear that exceeds the physiologic wear patterns associated with the attritional effects of food substances; the excessive wear of the teeth occurring as a result of continued afunctional gyrations of the mandible.

wear, interproximal, *n* a loss of tooth substance in contact areas through functional wear and friction, resulting in broadening and flattening of the contacts and a decrease in the mesiodistal dimension of the teeth and the dentition as a whole.

wear, occlusal, *n* attritional loss of substance on opposing occlusal units or surfaces. See also abrasion and attrition.

wear pattern, *n* See pattern, wear.

wear, physiologic, *n* attrition or abrasion of tooth substance occurring as a result of such conditions as the abrasive consistency of the normal diet or the slight buccolingual movement of the teeth possible in the masticatory process. It does not include the wear produced by such influences as habits or occlusal prematurities.

Weber's disease, *n.pr* See telangiectasia, hereditary hemorrhagic.

Weber-Dimitri disease, *n.pr* See disease, Sturge-Weber-Dimitri.

Wedelstaedt chisel (vēd′əlshtat), *n.pr* See chisel, Wedelstaedt.

wedge, *n* a small, pointed, triangular, contoured piece of wood used to seal the gingival margin of a cavity preparation before placement of an amalgam restoration.

wedge, step, *n* See penetrometer.

wedging, *n* packing or fixing tightly by driving in a wedge or wedges.

wedging effect, *n* See effect, wedging.

weekly permissible dose, *n* See dose, weekly permissible.

weight, *n* the product of the gravitational acceleration of one body and the mass of an attracted body; the measurement in pounds and ounces of how heavy an object is. In the metric system, weight (force) is measured in kg × m/sec².

weight, molecular **(mələk′yōōlur),** *n* the sum of the atomic weights of all atoms in a molecule.

weight, rubber dam, *n* a piece of metal varying in shape and weight, attached to a clip that is hung on the bottom of a placed rubber dam to keep the field of operation clear.

Weil's disease (vīlz), *n.pr* See disease, Weil's.

welding, *n* a process used to join metals.

welding, arc and gas, *n* See welding, fusion.

welding, cold, *n* property of welding at room temperature when clean surfaces are pressed into contact. This property is exhibited to the highest degree by gold in the form of foil or crystals.

welding, fusion, *n* a process in which parts are melted and fused together. Also called *arc and gas welding.*

welding, pressure, *n* a welding process in which the parts are not melted, although heat is usually re-

quired. Recrystallization across the interface occurs. Gold foil is welded by pressure without temperature elevation. Also called *resistance welding* and *spot welding.*

welding property, *n* the characteristic of certain materials, especially metals, to firmly unite together when subjected to heat or pressure in a suitable environment.

welding, resistance, *n* See welding, pressure.

welding, spot, *n* See welding, pressure.

Werlhof's disease (verl′hofs), *n.pr* See purpura, thrombocytopenic.

Wernicke-Korsakoff's syndrome (ver′nikē kŏr′səkôf), *n.pr* a disorder caused by a lack of thiamine due to long-term alcohol abuse in which the patient has difficulty in walking, seeing, or thinking clearly.

Western blot, *n pr* a confirmatory test for HIV exposure that identifies antibodies to HIV proteins and glycoproteins.

wet strength, *n* See strength, wet.

wetting agent, *n* See agent, wetting.

Wharton's duct, *n* See duct, Wharton's.

wheal (w(h)ēl), *n* edematous elevation of the skin or mucosa. See also urticaria.

wheel, Burlew, *n.pr* See Burlew wheel.

wheel stone, *n* See stone, wheel.

wheelchair, *n* a mobile chair equipped with large wheels and brakes used to transport patients or to allow disabled persons to move themselves from one place to another. Federal law requires handicapped access to public buildings with ramps, doors, elevators, restrooms, and drinking fountains designed and constructed to allow patients in wheelchairs proper access.

wheelchair transfer, *n* any of various techniques for assisting a wheelchair-bound patient from the wheelchair to the dental chair.

wheeze, *n* a whistling sound made during breathing that is caused by a foreign substance in the trachea or bronchus.

white blood cell (WBC), *n* See leukocyte and white blood cell count.

white blood cell count, *n* a diagnostic clinical laboratory test to determine the number and types of leukocytes present in a measured sample of blood. Overall the normal number of leukocytes ranges from 5,000 to 10,000/mm³. A differential white blood cell count identifies, counts, and determines the ratios of the various types of leukocytes present in a sample of blood. See also leukopenia and leukocytosis.

white lesions, *n.pl* lesions found on the mucosa that have a white coating. They require differential diagnosis because they may indicate trauma, infection, or a cancerous process.

white spot, *n* See enamel opacity.

whiting, *n* a grade of calcium carbonate used to polish dental surfaces.

whitlow, *n* an inflammation of the end of a finger or toe that results in suppuration.

whitlow, herpetic, *n* an infection caused by the herpes simplex virus that enters the body through small breaks in the skin; usually appears as cracks in the skin around the fingernails; dental personnel are at risk of contracting the virus from an infected patient by direct contact with saliva or a lesion on the lip.

whooping cough, *n* See pertussis.

Widman procedure, *n.pr* a surgical procedure in which a periodontal flap is made to gain better access to root surfaces for complete dèbridement and root planing.

wife, *n* a woman united to a man in lawful wedlock; a married woman whose husband is alive and from whom she is not divorced; a female spouse.

will, *n* a legal document detailing one's wishes in the disposal of one's body and property and the care of one's minor children and dependents.

will, living, *n* a document that details one's wishes regarding the degree and amount of health care desired if one becomes mentally incapacitated.

willfully, *adv* intentionally; purposefully.

Wilson, curve of, *n.pr* a lateral curve of the occlusal table formed by the lingual inclination of the posterior teeth. Because the lingual cusps are lower than the buccal cusps, they form a curve with their antimeres. See also curve of Wilson theory.

windchill factor, *n* the amount of chilling of the body because of exposure to wind or cold air currents, beyond that resulting from a cold ambient temperature.

window period, *n* the period of time between which a party is exposed to an infectious organism and that when that organism becomes detectable via a serum marker. See incubation period.

winking, jaw, *n* See syndrome, jaw-winking.

wire, *n* slender and pliable rod or thread of metal.

wire, arch, *n* wire used in orthodontics as a source of force to direct teeth to move in desired directions. The wire may be described according to the shape of its cross-section, such as ribbon, rectangular, or round.

wire, diagnostic, *n* See wire, measuring.

wire edge, *n* a thin, rough ridge created by particles that have been rearranged during hand instrument sharpening and appear on the surface adjoining the cutting edge.

wire, internal suspension, *n* one of a network of wires placed inside the oral cavity connecting the zygoma and mandibular arch bar, which are used to immobilize the upper jaw for healing after a LeFort I fracture. See also fracture, LeFort.

wire, Kirschner, *n.pr* a surgical steel wire of heavy gauge with pointed ends; used in the reduction and fixation of bone fragments by passing it through the cancellous portion of the bone and spanning the fracture site.

wire, ligature, *n* a soft, thin wire used to tie an arch wire to the band attachments.

wire, measuring, *n* a wire or other similar metal placed in a root canal to determine the length of the canal. A radiogram is used to make the determination.

wire, orthodontic, *n* stainless steel and wrought gold wire of various dimensions used in orthodontic treatment.

wire, Risdon **(riz'don),** *n.pr* a wire arch bar tied in the midline.

wire, separating, *n* wire threaded interproximally between two adjacent teeth and tightened by twisting the ends together to wedge the teeth slightly apart. Separating wire is used in preparation to adapt bands to teeth having tight contacts with adjacent teeth.

wire, transosseous (tranzos'ē-us), *n* a thin, flexible thread of metal that is laced through a hole drilled into the bone to bridge a fracture line and stabilize bone fragments. See also wire, Kirschner and wiring, perialveolar.

wire, wrought, n **1.** a wire formed by drawing a cast structure through a die; used in dentistry for partial denture clasps and orthodontic appliances. *n* **2.** a form of metal resulting from the swaging, rolling, and drawing of a metal ingot into a desired shape and size.

wiring, *n* an arrangement of a wire or wires.

wiring, circumferential, n the placement of a wire around a bone contiguous to the oral cavity, with the ends exiting in the oral cavity to maintain mandibular and maxillofacial surgical appliances. Also known as *circumferential mandibular wiring* and *circumzygomatic wiring.*

wiring, continuous loop, n a technique of wiring the teeth for the reduction and fixation of fractures. Also called *multiple loop wire.*

wiring, craniofacial suspension, n a method of wiring using areas of bones not contiguous with the oral cavity for the support of fractured jaw segments (e.g., piriform aperture, zygomatic arch, zygomatic process of the frontal bone).

wiring, Ivy loop, n.pr a method using a wire around two adjacent teeth, providing a loop useful for fixation of a fracture.

wiring, multiple loop, n See wiring, continuous loop.

wiring, perialveolar (per'ē alvē' əlur), n a method of wiring a splint to the maxilla by passing a wire through the bone from the buccal plate to the palate.

wiring, piriform aperture (pir'ifôrm), n a method of wiring using that area of the nasal bones to stabilize fractures of the jaws.

wisdom tooth, *n* a lay term for the third molar tooth, the last tooth in each quadrant of each dental arch. It appears in the oral cavity at about 18 years of age.

witch hazel, *n* a shrub, *Hamamelis virginiana,* indigenous to North America, from which an astringent extract is derived.

withdrawal (abstinence) syndrome, *n* somatic and psychosomatic symptoms recognizable after the abrupt termination of regular drug or other substance use. The types of symptoms are specific to the type of the withdrawn substance.

witness, *n* one who has knowledge of an event; a person whose declaration under oath is received as evidence for any purpose.

witness, expert, n a person whose education, training, and experience can provide the court with an assessment, opinion, or judgment within the area of his or her competence, which is not considered known or available to the general public.

witness, hostile, n witness who manifests so much hostility or prejudice under examination (in chief or direct) that the party who has called the witness is allowed to cross-examine the witness (i.e., to treat him or her as though he or she had been called by the opposite party).

witness, lay, n a witness who testifies only to firsthand knowledge of facts before judge and jury, different from an expert witness in that the witness is not allowed to testify to theories or hypothesize based on education or expertise.

witness marks, n.pl the small hemispheric depressions that may be prepared in the bone surface in lieu of abutment grooves as a guide for seating the abutment posts of the implant.

Wolff's law, *n.pr* See law, Wolff's.

Wolinella recta (wō'linel'ə rek'tə), *n* a microorganism associated with progressive periodontal destruction and refractory forms of periodontitis. A regimen combining antibiotic treatment, débridement, and home oral care seems to suppress or control periodontal infections. Also called *Campylobacter rectus.*

wooden interdental cleaner, *n* an implement made from birchwood and bass wood, used to clean between teeth, particularly when significant gum recession is indicated.

word processing (W/P), *n* the handling, manipulating, or performing of some operation or sequence of operations by a dedicated machine (usually by a microprocessor) on free text.

work hardening, *n* See hardening, work.

work sheet, *n* the office form used for a complete planning program for the completion of dental services.

work simplification, *n* the application of the principles of the scientific method to increase the ability to produce without sacrificing quality.

work stroke, *n* stroke used for removal of calculus or to reshape an overhanging margin.

working capital, *n* a firm's investment in short-term assets or cash, short-term securities, accounts receivable, and inventories. Gross working capital is defined as current assets minus current liabilities. If the term *working capital* is used without further qualification, it generally refers to gross working capital.

working contact, *n* See contact, working.

working end, *n* the section of an instrument that is used to accomplish the task for which the instrument is intended. A working end may be sharp (a blade) or dull (a nib).

Working end of periodontal probe.
(Bird/Robinson, 2002)

working occlusal surface, *n* See surface, working occlusal.

working occlusion, *n* See occlusion, working.

working side, *n* the lateral segment of a denture or dentition toward which the mandible is moved.

Workmen's Compensation Board of Industrial Commission, *n.pr* an administrative body that receives claims for injuries and refers them to certain physicians or dentists for treatment, if indicated, with the express or implied assurance to the claimant that the expense will be defrayed by the employer under the Workmen's Compensation Law. The determination of the Industrial Commission is subject to an appeal to court. The federal agency overseeing these matters is the Bureau of Employees Compensation.

World Health Organization (WHO), *n.pr* an agency of the United Nations concerned with worldwide and regional health problems. Its functions include furnishing technical assistance, stimulating and advancing epidemiologic investigation of diseases, recommending health regulations, promoting cooperation among scientific and professional health groups, and providing information and counsel relating to health matters.

worms, *n* a family of parasites characterized by a long body, either flat (platyhelminthes) or round (nematodes). They primarily reside in the intestinal tract, but some types can also survive in other major organs and tissue, such as the brain or muscles, respectively.

wound, *n* an injury to the body of a person, especially one caused by violence.

wound, incised, *n* in medical jurisprudence, a cut or incision on a human body; a wound made by a cutting instrument.

wound repair, *n* restoration of the normal structure after an injury.

wrist drop, *n* a condition caused by paralysis of the extensor muscles of the hand and fingers or by injury of the radial nerve, resulting in flexion of the wrist.

writ of execution, *n* a mandatory precept in writing to implement the judgment or decree of a court.

writing, *n* any written or printed paper or document (e.g., contract, deed).

wrong, *n* an injury; a tort; a violation of right or of law; an injustice; a violation of right resulting in damage to another.

wrongful death status, *n* a statute existing in all states that provides that the death of a person can give rise to a cause of legal action brought by the person's beneficiaries in a civil suit against the person or persons whose willful or negligent acts caused the death.

wrought clasp (wrôt), *n* See clasp, wrought.

wrought wire, *n* See wire, wrought.

X chromosome, *n* a sex chromosome that in humans and many other species is present in both male and female. The male somatic cell consists of one X chromosome and one Y chromosome; the female somatic cell carries two X chromosomes. All female gametes carry the X chromosome, whereas half of the male gametes possess the X chromosome and the other half the Y chromosome.

X-bite, *n* See *cross-bite.*

X-C-P film holder, *n.pr* See *film holder, Rinn X-C-P.*

xanthines (zan'thinz), *n.pl* a family of chemicals that includes caffeine, theophylline, and theobromine, which stimulate the central nervous system, act on the kidneys to produce diuresis, stimulate cardiac muscle, and relax smooth muscle.

xanthogranuloma (zan'tho-gran' yōō-lō'mǝ), *n* a benign lesion occurring in infancy, usually solitary and composed of lipid-laden histiocytes with varying numbers of Touton giant cells. In the oral cavity the lesion occurs most often on the tongue and regresses spontaneously.

xanthoma (zan-thō-mǝ), *n* a small yellow nodule, composed of lipid-laden macrophages, which generally occurs in subcutaneous tissue.

xanthoma palpebrarum **(pal'pǝ-brä'rǝm),** *n* a small, yellowish plaque on the eyelids resulting from an accumulation of lipids in reticuloendothelial cells. They frequently occur in persons with diabetes.

xanthomatosis (zan'thō-mǝ-tō'sis), *n* a disease characterized by the accumulation of excess lipids. See also *histiocytosis X.*

xanthosis, *n* **1.** a yellowish discoloration sometimes seen in degenerating tissues of malignant diseases. *n* **2.** also called carotenosis, a reversible yellow discoloration of the skin most commonly caused by the ingestion of large amounts of yellow vegetables containing carotene pigment, usually in the form of carrot juice. Xanthosis may be differentiated clinically from jaundice because the sclerae are colored yellow in jaundice but are not discolored in xanthosis.

xenograft, *n* tissue from another species used as temporary graft in certain cases, as in treating a severely burned patient when sufficient tissue from the patient or from a tissue bank is not available. It is quickly rejected but provides a cover of the burn for the first few days, reducing the amount of fluid loss from the open wound. Also called *heterograft.*

xenophobia, *n* an anxiety disorder characterized by a pervasive, irrational fear or uneasiness in the presence of strangers, especially foreigners, or in new surroundings.

xeroderma, *n* a chronic skin condition characterized by dryness and roughness.

xeroderma pigmentosum, *n* an eruption of exposed skin occurring in childhood and characterized by numerous pigmental spots resembling freckles, larger atrophic lesions eventually resulting in glossy white thinning of the skin surrounded by telangiectases, and multiple solar keratoses that undergo malignant changes at an early age. This results from a single-gene autosomal recessive disorder.

xerodermosteosis (zir'ō-dur-mos'tē-ō'sis), *n* See *syndrome, Sjögren's.*

xerogenic (zir'ō-jen'ik), *adj* indicates a substance that causes the mouth to be unusually dry.

xerography, *n* a dry radiologic process in which an image is made on a metal plate coated with powdered selenium. The plate is electrically charged in a dark room. Exposure to light or x-rays causes the charge to be redistributed in a pattern proportional to the intensity of exposure in various areas of the plate. When "developed" in a cloud of charged particles, the particles are attracted to the areas discharged by radiation, producing the equivalent of a photographic negative.

xerophthalmia (zir′of-thal′mē-ə), *n* dryness of the conjunctiva caused by functional or organic disorders of the lacrimal apparatus. It may be found in vitamin A deficiency or Sjögren's syndrome and may follow chronic conjunctivitis.

xeroradiography, *n* the use of xerography to produce an image electrically rather than chemically, permitting lower exposure times and lower energy levels of x-rays.

xerostomia (zir′ə-stō′mē-ə), *n* dryness of the mouth resulting from functional or organic disturbances of the salivary glands and lack of the normal secretion, primarily caused by prescribed medications. Dryness, loss of basic environment, and resultant overgrowth of oral microorganisms frequently lead to rampant caries. See also *hyposalivation.*

Xerostomia. (Neville/Damm/Allen/Bouquot, 2002)

xerotic keratitis, *n* an inflammation of the cornea resulting from dryness of the conjunctiva. Underlying causes may be autoimmune diseases or a deficiency of vitamin A.

X-linkage, *n* See *linkage, sex.*

x-ray, *n* a type of electromagnetic radiation characterized by wavelengths between approximately 10^3 Å and 10^{-4} Å, corresponding to photon energies of about 20 eV to 125 MeV. X-rays are invisible; penetrative, especially at higher photon energies; and travel with the same speed as visible light. Typical production involves bombarding a target of high atomic number with fast electrons in a high vacuum; they are also emitted as a product of some radioactive

disintegrations (specifically originating from the extranuclear part of the atom). X-rays were first discovered by Wilhelm C. Roentgen in 1895; hence the term *roentgen rays,* often applied to mechanically generated x-rays. Roentgen called them x-rays after the mathematic symbol x for an unknown.

x-ray, low-voltage filament circuit, *n* the lower-energy circuit in an x-ray machine that uses a step-down transformer to lower the line voltage to around 3 volts, just enough to heat the filament and produce an electron cloud.

x-ray, monochromatic, *n* an x-ray that has a single wavelength or an extremely narrow band of wavelengths.

x-ray beam, *n* the spatial distribution of radiation emerging from an x-ray generator or source.

x-ray beam, central, *n* the straight line passing through the center of the source and the center of the final beam-limiting diaphragm.

x-ray beam, edges, *n* the lines joining the center of the anterior face of the source to the diaphragm edges farthest from the source.

x-ray beam, field size, *n* the geometric projection, on a plane perpendicular to the central ray, of the distal end of the limiting diaphragm as seen from the center of the front surface of the source. The field is thus the same shape as the aperture of the collimator, and it can be defined at any distance from the source.

x-ray beam, principal plane, *n* a plane that contains the central ray and, in the case of rectangular section beams, is parallel to one side of the rectangle.

x-ray film, full-mouth, *n* See *survey, radiographic.*

x-ray mount, *n* See *mount, x-ray.*

x-ray tube, *n* an electronic tube in which x-rays can be generated.

X-ray tube. (Frommer, 2001)

x-ray tube, Coolidge, *n.pr* a vacuum tube in which x-rays are generated when the target (integral with the anode) is bombarded by electrons that are emitted from a heated filament (on the cathode) and accelerated toward the anode across a high-potential difference. Modern x-ray tubes are of this type. See also *tube, Coolidge.*

x-ray tube, Crookes', *n.pr* a vacuum discharge tube used by Sir William Crookes in early experimental work with cathode rays. Wilhelm C. Roentgen first discovered that in addition to the production of cathode rays, x-rays were emitted during the operation of these tubes.

x-ray tube, gas, *n* an early type of x-ray tube in which electrons were derived from residual gases within the tube.

x-ray unit, *n* See *unit, x-ray.*

xylene (zī′lēn), *n* a colorless, flammable fluid used as a solvent and clarifying agent in the preparation of tissue sections for microscopic study. Also called *xylol;* $C_6H_4[CH_3]_2$ *dimethylbenzene.*

Xylocaine, *n.pr* See *lidocaine.*

xylol (zī′lôl), *n* See *xylene.*

xylose, *n* wood or beechwood sugar; an aldopentose, isomeric with ribose, obtained by fermentation or hydrolysis of naturally occurring carbohydrate substances such as wood fiber.

xylulose, *n* a substance that appears in the urine of patients with essential pentosuria; its presence is diagnostic.

Y axis, *n* See *axis, Y.*

Y chromosome, *n* a sex chromosome that in humans and many other species is present only in the male, appearing singly in the normal male. It is carried as a sex determinant by one-half of the male gametes. None of the female gametes contain a Y chromosome.

yawn, *n* an involuntary act of opening the mouth wide and taking a deep breath. It tends to occur when a person is bored, drowsy, or depressed and may be accompanied by upper body movements to aid chest expansion.

yaws (yôz), *n* a disease caused by *Treponema pertenue.* It occurs in hot regions; raspberry-like excrescences occur on the hands, face, feet, and external genitalia.

yeast, *n* a general term denoting true fungi of the family *Saccharomycetaceae.* Because of their ability to ferment carbohydrates, some yeasts are important to the brewing and baking industries.

Yersinia, *n* a genus of motile and nonmotile, nonspore-forming bacteria containing gram-negative, unencapsulated, ovoid- to rod-shaped cells. These organisms are parasitic on humans and other animals.

Yersinia enterocolitica (yur-sin′ē-ə en′tər-ō-kō-lit′ik-ə), *n.pl* bacteria that causes *Yersinia enterocolitis,* contracted from contaminated food or water. Symptoms of infection often mimic acute appendicitis and are most common in children younger than age 7. A sister bacteria, *Yersinia pestis,* was the cause of the historic bubonic plague.

yield point, *n* See *point, yield.*

yield strength, *n* See *strength, yield.*

yin-yang, *n* **1.** Yin and Yang, in ancient Chinese thought, are the underlying and controlling elements of all nature. The aim of Chinese medicine is to produce a proper balance between them. *n* **2.** used in the Western world to express any dualistic, reciprocal control system in which one influence tends to promote things that the opposing influence tends to inhibit.

yoga, *n* a discipline that focuses on the body's musculature, posture, breathing mechanisms, and consciousness. The goal of yoga is attainment of physical and mental well-being through mastery of the body, achieved through exercise, holding of postures, proper breathing, and meditation.

yogurt, *n* a slightly acid, semisolid curdled milk preparation made from either whole or skimmed cow's milk and milk solids by fermentation with organisms from the genus *Lactobacillus.* It is rich in B-complex vitamins, and is a good source of protein.

It provides a medium in the gastrointestinal tract that retards the growth of harmful bacteria and aids in the absorption of minerals. Also spelled *yoghurt.*

yohimbine, *n* an alkaloid, the active principle comes from the bark of *Corynanthe johimbe.* It produces a competitive blockage of limited duration of α-adrenergic receptors. It has also been used for its alleged aphrodisiac properties.

yoke, *n* **1.** something that connects or binds. *n* **2.** assembly of metal clamps with adjustable screws that secure the cylinders to the apparatus or reducing valves. They are equipped with nipples that fit snugly into the inlet socket or part of the cylinder valve.

Young's modulus, *n* See *elasticity, modulus of.*

Young's rule, *n* See *rule, Young's.*

Y-plasty, *n* a method of surgical revision of a scar, using a Y-shaped incision to reduce scar contractures. See also *Z-plasty.*

ytterbium (Yb), *n* a metallic element of the lanthamide group with an atomic number of 70 and an atomic weight of 173.04.

yttrium (Y), *n* a scaly, grayish metallic element with an atomic number of 39 and an atomic weight of 88.9059. Radioactive isotopes of yttrium have been used in cancer therapy.

Z, *n* a symbol for atomic number.

zalcitabine, *n* *trade name:* Hivid; *drug class:* synthetic pyrimidine antiviral; *action:* converted by cellular enzymes to active drug; functions as antimetabolite to inhibit replication of HIV in vitro; *uses:* used in combination with zidovudine in advanced HIV infection, second-line monotherapy if AZT tolerant.

zero, *n* **1.** a symbol for nothing or for the starting point. **2.** the point on most scales from which measurements begin. **3.** absolute zero, the temperature at which there is no molecular movement, corresponding to −273.15 on the Kelvin scale.

zidovudine, *n* *trade names:* AZT, Retrovir; *drug class:* antiviral thymidine analog; *action:* inhibits replication of viral DNA; *uses:* symptomatic HIV infections (AIDS, ARC), confirmed *P. carinii* pneumonia, or absolute CD4 lymphocytes of less than 200 milliliters, prevention of HIV transmission from an infected mother to her baby.

zinc (Zn) (zingk), *n* a bluish-white chemical element used in medicine in the form of various salts and as a component in some silver amalgams.

zinc oxide, *n* a zinc compound used as a topical protectant, prescribed for a wide range of minor skin irritations.

zinc oxide and eugenol **(zingk ok´sīd yōō´jənol),** *n* two substances that react chemically to form a relatively hard mass. When modified by certain additives, the material is used for impression pastes, root canal fillings, surgical dressings, temporary filling materials, and cementing media.

zinc oxide-eugenol cement, See cement, dental, zinc oxide-eugenol.

zinc oxyphosphate **(zingk ok´sēfos´fāt),** *n* See cements.

zinc phosphate cement **(zingk fos´fāt),** *n* See cement, zinc phosphate.

zinc polycarbonate cement **(zingk pol´ēkär´bənāt),** *n* See cements.

Zinsser-Cole-Engman syndrome, *n.pr* See syndrome, Zinsser-Cole-Engman.

zirconium (Zr), *n* a metallic element with an atomic number of 40 and an atomic weight of 91.22. It is widely distributed in nature, although no concentrations are found in any one place.

ZOE, *n* See zinc oxide and eugenol.

Zollinger-Ellison syndrome, *n.pr* a condition characterized by severe peptic ulceration, gastric hypersecretion, elevated serum gastrin, and gastrinoma of the pancreas or the duodenum. It may occur in early childhood but is seen more frequently in people between 20 and 50 years of age. Two-thirds of the tumors are malig-

Z

nant. Total gastrectomy may be necessary, but the administration of cimetidine in large doses may control gastric hypersecretion and allow the ulcers to heal.

zolpidem, *n* *trade name:* Ambien; *drug class:* nonbarbiturate, nonbenzodiazepine sedative/hypnotic; *action:* presumed to interact with subunit of GABA-benzodiazepine receptor; *use:* insomnia.

zone (zōn), *n* a region or area with specific characteristics or boundary.

zone, incubation, n an area that provides a favorable environment for growth of microorganisms and is thus conducive to initiation or perpetuation of a pathologic process (e.g., gingival flap over a partly erupted third molar).

zone, neutral, n the potential space between the lips and cheeks on one side and the tongue on the other. Natural or artificial teeth in this zone are subject to equal and opposite forces from the surrounding musculature.

zone of reference, n the area of perceived pain referred by a trigger point. See also trigger point.

zonography, *n* an x-ray-imaging technique used to produce films of body sections similar to those made by tomography.

zoster, See herpes zoster.

zoster (shingles) (zos'tur), See herpes zoster.

Z-plasty, *n* a surgical procedure using the transposition of tissue flaps to ensure the release of contractures, as in the repair of a cleft lip or in ankyloglossia.

z-score, *n* a standard score based on the normal distribution; the difference between the obtained score and the mean, divided by the standard deviation. Standard scores computed for different variables are comparable; used to determine statistical significance in large samples.

zygoma, *n* **1.** a long, slender process of the temporal bone, arising from the lower part of the squamous portion of the temporal bone and passing forward horizontally to join with the malar or zygomatic bone. **2.** the zygomatic or malar bone that forms the prominence of the cheek.

zygomatic arch, *n* the arch formed by articulation of the temporal process of the zygomatic bone with the zygomatic process of the temporal bone.

zygomaxillare (zī'gōmaksəler'ē), *n* See ridge, key.

zygosity, *n* the characteristic or condition of a zygote. The term occurs primarily as a suffix combining form to denote genetic makeup, referring specifically to whether the paired alleles determining a particular trait are identical (homozygosity) or different (heterozygosity), or to the condition in twins of having developed from the fertilization of one ovum (monozygosity) or two (dizygosity).

zygote, *n* the developing ovum from the time it is fertilized until, as a blastocyst, it is implanted in the uterus.

Z

Symbols and Abbreviations*

Table A-1 Symbols

Symbol	Meaning
@	At
ʒ	Dram
fʒ	Fluid dram
℥	Ounce
f℥	Fluid ounce
O	Pint
lb	Pound
℞	Recipe; take
M	Misce; mix
A, Å	Angstrom unit
E_0	Electroaffinity
F_1	First filial generation
F_2	Second filial generation
mμ	Millimicron, micromillimeter
μg	Microgram
mEq	Milliequivalent
mg	Milligram
m%	Milligrams percent; milligrams per 100 ml
$Q\,O_2$	Oxygen consumption
m-	Meta-
o-	Ortho-
p-	Para-
Po_2	Partial pressure of oxygen
Pco_2	Partial pressure of carbon dioxide
μm	Micrometer
μ	Micron
μμ	Micromicron
+	Plus; excess; acid reaction; positive
−	Minus; deficiency; alkaline reaction; negative
±	Plus or minus; either positive or negative; indefinite
↑	Increased
↓	Decreased
→	Yields; leads to
←	Resulting from; secondary to
Δ	Change
#	Number; following a number, pounds
÷	Divided by
×	Multiplied by; magnification
=	Equals
≅	Approximately equals
≠	Not equal to
>	Greater than; from which is derived
<	Less than; derived from
≮	Not less than
≯	Not greater than
≦, ≤	Equal to or less than

*From *Mosby's medical, nursing, and allied health dictionary*, ed 6, St Louis, 2002, Mosby.

Continued

Table A-1   Symbols—cont'd

Symbol	Meaning
$\geqq$, $\geq$	Equal to or greater than
/	Divided by; per
$\sqrt{}$	Root; square root; radical
$\sqrt[2]{}$	Square root
$\sqrt[3]{}$	Cube root
∞	Infinity
:	Ratio; "is to"
$\therefore$	Therefore
$\circ$	Degree
%	Percent
π	3.1416—ratio of circumference of a circle to its diameter; pi
$\square$, $\male$	Male
O, $\female$	Female
$\rightleftharpoons$	A reversible reaction

Table A-2 Abbreviations

Note: Abbreviations in common use can vary widely from place to place. Each institution's list of acceptable abbreviations is the best authority for its records.

Abbreviation	Meaning	Abbreviation	Meaning	Abbreviation	Meaning
A	Accommodation; acetum; Angström unit; anode; anter or anterior; area	ADL	Activities of daily living	alt. noct.	Alternate nights (alternis noctes)
		ADS	Antidiuretic substance	Am	Mixed astigmatism
a	Accommodation; ampere; anterior; area	AF	Atrial fibrillation	AM	Morning
ā	Before	AFB	Acid-fast bacillus	ama	Against medical advice
		AFP	Alpha-fetoprotein	AMI	Acute myocardial infarction
A₂	Aortic second sound	A/G; A-G ratio	Albumin/globulin ratio	amp	Ampule; amputation
abd	Abdominal/abdomen			amp.	Ampere
ABG	Arterial blood gases	Ag	Silver, antigen	amt	Amount
ABO	Three basic blood groups	AgNO₃	Silver nitrate	ANA	Antinuclear antibody
AC	Alternating current; air conduction; axiocervical; adrenal cortex	ah	Hypermetropic astigmatism	ana	So much of each, or āā
		AHF	Antihemophilic factor	anat	Anatomy or anatomic
		AICD	Automatic implantable cardiac defibrillator	ant.	Anterior
acc.	Accommodation			AO	Anodal opening; atrioventricular valve openings
ACE	Adrenocortical extract; angiotensin-converting enzyme	AIDS	Acquired immunodeficiency syndrome	AOP	Anodal opening picture
ACh	Acetylcholine	aj	Ankle jerk	AOS	Anodal opening sound
ACH	Adrenocortical hormone	AK	Above the knee	A-P; AP; A/F	Anterior-posterior
ACLS	Advanced cardiac life support	Al	Aluminum	A.P.	Anterior pituitary gland
ACTH	Adrenocorticotropic hormone	Alb	Albumin	APA	Antipernicious anemia factor
AD	Right ear (auris dextra)	ALH	Combined sex hormone of the anterior lobe of the hypophysis	AQ	Achievement quotient
ADD	Attention deficit disorder			AR	Alarm reaction
add	Add to (adde)	ALS	Advanced life support, amyotrophic lateral sclerosis	ARC	Anomalous retinal correspondence, AIDS-related complex
ADDH	Attention deficit disorder, hyperactivity	ALT	Alanine aminotransferase (formerly SGPT)	ARD	Acute respiratory disease
ADH	Antidiuretic hormone	alt. dieb.	Every other day (alternis diebus)	arg	Silver
ADHD	Attention deficit-hyperactivity disorder	alt. hor.	Alternate hours (alternis horis)	As	Arsenic

Continued

Table A-2 Abbreviations—cont'd

Abbreviation	Meaning
As.	Astigmatism
AS	Left ear (*auris sinistra*)
ASCVD	Arteriosclerotic cardiovascular disease
ASD	Atrial septal defect
AsH	Hypermetropic astigmatism
ASHD	Arteriosclerotic heart disease
AsM	Myopic astigmatism
ASS	Anterior superior spine
AST	Aspartate aminotransferase (formerly SGOT)
Ast	Astigmatism
ATS	Anxiety tension state; antitetanic serum
AU	Angström unit
Au	Gold
A-V; AV; A/V	Arteriovenous; atrioventricular
Av	Average or avoirdupois
ax	Axis
B	Boron; bacillus
Ba	Barium
BAC	Buccoaxiocervical
Bact	Bacterium
BBB	Blood-brain barrier
BBT	Basal body temperature
BCLS	Basic cardiac life support
BE	Barium enema
Be	Beryllium
BFP	Biologically false positivity (in syphilis tests)
Bi	Bismuth
Bib	Drink
bid; b.i.d.	Twice a day (*bis in die*)
BK	Below the knee
BM	Bowel movement
BMR	Basal metabolic rate
BP	Blood pressure; buccopulpal
bp	Boiling point
BPH	Benign prostatic hypertrophy
bpm	Beats per minute
BRP	Bathroom privileges
BSA	Body surface area
BSE	Breast self-examination
BSP	Bromsulphalein
BUN	Blood urea nitrogen
BW	Birthweight
Bx	Biopsy
C	Carbon; centigrade; Celsius
$\bar{c}$	With
C_{alb}	Albumin clearance
C_{cr}	Creatinine clearance
C_{in}	Inulin clearance
CA	Chronologic age; cervicoaxial
Ca	Calcium; cancer; carcinoma
CABG	Coronary artery bypass graft
CABS	Coronary artery bypass surgery
$CaCO_3$	Calcium carbonate
CAD	Coronary artery disease
CAH	Chronic active hepatitis
Cal	Large calorie
cal	Small calorie
C&S	Culture and sensitivity
CAT	Computed (axial) tomography
cath.	Catheter
CBC or cbc	Complete blood count
CC	Chief complaint
cc	Cubic centimeter
CCl_4	Carbon tetrachloride
CCU	Coronary care unit; critical care unit
CF	Cystic fibrosis
cf	Compare or bring together
CFT	Complement-fixation test
Cg; Cgm	Centigram
CH	Crown-heel (length of fetus)
$CHCl_3$	Chloroform
CH_3COOH	Acetic acid
CHD	Congenital heart disease; coronary heart disease
ChE	Cholinesterase
CHF	Congestive heart failure
$C_6H_4N_4O_3$	Uric acid
CHO	Carbohydrate

C_2H_6O	Ethyl alcohol	DOA	Dead on arrival
CH_2O	Formaldehyde	DOB	Date of birth
CH_4O	Methyl alcohol	DOE	Dyspnea on exertion
CI	Cardiac index; cardiac insufficiency; cerebral infarction	DPT	Diphtheria-pertussis-tetanus
		dr	Dram
CK	Creatinine kinase	DRG	Diagnosis-related groups
Cl	Chlorine	DSD	Discharge summary dictated, dry sterile dressing
cm	Centimeter		
CMR	Cerebral metabolic rate	DT	Delirium tremens
CMV	Cytomegalovirus	DTR	Deep tendon reflex
CNS	Central nervous system	D5W	Dextrose 5% in water
c/o	Complaints of	Dx	Diagnosis
CO	Carbon monoxide; cardiac output	E	Eye
CO_2	Carbon dioxide	EAHF	Eczema, asthma, and hayfever
Co	Cobalt	EBV	Epstein-Barr virus
COLD	Chronic obstructive lung disease	EC	Electroconvulsive therapy
COPD	Chronic obstructive pulmonary disease	ECF	Extended care facility; extracellular fluid
CP	Cerebral palsy; cleft palate	ECG	Electrocardiogram, electrocardiograph
CPAP	Continuous positive airway pressure	ECHO	Echocardiography
		ECMO	Extracorporeal membrane oxygenation
CPC	Clinicopathologic conference		
CPD	Cephalopelvic disproportion	ECT	Electroconvulsive therapy
CPK	Creatinine phosphokinase	ED	Emergency department; erythema dose; effective dose
CPR	Cardiopulmonary resuscitation		
CR	Crown-rump length (length of fetus)	ED_{50}	Median effective dose
		EDE	Estimated date of delivery (formerly EDC, estimated date of confinement)
CS	Cesarean section		
CSF	Cerebrospinal fluid		
CSM	Cerebrospinal meningitis		
CT	Computed tomography	EEG	Electroencephalogram, electroencephalograph
Cu	Copper		

$CuSO_4$	Copper sulfate		
CV	Cardiovascular; closing volume		
CVA	Cerebrovascular accident; costovertebral angle		
CVP	Central venous pressure		
CVS	Chorionic villi sampling; clean voided specimen		
CXR	Chest x-ray		
cyl	Cylinder		
D	Dose; vitamin D; right (*dexter*)		
d	Day; diem		
D/H	Disordered action of the heart		
D & C	Dilation (dilatation) and curettage		
db, dB	Decibel		
DC	Direct current		
dc, DC, D/C	Discontinue		
DCA	Deoxycorticosterone acetate		
Deg	Degeneration; degree		
dg	Decigram		
DIC	Disseminated intravascular coagulation		
diff	Differential blood count		
dil	Dilute or dissolve		
dim	One-half		
DJD	Degenerative joint disease		
DKA	Diabetic ketoacidosis		
dL	Deciliter		
DM	Diabetes mellitus, diastolic murmur		
DNA	Deoxyribonucleic acid		
DNR	Do not resuscitate		

Continued

Table A-2 Abbreviations—cont'd

Abbreviation	Meaning	Abbreviation	Meaning	Abbreviation	Meaning
EENT	Eye, ear, nose, and throat	F & R	Force and rhythm (pulse)	GL	Greatest length (small flexed embryo)
EKG	Electrocardiogram, electrocardiograph	FAS	Fetal alcohol syndrome	GLA	Gingivolinguoaxial
ELISA	Enzyme-linked immunosorbent assay	FBS	Fasting blood sugar	GP	General practitioner; general paresis
		FD	Fatal dose; focal distance		
Em	Emmetropia	Fe	Iron	G6PD	Glucose-6-phosphate dehydrogenase
EMB	Eosin-methylene blue	$FeCl_3$	Ferric chloride		
EMC	Encephalomyocarditis	ferv.	Boiling	gr	Grain
EMF	Erythrocyte maturation factor	FEV	Forced expiratory volume	Grad	By degrees (*gradatim*)
EMG	Electromyogram	FH, Fhx	Family history	GRAS	Generally recognized as safe
EMS	Emergency medical service	FHR	Fetal heart rate	Grav I, II, III, etc.	Pregnancy one, two, three, etc. (*Gravida*)
ENT	Ear, nose, and throat	Fl, fld	Fluid	GSW	Gunshot wound
EOM	Extraocular movement	fl dr	Fluid dram	gt	Drop (*gutta*)
EPR	Electrophrenic respiration	fl oz	Fluid ounce	GTT	Glucose tolerance test
ER	Emergency room (hospital); external resistance	FR	Flocculation reaction	gtt	Drops (*guttae*)
		FSH	Follicle-stimulating hormone	GU	Genitourinary
ERG	Electroretinogram	ft	Foot	Gyn	Gynecology
ERPF	Effective renal plasma flow	FTT	Failure to thrive	H	Hydrogen
ERV	Expiratory reserve volume	FUO	Fever of unknown origin	H^+	Hydrogen ion
ESR	Erythrocyte sedimentation rate	fx	Fracture	H & E	Hematoxylin and eosin stain
ESRD	End-stage renal disease	Gm; g; gm	Gram	H & P	History and physical
EST	Electroshock therapy	GA	Gingivoaxial	HAV	Hepatitis A virus
Et	Ethyl	Galv	Galvanic	Hb; Hgb	Hemoglobin
ext	Extract	GB	Gall bladder	H_3BO_3	Boric acid
F	Fahrenheit; field of vision; formula	GBS	Gall bladder series	HBV	Hepatitis B virus
		GC	Gonococcus or gonorrheal	HC	Hospital corps
FA	Fatty acid	GDM	Gestational diabetes mellitus	HCG	Human chorionic gonadotropin
FANA	Fluorescent antinuclear antibody test	GFR	Glomerular filtration rate	HCHO	Formaldehyde
		GH	Growth hormone		
		GI	Gastrointestinal		

Continued

HCl	Hydrochloric acid	HTLV-III	Human T lymphotropic virus type III
HCN	Hydrocyanic acid	hx, Hx	History
H₂CO₃	Carbonic acid	Hy	Hyperopia
HCT	Hematocrit	I	Iodine
HD	Hearing distance	¹³¹I	Radioactive isotope of iodine (atomic weight 131)
HDL	High-density lipoprotein		
HDLW	Distance at which a watch is heard by the left ear	³²I	Radioactive isotope of iodine (atomic weight 132)
HDRW	Distance at which a watch is heard by the right ear	I & O	Intake and output
He	Helium	IB	Inclusion body
HEENT	Head, eye, ear, nose, and throat	IBW	Ideal body weight
Hg	Mercury	IC	Inspiratory capacity; intracutaneous
Hgb	Hemoglobin		
HHC	Home health care	ICP	Intracranial pressure
Hib	*Haemophilus influenzae* type 3	ICS	Intercostal space
HIV	Human immunodeficiency (AIDS) virus	ICSH	Interstitial cell-stimulating hormone
HME	Home medical equipment	ICT	Inflammation of connective tissue
HNO₃	Nitric acid	ICU	Intensive care unit
h/o	History of	Id.	The same (*idem*)
H₂O	Water	IDDM	Insulin-dependent diabetes mellitus
H₂O₂	Hydrogen peroxide		
HOP	High oxygen pressure	Ig	Immunoglobulin
HPI	History of present illness	IH	Infectious hepatitis
HR	Heart rate	IM	Intramuscular; infectious mononucleosis
H₂SO₄	Sulfuric acid		
HSV	Herpes simplex virus	IOP	Intraocular pressure
Ht	Total hyperopia	IPPB	Intermittent positive pressure breathing
HT, HTN	Hypertension		
		IQ	Intelligence quotient
		IRV	Inspiratory reserve volume
		IS	Intercostal space
		IU	Immunizing unit
		I.U.	International Unit
		IUD	Intrauterine device
		IV	Intravenous
		IVP	Intravenous pyelogram, intravenous push
		IVT	Intravenous transfusion
		IVU	Intravenous urogram/urography
		JRA	Juvenile rheumatoid arthritis
		K	Potassium
		k	Constant
		Ka	Cathode or kathode
		KBr	Potassium bromide
		kc	Kilocycle
		KCl	Potassium chloride
		kev	Kilo electron volts
		kg	Kilogram
		KI	Potassium iodide
		kj	Knee jerk
		km	Kilometer
		KOH	Potassium hydroxide
		KUB	Kidney, ureter, and bladder
		kv	Kilovolt
		KVO	Keep vein open
		kw	Kilowatt
		L	Left; liter; length; lumbar; lethal; pound

Table A-2 Abbreviations—cont'd

Abbreviation	Meaning	Abbreviation	Meaning	Abbreviation	Meaning
lab	Laboratory	LP	Lumbar puncture	MED	Minimal erythema dose; minimal effective dose
L & A	Light and accommodation	LPF	Leukocytosis-promoting factor		
L & D	Labor and delivery	LR	Lactated Ringer's	mEq	Milliequivalent
lat.	Lateral	LTD	Lowest tolerated dose	μEq	Microequivalent
lb	Pound (*libra*)	LTH	Luteotrophic hormone	mEq/L	Milliequivalent per liter
LB	Large bowel (x-ray film)	LUE	Left upper extremity	ME ratio	Myeloid/erythroid ratio
LBW	Low birth weight	LUL	Left upper lobe	Mg	Magnesium
LCM	Left costal margin	LUQ	Left upper quadrant	mg	Milligram
LD	Lethal dose; perception of light difference	LV	Left ventricle	μg	Microgram
		LVH	Left ventricular hypertrophy	MHD	Minimal hemolytic dose
LDL	Low-density lipoprotein	L & W	Living and well	MI	Myocardial infarction
LE	Lower extremity; lupus erythematosus	M	Myopia; meter; muscle; thousand	MID	Minimum infective dose
		m	Meter	ML	Midline
le	Left extremity	MA	Mental age	mL	Milliliter
l.e.s.	Local excitatory state	Mag	Large (*magnus*)	MLD	Median or minimum lethal dose
LFD	Least fatal dose of a toxin	MAP	Mean arterial pressure	MM	Mucous membrane
LGA	Large for gestational age	MBD	Minimal brain dysfunction	mm	Millimeter; muscles
LH	Luteinizing hormone	mc; mCi	Millicurie	mm Hg	Millimeters of mercury
Li	Lithium	μc	Microcurie	mmm	Millimicron
LIF	Left iliac fossa	mcg	Microgram	MMR	Maternal mortality rate; measles-mumps-rubella
lig	Ligament	MCH	Mean corpuscular hemoglobin		
Liq	Liquor	MCHC	Mean corpuscular hemoglobin concentration	mμ	Millimicron
LLE	Left lower extremity			μm	Micrometer
LLL	Left lower lobe	MCV	Mean corpuscular volume	$\mu\mu$	Micromicron
LLQ	Left lower quadrant	MD	Muscular dystrophy	Mn	Manganese
LMP	Last menstrual period	MDI	Medium-dose inhalants; metered-dose inhaler	mN	Millinormal
LNMP	Last normal menstrual period			MRI	Magnetic resonance imaging
LOC	Level/loss of consciousness	Me	Methyl	MS	Multiple sclerosis

Abbr.	Meaning	Abbr.	Meaning	Abbr.	Meaning
MSL	Midsternal line	NICU	Neonatal intensive care unit	OT	Occupational therapy
MT	Medical technologist; membrane tympani	NIDDM	Noninsulin-dependent diabetes mellitus	OTC	Over-the-counter
mu	Mouse unit	NIH	National Institutes of Health	OTD	Organ tolerance dose
MVA	Motor vehicle accident	NKA	No known allergies	OU	Each eye (oculus uterque)
MW	Molecular weight	rm	Nanometer	oz; ℥	Ounce
My	Myopia	NMR	Nuclear magnetic resonance	P	Phosphorus; pulse; pupil
N	Nitrogen	N.O.	Nursing order	p	After
n	Normal	NPN	Nonprotein nitrogen	P_2	Pulmonic second sound
N/A	Not applicable	NPO n.p.o.	Nothing by mouth (non per os)	P-A; P*A; PA	Posterior-anterior
Na	Sodium	NRC	Normal retinal correspondence	PAB; PABA	Para-aminobenzoic acid
NaBr	Sodium bromide	NS	Normal saline	PALS	Pediatric Advanced Life Support
NaCl	Sodium chloride	NSAID	Nonsteroidal anti-inflammatory drug	P & A	Percussion and auscultation
Na_2CO_3	Sodium carbonate			Pap test	Papanicolaou smear
$Na_2C_2O_4$	Sodium oxalate	NSR	Normal sinus rhythm	Para I, II, III, etc.	Unipara, bipara, tripara, etc.
NAD	No appreciable disease	NTP	Normal temperature and pressure	PAS; PASA	Para-aminosalicylic acid
NaF	Sodium fluoride	NYD	Not yet diagnosed	PAT	Paroxysmal atrial tachycardia
$NaHCO_3$	Sodium bicarbonate	O	Oxygen; oculus; pint	Pb	Lead
Na_2HPO_4	Sodium phosphate	O_2	Oxygen; both eyes	PBI	Protein-bound iodine
NaI	Sodium iodide	O_3	Ozone	PCA	Patient-controlled analgesia
N & V, N/V	Nausea and vomiting	OB	Obstetrics	PCP	Phencyclidine, *Pneumocystis carinii* pneumonia, primary care physician, pulmonary capillary pressure
$NaNO_3$	Sodium nitrate	OBS	Organic brain syndrome		
Na_2O_2	Sodium peroxide	OD	Optical density; overdose; right eye (*Oculus dexter*)		
NaOH	Sodium hydroxide			PCV	Packed cell volume
Na_2SO_4	Sodium sulfate	OOB	Out of bed	PCWP	Pulmonary capillary wedge pressure
n.b.	Note well	OPD	Outpatient department		
NCA	Neurocirculatory asthenia	OR	Operating room	PD	Interpupillary distance
Ne	Neon	ORIF	Open reduction and internal fixation	pd	Prism diopter; pupillary distance
NG, ng	Nasogastric	OS	Left eye (*oculus sinister*)	PDA	Patent ductus arteriosus
NH_3	Ammonia	Os	Osmium		
Ni	Nickel				

Continued

Table A-2 Abbreviations—cont'd

Abbreviation	Meaning	Abbreviation	Meaning	Abbreviation	Meaning
PDR	*Physician's Desk Reference*	PMH	Past medical history	PVC	Premature ventricular contraction
PE	Physical examination	PMI	Point of maximal impulse	Px	Pneumothorax
PEEP	Positive end expiratory pressure	PMN	Polymorphonuclear neutrophil leukocytes (polys)	PZI	Protamine zinc insulin
PEFR	Peak expiratory flow rate			Q	Electric quantity
PEG	Pneumoencephalography	PMS	Premenstrual syndrome	q	Every
PERRLA	Pupils equal, regular, react to light and accommodation	PN	Percussion note	qns	Quantity not sufficient
		PND	Paroxysmal nocturnal dyspnea	q.o.d.	Every other day
PET	Positron emission tomography	PNH	Paroxysmal nocturnal hemoglobinuria	qt	Quart
PFF	Protein-free filtrate			Quat	Four (*quattuor*)
PGA	Pteroylglutamic acid (folic acid)	PO; p.o.	Orally (*per os*)	R	Respiration; right; *Rickettsia;* roentgen
PH	Past history	PPD	Purified protein derivative (TB test)		
pH	Hydrogen ion concentration (alkalinity and acidity in urine and blood analysis)			R	Take
		ppm	Parts per million	RA	Rheumatoid arthritis
		Pr	Presbyopia; prism	Ra	Radium
Pharm; Phar.	Pharmacy	PRN, p.r.n.	As required (*pro re nata*)	rad	Unit of measurement of the absorbed dose of ionizing radiation; root
PI	Previous illness; protamine insulin	pro time	Prothrombin time		
PICC	Percutaneously inserted central catheter	PSA	Prostate-specific antigen	RAI	Radioactive iodine
		PSP	Phenolsulfonphthalein	RAIU	Radioactive iodine uptake
PID	Pelvic inflammatory disease	pt	Pint	RBC; rbc	Red blood cell; red blood count
PK	Psychokinesis	Pt	Platinum; patient	RCD	Relative cardiac dullness
PKU	Phenylketonuria	PT	Prothrombin time; physical therapy	RCM	Right costal margin
PL	Light perception			RDA	Recommended daily/dietary allowance
PM	Postmortem; evening	PTA	Plasma thromboplastin antecedent		
PMB	Polymorphonuclear basophil leukocytes	PTC	Plasma thromboplastin component	RDS	Respiratory distress syndrome
		PTT	Partial thromboplastin time	RE	Right eye; reticuloendothelial tissue or cell
PME	Polymorphonuclear eosinophil leukocytes	Pu	Plutonium		
		PUO	Pyrexia of unknown origin		

Continued

Re	Rhenium	RU	Rat unit	SLP	Speech-language pathology
re	Right extremity	RUE	Right upper extremity	Sn	Tin
Rect	Rectified	RUL	Right upper lobe	SNF	Skilled nursing facility
Reg umb	Umbilical region	RUQ	Right upper quadrant	SOB	Shortness of breath
RES	Reticuloendothelial system	S	Sulfur	sol	Solution, dissolved
Rh	Symbol of rhesus factor; symbol for rhodium	S.	Sacral	SP	Spirit
		s̄	Without	sp. gr. SG, s.g	Specific gravity
RhA	Rheumatoid arthritis	S-A; S/A; SA	Sinoatrial	sph	Spherical
RHD	Relative hepatic dullness; rheumatic heart disease			SPI	Serum precipitable iodine
RLE	Right lower extremity	SAS	Sodium acetate solution	spir	Spirit
RLL	Right lower lobe	SB	Small bowel (x-ray film); sternal border	SR	Sedimentation rate
RLQ	Right lower quadrant			Sr	Strontium
RM	Respiratory movement	Sb	Antimony	s/s	Signs and symptoms
RML	Right middle lobe of lung	SC	Closure of semilunar valves	SSS	Specific soluble substance, sick sinus syndrome
Rn	Radon	SD	Skin dose		
RNA	Ribonucleic acid	Se	Selenium	sss	Layer upon layer (*stratum super stratum*)
R/O	Rule out	Sed rate	Sedimentation rate		
ROM	Range of motion	SGA	Small for gestational age	St	Let it stand (*stet; stent*)
ROS	Review of systems	SGOT	Serum glutamic oxaloacetic transaminase	Staph	*Staphylococcus*
RPF	Renal plasma flow			stat	Immediately (*statim*)
RPM; rpm	Revolutions per minute	SGPT	Serum glutamic pyruvic transaminase	STD	Sexually transmitted disease; skin test dose
RPR	Rapid plasma reagin	SH	Serum hepatitis		
RPS	Renal pressor substance	SI	International system of units (stroke index)	STH	Somatotrophic hormone
RQ	Respiratory quotient			Strep	*Streptococcus*
RR	Recovery room; respiratory rate	S.I.	Soluble insulin	STS	Serologic test for syphilis
RT	Radiation therapy; reading test; respiratory therapy	Si	Silicon	STU	Skin test unit
		SIDS	Sudden infant death syndrome	SV	Stroke volume; supraventricular
R/T	Related to	SLE	Systemic lupus erythematosus	sv	Alcoholic spirit (*spiritus vini*)

Table A-2 Abbreviations—cont'd

Abbreviation	Meaning	Abbreviation	Meaning	Abbreviation	Meaning
Sx	Symptoms	TCA	Tetrachloracetic acid	TPN	Total parenteral nutrition
Sym	Symmetrical	Te	Tellurium; tetanus	TPR	Temperature, pulse, and respiration
T	Temperature; thoracic	TEM	Triethylene melamine		
t	Temporal	TENS	Transcutaneous electrical nerve stimulation	tr	Tincture
T_3	Triiodothyronine			Trans D	Transverse diameter
T_4	Thyroxine	Th	Thorium	TRU	Turbidity reducing unit
TA	Toxin-antitoxin	TIA	Transient ischemic attack	TS	Test solution
Ta	Tantalum	TIBC	Total iron-binding capacity	TSE	Testicular self-examination
TAB	Vaccine against typhoid, paraty-phoid A and B	Tl	Thallium	TSH	Thyroid-stimulating hormone
		TM	Tympanic membrane	TSP	Trisodium phosphate
Tab	Tablet	Tm	Thulium; symbol for maximal tubular excretory capacity (kidneys)	TST	Triple sugar iron test
TAH	Total abdominal hysterectomy			TUR; TURP	Transurethral resection
TAM	Toxoid-antitoxoid mixture			Tx	Treatment
T & A	Tonsillectomy and adenoidectomy	TMJ	Temporomandibular joint	U	Uranium; unit
TAT	Toxin-antitoxin, tetanus antitoxin	TNT	Trinitrotoluene	UA	Urinalysis
TB	Tuberculin; tuberculosis; tubercle bacillus	TNTM	Too numerous to mention	UBI	Ultraviolet blood irradiation
		TP	Tuberculin precipitation	UE	Upper extremity
Tb	Terbium	TPI	*Treponema pallidum* immobiliza-tion test for syphilis	UIBC	Unsaturated iron-binding capacity

Umb; umb	Umbilicus
URI	Upper respiratory infection
US	Ultrasonic
USP	*U.S. Pharmacopeia*
UTI	Urinary tract infection
UV	Ultraviolet
V	Vanadium; vision; visual acuity
v	Volt
VA	Visual acuity
V & T	Volume and tension
VC	Vital capacity
VD	Venereal disease
VDA	Visual discriminatory acuity
VDG	Venereal disease—gonorrhea
VDM	Vasodepressor material
VDRL	Venereal Disease Research Laboratories (sometimes used loosely to mean venereal disease report)
VDS	Venereal disease—syphilis
VEM	Vasoexciter material
Vf	Field of vision
VHD	Valvular heart disease
VIA	Virus inactivating agent
VLEW	Very low birth weight
VLDL	Very low-density lipoprotein
VMA	Vanillylmandelic acid
vol	Volume
VR	Vocal resonance
VS	Volumetric solution
VS, v.s.	Vital signs
Vs	Venisection
VsB	Bleeding in arm (*venaesectio brachii*)
VSD	Ventricular septal defect
VW	Vessel wall
VZIG	Varicella zoster immune globulin
W	Tungsten
w	Watt
WBC, wbc	White blood cell; white blood count
WD	Well developed
WL	Wavelength
WN	Well nourished
WNL	Within normal limits
WR	Wassermann reaction
wt	Weight
X-ray	Roentgen ray
y, yr	Year
yo	Years old
Z	Symbol for atomic number
Zn	Zinc
Zz	Ginger

American Dental Association (ADA) Dental Codes*

Table B-1 Coding system

CDT-4 is organized by a numbered system with twelve categories. The categories are as follows:

	Category of service	Code series
I.	Diagnostic Services	D0100-D0999
II.	Preventive Services	D1000-D1999
III.	Restorative Services	D2000-D2999
IV.	Endodontics	D3000-D3999
V.	Periodontics	D4000-D4999
VI.	Prosthodontics, removable	D5000-D5899
VII.	Maxillofacial Prosthetics	D5900-D5999
VIII.	Implant Services	D6000-D6199
IX.	Prosthodontics, fixed	D6200-D6999
X.	Oral and Maxillofacial Surgery	D7000-D7999
XI.	Orthodontics	D8000-D8999
XII.	Adjunctive General Services	D9000-D9999

Note how the coding system is arranged so that each procedure is identified by five numbers. Each number begins with D, which tells the payer that the service is a dental procedure. The dental category—such as orthodontics or periodontics—of the service is indicated by the second numeral of each code; unclassifiable services are coded with the number 9 as the second digit. *CDT-4* is functional for all services that can be performed by a licensed dentist.

*From: *CDT-4 users manual: the comprehensive guide to accurate claims reporting*, ed 4, 2003, American Dental Association.

Anxiety and Pain Management*

Table C-1 Mandibular injections

Injection	Needle	Structures anesthetized	Penetration site	Terminal deposition site	Amount deposited
Inferior alveolar (IA) and Lingual (L)	Long	1. Mandibular teeth 2. Facial gingiva of mandibular anterior teeth and first premolar 3. Skin of chin 4. Lower lip 5. Lingual gingiva of mandibular teeth 6. Floor of mouth 7. Anterior ⅔ of tongue	Pterygotemporal depression; place thumb in coronoid notch and roll medially to temporal crest	Approach from opposite canine/premolar area; needle path is parallel to occlusal plane of mandibular teeth and 6–10 mm superior; site is directly above mandibular foramen between sphenomandibular ligament and ramus of mandible; approximately ¾ of long needle is inserted	⅞ cartridge (1.5 mL) Wait 1–5 minutes
Buccal (B)	Long	1. Facial gingiva of mandibular molars 2. Skin of cheek	Mucobuccal fold, 2–3 mm posterior to distobuccal root of last molar adjacent to retromolar pad	2–3 mm penetration; needle is held parallel and inferior to horizontal plane of occlusal surfaces when directed toward penetration site	⅛ cartridge (0.3 mL) Wait 1–5 minutes
Mental (M)	Short	1. Facial gingiva of mandibular anterior teeth and first premolar 2. Skin of chin 3. Lower lip	Vertical approach: Mucobuccal fold between first and second premolars Horizontal approach: Mucobuccal fold at apex of first premolar	Directly over mental foramen	⅓ cartridge (0.6 mL) Wait 1–5 minutes

*From Darby ML: Mosby's comprehensive review of dental hygiene ed 5, St Louis, 2002, Mosby.

Table C-2 Maxillary injections

Injection	Needle	Structures anesthetized	Penetration site	Terminal deposition site	Amount deposited
Anterior-superior alveolar (ASA)	Short	1. Facial gingiva of maxillary anterior teeth 2. Maxillary anterior teeth	Mucolabial fold anterior and parallel to canine eminence	Apex of the canine tooth	½–⅔ cartridge (0.9–1.2 mL) Wait 1–5 min
Middle superior alveolar (MSA)	Short	1. Facial gingiva of maxillary premolars and mucobuccal root of first molar 2. Maxillary premolars and mucobuccal root of first molar	Mucobuccal fold parallel to apex of second premolar	3–5 mm superior to apex of the second premolar	½ –⅔ cartridge (0.9–1.2 mL) Wait 1–5 min
Infraorbital (IO)	Long	1. Facial gingiva of maxillary anteriors, premolars, and mucobuccal root of first molar 2. Maxillary anteriors, premolars, and mucobuccal root of first molar 3. Side of nose 4. Upper lip 5. Lower eyelid	Mucobuccal fold parallel to apex of first premolar	Infraorbital foramen; keep needle parallel with tooth; approximately ½ of long needle	½–⅔ cartridge (0.9–1.2 mL) Wait 1–5 min
Posterior-superior alveolar (PSA)	Short	1. Facial gingiva of maxillary molars, except for mucobuccal root of first molar 2. Maxillary molars, except for the mucobuccal root of first molar	Within the soft tissue depression just distal to the maxillary second molar	Insert needle 45 degrees to mid-sagittal plane and 45 degrees to horizontal plane of maxillary occlusal surfaces Approximately ½ of short needle	½–1 cartridge (0.9–1.8 mL) Wait 1–5 min
Greater palatine (GP)	Short	1. Lingual gingiva of maxillary posterior teeth 2. Palatal mucosa to the midline	Pressure anesthesia (1 min); 2–3 mm anterior to the greater palatine foramen	Approximately 2 mm (until bevel is covered)	¼–⅓ cartridge (0.45–0.6 mL) Wait 1–5 min
Nasopalatine (NP)	Short	1. Lingual gingiva of maxillary anterior teeth 2. Palatal mucosa in the premaxillary area	Pressure anesthesia (1 min); incisive papilla at base and into fattest portion	Approximately 2 mm (until bevel is covered)	½ cartridge (0.45 mL) Wait 1–5 min

Table C-3 Comparison of traditional syringe and wand

	Traditional	Wand
Grasp and needle control	• Palm grasp • Relies on large muscles of wrist, forearm, and shoulder • Weighs 80 g • Held 9 inches from the insertion point	• Pen grasp • Control is transferred to the small muscles of the fingers and thumb • Weighs a few grams • Held within 2 inches of the insertion point
Fluid delivery Fluid metering	• The thumb is used to start and stop the flow of solution • Pressure and volume cannot be separated, thus it is operator dependent	• Uses a foot control to deliver a constant flow of solution • Maintains constant pressure and controlled volume
Aspiration	• Relies on operator control	• Aspirates automatically (on demand) by releasing the foot control
Needles	• Threaded hub 25 ga, long and short 27 ga, long and short	• Luer-Lok hub smaller gauge and length preferred 30 ga, 1/2 inch 30 ga, 1 inch 27 ga, 1 1/4 inch
Path of insertion	• Linear insertion (straight push through the tissues, causing needle deflection)	• Bi-rotational insertion (180 degrees) between the thumb and index finger to overcome needle deflection

Table C-4 Comparison of frequently used local anesthetic agents in dentistry

Generic name	Commercial name	Color code	Concentrations (%)	Chemical classification	Vasoconstrictor	Cartridge vol. (mg)	Concentrations of vasoconstrictor	Onset of action	Maximum safe dose for normal adult patient — mg; mL	No. cartridges
Lidocaine	Xylocaine	Green Red	2	Amide	Epinephrine	36	1:50,000 1:100,000	2 min	300 mg; 15 mL	8.3
Mepivacaine	Carbocaine	Brown Beige	2 3	Amide Amide	Neo-cobefrin	36	1:20,000 —	1½–2 min	300 mg; 15 mL 360 mg; 12 mL	8.3 6.6
Prilocaine	Citanest Forte Citanest	Yellow Black	4	Amide Amide	Epinephrine	54 72	1:200,000 —	2–4 min	400 mg; 10 mL 400 mg; 10 mL	5.5 5.5

	Approximate duration		Toxicity	Method of metabolism
	Without vasoconstrictor	With vasoconstrictor		
	Pulpal = 5–10 min Soft tissue = 60–120 min	Pulpal = 60 min Soft tissue = 3–5 hr	2.0	Liver
	Pulpal = 20–40 min Soft tissue = 2–3 hr	Pulpal = 60 min Soft tissue = 3–5 hr	1.5–2.0 1.5–2.0	Liver Liver
	Pulpal = 40–60 min Soft tissue = 2–4 hr	Pulpal = 60–90 min Soft tissue = 3–8 hr	1.0 1.0	Liver and lung Liver and lung

APPENDIX D

Clinical Oral Structures*

Table D-1 Oral structures

Structure	Clinical description	Clinical consideration
Lips and Cheeks		
Philtrum	Midline vertical depression of the skin between the nose and upper lip	Common location for cleft lip
Vermilion zone	Transition area between skin of the face and oral mucosa of the lips; medium pink in light-skinned persons and pigmented with melanin in darker-skinned individuals	The junction between the vermilion zone and the skin of the face is frequently the site of herpetic lesions; lower lip is frequent site of oral cancer
		Fordyce's granules or spots (small white spots of ectopic sebaceous material) may be present
Labial commissure	Junction of the upper and lower lips at the corner of the mouth	Frequent site of chafing, herpetic lesions, and cracking (angular cheilitis); avoid pulling with instrument handle
Vestibule	Space bounded by the cheeks, lips, and facial surfaces of the teeth and gingiva	Frequent site of aphthous ulcers
Labial mucosa	Mucosal lining of the inner lip; vascular; small elevations are external manifestation of numerous labial salivary glands	Frequent site of mucoceles, mucus-retention cysts, aphthous ulcers, and scars
Labial frenum (maxillary and mandibular)	Fold of tissue at the midline (maxillary and mandibular) between the inner surface of the lip and the alveolar mucosa	Maxillary fold is sometimes overdeveloped, which results in a space between the central incisors called a *diastema*
		Maxillary fold frequently has an extra flap of tissue
		If overextended onto the attached gingiva mandibular fold may cause recession
Buccal mucosa	Mucus membrane lining of the inner cheek	Frequent site of linea alba, cheek bites, and Fordyce's granules

Continued

*From Darby ML: *Mosby's comprehensive review of dental hygiene*, ed 5, St Louis, 2002, Mosby.

721

Table D-1 Oral structures—cont'd

Structure	Clinical description	Clinical consideration
Buccal frena (muscle attachments)	Folds of epithelium between the cheek and attached gingiva (maxillary and mandibular) in the first premolar area	Overextension may cause gingival recession
Alveolar mucosa	Thin movable mucosal lining covering the alveolar bone; between the attached gingiva and mucobuccal fold on the facial of the maxillary and mandibular arches; and between the attached gingiva and floor of the mouth on the lingual aspect of the mandibular arch	Very thin and fragile epithelium Frequent site of aphthous ulcers Mandibular lingual lining is the site of tori (bony projections), which may interfere with exposing radiographs or taking impressions
Muco-buccal fold	Fold or "gutter" area between the alveolar and buccal or labial mucosa	The height of the mucobuccal fold above a maxillary tooth area to be anesthetized is the needle insertion area The mental foramen of the mandible can be palpated in the mucobuccal fold area, facial to the mandibular premolars; this is the needle insertion site for a mental nerve block
Parotid papilla	Flap of tissue on the cheek opposite the maxillary first molars; contains the opening of Stenson's duct, which carries saliva from the parotid gland	Large amounts of mainly serous saliva come from this duct The opening often can be seen as a dark spot
Tongue		
	The tongue is a flat, muscular organ of speech and taste; the lateral border and undersurface are frequent sites of oral cancer	
Median sulcus	Midline depression on the dorsum of the tongue	Presence and depth vary Additional deep depressions are called *fissures*; a fissured tongue
Fungiform papillae	Mushroom-shaped, red to dark brown elevations scattered over the anterior third of the dorsum of the tongue	In darker-skinned individuals these may contain melanin pigmentation Function in taste sensations of sweet, sour, and salt
Filiform papillae	Fringelike keratinized projections concentrated in the middle third of the dorsum of the tongue	Readily collect plaque and stain Moving patches devoid of these papillae is called a *geographic tongue*

Circumvallate papillae	8–10 large papillae arranged in an inverted V-shaped row posterior to the filiform papillae	Function in taste sensation of bitter Ducts of von Ebner's salivary glands open around them and secrete serous saliva
Foliate papillae	Vertical ridges on the lateral borders of the tongue	Function in taste sensation of sour
Lingual tonsils	Mass of lymphoid tissue on the base of the tongue, posterior to the circumvallate papillae	May be a site of precancerous or cancerous findings (white or red areas, ulcers, masses, pigmentations)
Lingual frenum	Thin fold of epithelium attaching the under surface of the tongue to the floor of the mouth	Difficult to observe: extend and move the tongue to the right and left to examine A short frenum limits movement (*ankyloglossia*, tongue-tied) and makes exposing of radiographs and taking impressions difficult
Sublingual folds	Two ridges of tissue on the floor of the mouth arranged in a V-shaped direction, from the lingual frenum to the base of the tongue	Contains Wharton's duct from the submandibular (also called *submaxillary*) salivary gland; and the Bartholin and Rivinis ducts and openings of the sublingual salivary glands
Sublingual caruncle	Round elevation of the floor of the mouth on either side of the lingual frena Contains the opening for Wharton's ducts	Limited amounts of mixed saliva secreted here Wharton's duct carries large amounts of saliva from the submandibular (also called *submaxillary*) salivary gland
Lingual veins	Blue line on the under surface of the tongue on either side of the lingual frenum	With age this vein becomes more prominent in size and color; varicosities may be present
Plica fimbriatae	Fringe like projections on the under surface of the tongue, lateral to the lingual vein	May be darker colored, with more melanin pigmentation

Palate

Anterior two thirds of the roof of the mouth is hard palate; posterior third is soft palate; a frequent site of oral cancer

Incisive papillae	Midline pad of tissue lingual to the maxillary central incisors	Often burned or traumatized when eating Protect the nasopalatine nerve, which enters through the underlying *incisive foramen*; the palatal mucosa immediately lateral to the papilla is the needle insertion site for nasopalatine nerve-block anesthesia

Continued

Table D-1 Oral structures—cont'd

Structure	Clinical description	Clinical consideration
Rugae	Firm irregular ridges of masticatory mucosa on the anterior half of the hard palate	If prominent, rugae may be burned or traumatized more easily
Palatine fovea	Small dimple on either side of the midline at the junction of the hard and soft palates	Touching the posterior area of this may initiate the gag reflex
Palatal salivary duct openings	Small dark spots scattered on the hard and soft palates	Represent the duct openings of the minor palatal salivary glands
Palatine raphe	Hard linear elevation along the midline of the hard palate; external manifestation of the palatine suture, which joins the right and left maxillary and palatine bones	Excess bone (tori) or a deep depression may be present here; Site of hyperkeratinization or associated nicotinic stomatitis
Maxillary tuberosity	Protuberance of the alveolar bone distal to the last maxillary molar	Erupting third molar may be present here
	Tonsillar Region	
Retromolar Area	Triangular area of bone and pad of tissue distal to the last mandibular molar	Erupting third molar may be present, and a flap of tissue (operculum) often is associated with an infection in this area
Pterygomandibular raphe	Fold of tissue from the retromolar area to an area near the maxillary tuberosity; separates the soft palate from the cheek; lies medial to the posterior border of the ramus of the mandible	Covers a ligament from the mandible to the sphenoid bone; Used as a guide to identify the posterior border of the ramus of the mandible when targeting the area for needle insertion for inferior alveolar-nerve anesthesia

Anterior or glossopalatine arch	Thin fold of epithelium extending laterally and inferiorly from both sides of the soft palate to the base of the tongue
	Marks the entry into the pharynx; the anterior boundary of the tonsillar recess
Posterior or pharyngopalatine arch	Thin fold of epithelium that is more posterior and narrower than the anterior arch
	Marks the posterior boundary of the palatine tonsillar recess
Tonsillar recess	Recessed area between the anterior and posterior arches
Palatine tonsils	Globules of lymphoid tissue in the tonsillar recess
	May or may not contain palatine tonsils
	Vary greatly in size
	Not visible if removed or atrophied, or may be so large the fauces is very narrow
Uvula	Fleshy tissue suspended from the midline of the posterior border of the soft palate
	Closes the opening to the nasopharynx when swallowing
	Varies in size and shape
Pharyngeal tonsils	Globules of lymphoid tissue on the oropharyngeal wall
	Lay term is *adenoids*
	Appear as globules of reddish-orange tissue
	Mucosal secretions from the sinuses may be seen here
Fauces or *faucial isthmus*	Isthmus (narrowing) of the space from the oral cavity into the pharynx

Dental Professional Organizations

Table E-1 Dental professional organizations

Abbreviation	Organization	Website
AADS	American Association for Dental Schools	http://www.aads.jhu.edu
AAE	American Association of Endodontists	http://www.aae.org
AAO	American Association of Orthodontists	http://www.braces.org
AAOMP	American Association of Oral and Maxillofacial Pathology	http://www.aaomp.org
AAOMR	American Association of Oral and Maxillofacial Radiology	http://www.aaomr.org
AAOMS	American Association of Oral and Maxillofacial Surgeons	http://www.aaoms.org
AAP	American Academy of Periodontology	http://www.perio.org
AAPD	American Academy of Pediatric Dentistry	http://www.aapd.org
AAPHD	American Association of Public Health Dentistry	http://www.aaphd.org
ABPD	American Board of Pediatric Dentistry	http://www.abpd.org
ACP	American College of Prosthodontics	http://www.prosthodontics.org
ADA	American Dental Association	http://www.ada.org
ADAA	American Dental Assistants' Association	http://www.dentalassistant.org
ADHA	American Dental Hygienists' Association	http://www.adha.org
AGD	Academy of General Dentistry	http://www.agd.org
ASDA	American Student Dental Association	http://www.asdanet.org
ASDA	American Society of Dentist Anesthesiologists	http://www.asdahq.org
IADR	International Association of Dental Research	http://www.iadr.com
IAO	International Association for Orthodontics	http://www.iaortho.com
WFO	World Federation of Orthodontists	http://www.wfo.org

Table E-2 Federal and international organizations

Abbreviation	Organization	Website
CDC	Centers for Disease Control and Prevention	http://www.cdc.gov
FDA	Food and Drug Administration	http://www.fda.gov
Library of Congress	THOMAS	http://thomas.loc.gov
NHIC	National Health Information Center	http://www.health.gov/nhic
NIDRC	National Institute of Dental Research and Craniofacial	http://www.nidcr.nih.gov
NIH	National Institutes of Health	http://www.nih.gov
NLM	National Library of Medicine	http://www.nlm.nih.gov
NOHIC	National Oral Health Information Clearinghouse	http://www.nohic.nidcr.nih.gov
OSHA	Occupational Safety and Health Administration	http://www.osha.gov
WHO	World Health Organization	http://www.who.int/en

Health Insurance Portability and Accountability Act of 1996

The Health Insurance Portability and Accountability Act (HIPAA) of 1996 was signed into law by President Bill Clinton on August 21, 1996. Conclusive regulations were issued on August 17, 2000, to be instated by October 16, 2002. HIPAA requires that the transactions of all patient healthcare information be formatted in a standardized electronic style. In addition to protecting the privacy and security of patient information, HIPAA includes legislation on the formation of medical savings accounts, the authorization of a fraud and abuse control program, the easy transport of health insurance coverage, and the simplification of administrative terms and conditions.

HIPAA encompasses three primary areas, and its privacy requirements can be broken down into three types: privacy standards, patients' rights, and administrative requirements.

1. Privacy Standards. A central concern of HIPAA is the careful use and disclosure of protected health information (PHI), which generally is electronically controlled health information that is able to be distinguished individually. PHI also refers to verbal communication, although the HIPAA Privacy Rule is not intended to hinder necessary verbal communication. The U.S. Department of Health and Human Services (USDHHS) does not require restructuring, such as soundproofing, architectural changes, and so forth, but some caution is necessary when exchanging health information by conversation.

An Acknowledgement of Receipt Notice of Privacy Practices, which allows patient information to be used or divulged for treatment, payment, or health care operations (TPO), should be procured from each patient. A detailed and time-sensitive authorization can also be issued, which allows the dentist to release information in special circumstances other than TPOs. A *written consent* is also an option. Dentists can disclose PHI *without* acknowledgement, consent, or authorization in very special situations, for example, perceived child abuse, public health supervision, fraud investigation, or law enforcement with valid permission (i.e., a warrant). When divulging PHI, a dentist must try to disclose only the *minimum necessary* information, to help safeguard the patient's information as much as possible.

It is important that dental professionals adhere to HIPAA standards because healthcare providers (as well as healthcare clearinghouses and healthcare plans) who convey *electronically* formatted health information via an outside billing service or merchant are considered *covered entities*. Covered entities may be dealt serious civil and criminal penalties for violation of HIPAA legislation. Failure to comply with HIPAA privacy requirements may result in civil penalties of up to $100 per offense with an annual maximum of $25,000 for repeated failure to comply with the same requirement. Criminal penalties resulting from the illegal mishandling of private health information can range from $50,000 and/or 1 year in prison to $250,000 and/or 10 years in prison.

2. Patients' Rights. HIPAA allows patients, authorized representatives, and parents of minors, as well as minors, to become more aware of the health information privacy to which they are entitled. These rights include, but are not limited to, the right to view and copy their health information, the right to dispute alleged breaches of policies and regulations, and the right to request alternative forms of communicating with their dentist. If any health information is released for any reason other than TPO, the patient is entitled to an account of the transaction. Therefore it is important for dentists to keep accurate records of such information and to provide them when necessary.

The HIPAA Privacy Rule determines that the parents of a minor have access to their child's health information. This privilege may be overruled, for example, in cases where there is suspected child abuse or the parent consents to a term of confidentiality between the dentist and the minor. The parents' rights to access their child's PHI also may be restricted in situations when a legal entity, such as a court, intervenes and when a law does not require a parent's consent. For a full list of patient rights provided by HIPAA, be sure to acquire a copy of the law and to understand it well.

3. Administrative Requirements. Complying with HIPAA legislation may seem like a chore, but it does not need to be so. It is recommended that you become appropriately familiar with the law, organize the requirements into simpler tasks, begin compliance early, and document your progress in compliance. An important first step is to evaluate the current information and practices of your office.

Dentists will need to write a *privacy policy* for their office, a document for their patients detailing the office's practices concerning PHI. The American Dental Association's (ADA) *HIPAA Privacy Kit* includes forms that you (the dentist) can use to customize your privacy policy. It is useful to try to understand the role of healthcare information for your patients and the ways in which they deal with the information while they are visiting your office. Train your staff; make sure they are familiar with the terms of HIPAA and your office's privacy policy and related forms. HIPAA requires that you designate a *privacy officer*, a person in your office who will be responsible for applying the new policies in your office, fielding complaints, and making choices involving the minimum necessary requirements. Another person with the role of *contact person* will process complaints.

A *Notice of Privacy Practices*—a document detailing the patient's rights and the dental office's obligations concerning PHI—also must be drawn up. Further, any role of a third party with access to PHI must be clearly documented. This third party is known as a *business associate* (BA) and is defined as any entity who, on behalf of the dentist, takes part in any activity that involves exposure of PHI. The *HIPAA Privacy Kit* provides a copy of the USDHHS "Business Associate Contract Terms," which provides a concrete format for detailing BA interactions.

The main HIPAA privacy compliance date, including all staff training, was April 14, 2003, although many covered entities who submitted a request and a compliance plan by October 15, 2002, were granted 1-year extensions. Contact your local branch of the ADA for details. It is recommended that dentists prepare their offices ahead of time for all deadlines, which include preparing privacy polices and forms, business associate contracts, and employee training sessions.

For a comprehensive discussion of all of these terms and requirements, a complete list of HIPAA policies and procedures, and a full collection of HIPAA privacy forms, contact the ADA for a *HIPAA Privacy Kit*. The relevant ADA website is www.ada.org/goto/hipaa. Other websites that may contain useful information about HIPAA are the following:

- USDHHS Office of Civil Rights www.hhs.gov/ocr/hipaa
- Work Group on Electronic Data Interchange www.wedi.org/SNIP
- Phoenix Health www.hipaadvisory.com
- USDHHS Office of the Assistant Secretary for Planning and Evaluation http://aspe.os.dhhs.gov/admnsimp/

Sources used:
1. *HIPAA Privacy Kit*
2. http://www.ada.org/prof/prac/issues/topics/hipaa/index.html

Infection Control

One of the most important areas in dentistry today is infection control, maintaining a healthy, disease-free work zone that protects both patients and dental workers. The process encompasses not only common communicable infections, such as influenza and strep throat, and long-term life-threatening illnesses, such as human immunodeficiency virus (HIV) and hepatitis, but also the handling of biohazard and hazardous materials. Two national organizations, the Occupational Safety and Health Administration (OSHA) and the Centers for Disease Control and Prevention (CDC), are committed to protecting dental hygienists and technicians from these daily risks and produce a number of publications that focus on making dentistry a healthy and safe environment in which to work. Here are links to these governing bodies and the informational materials with which every dental professional should be familiar.

Table G-1 Infection control resources

Organization	Website	Description
OSHA	http://www.osha.gov	This is the link to the main OSHA website. There is a search function available to quickly locate whatever information you need.
OSHA on dentistry	http://www.osha.gov/SLTC/ dentistry/index.html	Covering all of the risks in and requirements for dental offices, OSHA provides dentistry with its own articles that educate a dental professional about topics including potential hazards, workplace violence, and noise control.
OSHA standards for bloodborne pathogens	http://www.osha.gov/pls/ oshaweb/owadisp.show_ document?p_table= STANDARDS&p_id=10051	This explains OSHA's requirements for businesses that work with potential infectious agents, such as blood and needles, to have a plan to protect their employees.

Continued

Table G-1 Infection control resources—cont'd

Organization	Website	Description
OSHA plan for safe healthcare facilities	http://www.osha.gov/SLTC/ healthcarefacilities/ index.html	This link covers how to establish a safe healthcare facility. The page covers identifying potential hazards, developing plans to address those hazards, and providing training for employees about the risks in their work environment.
OSHA guidelines for exposure to anesthetic gases	http://www.osha.gov/dts/ osta/anestheticgases/ anesthetic_gases.html	Focusing on educating employees about the damaging materials around them, this page describes and teaches dental professionals about the risks and realities of contact with the inhaled anesthetics in their dental office.
OSHA and needlestick prevention	http://www.osha.gov/SLTC/ needlestick/index.html	In compliance with the 2000 Needlestick Safety and Prevention Act, OSHA is raising the awareness of needlestick safety. This page is devoted to keeping healthcare workers informed of new techniques and procedures to protect them from needlesticks.
CDC	http://www.cdc.gov	The link to the main CDC website has the latest information in the healthcare world as well as a wealth of information and resource materials on training and employment.
CDC's recommendations for infection control	http://www.cdc.gov/ OralHealth/ infection_control/ guidelines/comments.htm http://www.cdc.gov/mmwr/ preview/mmwrhtml/ 00021095.htm	This is a draft of the updated recommendations for dental practices' guidelines for infection control. The older version from 1993 is available at the second link.
CDC on exposure to blood	http://www.cdc.gov/ncidod/ hip/Blood/exp_blood.htm	This electronic pamphlet covers all of the bases that a healthcare worker needs to know about blood exposure. It gives detailed answers to questions about HIV and hepatitis.

APPENDIX H

Legal and Ethical Issues

Table H-I Differentiating between ethics and law*

	Ethics	Law
Definition	Individual interpretation of the nature of right and wrong and rules of conduct	Rules and regulations by which society is governed, set forth in a formal and legally binding manner
Source	Internalized; individual nature and beliefs	Externalized rules and regulations of society
Emphasis	Individual moral behavior for the good of the individual within society	Social behaviors that are good for society as a whole
Conduct	Motives and reasons why the individual behaves the way he or she does	Overt conduct of the individual; what a person actually did or failed to do
Sanctions	Professional organization—expulsion from the organization	Judicial and administrative bodies—criminal sanctions such as fines and imprisonment imposed by the courts; civil sanctions such as monetary damages imposed by the courts; disciplinary sanctions such as fines, license suspension, or license revocation by a board of dentistry

*From Darby ML: *Mosby's comprehensive review of dental hygiene*, ed 5, St Louis, 2002, Mosby.

Table H-2 Historical court cases

Category of law	Court case	Issue	Decision in favor of	Precedent established
Civil/affirmative action/age discrimination	M. Bennett v Hardy (1990)	Unlawful discharge	Defendant	Burden of proof was lacking.
Civil/contract/disability	Hansen v Gordon (1992)	Work-related impairment	Plaintiff	Disease impairment covered under worker's compensation.
Civil/contract/employment rights	Murphy v Birdtree Dental (1997)	Breach of contract	Plaintiff	Contractual right confirmed by policy handbook.
Civil/contract/insurance coverage	Hawkins v Berkshire Life Ins. Co. (1999)	Full disclosure	Defendant	Contract void if full disclosure is not given.
Civil/contract/insurance coverage	Freidin v Pan-Am Ins. (1992)	Full disclosure	Plaintiff	Facts did not support claims of the defendant.
Civil/contract/unemployment benefits	Stagner v Highfill (1990)	Work rules	Defendant	Reasonable work rules are contractually valid.
Civil/malpractice/breach of practice act*	Edwards v Pennsylvania Dental Examining Board (1983)	Unlawful action	Pennsylvania Dental Examining Board	Police power of the state upheld.
Civil/malpractice/breach of practice act*	Bach v Florida State Board of Dentistry (1979)	Unlawful action	Florida State Board of Dentistry	Police power of the state upheld.
Civil/malpractice/breach of practice act*	Barletta v State of LA/School of Dentistry (1988)	Unlawful action	Defendant	Due process affirmed.
Civil/malpractice/breach of practice act*	Oppenheim, Sloan v Pennsylvania Dental Examining Board (1983)	Unlawful action	Pennsylvania Dental Examining Board	Police power of the state upheld.
Civil/malpractice/negligence/personal injury	Myers v Dunscombe (1983)	Unlawful action	Defendant	Police power of the state upheld.

Civil/restraint of trade	CDA v CDHA (1990)	Freedom of association	Defendant	Collective bargaining right in professional organizations affirmed.
Civil/state practice act	Fosket v State Board of Dentistry (1977)	Independent practice	Defendant	Police power of the state upheld.
Civil/tort/negligence/ personal injury	Campbell v Pommier (1985)	Reasonable care	Defendant	Burden of proof lies with plaintiff.
Civil/tort/negligence/ personal injury	Sirkin and Levine v Timmons (1994)	Work environment risk	Plaintiff	Reasonable precautions required of employers.
Civil/tort/negligence/ personal injury	Flor v Holguin (2000)	Work environment risk	Plaintiff	Reasonable precautions required of employers.
Civil/tort/negligence/ personal injury	Kilburn v US (1991)	Full disclosure	Defendant	Plaintiff did not show probable cause.
Civil/tort/negligence/ personal injury	Ryan v Hiller (1994)	Dual capacity doctrine	Defendant	Transporting an employee to another office is work-related.
Civil/tort/negligence/ personal injury	Parker v Frelich (2002)	Respondent superior	Plaintiff	Liability is assumed if not explicitly informed of independence.
Civil/tort/negligence/ personal injury	Austin v AANS (2001)	Expert testimony	Plaintiff	Misrepresentation is actionable.
Civil/tort/work-related injury	Colwell v Trotman (1980)	Working conditions	Plaintiff	
Civil/vendor-proximate cause/injury	Falcone v Baxter Healthcare Corp. et al. (1996)	Defective product	Remanded to State Court	Two employers may be jointly liable.

*Although these cases were adjudicated in civil court, criminal charges of fraud and/or assault could have been levied. The reason for adjudication in civil court was the possibility of restitution or remuneration rather than only retribution.
Furthermore, the burden of proof is higher in a criminal proceeding (beyond a reasonable doubt) than in a civil proceeding (by the preponderance of evidence).

How Dental Terms Are Made and Read

Dental terminology is a hybrid speech. Most of the words also are common to medical terminology and as such are largely made up of Greek and Latin stems, prefixes, and suffixes. However, many words have been borrowed from other languages as well. Dental terminology also is dynamic in the sense that many new words are coined as necessity demands. Generally, technical words can be analyzed for their meanings by dividing them into their component parts and determining the meaning of each part.

To build or analyze any vocabulary, the five elements that can be used to form words must be understood: the word root, combining vowel, combining form, prefix, and suffix.

WORD ROOT

The word root is the basic core of any word and gives it its primary meaning. (Some compound words may be made up of more than one root.) For instance, in the words *stomatitis, adenitis,* and *pulpitis* the word roots are *stomat* (meaning "mouth"), *aden* (meaning "gland"), and *pulp* (meaning "the soft tissue within a tooth").

COMBINING VOWEL

Certain combinations of word roots are difficult to pronounce, especially when the first word root ends in a consonant and the second begins with a consonant. This awkwardness of pronunciation necessitates the insertion of a vowel called a combining vowel. Usually the combining vowel is an *o,* although *a, e, i, u,* and *y* may be encountered occasionally. Combining vowels are encountered in everyday words. Instead of joining the two word roots *speed* and *meter* directly, the combining vowel *o* is inserted to create *speedometer.* Another example is *megal* and *glossia,* which become *megaloglossia.*

COMBINING FORM

The combination of word root plus combining vowel is known as the combining form.

Word root	+	Combining vowel	=	Combining form
-gnath-		O		-gnatho-
-micr-		O		-micro-
-dent-		O		-dento-
-arthr-		O		-arthro-

SUFFIX

A suffix is a syllable or syllables added at the end of a word root or combining form to change the meaning of the root, give it grammatical function, or form a new word. *Play, read,* and *speak* are word roots; by adding the suffix *-er* (meaning "one who") the words are changed to "one who plays," "one who reads," and "one who speaks." If the suffix *-able* (meaning "capable of being") were added, the words mean "capable of being played," "capable of being read," and "capable of being spoken." In the words *microtome, dermatome,* and *arthrotome,* -tome is a suffix meaning "instrument for cutting." Notice that the suffix is added to the combining form rather than the word root:

Word root	+	Combining vowel	+	Suffix	=	Meaning
micr-		O		-tome		instrument to cut very fine sections
derm-		O		-tome		instrument to cut skin
arthr-		O		-tome		instrument to cut joints

PREFIX

A prefix is a syllable or syllables placed before a word or word root to alter its meaning or create a new word. If the prefixes *over-, re-,* and *out-* are added before the words *play, read,* and *speak,* three new words are created—*overplay, reread,* and *outspeak.* Any number of these five elements can be combined to form new words.

Auto-bi-o-graph-ic-al		*Sub-strat-o-spher-e*		*Electr-o-cardi-o-gram*	
auto-	prefix	sub-	prefix	electr-	word root
-bi-	word root	-strat-	word root	-o-	combining vowel
-o-	combining vowel	-o-	combining vowel	-cardi-	word root
-graph-	word root	-spher-	word root	-o-	combining vowel
-ic	suffix	-e	suffix	-gram	suffix
-al	suffix				

WORD AND ROOT ORDER

The order in which the various elements of compound words are placed is of great importance. Observe the consequences if the order of the elements in the following words were reversed:

leg iron	became	iron leg
motorboat	became	boat motor
snake poison	became	poison snake
pig iron	became	iron pig
zoo animal	became	animal zoo
eyeglass	became	glass eye
house dog	became	dog house

In all of these instances the order of the elements may be reversed and still arrive at a sensible word, although the subject in each example has changed. Other compound words such as the following may become nonsensical if the order of their elements is changed:

shoulder blade	cannot become	blade shoulder
nerve tonic	cannot become	tonic nerve
chickenpox	cannot become	pox chicken
headache	cannot become	achehead

The following is a list of combining forms for anatomic structures and body fluids, prefixes, suffixes, verbs, and adjectives. Although the combining form generally appears at the beginning of a term, it may appear within a term or at the end of it.*

---

*From Young CG, Austin MG: *Learning medical terminology step by step,* ed 4, St Louis, 1979, Mosby.

adeno- gland
adreno- adrenal gland
angio- vessel
ano- anus
arterio- artery
arthro- joint
balano- glans penis
blepharo- eyelid
broncho- bronchus (windpipe)
cantho- canthus (angle at either end of slit between eyelids)
capit- head
cardi-, cardio- heart
carpo- wrist
cephalo- head
cerebello- cerebellum (part of brain)
cerebro- cerebrum (part of brain)
cheilo- lip (mouth)
chole- bile (NOTE: *chole-* + *cyst* meaning "bladder," = gallbladder; *chole-* + *doch,* meaning "duct," = choledocho, or common bile duct.)
chondro- cartilage
chordo- cord or string (generally used in connection with the vocal cord or spermatic cord)
cilia- hair (Latin)
cleido- collarbone
coccygo- coccyx (end bone of the spinal column)
colpo- vagina
cordo- cord (usually vocal cord)
coxa- hip (Latin)
cranio- head
cysto- sac, cyst, or bladder (most often used in connection with the urinary bladder)
cyto- cell
dacryo- tear (used commonly in relation to tear duct or sac)
dento-, donto- tooth
derma- skin
duodeno- duodenum (part of small intestine)
emia- blood
encephalo- brain
entero- intestines
fascia- sheet or band of fibrous tissue (Latin)
fibro- fibers

gastro- stomach
genu- knee (Latin)
gingivo- gums
glomerulo- glomerulus (often a structure of the kidney)
glosso- tongue
gnatho- jaw
hem-, hema-, hemo-, hemato- blood
hepato- liver
hilus- pit or depression in an organ where vessels and nerves enter (Latin)
histio- tissue
hystero- uterus (NOTE: This term may also pertain to hysteria.)
ileo- ileum (part of small intestine)
ilio- flank or ilium (bone of pelvis)
jejuno- jejunum (part of small intestine)
kerato- cornea or horny layer of the skin
labio- lips (either of mouth or vulva)
lacrimo- tears (used also in connection with tear ducts or sacs)
laparo- loin or flank (also refers to abdomen)
laryngo- larynx
linguo- tongue
lympho- lymph
masto- breast
meningo- meninges (coverings of the brain and spinal cord)
metra-, metro- uterus
morpho- form
myelo- bone marrow and spinal cord (NOTE: Use of this term will determine which tissue is meant.)
myo- muscle (NOTE: The Latin word for muscle is *mus.*)
myringo- eardrum
naso- nose
nephro- kidney
neuro- nerve
oculo- eye
odonto- tooth
omphalo- navel or umbilicus
onycho- nails
oophoro- ovary
ophthalmo- eye
ora-, oro- mouth

orthio-, orchido- testis
os- bone or mouth
osteo- bone
oto- ear
ovario- ovary
palato- palate of mouth
palpebro- eyelid
pectus- breast, chest, or thorax (Latin)
pharyngo- pharynx
phlebo- vein
pllo- hair
pleuro- pleura of lung (relates also to side or rib)
pneumo-, pneumono- lungs (also used in referring to air or breath)
procto- rectum
pyelo- pelvis of kidney
pyloro- pylorus (part of stomach just before duodenum)
rhino- nose
sacro- sacrum
salpingo- fallopian tube or oviduct

sialo- saliva (used in connection with a salivary duct or gland)
splanchno- viscera
spleno- spleen
sterno- sternum
stoma- mouth
tarso- instep of foot; ankle (also edge of eyelid)
teno-, tenonto- tendon
thoraco- thorax or chest
thyro- thyroid
trachelo- neck, particularly the neck of the uterus or bladder
tracheo- trachea
unguis- nail
uretero- ureter
urethro- urethra
uro- urine, urinary
utero- uterus
vaso- vessel
veno- vein
ventriculo- ventricle of heart or brain
viscero- viscera

PREFIXES

Prefixes, the most frequently used elements in the formation of medical-dental words, are one or more syllables (prepositions or adverbs) placed before words or roots to show various kinds of relationships. They are never used independently, but when added before verbs, adjectives, or nouns, they modify the meaning. Most prefixes are a part of words in ordinary speech and do not refer specifically to medical-dental or scientific terminology, but many also occur frequently in medical terminology. Studying them is an important step in learning medical terms and building a medical-dental vocabulary.

Prefix	Translation	Examples
a (an before vowel)	Without, lack of	Apathy (lack of feeling), apnea (without breath), aphasia (without speech), anemia (lack of blood)
ab-	Away from	Abductor (leading away from), aboral (away from mouth)
ad-	To, toward, near to	Adductor (leading toward), adhesion (sticking to), adnexa (structures joined to), adrenal (near the kidney)
ambi-	Both	Ambidextrous (ability to use hands equally), ambilaterally (both sides)
amphi-	About, on both sides, both	Amphibious (living on both land and water)
ampho-	Both	Amphogenic (producing offspring of both sexes)
ana-	Up, back, again, excessive	Anatomy (a cutting up), anagenesis (reproduction of tissue), anasarca (excessive serum in cellular tissues of body)
ante-	Before, forward	Antecubital (before elbow), anteflexion (forward bending)
anti-	Against, opposed to, reversed	Antiperistalsis (reversed peristalsis), antisepsis (against infection)

apo-	From, away from	Aponeurosis (away from tendon), apochromatic (abnormal color)
bi-	Twice, double	Biarticulate (double joint), bifocal (two foci), bifurcation (two branches)
cata-	Down, according to, complete	Catabolism (breaking down), catalepsia (complete seizure), catarrh (flowing down)
circum-	Around, about	Circumflex (winding about), circumference (surrounding), circumarticular (around joint)
com-	With, together	Commissure (sending or coming together)
con-	With, together	Conductor (leading together), concrescence (growing together), concentric (having a common center)
contra-	Against, opposite	Contralateral (opposite side), contraception (prevention of conception), contraindicated (not indicated)
de-	Away from	Dehydrate (remove water from), decompensation (failure of compensation)
di-	Twice, double	Diplopia (double vision), dichromatic (two colors), digastric (double stomach)
dia-	Through, apart, across, completely	Diaphragm (wall across), diapedesis (ooze through), diagnosis (complete knowledge)
dis-	Reversal, apart from, separation	Disinfection (apart from infection), disparity (apart from equality), dissect (cut apart)
dys-	Bad, difficult, disordered	Dyspepsia (bad digestion), dyspnea (difficult breathing), dystopia (disordered position)
e-, ex-	Out, away from	Enucleate (remove from), eviscerate (take out viscera or bowels), exostosis (outgrowth of bone)
ec-	Out from	Ectopic (out of place), eccentric (away from center), ectasia (stretching out or dilation)
ecto-	On outside, situated on	Ectoderm (outer skin), ectoretina (outer layer of retina)
em-, en-	In	Empyema (pus in), encephalon (in the head)
endo-	Within	Endocardium (within heart), endometrium (within uterus), endodont (within tooth)
epi-	Upon, on	Epidural (upon dura), epidermis (on skin)
exo-	Outside, on outer side, outer layer	Exogenous (produced outside), exocolitis (inflammation of outer coat of colon)
extra-	Outside	Extracellular (outside cell), extrapleural (outside pleura)
hemi-	Half	Hemiplegia (partial paralysis), hemianesthesia (loss of feeling on one side of body)
hyper-	Over, above, excessive	Hyperemia (excessive blood), hypertrophy (overgrowth), hyperplasia (excessive formation)
hypo-	Under, below, deficient	Hypotension (low blood pressure), hypothyroidism (deficiency or underfunction of thyroid)
im-, in-	In, into	Immersion (act of dipping in), infiltration (act of filtering in), injection (act of forcing liquid into)
im-, in-	Not	Immature (not mature), involuntary (not voluntary), inability (not able)
infra-	Below	Infraorbital (below eye), infraclavicular (below clavicle or collarbone)
inter-	Between	Intercostal (between ribs), intervene (come between)
intra-	Within	Intracerebral (within cerebrum), intraocular (within eyes), intraventricular (within ventricles)
intro-	Into, within	Introversion (turning inward), introduce (lead into)
meta-	Beyond, after, change	Metamorphosis (change of form), metastasis (beyond original position), metacarpal (beyond wrist)

opistho-	Behind, backward	Opisthotic (behind ears), opisthognathous (behind jaws)
para-	Beside, by side	Paraplegia (paralysis of both sides), paracentesis (puncture along side of), parathyroid (beside thyroid)
per-	Through, excessive	Permeate (pass through), perforate (bore through), peracute (excessively acute)
peri-	Around	Periosteum (around bone), periatrial (around atrium), peribronchial (around bronchus)
post-	After, behind	Postoperative (after operation), postpartum (after childbirth), postocular (behind eye)
pre-	Before, in front of	Premaxillary (in front of maxilla), preoral (in front of mouth)
pro-	Before, in front of	Prognosis (foreknowledge), prophase (appear before)
re-	Back, again, contrary	Reflex (bend back), revert (turn again to), regurgitation (backward flowing, contrary to normal)
retro-	Backward, located behind	Retrocervical (located behind cervix), retrograde (going backward), retrolingual (behind tongue)
semi-	Half	Semicartilaginous (half cartilage), semilunar (half moon), semiconscious (half conscious)
sub-	Under	Subcutaneous (under skin), subarachnoid (under arachnoid), subungual (under nail)
super-	Above, upper, excessive	Supercilia (upper brows), supernumerary (excessive number), supermedial (above middle)
supra-	Above, upon	Suprarenal (above kidney), suprasternal (above sternum), suprascapular (on upper part of scapula)
sym-, syn-	Together, with	Symphysis (growing together), synapsis (joining together), synarthrosis (articulation of joints together)
trans-	Across, through	Transection (cut across), transduodenal (through duodenum), transmit (send beyond)
ultra	Beyond, in	Ultraviolet (beyond violet end of spectrum), ultraligation (ligation of vessel beyond point of origin), ultrasonic (sound waves beyond the upper frequency of hearing by human ear)

SUFFIXES

Suffixes are the one or more syllables or elements added to the root, or stem, of a word (the part that indicates the essential meaning) to alter the meaning or indicate the intended part of speech.

To make it pronounceable the last letter or letters of the root to which the suffix is attached may be changed. The last vowel may be changed to an *o*, or *o* may be inserted if it is not already present before a suffix beginning with a consonant, as in *cardiology*. The final vowel in the root may be dropped before a suffix beginning with a vowel, as in *neuritis*.

Most suffixes are in common use in English, but some are peculiar to medical science. The suffixes most commonly used to indicate disease are *-itis*, meaning "inflammation," *-oma*, meaning "tumor," and *-osis*, meaning "a condition," usually morbid. The following suffixes occur often in medical-dental terminology, but they are also in use in ordinary language:

Suffix	*Use*	*Examples*
-ise, -ate	Added to nouns or adjectives to make verbs expressing to use and to act like; to subject to; make into	Visualize (able to see), impersonate (act like), hypnotize (put into state of hypnosis)

-ist, -or, -er	Added to verbs to make nouns expressing agent or person concerned or instrument	Anesthetist (one who practices the science of anesthesia), dissector (instrument that dissects or person who dissects), donor (giver)
-ent	Added to verbs to make adjectives or nouns of agency	Recipient (one who receives), concurrent (happening at the same time)
-sia, -y	Added to verbs to make nouns expressing action, process, or condition	Therapy (treatment), anesthesia (process or condition of feeling)
-ia, -ity	Added to adjectives or nouns to make nouns expressing quality or condition	Septicemia (poisoning of blood), disparity (inequality), acidity (condition of excess acid), neuralgia (pain in nerves)
-ma, mata, -men, -mina, -ment, -ure	Added to verbs to make nouns expressing result of action or object of action	Trauma (injury), foramina (openings), ligament (tough fibrous band holding bone or viscera together), fissure (groove)
-ium, -olus, -olum, -culus, -culum, -cule, -cle	Added to nouns to make diminutive nouns	Bacterium, alveolus (air sac), follicle (little bag), cerebellum (little brain), molecule (little mass), ossicle (little bone)
-ible, -ile	Added to verbs to make adjectives expressing ability or capacity	Contractile (ability to contract), edible (capable of being eaten), flexible (capable of being bent)
-al, -c, -ious, -tic	Added to nouns to make adjectives expressing relationship, concern, or pertaining to	Neural (referring to nerve), neoplastic (referring to neoplasm), cardiac (referring to heart), delirious (suffering from delirium)
-id	Added to verbs or nouns to make adjectives expressing state or condition	Flaccid (state of being weak or lax), fluid (state of being fluid or liquid)
-tic	Added to verbs to make adjectives showing relationships	Caustic (referring to burn), acoustic (referring to sound or hearing)
-oid, -form	Added to nouns to make adjectives expressing resemblance	Polypoid (resembling polyp), plexiform (resembling a plexus), fusiform (resembling a fusion), epidermoid (resembling epidermis)
-ous	Added to nouns to make adjectives expressing material	Ferrous (composed of iron), serous (composed of serum), mucinous (composed of mucin)

The following verbs or combining forms of verbs are derived from Greek or Latin. They may be attached to other roots to form words, or suffixes and prefixes may be added to them to form words. In the following examples, the part or root of the word to which the verb is attached is italicized and the meaning, if not clear, is given in parentheses:

Root	Translation	Examples
-algia-	Pain	*Cardi*algia (heart), *gastr*algia (stomach), *neur*algia (nerve)
-dynia-	Pain	*Masto*dynia (breast), *pleuro*dynia (chest), *esophago*dynia (esophagus), *coccygo*dynia (coccyx)
-audi-, -audio-	Hear, hearing	Audio*meter* (measure), audio*phone* (voice instrument for deaf)
-bio-	Live	*Bio*logy (study of living), *bio*statistics (vital statistics), *bio*genesis (origin)
cau-, -caus-	Burn	*Caus*tic (suffix added to make adjective), *cau*terization; *caus*algia (burning pain), *electrocautery*

-centesis-	Puncture, perforate	Thoracentesis (chest), pneumocentesis (lung), arthrocentesis (joint), enterocentesis (intestine)
-clas-, -claz-	Smash, break	Osteoclasis (bone), odontoclasis (tooth)
-duct-	Lead	Ductal (suffix added to make adjective), oviduct (egg uterine tube or fallopian tube), periductal (peri means "around"), abduct (prefix meaning lead away from)
-ecta-, -ectas-	Dilate	Venectasia (dilation of vein), cardiectasis (heart), ectatic (suffix added for adjective)
-edem-	Swell	Myoedema (muscle), lymphedema (lymph) (a is a suffix added to make a noun)
-esthes-	Feel	Esthesia (suffix added to make noun), anesthesia (an is a prefix)
-fiss-	Split	Fissure, fission (suffixes added to make nouns)
-flex-, -flec-	Bend	Flexion (suffix added to make noun), flexor (suffix added), anteflect (prefix added meaning "before" bending forward)
-flu-, -flux-	Flow	Fluctuate, fluxion, affluent (abundant flowing)
geno-, -genesis-	Produce, origin	Genotype, homogenesis (same origin), pathogenesis (disease, origin of disease), heterogenesis (prefix added meaning "other," alteration of generation)
-iatro-, -iatr-	Treat, cure	Geriatrics (old age), pediatrics (children)
-kine , kino-, -kineto-, -kinesio	Move	Kinetogenic (producing movement), kinetic (suffix added to make adjective), kinesiology (study)
-liga-	Bind	Ligament (suffix added to make noun) ligate, ligature
-logy-	Study	Parasitology (parasites), bacteriology (bacteria), histology (tissues)
-lysis-	Breaking up, dissolving	Hemolysis (blood), glycolysis (sugar), autolysis (self-destruction of cells)
-morph-, -morpho-	Form	Morphology, amorphous (not definite form), pleomorphic (more, occurring in various forms), polymorphic (many)
-olfact-	Smell	Olfactophobia (fear), olfactory (suffix added to make adjective)
-op-, -opto-	See	Amblyopia (dull, dimness of vision), presbyopia (old, impairment of vision in old age), optic, myopia (myo, to wink, half close the eyes)
-palpit-	Flutter	Palpitation
-par-, -partus-	Labor	Postpartum (after birth), parturition (act of giving birth) (NOTE: para I, II, III, IV, etc., are symbols for number of births.)
-pep-	Digest	Dyspepsia (bad, difficult), peptic (suffix added to make adjective)
-pexy-	Fix	Mastopexy (fixation of breast), nephrosplenopexy (surgical fixation of kidney and spleen)
-phag-, -phago-	Eat	Phagocytosis (eating of cells), phagomania (madness, mad craving for food or to eat), dysphagia (difficult eating or swallowing)
-phan-	Appear, visible	Phanerosis (act of becoming visible), phantasia, phantasy
-phas-	Speak, utter	Aphasia (unable to speak), dysphasia (difficulty in speaking)
-phil-	Like, love	Hemophilia (blood, a hereditary disease characterized by delayed clotting of blood), acidophilia (acid stain, liking or straining with acid stains), philanthropy (love of mankind)
-phobia-	Fear	Hydrophobia (fear of water), photophobia (fear of light), claustrophobia (closeness, fear of close places)
-phrax-, -phrag-	Fence off, wall off	Diaphragm (across, partition separating thorax from abdomen), phragmoplast (formed)
-plas-	Form, grow	Neoplasm (new growth), rhinoplasty (nose operation for formation of nose), otoplasty (ear), choledochoplasty (common bile duct)
-plegia-	Paralyze	Paraplegia (paralysis of lower limbs), ophthalmoplegia (eye), hemiplegia (partial paralysis)

-pne-, -pneo-	Breathe	*Dyspnea* (difficult breathing), *apnea* (lack of breathing), *hyperpnea* (overbreathing)
-poie-	Make	*Hematopoiesis* (blood), *erythropoiesis* (red blood cells), *leukopoiesis* (making white cells)
-ptosis-	Fall	*Proctoptosis* (anus, prolapse of anus), *splanchnoptosis* (viscera)
-rrhagia-	Burst forth, pour	*Menorrhagia* (abnormal bleeding during menstruation), *menometrorrhagia* (abnormal uterine bleeding), *hemorrhage* (blood)
-rrhaphy-	Suture	*Hemiorrhaphy* (suturing or repair of hernia), *hepatorrhaphy* (liver), *nephrorrhaphy* (kidney)
-rrhea-	Flow, discharge	*Leukorrhea* (white discharge from vagina), *galactorrhea* (milk discharge), *rhinorrhea* (nasal discharge)
-rrhexis-	Rupture	*Enterorrhexis* (intestines), *metrorrhexis* (uterus)
-schiz-	Split, divide	*Schizophrenia* (mind, split personality), *schizonychia* (nails), *schizotrichia* (hair)
-scope-	Examine	*Microscopic, cardioscope, endoscope* (*endo* means "within," an instrument for examining the interior of a hollow internal organ)
-stasis-	Stop, stand still	*Hematostatic* (pertaining to stagnation of blood), *epistasis* (checking or stopping of any discharge)
-stazien-	Drop	*Epistaxis* (nosebleed)
-teg-, -tect-	Cover	*Tegmen, tectum* (rooflike structure), *integument* (skin covering)
-therap-	Treat, cure	*Therapy, neurotherapy* (nerves), *chemotherapy* (chemicals), *physiotherapy*
-tomy-	Cut, incise	*Phlebotomy* (incision of vein), *arthrotomy* (joint), *appendectomy* (*ectomy*, meaning "cutout," excision of appendix), *oophorectomy* (excision of ovary), *ileocecostomy* (*ostomy*, meaning "creation of an artifical opening," *os*, meaning "opening or mouth"; ileocecostomy is an anatomosis of ileum and cecum)
-topo-	Place	*Topography, toponarcosis* (numbing, hence numbing of a part or localized anesthesia)
-tropho-	Nourish	*Hypertrophy* (enlargement or overnourishment), *atrophy* (undernourishment), *dystrophy* (difficult or bad)
-volv-	Turn	*Involution, volvulus* (twisting of an organ, as in intestinal obstruction with twisting of the bowel or twisting of the esophagus)

The following roots and combining forms are derived from Greek or Latin adjectives. Adjectives appear most often in compounds and are joined to nouns or verbs. Suffixes may be added to make them into nouns.

In the following examples, the part or root of the word that the adjective modifies is italicized, and the meaning, if not clear, is given in parentheses:

Root	Translation	Examples
-auto-	Self	*Autoinfection, autolysis, autopathy* (disease), *autopsy* (view, postmortem examination)
-brachy-	Short	*Brachycephalia* (head), *brachydactylia* (fingers), *brachychelia* (lip), *brachygnathous* (jaw)
-brady-	Slow	*Bradypnea* (breath), *bradypragia* (action), *bradyuria* (urine), *bradypepsia* (digestion)
-brevis-	Short	*Brevity, breviflexor* (short flexor muscle)
-cavus-	Hollow	*Cavity, cavernous, vena cava* (vein)
-coel-	Hollow	*Coelarium* (lining membrane of body cavity), *coelom* (body cavity of embryo)
-cryo-	Cold	*Cryotherapy, cryotolerant, cryometer*

-crypto-	Hidden, concealed	Cryptorchid (testis), cryptogenic (origin obscure or doubtful), cryptophthalmos (eye)
-dextro-	Right	Ambidextrous (using both hands with equal ease), dextrophobia (fear of objects on right side), dextrocardia (heart)
-dys-	Difficult, bad, disordered, painful	Dysarthria (speech), dyshidrosis (sweat), dyskinesia (motion), dystocia (birth), dysphasia (speech), dyspepsia (digestion)
-eu-	Well, good	Euphoria (well-being), euphagia, eupnea (breath), euthyroid (normal thyroid), eutocia (normal birth)
-eury-	Broad, wide	Eurycephalic (head), euryopia (vision), eurysomatic (body, squat thickset body)
-glyco-	Sugar, sweet	Glycohemia (sugar in blood), glycopenia (poverty of sugar, low blood sugar level)
-gravis-	Heavy	Gravida (pregnant woman), gravidism (pregnancy)
haplo-	Single, simple	Haploid (having a single set of chromosomes), haplodont (teeth without simple crowns), haplopathy (simple, uncomplicated disease)
-hetero-	Other, different	Heterogeneous (kind, dissimilar elements), heteroinoculation, heterology (abnormality of structure), heterointoxication
homo-	Same	Homogeneous (same kind or quality throughout), homozygous (possessing identical pair of genes), homologous (corresponding in structure)
hydro	Wet, water	Hydronephrosis (kidney, collection of urine in kidney pelvis), hydropneumothorax (fluid in chest), hydrophobia (fear of water, water causes painful reaction in this disease)
-iso-	Equal	Isocellular (similar cells), isodontic (all teeth alike), isocytosis (equality of size of cells), isochromatic (having same color throughout)
-latus-	Broad	Latitude, latissimus dorsi (muscle adducting humerus)
-leio-	Smooth	Leiomyosarcoma (smooth muscle, fleshy malignant tumor), leiomyofibroma (tumor of muscle and fiber elements), leiomyoma (tumor of unstriped muscle)
-lepto-	Slender	Leptosomatic (body), leptodactylous (fingers)
-levo-	Left	Levocardia (heart), levorotation (turning to left)
-longus-	Long	Adductor longus (muscle of thigh), longitude
-macro-	Large, abnormal size	Macrocephalic (head), macrocheiria (hands), macromastia (breast), macronychia (nails)
-magna-	Large, great	Magnitude, adductor magnus (thigh muscle)
-malaco-	Soft	Malacia (softening), osteomalacia (bones)
-malus-	Bad	Malady, malaise, malignant, malformation
medius-	Middle	Median, medium, gluteus medius (femur muscle)
mega	Great	Megacolon (large colon), megacephaly (head)
-megalo-	Huge	Megalomania (delusion of grandeur), hepatomegaly (enlarged liver), splenomegaly (enlarged spleen)
-meso-	Middle, mid	Mesocarpal (wrist), mesoderm (skin), mesothelium (a lining membrane of cavities)
-micro-	Small	Microglossia (tongue), microblepharia (eyelids), microorganism, microphonia (voice)
-minimus-	Smallest	Gluteus minimus (smallest muscle of hip), adductor minimus (muscle of thigh)
-mio-	Less	Miolecithal (egg with little yolk), miopragia (perform, decreased activity)
-mono-	One, single, limited to one part	Monochromatic (color), monobrachia (arm)
-multi-	Many, much	Multipara (bear, woman who has borne many children), multilobar (numerous lobes), multicentric (many centers)
-necro-	Dead	Necrosed, necrosis, necropsy (postmortem examination), necrophobia (fear of death)
-neo-	New	Neoformation, neomorphism (form), neonatal (first 4 weeks of life), neopathy (disease)

-oligo-	Few, scanty, little	Oligophrenia (mind), oligopnea (breath), oliguria (urine), oligodipsia (thirst)
-ortho-	Straight, normal, correct	Orthodontic (teeth, normal), orthogenesis (progressive evolution in a given direction), orthograde (walk, carrying body upright), orthopnea (breath, unable to breathe unless in an upright position)
-oxy-	Sharp, quick	Oxyesthesia (feel), oxyopia (vision), oxyosmia (smell)
-pachy-	Thick	Pachyderm (skin), pachysulemia (blood), pachypleuritis (inflammation of pleura), pachycholia (bile), pachyotia (ears)
-paleo-	Old	Paleogenetic (origin in the past), paleopathology (study of diseases in mummies)
-platy-	Flat	Platybasia (skull base), platycoria (pupil), platycrania (skull)
-pleo-	More	Pleomorphism (forms), pleochromocytoma (tumor composed of different colored cells)
-poikilo-	Varied	Poikiloderma (skin mottling), poikilothermal (heat, variable body temperature)
-poly-	Many, much	Polyhedral (many bases or faces), polymastia (more than two breasts), polymelia (supernumerary limbs), polymyalgia (pain in many muscles)
-pronus-	Face down	Prone, pronation
-pseudo-	False, spurious	Pseudostratified (layered), pseudocirrhosis (apparent cirrhosis of liver), pseudohypertrophy
-sclero-	Hard	Sclerosis (hardening), arteriosclerosis (artery), scleronychia (nails), scleroderma (skin)
-scolio-	Twisted, crooked	Scoliodontic (teeth), scoliosis, scoliokyphosis (curvature of spine)
-sinistro-	Left	Sinistrocardia, sinistromanual (left handed), sinistraural (hearing better in left ear)
-steno-	Narrow	Stenosis, stenostomia (mouth), mitral stenosis (mitral valve in heart)
-stereo-	Solid, three dimensions	Stereoscope, stereometer
-supinus-	Face up	Supine, supination, supinator longus (muscle in arm)
-tachy-	Fast, swift	Tachycardia (heart), tachyphrasia (speech)
-tele-	End, far away	Telepathy, telecardiogram
-telo-	Complete	Telophase
-thermo-	Heat, warm	Thermal, thermometer, thermobiosis (ability to live in high temperature)
-trachy-	Rough	Trachyphonia (voice), trachychromatic (deeply staining)
-xero-	Dry	Xerophagia (eating of dry foods) xerostomia (mouth), xeroderma (skin)

PRONUNCIATION OF MEDICAL-DENTAL TERMS

Medical terms are hard to pronounce, especially if a person has read them but never heard them spoken. Following are some helpful shortcuts:

ch is sometimes pronounced like *k*. Examples: chromatin, chronic.

ps is pronounced like *s*. Examples: psychiatry, psychology.

pn is pronounced with only the *n* sound. Example: pneumonia.

c and *g* are given the soft sound of *s* and *j*, respectively, before *e, i,* and *y* in words of both Greek and Latin origin. Examples: cycle, cytoplasm, giant, generic.

c and *g* have a harsh sound before other letters. Examples: gastric, gonad, cast, cardiac.

ae and *oe* are pronounced *ee*. Examples: coelom, fasciae.

i at the end of a word (to form a plural) is pronounced *eye*. Examples: alveoli, glomeruli, fasciculi.

e and *es,* when forming the final letters or letter of a word, are often pronounced as separate syllables. Examples: rete (reetee), nares (nayreez).

PLURALS

In most English words the plurals are formed by merely adding an *s* or *es,* but in Greek and Latin the plural may be designated by changing the ending.

> *-ae,* as in fasciae (singular form, fascia). *-ia,* as in crania (singular form, cranium).
>
> *-i,* as in glomeruli (singular form, glomerulus). When the singular form ends in *us,* the plural form is made by adding *i* and dropping the *us.*
>
> *-ata,* as in adenomata (singular form, adenoma).

SPELLING

The aforementioned rules for pronunciation and the formation of plurals are essential for spelling, but the professional should consult a medical dictionary if unsure. Phonetic spelling has no place in medicine, because a misspelled word may give the wrong meaning to a diagnosis. Furthermore, some terms are pronounced alike but spelled differently, for example, ileum is a part of the intestinal tract, but ilium is a pelvic bone.

Nutrition and Nutritional Counseling

Table J-1 Body Mass Index classification chart

	Obesity class	Body Mass Index (BMI) (1 kg/m^2)
Underweight	—	<18.5
Normal	—	18.5–24.9
Overweight	—	25.0–25.9
Obesity	I	30.0–34.9
	II	35.0–39.9
Extreme obesity	III	>40

Adapted from National Institutes of Health: Clinical guidelines on the identification, evaluation, and treatment of overweight and obesity in adults: Obesity Initiative. Washington, DC, NIH 1998.

Table J-2 Effects of nutrients on oral tissues and their role in tooth formation

Nutrients	Effects on oral soft and hard tissue	Role in tooth formation
Vitamin A	• Synthesis and function of epithelial cells • Maintenance of the integrity of the sulcus • Normal growth and function of salivary glands • Essential for activity of epiphyseal cartilage cells and normal endochondral bone growth	• Normal growth of dentin and enamel • Normal growth of periodontal tissues and maintenance of epithelium
Vitamin D	• No effects noted	• Controls calcification of dentin and enamel by regulating calcium absorption at the intestines
Vitamin C	• Synthesis of connective tissue • Essential for integrity of capillaries and oral mucosa • Needed for normal bone matrix formation • Needed for normal phagocytic function and antibody synthesis in host defense system	• Integrity of blood vessels in gingival and pulpal tissues • Hydroxylation of proline and lysine in collagen synthesis • Normal formation of dentin
B-complex vitamins		
Niacin	• Integrity of oral tissues	• No effects noted
Folacin	• Normal synthesis of protein compounds in oral tissues (e.g., hemoglobin and enzymes)	• No effects noted
Thiamin	• Normal energy metabolism during development and maintenance of oral tissue	• No effects noted
Riboflavin	• Energy metabolism of oral tissues	• No effects noted
Pyridoxine	• Normal carbohydrate metabolism and hemoglobin synthesis in oral tissues	• No effects noted
Cobalamin	• Integrity of nerve tissue and normal red blood cell formation in oral tissues	• No effects noted
Calcium-phosphorus ratio	• No effects noted	• Normal tooth and bone mineralization
Fluoride	• No effects noted	• Forms dentin and enamel
Iron	• Normal hemoglobin formation and carbon dioxide transport to tissue	• No effects noted
Fiber	• Stimulates salivary flow and maintains integrity of periodontal tissues	• No effects noted
Protein	• Synthesis of antibodies and leukocytes • Synthesis of epithelial and connective tissues in the healing process • Maintains integrity of periodontal tissues	• Formation of matrix of dentin and enamel • Collagen formation

Data from DePaola DP, Faine MP, Palmer CA: Nutrition in relation to dental medicine. In Shils ME, et al (eds): Modern nutrition in health and disease, ed 9. Baltimore, Williams & Wilkins, 1998, p 1114; and from Lee M, Stanmeyer W, Weight A: Nutrition and dental health. Chapel Hill, Health Sciences Consortium, 1982.

Table J-3 Dietary Reference intake, adequate intake, and tolerable upper limits of nutrients specific to bone health

Nutrient	Dietary Reference Intake (DRI)/Recommended Dietary Allowance (RDA)§	Therapeutic range‡ (adequate intake)	Tolerable upper limit
Calcium (g/d)	—	*210–1300	2.5 for children and adults
Phosphorous (g/d)	460–1250 for most healthy children and adults	*100–275	†3–4 for healthy individuals
Magnesium (mg/d)	80–420 for most healthy children and adults	*30–75	†65–350 for healthy individuals
Vitamin D (μg/d)	—	*5–15	†25–50 for healthy individuals
Fluoride (mg/d)	—	*0.01–4	†0.7–10 for healthy individuals

From Darby ML: *Mosby's comprehensive review of dental hygiene,* ed 5, St Louis, 2002, Mosby.

*Lower number represents the adequate intake for infants and children, and the higher range of numbers will vary depending on life stage and gender group. Refer to the National Academy Press website (http://www.nap/edu/info/browse.htm) for more in-depth information. The therapeutic range, also referred to as adequate intake, is the dose at which there may be physiological benefits for healthy individuals and decreased risk for toxicity.

†Lower number represents upper limit for infants and children, and higher number represents upper limit for males and females (pregnant and lactating). The tolerable upper limit is the highest level of daily nutrient intake that is likely to pose no risk of adverse health effects.

‡Adequate intake (AI), also known as a therapeutic range, is the mean intake for healthy individuals that is used when an RDA cannot be determined.

§Recommended dietary allowance values meet the needs of 97% to 98% of individuals in a group. Daily reference intake values are groups of values that provide quantitative estimates of nutrient intake for planning and assessing diets for all healthy individuals.

Pharmacology

Box K-1 Formulas for drug calculations

Surface area rule:

$$\text{Child dose} = \frac{\text{Surface area } (m^2)}{1.73 \text{ m}^2} \times \text{Adult dose}$$

Calculating strength of a solution:

Solution Strength.   Desired Solution·

$$\frac{x}{100} = \frac{\text{Amount of drug desired}}{\text{Amount of finished solution}}$$

Calculating flow rate for IV:

$$\text{Rate of flow} = \frac{\text{Amount of fluid} \times \text{Administration set calibration}}{\text{Running time}}$$

$$\frac{x}{1} = \frac{(\text{ml}) \, (\text{gtt/min})}{\text{min}}$$

Calculation of medication dosages:
Formula method:

$$\frac{\text{Amount ordered}}{\text{Amount on hand}} \times \text{Vehicle} = \text{Number of tablets, capsules, or amount of liquid}$$

Vehicle is the drug form or amount of liquid containing the dosage. Amounts used in calculation by formula must be in same system.

Ratio—proportion method:

1 tablet:tablet in mg on hand::x tablet order in mg
Know or have::Want to know or order

Multiply means and extremes, divide both sides by known amount to get x. Amounts used in equation must be in same system.

Dimensional analysis method:

$$\text{Order in mg} \times \frac{1 \text{ tablet or capsule}}{\text{What 1 tablet or capsule is in mg}} = \text{Tablets or capsules to be given}$$

If amounts are in different systems:

$$\text{Order in mg} \times \frac{1 \text{ tablet or capsule}}{\text{What 1 tablet or capsule is in g}} \times \frac{1}{1000 \text{ mg}}$$
$$= \text{Tablets or capsules to be given}$$

From Skidmore-Roth L: *Mosby's 2003 nursing drug reference,* St Louis, 2003, Mosby.

Table K-1 Common abbreviations used in writing prescriptions

Abbreviation	Derivation	Meaning	Abbreviation	Derivation	Meaning
āā	ana	of each	o.m.	omni mane	every morning
a.	ante	before	o.n.	omni nocte	every night
a.c.	ante cibum	before meals	o.s.	oculus sinister	left eye
ad	ad	to, up to	os	os	mouth
A.D.	auris dextra	right ear	o.u.	oculus uterque	each eye
ad lib.	ad libitum	freely as desired	oz	uncia	ounce
agit. ante sum.	agitare ante	shake before taking	p.c.	post cibum	after meals
A.L.	auris laeva	left ear	per	per	through or by
alt. dieb.	alternis diebus	every other day	pil.	pilula	pill
alt. hor.	alternis horis	alternate hours	p.o.	per os	orally
alt. noct.	alternis noctibus	alternate nights	p.r.		by rectum
aq.	aqua	water	p.r.n.	pro re nata	when required or as needed
aq. dest.	aqua destillata	distilled water	q	quaque	every
b.i.d.	bis in die	two times a day	q.d.	quaque die	every day or once per day
b.i.n.	bis in nocte	two times a night	q.h.	quaque hora	every hour
c., c̄	cum	with	q. 2 h.		every two hours
Cap.	capiat	let him take	q. 3 h.		every three hours
caps.	capsula	capsule	q. 4 h.		every four hours
c.m.s.	cras mane sumendus	to be taken tomorrow morning	q. 6 h.		every 6 hours
c.n.	cras nocte	tomorrow night	q.i.d.	quater in die	four times a day
c.n.s.	cras nocte sumendus	to be taken tomorrow night	q.o.d.		every other day
comp.	compositus	compound	q.l.	quantum libet	as much as desired
Det.	detur	let it be given	q.n.	quaque nocte	every night

Dieb. tert.	diebus tertiis	every third day
dil.	dilutus	dilute
elix.	elixir	elixir
ext.	extractum	extract
fld.	fluidus	fluid
Ft.	fiat	make
g	gramme	gram
gr	granum	grain
gt	gutta	a drop
gtt	guttae	drops
h.	hora	hour
h.d.	hora decubitus	at bedtime
h.s.	hora somni	hour of sleep (bed-time)
M.	misce	mix
m.	minimum	a minim
mist.	mistura	mixture
non rep.	non repetatur	not to be repeated
noct.	nocte	in the night
O	octarius	pint
o.d.	oculus dexter	right eye
ol.	oleum	oil
o.d.	omni die	every day
o.h.	omni hora	every hour
q.p.	quantum placeat	as much as desired
q.v.	quantum vis	as much as you please
q.s.	quantum sufficit	as much as is required
R	recipe	take
Rep.	repetatur	let it be repeated
s, s̄	sine	without
seq. luce.	sequenti luce	the following day
Sig. or S.	signa	write on label
sl.		sublingual
s.o.s.	si opus sit	if necessary
sp.	spiritus	spirits
supp.		suppository
ss	semis	a half
stat.	statim	immediately
syr.	syrupus	syrup
t.d.s.	ter die sumendum	to be taken three times daily
t.i.d.	ter in die	three times a day
t.i.n.	ter in nocte	three times a night
tr. or tinct.	tinctura	tincture
ung.	unguentum	ointment
ut. dict. or u.d	ut dictum	as directed
vin.	vini	of wine

Adapted from *Mosby's medical, nursing, & allied health dictionary*, ed 6, St Louis, 2002, Mosby; Daniel SJ, Harfst SA: *Mosby's dental hygiene: Concepts, cases, and competencies*, St Louis, 2002, Mosby.

Table K-2 Use of drugs in pediatric dentistry

Drug	Route	Dose	Frequency	Notes
Antibiotics				
Amoxycillin	PO	25-50 mg/kg/day	tds	Syrup or chewable tablets for young children
	IV	100-400 mg/kg/day	tds	Endocarditis prophylaxis.
	PO, IV	50 mg/kg up to adult dose 3 g	1 hour before	For highly susceptible patients, half dose 6 hours later
Amoxycillin plus clavulanic acid	PO	20-40 mg/kg/day	tds	For beta-lactam resistant organisms only
Ampicillin	IV	50-100 mg/kg/day	qid	Endocarditis prophylaxis
Benzylpenicillin	IV	50 mg/kg	stat	First IV drug of choice for odontogenic infections
	IV	15-350 mg/kg/day	qid	
		20,000-500,000 U/kg/day		
Penicillin VK	PO	<5 years	qid	Give 1 hour before meals
		500 mg/day		
		>5 years 1-2 g/day		
Cephalexin	PO	25-50 mg/kg/day	qid	
Cephalothin IV	IV	40-80 mg/kg/day	qid	Not in pregnancy
Cephalozin	IV	25-50 mg/kg/day		
Erythromycin	PO	25-40 mg/kg/day	qid	Ethylsuccinate is readily absorbed
Metronidazole	IV	22.5 mg/kg/day	tds	Not in pregnancy
	PO	10-15 mg/kg/day	tds	
Gentamicin	IV	2.5 mg/kg (children) up to 80 mg maximum	stat	Endocarditis prophylaxis, highly susceptible patients. In conjunction with ampicillin. Follow-up dose of ampicillin or amoxycillin required 6 hours later

Antibiotics				
Clindamycin	PO, IV	15-40 mg/kg/day	qid	Risk of pseudomembranous colitis
	PO, IV	10 mg/kg up to adult dose 600 mg	oral 1 hour before, IV stat	Endocarditis prophylaxis, susceptible patients
				Follow-up dose half initial dose, 6 hours later (5 mg/kg up to 300 mg)
Vancomycin	IV	20 mg/kg up to adult dose 1 g	infused over 1 hour	Endocarditis prophylaxis, susceptible patients allergic to penicillin
Antifungals				
Nystatin	Tablets	500,000 U	tds	
	Mixture	100,000 U/mL	6-hrly	
Amphotericin B	Lozenges	10 mg	6-hrly	Apply to affected area
	Suspension	100 mg/mL	6-hrly	Apply to affected area
	Ointment	3%	6-hrly	Apply to affected area
				Apply to affected area
Analgesics and sedatives				
Aspirin				Should not be used in children under 12 years of age because of the risk of Reye's syndrome
Paracetamol	PO, PR	15 mg/kg	4-hrly	Hepatotoxic if overdose
Codeine phosphate	PO	1-1.5 mg/kg single dose	4-6 divided doses	Similar side-effects to narcotics, including nausea and constipation
		1-3 mg/kg/day		Maximum 100 mg
Pethidine	IV, IM	1 mg/kg	3-4 hrly	Should only be used in admitted patients
Morphine	IV, IM	0.1-0.2 mg/kg	6-hrly	May be repeated at 2-3-minute intervals if necessary
Naloxone	IM, IV	1-10 µg/kg	stat	Sedation, may be given intranasally
Midazolam	IV, IM	0.1-0.2 mg/kg	single dose	Sedation
Chloral hydrate	PO	30-50 mg/kg/day, 15-20 mg/kg single dose	4-6 hrly	

Continued

Table K-2 Use of drugs in pediatric dentistry—cont'd

Drug	Route	Dose		Frequency	Notes
Trimeprazine	PO	3-4 mg/kg		single dose	Vallergan, sedation
Metoclopramide	PO, IM	3-5 years	2 mg	single dose	Single dose after narcotic if vomiting or nausea. Maxolon. Dystonic reactions may occur
		5-9 years	2.5 mg		
		9-14 years	5 mg		
		15-19 years	10 mg		
Other medications					
Kenalog in Orabase	Ointment	Triamcinolone 0.1%		4-6 hrly	Recurrent severe oral ulceration in children, apply to ulcer but do not rub ointment in
Ipecac syrup	PO	0-1 years	5-10 mL	>12 years or adult 30 mL	Give copious water. Used for ingestion of non-corrosive poisons. For information contact Poisons Information Service
		1-12 years	15 mL		
ε aminocaproic acid	IV	30 mg/kg			Antifibrinolytic, loading dose of 100 mg/kg
Tranexamic acid	PO	15-20 mg/kg		qid	Antifibrinolytic
DDAVP	IV	0.3 µg/kg			Infused over 1 hour before surgery
Heparin	IV	50-100 U/kg		4-6 hrly	Anticoagulant
Tetanus toxoid	IM	0.5 mL		single dose	If immunization protocol not complete, course should be given. Otherwise, a booster may be required for tetanus-prone wounds if >2 years since last booster

From Cameron AC, Widmer RP: *Handbook of pediatric dentistry,* ed 2, London, 2003, Mosby.
The table which forms Table K-2 is a guide to the administration of commonly used drugs in pediatric dentistry. Medications for children should always be prescribed in relation to weight. It is of utmost importance that clinicians understand the contraindications and precautions relevant to the drugs they are prescribing and should consult prescribing information supplied by the pharmaceutical manufacturers and relevant pharmacopeia. In the table, PO = oral, IV = intravenous, IM = intramuscular, tds = ×3 daily, qid = ×4 daily and stat = immediately.

APPENDIX L

Radiology and Radiography*

Box L-1 Criteria for intraoral radiographs

1. The radiograph should show proper definition and detail and a degree of density and contrast so that all structures can be delineated easily.
2. The structures should not be distorted either by elongation or by foreshortening.
3. The radiograph should show the teeth from the occlusal or incisal edges to 2 to 3 mm beyond their apices.
4. In a full-mouth survey, the entire alveolar processes of the mandible and maxilla must be seen—as far distal as the tuberosity in the maxilla and the beginning of the ascending ramus in the mandible.
5. All interproximal surfaces of the teeth should be seen without overlapping, providing the teeth are not overlapped in the mouth.
6. The x-ray beam should be centered on the film so that there are no unexposed parts of the film ("cone cuts" or "collimator cutoff").
7. The radiograph should not be cracked or bent or have any other artifacts.
8. The radiograph should be processed properly.

Box L-2 Common errors

Patient positioned too far forward. If the patient is positioned in front of the focal plane, the upper and lower anterior teeth appear blurred and narrow. The spinal column is superimposed on the ramus, and the premolars are overlapped.
Remedy. The patient's teeth or edentulous ridges must be in the proper position in the anterior-posterior plane. Check the position of the teeth on the bite block or bite stick and the position of the patient's chin on the rest. Make sure the distance setting is correct.
Patient positioned too far back. If the patient is positioned in back of the focal plane, the upper and lower anterior teeth appear blurred and widened. Increased ghosting of the mandible also appears.
Remedy. The patient's teeth or ridges must be in the proper position on the bite block or bite stick. Check the position of the chin rest and the chin for the correct distance in the posterior-anterior plane.
Patient's head tilted up. If the patient's head is tilted up, the forehead is too far back, and the chin is too far forward. This position causes the upper incisors to be out of focus, and the radiopaque hard palate is superimposed over the apices of the upper teeth. The condyles may be off the film.
Remedy. The reference lines on the patient's face, the Frankfort plane or the ala-tragus line, should be aligned parallel to the floor.
Patient's head tilted down. If the patient's head is tilted down, then the chin is back, and the forehead is forward. This position causes the lower incisors to be blurred. The radiopaque image of the hyoid bone is superimposed on the anterior part of the mandible. The superior portions of the condyles may be cut off the film, and the premolars are overlapped.
Remedy. The reference lines on the patient's face, the Frankfort plane or the ala-tragus line, should be aligned parallel to the floor.

Continued

*From Frommer HH: *Radiology for dental auxiliaries,* ed 7, St Louis, 2001, Mosby.

Box L-2 Common errors—cont'd

Patient moved during exposure. If the patient moves anytime during the exposure, the part of the film that was being exposed at that time appears blurred. This effect differs from intraoral radiography, in which patient movement blurs the entire film.

Remedy. Talk to patients during the exposure, reminding them not to move.

Large radiolucent area below the palate. If patients do not hold the tongue against the roof of the mouth, an airspace is created that produces a black shadow on the radiograph.

Remedy. Remind patients during the exposure to keep the tongue against the roof of the mouth.

Patient does not sit or stand erect. If the patient slumps, either standing or sitting, the spinal column causes a triangular radiolucency to be superimposed on the anterior teeth.

Remedy. When positioning patients, keep their spines erect. If patients are seated, the operator can place a cushion or support in the small of the back to help them to sit upright.

Failure to remove metal objects such as dentures, jewelry, and eyeglasses from the face, head, and mouth. These metal objects, if not removed, cause radiopaque ghosting on the opposite side of the film and may obscure structures, making the film undiagnostic.

Remedy. Remove all dentures from the patient's mouth as done in intraoral radiography. All objects must be removed from the face as well.

Lead apron placed too high on the patient. The lead apron cannot be placed on the patient above the level of the clavicles because it will create a large radiopacity on the film.

Remedy. Keep the lead apron low on the patient and never use a thyroid collar when taking a panoramic radiograph.

Film cassette slowing down because of patient contact. If the film cassette is slowed down or stopped for an instant during the exposure travel around the patient, black vertical bands show up on the film as a result of the localized overexposure.

Remedy. Position the patient carefully. With large-framed patients, the operator should run the machine first without radiation to acquaint the patient with the procedure and to check on the patient's position.

Box L-3 Time and temperature chart

Temperature of Developer	Time in Developer
80° F	2½ minutes
75° F	3 minutes
70° F	4 minutes (optimum)
68° F	4½ minutes
60° F	6 minutes

Tooth Numbering Systems and Explanation for Mounting Radiographs

TOOTH NUMBERING

According to a resolution passed by the 1968 American Dental Association (ADA) House of Delegates, teeth should be numbered as follows:

Permanent Dentition

Permanent teeth should be numbered from 1 to 32, starting with the patient's upper right third molar (1), following around the upper arch to the patient's upper left third molar (16), descending to the patient's lower left third molar (17), and following around the lower arch to the patient's lower right third molar (32).

Primary Dentition

In the same manner as described for permanent dentition, primary teeth should be lettered with uppercase letters A through T, with A being the patient's upper right second primary molar and T being the patient's lower right second primary molar.

MOUNTING RADIOGRAPHS

According to the same resolution from the 1968 ADA House of Delegates, radiographs should be mounted as follows:

Looking at the teeth from outside the mouth, radiographs should be viewed in the same manner, and so mounted.

NOTE: The raised dot in the film should be toward you when mounting radiographs.

PERMANENT DENTITION

	Upper teeth	*Erupt*
	Central incisor	7 to 8 yr
	Lateral incisor	8 to 9 yr
	Canine (cuspid)	11 to 12 yr
	First premolar (first bicuspid)	10 to 11 yr
	Second premolar (second bicuspid)	10 to 12 yr
	First molar	6 to 7 yr
	Second molar	12 to 13 yr
	Third molar (wisdom tooth)	17 to 21 yr

	Lower teeth	*Erupt*
	Third molar (wisdom tooth)	17 to 21 yr
	Second molar	11 to 13 yr
	First molar	6 to 7 yr
	Second premolar (second bicuspid)	11 to 12 yr
	First premolar (first bicuspid)	10 to 12 yr
	Canine (cuspid)	9 to 10 yr
	Lateral incisor	7 to 8 yr
	Central incisor	6 to 7 yr

PRIMARY DENTITION

Upper teeth	Erupt	Shed
Central incisor	8 to 12 mo	6 to 7 yr
Lateral incisor	9 to 13 mo	7 to 8 yr
Canine (cuspid)	16 to 22 mo	10 to 12 yr
First molar	13 to 19 mo	9 to 11 yr
Second molar	25 to 33 mo	10 to 12 yr
Lower teeth	Erupt	Shed
Second molar	23 to 31 mo	10 to 12 yr
First molar	14 to 18 mo	9 to 11 yr
Canine (cuspid)	17 to 23 mo	9 to 12 yr
Lateral incisor	10 to 16 mo	7 to 8 yr
Central incisor	6 to 10 mo	6 to 7 yr

Illustration Credits

Bath-Balogh M, Fehrenbach MJ: *Illustrated dental embryology, histology, and anatomy*, Philadelphia, 1997, Saunders.

Bird DL, Robinson DS: *Torres & Ehrlich modern dental assisting,* ed 7, St Louis, 2002, Saunders.

Callen PW (ed): *Ultrasonography in obstetrics and gynecology*, ed 4, Philadelphia, 2000, Saunders.

Cameron AC, Widmer RP: *Handbook of pediatric dentistry*, ed 2, London, 2003, Mosby International Ltd.

Christensen GJ: *A consumer's guide to dentistry,* ed 2, St Louis, 2002, Mosby.

Daniel SJ, Harfst SA: *Mosby's dental hygiene: concepts, cases and competencies*, St Louis, 2002, Mosby.

Frommer H: *Radiology for dental auxiliaries*, ed 7, St Louis, 2001, Mosby.

Genco RJ, Goldman HM, Cohen DW: *Contemporary periodontics*, St Louis, 1990, Mosby.

Habif TP: *Clinical dermatology*, ed 3, St Louis, 1996, Mosby.

Haring J, Jansen L: *Dental radiography: principles and techniques*, ed 2, Philadelphia, 2000, Saunders.

Hatrick CD, Eakle S, Bird WF: *Dental materials—clinical applications for dental assistants and dental hygienists*, St Louis, 2003, Saunders.

Hockenberry MJ, Wilson D, Winkelstein ML, et al: *Wong's nursing care of infants and children*, ed 7, St Louis, 2003, Mosby.

Ibsen OAC, Phelan JA: *Oral pathology for the dental hygienist*, ed 4, Philadelphia, 2004, Saunders.

Jarvis C: *Physical examination and health assessment*, ed 3, Philadelphia, 2000, Saunders.

Kerr DA, Ash MM, Millard HD: *Oral diagnosis*, ed 3, St Louis, 1983, Mosby.

Kinn ME, Woods M: *The medical assistant: administrative and clinical*, ed 8, Philadelphia, 1999, Saunders.

Leonard PC: *Building a Medical Vocabulary,* ed 5, Philadelphia, 2001, Saunders.

Liebgott B: *The anatomical basis of dentistry,* ed 2, St Louis, 2001, Mosby.

Moore KL, Persaud TVN: *Before we are born: essentials of embryology and birth defects*, ed 6, Philadelphia, 2003, Saunders.

Neville BW, Damm DD, Allen CM, et al: *Oral & maxillofacial pathology*, ed 2, Philadelphia, 2002, Saunders.

Newman MG, Takei H, Carranza FA: *Carranza's clinical periodontology*, ed 9, Philadelphia, 2002, Saunders.

Potter PA, Perry AG: *Fundamentals of nursing,* ed 5, St Louis, 2001, Mosby.

Proffit WR, Fields HW: *Contemporary Orthodontics*, ed 3, St Louis, 2000, Mosby.

Proffit WR, White RP, Sarver DM: *Contemporary treatment of dentofacial deformity*, St Louis, 2003, Mosby.

Regezi JA, Sciubba JJ, Jordan RCK: *Oral pathology–clinical pathologic correlations,* ed 4, St Louis, 2003, Saunders.

Regezi JA, Sciubba JJ, Pogrel MA: *Atlas of oral and maxillofacial pathology,* Philadelphia, 2000, Saunders.

Roberson TM, Heymann HO, Swift EJ: *Sturdevant's art and science of operative dentistry*, ed 4, St Louis, 2001, Mosby.

Rosenstiel SF, Land MF, Fujimoto J: *Contemporary fixed prosthodontics*, ed 3, St Louis, 2001, Mosby.

Sapp JP, Wysocki GP, Eversole LR: *Contemporary oral and maxillofacial pathology*, ed 2, St Louis, 2003, Mosby.

Sams WM, Lynch P (eds): *Principles of dermatology*, New York, 1990, Churchill Livingstone.

Seidel HM, Ball JW, Dains JE, et al: *Mosby's guide to physical examination*, ed 5, St Louis, 2003, Mosby.

Stepp CA, Woods M: *Laboratory procedures for medical office personnel*, Philadelphia, 1998, Saunders.

Thibodeau GA, Patton KT: *Anatomy and physiology*, ed 5, St Louis, 2003, Mosby.

Thibodeau GA, Patton KT: *The human body in health and disease*, ed 3, St Louis, 2002, Mosby.

Tyldesley WR: *Colour atlas of orofacial diseases*, ed 2, St Louis, 1991, Mosby [Wolfe], 1991, WR Tyldesley.

Whaites E: *Essentials of dental radiography and radiology*, ed 3, London, 2002, Churchill Livingstone.

Zakus SM: *Mosby's clinical skills for medical assistants*, ed 4, St Louis, 2001, Mosby.

Zitelli BJ, Davis HW: *Atlas of pediatric physical diagnosis*, ed 4, St Louis, 2002, Mosby.